D1604606

Peripheral Vascular Disease

Basic Diagnostic and Therapeutic Approaches

Peripheral Vascular Disease

Basic Diagnostic and Therapeutic Approaches

Editor

George S. Abela, M.Sc., M.B.A., M.D.
Professor and Chief
Division of Cardiology
Michigan State University
East Lansing, Michigan

LIPPINCOTT WILLIAMS & WILKINS
A **Wolters Kluwer** Company

Philadelphia • Baltimore • New York • London
Buenos Aires • Hong Kong • Sydney • Tokyo

Acquisitions Editor: Ruth W. Weinberg
Developmental Editor: Erin McMullan
Production Editor: Rakesh Rampertab
Manufacturing Manager: Benjamin Rivera
Cover Designer: Brian Crede
Compositor: TechBooks
Printer: Edwards Brothers

© 2004 by LIPPINCOTT WILLIAMS & WILKINS
530 Walnut Street
Philadelphia, PA 19106 USA
LWW.com

Printed in the USA

Library of Congress Cataloging-in-Publication Data

Peripheral vascular disease : basic diagnostic and therapeutic approaches /
[edited by] George S. Abela.—1st ed.
    p.   ; cm.
Includes bibliographical references and index.
ISBN 0-7817-4383-4
1. Peripheral vascular diseases.   2. Blood-vessels—Diseases.   3. Extremities
(Anatomy)—Diseases.   I. Abela, George S.
[DNLM: 1. Peripheral Vascular Diseases—diagnosis.   2. Peripheral
Vascular Diseases—therapy. WG 500 P4425 2004]
    RC694.P484 2004
    616.1'31—dc22
                                                              2004010609

10 9 8 7 6 5 4 3 2 1

This book is dedicated to the memory of Jeffrey M. Isner, M.D.,
a good friend and pioneer in the field of peripheral vascular disease.
He will be remembered as a wonderful human being.

Contents

Contributors

George S. Abela, M.D., M.Sc., M.B.A, *Division of Cardiology, Michigan State University, East Lansing, Michigan; Department of Internal Medicine, Cardiology, East Lansing, Michigan and Sparrow Hospital, Lansing, Michigan*

Alex Abou-Chebl, M.D., *Interventional Neurology, The Cleveland Clinic Foundation, Cleveland, Ohio*

Timothy Alikakos, M.D., F.A.C.C., *Division of Interventional Cardiology, Department of Cardiology, The Lahey Clinic Medical Center, Burlington Massachusetts; Department of Cardiology, Interventional Cardiology, Condell Medical Center, Libertyville, Illinois*

Gary J. Arnold, M.D., *University of Louisiana at Lafayette, Lafayette, Louisiana*

Gérald, Barbeau, M.D., *Department of Medicine, Laval University; Cardiologist, Department of Medicine, Laval Hospital, Ste-Foy, Quebec, Canada*

Joel M. Cohn, M.D., *Michigan State University and Thoracic and Cardiovascular Institute, East Lansing, Michigan*

Patricia M. Dear, R.N., C.R.R.N., *Alpha Quest LLC, Atlanta, Georgia*

Anthony C. DeFanco, M.D., *Michigan State University, East Lansing, Michigan; Division of Cardiology, McLaren Regional Medical Center, Flint, Michigan*

Michael G. Dickinson, M.D., *Department of Medicine, Division of Cardiology, Michigan State University, East Lansing, Michigan*

Donald J. DiPette, M.D., *Department of Medicine, Texas A&M; Department of Medicine, Scott and White Memorial Hospital, Temple, Texas*

Linda K. East, B.Sc., C.C.V.T., *Michigan State University, East Lansing, Michigan*

Kim A. Eagle, M.D., *University of Michigan Medical School; Cardiovascular Center, University of Michigan Health Systems, Ann Arbor, Michigan*

Andrew C. Eisenhauer, M.D., *Harvard Medical School, Boston, Massachusetts; Director, Interventional Cardiovascular Medicine, Brigham and Women's Hospital, Boston, Massachusetts*

Fernando Elijovich, M.D., F.A.H.A, *The Center for Hypertension and Cardiovascular Medicine, Department of Medicine, Lenox Hill Hospital, New York, New York*

William J. Ennis, D.O., M.B.A, F.A.C.O.S., *Department of Surgery, Midwestern University; Wound Treatment Program, Advocate Christ Hospital and Medical Center, Oak Lawn, Illinois*

Mahmoud Eslami-Farsani, M.D., *University of Southern California, Los Angeles, California; Interventional Cardiologist, Cardiology Specialists of Orange County, Santa Ana, California*

James J. Ferguson, III, M.D., *Department of Medicine, Baylor College of Medicine; Texas Heart Institute, Houston, Texas*

Malcolm T. Foster, III, M.D., *Department of Medicine, Michigan State University, Baptist Heart Institute, Baptist Hospital, Knoxville, Tennessee*

Julia Gates, M.D., *Tufts University School of Medicine, Boston, Massachusetts; Department of Radiology, West Roxbury Veterans Administration Hospital, Boston, Massachusetts*

Ved V. Gossain, M.D., *Division of Endocrinology and Metabolism, Department of Medicine, Michigan State University, East Lansing, Michigan; Department of Medicine, Sparrow Health System, Lansing, Michigan*

Patricia A. Gum, M.D., *Department of Cardiology, The Medical Center of Plano, Plano, Texas*

Elie Hage-Korban, M.D., *Department of Medicine, Jackson General Madison, Jackson, Tennessee*

George G. Hartnell, M.D., *Department of Radiology, Tuffs University School of Medicine, Boston, Massachusetts; Department of Radiology, Bay State Medical Center, Springfield, Massachusetts*

Richard Henry, M.D., *Department of Medicine, Division of Cardiology, Michigan State University, East Lansing, Michigan*

Greg Houlihan, M.D., *Department of Medicine, Division of Cardiology, Michigan State University, East Lansing, Michigan*

Zeeshan S. Husain, D.P.M., A.A.C.F.A.S., *Department of Orthopedics, Detroit Medical Center, Detroit, Michigan*

Ayman Iskander, M.D., *Department of Medicine/Cardiology, Tufts University School of Medicine, Boston, Massachusetts; Interventional Cardiology, Lahey Clinical Medical Center, Burlington, Massachusetts*

James D. Joye, M.D., *Cardiac Catheterization Labs, El Camino Hospital, Mountain View, California*

Douglas S. Jacoby, M.D., *Department of Medicine, University of Pennsylvania, Philadelphia, Pennsylvania*

SriCharan C. Kantipudi, M.D., *Department of Medicine, Division of Cardiology, Michigan State University, East Lansing, Michigan; Department of Cardiology, Sparrow Health System, Lansing, Michigan*

Charles G. Kissel, D.P.M, F.A.C.F.A.S., *Department of Medicine, Wayne State University; Department of Orthopedics, Detroit Medical Center, Detroit, Michigan*

Zvonimir Krajcer, M.D., *University of Texas, Baylor College of Medicine; Department of Cardiology, Texas Heart Institute & St Luke's Episcopal Hospital, Houston, Texas*

Urma Krishnan, M.D., F.A.C.C., *Cardiac Study Center, Tacoma, Washington*

Cheryl L. Laffer, M.D., Ph.D., F.A.H.A., *The Center for Hypertension and Cardiovascular Medicine, Lenox Hill Hospital, New York, New York*

John R. Laird, M.D., *Department of Cardiology, Georgetown University Medical Center; Cardiovascular Research Institute Washington Hospital Center, Washington, DC*

Glenn M. LaMuraglia, M.D., *Harvard Medical School, Boston; Division of Vascular and Endovascular Surgery, Massachusetts General Hospital, Boston, Massachusetts*

Hongbao Ma, Ph.D., *Department of Medicine, Michigan State University, East Lansing, Michigan*

James J. Maciejko, M.S., Ph.D., *Department of Internal Medicine, Wayne State University; Preventive Cardiology, St. John's Hospital, Detroit, Michigan*

Alok Maheshwari, M.D., *Department of Medicine, Division of Cardiology, Michigan State University, East Lansing, Michigan*

Keith A. Mauney, R.N., R.C.U.T., R.V.T., *Keith Mauney and Associates Ultrasound Training Institutes, Dallas, Texas*

Peter A. McCullough, M.D., M.P.H, *Division of Nutrition and Preventative Medicine, William Beaumont Hospital, Royal Oak, Michigan*

Vallerie V. McLaughlin, M.D., *Division of Cardiovascular Medicine, University of Michigan, Ann Arbor, Michigan*

Avanti Mehrotra, M.D., *Department of Medicine, Division of Hematology-Oncology, Michigan State University, East Lansing, Michigan*

Patricio Meneses, Ph.D., *Wound Treatment Program, Department of Surgery, Advocate Christ Medical Center, Oak Lawn, Illinois*

Mary A. Metler, *Department of Medicine, Michigan State University, East Lansing, Michigan*

Raghu R. Midde, M.D., *Department of Cardiovascular Medicine, Stanford University, Stanford, California; Department of Medicine, Kaiser Permanente, Redwood City, California*

Emile R. Mohler, III, M.D., *Department of Medicine, University of Pennsylvania School of Medicine; Department of Vascular Medicine, University of Pennsylvania Health System, Philadelphia, Pennsylvania*

Mehran Moussavian, D.O., *Department of Cardiology, Community Memorial Hospital, Ventura, California*

Debabrata Mukherjee, M.D., M.S., F.A.C.C., *Division of Cardiology, University of Michigan; Director, Peripheral Vascular Interventions, Cardiology, Division of Cardiology, University of Michigan Hospital System, Ann Arbor, Michigan*

Mohanram Narayanan, M.D. F.A.C.P., *Department of Medicine, Texas A&M University; Division of Nephrology and Hypertension, Scott and White Clinic, Temple, Texas*

Giuseppe R. Nigri, M.D., Ph.D., *Department of Surgery, Harvard Medical School; Resident in General Surgery, Massachusetts General Hospital, Boston, Massachusetts*

Mary Noel, M.Ph., Ph.D., R.D., *Department of Family Practice, Michigan State University, East Lansing, Michigan*

Dana A. Ohl, M.D., *Professor of Urology, Michigan Urology Center, University of Michigan, Ann Arbor, Michigan*

Susanne A. Quallich, A.P.R.N., B.C., N.P.-C., C.U.N.P., *Michigan Urology Center, University of Michigan, Ann Arbor, Michigan*

John Penner, M.D., *Professor and Chief Division of Thrombosis and Homeostasis, Michigan State University, East Lansing, Michigan*

Thomas C. Piemonte, M.D., *Clinical Instructor of Medicine, Harvard Medical School, Boston, Massachusetts; Director of Interventional Cardiovascular Medicine, Lahey Clinic, Burlington, Massachusetts*

Alejandro R. Prieto, M.D, *Department of Medicine, Michigan State University, East Lansing, Michigan*

Catherine R. Ratliff, Ph.D., G.N.P, *Department of Plastics, School of Nursing; University of Virginia, Charlottesville, Virginia*

Charles A. Reasner, II, M.D., *Department of Medicine, Division of Cardiology, University of Texas Health Science Center, Texas Diabetes Institute, University of Texas at San Antonio, San Antonio, Texas*

Stanley G. Rockson M.D., *Division of Cardiovascular Medicine, Stanford University School of Medicine, Stanford, California*

Michael S. Schey, D.P.M., F.A.C.F.A.S., *Department of Orthopedics, Detroit Medical Center, Detroit, Michigan*

James A. Shaw, M.B.B.S., Ph.D., *Cardiology Division, Baker Heart Institute; Department of Cardiology, Alfred Hospital, Prahran, Australia*

Peter Sheehan, M.D., *Department of Medicine, New York University School of Medicine; Diabetes Foot and Ankle Center, Department of Orthopaedics, Hospital for Joint Diseases, New York, New York*

John A. Spittell, M.D., *Professor Emeritus, Mayo Clinic, Rochester, Minnesota*

Peter C. Spittell, M.D., *Department of Cardiovascular Diseases, Mayo Clinic; Mayo College of Medicine, Rochester, Minnesota*

Martin J. Stevens, M.D., *Internal Medicine, University of Michigan, Ann Arbor, Michigan*

Patricia Thorpe, M.D., *University of Iowa, Iowa City, Iowa*

Craig M. Walker, M.D., *Department of Medicine/Cardiology, Tulane University, New Orleans, Louisiana; Terrebonne General Hospital, Houma Louisiana; South West Medical Center, Layfayette, Louisiana; Cardiovascular Institute of the South, Houma, Louisiana*

Ralph E. Watson, M.D. F.A.C.P., *Department of Medicine, Division of Internal Medicine, Michigan State University, East Lansing, Michigan*

Christopher J. White, M.D., *Department of Cardiology, Ochsner Clinic Foundation, New Orleans, Louisiana*

Terence Whiteman, M.D., *Department of Medicine, Division of Cardiology, Michigan State University, East Lansing, Michigan; Department of Medicine, Sparrow Hospital, Lansing, Michigan*

Terry L. Woodward, Ph.D., M.B.A., *Department of Physiology, Michigan State University, East Lansing, Michigan; Venture Capital, Teachers Merchant Bank, Toronto, Ontario, Canada*

Jay S. Yadav, M.D., F.A.C.C., F.S.C.A.I., *Department of Cardiovascular Medicine, Cleveland Clinic, Cleveland, Ohio*

Foreword

It is a pleasure to write a foreword to Dr. George Abela's book, *Peripheral Vascular Disease: Basic Diagnostic and Therapeutic Approaches*. In addition to the usual considerations, the refreshingly different approach to the major topic of the book, occlusive peripheral arterial disease, is undoubtedly related to Dr. Abela's clinical and teaching experience. Unique in the book is the inclusion of chapters devoted to important comorbid conditions and complications of occlusive peripheral arterial disease—diabetes, insulin resistance, hypertension, obesity, and peripheral neuropathy—any and all of which can influence prognosis and complicate successful management of these patients. Clinicians, physicians in training, and students, particularly those with a serious interest in peripheral vascular disease, will find this book a useful addition to this increasingly important field—vascular medicine.

John A. Spittell, Jr., MD, MACP, FACC
Professor of Medicine (emeritus)
Mayo College of Medicine
Consultant (emeritus) Cardiovascular Disease
Mayo Clinic
Rochester, Minnesota

Preface

For many decades, peripheral vascular therapy lay dormant with a simple regimented approach that included either conservative management or surgery. However, technological advances of both diagnostic techniques with computerized tomographic and magnetic resonance angiography as well as refined interventional tools with stents have found their way to applications from cerebral to foot vessels. With this new frontier, medical therapy has also evolved to include more effective antiplatelet, lipid lowering, red blood cell modifying, insulin sensitizing and lytic agents in peripheral vascular disease. These evolving technologies have propelled a new paradigm shift in how vascular disease is viewed.

The need to educate trainees in the field of vascular disease is critical since this rapidly evolving area demands highly specialized skills. It is important that trainees be exposed to the basic elements of the field and recognize what they may offer to their patients. This book attempts to provide the residents, fellows in training, and professionals interested in vascular disease a practical reference with guidelines that range from the essentials of the physical exam to the most sophisticated technologic developments in diagnostics and therapeutics of peripheral vascular disease.

The aim is to provide a timely, practical, and comprehensive compilation of developments in this field using multidisciplinary perspectives. This is critical since much of the expertise is highly specialized and no single medical specialty can claim it entirely. Consequently, a dynamic interaction between various specialty groups is needed to integrate skills to provide comprehensive care in peripheral vascular disease.

The book is divided into ten parts each of which takes the reader to another level of intensity relative to understanding and treatment. **Part I**—*Anatomy, Etiology, Signs, and Symptoms of PVD* consists of four chapters that describe the basic elements related to vascular injury and repair atherosclerosis as a systemic disease, history and physical exam of the arterial and venous system and symptoms of claudication in PVD. **Part II**—*Risk Factors for PVD* consists of eleven chapters that address risks and unique clinical presentations of PVD. These include a chapter on PVD in diabetes, metabolic syndrome, uncommon types of occlusive arterial disease, the latest recommendations on hypertension, obesity and its management, peripheral neuropathy, and erectile dysfunction. **Part III**—*Medical treatment of PVD* includes treatment of hyperlipidemia with drugs and exercise, modification of risk factors and anticoagulants. **Part IV**—*Diagnosis and Intervention in PVD* describes non invasive testing, optimal endovascular therapy, novel imaging methods, physiology of renal artery stenosis and its treatment, subclavian disease, treatment of cerebral disease and intracranial interventions, ilio-femoral disease and complications with interventions and transradial catheterization techniques, and renal injury from contrast agents. **Part V**—*Surgical Treatment in PVD* describes pre and post-operative management, surgery, stent grafts and foot care. **Part VI**—*Systemic Manifestations of PVD* describes wound healing and management of ulcers. **Part VII**—*Novel Developments in the Treatment of PVD* includes excimer laser revascularization and stent selection. **Part VIII**—*Training Cardiovascular Fellows, Medicine Residents and Housestaff* describes technical training requirements for practice and credentialing. **Part IX**—*Venous Disease* describes deep venous thrombosis and pulmonary embolism, venous insufficiency and pulmonary hypertension. Finally, **Part X**—*Impact of PVD* describes the economic effects of PVD and billing and coding of clinical charges.

It is expected that the contributions of this multi-disciplinary textbook will provide for a thorough understanding of the field of peripheral vascular disease and its treatment as well as the requirements and credentialing process needed.

George S. Abela
Editor

Acknowledgement

It is important to recognize that this work is a product of extensive efforts of individuals who took precious time to share knowledge with others in order to enhance the care of patients and alleviate human suffering. These efforts are most noble and the authors and other helpers are to be most highly commended and their names are listed in the text. A special acknowledgement is due to Hongbao Ma and Linda East who participated in extra effort in helping to proof read the manuscripts and help in the development of the summary bullets at the beginning of each chapter. I am greatly appreciative of their dedication and effort. Also, special thanks is due to Drs. Michael Dickinson, James Joye, Elie Hage-Korban, Andrew Prieto, who contributed two chapters and especially Dr. Christopher White for filling in at the last moment with an additional chapter. Recognition is due to the valuable contributions of fellows from our training program at Michigan State University. Finally, I would like to thank Ruth Weinberg and Erin McMullan with Lippincott Williams & Wilkins for their support and patience in the development of this book. Gratitude and thanks is due to all.

CHAPTER 1

Anatomy, Physiology, and Response to Vascular Injury

Anthony C. DeFranco, Hongbao Ma, SriCharan C. Kantipudi, and George S. Abela

---

Key Points

- Arteries have two major properties: elasticity and contractility. The elastic recoil of arteries forces blood forward.
- Normal endothelial function includes a barrier to prevent thrombosis and production of vasoreactive substances.
- Arterial remodeling is an adaptive change in the vessel lumen area that increases lumen size to accommodate atheroma (positive remodeling) or scars down the arterial lumen (negative remodeling).
- Increase in arterial flow stimulates nitric oxide production and enhances vascular dilation.
- Lipid challenges may interfere with normal vascular tone regulation.
- Brachial artery reactivity can be used to evaluate the status of vascular tone and may eventually serve to risk-stratify patients for future cardiovascular events.

INTRODUCTION

Understanding the anatomy and physiology of the arterial system is critical to understanding vascular disease processes and the therapeutic interventions used to address the altered functions. This chapter connects this basic knowledge to the response to injury, the repair of the vascular system, and the complex autocrine and paracrine dynamics that regulate the arterial circulation.

BASIC GROSS ANATOMY OF THE PERIPHERAL ARTERIAL CIRCULATION

Blood vessels form a network of tubes that transport blood from the heart to the tissues of the body and then return it to the heart (1). This was first described by William Harvey in 1628 (2). Arteries are vessels that carry blood from the heart to the tissues. Large, elastic arteries leave the heart and divide into medium-size muscular arteries, which branch out into the various regions of the body. Medium-size arteries then divide into small arteries, which divide into smaller arteries and ar-

terioles. In the tissues, the arterioles branch into countless microscopic vessels called capillaries. Through the walls of the capillaries, substances such as O_2/CO_2 and nutrient/waste are exchanged between the blood and body tissues. In the tissues, some capillaries reunite to form small veins called venules. The venules merge to form progressively larger veins. The veins deliver blood from tissue back to the heart. Because blood vessels also require O_2 and nutrients, they also have blood vessels in their walls, called vaso vasora.

Human arterial circulatory routes are shown in Fig. 1.1. The principal human veins are shown in Fig. 1.2.

Three arteries originate from the aortic arch: the brachiocephalic, which supplies part of the neck, head, brain, and right arm; the left common carotid, which supplies part of the neck, head, and brain; and the left subclavian, which supplies the left arm. The brachiocephalic divides into the right subclavian and the right common carotid arteries. The right subclavian gives rise to the right vertebral artery, and the left subclavian gives rise to the left vertebral artery. The continuation of the subclavian into the axilla is called the axillary artery, which continues into the arm as the brachial

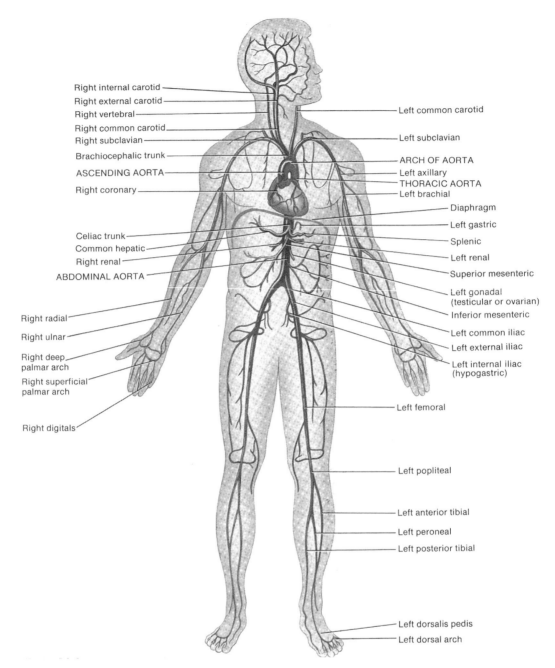

FIG. 1.1. Human arterial circulation including cerebral area, neck, torso, arms, and legs. (From Tortora GJ, Anagnostakos NP. *Principles of anatomy and physiology*, 6th ed. New York: Harper & Row, 1990, p. 498, with permission.)

artery, then divides into medial ulnar and lateral radial arteries, which go to the arm and the fingers.

The right and left common carotid arteries pass upward into the neck. These divide into the external and internal carotid arteries. The external carotids supply blood to the thyroid gland, tongue, face, throat, ear, scalp, and dura mater. The internal carotids supply blood to the brain, eyes, forehead, and nose.

The aorta continues after a downward turn (descending aorta) and enters the abdomen through the diaphragm. The vessel becomes the abdominal aorta, which travels in the retroperitoneal space, and at the mid-abdominal level it forks into the right and left common iliac arteries. Before it branches, it gives rise to the celiac, superior, and inferior mesenteric arteries and the spinal artery.

Each of the two common iliac vessels further divides into internal and external iliac arteries. The internal iliac arteries provide blood to the pelvis, including parts of the rectum, the sexual organs, and the buttocks. The external iliac arteries provide blood to the legs. The external iliac turns into the femoral artery, which further splits into superficial and deep femoral arteries. The superficial femoral artery

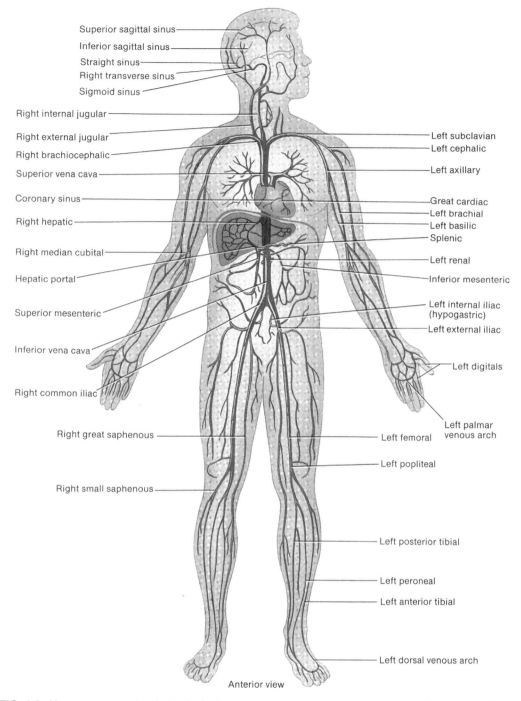

FIG. 1.2. Human venous circulation including cerebral, area neck, torso, arms, and legs. (From Tortora GJ, Anagnostakos NP. *Principles of anatomy and physiology,* 6th ed. New York: Harper & Row, 1990, p. 503, with permission.)

continues above the knee to form the popliteal artery. The popliteal spans the knee joint. In the lower leg, the popliteal becomes the tibioperoneal trunk, whose branches further supply the ankle and the foot via the posterior tibial and dorsalis pedis arteries (3).

The venous structures generally parallel the arterial structures. Smaller vessels in the periphery begin the long trek back to the heart and the lungs. The vessels of the head and the upper part of the body empty into the superior vena cava;

the vessels of the lower half of the body empty into the inferior vena cava. The inferior and superior vena cavae empty into the right atrium, which completes the vascular circuit back to the heart (4).

HISTOLOGY OF ARTERIES AND VEINS

Arteries have walls constructed of three coats or tunics and a hollow core (lumen) through which blood flows (5). The

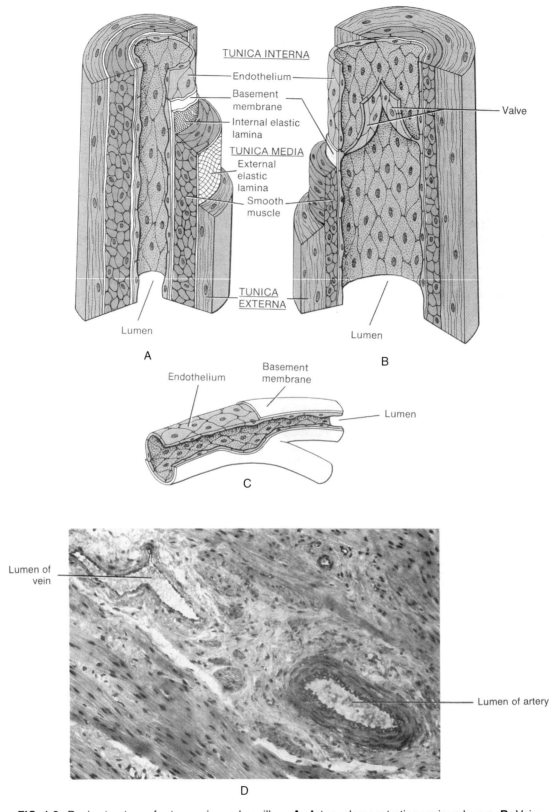

FIG. 1.3. Basic structure of artery, vein, and capillary. **A:** Artery, demonstrating various layers. **B:** Vein, demonstrating various layers. **C:** Capillary. **D:** Histologic cross section of artery (*right*) and vein (*left*) demonstrating differences in wall thickness between the two vessels. (From Tortora GJ, Anagnostakos, NP. *Principles of anatomy and physiology,* 6th ed. New York: Harper & Row, 1990, p. 607, with permission & courtesy of Andrew Kuntzman.)

inner coat of an arterial wall (the tunica interna) is composed of a lining of endothelium, which is in contact with the blood; a basement membrane; and a layer of elastic tissue called the internal elastic lamina. The middle coat (tunica media) is usually the thickest layer and consists of smooth muscle as well as collagenous and elastic fibers. The outer coat (tunica externa) is composed principally of elastic and collagenous fibers. An external elastic lamina may separate the tunica externa from the tunica media (Fig. 1.3).

Arteries have two major properties: elasticity and contractility. When the ventricles contract and eject blood into the large arteries, the arteries expand to accommodate the extra blood. Then, as the ventricles relax, the elastic recoil of the arteries forces the blood onward. The contractility of the artery comes from its smooth muscle cells.

The large arteries (elastic arteries) include the aorta and the brachiocephalic, common carotid, subclavian, vertebral, and common iliac arteries. The wall of elastic arteries is relatively thin and its tunica media contains more elastic fibers and fewer smooth muscle cells.

The medium-size arteries (muscular arteries) include the axillary, brachial, radial, intercostal, splenic, mesenteric, femoral, popliteal, and tibial arteries. Their tunica media contains more smooth muscle than elastic fibers and they are more important to the vasoconstriction and vasodilation involved in adjusting the flow of blood.

Ananastomoses are junctions of two or more vessels supplying the same body region. They give alternate routes for the blood to flow to a body part.

The exchange of nutrients and wastes between the blood and tissue cells occurs in capillary arteries. Capillary walls are composed of a single layer of endothelium cells and a basement membrane, which facilitate the exchange of substances.

Several capillaries unite to form small veins called venules. Venules collect blood from capillaries and drain it into veins. Veins are composed of essentially the same three types of coats as the arteries. The vein tunica interna and media are thinner and the tunica externa is thicker than those of accompanying arteries (6).

PHYSIOLOGY

Endothelium

Normal endothelial function is important in maintaining homeostasis. In addition to functioning as a physical and physiological barrier to prevent thrombotic and vasoactive substances from coming into contact with underlying smooth muscle cells, the endothelium possesses two crucial functions: as a secretory tissue and as an antithrombotic surface.

Endothelial Cell Function as a Secretory Tissue

Since Furchgott described the role of the endothelium in the relaxation of the vessel wall in response to acetylcholine in terms of a "substance" later called endothelial-derived relaxation factor, there have been important contributions by other investigators that have led to further understanding of the function of the endothelium (7,8).

In the secretory role, endothelial cells synthesize important vasoactive substances including endothelial-derived relaxation factor (EDRF), endothelial-derived hyperpolarizing factor (EDHF) (9), and prostacyclin, which act as vasodilators; and endothelin and endothelial-derived contracting factor (EDCF), which act as vasoconstrictors. Biological and chemical evidence supports the proposal that nitric oxide (NO), a potent vasodilator is a form of EDRF (10). Endothelial cells also make substances involved in the coagulation pathways, which include factor VIII antigen, von Willebrand's factor, and plasminogen activator. In addition, they produce collagen, elastin, glycosaminoglycans, and fibronectin, which are structural components of extracellular matrix (11). The endothelium manufactures and secretes heparan sulfates and growth factors, which regulate the smooth muscle cells. It also modifies the extracellular matrix by production of matrix metalloproteinases.

Endothelial cells regulate the metabolism of the plasma lipids. They bind the lipoprotein lipase by the heparin sulfates, and play a role in the transport and metabolism of low-density lipoprotein (LDL) and chylomicrons and release of free fatty acids. They possess receptors for LDL and thereby modify it (12). Normally the endothelial monolayer downregulates the LDL receptors. However, in a diseased state, the endothelium can facilitate the uptake of the LDL, leading to an increase in the cholesterol esters in the vessel wall. It clears and alters adenine nucleotides, nucleosides, bradykinin, angiotensin I, catecholamines, and serotonin in the circulation.

Role of Endothelium in the Thrombotic and Antithrombotic Balance

The negative charge on the surface of normal endothelial cells contributes to the antithrombotic surface, which prevents platelet adhesion and activation and resists coagulation. However, the same cells, when stimulated, can manufacture and secrete prothrombotic agents. Thus, the endothelium regulates a functional thrombosis/antithrombosis–thrombolytic balance.

On one hand, the endothelium produces prostacyclin, which inhibits platelet aggregation (13), and thrombomodulin, which activates protein C. The activated protein C inhibits plasminogen activator inhibitor-1 (PAI-1) and interacts with protein S to inactivate the activated factors V and VIII to limit thrombosis. Heparin-like molecules secreted by the endothelium adhere to anti-thrombin III to clear the thrombin. Another important function of the endothelium is to elaborate the tissue plasminogen activator, which enhances clot lysis. On the other hand, under inflammatory conditions, the endothelium can become potently prothrombotic. This is accomplished by an increase in expression of the tissue factor (14) and leukocyte adhesion molecules on the surface and a decrease in expression of thrombomodulin. Tissue factor activates the factors VII, IX, and X. Activated Xa assembles the prothrombinase complex, releasing thrombin, which in turn stimulates von Willebrand's factor, which, along with thrombospondin and fibronectin, furthers the thrombotic process.

Vascular Smooth Muscle

The smooth muscle cells contract and relax the arterial wall in response to hormonal stimulation and the endothelial cells. The vasoconstriction is facilitated by second-messenger pathways, which include G proteins. Growth factors such as platelet-derived growth factor (PDRF) activate similar signaling pathways. The cell growth takes place in two forms. Hypertrophy can occur in response to angiotensin II and thrombin and in large vessels due to hypertension. Hyperplasia can occur in response to growth factors like PDRF and fibroblast growth factor (FGF) after vascular injury.

Interaction of Endothelium with Vascular Smooth Cells

Endothelial cells play a dual role in the regulation of vascular tone.

Endothelial-Derived Relaxation Factor

In 1980, Furchgott first described the dilation of rabbit aortic rings in response to acetylcholine in the presence of the intact endothelium (7,8). The NO, which is believed to be the predominant form of EDRF, is synthesized from L-arginine by the enzymatic action of NO synthase. NO is unstable and has a mechanism of action different than that of prostaglandins, and is inhibited by methylene blue and oxygen free radicals. NO crosses the smooth muscle cell membrane and binds to the guanylate cyclase and increases the formation of cyclic GMP, which in turn reduces the intracellular calcium concentration, thereby causing dephosphorylation of the myosin light chain and ultimately relaxation (15). Other factors that can cause the release of EDRF by increasing the intracellular calcium concentration are norepinephrine, thrombin, ATP, bradykinin, vasopressin, ionophores, serotonin, histamine, and fatty acids.

Adenosine

Adenosine activates cAMP to relax the smooth muscle by binding to purinergic P1 receptors. Adenosine nucleotides (ADP and ATP) bind to P2 receptors and have a dual role. They stimulate the endothelial P2 receptors to release EDRF and prostacyclin, and act on P2 receptors on vascular smooth muscle to cause vasoconstriction. However, the endothelium can regulate these functions by converting ADP or ATP into adenosine through the ectonucleotidase enzymatic system.

Prostacyclin

Prostacyclin is produced by the endothelium and relaxes the vascular smooth muscle by increasing the levels of intracellular cAMP. It also works as a platelet suppressant and antithrombotic agent. Other factors that stimulate the synthesis of prostacyclin are PDGF, bradykinin, substance P, adenine nucleotides, and epidermal growth factor.

Endothelin

Endothelins occur in three types, of which endothelin-1 is the most potent vasoconstrictor. They work by the activation of phosphoinositide/protein kinase signaling pathway and play a role in nitroglycerin tolerance and as chemoattractants for monocytes.

Angiotensin-Converting Enzyme

Angiotensin-converting enzyme (ACE) is a protein expressed on the surface of endothelium, and converts angiotensin I to the potent vasoconstrictor angiotensin II and also deactivates bradykinin.

Regulation of Smooth Muscle Cell Growth

Even though the endothelium plays a dual role, its net effect is growth inhibitory. Two possible mechanisms are hypothesized on how the endothelium exerts a tonic inhibitory influence on smooth muscle cell growth. In one, it works as a physical barrier preventing blood-borne growth factors from coming into contact with underlying smooth muscle. The second mechanism is by secretion of growth-inhibiting factors like EDRF, heparin, heparin sulfates, and transforming growth factor-1. The growth factors eluted by endothelium are platelet-derived growth factor, interleukin-1, fibroblast growth factor, insulin-like growth factor-1, and endothelin.

Hemodynamic Influences on the Endothelium

Langille first showed that endothelium is essential for the compensatory arterial response to long-term changes in luminal blood flow rates (16). Shear stress, stretch of the vessel wall, and elevated pressure independently affect endothelial function and morphology.

RESPONSE TO VASCULAR INJURY

Arterial Remodeling

Remodeling is defined as a change in vessel area (i.e., within the external elastic membrane [EEM]) as atherosclerosis develops. Positive remodeling occurs when the area within the EEM area increases as atheroma develops. Glagov and colleagues first described these phenomena in peripheral specimens and then in coronary specimens in necropsy studies (17); subsequent intravascular ultrasound (IVUS) studies corroborated these observations in coronary (18–20) and peripheral arteries (21) in vivo. In positively remodeled segments, Glagov hypothesized that vessel expansion is "compensatory" because lumen size was relatively preserved

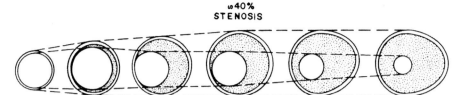

FIG. 1.4. The concept of vascular remodeling in atherosclerotic arteries is demonstrated sequentially in response to enlarging atherosclerotic plaques. In the early stages of plaque deposition, the lumen remains normal or enlarges slightly (*left*). When intimal plaque enlarges to involve the entire circumference of the vessel and produces more than 40% stenosis, the artery is no longer able to enlarge at a rate sufficient to prevent narrowing of the lumen. This leads to encroachment of the lumen. (From Glagov S, Weisenberg E, Zarms C, et al. Compensatory enlargement of human atherosclerotic coronary arteries. *N Engl J Med.* 1987;316:1371–1375, with permission.)

despite considerable amounts of atheroma compared to more normal segments in the same vessel. However, beyond a certain limit, in the range of 30% to 50% cross-sectional narrowing, this "compensatory" mechanism fails and luminal dimensions become progressively compromised, and hemodynamically significant obstruction occurs (Figs. 1.4 and 1.5).

Recently, histopathologic and IVUS studies have demonstrated that in *de novo* coronary lesions, remodeling can be negative as well as positive. At negatively remodeled sites, the cross-sectional area (CSA) within the external elastic lamina is significantly less than at an appropriate reference segment. Thus, at some sites in the peripheral (22) and coronary (23) circulations, stenoses are due to both atheroma accumulation and a decrease in the total vessel area.

Although the biological mechanisms responsible for positive and negative remodeling are unknown, the remodeling phenomenon has several critical implications. First, remodeling can conceal substantial atherosclerotic plaque burden even in the presence of angiographically normal coronary and peripheral vessels. Second, because of this, most contemporary studies of regression or stabilization of atherosclerosis use some modality that can accurately measure the effects of the intervention on remodeled segments, such as intravascular ultrasound or carotid B-mode ultrasound. Regression of disease, discussed later, may be a potential therapeutic strategy; however, studies designed to test whether arterial remodeling can be favorably affected are still in progress (24).

VASOREACTIVITY OF THE PERIPHERAL VASCULATURE

Vasoresponse of Normal Peripheral Endothelium

In the last decade, our understanding of the vascular biology of the human arterial system has experienced a fundamental paradigm shift in the concepts of arterial function and pathophysiology (Table 1.1). Arteries are no longer considered to be passive, fixed conduits that merely distribute blood to end organs. Instead, it is now recognized that the arterial system is

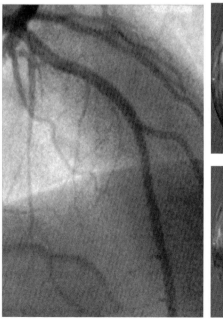

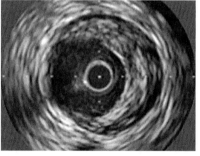
A

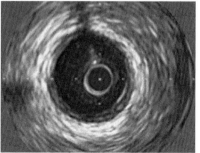
B

FIG. 1.5. Example of arterial remodeling illustrated by intravascular ultrasound in the coronary circulation. The external elastic membrane (EEM) cross-sectional area of the angiographically normal reference site **(A)** is nearly 50% larger than the EEM area of the distal site **(B)**, yet the lumen size is the same. Thus, there has been "expansion" or "compensatory remodeling" that has accommodated to the atheroma mass.

TABLE 1.1. *Factors affecting blood supply and symptoms in peripheral arterial disease*

Flow-limiting lesions ("fixed" stenoses, long lesions, tandem/multiple lesions, etc.)
Presence and extent of collateral circulation
Endothelial function/vasodilator reserve
Metabolic activity of the supplied territory
Impaired response to exogenous vasodilators
Enhanced vasoconstriction (serotonin, endothelin, angiotensin II, thromboxane)
Abnormal rheology
    Reduced red blood cell distensibility
    Increased leukocyte adhesion to the vessel wall
    Increased platelet adhesion and aggregation
    Increased fibrinogen levels
Acute vascular injury/plaque rupture
Thrombosis, embolization

a complex biomechanical system that responds dynamically to metabolic, biochemical, and hemodynamic changes in its local environment and that of the downstream tissues that it perfuses. The arterial endothelium is the largest paracrine organ in the body; it secretes many factors that regulate vascular tone, leukocyte and platelet interaction, thrombogenicity, lipid metabolism, and cell growth. Cell membrane receptors enable the endothelium to respond to an enormous number of external and internal stimuli; by means of these receptors, complex signal transduction mechanisms lead to the release of substances that regulate arterial constriction and dilation, thromboregulatory functions, and growth factors, which affect the arterial smooth muscle cells. The current paradigm of atherosclerosis considers that dysfunction of these processes contributes to or is the cause of the development of hypertension and atherosclerosis and exacerbates cardiac causes of heart failure.

Human arteries respond to physical and chemical stimuli to regulate arterial tone and adjust blood flow and distribution according to changes in the local environment. An increase in flow results in increased shear stress; shear results in an increase in endothelial release of NO, which causes acute vasodilation. This process is referred to as flow-mediated dilation (FMD). The exact mechanisms by which the endothelium senses and responds to acute changes in shear stress are the subject of intense investigation. The current working hypothesis is that acute (millisecond) changes in shear stress activate calcium-sensitive ionic channels in the endothelial cell membrane. These channels open in response to shear, hyperpolarize the cell membrane, augment the influx of calcium, and activate endothelial NO synthase (eNOS) (25–27). The result is an increase in the generation of NO and in FMD (28,29). This working hypothesis is supported by the observation that administration of an NO synthase (NOS) inhibitor or endothelial denudation abolishes FMD. Over longer time frames (minutes), shear stress induces phosphorylation of the eNOS enzyme, which results in an increase in its activity, generating higher net production of NO. Over even longer time periods, sustained or repeated shear stress (such

as with a regular exercise program of adequate intensity) may induce increased eNOS gene transcription, which increases the capability of the endothelium to generate NO. Thus, over the long term, arteries also adapt to chronic changes in local and regional hemodynamic stresses and to systemic conditions in an attempt to preserve optimal cross-sectional area, biomechanical characteristics, and optimal blood flow to downstream tissues. This observation is already influencing strategies to alleviate symptoms and reduce complications in patients with peripheral arterial disease, as is discussed later. In addition to NO, other mediators may also play a role in this response, such as prostanoids (30) or the as-yet-unidentified endothelium-derived hyperpolarizing factor.

Angiography has been the gold standard for the serial assessment of peripheral arterial disease and it remains a vital tool for clinical diagnosis and management; however, there are two fundamental limitations that impair its ability to accurately assess the relationship between disease severity and end-organ perfusion. First, although a flow-limiting stenosis is often the most important determinant of insufficient blood supply, stenosis severity is a relatively insensitive measure of the ability of the vessel to deliver blood to distal tissues. Conventionally, a 50%-diameter stenosis or a 75%-area stenosis has been the cutoff for a "hemodynamically significant" lesion, but this concept is now recognized to be overly simplistic and physiologically inaccurate. The impact of a particular lesion that extends into the arterial lumen depends on many factors, including the length of the lesion, the size and metabolic activity of the downstream tissues, the presence or absence of collateral flow and disease in other vessels, and, most importantly for this discussion, the endothelial function of the entire arterial territory. Even by the 1970s several important deficiencies of angiography were apparent. Studies documented high interobserver variability of angiogram interpretation (31). Major discrepancies were observed between the apparent severities of lesions as observed by angiograms and those observed histologically at postmortem (32–34). Angiography cannot visualize structures less than 0.2 mm, even though clinically relevant calcifications or thrombi may be of this size.

Second, even though angiographically visible stenoses are often the most important determinants of blood supply to downstream tissues, functional abnormalities in vasoreactivity may also adversely affect blood flow and transform an asymptomatic patient into a symptomatic one. Patients with peripheral arterial disease have impaired vasodilator reserve in both conduit and resistance vessels, as is discussed later. The immediate (millisecond to millisecond), intermediate (minute to minute), and long-term changes in arterial tone and thus lumen area are often below the level of sensitivity for quantitative angiography to detect any change in arterial caliber.

Direct measurements of coronary and peripheral arterial flow are accurate and have provided important insights into arterial physiology. The agent used most commonly to assess endothelial function is acetylcholine (Ach) infused at

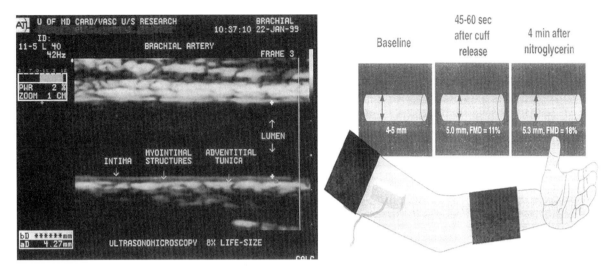

FIG. 1.6. Brachial artery reactivity study in a patient. Example of an ultrasound image obtained in the brachial fossa at baseline. (From Corretti MC, Anderson TJ, Benjamin EJ, et al. Guidelines for the ultrasound assessment of endothelial-dependent flow-mediated vasodilation of the brachial artery: a report of the International Brachial Artery Reactivity Task Force. *J Am Coll Cardiol* 2002;39(2):257–265, with permission.)

doses of 10^{-8} to 10^{-6} mol per L. In normal arteries, Ach causes the release of NO and results in vasodilation. However, in atherosclerotic vessels, Ach induces vasoconstriction. Atherosclerosis is associated with reduced NO release (35,36) (and perhaps increased NO degradation). The mechanism of this paradoxical vasoconstriction is thought to be smooth muscle cell activation, because in the presence of lower levels of NO, Ach exerts a greater net activation of smooth muscles cells in the arterial media via muscarinic receptors.

Early noninvasive studies of peripheral endothelial function (some of which are cited in what follows) utilized plethysmography. In this technique, the technician places pneumatic cuffs at the wrist and the upper arm and a strain gauge around the forearm of the patient. The wrist cuff is inflated to 200 mm Hg to prevent blood flow to the hand, the upper arm cuff is inflated to 40 mm Hg, and the resulting venous occlusion and forearm engorgement are recorded on the plethysmograph as a measure of resting blood flow. The upper arm cuff is inflated above systolic pressure for 5 to 10 minutes, and repeat measurements after deflation are used to estimate hyperemic blood flow. As one might expect, this technique is cumbersome and is now less commonly used than measurement of brachial artery reactivity.

Brachial Artery Reactivity Testing

Although invasive studies continue to provide invaluable data on arterial physiology, these tests are impractical for serial studies. A noninvasive test, brachial artery reactivity (BAR), has been developed as a surrogate. The advantages of this methodology are that it is simple, noninvasive, and practical for serial studies. A two-dimensional ultrasound image of the brachial artery is acquired in a longitudinal plane

above the antecubital fossa to allow accurate measurement of arterial diameter (Fig. 1.6). Skill and experience are required to select an image with clear definition of the anterior and posterior intimal interfaces of the lumen and the vessel wall during two-dimensioanl gray-scale imaging. Perivascular landmarks, such as veins and other structures, are used to maintain the same image location throughout the study. Time-averaging of the pulsed Doppler velocity signal allows estimation of basal blood flow. After baseline image acquisition, a blood pressure cuff is inflated either on the forearm or in the antecubital fossa to greater than 50 mm Hg above resting systolic pressure to occlude flow, typically for 5 minutes. The resulting downstream ischemia results in dilation of resistance vessels. When the cuff is deflated, this downstream vasodilation induces a high-flow state in the brachial artery, termed reactive hyperemia, and the resulting increase in shear stress causes brachial artery dilation. After cuff deflation, continuous two-dimensional longitudinal images are recorded for 1 to 2 minutes along with pulsed Doppler time-averaging of the mid-artery signal from the release of the blood pressure cuff for 15 seconds. Endothelial function can also be evaluated in the distribution of the femoral artery with a similar technique.

In individual with normal endothelial function, the brachial artery begins to dilate immediately after cuff deflation due to the increased velocity of blood flow and the increase in shear stress. Several studies suggest that the maximal increase in brachial artery diameter occurs 45 to 60 seconds after release (37–39). This response is dependent on endothelial production of nitric oxide, because studies document that it can be abolished after administration of NG-monomethyl-L-arginine (L-NMMA), a potent inhibitor of nitric oxide synthase (40,41). Flow-mediated vasodilation is usually reported as a percentage change in the poststimulus diameter compared to baseline. Celermajer et al. reported a mean flow-mediated dilation of approximately 10% in individuals between the ages of 8 and 57 years of age (42). The International Brachial Artery Reactivity Task Force recommends that baseline diameter and absolute change should also be reported (43). In some studies, data on the degree of brachial artery dilation are supplemented with additional endpoints, such as the time and duration of vasodilator response (44,45). In subjects with abnormal endothelial function, flow-mediated dilation is impaired or absent, as discussed later.

Although simple in concept, there are many technical and physiological aspects of the procedure that affect its accuracy and reproducibility. The International Brachial Artery Reactivity Task Force has recently published a set of guidelines in an attempt to standardize the technical aspects of the procedure (43). There are many variables that the operator must control. First, many variables affect flow-mediated dilation. The patient must fast for at least 8 to 12 hours before study; caffeine, tobacco, high-fat foods, and some vitamins affect the results. Sympathetic stimuli can profoundly affect the results; thus, patients must be studied in a quiet, temperature-controlled room. The task force recommends that vasoactive medications be withheld for a minimum of four half-lives. Even the patient's menstrual cycle can affect the results (46). Second, the ultrasound equipment utilized must be optimal; broad-band (7 to 12 MHz) linear-array transducers and a high-resolution scanner are optimal. Third, measurements must be electrocardiogram-gated. Fourth, the technician performing the procedure needs to have considerable facility and experience with the procedure because the time window for data acquisition after cuff deflation is very brief. Although occlusion above the brachial fossa elicits a greater reactive hyperemic response (enhanced dilation of the brachial artery, perhaps by recruitment of a larger number of resistance vessels downstream) and is the preferred technique, it is technically more challenging due to the resulting distortion of the brachial artery and more difficult ultrasonic imaging (38). If serial testing before and after challenge with an exogenous agent is part of the study protocol, at least 10 minutes between the baseline and the postchallenge study is required to reestablish baseline physiology. Despite these and other technical challenges, in experienced laboratories the accuracy, reproducibility, and safety of this technique are well established (47). Recently developed commercially available systems offer the promise of standardization and greater ease of use.

Vasoresponse of Abnormal Endothelium

Endothelial Function in Preclinical Vascular Disease

Even in the earliest phases of atherosclerosis, there is often endothelial dysfunction. Whether endothelial function is the result of atherosclerosis or its cause (or whether the two are interdependent) is a subject of much research. Endothelial dysfunction associated with vascular injury has been proposed as a precursor to atherosclerosis (48). Impaired endothelial function can be demonstrated in asymptomatic children and young adults who have risk factors for atherosclerosis, such as hypercholesterolemia and smoking (42). Accordingly, tests of endothelial function are in development to diagnose early disease and to monitor response to interventions, such as risk factor modification. Atherosclerotic vessels have abnormal flow-mediated dilation, which is associated with atherosclerotic risk factors and is thought to be a marker of preclinical disease (42,49). The end result is that these arteries vasoconstrict in response to stimuli that in normal arteries are vasodilatory, and, conversely, may dilate at times when vasoconstriction is the appropriate physiological response.

Recent necropsy and intravascular ultrasound studies document that atherosclerosis is present in a substantial percentage of children and young adults. Autopsy data from Korean and Vietnam War victims documented that advanced atherosclerotic lesions (greater than 50% stenosis) were present in approximately 20% of soldiers who died at an average age of less than 25 years (50). Stary reported from another necropsy series that 65% of children aged 12 to 14 years had the earliest signs of atherosclerosis (51). The Bogalusa Heart Study examined a large number of subjects who died of nonvascular causes at less than 40 years of age; this study documented a high prevalence of atherosclerosis in these young and middle-aged individuals (52). In an intravascular ultrasound study of transplanted hearts at the Cleveland Clinic Foundation, Tuzcu and colleagues corroborated these necropsy findings. Fifty-two percent of coronary arteries from asymptomatic teenagers and young adults (mean age 33.4 years) had atherosclerotic lesions (53). Thus, there is overwhelming evidence that the earliest morphological changes of atherosclerosis occur in young individuals.

Although there are few data correlating endothelial function in young individuals with documented vascular disease (either by invasive or noninvasive methodologies, such as electron beam tomography, carotid intima–media thickness, or magnetic resonance angiography), the Bogalusa Heart Study demonstrated a strong correlation between morphological changes of atherosclerosis with conventional atherosclerotic risk factors as assessed postmortem (52). Thus, it is not surprising that in middle-aged individuals with atherosclerotic risk factors or established vascular disease, endothelial dysfunction as assessed by brachial artery reactivity is common.

As a result of these observations, there is intense interest in determining whether brachial artery reactivity testing can be used as a screening tool to identify people with preclinical coronary and peripheral atherosclerosis to target risk factor intervention and reduce subsequent vascular events. In patients with coronary disease, several studies suggest that endothelial dysfunction is an independent predictor of subsequent cardiovascular events (54,55). In a pilot study, Schroeder and colleagues examined 122 consecutive participants with suspected coronary artery disease (CAD) by history followed by exercise stress testing and cardiac catheterization (56). One hundred and one patients had angiographic abnormality confirming the presence of disease; flow-mediated dilation was significantly higher in the group without than in the group with angiographic disease ($7.0 \pm 3.5\%$ vs. $3.8 \pm 4.1\%$, $p < 0.001$), for a sensitivity and specificity of 71% and 81%, respectively. However, the magnitude of the FMD abnormality did not discriminate the severity of the angiographic disease, and because IVUS studies have confirmed that some patients may have substantial atheroma burden in the absence of any angiographic abnormality, and coronary endothelial function was not assessed, some of the patients with angina but normal angiograms might still have had angina on the basis of endothelial dysfunction. Although BAR holds promise as a screening technique for the identification of vascular disease patients in the earliest stages of disease, this strategy requires more study before clinical application is appropriate. Brachial artery reactivity has also been suggested as a screening tool to identify the effect of various interventions on endothelial function, on the assumption that improvements might predict clinical improvement or a reduction in vascular events when such agents are tested in larger, subsequent trials powered for clinical endpoints (57).

Effect of Vascular Risk Factors on Peripheral Endothelial Function

Conventional atheroscleotic risk factors appear to increase the incidence of endothelial dysfunction. All conventional risk factors increase the oxidative stress on arterial endothelium, and the resulting increase in reactive oxygen species accelerates the degradation of nitric oxide. In a study of 500 individuals aged 5 to 73 years without known vascular disease, FMD was lower in the presence of hypercholesterolemia, smoking, hypertension, and a family history of premature vascular disease (58). An association between essential hypertension and endothelial dysfunction has been documented (59,60), suggesting the possibility that some abnormality of endothelial function may be the cause, rather than the result, of hypertension. Other studies have supported the association of uncontrolled vascular risk factors and an increased incidence of abnormal endothelial function using FMD techniques in either the brachial or the femoral distribution (61,62). Brachial artery reactivity and flow-mediated dilation are reduced by cigarette smoking (63), hypertension (64), hypercholesterolemia (65), and aging (62).

Endothelial Function in Established Vascular Disease

Given these abnormalities in endothelial function in patients with vascular risk factors but without overt vascular disease, it is not surprising that patients with established vascular disease also frequently demonstrate abnormal endothelial function, particularly if risk factors remain uncontrolled. Impaired brachial FMD has been shown to correlate with the extent of CAD and the maximum percentage diameter stenosis in any

of the major epicardial coronary arteries (66,67). Similarly, impaired FMD has been reported in an older population with symptomatic peripheral vascular disease (PVD) compared to age-matched controls without apparent PVD (68).

Flow-mediated dilation can also be studied after the administration of exogenous nitroglycerin (NTG); this agent potentiates the vasodilatory response. Several studies have demonstrated that most patients with established vascular disease still potentiate their FMD response. However, when conventional risk factors persist in such patients, the vasodilatory response to NTG is often impaired (69,70). Many conventional risk factors increase the oxidative stress on the endothelium, and the reactive oxygen species that result may lead to more rapid inactivation of endogenous NO and exogenously administered NTG (71).

Vasoresponse after Acute Oxidative Stress: Lipid Challenge in Normal Subjects

Acute ingestion of a high-fat meal results in an acute oxidative stress on human endothelium (72,73); because dietary fat intake is known to be a risk factor for the development of vascular disease, the possibility that acute and chronic dietary habits might lead to endothelial dysfunction and initiate or accelerate atherosclerosis is intriguing. In 1997 Vogel and colleagues reported provocative findings suggesting that acute intake of fat results in acute impairment of endothelial vasoreactivity (74). These investigators studied ten healthy, normocholesterolemic volunteers before and hourly for 6 hours after a single high- (50 g) or low-fat (0 g) meal with brachial artery reactivity. Flow-dependent vasoreactivity decreased from $21 \pm 5\%$ preprandially to $11 \pm 4\%$, $11 \pm 6\%$, and $10 \pm 3\%$ at 2, 3, and 4 hours after the high-fat meal, respectively, whereas a low-fat meal did not produce any changes in FMD (all $ps < 0.05$ compared with the low-fat meal); thus, on average, subjects demonstrated a 50% diminution of brachial artery reactivity. Mean change in postprandial flow-mediated vasoactivity at 2, 3, and 4 hours correlated with change in 2-hour serum triglycerides ($r = -0.51$, $p = 0.02$), suggesting that the fat content of the meal and the effect on postprandial triglyceride levels might be causative. These results suggest that a single high-fat meal transiently impairs endothelial function and might be the link between a high-fat diet and atherogenesis. In a slightly larger study of 20 patients, these investigators replicated these findings and, in addition, generated data to suggest that the detrimental effect of the high-fat meal could be blocked with pretreatment with the antioxidants vitamin C (1 g) and vitamin E (800 IU) (75) (Fig. 1.7). Other investigators have replicated these findings (76–89).

However, other studies have failed to demonstrate acute declines in arterial vasoreactivity following an acute lipid challenge (90–96), with some showing no change, a mixed response, or even vasodilation after fat challenge. Raitakari and colleagues studied 12 normal volunteers before, 3 hours after, and 6 hours after a high-fat meal (61 g) rich in saturated

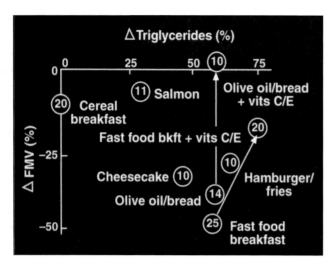

FIG. 1.7. Effect of lipid challenge in normal individuals. Three-hour postprandial changes in triglycerides and flow-mediated vasodilation (FMV) after specific meals. Changes are expressed on the *y* axis as percentage changes versus baseline (prechallenge) FMV. Pretreatment with vitamin E (800 U) and vitamin C (1 gm) restores FMV toward normal values despite fat ingestion. vits, vitamins; bkft, breakfast. (From Vogel R. Brachial artery ultrasound: a noninvasive tool in the assessment of triglyceride-rich lipoproteins. *Clin Cardiol* 1999;22[Suppl II]:II34–II39, with permission.)

fatty acids, 10 of whom were restudied after a similar meal rich in monounsaturated fatty acids (92). Brachial artery basal diameter (assessed by BAR), resting forearm blood flow, and postischemic hyperemia (assessed by plethysmography) increased after high-fat meals, and FMD was unchanged. Thus, in contrast to the previous studies, a high-fat meal was not associated with impaired conduit artery vasoreactivity.

The conflicting results may have several possible explanations. First, there appear to be wide differences among individuals in the FMD response to a high-fat meal, and many other subject-related factors may influence the results, predisposing studies with small numbers of participants vulnerable to Type 1 or Type 2 error. For example, baseline lipoprotein status may affect the results (97). Anderson and colleagues suggested that baseline high-density lipoprotein (HDL) is inversely related to post–high-fat-meal FMD changes (72). Together these observations suggest that baseline lipid status or other metabolic factors among the small numbers of participants in the preceding studies may have accounted for some of the differences. Second, the overall diet of the participants in the weeks before study may affect the response to fat challenge (98), as may consumption of folic acid (79) or a diet rich in fruit and vegetable extracts (89). Third, the biochemical form of the fat may affect the results [trans vs. non-trans (99); the proportion of omega-3-fatty acids (100); whether the fat has been heated to high temperature (101)]. Fourth, there are significant individual differences in the generation

of different lipoprotein subfractions after a fat challenge; individuals who generate higher levels of these remnants have been shown to have lower values for preprandial FMD and a larger diminution in postprandial FMD (102). Fifth, because BAR methodology is not yet standardized, methodological differences among protocols are an important confounder (38). Finally, and perhaps most importantly, all of these studies assume that their "normal control" individuals were truly without occult vascular disease.

In summary, acute and chronic dietary composition may play a role in the genesis of endothelial dysfunction, abnormal brachial artery vasoreactivity, and the development of atherosclerosis. Although it is tempting to speculate that this may be a critical factor in the development of disease later in life, the role of dietary-induced endothelial dysfunction, individual genetic variabilities in resistance to such stresses, and the optimal means of assessing it (whether by BAR or some other means) require further study. Ideally, larger studies with long-term follow-up should be performed to prove or disprove this hypothesis.

Vasoresponse after Risk Factor Modification

Hypercholesterolemia

Many studies have reported that risk factor modification and pharmacologic intervention in particular improve endothelial function. In the coronary circulation, serial study of endothelium-mediated dilation (assessed with Ach infusion and either quantitative angiography and/or intracoronary Doppler probes) has been shown to improve after treatment of atherosclerotic risk factors. For example, CAD patients treated for 6 months with cholesterol-lowering 3-hydroxymethylglutamyl coenzyme A reductase (HMG-CoA reductase, or "statin") therapy demonstrate improved or preserved endothelial function compared to patients treated without statins (105). Other trials of lipid lowering (106–108), estrogen replacement (109,110), and ACE inhibition (77) reported serial improvement in flow-mediated dilation. Probuchol, a potent antioxidant, may potentiate this improvement when added to a standard lipid-lowering regimen (111). Using serial positron emission tomography scanning, Gould and colleagues demonstrated significant improvements in myocardial perfusion after only 3 months of therapy (112,113). These observations have led to several large, multicenter clinical trials that are investigating whether intensive risk factor modification rather than revascularization in patients with established CAD can lead to improvements in ischemic episodes compared to conventional treatment (114).

Given that intravascular and necropsy studies demonstrate that substantial coronary atherosclerosis is uniformly present (even if angiographically occult) in patients with clinical PAD, it is somewhat surprising that there are relatively few prospective studies on the effects of HMG-CoA reductase inhibitors on outcomes in patients with peripheral arterial disease but without overt coronary disease. The recently completed Anglo-Scandanavian Cardiac Outcomes Trial lipid substudy enrolled 261 patients who were diagnosed with PAD but did not have known CAD, and randomized them to atorvastatin 10 mg (without titration to a specific LDL goal) versus placebo (115). In this subgroup, total vascular events were reduced by 20%, in accord with the results of the overall study; however, the 95% confidence intervals were wide (0.45 to 1.42) due to the small number of PVD patients (115). In the absence of additional data, most experts agree that the indications and treatment goals for cholesterol and other risk factors are the same for patients with PAD as for those with CAD. Nevertheless, a recent study documents that only a small fraction of PAD patients are at target levels of cholesterol, blood pressure, and diabetes control (116).

In the absence of large prospective studies, the correlation between coronary and peripheral reactivity in normal individuals and in individuals with risk factors or established vascular disease has led investigators to use peripheral vasoreactivity as a marker for treatment response. A striking finding from many of these studies is the short time period in which a favorable response can be demonstrated. For example, in patients with familial hypercholesterolemia a single LDL apheresis session can improve endothelial function in both the coronary and the peripheral circulation (117). In a small, single-center study of hypercholesterolemic patients, statin therapy improved forearm vasodilator response to acetylcholine infusion in only 4 weeks (118). In patients with acute myocardial infarction or unstable angina, and hypercholesterolemia, statin therapy resulted in a 42% relative improvement in brachial FMD in statin-treated versus placebo, treated patients in 6 weeks (119). Multicenter trials on this issue are nearing completion. The Reversal of Atherosclerosis with Lipitor trial is comparing the ability of a "conventional" (target LDL less than or equal to 100 mg per dL) versus an "aggressive" lipid-lowering strategy (anticipated LDL less than 70 mg per dL) to reduce coronary atheroma volume as measured by IVUS over an 18-month period. A brachial artery reactivity substudy of 220 patients who underwent serial study at 3-month intervals is nearing completion (120).

Angiotensin-Converting Enzyme Inhibition

Endothelial NO production is in part regulated by the renin–angiotensin system, although the details of mechanisms remain to be fully elucidated. In 129 normotensive patients with one- or two-vessel angiographic coronary disease, the Trial on Reversing ENdothelial Dysfunction investigators reported that the angiotensin-converting enzyme inhibitor (ACE-I) quinapril resulted in improved coronary endothelial function compared to placebo as assessed by brachial artery reactivity (121). Anderson and colleagues compared the effects on BAR of quinapril, enalapril, amlodipine, and losartan in 80 patients who had at least one epicardial coronary stenosis

of greater than 50% in a crossover design (122). The mean baseline FMD was $7.3 \pm 0.6\%$; quinapril resulted in an absolute increase in FMD of $1.8 \pm 1.0\%$ ($p < 0.02$), whereas the other agents did not result in any significant improvement (122). This observation, along with data from clinical endpoint studies such as the Heart Outcomes Prevention Evaluation (HOPE) Trial (123), has led some investigators to conclude that high tissue-ACE inhibition may be necessary to generate improvements in endothelial function and reduce clinical events (enalapril is a weaker inhibitor of tissue-specific ACE than is quinapril). In the HOPE Trial, 44% of the 9,297 patients had evidence of PAD as determined by an ankle–brachial index (ABI) of 0.9; ramipril reduced cardiovascular events to a similar degree as in patients with normal ABIs. However, the issues of tissue specificity and of whether angiotensin receptor blockers (ARBs) can also produce favorable effects on peripheral vasoreactivity require further study; some smaller studies have suggested that non–tissue-specific ACE and ARBs may improve flow-mediated dilation in diabetics (124–126).

Detrimental Response to Coronary Vasodilators

The ability of available coronary vasodilators to relieve symptoms in either intermittent claudication or critical limb ischemia is disappointing, with the vast majority of studies reporting no benefit. In fact, direct vasodilators theoretically may worsen ischemia in PAD. In coronary disease, these agents exert much of their favorable effect by dilating the systemic vasculature generally, thereby reducing afterload and myocardial oxygen consumption. However, in PAD, vasodilators have no such effect on reducing downstream oxygen consumption. In addition, exercise induces resistance vessels to dilate, whereas resistance vessels in nonexercising tissues remain in a more constricted state. Systemically administered vasodilators might preferentially dilate these territories, creating a "steal" phenomenon. Third, given that peripheral territories (unlike cardiac muscle) receive the majority of blood flow in systole, reduction of systolic pressure may reduce the driving force across peripheral stenoses, particularly long or sequentially diseased segments. Although it is not known whether effective control of hypertension prevents or slows the progression of PAD, attaining current blood pressure targets in hypertensive patients has such a profound effect on reducing overall cardiovascular mortality that these agents should not be withheld due to theoretical concerns of peripheral perfusion, and blood pressure targets should be routinely reached.

Beta-Blockers

Beta-blockers have the potential to perturb the balance of beta- and alpha-receptor activity, which theoretically can result in vasoconstriction. A recent meta-analysis of 11 trials concluded that beta-blockers do not worsen symptoms of intermittent claudication; because many patients with PAD suffer from known CAD as well, and because these drugs produce a reduction in cardiac death rates in CAD patients, they should not be withheld solely due to the presence of PAD. Nevertheless, clinicians encounter occasional patients whose symptoms are markedly worse when given beta-blockers (127).

Exercise

Exercise is clearly beneficial in patients with intermittent claudication and is discussed in greater detail in Chapter 12. Although the mechanism by which exercise improves symptoms has long been assumed to be the result of increased collateral development, it is also possible that improved peripheral vasoreactivity plays a role. Exercise training improves endothelium-dependent vasodilation in the coronary arteries in CAD patients (128) and in the peripheral circulation in patients with congestive heart failure (129,130). However, other mechanisms, such as favorable alterations in skeletal muscle metabolism, may also be operative (131,132). The relative contribution of each of these mechanisms is unknown.

L-Arginine

The essential amino acid L-arginine is the metabolic precursor to nitric oxide, and its administration can significantly improve vasoreactivity. After L-arginine administration, improvements in flow-mediated dilation can be demonstrated in hypercholesterolemic subjects and in cigarette smokers (104). Interestingly, preliminary studies suggest that L-arginine improves claudication distance in patients with PAD. These and other studies (104,133,134) taken together suggest that in addition to the effects of "fixed" stenoses, endothelial-dependent vasodilation is abnormal in PAD patients and pharmacologic therapies may improve perfusion and symptom status.

Manipulation of Other Endogenous Vasoactive Substances

In addition to nitric oxide, a variety of other vasoactive substances, some derived from the endothelium and others originating in local or distant tissues, influence endothelial function and vasomotor tone. Examples of such substances include prostacyclin, adenosine, prostanoids, serotonin, thrombin, thromboxane, endothelin, and catecholamines. Accordingly, many other pharmacologic agents are in the early stages of development to treat symptomatic peripheral arterial disease, and many such agents are targeted at vasoreactive pathways. Examples of such drugs include novel calcium-channel-blocking agents, angiogenic growth factors, and vasodilator prostaglandins. A serotonin antagonist, naftidrofuryl, has improved claudication symptoms in two studies and is available for clinical use in Europe (135). A multi-center, randomized trial suggests that a cofactor of fatty acid metabolism, proprionyl L-carnitine, can improve intermittent claudication symptoms (136).

Effect of Multiple-Risk-Factor Interventions

Finally, preliminary data suggest that by targeting multiple-risk-factor pathways, one may improve endothelial function further than by treating individual risk factors alone. Nazzaro and colleagues demonstrated that when ACE inhibition was combined with HMG-CoA reductase inhibition in hypercholesterolemic and hypertensive patients without known vascular disease, flow-mediated dilation was improved to a greater degree than with either agent alone (137). This study supports the concept of global risk and the importance of treating multiple risk factors to obtain the largest improvement in endothelial function and, perhaps, in symptom relief. Prospective studies with a larger number of patients are underway.

Atherosclerosis Regression, Disease Stabilization, and Vasoreactivity

Most vascular events are initiated by atheroma rupture or erosion (138), and some researchers have hypothesized that improvement in endothelial function after aggressive risk factor modification may be the mechanism by which rupture/erosion episodes and clinical events are reduced. Because the endothelium also regulates other functions, such as thrombosis, platelet and leukocyte interactions with the vessel wall, and growth factors that regulate smooth muscle cell proliferation and migration, the mechanisms by which an improvement in endothelial function and a reduction in events remain speculative.

Nevertheless, preliminary studies suggest that atheroma volume regression, as assessed either in the coronary circulation with IVUS or in the peripheral circulation with B-mode ultrasound, can occur in humans, and several studies that have coupled morphological and functional assessment indicate that both can improve. In the coronary circulation, lipid lowering is associated with reductions in plaque volume and improvements in lumen area as well as increased IVUS echogenicity (139), which is considered to be a measure of decreased lipid content and lower vulnerability to rupture. Favorable alterations in structure may be associated with improvements in vasoreactivity. Hamasaki et al. studied 101 patients with normal or only mildly diseased (less than 30% angiographic narrowing) left anterior descending coronary artery segments with intravascular ultrasound and assessed endothelial function with intracoronary acetylcholine (140). Patients with a history of total cholesterol greater than 240 mg per dL who had lowered their total cholesterol below this value with medical therapy and those whose initial values were below this level (not on treatment at the time of study) had both larger mean EEM CSA and a greater increase in acetylcholine-induced vasodilation than did patients with total cholesterol values greater than 240 mg per dL. In this study, mean plaque areas were similar in patients who did and did not have enhanced remodeling and improved endothelial function. Thus, coronary regression may involve favorable remodeling of the EEM CSA along with improved endothelial function, even without measurable differences in plaque volume. The extent to which these favorable, albeit preliminary, changes will be observed in the peripheral circulation is uncertain. In the Antioxidant Supplementation in Atherosclerosis Prevention Study, "aggressive" LDL lowering in patients with familial hypercholesterolemia resulted in regression of carotid intimal–medial thickness as assessed by B-mode ultrasound compared to "less aggressive" LDL lowering (141). Whether individuals with lower starting levels of cholesterol will experience slower disease progression, fewer plaque rupture events, and, perhaps, disease regression is unknown. Large-scale trials of coronary atherosclerosis regression are underway and are discussed in a later section.

Summary: Is Peripheral Arterial Vasoreactivity a New Vascular Risk Factor?

Can peripheral arterial endothelial function, as assessed by brachial artery reactivity, serve as a barometer for the health of the endothelium as a whole? Many studies have documented substantial reductions in major vascular events in both the coronary and the peripheral circulation with adequate control of conventional atherosclerotic risk factors. Endothelial dysfunction precedes the development of overt vascular disease by many years, and abnormal vasoreactivity can frequently be demonstrated in patients without overt clinical atherosclerosis. Risk factor modification (and perhaps treatment with ACE-I or other agents even in normotensive subjects) is associated with improvement in peripheral FMD. Preliminary evidence suggests that this improvement in peripheral FMD is often associated with an improvement in clinical status (111).

Taken together, these observations suggest that assessment of peripheral arterial vasoreactivity with BAR may be useful as a screening tool to detect individuals at higher risk for the development of overt vascular disease. Several studies suggest that peripheral vasoreactivity strongly correlates with clinical outcome. Schachinger and colleagues studied 147 patients at baseline with intracoronary Ach and NTG; during a median follow-up of 7.7 years, patients with abnormal responses had a significantly higher rate of vascular events (cardiovascular death, unstable angina, myocardial infarction, revascularization, or ischemic stroke) (55). Suwaidi and colleagues studied 157 patients with mild angiographic CAD (no lesion with greater than 40% narrowing). During a mean of 28 months follow-up, there were no events in the 32 patients with normal or only mildly abnormal coronary endothelial function, compared to a 14% event rate in the 83 patients with severely impaired coronary response to Ach (percentage change in flow less than 0%) (54).

Gokce and colleagues measured BAR in 199 patients prior to elective surgery for peripheral vascular disease; during a mean follow-up of 1.2 years, 18% had a major vascular event (death, myocardial infarction unstable angina, or stroke). Abnormal FMD was an independent predictor of events and conferred a ninefold higher risk (142). Taken together, these data suggest that noninvasive evaluation of peripheral vasoreactivity may become an inexpensive screening tool for identifying individuals at higher risk before the development of overt disease, so that risk factor modification or prophylactic prescription of therapeutic agents could be targeted to these individuals. Nevertheless, most of these studies have been performed in patients with a known disease, multiple uncontrolled risk factors, or a higher-than-average probability of significant occult vascular disease. Two central issues—whether screening for endothelial dysfunction in lower-risk populations will have incremental value to conventional risk factor assessment, and whether intervention (beyond current risk factor goals) will reduce subsequent events or slow disease progression—remain to be resolved. Until adequately designed studies with sufficient numbers of patients prove these relationships, and until the technical and reporting aspects of BAR are further refined, the technique will not be ready for use as a screening or monitoring tool in clinical practice.

Vasoresponse to Injury: Pathophysiologic Mechanisms

Developmental Biology of the Human Vasculature

Although a detailed discussion of arterial embryology is beyond the scope of this chapter, several concepts are vital to a discussion of the arterial response to injury. Human arteries in different beds are heterogeneous, with distinct morphology, physiology, and ability to respond to various pharmacologic agents. During human embryogenesis, all vascular endothelial cells and blood cells are thought to arise from the "blood islands" located at the periphery of the young embryo. However, in different regions of the body, different cell signal mechanisms from surrounding tissues induce considerable heterogeneity in endothelial cell surface receptors (143) and in other cellular functions. For example, the gene that codes for nitric oxide synthase in the coronary arteries has bed-specific regulation (144). Thus, despite their common origin, there is considerable variation in the phenotype of the mature endothelial cells. In contrast to endothelial cells, arterial smooth muscle cells arise from several different locations in the embryo; for example, in the upper part of the body, smooth muscle cells derive from neuroectoderm, whereas in the lower part of the body, a completely different germ layer, the mesoderm, is the source of smooth muscle cells (145). As with endothelial cells, smooth muscle cells demonstrate considerable phenotypic heterogeneity.

The clinical implications of this arterial heterogeneity may profoundly affect the propensity for atherosclerosis to develop in particular locations and may affect the response of different arterial beds to injury. Atheromatous lesions affect certain key locations preferentially and tend to form at flow dividers and branch points while sparing other characteristic locations (such as the internal thoracic artery) (146–148). The Pathobiologic Determinants of Atherosclerosis in Youth Study collected necropsy specimens from individuals under the age of 35 years who died of noncardiac causes. Fatty streaks and raised arterial lesions initially localize in the dorsal portion of the abdominal aorta, followed by lesion formation in the thoracic aorta (149,150). Right coronary fatty streaks usually follow the development of aortic lesions.

Spontaneous Arterial Injury: Plaque Rupture

The cause of most myocardial infarctions, nonhemorrhagic strokes, and episodes of acute limb ischemia is atherothrombosis. The role of spontaneous plaque rupture as the cause of most acute coronary syndromes is well established (138,151), whereas the frequency with which plaque rupture is responsible for acute events in the peripheral circulation is less well established. There are many reasons why the response to any injury may be different in different arterial beds, including the diverse embryogenesis, the size of the vessels, flow rates, the presence of stenotic regions, and the fact that coronary arteries receive most of their perfusion during diastole, in contrast to peripheral vessels. In addition, peripheral vessels are subject to different hemodynamic stresses. Larger arteries are subjected to larger degrees of circumferential stress, according to the law of Laplace. Accordingly, the large radius of the aorta may make it particularly prone to plaque rupture, and evidence from necropsy and magnetic resonance studies suggests that aortic plaque rupture is a very common occurrence. Even though aortic plaque ruptures are infrequently associated with complete thrombotic occlusion (presumably due to the large residual area even in moderately diseased aortas and the high flow rate), aortic thrombi are a clinically important source of many embolic episodes of acute limb ischemia and stroke. Recent data also suggest that plaque rupture is a common cause of a symptomatic carotid disease. Endarterectomy specimens demonstrate plaque rupture in 74% of symptomatic patients versus only 32% of asymptomatic patients, despite similar degrees of stenosis (152). As with plaque rupture sites in the coronaries, plaque rupture sites in the carotids demonstrate "vulnerable" features, such as thinning of the fibrous cap, lipid-rich or necrotic areas, and infiltration of activated inflammatory cells. Interestingly, the proportion of activated inflammatory cells (as assessed by HLA-DR expression) is higher in ruptured plaque than in specimens from asymptomatic patients (153). Although acute plaque rupture is thought to be an important mechanism for acute syndromes generally in the peripheral circulation, the exact incidence of this phenomenon is unknown (see Chapter 2).

Implications for Long-Term Success of Revascularization of Peripheral Vessels

Therapeutic Arterial Injury (Angioplasty): Outcome in Different Peripheral Territories

Although percutaneous and surgical interventions are discussed in other chapters, the relationships among peripheral arterial morphology and anatomy, vasoreactivity, and pharmacology have a profound impact on strategies for effective percutaneous revascularization. A summary of the literature is complicated by the variety of endpoints utilized; some studies use only angiographic patency rates, whereas others use surrogates of vessel patency or percentage stenosis by duplex ultrasound, ankle–brachial index, or simply the relief of symptoms. Nevertheless, three broad generalizations are warranted by the data. First, the efficacy of percutaneous interventions is better in vessels with good as opposed to poor runoff, that is, when distal vessels are widely patent. Second, the treatment of focal severe stenoses is more successful than the treatment of occlusions (154–156). Third, differences in the acute and long-term success rates of percutaneous interventions in different peripheral arterial territories are striking. For example, iliac artery balloon angioplasty results in a 4- to 5-year patency rate of 60% to 80% (157,158); stent placement improves these numbers to the range of 75% to 95% (159–161). In contrast, the efficacy of balloon angioplasty alone in the femoral and popliteal arteries is less satisfactory. Several registry series have documented 1-, 3-, and 5-year patency rates in the range of 60%, 50%, and 40%, respectively (162,163). Stent placement in the femoral circulation improves these outcomes. Similarly, stent placement in the subclavian and innominate is successful in greater than 85% of cases at 1 year in patients with suitable lesions (164–166).

Unfortunately, with more distal and smaller peripheral vessels, the response to therapeutic injury of angioplasty is far less satisfactory. Balloon angioplasty alone in the peroneal and tibial results in short-term patency rates of less than 50% (155,167–170). Although the results in the infrapopliteal arteries may be skewed by a higher proportion of high-risk patients with unfavorable anatomy and critical limb ischemia, taken together, these studies suggest that vessel size is inversely related to long-term procedural success, especially with balloon angioplasty. Whether the different embryologic origins of these vessels affect the response to therapeutic injury is unknown.

Studies using pre- and postprocedural intravascular ultrasound studies provide insight into the inverse relationship between vessel size and long-term success. Following balloon angioplasty of peripheral vessels, plaque fracture is the most common mechanism of lumen enlargement, followed by atheroma compression/redistribution and, to a lesser degree, vessel "stretch" (171,172). As noted previously, in at least 30% to 40% of advanced femoral arterial stenoses, the EEM area is *less* than that at the reference site (22); in these lesions with "vessel shrinkage," the relative contribution of stretching may be considerably more important (173). In coronary artery lesions treated with non-stent interventions, Mintz and colleagues used serial intravascular ultrasound in patients with restenosis to document that approximately three-fourths of late lumen loss was due to vessel contraction or shrinkage, whereas only approximately one-fourth was due to neointimal hyperplasia (174,175). Only small serial studies have been done on the peripheral circulation, but these support the notion that vessel constriction after non-stent peripheral interventions is also an important factor in restenosis (176). This observation supports the current widespread use of primary stent deployment because stents minimize or eliminate vessel contraction.

Intravascular Ultrasound Assessment of Peripheral Arterial Stenting

Despite the relatively high long-term patency rates in lesions treated with percutaneous peripheral interventions, a substantial minority of patients experience restenosis or complete occlusion and recurrent symptoms. Whether stent underdeployment, edge dissections, or other suboptimal results (which are frequently angiographically occult, but can be readily diagnosed by IVUS) contribute to the portion of peripheral interventions that fail is unknown. Whether routine or selective intravascular ultrasound utilization could improve clinical outcomes is also unknown. Data suggest that stent underdeployment is common (30% to 40%) and that IVUS can guide more aggressive deployment strategies and result in larger final stent cross-sectional areas (177). Single-center, nonrandomized series suggest that IVUS use in iliac lesions is associated with larger final stent dimensions and higher long-term patency rates (178). Importantly, different peripheral territories may undergo different mechanisms of restenosis after stenting. Using serial intravascular ultrasound, Leertouwer and colleagues demonstrated that renal artery stents suffered substantially less lumen loss from neointimal hyperplasia than did femoropopliteal stents (17% vs. 62%, $p < 0.001$) (178a). In current practice in the United States, IVUS is used in less than 10% of iliac and femoropopliteal interventions, yet the possibility that more liberal utilization would further improve outcomes is untested. Nevertheless, given the inherent limitations of angiography alone, several high-volume peripheral intervention centers report that selective IVUS utilization is invaluable for difficult or challenging cases or when measurements of arterial dimensions are uncertain (179–183).

In the carotid circulation, balloon angioplasty alone was rarely performed due to the potential catastrophic consequences of embolic or thrombotic events. However, carotid stenting in combination with distal protection against atheromatous emboli has recently been shown to be superior to conventional endarterectomy in a multicenter, randomized trial, due to a 50% reduction in acute neurological complications (184). Although many clinicians already consider stenting to be the preferred treatment for most patients with symptomatic carotid disease or critical stenoses, additional studies and appropriate reimbursement will be required before the strategy is universally adopted.

Implications for Restenosis Prevention and Treatment

In large and medium-size peripheral vessels (iliac, innominate, subclavian, femoral, and politeal vessels, carotids, and renals), most interventionalists in the United States treat focal stenoses with stents at the time of initial procedure to minimize the probability of restenosis. This is despite a Dutch study that suggested that provisional rather than routine stent placement is potentially more cost-effective in the iliacs (185), and a small, preliminary study that suggested that brachytherapy after balloon angioplasty of the femoral artery results in excellent 6-month patency and enhanced remodeling compared to use of balloon alone (186). An exception to routine stenting of noncoronary lesions is renal artery fibromuscular dysplasia, which often responds favorably to balloon angioplasty alone (187). In contrast to balloon angioplasty, stent restenosis is almost always due to neointimal hyperplasia [with the occasional exception of stent crush due to trauma in stents that are close to a vulnerable area (188)]. In the coronaries, stents covered with a polymer that contains and secretes one of several cell-cycle inhibitors (all are rapamycin derivatives) in the months after placement have reduced angiographic restenosis rates from the 20% to 40% range to the 0% to 5% range by virtue of their ability to inhibit neointimal hyperplasia, and are in widespread clinical use (189–191). Drug-eluting stents are in development for the periphery, but the larger deployed size of these stents (often greater than 5 to 8 mm) makes polymer adhesion to the struts technologically more challenging than with small (less than 3.5 mm) coronary stents. Furthermore, with clinical restenosis rates already less than 10% in many large peripheral vessels, cost-effectiveness would be unlikely unless the per-unit cost were substantially less than the $3,200 cost per stent in the coronaries. Carotid lesions might become an important exception: Even though restenosis occurs in less than 5% of stented targets, it is often difficult to treat by repeat percutaneous intervention and difficult or impossible to treat surgically (except by carotid bypass) due to the presence of the stent. For this situation, and for restenosis of bare-metal peripheral stents, radiation therapy is in development (192,193).

Vasoreactivity and the Treatment of Peripheral Arterial Disease in the Future

Although revascularization (either surgical or percutaneous) is the predominant strategy for treating severe peripheral arterial disease, the pharmacologic approach is yet to be fully exploited. Compared to the coronary vasculature, the pharmacologic treatment of peripheral disease is in its earliest stages. Angiogenic growth factors to induce next-generation pharmacologic neovascularization agents are in development. In addition, agents that enhance endothelial function offer another and potentially vital approach to treating these increasingly common diseases. In the coronary circulation, Gould, Lehrman, and others have demonstrated that tissue-level perfusion can be enhanced significantly solely with this approach (112,113,194). It is likely that such agents targeted toward the peripheral circulation will be developed to enhance peripheral perfusion by restoring or enhancing the ability of resistance vessels to regulate flow and deliver blood to downstream tissues, and, perhaps, decrease the incidence of plaque rupture and progression to occlusion. As the prevalence of peripheral arterial disease increases with the aging population, new approaches (such as brachytherapy or drug-eluting stents) will improve the success rates in smaller vessels and total occlusions and will improve long-term success of stenting even further. In the future, revascularization and pharmacologic therapy will be increasingly employed as combined rather than competitive strategies for improving peripheral perfusion, reducing symptoms, and reducing the burden of peripheral arterial disease in these patients.

REFERENCES

1. Tortora GJ, Anagnostakos NP. *Principles of anatomy and physiology,* 6th ed. New York: Harper & Row, 1990:605–653.
2. Harvey W. *Exercitatio anatomica du motu cordis et sanguinis in animalibus,* Leake CD, trans. Springfield, IL: Charles C Thomas, 1928.
3. Donnelly PJ, Wistreich GA. *Laboratory manual for anatomy and physiology.* New York: HarperCollins, 1993:481–515.
4. Schlant RC, Silverman ME, Roberts WC. Anatomy of the heart. In: Hurst JW, Schlant RC, Rackley CE, et al., eds. *The heart: arteries and veins,* 7th ed. New York: McGraw-Hill, 1990:28–35.
5. Ross MH, Reith EJ, Romrell LJ. *Histology.* Baltimore: Williams & Wilkins, 1989:283–305.
6. Moffett DF, Moffett SB, Schauf CL. *Human physiology.* St. Louis: Mosby–Year Book, 1993:299–405.
7. Furchgott RF, Zawadski JV. The obligatory role of endothelial cells in the relaxation of arterial smooth muscle cell by acetylcholine. *Nature* 1980;228:373–376.
8. Furchgott RF, Vanhoutte PM. Endothelium derived relaxing and contracting factors. *FASEB J* 1989;3:2007–2018.
9. Taylor SG, Weston AH. Endothelium derived hyperpolarizing factor: a new endogenous inhibitor from vascular endothelium. *Trends Pharmacol Sci* 1988;9:272–274.
10. Furchgott RF. Introduction to EDRF research. *J Cardiovasc Pharmacol* 1993;22[Suppl 7]:S1–S2.
11. Stato T, Arai K, Ishiharajima S, et al. Role of glycosaminoglycan and fibronectin in endothelial cell growth. *Exp Mol Pathol* 1987;47:202–210.
12. Vlodavsky I, Fielding PE, Johnson LK, et al. Inhibition of LDL uptake in endothelium correlates with a restricted surface receptor redistribution. *J Cell Physiol* 1979;100:481–495.
13. Gryglewski RJ, Botting RM, Vane JR. Mediators produced by the endothelial cell. *Hypertension* 1988;12:530–548.
14. Schorer AE, Moldow CF. Production of tissue factor. In: Ryan US, ed. *Endothelial cells.* Boca Raton, FL: CRC Press, 1988:85.
15. Rapoport RM, Draznin MB, Murad F. Endothelium dependent relaxation in rat aorta may be mediated through cyclic GMP dependent protein phosphorylation. *Nature* 1983;306:174–176.
16. Langille BL, O'Donnell F. Reductions in arterial diameter produced by chronic decreases in blood flow are endothelium dependent. *Science* 1986;231:405–407.
17. Glagov S, Weisenberg E, Zarins C, et al. Compensatory enlargement of human atherosclerotic coronary arteries. *N Engl J Med* 1987;316:1371–1375.
18. Schoenhagen P, Nissen SE, Tuzcu EM. Coronary arterial remodeling: from bench to bedside. *Curr Atheroscler Rep* 2003;5:150–154.
19. Schoenhagen P, Ziada KM, Vince DG, et al. Arterial remodeling and coronary artery disease: the concept of "dilated" versus "obstructive" coronary atherosclerosis. *J Am Coll Cardiol* 2001;38:297–306.
20. Schoenhagen P, Ziada KM, Kapadia SR, et al. Extent and direction of arterial remodeling in stable versus unstable coronary syndromes: an intravascular ultrasound study. *Circulation* 2000;101:598–603.
21. Hagenaars T, Gussenhoven EJ, Athanassopoulos P, et al. Intravascular ultrasound evidence for stabilization of compensatory enlargement of the femoropopliteal segment after endograft placement. *J Endovasc Ther* 2001;8:308–314.
22. Pasterkamp G, Wensing PJ, Post MJ, et al. Paradoxical arterial wall shrinkage may contribute to luminal narrowing of human atherosclerotic femoral arteries. *Circulation* 1995;91:1444–1449.
23. Mintz GS, Kent KM, Pichard AD, et al. Contribution of inadequate arterial remodeling to the development of focal coronary artery stenoses. An intravascular ultrasound study. *Circulation* 1997;95:1791–1798.
24. Hagenaars T, Gussenhoven EJ, Poldermans D, et al. Rationale and design for the SARIS trial; effect of statin on atherosclerosis and vascular remodeling assessed with intravascular sonography. *Cardiovasc Drugs Ther* 2001;15:339–343.
25. Olesen SP, Clapham DE, Davies PF. Haemodynamic shear stress activates a K+ current in vascular endothelial cells. *Nature* 1988;331:168–170.
26. Cooke JP, Rossitch Jr E, Andon NA, et al. Flow activates an endothelial potassium channel to release an endogenous nitrovasodilator. *J Clin Invest* 1991;88:1663–1671.
27. Miura H, Wachtel RE, Liu Y, et al. Flow-induced dilation of human coronary arterioles: important role of Ca(2+)-activated K(+) channels. *Circulation* 2001;103:1992–1998.
28. Pohl U, Holtz J, Busse R, et al. Crucial role of endothelium in the vasodilator response to increased flow *in vivo. Hypertension* 1986;8:37–44.
29. Joannides R, Haefeli WE, Linder L, et al. Nitric oxide is responsible for flow-dependent dilatation of human peripheral conduit arteries *in vivo. Circulation* 1995;91:1314–1319.
30. Sun D, Huang A, Smith CJ, et al. Enhanced release of prostaglandins contributes to flow-induced arteriolar dilation in eNOS knockout mice. *Circ Res* 1999;85:288–293.
31. Zir L, Miller S, Dinsmore R, et al. Interobserver variability in coronary angiography. *Circulation* 1976;53:627–632.
32. Arnett E, Isner J, Redwood C, et al. Coronary artery narrowing in coronary heart disease: comparison of cineangiographic and necropsy findings. *Ann Intern Med* 1979;91:350–356.
33. Isner J, Kishel J, Kent K. Accuracy of angiographic determination of left main coronary arterial narrowing. *Circulation* 1981;63:1056–1061.
34. Isner JM, Donaldsen RF. Coronary angiographic and morphologic correlaton. In: Waller BF, ed. *Cardiac morphology.* Philadelphia: Saunders, 1984:571–592.
35. Werns SW, Walton JA, Hsia HH, et al. Evidence of endothelial dysfunction in angiographically normal coronary arteries of patients with coronary artery disease. *Circulation* 1989;79:287–291.
36. Oemar BS, Tschudi MR, Godoy N, et al. Reduced endothelial nitric oxide synthase expression and production in human atherosclerosis. *Circulation* 1998;97:2494–2498.
37. Uehata A, Lieberman EH, Gerhard MD, et al. Noninvasive assessment of endothelium-dependent flow-mediated dilation of the brachial artery. *Vasc Med* 1997;2:87–92.
38. Vogel RA, Corretti MC, Plotnick GD. A comparison of brachial artery flow-mediated vasodilation using upper and lower arm arterial occlusion in subjects with and without coronary risk factors. *Clin Cardiol* 2000;23:571–575.
39. Corretti MC, Plotnick GD, Vogel RA. Technical aspects of evaluating brachial artery vasodilatation using high-frequency ultrasound. *Am J Physiol* 1995;268:H1397–H1404.
40. Lieberman EH, Gerhard MD, Uehata A, et al. Flow-induced vasodilation of the human brachial artery is impaired in patients less than 40 years of age with coronary artery disease. *Am J Cardiol* 1996;78:1210–1214.
41. Joannides R, Richard V, Haefeli WE, et al. Role of nitric oxide in the regulation of the mechanical properties of peripheral conduit arteries in humans. *Hypertension* 1997;30:1465–1470.

42. Celermajer DS, Sorensen KE, Gooch VM, et al. Non-invasive detection of endothelial dysfunction in children and adults at risk of atherosclerosis. *Lancet* 1992;340:1111–1115.
43. Corretti MC, Anderson TJ, Benjamin EJ, et al. Guidelines for the ultrasound assessment of endothelial-dependent flow-mediated vasodilation of the brachial artery: a report of the International Brachial Artery Reactivity Task Force. *J Am Coll Cardiol* 2002;39:257–265.
44. Leeson P, Thorne S, Donald A, et al. Non-invasive measurement of endothelial function: effect on brachial artery dilatation of graded endothelial dependent and independent stimuli. *Heart* 1997;78:22–27.
45. Stadler RW, Ibrahim SF, Lees RS. Measurement of the time course of peripheral vasoactivity: results in cigarette smokers. *Atherosclerosis* 1998;138:197–205.
46. Hashimoto M, Akishita M, Eto M, et al. Modulation of endothelium-dependent flow-mediated dilatation of the brachial artery by sex and menstrual cycle. *Circulation* 1995;92:3431–3435.
47. Hardie KL, Kinlay S, Hardy DB, et al. Reproducibility of brachial ultrasonography and flow-mediated dilatation (FMD) for assessing endothelial function. *Aust N Z J Med* 1997;27:649–652.
48. Ross R. Atherosclerosis: current understanding of mechanisms and future strategies in therapy. *Transplant Proc* 1993;25:2041–2043.
49. Corretti MC, Plotnick GD, Vogel RA. The effects of age and gender on brachial artery endothelium-dependent vasoactivity are stimulus-dependent. *Clin Cardiol* 1995;18:471–476.
50. Joseph A, Ackerman D, Talley JD, et al. Manifestations of coronary atherosclerosis in young trauma victims—an autopsy study. *J Am Coll Cardiol* 1993;22:459–467.
51. Stary HC. Evolution and progression of atherosclerotic lesions in coronary arteries of children and young adults. *Arteriosclerosis* 1989;9[1 Suppl]:I19–I32.
52. Berenson GS, Srinivasan SR, Bao W, et al. Association between multiple cardiovascular risk factors and atherosclerosis in children and young adults. The Bogalusa Heart Study. *N Engl J Med* 1998;338:1650–1656.
53. Tuzcu EM, Hobbs RE, Rincon G, et al. Occult and frequent transmission of atherosclerotic coronary disease with cardiac transplantation. Insights from intravascular ultrasound. *Circulation* 1995;91:1706–1713.
54. Suwaidi JA, Hamasaki S, Higano ST, et al. Long-term follow-up of patients with mild coronary artery disease and endothelial dysfunction. *Circulation* 2000;101:948–954.
55. Schachinger V, Britten MB, Zeiher AM. Prognostic impact of coronary vasodilator dysfunction on adverse long-term outcome of coronary heart disease. *Circulation* 2000;101:1899–1906.
56. Schroeder S, Enderle MD, Ossen R, et al. Noninvasive determination of endothelium-mediated vasodilation as a screening test for coronary artery disease: pilot study to assess the predictive value in comparison with angina pectoris, exercise electrocardiography, and myocardial perfusion imaging. *Am Heart J* 1999;138:731–739.
57. Vogel RA, Corretti MC. Estrogens, progestins, and heart disease: can endothelial function divine the benefit? *Circulation* 1998;97:1223–1226.
58. Celermajer DS, Sorensen KE, Bull C, et al. Endothelium-dependent dilation in the systemic arteries of asymptomatic subjects relates to coronary risk factors and their interaction. *J Am Coll Cardiol* 1994;24:1468–1474.
59. Perticone F, Ceravolo R, Pujia A, et al. Prognostic significance of endothelial dysfunction in hypertensive patients. *Circulation* 2001;104:191–196.
60. Cardillo C, Kilcoyne CM, Quyyumi AA, et al. Selective defect in nitric oxide synthesis may explain the impaired endothelium-dependent vasodilation in patients with essential hypertension. *Circulation* 1998;97:851–856.
61. Arcaro G, Zenere BM, Travia D, et al. Non-invasive detection of early endothelial dysfunction in hypercholesterolaemic subjects. *Atherosclerosis* 1995;114:247–254.
62. Gerhard M, Roddy MA, Creager SJ, et al. Aging progressively impairs endothelium-dependent vasodilation in forearm resistance vessels of humans. *Hypertension* 1996;27:849–853.
63. Celermajer DS, Sorensen KE, Georgakopoulos D, et al. Cigarette smoking is associated with dose-related and potentially reversible impairment of endothelium-dependent dilation in healthy young adults. *Circulation* 1993;88:2149–2155.
64. Laurent S, Lacolley P, Brunel P, et al. Flow-dependent vasodilation of brachial artery in essential hypertension. *Am J Physiol* 1990;258:H1004–1011.
65. Steinberg HO, Bayazeed B, Hook G, et al. Endothelial dysfunction is associated with cholesterol levels in the high normal range in humans. *Circulation* 1997;96:3287–3293.
66. Corretti MC, Plotnick GD, Vogel RA. Correlation of cold pressor and flow-mediated brachial artery diameter responses with the presence of coronary artery disease. *Am J Cardiol* 1995;75:783–787.
67. Neunteufl T, Katzenschlager R, Hassan A, et al. Systemic endothelial dysfunction is related to the extent and severity of coronary artery disease. *Atherosclerosis* 1997;129:111–118.
68. Yataco AR, Corretti MC, Gardner AW, et al. Endothelial reactivity and cardiac risk factors in older patients with peripheral arterial disease. *Am J Cardiol* 1999;83:754–758.
69. Adams MR, Robinson J, McCredie R, et al. Smooth muscle dysfunction occurs independently of impaired endothelium-dependent dilation in adults at risk of atherosclerosis. *J Am Coll Cardiol* 1998;32:123–127.
70. Bhagat K, Hingorani A, Vallance P. Flow associated or flow mediated dilatation? More than just semantics. *Heart* 1997;78:7–8.
71. Ohara Y, Peterson TE, Harrison DG. Hypercholesterolemia increases endothelial superoxide anion production. *J Clin Invest* 1993;91:2546–2551.
72. Anderson RA, Evans ML, Ellis GR, et al. The relationships between post-prandial lipaemia, endothelial function and oxidative stress in healthy individuals and patients with type 2 diabetes. *Atherosclerosis* 2001;154:475–483.
73. Nappo F, Esposito K, Cioffi M, et al. Postprandial endothelial activation in healthy subjects and in type 2 diabetic patients: role of fat and carbohydrate meals. *J Am Coll Cardiol* 2002;39:1145–1150.
74. Vogel RA, Corretti MC, Plotnick GD. Effect of a single high-fat meal on endothelial function in healthy subjects. *Am J Cardiol* 1997;79:350–354.
75. Plotnick GD, Corretti MC, Vogel RA. Effect of antioxidant vitamins on the transient impairment of endothelium-dependent brachial artery vasoactivity following a single high-fat meal. *JAMA* 1997;278:1682–1686.
76. Lundman P, Eriksson M, Schenck-Gustafsson K, et al. Transient triglyceridemia decreases vascular reactivity in young, healthy men without risk factors for coronary heart disease. *Circulation* 1997;96:3266–3268.
77. Wilmink HW, Banga JD, Hijmering M, et al. Effect of angiotensin-converting enzyme inhibition and angiotensin II type 1 receptor antagonism on postprandial endothelial function. *J Am Coll Cardiol* 1999;34:140–145.
78. Ong PJ, Dean TS, Hayward CS, et al. Effect of fat and carbohydrate consumption on endothelial function. *Lancet* 1999;354:2134.
79. Wilmink HW, Stroes ES, Erkelens WD, et al. Influence of folic acid on postprandial endothelial dysfunction. *Arterioscler Thromb Vasc Biol* 2000;20:185–188.
80. Cuevas AM, Guasch V, Castillo O, et al. A high-fat diet induces and red wine counteracts endothelial dysfunction in human volunteers. *Lipids* 2000;35:143–148.
81. Marchesi S, Lupattelli G, Schillaci G, et al. Impaired flow-mediated vasoactivity during post-prandial phase in young healthy men. *Atherosclerosis* 2000;153:397–402.
82. Schinkovitz A, Dittrich P, Wascher TC. Effects of a high-fat meal on resistance vessel reactivity and on indicators of oxidative stress in healthy volunteers. *Clin Physiol* 2001;21:404–410.
83. Gaenzer H, Sturm W, Neumayr G, et al. Pronounced postprandial lipemia impairs endothelium-dependent dilation of the brachial artery in men. *Cardiovasc Res* 2001;52:509–516.
84. Bae JH, Bassenge E, Lee HJ, et al. Impact of postprandial hypertriglyceridemia on vascular responses in patients with coronary artery disease: effects of ACE inhibitors and fibrates. *Atherosclerosis* 2001;158:165–171.
85. Zhao SP, Liu L, Gao M, et al. Impairment of endothelial function after a high-fat meal in patients with coronary artery disease. *Coron Artery Dis* 2001;12:561–565.
86. Hozumi T, Eisenberg M, Sugioka K, et al. Change in coronary flow reserve on transthoracic Doppler echocardiography after a single high-fat meal in young healthy men. *Ann Intern Med* 2002;136:523–528.

87. Ling L, Zhao SP, Gao M, et al. Vitamin C preserves endothelial function in patients with coronary heart disease after a high-fat meal. *Clin Cardiol* 2002;25:219–224.

88. Bae JH, Schwemmer M, Lee IK, et al. Postprandial hypertriglyceridemia-induced endothelial dysfunction in healthy subjects is independent of lipid oxidation. *Int J Cardiol* 2003;87:259–267.

89. Plotnick GD, Corretti MC, Vogel RA, et al. Effect of supplemental phytonutrients on impairment of the flow-mediated brachial artery vasoactivity after a single high-fat meal. *J Am Coll Cardiol* 2003;41:1744–1749.

90. Djousse L, Ellison RC, McLennan CE, et al. Acute effects of a high-fat meal with and without red wine on endothelial function in healthy subjects. *Am J Cardiol* 1999;84:660–664.

91. Gudmundsson GS, Sinkey CA, Chenard CA, et al. Resistance vessel endothelial function in healthy humans during transient postprandial hypertriglyceridemia. *Am J Cardiol* 2000;85:381–385.

92. Raitakari OT, Lai N, Griffiths K, et al. Enhanced peripheral vasodilation in humans after a fatty meal. *J Am Coll Cardiol* 2000;36:417–422.

93. Gokce N, Duffy SJ, Hunter LM, et al. Acute hypertriglyceridemia is associated with peripheral vasodilation and increased basal flow in healthy young adults. *Am J Cardiol* 2001;88:153–159.

94. Katz DL, Nawaz H, Boukhalil J, et al. Acute effects of oats and vitamin E on endothelial responses to ingested fat. *Am J Prev Med* 2001;20:124–129.

95. Sarabi M, Fugmann A, Karlstrom B, et al. An ordinary mixed meal transiently impairs endothelium-dependent vasodilation in healthy subjects. *Acta Physiol Scand* 2001;172:107–113.

96. Edwards C, Stewart RA, Ramanathan K, et al. Increased myocardial ischemia after food is not explained by endothelial dysfunction. *Am Heart J* 2002;144(5):E8 2002 Nov:789.

97. Vogel RA, Corretti MC, Plotnick GD. Changes in flow-mediated brachial artery vasoactivity with lowering of desirable cholesterol levels in healthy middle-aged men. *Am J Cardiol* 1996;77:37–40.

98. Fuentes F, Lopez-Miranda J, Sanchez E, et al. Mediterranean and low-fat diets improve endothelial function in hypercholesterolemic men. *Ann Intern Med* 2001;134:1115–1119.

99. de Roos NM, Bots ML, Katan MB. Replacement of dietary saturated fatty acids by trans fatty acids lowers serum HDL cholesterol and impairs endothelial function in healthy men and women. *Arterioscler Thromb Vasc Biol* 2001;21:1233–1237.

100. Vogel RA, Corretti MC, Plotnick GD. The postprandial effect of components of the Mediterranean diet on endothelial function. *J Am Coll Cardiol* 2000;36:1455–1460.

101. Williams MJ, Sutherland WH, McCormick MP, et al. Impaired endothelial function following a meal rich in used cooking fat. *J Am Coll Cardiol* 1999;33:1050–1055.

102. Funada J, Sekiya M, Hamada M, et al. Postprandial elevation of remnant lipoprotein leads to endothelial dysfunction. *Circ J* 2002;66:127–132.

103. Levine GN, Frei B, Koulouris SN, et al. Ascorbic acid reverses endothelial vasomotor dysfunction in patients with coronary artery disease. *Circulation* 1996;93:1107–1113.

104. Thorne S, Mullen MJ, Clarkson P, et al. Early endothelial dysfunction in adults at risk from atherosclerosis: different responses to L-arginine. *J Am Coll Cardiol* 1998;32:110–116.

105. Treasure CB, Klein JL, Weintraub WS, et al. Beneficial effects of cholesterol-lowering therapy on the coronary endothelium in patients with coronary artery disease. *N Engl J Med* 1995;332:481–487.

106. Koh KK, Cardillo C, Bui MN, et al. Vascular effects of estrogen and cholesterol-lowering therapies in hypercholesterolemic postmenopausal women. *Circulation* 1999;99:354–360.

107. Megnien JL, Simon A, Andriani A, et al. Cholesterol lowering therapy inhibits the low-flow mediated vasoconstriction of the brachial artery in hypercholesterolaemic subjects. *Br J Clin Pharmacol* 1996;42:187–193.

108. Cohen JD, Drury JH, Ostdiek J, et al. Benefits of lipid lowering on vascular reactivity in patients with coronary artery disease and average cholesterol levels: a mechanism for reducing clinical events? *Am Heart J* 2000;139:734–738.

109. Lieberman EH, Gerhard MD, Uehata A, et al. Estrogen improves endothelium-dependent, flow-mediated vasodilation in postmenopausal women. *Ann Intern Med* 1994;121:936–941.

110. Gerhard M, Walsh BW, Tawakol A, et al. Estradiol therapy combined with progesterone and endothelium-dependent vasodilation in postmenopausal women. *Circulation* 1998;98:1158–1163.

111. Anderson TJ, Meredith IT, Yeung AC, et al. The effect of cholesterol-lowering and antioxidant therapy on endothelium-dependent coronary vasomotion. *N Engl J Med* 1995;332:488–493.

112. Gould KL, Martucci JP, Goldberg DI, et al. Short-term cholesterol lowering decreases size and severity of perfusion abnormalities by positron emission tomography after dipyridamole in patients with coronary artery disease. A potential noninvasive marker of healing coronary endothelium. *Circulation* 1994;89:1530–1538.

113. Gould KL, Ornish D, Scherwitz L, et al. Changes in myocardial perfusion abnormalities by positron emission tomography after long-term, intense risk factor modification. *JAMA* 1995;274:894–901.

114. Chiquette E, Chilton R. Aggressive medical management of coronary artery disease versus mechanical revascularization. *Curr Atheroscler Rep* 2003;5:118–123.

115. Sever PS, Dahlof B, Poulter NR, et al. Prevention of coronary and stroke events with atorvastatin in hypertensive patients who have average or lower-than-average cholesterol concentrations, in the Anglo-Scandinavian Cardiac Outcomes Trial—Lipid Lowering Arm (ASCOT-LLA): a multicentre randomised controlled trial. *Lancet* 2003;361:1149–1158.

116. Mukherjee D, Lingam P, Chetcuti S, et al. Missed opportunities to treat atherosclerosis in patients undergoing peripheral vascular interventions: insights from the University of Michigan Peripheral Vascular Disease Quality Improvement Initiative (PVD-QI2). *Circulation* 2002;106:1909–1912.

117. Tamai O, Matsuoka H, Itabe H, et al. Single LDL apheresis improves endothelium-dependent vasodilatation in hypercholesterolemic humans. *Circulation* 1997;95:76–82.

118. O'Driscoll G, Green D, Taylor RR. Simvastatin, an HMG–coenzyme A reductase inhibitor, improves endothelial function within 1 month. *Circulation* 1997;95:1126–1131.

119. Dupuis J, Tardif JC, Cernacek P, et al. Cholesterol reduction rapidly improves endothelial function after acute coronary syndromes. The RECIFE (Reduction of Cholesterol in Ischemia and Function of the Endothelium) Trial. *Circulation* 1999;99:3227–3233.

120. Nissen SE. Rationale for a postintervention continuum of care: insights from intravascular ultrasound. *Am J Cardiol* 2000;86:12H–17H.

121. Mancini GB, Henry GC, Macaya C, et al. Angiotensin-converting enzyme inhibition with quinapril improves endothelial vasomotor dysfunction in patients with coronary artery disease. The TREND (Trial on Reversing ENdothelial Dysfunction) Study. *Circulation* 1996;94:258–265.

122. Anderson TJ, Elstein E, Haber H, et al. Comparative study of ACE-inhibition, angiotensin II antagonism, and calcium channel blockade on flow-mediated vasodilation in patients with coronary disease (BANFF study). *J Am Coll Cardiol* 2000;35:60–66.

123. Yusuf S, Sleight P, Pogue J, et al. Effects of an angiotensin-converting-enzyme inhibitor, ramipril, on cardiovascular events in high-risk patients. The Heart Outcomes Prevention Evaluation Study Investigators. *N Engl J Med* 2000;342:145–153.

124. Mullen MJ, Clarkson P, Donald AE, et al. Effect of enalapril on endothelial function in young insulin-dependent diabetic patients: a randomized, double-blind study. *J Am Coll Cardiol* 1998;31:1330–1335.

125. O'Driscoll G, Green D, Maiorana A, et al. Improvement in endothelial function by angiotensin-converting enzyme inhibition in non-insulin-dependent diabetes mellitus. *J Am Coll Cardiol* 1999;33:1506–1511.

126. Cheetham C, Collis J, O'Driscoll G, et al. Losartan, an angiotensin type 1 receptor antagonist, improves endothelial function in non-insulin-dependent diabetes. *J Am Coll Cardiol* 2000;36:1461–1466.

127. Tzemos N, Lim PO, MacDonald TM. Nebivolol reverses endothelial dysfunction in essential hypertension: a randomized, double-blind, crossover study. *Circulation* 2001;104:511–514.

128. Hambrecht R, Wolf A, Gielen S, et al. Effect of exercise on coronary endothelial function in patients with coronary artery disease. *N Engl J Med* 2000;342:454–460.

129. Hambrecht R, Fiehn E, Weigl C, et al. Regular physical exercise corrects endothelial dysfunction and improves exercise capacity in patients with chronic heart failure. *Circulation* 1998;98:2709–2715.

130. Hornig B, Maier V, Drexler H. Physical training improves endothelial function in patients with chronic heart failure. *Circulation* 1996;93:210–214.

131. Hiatt WR, Regensteiner JG, Hargarten ME, et al. Benefit of exercise conditioning for patients with peripheral arterial disease. *Circulation* 1990;81:602–609.

132. Hiatt WR, Regensteiner JG, Wolfel EE, et al. Effect of exercise training on skeletal muscle histology and metabolism in peripheral arterial disease. *J Appl Physiol* 1996;81:780–788.

133. Schellong SM, Boger RH, Burchert W, et al. Dose-related effect of intravenous L-arginine on muscular blood flow of the calf in patients with peripheral vascular disease: a $H_2^{15}O$ positron emission tomography study. *Clin Sci* (Lond) 1997;93:159–165.

134. Boger RH, Bode-Boger SM, Thiele W, et al. Restoring vascular nitric oxide formation by L-arginine improves the symptoms of intermittent claudication in patients with peripheral arterial occlusive disease. *J Am Coll Cardiol* 1998;32:1336–44.

135. Barradell LB, Brogden RN. Oral naftidrofuryl. A review of its pharmacology and therapeutic use in the management of peripheral occlusive arterial disease. *Drugs Aging* 1996;8:299–322.

136. Brevetti G, Diehm C, Lambert D. European multicenter study on propionyl-L-carnitine in intermittent claudication. *J Am Coll Cardiol* 1999;34:1618–1624.

137. Nazzaro P, Manzari M, Merlo M, et al. Distinct and combined vascular effects of ACE blockade and HMG–CoA reductase inhibition in hypertensive subjects. *Hypertension* 1999;33:719–725.

138. Virmani R, Burke AP, Farb A, et al. Pathology of the unstable plaque. *Prog Cardiovasc Dis* 2002;44:349–356.

139. Schartl M, Bocksch W, Koschyk DH, et al. Use of intravascular ultrasound to compare effects of different strategies of lipid-lowering therapy on plaque volume and composition in patients with coronary artery disease. *Circulation* 2001;104:387–392.

140. Hamasaki S, Higano ST, Suwaidi JA, et al. Cholesterol-lowering treatment is associated with improvement in coronary vascular remodeling and endothelial function in patients with normal or mildly diseased coronary arteries. *Arterioscler Thromb Vasc Biol* 2000;20:737–743.

141. Smilde TJ, van Wissen S, Wollersheim H, et al. Effect of aggressive versus conventional lipid lowering on atherosclerosis progression in familial hypercholesterolaemia (ASAP): a prospective, randomised, double-blind trial. *Lancet* 2001;357:577–581.

142. Gokce N, Keaney Jr JF, Hunter LM, et al. Predictive value of noninvasively determined endothelial dysfunction for long-term cardiovascular events in patients with peripheral vascular disease. *J Am Coll Cardiol* 2003;41:1769–1775.

143. Adams RH, Wilkinson GA, Weiss C, et al. Roles of ephrinB ligands and EphB receptors in cardiovascular development: demarcation of arterial/venous domains, vascular morphogenesis, and sprouting angiogenesis. *Genes Dev* 1999;13:295–306.

144. Guillot PV, Guan J, Liu L, et al. A vascular bed-specific pathway. *J Clin Invest* 1999;103:799–805.

145. Bergwerff M, Verberne ME, DeRuiter MC, et al. Neural crest cell contribution to the developing circulatory system: implications for vascular morphology? *Circ Res* 1998;82:221–231.

146. Ikari Y, McManus BM, Kenyon J, et al. Neonatal intima formation in the human coronary artery. *Arterioscler Thromb Vasc Biol* 1999;19:2036–2040.

147. Weninger WJ, Muller GB, Reiter C, et al. Intimal hyperplasia of the infant parasellar carotid artery: a potential developmental factor in atherosclerosis and SIDS. *Circ Res* 1999;85:970–975.

148. Schwartz SM. The intima: a new soil. *Circ Res* 1999;85:877–879.

149. Rainwater DL, McMahan CA, Malcom GT, et al. Lipid and apolipoprotein predictors of atherosclerosis in youth: apolipoprotein concentrations do not materially improve prediction of arterial lesions in PDAY subjects. The PDAY Research Group. *Arterioscler Thromb Vasc Biol* 1999;19:753–761.

150. Strong JP, Malcom GT, Oalmann MC, et al. The PDAY Study: natural history, risk factors, and pathobiology. Pathobiological Determinants of Atherosclerosis in Youth. *Ann NY Acad Sci* 1997;811:226–235; discussion 235–237.

151. Virmani R, Burke AP, Kolodgie FD, et al. Vulnerable plaque: the pathology of unstable coronary lesions. *J Interv Cardiol* 2002;15:439–446.

152. Carr S, Farb A, Pearce WH, et al. Atherosclerotic plaque rupture in symptomatic carotid artery stenosis. *J Vasc Surg* 1996;23:755–765; discussion 765–756.

153. Carr SC, Farb A, Pearce WH, et al. Activated inflammatory cells are associated with plaque rupture in carotid artery stenosis. *Surgery* 1997;122:757–763; discussion 763–764.

154. Gupta AK, Ravimandalam K, Rao VR, et al. Total occlusion of iliac arteries: results of balloon angioplasty. *Cardiovasc Intervent Radiol* 1993;16:165–177.

155. Pentecost MJ, Criqui MH, Dorros G, et al. Guidelines for peripheral percutaneous transluminal angioplasty of the abdominal aorta and lower extremity vessels. A statement for health professionals from a special writing group of the Councils on Cardiovascular Radiology, Arteriosclerosis, Cardio-Thoracic and Vascular Surgery, Clinical Cardiology, and Epidemiology and Prevention, the American Heart Association. *Circulation* 1994;89:511–531.

156. Motarjeme A, Gordon GI, Bodenhagen K. Thrombolysis and angioplasty of chronic iliac artery occlusions. *J Vasc Interv Radiol* 1995; 6[6 Pt 2 Suppl]:66S–72S.

157. Johnston KW. Iliac arteries: reanalysis of results of balloon angioplasty. *Radiology* 1993;186:207–212.

158. Tegtmeyer CJ, Hartwell GD, Selby JB, et al. Results and complications of angioplasty in aortoiliac disease. *Circulation* 1991; 83[2 Suppl]:I53–I60.

159. Henry M, Amor M, Ethevenot G, et al. Palmaz stent placement in iliac and femoropopliteal arteries: primary and secondary patency in 310 patients with 2–4-year follow-up. *Radiology* 1995;197:167–174.

160. Sullivan TM, Childs MB, Bacharach JM, et al. Percutaneous transluminal angioplasty and primary stenting of the iliac arteries in 288 patients. *J Vasc Surg* 1997;25:829–838; discussion 838–839.

161. Martin EC, Katzen BT, Benenati JF, et al. Multicenter trial of the wallstent in the iliac and femoral arteries. *J Vasc Interv Radiol* 1995;6:843–849.

162. Matsi PJ, Manninen HI. Complications of lower-limb percutaneous transluminal angioplasty: a prospective analysis of 410 procedures on 295 consecutive patients. *Cardiovasc Intervent Radiol* 1998;21:361–366.

163. Hunink MG, Donaldson MC, Meyerovitz MF, et al. Risks and benefits of femoropopliteal percutaneous balloon angioplasty. *J Vasc Surg* 1993;17:183–192; discussion 192–194.

164. Sullivan TM, Gray BH, Bacharach JM, et al. Angioplasty and primary stenting of the subclavian, innominate, and common carotid arteries in 83 patients. *J Vasc Surg* 1998;28:1059–1065.

165. Mathias KD, Luth I, Haarmann P. Percutaneous transluminal angioplasty of proximal subclavian artery occlusions. *Cardiovasc Intervent Radiol* 1993;16:214–218.

166. Millaire A, Trinca M, Marache P, et al. Subclavian angioplasty: immediate and late results in 50 patients. *Cathet Cardiovasc Diagn* 1993;29:8–17.

167. Bakal CW, Sprayregen S, Scheinbaum K, et al. Percutaneous transluminal angioplasty of the infrapopliteal arteries: results in 53 patients. *AJR Am J Roentgenol* 1990;154:171–174.

168. Bakal CW, Cynamon J, Sprayregen S. Infrapopliteal percutaneous transluminal angioplasty: what we know. *Radiology* 1996;200:36–43.

169. Matsi PJ, Manninen HI, Suhonen MT, et al. Chronic critical lower-limb ischemia: prospective trial of angioplasty with 1–36 months follow-up. *Radiology* 1993;188:381–387.

170. Dorros G, Jaff MR, Murphy KJ, et al. The acute outcome of tibioperoneal vessel angioplasty in 417 cases with claudication and critical limb ischemia. *Cathet Cardiovasc Diagn* 1998;45:251–256.

171. The SH, Gussenhoven EJ, Zhong Y, et al. Effect of balloon angioplasty on femoral artery evaluated with intravascular ultrasound imaging. *Circulation* 1992;86:483–493.

172. Losordo DW, Rosenfield K, Pieczek A, et al. How does angioplasty work? Serial analysis of human iliac arteries using intravascular ultrasound. *Circulation* 1992;86:1845–1858.

173. Pasterkamp G, Borst C, Gussenhoven EJ, et al. Remodeling of *de novo* atherosclerotic lesions in femoral arteries: impact on mechanism of balloon angioplasty. *J Am Coll Cardiol* 1995;26:422–428.

174. de Vrey EA, Mintz GS, von Birgelen C, et al. Serial volumetric (three-dimensional) intravascular ultrasound analysis of restenosis after directional coronary atherectomy. *Journal of the American College of Cardiology* 1998;32:1874–1880.

175. Mintz GS, Kimura T, Nobuyoshi M, et al. Intravascular ultrasound assessment of the relation between early and late changes in arterial area and neointimal hyperplasia after percutaneous transluminal coronary angioplasty and directional coronary atherectomy. *American Journal of Cardiology* 1999;83:1518–1523.

176. van Lankeren W, Gussenhoven EJ, Honkoop J, et al. Plaque area increase and vascular remodeling contribute to lumen area change after percutaneous transluminal angioplasty of the femoropopliteal artery: an intravascular ultrasound study. *J Vasc Surg* 1999;29:430–441.

177. Arko F, McCollough R, Manning L, et al. Use of intravascular ultrasound in the endovascular management of atherosclerotic aortoiliac occlusive disease. *Am J Surg* 1996;172:546–549; discussion 549–550.

178. Buckley CJ, Arko FR, Lee S, et al. Intravascular ultrasound scanning improves long-term patency of iliac lesions treated with balloon angioplasty and primary stenting. *J Vasc Surg* 2002;35:316–323.

178a. Leertouwer TC, Gussenhoven EJ, van Lankeren W, et al. Response of renal and femoropopliteal arteries to Palmaz stent implantation assessed with intravascular ultrasound. *J Endovasc Surg* 1999;6:259–264.

179. Nishanian G, Kopchok GE, Donayre CE, et al. The impact of intravascular ultrasound (IVUS) on endovascular interventions. *Semin Vasc Surg* 1999;12:285–299.

180. van Sambeek MR, Gussenhoven EJ, van Overhagen H, et al. Intravascular ultrasound in endovascular stent-grafts for peripheral aneurysm: a clinical study. *J Endovasc Surg* 1998;5:106–112.

181. White RA, Donayre CE, Kopchok GE, et al. Utility of intravascular ultrasound in peripheral interventions. *Tex Heart Inst J* 1997;24:28–34.

182. White RA, Donayre CE, Walot I, et al. Endoluminal graft exclusion of a proximal para-anastomotic pseudoaneurysm following aortobifemoral bypass. *J Endovasc Surg* 1997;4:88–94.

183. Muller-Hulsbeck S, Schwarzenberg H, Hutzelmann A, et al. Intravascular ultrasound evaluation of peripheral arterial stent-grafts. *Invest Radiol* 2000;35:97–104.

184. Yadav J. Presentation. Annual Scientific Sessions of the American Heart Association, November 9–12, 2003; Orlando, FL.

185. Bosch JL, Tetteroo E, Mali WP, et al. Iliac arterial occlusive disease: cost-effectiveness analysis of stent placement versus percutaneous transluminal angioplasty. Dutch Iliac Stent Trial Study Group. *Radiology* 1998;208:641–648.

186. Hagenaars T, Lim AP. IF, van Sambeek MR, et al. Gamma radiation induces positive vascular remodeling after balloon angioplasty: a prospective, randomized intravascular ultrasound scan study. *J Vasc Surg* 2002;36:318–324.

187. Tegtmeyer CJ, Selby JB, Hartwell GD, et al. Results and complications of angioplasty in fibromuscular disease. *Circulation* 1991;83 [2 Suppl]:I155–I161.

188. Rosenfield K, Schainfeld R, Pieczek A, et al. Restenosis of endovascular stents from stent compression. *Journal of the American College of Cardiology* 1997;29:328–38.

189. Degertekin M, Serruys PW, Foley DP, et al. Persistent inhibition of neointimal hyperplasia after sirolimus-eluting stent implantation: long-term (up to 2 years) clinical, angiographic, and intravascular ultrasound follow-up. *Circulation* 2002;106:1610–1613.

190. Serruys PW, Degertekin M, Tanabe K, et al. Intravascular ultrasound findings in the multicenter, randomized, double-blind RAVEL (RAndomized study with the sirolimus-eluting VElocity balloon-expandable stent in the treatment of patients with *de novo* native coronary artery Lesions) trial. *Circulation* 2002;106:798–803.

191. Sonoda S, Honda Y, Kataoka T, et al. Taxol-based eluting stents from theory to human validation: clinical and intravascular ultrasound observations. *J Invasive Cardiol* 2003;15:109–114.

192. Hansrani M, Overbeck K, Smout J, et al. Intravascular brachytherapy for peripheral vascular disease. *Cochrane Database Syst Rev* 2002:CD003504.

193. Pokrajac B, Wolfram R, Lileg B, et al. Endovascular brachytherapy in peripheral arteries: solution for restenosis or false hope? *Curr Treat Options Cardiovasc Med* 2003;5:121–126.

194. Lerman A, Burnett Jr JC, Higano ST, et al. Long-term L-arginine supplementation improves small-vessel coronary endothelial function in humans. *Circulation* 1998;97:2123–2128.

CHAPTER 2

Atherosclerotic Vascular Disease as a Systemic Process

George S. Abela, Alok Maheshwari, and SriCharan C. Kantipudi

Key Points

- Atherosclerotic vascular disease has become a global epidemic.
- "Vulnerable" plaque is the precursor of acute thrombosis and end-organ ischemia.
- Inflammation is a cause of atherosclerosis and destabilization of plaque. This may be the result of a cumulative process that leads to a chain reaction causing thrombosis.
- Clinical manifestation of peripheral atherosclerosis is less symptomatic than coronary artery events.
- New devices are being developed to detect plaques that undergo disruption; these include thermal detection, intravascular ultrasound, optical coherence tomography, angioscopy, magnetic resonance, and computerized tomography.
- Future evaluation of atherosclerosis by gene analysis and environmental stressors is being investigated.

HISTORICAL PERSPECTIVES

Atherosclerosis is the predominant form of arterial disease. The term is derived from the Greek words *athere*, which means porridge, and *sclerosis,* which means hardening (1). The term was coined to describe a cystic space containing a gruel-like substance. Atherosclerosis is not a condition of modern civilization as is often thought. Autopsy studies of ancient Egyptian mummies have revealed the presence of atherosclerosis in carotid and peripheral arteries (2). Furthermore, it is a misconception to assume that atherosclerosis is primarily a disease of industrialized societies. In the twenty-first century, atherosclerosis has become recognized not only as a leading cause of morbidity and mortality in industrialized societies, but also as a global epidemic (3).

Rudolph Virchow (1821 to 1902), who is acknowledged to be the father of cellular pathology, proposed that atherosclerosis was a direct result of an inflammatory process (4,5). He coined the term endarteritis deformans to indicate that reactive fibrosis in response to injury was due to the repair mechanism. Carl von Rokitansky (1804 to 1878) emphasized an alternate hypothesis for atherosclerosis, and suggested as the cause the layering or deposition of circulating blood elements

on the arterial lumen (6). A heated debate raged between the two giants of pathology, as illustrated by the following quote from Virchow's 1858 Lecture XVI at the Pathological Institute in Berlin:

> In this manner the view which was for a considerable time defended by Rokitansky also, that the affliction consists in a deposit upon the internal coat, is refuted. In a vertical section it is distinctly seen that the most external layers run in a curve over the whole swelling and return into the internal coat, and the old writers were quite right when they said—speaking of a stage in which the formation of the atheromatous depot had already made considerable progress—the internal coat over the whole of the depot could be stripped off in a piece (7).

PLAQUE DISRUPTION AND THROMBOSIS: "VULNERABLE" PLAQUE

Acute thrombosis is a major component of the arterial obstruction leading to acute cardiovascular events (8). This was a renewed discovery based on observations in patients undergoing emergency bypass surgery for myocardial infarction. In that study, patients in the Seattle area were brought to surgery for the treatment of their heart attacks (8). It was demonstrated that 110 of 126 patients (87%) had fresh thrombus obstructing the artery associated with the myocardial infarction. However, after 24 hours, fewer thrombi were noted during bypass surgery. Until that time, it had not been agreed that the primary mechanism of myocardial infarction was due to arterial thrombosis. This was despite literature from the turn of the twentieth century describing fresh thrombus in the coronary arteries at postmortem examination (9). A report by Fuster et al. suggested that acute coronary events did not seem to occur at the sites of severe arterial narrowing as anticipated by the earlier concept of myocardial infarction (10). Instead, collateral circulation seemed to develop in chronically narrowed arterial beds. In addition, angiographic studies demonstrated that the majority of coronary lesions that were the site of subsequent arterial thrombosis had been previously reported to have less than 50% luminal narrowing by angiography (Figs. 2.1 and 2.2) (11,12). In their pioneering work on angioscopy, Seeger and Abela demonstrated similar findings of a fresh thrombus overlying a ruptured plaque in a patient presenting with an acute ischemic leg syndrome (Fig. 2.3) (13). Sherman et al. demonstrated a high frequency of thrombus in the coronary circulation, using angioscopy in patients with unstable coronary syndromes (14). The clinical presentation of acute peripheral limb syndromes is less frequent than for coronary artery disease (15). This may be related to the larger size of peripheral arteries and better collateral circulation. However, the underlying mechanisms appear to be the same. In a recent report using intravascular ultrasound (IVUS), Hongo et al. demonstrated that plaque rupture in femoropopliteal arteries was common and frequently associated with positive remodeling (Fig. 2.4) (16).

Autopsy studies by Constantinides (17) and subsequently by Davies (18) demonstrated that the plaques responsible for myocardial infarctions or aortic plaques with thrombus formation often had a ruptured fibrous cap usually at the plaque shoulder region (Fig. 2.5). They also demonstrated that these lesions frequently had a rich lipid core, a reduced number of smooth muscle cells, and a thin fibrous cap (19). It is the cap that separates the highly thrombogenic plaque gruel from circulating blood elements. Within the plaque matrix, activated macrophages release various lytic enzymes such as collagenases and metalloproteinases. The progressive digestion of the cap eventually leads to plaque rupture and acute thrombosis (Fig. 2.6). In addition, a large lipid core rich in cholesterol seems to enhance the inflammatory process (20).

Attempts were made to correlate the pathological findings with the clinical discovery that there was an associated clustering of cardiovascular events (i.e., strokes and myocardial infarction) in early-morning hours, which was consistent with a circadian rhythm (21). Other associated triggers of cardiovascular events included sudden stressful exercise, sexual activity, and anger (22). The surge in catecholamine after the waking-up hours suggested that sudden rise in blood pressure could be responsible for plaque rupture leading to acute cardiovascular events. However, Loree et al., working with atherosclerotic plaque from human aorta,

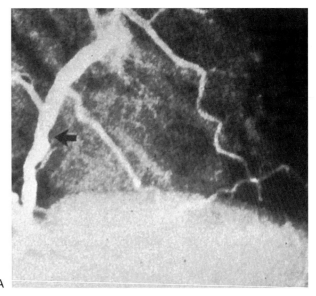

A

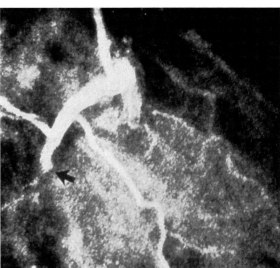

B

FIG. 2.1. Coronary angiogram demonstrating minimal irregularity leading to myocardial infarction. **A:** Initial coronary angiogram of the right coronary artery, demonstrating a luminal irregularity. **B:** Coronary angiogram of the same artery after an inferior infarction 13 days later, demonstrating a totally occluded mid-right coronary artery. (From Little WC, Constantinescu M, Applegate RJ, et al. Can coronary angiography predict the site of a subsequent myocardial infarction in patients with mild-to-moderate coronary artery disease? *Circulation* 1988;78:1157–1166, with permission.)

used finite-element analysis to evaluate stress and strain relationships within the arterial lumen (23). These studies suggested that it would require more than ten times the normal blood pressure levels to obtain the expected plaque rupture (23). These data did not support the concept that the surge in blood pressure was the cause of cardiovascular events. Instead, they implied that weakening of the plaque by biochemical enzymatic digestion was a more plausible mechanism. Given these observations and the triggers that sometimes preceded unstable cardiovascular syndromes, Muller

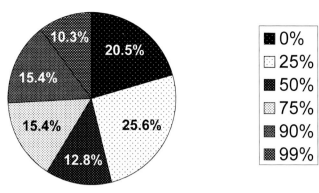

FIG. 2.2. The relationship between severity of stenosis and new myocardial infarction occurrence. More than half of the infarctions occurred at lesions that had less than 50% stenosis. (From Nobuyoshi, M, Tanaka M, Nosaka H, et al. *J Am Coll Cardiol* 1991;18:904–910, with permission.)

et al. proposed to describe atherosclerotic lesions that caused cardiovascular events as "vulnerable" plaque (24). In addition, epidemiologic studies of population cohorts demonstrated that increased myocardial infarctions occurred following great catastrophes such as the San Francisco earthquake of 1987 and the Scud missile attacks in the Gulf War of 1993 (25,26).

Despite early studies demonstrating plaque rupture as the primary histological finding in acute cardiovascular events,

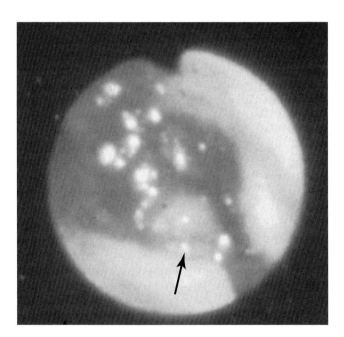

FIG. 2.3. (See Color Fig. 2.3.) Angioscopic view of thrombus totally occluding the superficial femoral artery in a patient presenting with acute limb ischemia. The thrombus is reddish brown superimposed on a yellow plaque with protruding lipid core (*arrow*) into the lumen. (From Seeger JM, Abela GS. Angioscopy as an adjunct to arterial reconstructive surgery. *J Vasc Surg* 1986;4:315–320, with permission.)

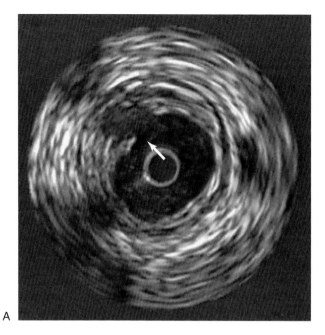

A

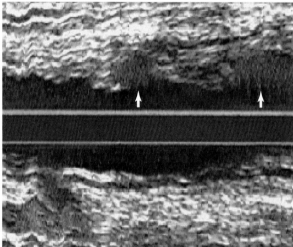

B

FIG. 2.4. A 64-year-old woman with chronic intermittent claudication, stable angina, history of coronary artery bypass grafting and hypertension, and hyperlipidemia. **A:** Intravascular ultrasound cross-sectional view of plaque rupture (*arrow*) in the femoropopliteal artery. **B:** Intravascular ultrasound pullback longitudinal view, demonstrating site of plaque rupture (*arrowheads*).

many thrombosed arteries did not have typical plaque rupture as described by Constatinides (17) and Davies (18). Thus, other mechanisms of plaque disruption and thrombosis were plausible. Barger et al. reported on the presence of extensive vasa vasora around the arterial plaques in human coronary arteries (27,28). These vessels penetrated into the mid layers of the plaque and were composed of fragile small vessels. It is hypothesized that these vessels are weak and may easily hemorrhage into the plaque, resulting in plaque disruption and thrombosis. Autopsy data support this hypothesis and demonstrate that hemorrhage into plaque occurs in

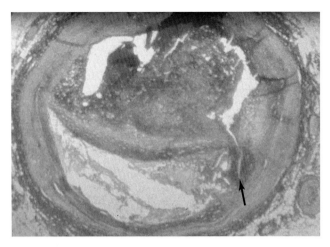

FIG. 2.5. Cross-sectional view of human coronary artery following rupture and thrombus formation. Rupture is clearly seen at the plaque margin site (*arrow*). This was obtained after serial sectioning by Dr. Paris Constantinides.

about 15% of cases in the absence of typical rupture (17). Barbieri and Abela used India ink to stain the vasa vasora of plaques in human femoral arteries at postmortem. This demonstrated a wide network of small vessels in the plaques of patients with peripheral vascular disease. Grossly, these had an appearance similar to retinopathy, and numerous small areas of hemorrhages could be readily seen (Fig. 2.7). Vasospasm is another mechanism that has been implicated in plaque disruption and thrombosis (12). In the presence of arterial spasm, the part of the arterial wall between the plaque and normal artery acts to create a fulcrum against which high shear stress develops, resulting in a tear or rupture of the plaque margins (Fig. 2.8).

In a postmortem study, van der Wall et al. reported that 40% of the patients with fatal myocardial infarction did not have the typical plaque rupture, but instead had a surface erosion of the plaque with an associated inflammatory cell reaction (29). Plaque erosion has been noted to occur more frequently in female patients (Fig. 2.9) (30). Furthermore, estrogens have been noted to enhance inflammation (31). These observations may have implications for the use of estrogens in the presence of atherosclerotic disease (32). In fact, inflammation induces tissue factor and endothelial tissue adhesion molecules (e.g., vascular cell adhesion molecule-1, VCAM-1) expression in association with elevated cholesterol (33,34). Multi-

TABLE 2.1. *Proposed circulating inflammatory markers*[a]

High-sensitivity C-reactive protein
Serum amyloid A
Interleukin-1
Interleukin-6
Vascular cell adhesion molecule-1
Tissue necrosis factor-α
Fibrinogen

[a]Data from Ridker PM, Hennekens CH, Buring JE, et al. *N Engl J Med* 2000;342:836–843.

ple inflammatory markers have been studied in association with vascular disease, but so far C-reactive protein (CRP) appears to be best correlated with cardiovascular events (35) (Table 2.1).

ATHEROSCLEROSIS AS A CHRONIC ARTERIAL INFLAMMATION

There has been recent interest in the role of inflammation as a major etiologic factor in the development and destabilization of arterial plaque. Destabilization of atherosclerotic plaque leading to acute cardiovascular events is being assessed by determining whether the expression of circulating markers of inflammation can be used to risk-stratify patients with vulnerable plaques prone to acute cardiovascular events.

C-reactive protein is an acute-phase reactant produced by the liver in response to circulating inflammatory molecules, namely interleukin-6 (IL-6) (36,37). The CRP blood test has been available for a very long time (37). However, recently a high-sensitivity CRP that is a nonspecific marker for low-grade inflammation has been correlated with cardiovascular events including unstable angina and myocardial infarction (35). Furthermore, it is being evaluated for correlation as an independent risk factor for coronary artery disease as well as peripheral vascular disease (Fig. 2.10) (38,39).

Recent studies have found elevated CRP levels in patients with acute coronary syndromes, suggesting its role as a predictor of mortality in the setting of myocardial infarction (40). In addition, the presence of established risk factors of coronary artery disease (i.e., diabetes, obesity, and smoking) has been associated with elevated CRP levels. Preliminary data suggest that lipid lowering with statins as well as weight loss and diabetes control lower CRP levels (36,41–44). Aspirin seems to improve outcomes in patients with elevated CRP levels while not necessarily impacting the levels (41). Elevated CRP levels have been implicated in interventional procedures, with evidence to suggest an association between early complications and late restenosis after angioplasty (45). More recently, CRP has been suspected to be an inducer of inflammation (37). Although CRP has been found to be a risk marker for peripheral arterial disease (39), it has not been found to be associated with deep venous thrombosis (41).

Plaque Disruption and Thrombosis: A Chain Reaction?

Concurrent local and remote systemic arterial bed effects have been associated with acute cardiovascular events. The common factor implicated in this widespread effect is arterial inflammation (46,47). Thus, plaque rupture in one coronary artery may be accompanied by additional ruptured plaques in the same or adjacent arterial beds. In addition, carotid artery plaque rupture has been noted in the presence of an acute myocardial event. This is consistent with data demonstrating a very strong linear correlation between cardiac events and plaque thickening of the walls of the carotid arteries (48).

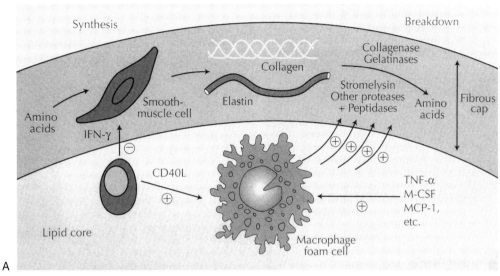

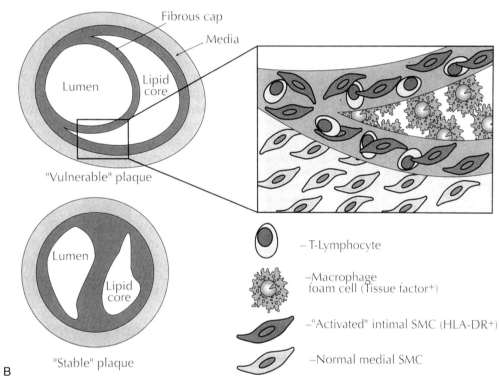

FIG. 2.6. The effect of inflammation on the mechanism of plaque rupture. **A:** The metabolism of collagen and elastin in the plaque cap. Vascular smooth muscle cells produce the structural proteins (i.e., collagen, matrix, and amino acids). Activated macrophages secrete proteinases that can break down the structural proteins. Interferon gamma (IFN-γ) from the lymphocytes inhibits collagen synthesis and activates the macrophages. TNF-α, tumor necrosis factor-α; M-CSF, macrophage colony-stimulating factor; MCP-1, monocyte chemotactic protein-1. **B:** The characteristics of vulnerable and stable plaques. Vulnerable plaques have a large lipid core and a thin fibrous cap. Stable plaques have a relatively thick fibrous cap. SMC, smooth muscle cell. (From Libby P. Molecular bases of the acute coronary syndromes. *Circulation* 1995;91:2844–2850, with permission.)

Further evidence for the hypothesis of plaque burden in the pathogenesis of acute events comes from the work of Goldstein et al., who demonstrated that plaque load in the coronary circulation was associated with greater event rates (49). In addition, a study of culprit coronary artery lesions demonstrated that the nonaffected coronary artery was involved in the in-

flammatory reaction as evidenced by neutrophil myeloperoxidase depletion in that vascular territory (50). Furthermore, it has been demonstrated that peripheral vascular disease is frequently associated with coronary artery disease (Fig. 2.11). These data lead one to speculate that the total plaque load in a particular individual may elicit a systemic inflammatory

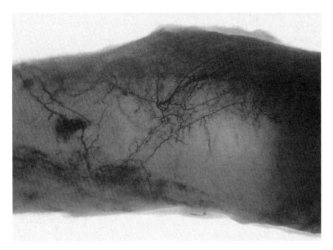

FIG. 2.7. (See Color Fig. 2.7.) Vasa vasorum in plaque removed from the superficial femoral artery of a patient at postmortem. The vasa vasorum is stained with India ink, demonstrating a profuse network of small vessels with areas of vessel disruption evidenced by leaking of the ink into the plaque. (Courtesy of Drs. Erico Barbieri and George Abela.)

response leading to a localized vascular destabilization event. This would be comparable to a chain reaction due to an inflammatory process provoked by a critical mass of plaque (5).

OTHER ISSUES RELATED TO ATHEROSCLEROSIS AND PLAQUE DISRUPTION: OXIDATIVE STRESS, INFECTION, AND CYCLOOXYGENASE-2 INHIBITORS

Antioxidized Low-Density Lipoprotein Antibodies

Enhanced lipid peroxidation has been associated with the development and acceleration of atherosclerosis. Oxidative

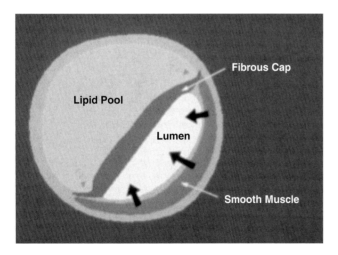

FIG. 2.8. Artery with plaque, illustrating thinning of the media beneath the plaque and contraction of the preserved media in the opposite wall, creating a sheer stress at the plaque margins. In the presence of arterial spasm, rupture is likely to occur at the plaque margin sites. (Courtesy of Dr. Richard Nesto.)

modification of LDL involves fatty acid oxidation, which generates hydroperoxides and active aldehydes such as malondialdehyde. The LDL lysine ring (on apolipoprotein B), when oxidized by malondialdehyde, can become antigenic and more attractive to the scavenger receptor present on the macrophages. Oxidized LDL levels are proportional to the levels of total LDL; however, small, dense LDL particles are more susceptible to oxidation than large, buoyant LDL particles (51). This may lead to considerable variability in individuals regarding cardiovascular events and the level of LDL.

Antibodies to oxidized LDL have been demonstrated in atherosclerotic plaques and in the plasma of patients with atherosclerosis (52,53). In one study, the titer of these antibodies distinguished between the absence and the presence of coronary disease (especially multivessel) and between patients with chronic coronary disease and those with acute coronary syndrome (52). The latter observation suggests that these antibodies may play a role in plaque instability.

In another study, antibodies to oxidized LDL were present in a higher titer in patients with peripheral arterial disease than in patients with unstable angina or stable angina and also correlated with the severity of atherosclerosis (54). Based on a study of 144 healthy adult men, Ridker et al. suggested that baseline levels of C-reactive protein predict future risk of developing symptomatic peripheral arterial disease (55).

Antioxidant treatment to prevent or retard atherosclerosis has been a subject of considerable interest. However, the results of trials with vitamin E, vitamin C, and beta-carotene supplementation have been negative or conflicting. One of the largest of these trials is the Heart Protection Study, which included 20,536 patients with a history of cardiovascular disease, diabetes mellitus, or hypertension. One arm of this lipid-lowering trial consisted in random assignment to supplementation with antioxidant vitamins (600 mg of vitamin E, 250 mg of vitamin C, and 20 mg of beta-carotene) or placebo. At 5-year follow-up, there was no difference among the groups in any endpoint, including all-cause cardiovascular mortality, nonfatal myocardial infarction or stroke, or incidence of cancer (56).

Infection

Chronic infection may contribute to atherosclerosis by a number of mechanisms, including direct vascular injury and induction of a systemic inflammatory state. The role of several putative infectious organisms in the pathogenesis has been investigated.

Chlamydia pneumoniae has been suggested as a possible contributor to atherosclerosis in some studies (57,58). However, a benefit from antibiotic therapy for *C. pneumoniae* in coronary artery disease has not been demonstrated. Cytomegalovirus (CMV) and other herpesviruses, such as herpes simplex virus, have been implicated in some studies in the development of atherosclerosis, restenosis, and transplant

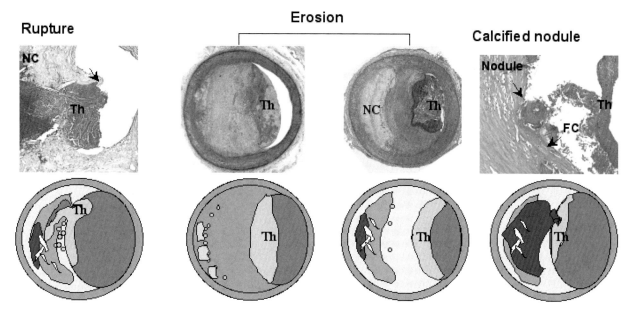

FIG. 2.9. (See Color Fig. 2.9.) Atherosclerotic lesions with luminal thrombi. Ruptured plaques (*arrow*) have thin, fibrous caps (*FC*) with luminal thrombi (*Th*) (**left**). These lesions often have a necrotic core (*NC*) containing large numbers of cholesterol crystals and thin, fibrous caps (less than 65 mm). The fibrous cap is thinnest at the site of rupture and consists of a few collagen bundles and rare smooth muscle cells. Plaque with thrombus at a site of surface erosion can also be detected (**middle**). Occasionally, plaques with calcified nodules protruding into the lumen can be seen at sites of plaque disruption (**right**). (From Virmani R, Kolodgie FD, Burke AP, et al. Lessons from sudden coronary death. A comprehensive morphological classification scheme for atherosclerotic lesions. *Arterioscler Thromb Vasc Biol* 2000;20:1262–1275, with permission.)

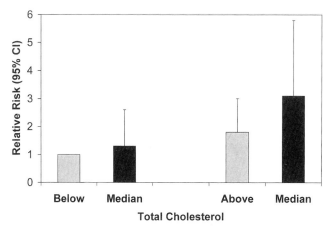

FIG. 2.10. Relative risk of developing peripheral arterial disease in apparently healthy middle-aged men by stratification using baseline levels of total cholesterol and C-reactive protein (CRP). CRP significantly improved the predictive value of models based on total cholesterol prediction alone. CI, confidence interval. (Adapted from Ridker PM, Stampfer MJ, Rifai N, et al. Novel risk factors for systemic atherosclerosis: a comparison of C-reactive protein, fibrinogen, homocyteine, lipoprotein (a), and standard cholesterol screening as predictors of peripheral vascular disease. *JAMA* 2001;285:2481–2485, with permission.)

vasculopathy (59–64). Serum anti-CMV antibody levels are significantly elevated in patients with coronary artery disease compared to controls (60,65) and in those with carotid intimal thickening (66). CMV infection might promote the development of atherosclerosis by several mechanisms. An association between CMV antibodies and elevated levels of C-reactive protein and IL-6 has been shown (67,68). CMV may increase the uptake of oxidized LDL in vascular smooth muscle cells (69) and increase the neointimal response to vascular injury (70). There some evidence linking *Helicobacter pylori* infection with atherosclerosis and premature myocardial infarction (71,72). However, this may be due to associated confounding factors like smoking, older age, and lower socioeconomic class (73).

It has been suggested that the "infectious burden" or "pathogen burden" (the number of pathogens to which an individual has been exposed) may correlate with the development and extent of atherosclerosis (63,64,74–76). In a report on 375 patients undergoing coronary angiography, the presence and severity of coronary disease were correlated with the pathogen burden more than with any single pathogen (63,64). Increasing pathogen burden in patients with known coronary heart disease is also associated with an increased risk of myocardial infarction and death (74). In a report on 228 young women with peripheral arterial disease (PAD), serological evidence of infection with *C. pneumoniae, H. pylori,* and CMV was sought. A positive association between infection burden and PAD was only seen in women with a high CRP level (77).

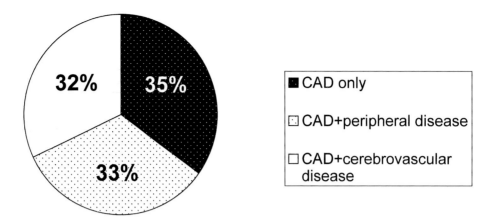

FIG. 2.11. Pie diagram demonstrating the coexistence of coronary artery disease (CAD), peripheral arterial disease, and atherothrombotic brain infarction in men and women 62 years of age and older. (Adapted from Aronow WS, Ahn C. Prevalence of coexistence of coronary artery disease, peripheral arterial disease, and atherothrombotic brain infarction in men and women ≥62 years of age. *Am J Cardiol* 1994;74:64–65, with permission.)

In a prospective study of 45,136 healthy males, it was found that incident tooth loss was significantly associated with PAD, especially among those with periodontal disease. These results suggest a potential oral infection–inflammation pathway (78). Circulating bacterial endotoxin can exhibit a variety of proatherogenic properties and endothelial dysfunction (79). Exposure to sustained high levels of endotoxin accelerates atherosclerosis in an animal model (80) and may also be a risk factor in humans, especially in those with chronic infections and in smokers (81). Heat-shock protein 60 (HSP60) is produced in response to variety of stress stimuli, including infection. HSP60 has cytokine-like activity and its levels correlate with other markers of inflammation and with the presence of atherosclerosis (82–85).

Cardiovascular Disease and Cyclooxygenase-2 Inhibitors

Selective cyclooxygenase-2 (COX-2) inhibition is associated with decreased production of prostacyclin or prostaglandin I2 (PGI2) by vascular endothelium. However, there is little or no inhibition of potentially prothrombotic platelet thromboxane A2 production (86). Prostacyclin is a part of the hemostatic defense mechanism and plays a role in limiting the consequences of platelet activation. Its reduction could therefore potentially predispose to endothelial injury (87).

There are conflicting data regarding worse cardiovascular outcomes with rofecoxib compared to naproxen and other nonsteroidal antiinflammatory drugs (NSAIDs). The VIGOR trial compared rofecoxib to naproxen in 8,076 patients with rheumatoid arthritis. Patients treated with rofecoxib had higher rate of nonfatal myocardial infarction, nonfatal stroke, transient ischemic attacks, and death from any vascular event (0.8% vs. 0.4%) and an increased incidence of myocardial infarction (0.4% vs. 0.1%) (88). In the CLASS trial, there was no significant difference in the cardiovascu-

lar event rate between celecoxib and the NSAIDs in 8,059 patients, most of whom had osteoarthritis (89).

COX-2 inhibitors were shown to increase blood pressure in the VIGOR trial. In this trial, more patients in the rofecoxib group developed hypertension than those in the naproxen group. The mean increase in systolic and diastolic blood pressure in the VIGOR trial with rofecoxib was 4.6 and 1.7 mm Hg, respectively, compared with 1.0- and 0.1-mm Hg increases in systolic and diastolic blood pressure, respectively, with naproxen. The elevation in blood pressure reported with use of COX-2 inhibitors may be potentially important in adverse cardiovascular outcomes (90).

A 2001 review found an increased relative risk (RR) for cardiovascular events with rofecoxib versus naproxen (RR=2.4; 95% confidence interval [CI]=1.39 to 4.0) (91). There was no difference in rates among the groups receiving celecoxib, ibuprofen, and diclofenac. Another review of data from rofecoxib studies included more than 28,000 patients and more than 14,000 patient-years of treatment. There was no increased risk of cardiovascular events or sudden deaths with rofecoxib compared to placebo (RR=0.84; 95% CI=0.51 to 1.38) (92). However, the risk of events was higher in rofecoxib- than naproxen-treated patients (RR=1.69; 95% CI=1.07 to 2.69). The latter two reviews suggest that the difference in cardiovascular risk may have been due to a protective effect of naproxen (93) rather than a deleterious effect of rofecoxib, although this has not been convincingly demonstrated.

A recent retrospective cohort study compared the rates of myocardial infarction and deaths due to coronary artery disease in 3,887 patients on high-dose rofecoxib (greater than 25 mg per day), 20,245 patients on lower-dose rofecoxib, 22,337 patients on celecoxib, 70,384 patients on naproxen, 59,007 patients on ibuprofen, and 202,916 patients not on an NSAID or a COX-2 inhibitor over a 2.5-year period (94). There was a trend toward increased risk for patients on high-dose rofecoxib compared to those who were not (RR=1.7; 95% CI=0.98 to 2.95), who had the same risk as those who used ibuprofen, naproxen, celecoxib, and lower-dose rofecoxib (less than or equal to 25 mg per day). The confidence in these findings is limited, however, because the increase in risk with high-dose rofecoxib was based on a small number of events.

POTENTIAL METHODS OF PLAQUE STABILIZATION

Statins and Fibrates

Statins can alter plaque composition and stabilize plaque. This may be achieved by reducing the inflammatory response in the plaque. CRP levels have been shown to be lowered by statin therapy (95). This pleiotropic antiinflammatory effect of statins may sometimes be sufficient to stabilize vulnerable lesions without the need to resort to intervention (96).

Fibrates have also been shown to have a pleiotropic anti-inflammatory effect mediated by the binding to the nuclear receptor peroxisome proliferator-activated receptor-α (PPAR-α) (97,98). Fibric acids (i.e., fenofibrate) activate PPAR-α, which in turn inhibits the tumor necrosis factor-α (TNF-α)-induced inflammation. This also reduces the expression of the cell adhesion molecule VACM-1 as well as tissue factor and T-cell activation (99,100). In addition, the thioglitizones bind the PPAR-α, which then inhibits macrophages (101). Although these are very impressive pharmacologic methods for stabilizing plaque by controlling inflammation, further work is pending to demonstrate the extent of clinical effectiveness of these approaches.

Effect of Hormone Replacement Therapy

Another important issue is whether hormone replacement therapy is a protective or a risk factor for cardiovascular events. Basic data have shown that estrogens weaken the atherosclerotic cap by enhancing metalloproteinase activity, which may lead to plaque rupture and thrombosis (31). In addition, estrogens are prothrombotic and enhance deep venous thrombosis and pulmonary embolism (102–104). In studies that used estrogens in male patients with prostate cancer, there was a significant increase in acute cardiovascular events, especially in patients with known coronary artery disease (105, 106). On the other hand, estrogens can have a beneficial effect by lowering the low-density lipoprotein moiety of cholesterol (107). In addition, they have been shown to improve arterial wall compliance in the carotid arteries and to improve vasodilation response in postmenopausal women (108–110). Conjugated estrogen, alone or combined with progestin therapy, reduces plasminogen activator inhibitor-1 (PAI-1) levels by about 50% in postmenopausal women (111). This is associated with enhanced systemic fibrinolysis. Thus, by lowering PAI-1, which acts to reduce thrombus breakdown, estrogens may reduce cardiovascular events. Taken orally, they increase the level of triglycerides and enhance inflammation as evidenced by increased CRP levels (106–113). However, whereas oral use of estrogen increases the CRP levels, transdermal use does not (114). These various effects need to be sorted out to determine which female patients would benefit the most from such interventions (see Chapter 12). The appropriate dose, type, and combination of hormones and the method of delivery need to be found in order to deliver the most benefit in conferring cardiovascular protection.

Role of Angiotensin-Converting Enzyme Inhibitors

Another potential means of plaque stabilization is angiotensin-converting enzyme (ACE) inhibition. There is clinical data to support this concept from the Heart Outcomes Prevention Evaluation trial, where myocardial infarction and death from cardiovascular causes were significantly reduced (115). Various mechanisms of this benefit have been hypothesized. One may be related to inhibition of the build-up of angiotensin II, which is an activator of PAI-1, thus enhancing thrombolysis (116). Another mechanism in plaque stabilization may involve the effect of ACE inhibition protein synthesis, which may alter plaque composition (117).

Models to for Evaluating Vulnerable Plaque

One way to elucidate the effect of inflammation is to use animal models of atherosclerosis. An atherosclerotic rabbit model developed by Constantinides and Chevarty (118) and modified by Abela et al. (119) provides a way to address some of these issues (Fig. 2.12). Bustos et al. demonstrated that hydroxy-methylglutamyl coenzyme A (HMG-CoA) reductase inhibitors can reduce neointimal inflammation in the atherosclerotic rabbit model (33). This was illustrated by reduction in macrophage infiltration as well as reduction in chemoattractant protein-1 (MCP-1) with atorvastatin. In addition, in vascular smooth muscle cells in culture, atorvastatin reduced MCP-1, and activity of nuclear factor-κB and TNF-α was downregulated. Other models of plaque rupture include the hypercholesterolemic double knockout (Apo E, LDLr) mouse that is fat feed and stressed. Also, the Dahl Salt-sensitive hypertensive rats transgenic for human cholesterol ester transfer protein has been proposed (119a).

GENETIC BASIS OF ATHEROSCLEROSIS

There has been considerable interest in recent years in the genetic basis of atherosclerosis. Clinicians regard family history of coronary artery disease as an important risk factor for vascular events. In view of the new genetic insight into this disease as a result of the Human Genome Project, there has been some excitement about the possibility of finding a gene that may be either responsible for or contributory to the pathogenesis of atherosclerosis. However, finding one particular gene or a group of genes linked directly to atherosclerosis has been elusive.

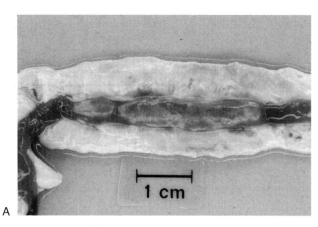

A

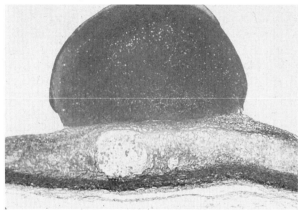

B

FIG. 2.12. (See Color Fig. 2.12.) Gross and histologic images of platelet-rich thrombi from an atherosclerotic model of plaque disruption and thrombosis. **A:** Large, white, platelet-rich thrombus with red thrombus attached on either side in the midthoracic aorta of an atherosclerotic rabbit triggered with Russell viper venom and histamine. **B:** Light micrograph of a thrombus attached to the thoracic aorta (Masson's trichrome, magnification 16 X). A cavity is noted below the thrombus, and the intimal surface is markedly thinned. (From Abela GS, Picon PD, Friedl SE, et al. Triggering of plaque disruption and arterial thrombosis in an atherosclerotic rabbit model. *Circulation* 1995;91:776–784, with permission.)

Risk Factors

Atherosclerosis has been regarded to be of multifactorial origin, with hypertension and diabetes mellitus being the most important risk factors (120). Both of these diseases have a strong hereditary component. Some of the inherited dyslipidemia syndromes are primary disorders of lipoprotein metabolism and include familial chylomicronemia, familial dysbetalipoproteinemia, familial combined hyperlipidemia, familial hypertriglyceridemia, familial hepatic lipase deficiency, familial hypercholesteremia, and familial defective apolipoprotein B-100 (121–124). Some of these disorders have been proven to be due to a single abnormal gene, whereas others are polygenic, and the basis for yet others is unknown.

Classical homozygous homocystinuria is associated with low or absent activity of cystathionine beta-synthase and leads to extremely high serum concentration of homocysteine. Disorders of remethylation involving vitamin B12 and methylenetetrahydrofolate reductase (MTHFR) can cause hyperhomocysteinemia (125). Apoprotein(a) and PAI-1 in addition to homocysteine are implicated in the possible inherited disorders that may play a role in the onset and progression of atherosclerosis.

Clinical Studies

The Atherosclerosis, Thrombosis, and Vascular Biology Italian Study provides no supporting evidence of an association between nine genetic polymorphisms encoding proteins involved in hemostasis and the occurrence of premature myocardial infarction or protection from it (126). These polymorphisms included genes for β-fibrinogen, factor V, prothrombin, factor VII, platelet glycoproteins Ia and IIIa, factor XIII, PAI-1, and MTHFR (126).

However, a positive parental history of stroke was associated with increased common and internal carotid artery intima–media thickness (IMT), and a positive parental history of myocardial infarction was associated with increased common carotid artery IMT. IMT is found to have a significant familial component that is independent of conventional risk factors (127).

Polymorphism Associations

With the use of refined molecular biology techniques and modern software assistance, several single-nucleotide polymorphisms (SNPs) have been isolated. SNPs are common but minute variations that occur in human DNA at a frequency of 1 every 1,000 bases. These variations can be used to track inheritance in families. The most notable of these is a variant allele of apolipoprotein E, which confers some additional risk independent of lipid levels. Others include polymorphisms of cholesteryl ester transfer protein and hepatic lipase. Newer promising polymorphisms are those of ATP-binding cassette transporter A1 (ABCA1), ABCC6, and peroxisome proliferator-activated receptor-alpha (128).

Recent evidence points to a significant association between severe vascular disease and the T786C polymorphism located in the promoter region of the endothelial nitric oxide synthase (eNOS) gene (129). The T786C promoter polymorphism decreases the transcription of this gene, and the G894T polymorphism in the same gene enhances the susceptibility of the gene to proteolytic cleavage. These functions lead to a relative nitric oxide deficiency and promote endothelial dysfunction (130). The T786C polymorphism reduces the forearm blood flow response to acetylcholine in white hypertensive patients (131). In patients with coronary and vascular disease, other risk factors such as smoking, obesity, hypercholesteremia, and older age were additive to the effect of the T786C polymorphism in predicting the prevalence of atherothrombotic disease (130). Current knowledge supports the concept that multiple genes determine the genetic component of atherosclerosis risk, with each one responsible for a limited portion of variability. Obviously, the influence of genetic factors is modified by various environmental risk factors.

As more and more suspect gene loci are added to the pool of possible culprits, and as newer and faster techniques decipher the functions of these genes, the explosion of this knowledge will help us to fathom better the profoundness and vastness of the human genome. The future promises to see a new era in which we may be able to localize genes responsible for the development of atherosclerosis and identify susceptible individuals earlier. This genetic research will spill over into the field of therapeutics and may provide a genetic solution for the difficult problem of systemic atherosclerosis.

APPROACHES FOR DETECTION OF VULNERABLE LESIONS

Various approaches are being investigated for detecting the presence of vulnerable plaque as the potential site of future cardiovascular events (Table 2.2). Most of these are invasive and part of interventional procedures.

Thermal Dispersion

Thermal dispersion has received much attention because it relies on the elevated local temperature induced by an active inflammation. Temperature elevation has been associated with increased inflammatory cell infiltration in human carotid arteries (132). However, this study was done *in vitro* after removal of the plaques from the carotid arteries during endarterectomy. There was a significant temperature dispersion in areas with dense macrophage cell accumulation. During coronary revascularization procedures in humans, Stefanadis et al. demonstrated increased local temperature at culprit lesions in coronary arteries of patients with unstable angina and myocardial infarction as compared to patients with stable angina and normal arteries (133). However, this method is limited by the huge thermal sink generated by flowing blood. This makes it technically difficult to detect very small temperature differences in the range of 0.1°C often needed for evaluation of thermal dispersion.

Intravascular Ultrasound

Another frequently used technique is intravascular ultrasound (IVUS). This technique is readily applicable, and can provide a cross-sectional view of the arterial wall and plaque (134–136). A potential limitation relates to the resolution by IVUS

TABLE 2.2. *Systems for detection of vulnerable plaque*

Invasive techniques
  Thermal detection
  Infrared detection
  Intravascular ultrasound
  Elastography
  Optical coherence tomography
  Angioscopy/colorimetry
Noninvasive techniques
  Magnetic resonance angiography
  Computerized tomography scanning

at 30 MHz of plaque caps that are 100 μm in size or smaller. Postmortem studies of plaque in patients who had plaque rupture in the coronary circulation often showed caps that were 75 μm thick (137). However, recent studies using IVUS in the femoropopliteal arteries of patients with claudication have demonstrated impressive evidence of plaque rupture and remodeling (16) (Fig. 2.4).

Angioscopy

Angioscopy in patients with cardiovascular events demonstrated that the majority of plaques with thrombosis are yellow (138) (Fig. 2.3). *In vitro* studies confirmed that the yellow saturation of plaques is due to a thin fibrous cap. This allows the lipid core, which is yellow, to reflect the yellow to the intimal surface of the artery (139). Postmortem studies of patients who had died of a coronary event showed yellow caps that were considerably thinner at the site of plaque rupture (140). Another advantage of angioscopy is that it can identify other surface pathologies in the peripheral circulation, including the presence of valves in veins used for *in situ* bypass surgery. In addition, other pathology, including thrombus, intimal flaps, and webs, can be detected (13). The disadvantages of angioscopy are the prolongation of the interventional procedure and occlusion of the blood flow necessary for visualization.

Optical Coherence Tomography

Optical coherence tomography is another optical system that allows visualization below the intimal surface (141). It can provide a high degree of resolution and can detect vulnerable lesions. However, it is also an invasive procedure and requires the interruption of blood flow to obtain images.

Magnetic Resonance Angiography

Magnetic resonance angiography is a noninvasive method and has significant advantages in detecting lipid–water interfaces. This allows the evaluation of the lipid core of a plaque with a high degree of accuracy (142). Although the motion of the heart limits the usefulness of this technique for the coronary circulation, potentially it could be used effectively in the peripheral circulation.

Overall, the development of noninvasive techniques for identifying vulnerable plaques is a very promising way to risk-stratify individuals at increased risk for cardiovascular events. Various approaches are being evaluated for this purpose.

SUMMARY

Vulnerable plaques seem to impart a higher risk for future thrombosis at a focal arterial site. However, systemic inflammation that may be low grade and ongoing may predispose to the development of an acute cardiovascular event. Risk factors such as obesity, chronic infections, and oxidative stress can heighten systemic inflammation. CRP seems to be a good marker for this process. Other markers (IL-1, IL-6, TNF-α, VCAM-1) seem to be less well correlated with acute cardiovascular events. This raises the question of whether a critical mass of body lipid (i.e., total body plaque load) can generate enough inflammation to eventually reach a critical level, which then sets off a chain reaction that causes an acute vascular event.

REFERENCES

1. Fulton JF. *Selected readings in the history of physiology*. Springfield, IL: Charles C Thomas, 1966:25.
2. Ruffer MA. On arterial lesions found in Egyptian mummies (1580 B.C.–525 A.D.) *J Pathol Bacteriol* 1911;15:453–462.
3. Yusuf S, Ounpuu S, Anand S. The global epidemic of atherosclerotic cardiovascular disease. *Med Princ Pract* 2002;11[Suppl 2]:3–8.
4. Acierno LJ. *The history of cardiology*. London: Parthenon, 1994:114.
5. Abela, GS. Atherosclerosis as an inflamatory arterial disease: "Déjà vu"? *ACC Curr J R* 2003;12:23–25.
6. Rokitansky C. *A manual of pathological anatomy,* Vol 1, Swaine W, transl. London: Sydenham Society, 1854:97.
7. Virchow R. *Cellular pathology as based upon physiological and Pathologicalp histology,* Chance F, transl. London: John Churchill, London, 1860:360.
8. DeWood MA, Spores J, Notske R, et al. Prevalence of total coronary occlusion during the early hours of transmural myocardial infarction. *N Engl J Med* 1980;303:897–902.
9. Herrick JB. Clinical features of sudden obstruction of the coronary arteries. *JAMA* 1912;59:2015–2020.
10. Fuster V, Badimon L, Badimon JJ, et al. The pathogenesis of coronary artery disease and the acute coronary syndromes. *N Engl J Med* 1992;326:242–250.
11. Little WC, Constantinescu M, Applegate RJ, et al. Can coronary angiography predict the site of a subsequent myocardial infarction in patients with mild-to-moderate coronary artery disease? *Circulation* 1988;78:1157–1166.
12. Nobuyoshi M, Tanaka M, Nosaka H, et al. Progression of coronary atherosclerosis: is coronary spasm related to progression? *J Am Coll Cardiol* 1991;18:904–910.
13. Seeger JM, Abela GS. Angioscopy as an adjunct to arterial reconstructive surgery. *J Vasc Surg* 1986;4:315–320.
14. Sherman CT, Litvack F, Grundfest W, et al. Coronary angioscopy in patients with unstable angina pectoris. *N Engl J Med* 1986;315:913–919.
15. Hetzer NR. The natural history of peripheral vascular disease. Implications for its management. *Circulation* 1991;83[Suppl I]:I12–I19.
16. Hongo Y, Hassan A, Sudhir K, et al. Incidence and characteristics of ruptured plaque in femoro-popliteal arteries. *J Am Coll Cardiol* 2003;41[Suppl A]:303A.
17. Constantinides P. Plaque fissures in human coronary thrombosis. *J Atheroscler Res* 1966;6:1–17.
18. Davies MJ, Thomas AC. Plaque fissuring: the cause of acute myocardial infarction causing sudden ischaemic death, and crescendo angina. *Br Heart J* 1985;53:363–373.
19. Davies MJ, Richardson PD, Woolf N, et al. Risk of thrombosis in human atherosclerotic plaques: role of extracellular lipid, macrophage, and smooth muscle cell content. *Br Heart J* 1993;69:377–381.
20. Libby P. Molecular bases of the acute coronary syndromes. *Circulation* 1995;91:2844–2850.
21. Muller JE, Tofler GH, Stone PH. Circadian variation and triggers of onset of acute cardiovascular disease. *Circulation* 1989;79:733–743.
22. Mittleman MA, Maclure M, Tofler GH, et al. Triggering of actue myocardial infarction by heavy physical exertion: prevention of triggering by regular exertion. *N Engl J Med* 1993;329:1677–1683.
23. Loree HM, Kamm RD, Stringfellow RG, et al. Effects of fibrous cap thickness on peak circumferential stress in model atherosclertic vessels. *Circ Res* 1992;71:850–858.
24. Muller JE, Abela GS, Nesto RW, et al. Triggers, acute risk factors and vulnerable plaques: the lexicon of a new frontier. *J Am Coll Cardiol* 1994;23:809–813.
25. Kloner RA, Leor J, Poole WK, et al. Population-based analysis of the effect of the Northridge earthquake on cardiac death in Los Angeles County, California. *J Am Coll Cardiol* 1997;30:1174–1180.
26. Meisel SR, Kutz I, Dayan KI, et al. Effect of Iraqi missile war on incidence of acute myocardial infarction and sudden death in Israeli civilians. *Lancet* 1991;338:660–661.
27. Barger AC, Beeuwkes III R, Lainey LL, et al. Hypothesis: vasa vasorum and neovascularization of human coronary arteries: a possible role in the pathophysiology of atherosclerosis. *N Engl J Med* 1984;310:175–177.
28. Barger AC, Beeuwkes R III. Rupture of coronary vas vsorum as a trigger of acute myocardial infarction. *Am J Cardiol* 1990;66:41G–43G.
29. van der Wall A, Becker AE, van der Loos C, et al. Site of intimal rupture or erosion of thrombosed coronary atherosclerotic plaques is characterised by an inflammatory process irrespective of the dominant plaque morphology. *Circulation* 1994;89:36–44.
30. Virmani R, Burke AP, Farb A. Plaque rupture and plaque erosion. *Thromb Haemost* 1999;82[Suppl 1]:1–3.
31. Zanger D, Yang BK, Ardans J, et al. Divergent effects of hormone therapy on serum markers of inflammation in postmenopausal women with coronary artery disease on appropriate medical management. *J Am Coll Cardiol* 2000;36:1797–1802.
32. Investigators. Risks and benefits of estrogen plus progestin in healthy postmenopausal women: principal results from the Women's Health Initiative randomised controlled trial. *JAMA* 2002;288:321–333.
33. Bustos C, Hernandez-Presa MA, Ortego M, et al. HMG-CoA reductase inhibition by atorvastatin reduces neointimal inflammation in a rabbit model of atherosclerosis. *J Am Coll Cardiol* 1998;32:2057–2064.
34. Cybulsky MI, Gimbrone MA. Endothelial expression of a mononuclear leukocyte adhesion molecule during atherogenesis. *Science* 1991;251:788–791.
35. Ridker PM, Hennekens CH, Buring JE, et al. C-reactive protein and other markers of inflammation in the prediction of cardiovascular disease in women. *N Engl J Med* 2000;342:836–843.
36. Libby P, Ridker P. Novel inflammatory markers of coronary risk: theory versus practice. *Circulation* 1999;100:1148–1150.
37. Ablij HC, Meinders AE. C-reactive protein: history and revival. *Eur J Intern Med* 2002;13:412–422.
38. Ridker PM, Rifai N, Rose L, et al. Comparison of C-reactive protein and low-density lipoprotein cholesterol levels in the prediction of first cardiovascular events. *N Engl J Med* 2002;347:1557–1565.
39. Ridker PM, Stampfer MJ, Rifai N. Novel risk factors for systemic atherosclerosis: a comparison of C-reactive protein, fibrinogen, homocyteine, lipoprotein (a), and standard cholesterol screening as predictors of peripheral vascular disease. *JAMA* 2001;285:2481–2485.
40. Morrow DA, Rifai N, Antman EM, et al. C-reactive protein is a potent predictor of mortality independently of and in combination with troponin T in acute coronary syndromes: a TIMI 11A substudy. *J Am Coll Cardiol* 1998;31:1460–1465.
41. Ridker P, Cushman M, Stampfer MJ, et al. Inflammation, aspirin, and the risk of cardiovascular disease in apparently health men. *N Engl J Med* 1997;336:973–979.
42. Yudkin JS, Stehouwer CDA, Emeis JJ, et al. C-reactive protein in healthy subjects: Associations with obesity, insulin resistance, and endothelial dysfunction: potential role for cytokines originating from adipose tissue? *Atheroscler Thromb Vasc Biol* 1999;19:972–978.
43. Das I. Raised C-reactive protein levels in serum from smokers. *Clin Chim Acta* 1985;153:9–13.
44. McLaughlin T, Abbasi F, Lamendola C, et al. Differentiation between obesity and insulin resistance in the association with C-reactive protein. *Circulation* 2002;106:2908–2912.
45. Buffon A, Liuzzo G, Biasucci LM, et al. Preprocedural serum levels of C-reactive protein predict early complications and late restenosis after coronary angioplasty. *J Am Coll Cardiol* 1999;34:1512–1521.
46. Fujimori Y, Morio H, Terasawa K, et al. Multiple plaque ruptures in patients with acute myocardial infarction: an angioscopic evidence of systemic cause of plaque instability. *J Am Coll Cardiol* 2002;37:307A.
47. Rossi A, Franceschini L, Fusaro M, et al. Carotid atherosclerotic plaque instability in patients with acute myocardial infarction. *J Am Coll Cardiol* 2002;37:308A.
48. Salonen JT, Salonen R. Ultrasonographically assessed carotid morphology and the risk of coronary heart disease. *Atheroscler Thromb* 1991;5:1245–1249.
49. Goldstein JA, Demetriou D, Grines CL, et al. Multiple complex coronary plaques in patients with acute myocardial infarction. *N Engl J Med* 2000;343:915–922.
50. Buffon A, Biasucii LM, Liuzzo G, et al. Widespread coronary inflammation in unstable angina. *N Engl J Med* 2002;347:5–12.
51. Tribble DL, Holl LG, Wood PD, et al. Variations in oxidative

susceptibility among six low density lipoprotein subfractions of differing density and particle size. *Atherosclerosis* 1992;93:189–199.

52. Inoue T, Uchida T, Kamishirado H, et al. Clinical significance of antibody against oxidized low density lipoprotein in patients with atherosclerotic coronary artery disease. *J Am Coll Cardiol* 2001;37: 775–779.

53. Bui MN, Sack MN, Moutsatsos G, et al. Auto-antibody titers to oxidized LDL in patients with coronary atherosclerosis. *Am Heart J* 1996;131:663–667.

54. Monaco C, Crea F, Niccoli G, et al. Autoantibodies against oxidized low density lipoproteins in patients with stable angina, unstable angina or peripheral vascular disease; pathophysiological implications. *Eur Heart J* 2001;22:1572–1577.

55. Ridker PM, Cushman M, Stampfer MJ, et al. Plasma concentration of C-reactive protein and risk of developing peripheral vascular disease. *Circulation* 1998;97:425–428.

56. Heart Protection Study Collaborative Group MRC/BHF Heart Protection Study of antioxidant vitamin supplementation in 20536 high-risk individuals: a randomised placebo-controlled trial. *Lancet* 2002;360:23–33.

57. Capron L. *Chlamydia* in coronary plaques—hidden culprit or harmless hobo. *Nat Med* 1996;2:856–857.

58. Muhlestein JB, Hammond EH, Carlquist GF, et al. Increased incidence of *Chlamydia* species within the cornary arteries of patients with severe atherosclerosis versus other forms of cardiovascular disease. *J Am Coll Cardiol* 1996;27:1555–1561.

59. Adler SP, Hur JK, Wang JB, et al. Prior infection with cytomegalovirus is not a major risk factor for angiographically demonstrated coronary artery atherosclerosis. *J Infect Dis* 1998;177:209–212.

60. Blum A, Giladi M, Weinberg M, et al. High anti-cytomegalovirus (CMV) IgG antibody titer is associated with coronary artery disease and may predict postcoronary balloon angioplasty restenosis. *Am J Cardiol* 1998;81:866–868.

61. Ridker PM, Hennekens CH, Stampfer MJ, et al. Prospective study of herpes simplex virus, cytomegalovirus, and the risk of future myocardial infarction and stroke. *Circulation* 1998;98:2796–2799.

62. Sorlie PD, Nieto FJ, Adam E, et al. A prospective study of cytomegalovirus, herpes simplex virus 1, and coronary heart disease: the Atherosclerosis Risk in Communities (ARIC) study. *Arch Intern Med* 2000;160:2027–2032.

63. Zhu J, Nieto FJ, Horne BD, et al. Prospective study of pathogen burden and risk of myocardial infarction or death. *Circulation* 2001;103:45.

64. Rupprecht HJ, Blankenberg S, Bickel C, et al. Impact of viral and bacterial infectious burden on long-term prognosis in patients with coronary artery disease. *Circulation* 2001;104:25–31.

65. Adam E, Melnick JL, Probtsfield JL, et al. High level of cytomegalovirus antibody in patients requiring vascular surgery for atherosclerosis. *Lancet* 1987;2:291–293.

66. Nieto FJ, Adam E, Sorlie P, et al. Cohort study of cytomegalovirus infection as a risk factor for carotid intimal–medial thickening. A measure of subclinical atherosclerosis. *Circulation* 1996;94:922–927.

67. Muhlestein JB, Horne BD, Carlquist JF, et al. Cytomegalovirus seropositivity and C-reactive protein have independent and combined predictive value for mortality in patients with angiographically demonstrated coronary artery disease. *Circulation* 2000;102:1917–1923.

68. Blankenberg S, Rupprecht HJ, Bickel C, et al. Cytomegalovirus infection with interleukin-6 response predicts cardiac mortality in patients with coronary artery disease. *Circulation* 2001;103:2915–2921.

69. Zhou YF, Guetta E, Yu ZX, et al. Human cytomegalovirus increases modified low density lipoprotein uptake and scavenger receptor mRNA expression in vascular smooth muscle cells. *J Clin Invest* 1996;98:2129–2138.

70. Zhou YF, Shou M, Guetta E, et al. Cytomegalovirus infection of rats increases the neointimal response to vascular injury without consistent evidence of direct infection of the vascular wall. *Circulation* 1999;100:1569–1575.

71. Patel P, Mendall MA, Carrington D, et al. Association of *Helicobacter pylori* and *Chlamydia pneumoniae* infections with coronary heart disease and cardiovascular risk factors. *BMJ* 1995;311:711–714.

72. Gunn M, Stephens JC, Thompson JR, et al. Significant association of cagA positive *Helicobacter pylori* strains with risk of premature myocardial infarction. *Heart* 2000;84:267–271.

73. Danesh J, Peto R. Risk factors for coronary heart disease and infection with *Helicobacter pylori*: meta-analysis of 18 studies. *BMJ* 1998;316:1130–1132.

74. Prasad A, Zhu J, Halcox JP, et al. Predisposition to atherosclerosis by infections: role of endothelial dysfunction. *Circulation* 2002;106:184–190.

75. Anderson JL, Carlquist JF, Muhlestein JB, et al. Evaluation of C-reactive protein, an inflammatory marker, and infectious serology as risk factors for coronary artery disease and myocardial infarction. *J Am Coll Cardiol* 1998;32:35–41.

76. Mayr M, Kiechl S, Willeit J, et al. Infections, immunity, and atherosclerosis: associations of antibodies to *Chlamydia pneumoniae, Helicobacter pylori,* and cytomegalovirus with immune reactions to heat-shock protein 60 and carotid or femoral atherosclerosis. *Circulation* 2000;102:833–839.

77. Bloemenkamp DG, Mali WP, Tanis BC, et al. *Chlamydia pneumoniae, Helicobacter pylori* and cytomegalovirus infections and the risk of peripheral arterial disease in young women. *Atherosclerosis* 2002;163:149–156.

78. Hung HC, Willett W, Merchant A, et al. Oral health and peripheral arterial disease. *Circulation* 2003;107:1152–1157.

79. Bhagat K, Moss R, Colier J, et al. Endothelial "stunning" following a brief exposure to endotoxin: a mechanism to link infection and infarction? *Cardiovasc Res* 1996;32:822–829.

80. Lehr HA, Sagban TA, Ihling C, et al. Immunopathogenesis of atherosclerosis: endotoxin accelerates atherosclerosis in rabbits on hypercholesterolemic diet. *Circulation* 2001;104:914–920.

81. Wiedermann CJ, Kiechl S, Dunzendorfer S, et al. Association of endotoxemia with carotid atherosclerosis and cardiovascular disease. Prospective results from the Bruneck study. *J Am Coll Cardiol* 1999;34:1975–1981.

82. Xu Q, Schett G, Perschinka H, et al. Serum soluble heat shock protein 60 is elevated in subjects with atherosclerosis in a general population. *Circulation* 2000;102:14–20.

83. Zhu J, Quyyumi AA, Rott D, et al. Antibodies to human heat-shock protein 60 are associated with the presence and severity of coronary artery disease: evidence for an autoimmune component of atherogenesis. *Circulation* 2001;103:1071–1075.

84. Burian K, Kis Z, Virok D, et al. Independent and joint effects of antibodies to human heat-shock protein 60 and *Chlamydia pneumoniae* infection in the development of coronary atherosclerosis. *Circulation* 2001;103:1503–1508.

85. Pockley AG. Heat shock proteins, inflammation, and cardiovascular disease. *Circulation* 2002;105:1012–1017.

86. Caughey GE, Cleland LG, Penglis PS, et al. Roles of cyclooxygenase (COX)-1 and COX-2 in prostanoid production by human endothelial cells: selective upregulation of prostacyclin synthesis by COX-2. *J Immunol* 2001;167:2831–2838.

87. Cheng Y, Austin SC, Rocca B, et al. Role of prostacyclin in the cardiovascular response to thromboxane A2. *Science* 2002;296:539–541.

88. Bombardier C, Laine L, Reicin A, et al. Comparison of upper gastrointestinal toxicity of rofecoxib and naproxen in patients with rheumatoid arthritis. VIGOR Study Group. *N Engl J Med* 2000;343:1520–1528.

89. Silverstein FE, Faich G, Goldstein J, et al. Gastrointestinal toxicity with celecoxib vs nonsteroidal anti-inflammatory drugs for osteoarthritis and rheumatoid arthritis. The CLASS study: A randomized controlled trial. *JAMA* 2000;284:1247–1255.

90. Muscara MN, Vergnolle N, Lovren F, et al. Selective cyclo-oxygenase-2 inhibition with celecoxib elevates blood pressure and promotes leukocyte adherence. *Br J Pharmacol* 2000;129:1423–1430.

91. Mukherjee D, Nissen SE, Topol EJ. Risk of cardiovascular events associated with selective COX-2 inhibitors. *JAMA* 2001;286:954–959.

92. Konstam MA, Weir MR, Reicin A, et al. Cardiovascular thrombotic events in controlled, clinical trials of rofecoxib. *Circulation* 2001;104:2280–2288.

93. Van Hecken A, Schwartz JI, Depre M, et al. Comparative inhibitory activity of rofecoxib, meloxicam, diclofenac, ibuprofen, and naproxen on COX-2 versus COX-1 in healthy volunteers. *J Clin Pharmacol* 2000;40:1109–1120.

94. Ray W, Stein C, Daugherty J, et al. COX-2 selective non-steroidal anti-inflammatory drugs and risk of serious coronary heart disease. *Lancet* 2002;360:1071–1073.

95. Ridker PM, Rifai N, Pfeffer MA, et al. Long-term effects of pravastatin on plasma concentration of C-reactive protein. The Cholesterol and Recurrent Events (CARE) investigators. *Circulation* 2000;100:230–235.

96. Pitt B, Waters D, Brown WV, et al. Aggressive lipid-lowering therapy compared with angioplasty in stable coronary artery disease.

Atorvastatin versus Revascularization Treatment Investigators. *N Engl J Med* 1999;341:70–76.

97. Neve BP, Corseaux D, Chinetti G, et al. PPARα agonists inhibit tissue factor expression in human monocytes and macrophages. *Circulation* 2001;103:213–219.

98. Marx N, Mackman N, Schonbeck U, et al. PPARα activators inhibit tissue factor expression and activity in human monocytes. *Circulation* 2001;103:207–212.

99. Marx N, Sukhova G, Collins T, et al. PPARα activators inhibit cytokine-induced vascular cell adhesion molecule 1 expression in human endothelial cells. *Circulation* 1999;99:3125–3131.

100. Marx N, Kehrle B, Kohlhammer K, et al. PPAR activators as anti-inflammatory mediators in human T lymphocytes: implications for atheroslcreosis and transplantation-associated atheroslcerosis. *Circ Res* 2002;90:703–710.

101. Ricote M, Li AC, Willson TM, et al. The peroxisome proliferator–activator receptor-α is a negative regulator of macrophage activation. *Nature* 1998;391:82–86.

102. Daly E, Vessey MP, Hawkins MM, et al. Risk of venous thrombolism in users of hormone replacement therapy. *Lancet* 1996;348:977–980.

103. Grodstein F, Stampfer MJ, Goldhaber SZ, et al. Prospective study of exogenous hormones and risk of pulmonary embolism in women. *Lancet* 1996;348:983–987.

104. Rabbani LE, Seminario NA, Sciacca RR, et al. Oral conjugated equine estrogen increases plasma von Willebrand factor in postmenopausal women. *J Am Coll Cardiol* 2002;40:1991–1999.

105. Glashan RW, Robinson MR. Cardiovascular complications in the treatment of prostatic carcinoma. *Br J Urol* 1981;53:624–627.

106. Lundgren R, Sundin T, Colleen S, et al. Cardiovascular complications of estrogen therapy for non-disseminated prostatic carcinoma. A preliminary report from a randomised multicenter study. *Scand J Urol Nephrol* 1986;20:101–105.

107. Kuller LH, Women's Health Initiative. Hormone replacement therapy and risk of cardiovascular disease: implications of results of the Women's Health Initiative. *Atheriosler Thromb Vasc Biol* 2003;23: 11–16.

108. Bui MN, Arai AE, Hathaway L, et al. Effect of hormone replacement therapy on carotid arterial compliance in healthy postmenopausal women. *Am J Cardiol* 2002;90:82–85.

109. Virdis A, Ghiadoni L, Pinto S, et al. Mechanisms responsible for endothelial dysfunction associated with acute estrogen deprivation in normotensive women. *Circulation* 2000;101:2258–2263.

110. Pinto S, Virdis A, Ghiadoni L, et al. Endogenous estrogen and actelycholine-induced vasodilatation in normotensive women. *Hypertension* 1997;29:268–273.

111. Koh KK, Mincemoyer R, Bui MN, et al. Effects of hormone-relacement therapy on fibrinolysis in postmenopausal women. *N Engl J Med* 1997;336:683–690.

112. Ridker PM, Hennekens CH, Rifai N, et al. Hormone replacement therapy and increased plasma concentration of C-reactive protein. *Circulation* 1999;100:713–716.

113. Cushman M, Legault C, Barrett-Connon E, et al. Effect of postmenopausal hormones on inflammation-sensitive proteins: the Postmenopausal Estrogen/Progestin Interventions (PEPI) Study. *Circulation* 1999;100:717–722.

114. Giltay EJ, Gooren LJ, Emeis JJ, et al. Oral ethinyl estradiol, but not transdermal 17 beta-estradiol, increases plasma C-reactive protein levels in men. *Thromb Haemost* 2000;84:359–360.

115. Yusuf S, Sleight P, Pogue J, et al. Effects of an angiotensin-converting-enzyme inhibitor, ramipril, on cardiovascular events in high-risk patients. The Heart Outcomes Prevention Evaluation Study investigators. *N Engl J Med* 2000;342:145–153.

116. Felmeden DC, Lip GY. The renin–angiotensin aldosterone system and fibrinolysis. *J Renin Angiotensin Aldosterone Syst* 2000;1:240–244.

117. Lonn EM, Yusuf S, Jha P, et al. Emerging role of angiotensin-converting enzyme inhibitors in cardiac and vascular protection. *Circulation* 1994;90:2056–2069.

118. Constantinides P, Chakravarti RN. Rabbit arterial thrombosis production by systemic procedures. *Arch Pathol* 1961;72:197–208.

119. Abela GS, Picon PD, Friedl SE, et al. Triggering of plaque disruption and arterial thrombosis in an atherosclerotic rabbit model. *Circulation* 1995;91:776–784.

119a. Lowe HC, Jang I-K, Khachigian LM. Animal models of vulnerable plaque: clinical context and current status. *Thromb Haemost* 2003;90: 774–780.

120. D'Agostino RB, Russel MW, Huse DM, et al. Primary and subsequent coronary risk appraisal: New results from the Framingham study. *Am Heart J* 2000;139:272–281.

121. Davignon J, Gregg RE, Sing CF. Apolipoprotein E polymorphism and atherosclerosis. *Arteriosclerosis* 1988;8:1–21.

122. Goldstein JL, Hobbs HH, Brown MS. Familial Hypercholesterolemia. In *The Metabolic and Molecular Basis of Inherited Disease* (vol. II; 7th edition). eds. Scriver CR, Beaudet AL, Sly WS, Valle D. New York: McGraw-Hill, 1995:1981–2030.

123. Kwiterovich Jr PO. Genetics and molecular biology of familial combined hyperlipidemia. *Curr Opin Lipidol* 1993;4:133–143.

124. Innerarity TL, Mahley RW, Weisgraber KH, et al. Familial defective apolipoprotein B-100: a mutation of apolipoprotein B that causes hypercholesteremia. *J Lipid Res* 1990;31:1331–1349.

125. Rader DJ. Lipid disorders. In *Textbook of cardiovascular medicine*, 2nd ed. Topol EJ, Prystowsky EN, Califf RM, et al., eds. Philadelphia: Lippincott Williams & Wilkins, 2002:43–73.

126. Atherosclerosis, Thrombosis, and Vascular Biology Italian Study Group. No evidence of association between prothrombotic gene polymorphisms and the development of acute myocardial infarction at a young age. *Circulation* 2003;107:1117–1122.

127. Jerrard-Dunne P, Markus HS, Steckel DA, et al. Early carotid atherosclerosis and family history of vascular disease. *Arterioscler Thromb Vasc Biol.* 2003;23:302–306.

128. Ordovas J. Cardiovascular disease genetics: a long and winding road. *Curr Opin Lipidol* 2003;14:47–54.

129. Rossi GP, Cesari M, Zanchetta M, et al. The T786C endothelial nitric oxide synthase genotype is a novel risk factor for coronary artery disease in Caucasian patients of the GENICA study. *J Am Coll Cardiol* 2003;41:930–937.

130. Loscalzo J, Functional polymorphisms in a candidate gene for atherothrombosis. *J Am Coll Cardiol* 2003;41:946–948.

131. Rossi GP, Taddei S, Virdis A, et al. The T786C and Glu298Asp polymorphisms of the endothelial nitric oxide gene affect the forearm blood flow responses of Caucasian hypertensive patients. *J Am Coll Cardiol* 2003;41:938–945.

132. Casscells W, Hathorn B, David M, et al. Thermal detection of cellular infiltrates in living atherosclerotic plaques: possible implications for plaque rupture and thrombosis. *Lancet* 1996;347:1447–1451.

133. Stefanadis C, Diamantopoulos L, Vlachopoulos C, et al. Thermal heterogeneity within human atherosclerotic coronary arteries detected *in vivo:* a new method of detection by application of a special thermographic catheter. *Circulation* 1999;99:1965–1971.

134. Hodgson M, Reddy KG, Suneya R, et al. Intracoronary ultrasound imaging: correlation of plaque morphology with angiography, clinical syndrome and procedural results in patients undergoing coronary angioplasty. *J Am Coll Cardiol* 1993;21:35–44.

135. Mecley M, Rosenfield K, Kaufman J, et al. Atherosclerotic plaque hemorrhage and rupture associated with crescendo caludication. *Ann Intern Med* 1992;117:663–666.

136. Yamagishi M, Terashima M, Awano K, et al. Morphology of vulnerable coronary plaque: insights from follow-up of patients examined by intravascular ultrasound before an acute coronary syndrome. *J Am Coll Cardiol* 2000;35:106–111.

137. Burke A, Farb A, Malcom GT, et al. Coronary risk factors and plaque morphology in men with coronary disease who died suddenly. *N Engl J Med* 1997;336:1276–1282.

138. Mizuno K, Miyamoto A, Satomura K. Angioscopic coronary macro-morphology in patients with acute coronary disorders. *Lancet* 1991; 337:809–812.

139. Miyamoto A, Prieto AR, Friedl SE, et al. Atheromatous plaque cap thickness can be determined by quantitative color analysis during angioscopy: implications for identifying the vulnerable plaque. *Clin Cardiol* 2004;27:9–15.

140. Uchida Y, Nakamura F, Tomaru T, et al. Prediction of acute coronary syndromes by percutaneous coronary angioscopy in patients with stable angina. *Am Heart J* 1995;130:195–203.

141. Jang IK, Bouma BE, Kang DH, et al. Visualization of coronary atherosclerotic plaques in patients using optical coherence tomography: comparison with intravascular ultrasound. *J Am Coll Cardiol* 2002;39:604–609.

142. Toussaint JF, Southern JF, Fuster V, et al. Water diffusion properties of human atherosclerosis and thrombosis measured by pulse field gradient nuclear magnetic resonance. *Arterioscler Thromb Vasc Biol* 1997;17:542–546.

CHAPTER 3

Peripheral Vascular Assessment

History Taking and Physical Examination of the Arterial and Venous Systems

Gary J. Arnold

Key Points

- Astute clinicians performing a complete history and physical exam can accurately diagnose peripheral vascular disease without extensive testing modalities.
- Patients today have a more sophisticated knowledge base, requiring clinicians to form a partnership with them.
- Many symptoms are well known to be associated with vascular diseases, but none is individually diagnostic.
- Symptoms of vascular disease may include dyspnea, chest pain, weakness, fatigue, edema, syncope, extremity pain, cough, hoarseness, hemoptysis, and neurological manifestations.
- Palpation is an important tool for assessing cardiovascular hemodynamics and static vascular conditions.
- The main aspects of evaluation include physical examination, palpation, and auscultation.

Today's clinician is armed with an impressive arsenal of technologically advanced instrumentation to help in reaching diagnostically sophisticated conclusions with regard to peripheral vascular diseases. The advances in ultrasonic, radiological, and nuclear technology during the last three decades are and will remain essential components of the total assessment of patients with peripheral arterial and peripheral venous diseases. The impressive graphics that result from these technologies provide the clinician with images of static as well as dynamic pathophysiologic processes that often lead to amazing precision in diagnosis, therapeutic planning, and gratification in outcomes.

As a result of these benefits of technology, however, there has been an increasing reliance by clinicians on the use of these methods to arrive at vascular diagnoses and a gradual abandonment of basic history taking and physical examina-

tion as assessment mechanisms. Proponents of the expanded use of technology are quick to point out the increased accuracy of tests over physical examination. Although this is often true, this comparison is somewhat of a self-fulfilling prophecy in that the temptation to rush to technology has lured the clinician into becoming less accurate in the techniques of interviewing and physical assessment. The astute clinician, however, knows that, especially with regard to vascular diseases, attentive interrogation during history taking and care and precision in physical examination techniques can be very accurate, even when used as the only means of patient evaluation. It is only by becoming better at interviewing and examining patients with vascular diseases that a clinician can optimize the use of available technologies, improving their selectivity and specificity, reducing their risks and costs, and enhancing their contribution to patient care.

TABLE 3.1. *Analysis of a vascular symptom*[a]

Location	The anatomic region where the symptom is noted to have the greatest intensity and also the anatomic regions to which the symptom radiates or other areas where the symptom is noted but at lower intensity
Quality	A description of the sensations experienced as a result of the symptom; may include a variety of adjectival descriptors and comparisons to nonmedical events
Quantity (or severity)	A description of the intensity of the symptom and any variations in intensity (progression or diminution) over time
Timing	A documentation of the temporal sequencing of the symptom including date and time of its onset, its duration, and, if intermittent, its frequency
Setting	A description of the environment or the circumstances in which the symptoms are usually noted; may include geographic physical locations, occupational or domestic situations, interpersonal relationships, or unique psychological or emotional states
Aggravating factors	A documentation of any physical activities, body positions, ambient temperature conditions, dietary factors, or medications that typically initiate or intensify the symptom
Alleviating factors	A documentation of any physical activity (or cessation of activity), change in body position, change in emotional state, or medication that typically eliminates or diminishes the intensity of the symptom
Associated manifestations	A documentation of any other symptoms, vascular or nonvascular, that seem to have a temporal relationship with the index symptom
Degree of disability	A description of how the symptom has affected the patient physically, socially, psychologically, emotionally, and financially

[a]For each vascular symptom elicited during the history, the additional details that must be discovered to establish the extent and urgency of the problem and to place the patient into a clinical disease pattern can be revealed by further inquiry. As each symptom is revealed, it is regarded as an index symptom, which is further analyzed by the characteristics listed here.

HISTORY TAKING

All clinicians, from novice to expert, understand the importance of history taking as a data-gathering mechanism and are well versed in the components of a complete history. What is often overlooked is the opportunity for the interview to be the basis for an honest and effective partnership in therapeutic decision making. Patients today are very knowledgeable about many of the aspects of vascular diseases and are well aware of their potentially disastrous outcomes. The communication process utilized in history taking requires special proficiency to establish a personal bond between clinician and patient and to create an environment of mutual trust that becomes crucial when discussing diseases and planning therapies that carry such risks as disability, dismemberment, and even death. History taking, typically the first occasion for interaction between clinician and patient, is an ideal opportunity for the clinician to practice the art and the science of medicine.

For the clinician to develop a professional, trusting, and empathetic relationship with the patient while efficiently and scientifically eliciting important clues about the illness requires skill, understanding, and patience. Proficiency in the vascular interview requires a broad knowledge base in vascular pathophysiology, permitting the clinician to deduce symptoms in a smooth and logical manner, recognizing both the classic symptoms of peripheral vascular conditions as well as the many variants of symptom patterns common in these diseases. As information is revealed, the essential additional details that so accurately characterize vascular diagnoses can be discovered with careful symptom analysis (Table 3.1). The emerging picture implied by these symptom details, especially temporal and causal relationships, allows for effective clinical reasoning and organization of information into a coherent picture of presumed vascular pathophysiology as well as for prioritization of the urgency for therapeutic interventions. The clinician must always be aware of the hidden as well as the obvious concerns that a patient may have regarding his or her health and the psychological, sociological, and financial consequences of any potential disability. Mastery of the art and science of the vascular interview is achieved by adhering to the basic principles of medical history taking and applying them to the vascular patient (1–4).

The cardinal symptoms associated with peripheral arterial and peripheral venous diseases are few in number (Table 3.2) (3,5). Although it is clear that each of these symptoms is well known to be associated with many different vascular diseases, it should also be apparent that none of them is

TABLE 3.2. *Cardinal symptoms of peripheral vascular disease*[a]

Dyspnea
Chest pain or discomfort
Weakness or fatigue
Peripheral edema
Syncope
Extremity pain or discomfort
Cough, hoarsness, or hemoptysis
Neurological manifestations

[a]Although there are many variations in the manner in which patients express symptoms, the majority of peripheral vascular complaints fall into relatively few major symptom categories.

individually diagnostic of any single disease. By definition, peripheral arterial diseases include those of the ascending aorta, the aortic arch and its branches, the descending aorta and its branches, and all muscular arteries. Peripheral venous diseases include conditions affecting all major venous channels in the neck, the trunk, and the extremities. Those pulmonary vascular conditions not of cardiac origin are also considered to be peripheral vascular diseases. To become a skilled interviewer, each clinician needs to develop a personal style of history taking relative to these structures, which will be tailored to individual patients. All clinicians, however, must fully understand the multiple symptom patterns that can result from such a large group of diseases and the numerous and often subtle ways that patients have in expressing them.

Dyspnea is defined as an uncomfortable awareness of difficulty with breathing or a sensation of breathlessness. When caused by cardiovascular conditions, it is most often associated with cardiac decompensation with or without pulmonary edema, but can also be associated with some peripheral arterial and venous diseases (3,6). When dyspnea is associated with peripheral vascular diseases, it results from conditions causing pulmonary arterial hypertension, acute elevation of systemic arterial blood pressure, or vascular compression of the left main stem bronchus. On occasion, it is also associated with decreased cardiac output, rendering respiratory musculature ischemic. Dyspnea may also result from the increased physical effort required by many patients to compensate for the deconditioning that results from generalized chronic vascular disease.

When patients are aware of their dyspnea, they will express it as "shortness of breath" or "difficulty catching my breath." Because most cardiovascular diseases develop slowly, over several weeks, months, or years, many patients develop dyspnea slowly and can describe it only as decreased exercise tolerance, the inability to speak or sing without taking several breaths, the need for frequent rest periods, or being "out of shape." The astute clinician should recognize these subtle statements as possible characterizations of early dyspnea. As the vascular disease progresses, dyspnea becomes unmistakable and persistent and may be clearly worsened by physical exertion. Like cardiac dyspnea, the breathlessness of peripheral vascular disease is accompanied by cough, fatigue, and weakness. Unlike the dyspnea of heart failure, however, dyspnea of peripheral vascular origin is usually not worsened by recumbency (3).

Chest pain, as a symptom of peripheral vascular disease, is uncommon and results from relatively few conditions. Like myocardial ischemic pain, the noncardiac causes of chest pain are of vital diagnostic importance because of the ominous consequences attendant to their lack of recognition. Their diagnoses and differentiation from angina require extensive symptom analysis with careful attention to location, radiation, quality, quantity, timing, aggravating and alleviating factors, and associated symptoms. Chest pain that accompanies arterial and venous conditions is varied and is generally described in three different patterns (3). One pain pattern is associated with vascular conditions that are of relatively slow onset and progression, and it is described as vague, dull pain or discomfort located roughly in the center of the chest with no radiation to other areas. These pains tend to be gradual in onset, become persistent, and have no relationship to physical effort or body position. There are usually no associated symptoms other than occasional dyspnea. A second pattern of noncardiac chest pain is typically associated with acute arterial conditions and is sudden in onset, is severe and unrelenting in nature, and frequently migrates to involve different parts of the chest (7,8). This type of pain is commonly described by patients as "tearing" or "ripping" and reported to radiate to the neck, the jaw, the left shoulder, and the intrascapular area of the back. It is not associated with physical effort and is not relieved by rest or changes in body position. The third pattern is variable in severity and location, is usually sharp and sudden in onset, and frequently involves the peripheral parts of the chest. It is pleuritic in nature and is accompanied by severe dyspnea (9). This pattern is also unrelated to physical effort and body position. Patients presenting with any of these pain patterns will not report any aggravating or alleviating factors and will typically not describe any particular setting for the pain. Differentiation of these causes of chest pain may require correlation with the physical signs of these conditions or a battery of tests including electrocardiogram, chest x-ray, pulmonary function studies, pulmonary angiogram, lung scan, aortogram, computerized tomography, magnetic resonance imaging, and transesophageal echocardiogram.

Weakness and fatigue are the least specific of all the vascular symptoms, being common features of many nonvascular medical conditions and diagnoses. They are, however, prominent symptoms associated with vascular disease and are important to document and quantify because they correlate well with the extent of the disease and the degree of disability it produces (6,10). Weakness or easy fatigability as they relate to vascular disease can be either generalized as a constitutional symptom or localized to selected individual muscles or muscle groups. Localized muscle weakness may result from selected impairment of blood flow to the affected muscles or it may be the consequence of a neurological deficit resulting from occlusive or hypertensive cerebral vascular disease. It should be noted, however, that these two types of weaknesses could coexist in the same patient. The concept of generalized weakness might be expressed in numerous ways. Some patients may describe themselves as becoming easily fatigued, lacking the stamina to maintain physical activities requiring exertion. Others may express it as lack of energy or tiredness or heaviness in the limbs, generally indicating the inability to even begin any form of physical activity. The magnitude of the weakness becomes more intense as the vascular condition deteriorates, and the astute clinician will use directed questions in an attempt to quantify the extent and the progression of the weakness as a gauge of disease severity.

Generalized weakness is most often associated with diffuse vascular disease resulting in impaired perfusion of peripheral tissues. This, in turn, results in hypoxia and a generalized reduction in metabolic rates in all affected muscle groups. Most cases of generalized weakness are secondary to diffuse arterial occlusive diseases, but severe impairment of the venous circulation can have the same effect. Its relationship to physical exertion gives it a close association with dyspnea, also contributing to tissue hypoxia. Although less common, generalized muscle weakness can be secondary to the neurological impairment that accompanies deficient arterial blood flow to the vertebrobasilar arterial system of the brain.

Localized muscle weakness, on the other hand, can result from impaired blood flow to selected muscle groups as the result of isolated arterial disease, but is more likely the result of impaired blood flow to the carotid arterial system and ischemia to the motor cortex of the brain.

Edema, as an accumulation of interstitial fluid, is most often apparent to patients in their legs, but may also be noted in the upper extremities in selected venous conditions, where it is almost always noted unilaterally. Edema is most often described as "swelling in the legs" or as a "swollen" or "stiff" hand or arm. It should be remembered, however, that edema can represent either systemic dysfunction of the heart or abnormalities of the peripheral venous circulation. Less often, edema is a secondary manifestation of peripheral arterial disease and an ischemic extremity. In contrast to the edema of heart failure, which is generalized, includes the lung, and may be reflected as ascites and sacral edema, the edema associated with venous disease of the legs is usually relatively rapid in onset and limited to swelling in one or both lower extremities. Patients with severe arterial insufficiency of the lower extremities can also present with edema in one or both legs. While attempting to control their ischemic rest pain with minimal exercise and voluntary foot dependency at night, they create inadequate venous return from the dependent parts. Although there are numerous noncardiovascular causes for edema, both generalized and localized, symptom analysis for their etiologies is beyond the scope of this chapter.

The phrase "swelling of the legs" can be a common description in a patient's narrative, but a patient might express dependent edema in the legs in a number of other subtle ways. Descriptions of periodic tiredness or aching in the legs, especially at the end of the day or after standing up for long periods, can be indicative of edema. Patients might complain about their shoes fitting too tightly or choose only to wear loose-fitting footwear or no shoes at all. In the upper extremities, patients may be aware only of rings or wrist watches fitting too tightly, the inability to button a shirt sleeve, or loss of fine motor control of the hand.

An important clue to the nature of edema can be obtained by an analysis of the alleviating factors noted by the patient. In dependent edema due to peripheral venous disease or early heart failure, patients seek relief with leg elevation or recumbency. In severe heart failure, however, patients may avoid recumbency because lying supine may worsen the symptom of

dyspnea due to redistribution of fluid from the lower extremities into the pulmonary circulation. This redistribution of fluid will relieve dependent edema, but can initiate or worsen pulmonary edema. Whereas patients with lower extremity edema from venous disease seek relief by leg elevation, patients with ischemic rest pain secondary to arterial insufficiency avoid leg elevation and active movement of the legs and feet because these would further compromise arterial blood flow to the feet. This self-imposed dependency of the lower extremities in arterial insufficiency results in edema that is not associated with cardiac decompensation or peripheral venous disease.

Syncope, or transient and complete loss of consciousness, has multiple noncardiovascular etiologies, but is a prominent and often ominous symptom that has several cardiovascular implications (3). Syncope, or its less complete variants presyncope, lightheadedness, and dizziness, can be a manifestation of relatively benign vasovagal reflexive responses (or vasomotor syncope), a symptom reflecting cerebrovascular arterial insufficiency, or an indication of serious cardiac dysfunction (cardiogenic syncope). Whether reported by patients as dizziness, lightheadedness, or fainting, it is important for the clinician to do careful symptom analysis to distinguish these different forms of vascular-related losses of consciousness. It is also important to differentiate them from such nonvascular causes of syncope as epilepsy, reflex (or cough) syncope, or hypoglycemia. Most important in the symptom analysis are details relating to the setting, duration, aggravating factors, and associated symptoms. In addition, eyewitness accounts to the event from family and friends may provide additional details that are not available from the patient.

Vasomotor syncope, although associated with vascular events such as bradycardia and peripheral vasodilatation, is not truly a cardiac event and is not related to heart or vascular disease. Patients can accurately describe it as being sudden in onset, predictable, and recurrent. The narrative very clearly identifies the events as typically precipitated by visually shocking sights (i.e., the sight of blood), pain, threats, anxiety, fasting, deconditioning, fatigue, or warm environments. These events are short in duration and commonly are limited to presyncope, frequently not progressing to complete loss of consciousness.

Syncope associated with cerebrovascular disease is typically part of a larger pattern of neurologic manifestations of compromised cerebral blood flow. It is caused by abrupt cessation of arterial blood flow to selected areas of the brain either from occlusive embolic or thrombotic events or from vasospasm associated with arterial hypertension. Syncope from cerebrovascular insufficiency is discussed later under neurologic manifestations.

Extremity pain, as a vascular symptom, can be the result of arterial insufficiency of the lower or upper extremities or increased venous pressure in the lower extremities secondary to venous diseases. Although the term *claudication* is frequently used as a cardinal symptom in peripheral arterial diseases in

TABLE 3.3. *Lower extremity pain symptom analysis[a]*

	Chronic arterial occlusion	Arterial rest pain	Venous insufficiency
Setting	Can occur in a variety of occupational and environmental settings; no relationship to psychological or emotional states	Occurs typically at bedtime, but common in any recumbency; psychological or emotional stressors may intensify the pain	Occurs typically in any setting requiring an upright position, especially standing still; no relationship to psychological or emotional states
Location	Typically in large muscle masses, especially the calves; may also occur in the thigh, hip, and buttocks	Commonly in the toes and forefoot, but may also involve the lower leg	Usually involves the feet and lower legs; rarely noted above the knee
Quality	Defined as claudication and typically described as cramping, aching, and heaviness and occasionally as pain	Usually described as stinging, burning, or stabbing	Commonly described as boring, tightness, and heaviness and occasionally as if the skin of the leg will break open
Quantity	Early claudication is described as mild, but intensity becomes moderately severe in significant occlusive disease	Typically described as severe, but there may be a past history of claudication of less intensity	Intensity varies from mild to severe depending on the degree and duration of venous insufficiency
Aggravating factors	Symptoms initiated and intensified by physical exercise, especially walking fast up an incline	Onset and severity of pain related to leg elevation, even if only to trunk level; cool ambient temperatures	Onset and severity of pain related to leg dependency, especially if standing idle
Alleviating factors	Slowing the pace of walking or, if severe, ceasing walking and resting	Placing feet in dependent position	Walking if insufficiency is minimal; leg elevation and wearing external support if condition is severe
Associated manifestations	Affected muscle weakness, fatigability, and atrophy; poor muscle control; loss of hair growth on extremity	Coldness, numbness, and paresthesias of the toes; cyanosis and ischemic ulcerations of the foot	Inability to find comfortable footwear because of swelling (edema); pruritis and scaly condition of skin

[a]Lower extremity pain or discomfort is a common peripheral vascular symptom, but may be caused by chronic arterial occlusive diseases or venous insufficiency. Careful symptom analysis of lower extremity pain will help to differentiate between these conditions.

the lower extremity, it does not adequately describe the pain of venous disease in the lower extremity and may not accurately express the discomfort noted in the upper extremity. In analyzing extremity pain, special note should be made as to its setting, location, quality, quantity, aggravating and alleviating factors, and associated manifestations (Table 3.3).

As the preeminent symptom of arterial insufficiency of the lower extremity, the term claudication is frequently incorrectly limited to use as a descriptor of pain (4,11). Experienced clinicians are alert to the more subtle expressions of claudication offered by patients in which the terms "cramping," "aching," "tiredness in the legs," and "leg heaviness" accurately identify this as a symptom of arterial insufficiency. The description offered by patients may be used to quantify the extent of the ischemia. Terms such as "tiredness" and "heaviness" typically represent minimal ischemic changes, whereas the words "pain" and "cramping" usually indicate more extensive impairment of arterial blood flow (8). Inquiry as to the setting and the aggravating factors of the pain will further clarify it as claudication. Claudication, by definition, is extremity pain initiated by muscular activity of the limb such as walking when it involves the lower extremity, and which is relieved by reducing or ceasing the physical

activity (11). The quantity of discomfort reported by patients is proportional to both the distance walked and the speed of walking, with patients describing prolonged or rapid walking or walking up an incline as most likely to produce the sensation. Early in the disease, simply slowing the pace of walking provides relief. When advanced, however, ischemic discomfort is only relieved by cessation of walking. This activity–symptom–rest response relationship defines the periodic and predictable nature of the discomfort, leading to the term intermittent claudication. Although much less common, vigorous physical exercise of the arms can provoke claudication in one or both arms in cases of impaired arterial flow to these sites.

Inquiry into the location of the claudication gives clues to the site of arterial compromise (12,13). Most commonly, patients describe claudication in the calf muscles because the most likely site of arterial occlusive disease is the femoral artery. It can also be limited to the feet, indicating partial arterial occlusion at or below the popliteal artery, or in the thighs and buttocks, indicating aortoiliac occlusion. Thigh and buttock claudication is more likely to be described as aching and may go unrecognized as claudication. In addition to the discomfort, patients may be aware of muscle weakness, especially of the muscles of the feet. Although patients may not normally have good control of the intrinsic muscles of the feet, if they are aware of a loss of ability to flare the toes, ischemic changes in the feet should be suspected. Loss of fine motor control of these muscles may be noted even before the claudication. This is especially true of the motor functions of the hand in upper extremity disease. In men with aortoiliac occlusive disease, impotence may be an associated manifestation in aortoiliac occlusion, and inquiry into this aspect of sexual functioning should be a part of the interview of all male cardiovascular patients (see Chapter 11).

Patients with severe arterial insufficiency of the lower extremities may also describe foot and leg pain that occurs at rest, especially at night when reclined (4,8,13). They frequently will provide a history of past claudication that had progressed, but will deny claudication now because of a self-imposed sedentary lifestyle. Most often involving the toes and the forefoot and nocturnal in timing, rest pain is classically described as "stinging," "burning," or "stabbing," and is clearly aggravated by elevation of the feet in bed. Patients note that relief is obtained only by placing the feet on the floor or by dangling them off the side of the bed (14). If rest pain develops gradually, patients may realize that they can only get restful sleep sitting up in a chair, not aware that this is because their feet are dependent in this position. Rest pain is not related to physical exercise of the lower extremity muscles and is commonly associated with coldness, numbness, or paresthesias of the toes.

In distinction to claudication and extremity rest pain, which are typically associated with chronic arterial disease, the pain of a sudden arterial occlusion is usually acute in onset, very severe and excruciating, and continuous, at least for a few hours. If the acute occlusion is unresolved, the initial pain period is followed by numbness as ischemic neuropathy ensues. There is no reported association with physical exertion and no relief with rest or positional changes.

Extremity pain resulting from venous diseases of the lower limbs is less readily identifiable than that associated with arterial disease (4). There are some recognizable patterns in the pain from venous diseases that can distinguish it from other causes. The discomfort secondary to venous disease is caused primarily by conditions of increased venous pressure secondary either to thrombotic obstruction of iliofemoral veins or to the influences of gravity in patent veins with incompetent valves. As such, the discomfort is frequently described as boring and continuous, deep inside the legs, as if they would "break open," but terms like "tightness" and "heaviness" are also used. Inquiry into the setting and the location are useful, with the discomfort being clearly present more when the legs are in a dependent position and to be more severe below the knees with gradual diminution from the lower thighs to the groin. Aggravating factors are commonly reported to be prolonged standing and walking, and even prolonged inactive sitting with the legs in a dependent position. Alleviating factors are readily recognized as rest, with the legs elevated, or the wearing of suitable external elastic compression of the affected legs in the form of support stockings. Other characteristics of venous extremity pain that can identify it as caused by insufficient venous blood flow include the associated manifestations of edema (or swelling), cutaneous evidence of venous stasis (as discussed later), or, in the absence of edema, distended and painful superficial veins.

Cough, hoarseness, and hemoptysis are more often than not associated with conditions originating in the respiratory system, but can be symptoms of vascular diseases, including some life-threatening conditions (13). Cough, as a vascular symptom, is typically described as dry or nonproductive and most often occurring at night (10). As with all vascular symptoms, the importance of cough is most recognizable by its associated manifestations, which include other symptoms of increased pulmonary arterial pressure or increased left atrial or left ventricular pressure. The most common associated manifestations reported by patients with a vascular cause for cough is the coughing up of blood, dyspnea, and chest pain. Lying adjacent to the trachea, the ascending aorta, if dilated, can exert pressure on the trachea or bronchi, triggering a cough reflex (7,8). In addition, any dilatation of the aortic arch can place a stretch on the recurrent laryngeal nerve as it loops under the aorta, which can result in a cough response or hoarseness.

Neurological manifestations reported during an interview are likely to be caused by some unrelated neurological disease, but careful effort should be made to investigate possible vascular explanations for them. Depending on the precise mechanism and the area of the central nervous system affected, patients may present with a variety of symptoms of neurological deficits that are secondary to focal ischemic injury in the brain (15,16). The majority of neurological symptoms (i.e., brain attack) derived from vascular diseases are caused by embolic occlusions of cerebral arteries originating from ulcerated plaques in the internal carotid or vertebral arteries or the proximal aorta, or from diseases affecting the left atrium or left ventricle. Less commonly, severe hypertension may be the explanation for the focal ischemic changes.

Whereas patients are usually the major historians for most of the other vascular symptoms, families or friends may provide more complete and accurate details of the neurological manifestations associated with vascular events because confusion and loss of consciousness may be prominent features. Symptom analysis should focus on location, timing (including duration), quality, quantity, and degree of disability. In analyzing the timing of neurological symptoms, clinicians should make special effort to differentiate transient ischemic attacks (TIAs) from the comparatively more severe stroke in evolution and completed stroke. This distinction is important because it will dictate the type and the urgency of any interventional therapy.

By definition, TIAs are obvious or subtle neurological deficits that occur suddenly and typically last less than 1 hour, although some authorities include durations of up to 24 hours as being "transient" (15–17). Included in this definition is the complete resolution of the deficits with no residual neurological symptoms. Patients or their families may describe several patterns of symptoms depending on the cerebrovascular system and the area of brain affected (15,16, 18,19). If the internal carotid artery system is the site of the transient embolic occlusion, the symptom of monocular blindness (amaurosis fugax) may be described as "suddenly losing vision in one eye" or the sensation of "a veil falling over one eye." In addition, the attack may include a description of hemiparesis as "weakness on one side or one arm or leg" or aphasia as evidenced by such comments as "couldn't speak" or "couldn't find the words," and paresthesias, frequently noted as "pins and needles or numbness" on the affected side. Occasionally dysarthria is reported as "slurred speech" or "speaking but couldn't understand what he or she was saying."

When the occlusive phenomenon involves the vertebrobasilar arterial system, the symptoms reported are somewhat different (15,16,18,19). Although hemiparesis, dysarthria, and paresthesias may also be reported, more likely expressions of ischemia affecting this arterial system include statements indicating confusion, dizziness, nausea, and vomiting. Another commonly reported symptom is ataxia or "walking like a drunk." Disturbances of vision are more likely to be bilateral and may include diplopia, described as "seeing double."

PHYSICAL EXAMINATION

As important as history taking is in establishing a basis for a presumptive vascular diagnosis, physical examination, when performed thoroughly and with attention to detail, will lead to remarkable accuracy in defining specific vascular disease processes and more appropriate application of technology and therapeutic interventions. As noted with regard to history taking, an analysis of the fine points in a patient's responses during the interview frequently allows conclusions that correlate closely with structural and functional alterations of the vascular system. So, too, does a peripheral vascular physical examination, carried out with care and thoughtfulness, ensure accuracy in the diagnosis and equivalence with the extent and the severity of associated pathophysiologic processes.

Although each clinician will develop an examination technique that is individual and personal, the method employed should utilize assessment skills in an efficient, effective, and decisive manner. Of the four basic examination techniques, inspection, palpation, and auscultation are directly applicable to vascular diagnoses. Efficiency and effectiveness are enhanced by appreciating the importance not only of the sequence in which the basic techniques are employed, but also the implications that each technique has for the others. When performed attentively, inspection, as the most appropriate initial technique, can reveal physical manifestations that become inferences for potential significant findings detectable later on palpation or auscultation. Similarly, discoveries made by palpation can alert the clinician to conditions in which auscultatory findings can be anticipated and that might otherwise

be overlooked. Although the setting and the objectives for the examination may require deviation from a planned examination approach, at least within each region of the body, optimal examination procedures should be maintained. The closer the adherence to the proper sequencing of inspection, palpation, and auscultation and the more deliberate the clinical reasoning employed during each stage, the more accurate and definitive will be the presumptive diagnoses at the conclusion of the examination.

Inspection

General Inspection

Astute clinicians begin inspection by making general observations during the interview (10,20). Even with the patient clothed, clues relating to vascular diseases can be noted. Inspection for the general state of nutrition might reveal evidence of recent weight loss or even inanition, often associated with severe generalized vascular diseases, or obesity with its well-known cardiac and vascular implications. A patient's general demeanor during the interview might reveal confusion, anxiety, depression, or despair, all common emotions associated with cardiovascular diagnoses. Observations of gait might reveal limping secondary to neurological deficits resulting from cerebrovascular ischemia or infarction. During the interview, taking note of the patient's general level of activity might reveal generalized weakness, fatigue, or effort intolerance as manifestations of many severe vascular conditions. Observing the patient's vocalizations might reveal abnormal voice characteristics including hoarseness associated with cigarette smoking and its obvious implications, or lack of vocal volume, breathlessness, cough, or the inability to speak in long phrases as characteristic of vascular conditions also associated with dyspnea.

With the patient partially disrobed, ideally in a room affording privacy and with an ambient temperature of 72°F (22°C), additional general observations should be made with reference to body habitus. Care should be taken not to overlook such body conformations as mesomorphism, often associated with atherosclerotic disease, or the genetically induced features of Marfan's or Turner's syndromes. Although variable in expression, the physical features of Marfan's syndrome, including tall stature, extended arm span, arachnodactyly, pectus deformities, and joint hyperextensibility, are easily recognizable on general inspection and should be correlated with possible aortic abnormalities and the potential for aortic dissection. In contrast, Turner's syndrome, identified in female patients by such structural features as short stature, neck webbing, wide chest, agenesis of the breasts, and metacarpal abnormalities, may be associated with aortic coarctation.

Head

Inspection of the head should seek evidence of *head bobbing* (de Mosset's sign), possibly indicating aortic regurgitation, but also a sign of markedly widened pulse pressures noted in systolic hypertension (10). Facial asymmetries caused by paresis or paralysis related to seventh cranial nerve deficits may be secondary to cerebrovascular disease, either TIA, stroke in evolution, or completed stroke.

Eyes

Both external and funduscopic examination of the eyes can reveal clues to cardiovascular diagnoses. External inspection should note the presence of *lid xanthelasmae,* inconsistently associated with atherosclerotic disease, *corneal arcus,* significant if present in patients under 40 years of age and possibly a manifestation of hyperlipidemia and atherosclerosis, *conjunctival hemorrhages and petechiae,* possibly indicative of bacterial endocarditis, and *blue sclera,* occasionally noted in Marfan's syndrome. Inspection of the lens might reveal *congenital cataracts,* frequently associated with patent ductus arteriosis, or *iridodonesis* (dislocation or subluxation of the lens), a common feature of Marfan's syndrome. The presence of *exophthalmia* may indicate thyrotoxicosis and its associated cardiovascular manifestations. Even noting a blank stare with infrequent blinking responses may provide clues to low-cardiac-output states such as shock and congestive heart failure.

Funduscopic examination is useful as a visualization of the arteriolar manifestations of hypertension and arteriosclerosis. Chronic or severe hypertension would be identified as a generalized attenuation of retinal arterioles or possibly localized arteriolar spasms, constrictions, or tortuosity. There may also be tapering of retinal venules, "cotton wool patches," and even papilledema in severe hypertension. Arteriosclerosis is associated with arteriovenous nicking or right-angle conformations at arteriovenous crossings. The clinician may also note an increase in the arteriolar light reflex and copper or silver wiring effects on the retinal arterioles in arteriosclerosis.

Mouth

Inspection of the mouth region, both externally and internally, can reveal clues to vascular diagnoses. Externally, *telangiectasias* on the lip are associated with pulmonary arteriovenous fistulas. Internally, there may be an indication of *nicotine staining* of the teeth, hard palate, and mucosa as clues to a significant tobacco history. An additional color variation of the tongue includes *pallor* as a manifestation of anemia and its associated vascular implications.

Neck

Inspection of the neck should include observations of both carotid arterial and jugular venous characteristics. Carotid arterial pulsations should be noted for intensity (or amplitude), rate, and cadence (21). The intensity of the arterial pulsations may be increased in hyperdynamic circulatory states. Decreased amplitude of the carotid arterial pulse may reflect low-cardiac-output states, occlusive disease of the aortic arch, carotid arterial occlusions, or hypotension. Variable intensities on alternate systoles may be recognizable as a manifestation of congestive heart failure or as a bigeminal arrhythmia. Timing characteristics of the pulsations, both rate and cadence, should be noted and might reveal abnormal electrical patterns that will be further defined by palpation and auscultation techniques and electrocardiographic testing.

Venous observations include assessments of venous filling in the upright, semi-Fowler, and supine positions and also notation of the pattern or waveforms of venous pulsations (10,20,22). More predictive of cardiac than peripheral vascular diseases, evaluation of the jugular veins is nonetheless part of the peripheral vascular examination. These observations are best made in the internal jugular vein on the right side of the neck. With the patient positioned in a supine position and with the neck slightly extended and rotated to the left, the examiner gradually raises the head of the examination table until he or she notes pulsations in the right internal jugular vein just above the medial end of the clavicle. In patients with normal central venous pressure, maximal visibility of venous pulsations typically occurs with the patient lying supine and with a 30- to 40-degree elevation of the trunk. An assessment of venous waveforms can be made by evaluating the amplitude of the "a" and "v" waves primarily and also of the depth of the "x" and "y" troughs following these waves. Proper identification of the components of the venous waveform is aided by correlation with the auscultated first heart sound or the palpated brachial artery pulse. The "a" component of the venous waveform occurs simultaneously with or immediately precedes the S_1 heart sound or the palpable brachial arterial impulse.

Additional elevation of the trunk to the 90-degree upright position allows for assessment of the degree of venous distension of the internal jugular vein and also of the external jugular and other veins in the neck. To accurately assess the clinical correlates of jugular venous distension, the examiner must ensure that the patient is breathing freely through the mouth without performing a Valsalva maneuver. Normally, in this position, the internal and external jugular veins are collapsed with no visible distension or pulsation.

Chest

Inspection of the chest is best performed with the patient in both the upright and the supine positions and should include assessments of general contour, sternal and spinal deformities, and anterior chest motions. The examiner should evaluate the chest contours from the front and side of the patient and also from the foot of the examining table with the patient supine. In evaluating general contour, special attention should be made for any increase in anteroposterior diameter common with chronic obstructive pulmonary disease and its possible association with heart failure. Other contour variations that may be observed include fixed asymmetrical precordial bulging of the anterior chest, which may be associated with congenital cardiac defects in children or with slowly expanding ventricular aneurysms in adults. Both of these cardiac defects have a high correlation with major peripheral arterial defects. Congenital sternal deformities may be observed by noting the position of the sternum relative to the anterior ribs. *Pectus excavatum* (funnel chest) exists when the level of the sternum is posterior to the level of the anterior ribs, whereas *pectus carinatum* (pigeon chest) is a more anterior projection of the sternum in front of the anterior ribs. These pectus deformities are a common finding in Marfan's syndrome and its associated aortic abnormalities. Examination of the thoracic spine should note any degree of *kyphosis,* which may be associated with chronic obstructive pulmonary disease.

Complete inspection of the anterior chest for motion is best performed with the patient in the supine, upright, and left lateral decubitus positions when doing a cardiac examination. Unlike chest inspection for cardiac disease states, which makes observations for pulsations, retractions, and heaves (or lifts), when limited to peripheral vascular assessment, the chest examination can be accomplished in the upright position and should make note of pulsations in the aortic, pulmonic, sternoclavicular, and epigastric areas. Pulsations in these areas are best observed with the lights in the examination room dimmed and by shining a penlight tangentially across the area of interest.

Prominent pulsations noted in the right second intercostals space (ICS) (or the aortic area) are usually associated with aortic regurgitation and poststenotic dilatation of the ascending aorta and with ascending aortic aneurysms. Visible pulsations in the left third ICS (or the pulmonic area) can be normal in children and even in adults with thin chest walls. Disease states associated with pulmonic pulsations are associated with conditions causing pulmonary artery dilatation and include pulmonary arterial hypertension, pulmonary embolism, and a variety of cardiac structural defects. Pulsations observed in the sternoclavicular area are usually associated with dilated or dissecting ascending aortas, tortuous innominate artery, and right-sided aorta. Epigastric pulsations can be associated with abdominal aortic aneurysms.

Upper Extremities and Hands

Physical manifestations of vascular conditions might be noted on inspection of the upper extremities and hands (23). Finger inspection should include observations for impaired perfusion involving the fingers, with the most significant findings involving the fingertips and becoming less evident toward the palm. The changes can be transient and patchy and are manifested by successive pallor, cyanosis, and rubor of one or more fingers, especially if the hands are exposed to ambient cooling. The changes may also be permanent and manifested by ulcerations and localized gangrenous changes on the tips of the fingers and at the edge of the nail beds; pitted scars where previous ulcerations have healed; taut, shiny, and atrophic skin; and loss of hair growth. Further inspection should note the presence of the *arachnodactyly* of Marfan's

syndrome, the *clubbing* associated with chronic obstructive pulmonary disease and with ischemic heart disease, *splinter hemorrhages* in the nail beds, and the tell-tale *nicotine staining* of the proximal portions of the index and long fingers implying a significant cigarette smoking history. Inspection of the palmar surfaces should note the presence of tender 3- to 15-mm-diameter papular lesions on the palms or fingertips that are reddish-purple in color and do not blanche with pressure (Osler's nodes) or nontender, macular lesions on the palms that are 5 mm in diameter and are pink to tan in color and nonblanching (Janeway lesions).

Inspection on the dorsum of the hands should make note of extensor tendon *xanthomas,* which have a possible association with atherosclerotic vascular disease. These lesions are best observed by having the patient alternately flex and extend the fingers while noting on the dorsum of the hand the subcutaneous movement of the xanthomatous nodules attached to the extensor tendons. With the aid of a magnifying glass, the nail beds should be inspected for the presence of *capillary pulsations,* which might indicate significant aortic regurgitation or the widened pulse pressure in some cases of systolic hypertension.

Upper extremity and hand inspection should also include an evaluation of the degree of venous filling or distension, making a comparison of the two extremities for asymmetry. If there is venous distension, an assessment for venous pulsations should also be made. In addition, the upper extremities should be evaluated for the presence of edema and for traumatic scars or other evidence of penetrating trauma near major arterial and venous structures.

Transient and patchy ischemia of the fingers is typical of Raynaud's disease and many diseases and conditions associated with secondary Raynaud's phenomenon. When the changes on the fingers are permanent or appear chronic, thromboangiitis obliterans (Buerger's disease) is more likely. Other conditions causing impaired perfusion of the upper extremities and hands include microembolic arterial occlusion, cryoglobulinemia, exposure to vasospastic drugs, and some connective tissue diseases. Asymmetrical nonpulsatile venous distension (and rarely bilateral venous distension) could indicate venous thromboses of axillary or subclavian veins or obstruction of the superior vena cava. The presence of pulsatile venous distension is suggestive of arteriovenous fistulae resulting from recent or old penetrating trauma or other nontraumatic conditions.

Lower Extremities

Inspection of the lower extremities for manifestations of vascular conditions may be noted on both the arterial side and the venous side of the circulation. Most of the evidence for these conditions will be obvious on inspection only, but palpation techniques can be combined with inspection as an additional method of assessment. Examination of the lower extremities for arterial compromise should include both static inspection and dynamic inspection (12,24,25). An important aspect

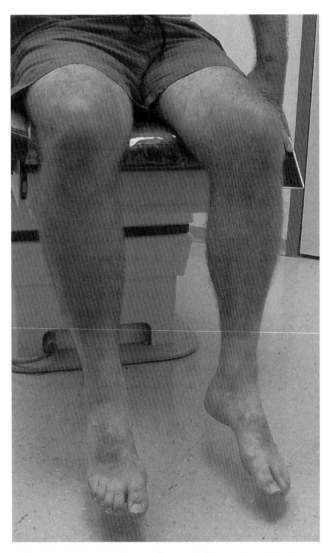

FIG. 3.1. Patient positioned for static inspection of the lower extremities.

and muscles. Absence of hair growth on the dorsum of the foot and toes, especially when it was previously present, suggests arterial insufficiency. Atrophy of the skin or muscles of the lower extremities or loss of subcutaneous tissues below the level of the knee is associated with progressive loss of arterial perfusion. Other skin changes indicating poor arterial perfusion are tight, shiny skin overlying the anterior tibia, evidence of poor healing of skin trauma, and skin ulcerations that appear chronic in nature. Special attention should be paid to the most likely areas for arterial ulcerations (Fig. 3.2). These include the tips of the toes, the dorsum of the feet, over the metatarsal heads and the heels, and overlying the malleoli. When ulcers are present, notation of their base, their border, and the surrounding skin should be assessed, with arterial ulcers having bases that are flat and pale in color and occasionally covered by an eschar. Their borders are sharp, appearing to be "punched out," and the surrounding skin is pale and nonpigmented (23). Inspection of the condition of the toenails may reveal thickened, textured, and ridged nail plates, which can be associated with chronic arterial compromise.

Static inspection of the lower extremities is particularly important in the days and weeks following any angiographic or surgical endovascular manipulation of proximal (aortic) ulcerative atheromatous disease. Cholesterol embolization from these lesions causes partial occlusion of small arteries, resulting in a diffuse, lacelike pattern of reddish-blue superficial tissue infarcts called livedo reticularis, which is most conspicuous with leg dependency. These patchy necrotic areas, eventually accompanied by punctate ulcerations, are most commonly noted on the volar aspect of the feet and toes, but, with extensive embolization, can involve the legs and thighs.

The technique for dynamic inspection of the lower extremity arterial supply involves exposure of both legs at 72°F for at least 10 minutes with the patient lying supine (12,24,25). After notation of the color of the extremities, the examiner then passively elevates both legs about 12 in. for 1 minute and

to lower extremity evaluation is comparisons between both lower extremities. Asymmetrical findings are almost always present in patients with arterial or venous insufficiency; rarely is the degree of vascular disease involving the extremities bilaterally symmetrical.

Static inspection for arterial insufficiency should be done after the patient has dangled both lower extremities over the side of the table for several minutes and at a room temperature of about 72°F (Fig. 3.1). Inspection for color variations, specifically *cyanosis* and *pallor,* combined with palpation for skin temperature, should be done, with all of these findings more significant when observed in the peripheral parts of the legs, feet, and toes. Maintaining an ambient temperature of 72°F will eliminate cyanosis secondary to peripheral vasoconstriction. Other static observations should be made for the distribution of hair growth, especially on the dorsum of the feet and toes and the condition of the skin, subcutaneous fat,

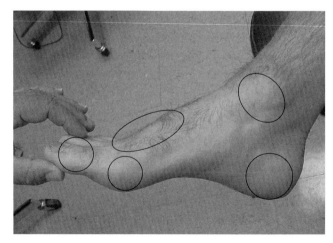

FIG. 3.2. Likely locations for arterial ulcerations.

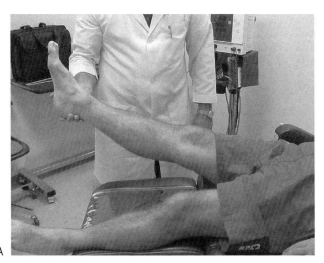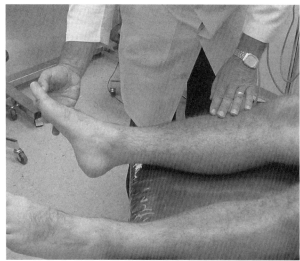

FIG. 3.3. Dynamic inspection of the lower extremities. **A:** Detection of elevation pallor. **B:** Observation of reperfusion time upon dependency.

again notes the color for *elevation pallor* (Fig. 3.3). Whereas slight elevation pallor may be observed in normal individuals, significant pallor after 10 to 20 seconds of elevation is indicative of arterial occlusive disease. If elevation pallor is observed, the legs are again lowered to the flat position and the time to return of normal color is noted. Color should return in normal individuals in less than 10 seconds, but a reperfusion time greater than 45 seconds indicates significant arterial insufficiency (24,25). If elevation pallor is not present, this maneuver should be repeated after the patient actively exercises the legs by flexing and extending the feet for 30 to 60 seconds. Elevation after exercise may reveal pallor on elevation that is not evident on passive testing. Confirmatory evidence for poor arterial perfusion is assessed by compressing the skin of the toes or distal feet for a few seconds to induce blanching and noting the time for capillary refilling. Capillary refilling time greater than 2 seconds is suggestive of arterial insufficiency (25).

Static inspection of the lower extremities also includes an assessment of the adequacy of the venous circulation, which has implications for both venous disease and cardiac functioning. From these standpoints, initial inspection should be made for evidence of edema. For the detection of mild cases of edema, the examiner should focus attention on the distal parts of the lower extremities, especially from the shoe-top area to just proximal to the ankle. Notations in these areas should include evidence of indented impressions made by footwear and socks or stockings, variations in skin color, especially cyanosis, the presence of irregular areas of brownish pigmentation, purpura and petechiae, and the condition of the skin, especially ulcerations (4). Comparisons of both lower extremities should be made for symmetry. In contrast to ulcerations of arterial origin, venous ulcers tend to be shallow and located on the medial side of the lower leg just above the

malleolus, but in severe cases can be located anywhere from mid-calf to mid-foot. The margins are irregular, undermined, and nodular, and frequently stand proud of the surrounding edematous skin. The surrounding skin is commonly heavily pigmented and often is covered with a scaly eruption. The base is moist, yellowish, and often covered with a seropurulent exudate.

Another dynamic inspection technique uses venous findings to indicate the adequacy of arterial blood flow. Again with the patient supine, the lower extremities are elevated for 1 minute to allow all blood to drain from the superficial veins. The patient is then allowed to sit up, suddenly dangling both legs over the side of the examining table. The time it takes to refill the superficial veins is noted, with a venous filling time greater than 20 to 30 seconds indicating significant arterial insufficiency.

Observable evidence of chronic arterial insufficiency is typically noted in peripheral atherosclerotic diseases (arteriosclerosis obliterans), thromboangiitis obliterans (Buerger's disease), and occasionally in aortic coarctation, other forms of congenital arterial narrowing, and various forms of arteritis. These conditions can involve both the lower and the upper extremities. When limited to the upper extremity, Takayasu's arteritis (aortic arch syndrome), subclavian steel syndrome, and dissecting aneurysm of the ascending aorta are most likely. Sudden arterial occlusion is typically associated with arterial emboli originating in the heart or some proximal arterial site. Acute arterial thrombosis may also result in sudden observable changes in perfusion. Acute thrombosis is associated with atherosclerotic disease, thromboangiitis obliterans, hypercoagulable states (polycythemia vera, thrombocytosis, etc.), arterial trauma, arterial spasm, and aortic dissection. Evidence of poor venous perfusion detected on inspection can be noted in chronic venous insufficiency, acute and chronic thrombophlebitis, and varicose vein disease.

Palpation

Palpation offers the clinician a mechanism not only for assessing static vascular states, but also for obtaining valuable information on the patient's cardiovascular hemodynamics. Many of the clues elicited during inspection can be confirmed with deliberate and thoughtful palpation techniques. When used properly, palpation can discover the adequacy of peripheral perfusion, the size, movements, and functioning of many cardiac structures, the status of the electrical activity of the heart, and the hemodynamics of blood flow. To these ends, palpation is used to detect peripheral arterial pulsations, the degree of edema formation, vibrations (thrills), and extremity surface temperature.

To maximize the detection of these physical properties, it is important for the clinician to appreciate the specialized sensory functions of the hand. Pulsations and evaluation for edema are best detected with the volar tips of the fingers, vibrations with the palmar surface overlying the distal metacarpals, and temperature by the dorsal aspects of the fingers. Many examiners find that the sensitivity of their nondominant hand is greater.

Precordium

Optimal detection of pulsations associated with peripheral arterial diseases is achieved by palpating selected areas on the anterior chest. Special attention should be given with the fingertips to the area above the suprasternal notch, the right sternoclavicular area, both supraclavicular areas, the aortic area at the right second and third ICS, the pulmonic area at the second left ICS, and the subxiphoid (or epigastric) area. For most areas, a complete description of a pulsation (or impulse) includes its location and its intensity or amplitude.

Prominent pulsations in the second left ICS are indicative of pulmonary hypertension. Those located in the aortic area, the right sternoclavicular area, or the supraclavicular areas may indicate aortic root dilatation, ascending aortic aneurysms, arterial hypertension, or coarctation of the aorta. When limited to the supraclavicular areas, subclavian or axillary aneurysms and occasionally carotid artery aneurysms must be considered. Prominent subxiphoid or epigastric pulsations are associated with descending or abdominal aneurysms.

Palpable vibrations (or *thrills*) will be detected in the same anatomic areas as pulsations. By using the base of the metacarpal heads, however, the areas to be examined will be slightly larger. The examiner should place a relaxed hand directly over the target areas, being careful not to arch the palm. If detected, thrills should be characterized as to intensity, location or site of maximal intensity, timing relative to left

ventricular systole, duration (as a percentage of the cardiac cycle), and direction of radiation. Although thrills associated with peripheral vascular conditions can be detected in the major arterial structures in the chest, they must be differentiated from thrills of intracardiac origin.

Peripheral Arteries

Palpation of peripheral arteries, carefully performed, not only can detect the rate, rhythm, amplitude, and symmetry of the pulse, but also can be used to evaluate the texture of the vessel (20). Palpation of arterial pulses can also reveal information about cardiac functioning. Best detected with a single fingertip (the thumb is also acceptable), the palpable pulse is the examiner's confirmation that the target artery has been located and is being evaluated. Once detected, the rate and the rhythm of the peripheral pulse can be correlated with cardiac apical rate and rhythm as a manifestation of cardiac electrical activity and contractile force. Carotid arterial pulsations normally occur almost simultaneously with cardiac apical impulses and provide the most accurate correlative information between peripheral and central hemodynamics. When rhythm disturbances are detected on peripheral arterial palpation, the cadence of the abnormal rhythm should be noted, paying special attention to any recurring timing patterns and to variations in the intensity of the pulsations within these patterns. The rate and rhythm of peripheral arterial pulsations should be correlated with the palpable apical pulse, with care taken to note evidence of pulse deficit.

Complete assessment of an arterial pulsation should include an analysis of the waveform, noting the rate of rise of the upstroke, the apparent height (amplitude) of the pulse, the duration or width of the impulse at its peak, and the rate of fall of the downstroke (10,12). In assessing the arterial waveform, conclusions can be drawn regarding cardiac as well as peripheral arterial disease. The amplitude and the shape of the waveform correlate with such cardiac functions as myocardial contractility, intracardiac pressure gradients across the ventricular septum, and the hemodynamics across the aortic and mitral valves. Assessment of peripheral arteries by waveform analysis provides clues to the patency of the arterial tree and correlates with both congenital and acquired occlusive conditions proximal to the point of palpation.

Additional evidence for arterial patency can be obtained by making horizontal and vertical comparisons of the pulse at two different sites simultaneously (4). A horizontal comparison of distal arterial hemodynamics is made by simultaneously palpating the amplitude and the timing of the pulsations of symmetrical arteries in the lower or in the upper extremities (Fig. 3.4). Any detectable decrease in amplitude or delay in timing in one artery compared to the corresponding location on the contralateral artery indicates the presence of some type of occlusion in the affected extremity, resulting in reduced volumes of blood delivered to that site. Vertical comparison of pulsations is made by simultaneously

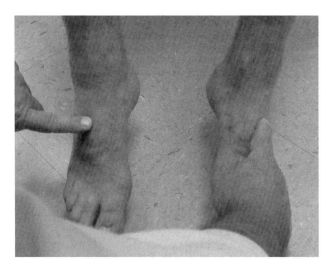

FIG. 3.4. Horizontal comparison of dorsalis pedis pulses.

palpating a proximal and distal artery in the same extremity or by palpating a radial and femoral artery and again noting pulse amplitude and timing. A marked difference in pulse amplitude or delay indicates some degree of arterial occlusion between the two points. Occasionally, asymmetry in distal pulsations becomes manifest only after exercise. Observations should be made both at rest and after 30 to 60 seconds of active flexion and extension of the ankles.

Similar horizontal and vertical comparisons of extremity perfusion can be made by simultaneously comparing surface temperature at selected points on the same or on both extremities. For any difference in temperature, detected with the dorsal surface of the examiner's fingers, conclusions can be drawn regarding the site of an occlusion in the arterial supply to that extremity.

Two specialized arterial palpation techniques are used to evaluate the adequacy of arterial flow in the upper extremities. The *Allen test* is used to assess the patency of the radial and the ulnar arteries (24,26). It combines a palpation technique with an inspection technique (Fig. 3.5). The patient is asked to tightly clench the fist to produce blanching of the palm. With the fist still tightly clenched, the examiner then occludes both radial and ulnar arterial flow by digitally compressing each artery with a thumb or forefinger. With the arteries still compressed, the examiner asks the patient to unclench the fist and after releasing compression on one of the arteries, notes the time to return of color to the palm. This step is repeated with release of the other artery. Failure of the color to return or a delay in return of color beyond 6 seconds indicates occlusion or narrowing of the artery not being compressed.

A second palpation technique used to assess upper extremity arterial flow patterns involves palpating the radial or brachial pulse amplitude while the patient's arm is abducted (hyperabduction maneuver) or when the patient's neck

is extended and rotated to the contralateral side (scalene or Adson's maneuver) (Fig. 3.6) (24). In both of these tests, the amplitude or intensity of the pulse is assessed first with the patient sitting up, looking straight ahead, and with the arm relaxed at the side. The amplitude of the pulse is again assessed as the patient's arm or neck is passively moved to the appropriate positions. Any decrease in the amplitude of the pulse is suggestive of positional compression of the axillary or subclavian artery on the affected side. It should be stressed that a positive result from these tests does not necessarily indicate the presence of arterial disease, because positional compression of normal arteries can occur.

Extremities

Palpation is also an essential technique in the assessment of peripheral edema. Accurate documentation of edema involves both static inspection of any structural distortion and dynamic inspection of physical changes produced by digital palpation. Static inspection should make note of the anatomic regions involved, the symmetry of the edematous parts, and the extent of the edema relative to a fixed anatomic reference (e.g., the malleolus in the lower extremity). Once static inspection reveals the presence of edema, clues can be gathered as to its cause, amount, and degree of pitting.

Proper technique in the evaluation of edema is essential for its precise quantification (12). The skin overlying a bony prominence in the edematous part of the extremity should be compressed with three fingers, holding the pressure for 10 seconds. After releasing the compressive palpation, a light source, directed tangentially, should be used to detect whether there is evidence of a persistent indented distortion of the skin and subcutaneous tissues left by the fingertips. If present, the depth of the impression or "pit" should be determined in millimeters, usually by gross estimation. When assessing edema, the actual measurement of the depth of the pit together with other physical observations of the extremity provides the most accurate description. Use of the 1+ to 4+ grading scale for pitting edema is often inaccurate and should be avoided. If a grading scale is used, the grades should accurately reflect the actual physical characteristics observed. In addition, pitting edema is further characterized according to its time to disappearance. Edema in which the pits disappear in less than 40 seconds is referred to a "fast edema" and is often linked to hypoalbuminemic states. Pitting that remains evident for greater than 1 minute is called "slow edema" and is usually associated with cardiovascular etiologies including venous conditions.

Slow dependent edema of venous origin in the lower extremities is associated with saphenofemoral incompetence or perforator vein incompetence and varicose veins, deep venous thrombosis of the iliac or femoral veins, chronic venous insufficiency, or extrinsic compression of veins in the upper thigh or pelvic areas. When located in the upper extremity,

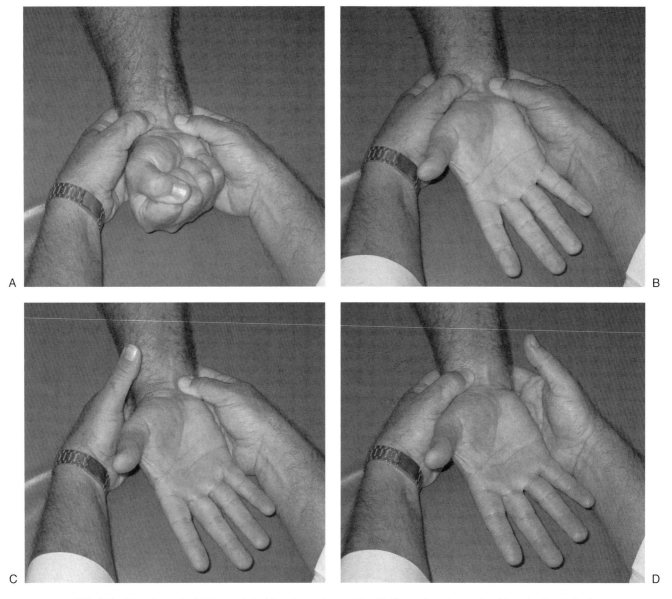

FIG. 3.5. Allen test. **A:** Fist clench to blanche palmar skin. **B:** Open hand remains blanched with both arteries occluded. **C:** Checking patency of radial artery. **D:** Checking patency of ulnar artery.

it is usually the result of acute axillary or subclavian venous thrombosis.

Abdomen

Depending on the size of the patient's abdomen, palpation can assess the intensity of the aortic pulsation as well as the diameter of the abdominal aorta. Whereas pulsations located in the midline between the xiphoid and the umbilicus are easily palpated and are frequently seen projecting anteriorly in normal individuals, abnormal dilatation of the aorta can be palpated by using the fingers of both hands to identify each side of the aorta by its pulsation. Care should be taken to note whether the pulsations seem expansile (i.e., moving laterally as well as anteriorly) or can be identified on the right side of the midline.

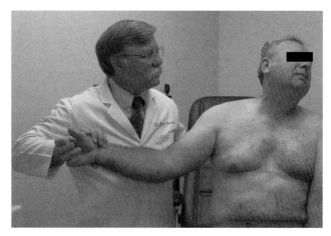

FIG. 3.6. Adson's maneuver.

Expansile pulsations, especially if noted to the right of the midline, indicate a dilated aorta or possibly an aortic aneurysm. Tenderness of a dilated or aneurysmal aorta suggests an aortic aneurysm in the process of rupturing. Decreased intensity of abdominal aortic pulsations suggests atherosclerotic disease, hypovolemia, hypotension, or possible coarctation of the aorta.

Auscultation

As a vascular assessment technique, auscultation requires the most skill. Accurate diagnosis demands extraordinary focus on the part of the examiner to detect the often very subtle sounds originating in peripheral vessels. Once detected, these sounds require further analysis as to amplitude, pitch, and timing. Using the clues elicited during the preceding inspection and palpation examinations, the examiner is alerted to possible vascular diagnoses that may be confirmed by additional auscultatory findings. Complete auscultation should include assessments of both peripheral arterial bruits and peripheral venous hum sounds.

Auscultation of peripheral arteries provides the clinician with information about arterial pressures and blood flow hemodynamics. For arterial blood pressure determinations, accuracy depends on proper equipment and technique (10,12). When recording blood pressure determinations with a sphygmomanometer, it should be remembered that readings are affected by patient position, arm and leg position, cuff size and placement, stethoscope placement, the length of time the artery is occluded, and the rate of deflation of the cuff. A comparison of blood pressures in both arms should be done to discover unsuspected unilateral occlusion of arterial flow to an upper extremity. With use of the bell of the stethoscope, standard blood pressure determinations are made in the brachial and often in the femoral arteries. In addition, with a Doppler device, comparative blood pressures can be determined in the brachial and in the dorsalis pedis or posterior tibial arteries, providing valuable information about peripheral blood flow and circulatory hemodynamics in the lower extremities. Called the ankle–brachial index (ABI), a vertical assessment of arterial flow in each lower extremity is determined by dividing the dorsalis pedis or posterior tibial Doppler systolic pressure by the brachial Doppler systolic pressure. An ABI of less than 0.95 is usually indicative of arterial occlusive disease in the iliac, the femoral, or the popliteal artery, with numbers less than 0.5 associated with severe arterial insufficiency (13). For these measurements to be valid, the peripheral arteries must be compressible. An additional index, the toe–ankle index, can be determined to evaluate the status of patency of the arterial supply below the ankle. A toe Doppler is used, and the systolic Doppler pressure of the digital artery of the great toe is divided by the systolic Doppler pressure of the dorsalis pedis (or posterior tibial) artery. A number below 0.64 is associated with arterial occlusive diseases involving the ankle arteries.

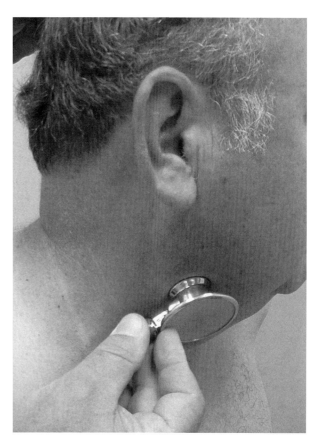

FIG. 3.7. Auscultation of the carotid artery.

Auscultation for altered arterial blood flow hemodynamics should be performed directly over the carotid, temporal, brachial, renal, abdominal aorta, iliac, popliteal, and femoral arteries. Again using the bell, the examiner should note the presence of bruits as indications of turbulent blood flow caused by occlusive diseases or vessel tortuosity (Fig. 3.7). Any bruits should be characterized as to pitch, timing (systolic, diastolic, or both), location, configuration, and intensity. When caused by stenosis or extrinsic compression, arterial bruits tend to be low pitched when located in large-diameter vessels like the aorta and high pitched in smaller-diameter arteries. They are always maximally audible during systole, with possible extension into early diastole, are of variable intensity depending on the diameter of the affected vessel, and have a crescendo–decrescendo (diamond-shaped) configuration. In locating a bruit, the examiner should determine the most proximal site on an artery where a bruit is audible. Arterial bruits are located at the site of arterial narrowing, but are audible for several centimeters downstream from the site of occlusion. It is typical to hear bruits for 4 to 6 cm distal to the point of narrowing in most muscular arteries and for as much as 15 cm in the aorta. By "inching" upstream, the examiner can locate the point of arterial narrowing as the most proximal point at which the bruit is audible.

When auscultating, the examiner should use care to exert minimal pressure with the stethoscope so as not to artificially compress the vessel, creating bruits in otherwise normal vessels. In addition, because carotid bruits can be short, soft, and localized, when examining each carotid, auscultation should be performed along the entire length of the artery from just above the clavicle to the bifurcation at the border of the mandible. It is useful to ask the patient to briefly stop breathing to eliminate audible interference from tracheal breath sounds. Any bruits detected in the carotid artery should be carefully distinguished from transmitted aortic valve murmurs.

Arterial bruits with the typical diamond-shaped configuration and with systolic accentuation are most often detected in arteriosclerosis obliterans involving the carotid, renal, aorta, iliac, and femoral arteries. Continuous bruits are noted in patent ductus arteriosus or some other type of abnormal aortopulmonary communication like large arteriovenous shunts, abnormal communication between the aorta and a right-sided cardiac chamber, and in other abnormal flow patterns in either arteries or veins such as coarctation of the aorta or pulmonary artery.

Auscultation is also used to evaluate the hemodynamics of blood flow in peripheral veins (12). An audible venous hum, commonly referred to as a continuous venous murmur, should be evaluated for pitch, location, and timing. It is typically a low-pitched, continuous sound heard throughout the cardiac cycle with an increase in intensity beginning just after the second heart sound and lasting for the remainder of diastole. Most venous hums are physiological in nature and have no clinical significance except to be differentiated from the bruits associated with arterial occlusive diseases. They are commonly audible in the supraclavicular areas in children and can be induced in this location in adults by extending the neck and rotating the head to the contralateral side. They are also commonly heard in adults overlying the internal jugular veins. On rare occasions, venous hums can indicate significant alterations of venous hemodynamics secondary to disease states and trauma.

Pathophysiologic venous hums may be detected in peripheral veins in the extremities secondary to arteriovenous fistulae, especially when the veins are distended and pulsatile. They may also be noted in the epigastric or right upper abdominal quadrant in cases of hepatic cirrhosis and in the neck in association with the hyperdynamic state of hyperthyroidism.

REFERENCES

1. Naumberg EH. Interviewing and the health history. In: Bickley LS, Szilagyi PG, eds. *Bates' guide to physical examination and history Taking,* 8th ed. Philadelphia: Lippincott Williams & Wilkins, 2003:21–49.
2. Swartz MH. *Textbook of physical diagnosis: history and examination,* 4th ed. Philadelphia: WB Saunders, 2002:3–34.
3. Braunwald E. Examination of the patient. In: Braunwald E, Zipes DP, Libby P, eds. *Heart Disease: a textbook of cardiovascular medicine,* Vol. 2, 6th ed. Philadelphia: WB Saunders, 2001:27–44.
4. Rutherford RB. Initial patient evaluation. In: Rutherford RB, ed. *Vascular surgery,* 5th ed. Philadelphia: WB Saunders, 2001:1–13.
5. Smith KW. Approach to the patient with cardiovascular disease. In: Wyngarden JB, Smith LH, Bennett JC, eds. *Cecil textbook of medicine,* 19th ed. Philadelphia: WB Saunders, 1992:147–148.
6. Nielsen CD, Malone DP. Pulmonary heart disease. In: Taylor GJ, ed. *Primary care management of heart disease.* St. Louis: Mosby, 2000:404–413.
7. Cohen LS. Diseases of the aorta. In: Wyngarden JB, Smith LH, Bennett JC, eds. *Cecil textbook of medicine,* 19th ed. Philadelphia: WB Saunders, 1992:350–355.
8. Zabalgoitia M, O'Rourke RA. Diseases of the aorta. In: Stein JH, ed. *Internal medicine,* 4th ed. St. Louis: Mosby, Inc., 1994:285–293.
9. Shabetai R. Diseases of the pericardium. In: Wyngarden JB, Smith LH, Bennett JC, eds. *Cecil textbook of medicine,* 19th ed. Philadelphia: WB Saunders, 1992:343–350.
10. Braunwald E, Perloff JK. Physical examination of the heart and circulation. In: Braunwald E, Zipes DP, Libby P, eds. *Heart disease: a Textbook of cardiovascular medicine,* Vol.1, 6th ed. Philadelphia: WB Saunders, 2001:45–81.
11. Kontos HA. Vascular diseases of the limbs. In: Wyngarden JB, Smith LH, Bennett JC, eds. *Cecil textbook of medicine,* 19th ed. Philadelphia: WB Saunders, 1992:355–368.
12. Seidel HM, Ball JW, Dains JE, et al. *Mosby's guide to physical examination,* 5th ed. St. Louis: Mosby, 2003.
13. Craeger MA, Libby P. Peripheral arterial disease. In: Braunwald E, Zipes DP, Libby P, eds. *Heart disease: a textbook of cardiovascular medicine,* Vol. 2, 6th ed. Philadelphia: WB Saunders, 2001:1457–1484.
14. Hartmann JR, Roth H. Peripheral arterial disease. In: Taylor GJ, ed. *Primary care management of heart disease.* St. Louis: Mosby, 2000:384–391.
15. Pulsinelli WA, Levy DE. Ischemic cerebrovascular diseases. In: Wyngarden JB, Smith LH, Bennett JC, eds. *Cecil textbook of medicine,* 19th ed. Philadelphia: WB Saunders, 1992:2152–2162.
16. Brust JCM. Cerebral infarction. In: Rowland LP, ed. *Merritt's neurology,* 10th ed. Philadelphia: Lippincott Williams & Wilkins, 2000:231–240.
17. Carter TD, VanBakel AB. Cerebrovascular disease. In: Taylor GJ, ed. *Primary care management of heart disease.* St. Louis: Mosby, 2000:392–403.
18. Caplan LR. Cerebrovascular disease. In: Stein JH, ed. *Internal medicine,* 4th ed. St. Louis: Mosby, 1994:1074–1087.
19. Victor M, Ropper AH. Cerebrovascular diseases. In: *Adams and Victors principles of neurology,* 7th ed. New York: McGraw-Hill, 2001:821–924.
20. Perloff JK. Physical examination of the cardiovascular system. In: Stein JH, ed. *Internal medicine,* 4th ed. St. Louis: Mosby, 1994:32–45.
21. Bickley LS, Szilagyi PG. *Bates' guide to physical examination and history Taking,* 8th ed. Philadelphia: Lippincott Williams & Wilkins, 2003:266–270.
22. Bickley LS, Szilagyi PG. *Bates' guide to physical examination and history taking,* 8th ed. Philadelphia: Lippincott Williams & Wilkins, 2003:256–258.
23. Johnson KW. Neurovascular conditions involving the upper extremity. In: Rutherford RB, ed. *Vascular surgery,* 5th ed. Philadelphia: WB Saunders, 2001:1111–1122.
24. Spittell PC, Spittell Jr JA. Diseases of the peripheral arteries and veins. In: Stein JH, ed. *Internal medicine,* 4th ed. St. Louis: Mosby, 1994:293–302.
25. Swartz MH. *Textbook of physical diagnosis: history and examination,* 4th ed. Philadelphia: WB Saunders, 2002:391–406.
26. Bickley LS, Szilagyi PG. *Bates' guide to physical examination and history taking,* 8th ed. Philadelphia: Lippincott Williams & Wilkins, 2003:457.

CHAPTER 4

Intermittent Claudication

Raghu R. Midde and Stanley G. Rockson

Key Points

- Intermittent claudication (IC) is the hallmark of patients with peripheral arterial disease (PAD).
- Frequency of IC increases markedly with age.
- As the degree of stenosis increases, flow decreases and distal perfusion is not maintained. Metabolites, produced by anerobic metabolism, trigger the claudication symptoms.
- Collateral circulation may help to minimize symptoms, but the development of collaterals varies greatly from patient to patient.
- Age and gender are the most important risk factors for IC. Other risk factors include tobacco use, hypertension, diabetes, hyperhomocyteinemia, and high cholesterol.
- Mortality as a direct result of PAD occurs in less than 10% of cases.
- There are five distinct outcomes of IC: improvement, stabilization, worsening without revascularization required, worsening with revascularization required, and amputation.
- Where feasible, all patients with IC should participate in a supervised exercise program.

Peripheral arterial disease (PAD), one of several clinical manifestations of atherosclerosis, is a highly prevalent condition that is associated with a substantial risk of morbidity and death, and a marked reduction in ambulatory capacity and quality of life (1). The disease has significant socioeconomic, functional, and prognostic implications, particularly because it predominantly affects those in the rapidly expanding segment of the population above age 65 years (2,3).

Intermittent claudication (IC) is the symptomatic hallmark and most frequent presenting clinical feature in patients with PAD (4). The word claudication is derived from the Latin word *claudicare,* meaning "to limp." In current clinical use, claudication is defined as an ache or a sensation of fatigue or pain in the affected leg. The symptom typically arises after a reproducible degree of effort, often culminating in the cessation of activity and, thereafter, is relieved within minutes of rest.

Although clinical identification of the claudicant is improving within the medical community, this symptomatic presentation remains substantially underdiagnosed, introducing a barrier to effective secondary prevention of the ischemic cardiovascular and cerebrovascular complications of the associated systemic atherosclerosis (5). Enhanced recognition of claudication, with its natural history, risk factors, and comorbidities, should lead to more effective management of these patients while providing access to a variety of emerging, novel therapies (6).

INCIDENCE AND PREVALENCE

The prevalence of intermittent claudication has been used epidemiologically as a marker that establishes the frequency of peripheral arterial insufficiency within defined patient populations. These estimates depend, however, on the demographic attributes of the specific population under study, such as age, gender, and geography. In addition, the results are dependent on the methods used to determine the frequency of IC. For instance, studies that rely on questionnaires tend to overestimate the frequency of symptomatic PAD with symptoms, inasmuch as patients with nonvascular complaints that resemble claudication can be erroneously identified as having PAD (7).

More recent studies have established that reliance on a classic history of claudication alone to identify PAD may lead to extraordinary underrecognition of the diagnosis. The large cohort of asymptomatic patients are likely to have come to clinical identification only through the use of an objective method, such as measurement of Doppler systolic ankle pressures (4,5). Using noninvasive testing, Criqui et al. established a two- to threefold higher prevalence of PAD when compared to the use of subjective claudication as a diagnostic discriminator (7). Thus, in patients aged 45 to 74 years, a detectable reduction of systolic ankle pressure occurred in 6.9% of patients, whereas only 22% of these individuals complained of claudication (4).

The frequency of IC increases substantially with advancing age: estimates range from 0.6% in those aged 45 to 54 years, to 2.5% in those aged 55 to 64 years, to 8.8% in patients aged 65 to 74 years (8). The mean incidence of IC derived from five large population-based studies by Dormandy et al. ranged from 2 per 1,000 men per year in the 30- to 34-year age group to 7 per 1,000 in those greater than 65 years of age (9). The Rotterdam Study, a population-based analysis of 7,715 patients, documented a frequency of IC ranging from about 1% in those aged 55 to 60 years to 4.6% in those between 80 and 85 years (10). Despite this rather low frequency of IC, 16.9% of men and 20.5% of women aged 55 years and older had PAD as defined by an ankle–brachial index of less than 0.90 in either leg. This observation confirms that most patients with significant PAD are symptom free (11).

ETIOLOGY AND PATHOGENESIS

Symptomatic claudication is caused primarily by an inadequate blood supply to the extremity. Inadequate perfusion occurs as a consequence of a flow-limiting lesion within a conduit artery, most typically atherosclerotic. A blood pressure gradient develops at rest if the stenosis reduces the luminal diameter by greater than 50%, because kinetic energy is lost as turbulence develops. This pressure gradient increases in a nonlinear manner, which underscores the importance of a modest stenosis at high blood flow rates. A lesion that does not occasion a resting gradient may provoke a gradient during exercise, consequent to the higher cardiac output and lowered vascular resistance. Thus, as the degree of stenosis increases, flow progressively decreases and distal perfusion pressure is no longer maintained. The ensuing reduction in blood supply is not sufficient to meet the increased metabolic demands of the exercising muscle. Consequently, anaerobic metabolism produces increasing concentrations of lactate and other metabolites, such as acylcarnitines, adenosine diphosphates, and hydrogen ions. Activation of local sensory receptors, invoked by the accumulation of these metabolites, elicits the symptoms of claudication. The increase in intramuscular pressure during exercise may exceed the arterial pressure distal to the stenotic lesion, further reducing the blood flow and exacerbating the perceived discomfort (11).

At the organ tissue level, evidence of distal axonal degeneration, affecting primarily the type II or glycolytic, fast twitch fibers, has been found in patients with PAD. The injury is thought to be mediated at the cellular level through increased oxidative stress, generation of oxygen free radicals, and lipid peroxidation secondary to reperfusion of the ischemic tissue. The muscle fiber atrophy that ensues leads to decreased muscle strength and further compromises the exercise performance (6).

Formation of collateral channels for blood flow is a likely compensatory mechanism for the inadequate blood supply. These collaterals may develop from the enlargement of preexisting, minute anastomoses of arterial branches with distal vessels. De novo angiogenesis, alternatively, theoretically may be responsible for some collateral formation. Whereas postnatal angiogenesis may be enough to meet the metabolic needs during rest or moderate exertion, it may not be adequate to meet the demands during more intense exercise. The extent of collateralization varies greatly from patient to patient. For any stenotic lesion of a defined severity, one individual may experience disabling claudication, whereas another may be thoroughly asymptomatic. Multiple vessel involvement, accompanied by inadequate collateral formation, may result in the more severe manifestations of ischemia, including rest pain and threatened loss of limb (2). An increased mitochondrial volume and enzymatic activity, possibly reflecting a metabolic adaptation to the reduced blood supply, has been observed in the skeletal muscle of patients with claudication. This response is further augmented through exercise and aids in the maximal extraction and utilization of oxygen delivered to the ischemic tissue by the compromised vasculature. Thus, although it might be conjectured that symptomatic improvement in peripheral ischemia through exercise rehabilitation occurs through a stimulation of collateral new vessel formation, it is at least as likely that an augmentation of mitochondrial responses reduces symptoms through the enhanced efficiency of oxidative metabolism in the ischemic muscle (12).

As the disease progresses, the microcirculation eventually becomes compromised, leading to critical limb ischemia. Although an initial compensatory vasodilatation takes place during tissue hypoxia, this response is ultimately impaired by a cascade of pathological alterations. Sluggish blood flow reduces shear stress, thereby promoting leukocyte adherence and platelet aggregation. The complement and the clotting factors are activated, leading to neutrophil activation and release of oxygen free radicals. This promotes further cellular injury and increased permeability, leading to interstitial edema and further limitation of nutrient transfer. Thus, in advanced, severe peripheral arterial disease with sustained ischemia, the escalating pattern of increased blood viscosity, enhanced aggregability, and vascular stasis together with eventual microvascular occlusion leads to critical limb ischemia and frequently limb loss (2).

RISK FACTORS

The risk factors for the claudicant are identical to those that confer risk for atherosclerosis in the coronary, cerebrovascular, and systemic circulations. Age and gender are among the most important of these. Atherosclerosis of the lower extremities is more common in the elderly (4), and the hormonally mediated protective effects in women are ultimately effaced in the more advanced decades of life, reflected in part in the more recently documented gender equality for claudicants in the population at large (6). PAD is observed with substantial frequency in all races and geographic areas, although some data indicate that isolated PAD is particularly common in blacks (13–15).

Tobacco use is one of the most prevalent risk factors associated with PAD: Nearly 80% of patients with claudication acknowledge the use of tobacco (2). IC has been reported to be three times higher in smokers than in nonsmokers, a relation first identified by Erb in 1911 (16). The Framingham Study reported the risk of PAD in smokers to be twice that in nonsmokers (17,18). On average, they experience the onset of claudication at least 10 years earlier than nonsmokers. Deranged endothelium-nitric oxide-dependent vasodilatation has been implicated as the possible mechanism for the development and progression of atherosclerosis in these individuals (19). The increased risk is correlated with the number of cigarettes smoked (17). Poor long-term outcomes have been observed in persistent smokers, with a significant increase in the incidence of amputation for ischemic gangrene, and impaired viability of both peripheral and coronary saphenous vein grafts. On the other hand, cessation of smoking has been associated with a rapid decrease in the risk of IC (20).

Hypertension may have both cause and effect relationships to PAD. It is well established that aggressive control of blood pressure in a newly diagnosed hypertensive patient occasionally will symptomatically unmask an unrecognized lesion converted to hemodynamic significance (6). It is also well known that uncontrolled hypertension promotes vascular complications, thus predisposing to a higher incidence of coronary and cerebrovascular events (i.e., myocardial infarction and stroke). The Framingham Study reported a 2.5-fold increase in the risk of PAD in men and a 3.9-fold increased risk in women with hypertension (17).

The contributory role of diabetes is well established (21,22). The risk of PAD increases three- to fourfold in patients with diabetes (7). In the Framingham cohort, glucose intolerance contributed more as a risk factor for claudication than it did for coronary artery disease or stroke (7,17,18,23–25). A recent study demonstrated that diet-controlled diabetes was not a significant risk factor, but that diabetes requiring either oral or insulin therapy was a strong predictor for the development of PAD (26). A 2.9-fold increase in the risk for development of ischemic ulceration and a 1.7-fold increased risk for development of ischemic rest pain in diabetics with claudication as compared to nondiabetics were reported (8).

Although data regarding the relationship between hyperlipidemia and PAD have at times been contradictory, the ratio of high-density lipoprotein (HDL) to total cholesterol has been identified as an accurate marker for the development of PAD (5,27,28). Hypertriglyceridemia and lipoprotein(a)

have been shown to be independently associated with lower extremity PAD (29).

Hyperhomocysteinemia is demonstrable in roughly 30% of patients with premature PAD, a relationship that is more robust than the one observed in coronary artery disease (odds ratio 6.8 vs 1.6, respectively) (30). Increased fibrinogen (31) concentrations and elevated hematocrit (32) have also been associated with increased risk of PAD with claudication.

Considered in aggregate, the Clopidogrel versus Aspirin in Patients at Risk of Ischemic Events (CAPRIE) trial has shown that smoking (current 38%, former 53%), hypertension (51%), hypercholesterolemia (45%), and gender (male:female = 3:1), were the most frequent comorbid risk factors (33). The concurrence of multiple risk factors in a single patient dramatically escalates the risk of PAD (4). For example, the combination of any risk factor with smoking nearly triples the likelihood of developing PAD (18,34).

COMORBIDITIES

There is a significant overlap in the incidence of intermittent claudication and both coronary and cerebrovascular atherosclerosis. In a Cleveland Clinic study involving preoperative coronary angiography for patients undergoing peripheral vascular surgery, only 10% with IC had normal coronaries, whereas 28% had severe triple-vessel disease requiring surgery or deemed inoperable (35).

The CAPRIE trial has clearly demonstrated that, in 20,000 patients with atherosclerosis of coronary, cerebrovascular, and peripheral arteries, approximately one-third had intermittent claudication as their presenting symptom. Approximately 41% of the patients with PAD had concurrent coronary artery or cerebrovascular disease and 8.6% had disease in all three vascular beds (33). Similarly, the Trans-Atlantic Inter-Society Consensus document compiled data from all the available studies and concluded that almost 60% of patients with PAD have significant coronary and/or cerebrovascular disease and about 40% of those with CAD of cerebrovascular disease will also have PAD (36,37).

NATURAL HISTORY

The natural history of lower extremity PAD has been studied extensively in multiple trials, both with regard to systemic morbidity and mortality and to the progression of the disease in the leg.

Even in patients without overt claudication, the mortality risk of those with PAD exceeds that of the patients without the disease. This has been well demonstrated by the classic study of Criqui et al. (38). Mortality, however, is rarely a direct result of lower extremity arterial disease itself. The risk of mortality increases with symptomatic disease and in those with critical limb ischemia. Approximately 55% of the patients die from coronary artery disease and its complications. Cerebrovascular disease accounts for 10% of the mortality, and 25% of the deaths are related to nonvascular causes.

Mortality as a direct result of PAD is observed in less than 10% of the patients. In these patients, a ruptured aortic aneurysm is the most common cause of death.

The Basle Study demonstrated angiographic progression of disease in 63% of patients over the 5 years that followed the initial diagnosis (34). The symptoms that compromise mobility and impair the activities of daily life, however, fail to develop in 66% of the surviving population over this same time period.

Studies conducted before the 1980s documented a low incidence of disease progression in patients with intermittent claudication. A 10-year cumulative amputation rate of approximately 11% was observed (39). However, there is no evidence in these studies that symptoms identified as claudication arose as a direct result of vascular insufficiency. Studies done in the 1980s conventionally utilized measurement of the ankle–brachial index. In this context, 30% to 40% of the patients had symptomatic and/or objective deterioration over time, but the amputation rate nevertheless remained low for these study subjects.

In general, studies done over the past four decades suggest that only one-fourth of the patients with intermittent claudication will ever deteriorate. When encountered, deterioration occurs most frequently during the first year following diagnosis. Thereafter, the disease worsens in approximately 2% to 3% of the patients annually. New vessel formation, metabolic adaptation of the ischemic muscle, or gait alteration to favor nonischemic muscle groups are some of the proposed mechanisms that might predispose to symptom stabilization (36,40).

The most important predictor of clinical outcome in all studies has been the severity of objectively determined arterial occlusive disease on initial evaluation. Thus, in summary, the claudicant can expect one of five distinct outcomes: improvement, stabilization of the disease, worsening of the disease with no revascularization required, worsening of the disease with vascularization required, or the requirement for an amputation (26).

A recent large serial study conducted by Aquino et al. involving 1,244 patients with claudication documented an average rate decline in the ankle–brachial index of 0.014 per year and a decline in the walking distance of 9.2 yards annually (26).

CLINICAL EVALUATION AND DIAGNOSIS

A complete medical history, beyond what is elicited specifically to evaluate dynamic limb pain, is mandatory for proper evaluation and management of the claudicant. The initial history should include the distance walked and the speed and incline of ambulation that produce the symptoms. These variables serve as a baseline measure of disability and assist in the future monitoring of the therapeutic efficacy. In view of the association of PAD with systemic atherosclerosis, detailed information on the signs and symptoms of coronary and cerebrovascular disease should be elicited. Existing risk factors as well as plans for subsequent risk factor modification and systemic therapy should be noted. Identification and proper management of other comorbid conditions, such as congestive heart failure, anemia, and chronic obstructive lung disease, can significantly alleviate lower extremity symptoms (6).

Intermittent claudication is the hallmark symptom of peripheral arterial insufficiency, classically described as a sensation of fatigue or cramping of the lower extremity during walking. It usually begins after a reproducible level of exertion, and resolves promptly within minutes of cessation of effort either by sitting or standing still. The location of pain is related to the level of arterial stenosis. Ankle or foot claudication is caused by tibial and peroneal artery disease. Superficial femoral disease or popliteal artery involvement typically elicits claudication in the calf muscles. Iliofemoral disease or obstruction of the aorta leads to claudication in the buttocks, hips, or thighs.

Several standard questionnaires have been developed to aid in the identification and severity assessment of claudication. The Rose Questionnaire, which gives an assessment of the symptoms at various levels of exertion, was developed to diagnose angina and IC in epidemiologic surveys. The San Diego Questionnaire and the Edinburgh Questionnaire are modifications of the Rose Questionnaire. The Medical Outcomes Short Form 36 Questionnaire evaluates the functional status and well-being of patients with chronic conditions (41). The walking impairment questionnaire is the most recent; it asks about the symptoms and assigns a point score to elicited responses regarding them (42).

Treadmill exercise testing is also used to evaluate the extent of the peripheral arterial stenosis and provide objective evidence of the patient's walking capacity. The initial claudication distance (ICD) is defined as the point at which symptoms of claudication first developed, and the absolute claudication distance (ACD) is the point at which the patient is no longer able to continue walking because of severe leg discomfort. These provide a useful, quantitative assessment of the patient's disability that can be monitored after therapeutic interventions. Reproducibility of repeated treadmill tests is reportedly better with progressive-grade than with constant-grade protocols (43–46). Additionally, the treadmill testing also provides adjunctive information regarding the presence of cardiac ischemia.

The diagnosis of PAD must be established in a thorough manner, beginning with a complete history and physical examination and progressing to objective documentation of disability and the severity of symptoms (measurement of ankle–brachial index and quantitative assessment of exercise performance, along with utilization of a variety of vascular imaging modalities, as clinically required). An assessment of associated risk factors is required. Routine laboratory tests including complete blood count, serum chemistry, lipid profile, and renal parameters are obtained. In some special situations, for example, premature atherosclerosis in a young patient or in patients requiring repeated interventional therapy, additional investigations are undertaken to identify hypercoagulable states (antiphospholipid antibody, antithrombin III antibodies, protein C and S deficiencies). Hyperhomocysteinemia and elevated lipoprotein(a) levels should also be excluded, where appropriate.

PHYSICAL EXAMINATION

The physical exam centers on, but is not limited to, the circulatory system. The general examination may reveal hypertension, arrhythmias, abnormal heart sounds, anemia, or aneurysms. Blood pressure is measured in both upper extremities, and any observed gradients are noted. Such observations may identify the presence of subclavian stenosis. Although uncommon, this condition is often associated with significant carotid arterial disease. A careful pulse examination in all extremities is performed. It is most practical to grade pulses according to whether they are absent (0), diminished (1), or normal (2). A very prominent pulse should be noted, and the abdomen palpated for evidence of a pulsatile mass. Auscultation for bruits is an integral part of the circulatory examination and includes the neck, abdomen, flank, and groin. Provocatory maneuvers such as brief exercise may add further information. A previously appreciated pulse may disappear or bruits may accentuate. A presumptive diagnosis of PAD frequently can be made simply on the basis of location and severity of claudication as well as the pulse examination (6).

A careful physical exam is essential to permit assessment of the anatomic level and severity of the arterial stenosis. Patients with aortoiliac disease have an attenuated femoral at times accompanied by an audible femoral bruit, due to accelerated blood flow velocity and turbulence at the site of stenosis. Similarly, with disease in the superficial femoral artery, there will be a normal femoral pulse, but popliteal and tibial pulses will be diminished or absent. Symptoms of calf claudication in the presence of preserved femoral and popliteal pulses but absent pedal pulses likely indicate tibioperoneal disease, seen commonly in diabetics (6).

Patients with PAD can be classified according to their symptomatic severity and to the abnormalities detected on physical exam. Two PAD classification systems are commonly employed: the Fontaine, which grades the symptoms from absent to critical, and the Rutherford, which consists of three grades and six categories of chronic limb ischemia.

Objectively quantitation of the presence and the severity of PAD with measurement of the ankle–brachial index (ABI), using a handheld Doppler probe, further enhances the physical examination. The ABI is expressed as a ratio of the ankle systolic pressure, measured at the malleolar level, and the greater of the two brachial systolic pressures. An ABI of greater than or equal to 1.0 is considered normal, whereas a value of less than 0.9 is indicative of mild disease. A value of less than or equal to 0.5 suggests severe disease. It must be emphasized, however, that the diagnostic accuracy of these maneuvers depends on the normal compressibility of the in-frapopliteal vessels. In the elderly and especially in diabetics, vascular calcification impairs the normal elasticity of the arterial wall. Consequently, the high pressures required to compress these inelastic vessels lead to an overestimation of the true arterial pressure. In such patients, pulse volume recordings will be able to document an attenuation of pulse volume compatible with arterial insufficiency.

Ancillary physical findings sometimes help to underscore the discrepancy between the spuriously normal or elevated ABI and the presence of significant limb ischemia. Pallor on elevation, dependent rubor, and cutaneous changes represent the physical changes of ischemia. Pallor at rest, without limb elevation, signals the presence of critical limb ischemia. The rapidity with which the pallor occurs is used as a semiquantitative bedside assessment of severity. With the patient supine and the leg held at a 60-degree angle, pallor will occur within 25 seconds with severe disease, within 30 seconds with moderate insufficiency, and within 60 seconds in the presence of mild arterial disease. Rubor on dependency can also be readily observed in patients with significant perfusion deficits. Additionally, during dependency after elevation, an observed delay in the venous filling time can be an additional semiquantitative indicator of disease severity. Filling times of 20 to 45 seconds denote the presence of more severe disease. In such patients, capillary refill (the return of color to the skin after blanching) will be sluggish as well.

Cutaneous changes in the affected extremity indicate the presence of significant longstanding arterial disease. Trophic changes in the skin along with hair loss and subcutaneous atrophy become evident. Livedo reticularis or cyanosis of one or more of the digits suggests a recent atheroembolic event. These findings should raise the suspicion of advanced aortic atherosclerotic disease or aneurysm, particularly if the changes are present in both lower extremities.

Ulceration of the skin is a cause for significant concern in these patients because it denotes the presence of critical degrees of ischemia. The arterial ulcer is characteristically sharply demarcated. It is typically covered with a dark, thick eschar, which, when removed, discloses a very avascular ulcer base with minimal granulation tissue. These ulcers usually occur in regions of contact or pressure or at acral parts of the extremity, and should be easily distinguished from other forms of cutaneous ulceration. Venous stasis ulcers, for example, typically have irregular borders. They are shallow and most often located about the medial malleolus, and are accompanied by chronic pigmentary changes ascribable to hemosiderin deposits in the skin. In contradistinction to the ischemic ulcer, these lesions are well perfused, with adequate granulation at the base. Finally, the neurotrophic ulcer crater is quite deep and well perfused; although surrounded by inflammatory changes, the lesion is typically painless.

DIFFERENTIAL DIAGNOSIS

Dynamic extremity pain need not always be intermittent claudication. Nonvascular causes of exertional leg pain should be considered in the differential diagnosis of true claudication. Nonatherosclerotic vascular considerations include a variety of vasculitides, arterial entrapment syndromes, cysts, irradiation, prior trauma, coarctation, and venous insufficiency. The nonvascular diagnoses feature lumbosacral radiculopathy, arthritis of the hips and knees, and various skeletal muscle disorders.

Venous claudication in patients with venous regurgitation typically presents with discomfort during exertion that can mimic calf claudication. The manifestations of peripheral edema, stasis, pigmentation, and varicosities help to identify venous insufficiency. A symptomatic Baker's cyst or a chronic compartment syndrome can similarly cause discomfort at the level of the calf. The nature and the location of the pain (characteristically a tight, bursting type of discomfort), often associated with a particular position, should lead to the proper diagnosis.

Arthritis of the hips and knees can also present with leg discomfort and pain on ambulation. This condition produces a persistent, aching pain, typically localized to the affected joint, and commonly precipitated by variable intensities of exercise. Furthermore, arthralgia should be reproducible with range-of-motion examinations.

Lumbosacral radiculopathy, usually a consequence of degenerative disc disease or spinal stenosis, elicits a similar quality of pain on walking very short distances, but is relieved only by sitting or leaning against a support. This has been termed neurogenic or pseudoclaudication. It is common in the elderly and often coexists with PAD in this group of individuals.

The differential diagnosis of critical limb and digital ischemia includes connective tissue disorders like lupus erythematosus and scleroderma, vasculitides such as thromboangiitis obliterans, atheroembolism, diabetic sensory neuropathy, reflex sympathetic dystrophy, acute gouty arthritis, and trauma.

LABORATORY STUDIES

Segmental Pressure Analysis

Measurement of systolic blood pressure at selected segments of each extremity to evaluate the presence and severity of stenoses in the peripheral arteries is one of the most useful and simplest noninvasive tests. The blood pressure cuffs are applied at the thigh, above and below the knee, and above the ankle. After quantification of any pressure gradients a hemodynamically significant stenosis can be suspected with any segmental pressure decrement of greater than 15%. Segmental pressure analysis is often supplemented by color flow Doppler ultrasound of the major conduit vessels. The Doppler probe is placed over an artery distal to the cuff to assess the blood flow. In the lower extremities the probe is usually placed over the posterior tibial artery as it courses inferior and posterior to the medial malleolus. It is also convenient to place the probe over the dorsalis pedis artery on the dorsum of the metatarsal arch. In the upper extremity, the brachial artery, in the antecubital fossa, and the radial and ulnar arteries, at the wrist, are convenient imaging targets.

Pulse Volume Recording

Pulse volume recordings are obtained with transducers placed along specific locations on the limb to record segmental pulse volumes at the thigh, calf, ankle, and toes. The arterial waveform morphology can be analyzed when the volumetric changes are displayed on a graphic recorder. With a significant stenosis, the amplitude of the pulse volume is reduced and the normal dicrotic notch disappears, with conversion from the normal biphasic waveform to an abnormal monophasic pattern.

Duplex Ultrasound Imaging

Duplex imaging provides a direct noninvasive means of assessing both the anatomic characteristics of peripheral arteries and the functional significance of arterial stenosis. Acoustic properties of the vascular wall differ from those of the surrounding tissue, which enables them to be imaged easily. Normal arteries have laminar flow, with the highest velocity at the center of the artery. The representative image is usually homogeneous with relatively constant hue and intensity. In the presence of stenosis, as the blood flow velocity through the narrowed lumen increases, progressive desaturation of the color display can be noted and flow disturbance distal to the lesion causes changes in hue and color. A twofold or greater increase in peak systolic velocity at the sight of the lesion indicates a greater than or equal to 50% decrease in the diameter. No signal is obtained if the artery is occluded. The specificity and sensitivity of duplex imaging are 95% and 85%, respectively, in identifying arterial stenosis (47–50).

Treadmill Testing

Treadmill exercise testing is used to evaluate the clinical significance of PAD and to provide objective evidence of the patient's walking capacity. It provides a quantitative assessment of the patient's disability as well as a baseline with which further disease progression can be monitored after therapy. A greater than or equal to 25% decrease in ABI after exercise in a patient with claudication is considered diagnostic and implicates PAD as the cause of symptoms. Treadmill testing also gives adjunctive information regarding the presence of myocardial ischemia.

Magnetic Resonance Angiography

Magnetic resonance angiography (MRA) is a noninvasive means of visualizing the peripheral arteries and the aorta. Sensitivities of 95% to 100% and specificities of 96% to 100% have been reported in various comparative studies (51–54). Resolution of the vascular anatomy with gadolinium-enhanced MRA approaches that of conventional contrast digital subtraction angiography. Its current utility may be greatest for the evaluation of symptomatic patients to assist decision making prior to performance of an endovascular intervention or in patients at risk for renal, allergic, or other complications during conventional angiography. It will likely play a much greater role in the evaluation of claudicants in the future.

Contrast Angiography

Conventional angiography is indicated for evaluation of arterial anatomy prior to a revascularization procedure or sometimes when the diagnosis is in doubt. It remains the gold standard with which all other tests must be compared. It is, however, a semiinvasive modality and its use should be confined to those patients for whom a surgical or percutaneous intervention is contemplated.

MANAGEMENT

Although the claudicant presents to the physician with complaints that refer to the lower extremity, primary therapeutic measures are equally directed toward treating the generalized atherosclerotic process.

Risk factor modification is a priority in the initial management of the claudicant. Abstinence from smoking should be strongly encouraged, with the aid of nicotine replacement, antidepressant drugs like bupropion, and behavior modification measures as required. Cessation of smoking has been associated with a rapid decrease in the risk of developing IC (20).

Numerous large clinical trials over the last decade have demonstrated the benefits of cholesterol-lowering therapy in patients with coronary artery disease. By inference from these important observations regarding the success of secondary prevention of coronary atherosclerosis, the current recommendation in patients with PAD is to reduce serum low-density lipoprotein (LDL) cholesterol to less than 100 mg per dL, reduce the serum triglyceride levels to less than 150 mg per dL, and raise the serum HDL cholesterol levels.

Although data are not sufficient to conclude whether aggressive control of blood pressure will alter the progression of PAD or the development of IC, the fact that successful therapy significantly reduces vascular complications, including myocardial infarction (MI) and stroke, is well established.

Treatment of the patient's claudication should be based on the severity of the symptoms. A supervised exercise program should be initiated in all patients presenting with claudication. Patients with mild to moderate symptoms usually experience the greatest functional improvement with therapeutic exercise. Pain-free walking distance can be expected to double after 3 months of sustained exercise training (55–58). It also improves the overall cardiovascular function and enhances the efficiency of the oxidative metabolism of the exercising muscle.

A rigorous exercise training program may be as beneficial as bypass surgery and may be more beneficial than angioplasty (59). A meta-analysis of randomized trials found that exercise training increased maximal treadmill walking distance by 179 m (95% confidence interval = 60 to 298) (60,61). This degree of improvement should translate into longer walking distances on level ground.

The best results of exercise therapy require a motivated patient in a supervised setting, typically modeled after cardiac rehabilitation. The training should also be maintained on a regular basis to reap the benefits of the therapeutic intervention (62).

DRUG THERAPY FOR CLAUDICATION

Aspirin

Aspirin may favorably affect the peripheral circulation and reduce the subsequent need for peripheral, arterial surgery.

The Antiplatelet Trialists' Collaboration found that the risk of MI, stroke, or death from vascular causes after a mean follow-up of 27 months was 9.7% in patients who received antiplatelet therapy, as compared with 11.8% in control patients. This 18% reduction was statistically nonsignificant. Despite the lack of statistical significance, aspirin improved vascular-graft patency in patients with PAD who were treated with bypass surgery (saphenous vein or prosthetic graft) or peripheral angioplasty, followed over a period of 19 months (63).

Clopidogrel

Clopidogrel is a thienopyridine drug and has fewer side effects than its congener, ticlopidine. The CAPRIE trial compared 75 mg of clopidogrel per day with 325 mg of aspirin per day in greater than 19,000 patients with a history of MI, stroke, or PAD. In the subgroup of patients with PAD (6,452 patients), the primary endpoint of fatal or nonfatal MI, fatal or nonfatal stroke, or death from other vascular causes occurred at an annual rate of 4.9% in those taking aspirin and 3.7% in those taking clopidogrel, a reduction of 23.8%. This reduction was greater than that in the subgroups of patients with MI or stroke (33).

Pentoxifylline

Pentoxifylline is a methylxanthine derivative approved in 1984 for the treatment of claudication. It is said to improve rheologic effects on erythrocyte deformability, give lower plasma fibrinogen levels, and provide mild platelet antiaggregatory effects. Several randomized trials concluded that pentoxifylline conferred marginal benefits over placebo in improving the walking distance. The data are not sufficient to warrant broad utilization (64–67).

Cilostazol

Cilostazol is a vasodilatory phosphodiesterase inhibitor, which also inhibits platelet aggregation, the formation of arterial thrombi, and vascular smooth-muscle proliferation. It was approved in 1999 by the U.S. Food and Drug Administration for the treatment of claudication. Four randomized, placebo-controlled trials of cilostazol have been published, representing the enrollment of 1,534 patients with claudication (68–69). In all four trials, cilostozol (100 mg twice daily) improved both pain-free and maximal treadmill walking distance as compared with placebo.

REFERRAL FOR ARTERIOGRAPHY AND REVASCULARIZATION

Endovascular or surgical intervention is warranted when noninvasive therapy fails and the patient continues to have disabling symptoms limiting his or her ambulatory capacity, thereby compromising the quality of life. In general, excellent long-term patency rates are achievable with percutaneous angioplasty and stenting above the inguinal ligament. In contrast, the results are not as promising with interventions in the superficial femoral artery (30% to 40% restenosis) and below the knee (40% to 50% restenosis). Unfavorable vascular anatomy (poor runoff, long stenotic segments), diabetes, and severe ischemia reduce the likelihood of a successful outcome. However, as newer technology emerges, it is likely that peripheral intervention will play a much bigger role in the future.

REFERENCES

1. Hiatt WR. Medical treatment of peripheral arterial disease and claudication. *N Engl J Med* 2001;344:1608–1621.
2. Rockson SG, Cooke JP. Peripheral arterial insufficiency: Mechanisms, natural history and therapeutic options. In: Schrier RW, Baxter JD, Dzau VJ, et al., eds. *Advances in internal medicine,* Vol. 43. St. Louis: Mosby, 1998:253–277.
3. Ouriel K. Peripheral arterial disease. *Lancet* 2001;358(9289):1257–1264.
4. Hirsch AT, Criqui MH, Comerota AJ, et al. Peripheral arterial disease detection, awareness, and treatment in primary care. *JAMA* 2001;286:1317–1324.
5. Schneider FA, Comerota AJ. Intermittent claudication: magnitude of the problem, patient evaluation, and therapeutic strategies. *Am J Cardiol* 2001;87[Suppl]:3D–13D.
6. Hiatt WR, Hoag S, Hammen RF. Effect of diagnostic criteria on the prevalence of peripheral arterial disease. *Circulation* 1995;92:1472–1479.
7. Criqui MH, Denenberg JO, Langer RD, et al. The epidemiology of peripheral arterial disease: importance of identifying the population at risk. *Vasc Med* 1997;2:221–226.
8. Stoffers HE, Rinkens PE, Kester AD, et al. The prevalence of asymptomatic and unrecognized peripheral arterial occlusive disease. *Int J Epidemiol* 1996;25:282–290.
9. Dormandy J, Heeck L, Vig S. Intermittent claudication: underrated risks. *Semin Vasc Surg* 1999;12:96–108.
10. Meijer WT, Hoes AW, Rutgers D, et al. Peripheral arterial disease in the elderly: the Rotterdam Study. *Arterioscler Thromb Vasc Biol* 1998;18:185–192.
11. Coffman JD. Pathophysiology of obstructive arterial disease. *Herz* 1988;13:343–350.
12. Newman AB, Sutton-Tyrrell K, Rutan GH, et al. Lower extremity arterial disease in elderly patients with systolic hypertension. *J Clin Epidemiol* 1991;44:15–20.
13. Newman AB, Tyrrell KS, Kuller LH. Mortality over four years in SHEP participants with a low ankle–arm index. *J Am Geriatr Soc* 1997;45:1472–1478.
14. Erb W. Klinische Beiträge zur Pathologie des Intermittierenden Hinkens. *Münch Med Wochenschr* 1911;2:2487.
15. Kannel WB, McGee DL. Update on some epidemiological features of intermittent claudication. *J Am Geriatr Soc* 1985;33:13–18.
16. Murabito JM, D'Agostino RB, Silbershatz H, et al. Intermittent claudication: a risk profile from the Framingham Heart Study. *Circulation* 1997;96:44–49.
17. Celermajer DS, Sorensen KE, Georgakopoulos D, et al. Cigarette smoking is associated with dose-related and potentially reversible impairment of endothelium-dependent dilation in healthy young adults. *Circulation* 1993;88:2149–2155.
18. Bainton DF, Sweetman P, Baker I, et al. Peripheral arterial disease: consequences for survival and association with risk factors in the Speedwell Prospective Heart Disease Study. *Br Heart J* 1994;72:128–132.
19. O'Riordan DS, O'Donnell JA. Realistic expectations for the patient with intermittent claudication. *Br J Surg* 1991;78:861–863.
20. Cronenwett JL, Warner KG, Zelenock GB, et al. Intermittent claudication: current results of nonoperative management. *Arch Surg* 1984;119:430–436.
21. Newman AB, Siscovick DS, Manolio TA, et al. Ankle–arm index as a marker of atherosclerosis in the Cardiovascular Health Study. Cardiovascular Heart Study (CHS) Collaborative Research Group. *Circulation* 1993;88:837–845.
22. Fowkes FG, Housley E, Riemersma RA, et al. Smoking, lipids, glucose intolerance, and blood pressure as risk factors for peripheral atherosclerosis compared with ischemic heart disease in the Edinburgh Artery Study. *Am J Epidemiol* 1992;135:331–340.
23. Gordon T, Kannel WB: Predisposition to atherosclerosis in the head, heart, and legs. The Framingham Study. *JAMA* 1972;221:661–666.
24. Aquino R, Johnnides R Makaroun M, et al. Natural history of claudication. *J Vasc Surg* 2001;34:962–970.
25. Pujia A, Gnasso A, Mancuso G, et al. Arteriopatia asintomatica degli arti inferiori. Prevalenza e fattori di rischio in una popolazione del sud Italia. *Minerva Cardioangiol* 1993;41:130–138.
26. Zimmerman BR, Palumbo PJ, O'Fallon WM, et al. A prospective study of peripheral occlusive arterial disease in diabetes. III: Initial lipid and lipoprotein findings. *Mayo Clin Proc* 1981;6:233–242.
27. Cheng SW, Ting AC, Wong J. Lipoprotein (a) and its relationship to risk factors and severity of atherosclerotic peripheral vascular disease. *Eur J Vasc Endovascular Surg* 1997;14:17–23.
28. Clarke R, Daly L, Robinson K, et al. Hyperhomocystinaemia: an independent risk factor for vascular disease. *N Engl J Med* 1991;324:1149–1155.
29. Kannel WB, D'Agostino RB, Belanger AJ. Update on fibrinogen as a cardiovascular risk factor. *Ann Epidemiol* 1992;2:45–466.
30. Handa K, Takao M, Nomoto J, et al. Evaluation of the coagulation and fibrinolytic systems in men with intermittent claudication. *Angiology* 1996;47:543–548.
31. CAPRIE Steering Committee. A randomised, blinded, trial of clopidogrel versus aspirin in patients at risk of ischaemic events (CAPRIE). *Lancet* 1996;348:1329–1339.
32. DaSilva A, Widmer LK, Ziegler HW, et al. The Basle Longitudinal Study; report on the relation of initial glucose level to baseline ECG abnormalities, peripheral artery disease, and subsequent mortality. *J Chronic Dis* 1979;32:797–803.
33. Hertzer NR, Beven EG, Young JR, et al. Coronary artery disease in peripheral vascular patients: a classification of 1000 coronary angiograms and results of surgical management. *Ann Surg* 1984;199:223–233.
34. Trans-Atlantic Inter-Society Consensus (TASC) Working Group. Management of peripheral arterial disease (PAD). *J Vasc Surg* 2000;31:S5–S44, S54–S74, S77–S122.
35. Aronow WS, Ahn C. Prevalence of coexistence of CAD, peripheral arterial disease, and atherothrombotic brain infarction in men and women less than 62 years of age. *Am J Cardiol* 1994;74:64–65.
36. Criqui MH, Langer RD, Fronek A, et al. Mortality over a period of ten years in patients with peripheral arterial disease. *N Engl J Med* 1992;326:381–386.

37. McAllister FF. The fate of patients with intermittent claudication managed nonoperatively. *Am J Surg* 1976;132:593–595.
38. Jelnes R, Gaardstring O, Hougaard Jensen K, et al. Fate of intermittent claudication: outcome and risk factors. *Br Med J* 1986;293:1137–1140.
39. Stewart AL, Greenfield S, Hays RD, et al. Functional status and well-being of patients with chronic conditions. Results from the Medical Outcomes Study. *JAMA* 1989;262:907–913.
40. Regensteiner JG, Steiner JF, Panzer RJ, et al. Evaluation of walking impairment by questionnaire in patients with peripheral arterial disease. *J Vasc Med Biol* 1990;2:142–152.
41. Gardner AW, Skinner JS, Cantwell BW, et al. Progressive vs single-stage treadmill tests for evaluation of claudication. *Med Sci Sports Exerc* 1991;23:402–408.
42. Labs KH, Nehler MR, Roessner M, et al. Reliability of treadmill testing in peripheral arterial disease: A comparison of a constant load with a graded load treadmill protocol. *Vasc Med* 1999;4:239–246.
43. Gardner AW, Skinner JS, Vaughan NR, et al. Comparison of three progressive exercise protocols in peripheral vascular occlusive disease. *Angiology* 1992;43:661–671.
44. Chaudhry H, Holland A, Dormandy J. Comparison of graded versus constant treadmill test protocols for quantifying intermittent claudication. *Vasc Med* 1997;2:93–97.
45. Ranke C, Creutzig A, Alexander K. Duplex scanning of the peripheral arteries: Correlation of the peak velocity ratio with angiographic diameter reduction. *Ultrasound Med Biol* 1992;18:433–440.
46. Sacks D, Robinson ML, Marinelli DL, et al. Peripheral arterial Doppler ultrasonography: diagnostic criteria. *J Ultrasound Med* 1992;11:95–103.
47. Pemberton M, London NJ. Colour flow duplex imaging of occlusive arterial disease of the lower limb. *Br J Surg* 1997;84:912–919.
48. Whelan JF, Barry MH, Moir JD. Color flow Doppler ultrasonography: comparison with peripheral arteriography for the investigation of peripheral vascular disease. *J Clin Ultrasound* 1992;20:369–374.
49. Poon E, Yucel EK, Pagan-Marin H, et al. Iliac artery stenosis measurements: comparison of two-dimensional time-of-flight and three-dimensional dynamic gadolinium-enhanced MR angiography. *AJR Am J Roentgenol* 1997;169:1139–1144.
50. Ho KY, de Haan MW, Kessels AG, et al. Peripheral vascular tree stenoses: Detection with subtracted and nonsubtracted MR angiography. *Radiology* 1998;206:673–681.
51. Quinn SF, Sheley RC, Semonsen KG, et al. Aortic and lower-extremity arterial disease: Evaluation with MR angiography versus conventional angiography. *Radiology* 1998;206:693–701.
52. Rofsky NM, Johnson G, Adelman MA, et al. Peripheral vascular disease evaluated with reduced-dose gadolinium-enhanced MR angiography. *Radiology* 1997;205:163–169.
53. Vogt M, Wofson S, Kuller L. Lower extremity arterial disease and the aging process: a review. *Clin Epidemiol* 1994;45:529.
54. Duprez D, Clement D. Medical treatment of peripheral vascular disease: good or bad. *Eur Heart J* 1992;13:149–151.
55. Ernst E, Fialka V. A review of the clinical effectiveness of exercise therapy for intermittent claudication: The Framingham Study. *J Am Geriatr Soc* 1985;33:13.
56. Regensteiner JG, Hiatt WR. Exercise rehabilitation for patients with peripheral arterial disease. *Exerc Sport Sci Rev* 1995;23:1–24.
57. Regensteiner JG, Steiner JF, Hiatt WR. Exercise training improves functional status in patients with peripheral arterial disease. *J Vasc Surg* 1996;23:104–115.
58. Lundgren F, Dahllof A, Lundholm K, et al. Intermittent claudication—surgical reconstruction or physical training? A prospective randomized trial of treatment efficiency. *Ann Surg* 1989;209:346–355.
59. Creasy TS, McMillan PJ, Fletcher EWL, et al. Is percutaneous transluminal angioplasty better than exercise for claudication? Preliminary results from a prospective randomised trial. *Eur J Vasc Surg* 1990;4:135–140.
60. Regensteiner JG, Meyer TJ, Krupski WC, et al. Hospital vs home-based exercise rehabilitation for patients with peripheral arterial occlusive disease. *Angiology* 1997;48:291–300.
61. Goldhaber SZ, Manson JE, Stampfer MJ, et al. Low-dose aspirin and subsequent peripheral arterial surgery in the Physicians' Health Study. *Lancet* 1992;340:143–145.
62. Girolami B, Bernardi E, Prins MH, et al. Treatment of intermittent claudication with physical training, smoking cessation, pentoxifylline, or nafronyl: a meta-analysis. *Arch Intern Med* 1999;159:337–345.
63. Hood SC, Moher D, Barber GG. Management of intermittent claudication with pentoxifylline: meta-analysis of randomized controlled trials. *CMAJ* 1996;155:1053–1059.
64. Ernst E. Pentoxifylline for intermittent claudication: a critical review. *Angiology* 1994;45:339–345.
65. Radack K, Wyderski RJ. Conservative management of intermittent claudication. *Ann Intern Med* 1990;113:135–146.
66. Dawson DL, Cutler BS, Hiatt WR, et al. A comparison of cilostazol and pentoxifylline for treating intermittent claudication. *Am J Med* 2000;109:523–530.
67. Dawson DL, Cutler BS, Meissner MH, et al. Cilostazol has beneficial effects in treatment of intermittent claudication: results from a multicenter, randomized, prospective, double-blind trial. *Circulation* 1998;98:678–686.
68. Money SR, Herd JA, Isaacsohn JL, et al. Effect of cilostazol on walking distances in patients with intermittent claudication caused by peripheral vascular disease. *J Vasc Surg* 1998;27:267–274.
69. Beebe HG, Dawson DL, Cutler BS, et al. A new pharmacological treatment for intermittent claudication: results of a randomized, multicenter trial. *Arch Intern Med* 1999;159:2041–2050.

CHAPTER 5

Peripheral Arterial Disease in Patients with Diabetes

Peter Sheehan

Key Points

- Peripheral arterial disease (PAD) is a manifestation of atherosclerosis and a hallmark for atherothrombotic disease. It is associated with a high risk for cardiovascular events.
- The genesis of atherosclerosis can pre-date the diagnosis of diabetes.
- PAD in diabetes is exceedingly prevalent and largely undetected due to the silent nature of its progression.
- Many diabetic patients may be asymptomatic or have atypical symptoms for claudication. Most symptoms are not volunteered and need to be asked about specifically.
- The ankle–brachial index may be unrealiable in diabetic patients due to calcified arteries. A toe pressure is the next appropriate test.
- Diabetic patients should be on an antiplatelet treatment and maintain a low-density lipoprotein level of less than 100 mg per dL.
- The loss of normal nitric oxide homeostasis can result in a potential cascade of vascular events.
- Diagnosis of PAD identifies patients with high risk for myocardial infarction, stroke, and death, and places emphasis on aggressive risk factor interventions.
- The complexity of the management of patients with diabetes and PAD requires a multidisciplinary approach.

INTRODUCTION

Diabetes mellitus is increasing in prevalence in near-epidemic proportions. In the United States, the prevalence has surpassed 7.3% of adults, a 48% increase from the 4.8% prevalence reported a decade ago (1). The number of people with diabetes in the United States exceeds 17 million; greater than 90% of this is type 2 diabetes (2).

The three factors most strongly associated with the rapid and dramatic increase in the number of people with diabetes in the United States are the increasing prevalence of obesity, the changing demographic and ethnic distribution of the population, and the aging of the population. Type 2 diabetes is an inherited metabolic disorder in which insulin resistance plays a primary role in pathophysiology. It is more common in certain ethnic groups, is brought on by aging, and is made precocious by obesity. The highest incidence worldwide is seen in Native Americans, but high rates are also seen in His-

panics, Polynesians, and people of Asian, South Asian, and African descent (3). Indeed, the country with the most people with diabetes is India, with greater than 40 million people afflicted.

Whites are in the lowest risk group for type 2 diabetes. The prevalence in the United States is increasing as the expansion of Hispanic, Asian, and African-American populations is occurring. In addition, Americans are more obese, with greater than 20% of adults having a body mass index greater than 30 (4). An additional factor is the aging of the large segment of the population born after World War II. The interplay of these three factors has led to the rapid expansion of the population of people diagnosed with type 2 diabetes in the United States. Unfortunately, the real impact of this epidemic has yet to be felt. The marked increase in the incidence of diabetes in the 1990s will manifest clinically in this decade as these people with diabetes present with the long-term complications of this devastating metabolic condition. The commonest and most life-threatening complication of type 2 diabetes is cardiovascular disease. With involvement of the coronary, cerebral, and peripheral vascular beds, this translates into increased risk of myocardial infarction, stroke, and amputation. It is imperative that clinicians prepare for this next wave of diabetic complications as these patients move into their second decade of disease.

Diabetes is a cardiovascular disease equivalent (5) and affects nearly every vascular bed; however, the pervasive influence of diabetes on the atherothrombotic milieu of the peripheral vasculature is unique. The abnormal metabolic state accompanying diabetes results in changes in the state of arterial structure and function. The onset of these changes may even pre-date the clinical diagnosis of diabetes. Whereas peripheral arterial disease (PAD) is common in diabetes, it is unique in its biology, presentation, and assessment and management compared to the PAD seen in other risk groups such as smokers and hypertensives. Thus, recommendations and guidelines used in the care of the patient with PAD and diabetes may differ from those used for the general population with PAD.

Recently, there have been attempts to make the evaluation and care for these patients more uniform. One such effort was a consensus development conference on PAD in patients with diabetes held jointly by the American Diabetes Association (ADA) and the American College of Cardiology (6). One key issue is the great need for diagnosis because this will identify patients with major cardiovascular risk, significant excess mortality, risk of disability and amputation. Increasing awareness of PAD in clinicians and patients should lead to improvements in assessment, management, and outcomes for this high-risk group.

This chapter discusses what is known and what needs to be learned about PAD and its unique and devastating consequences in patients with diabetes. The focus of the discussion is PAD, defined as lower extremity occlusive disease, and its prevalence and impact, biology, and assessment and management. It should become clear that diabetes stands alone in its power as a risk factor and in its unusual effects on the peripheral vasculature.

EPIDEMIOLOGY AND NATURAL HISTORY OF PERIPHERAL ARTERIAL DISEASE IN DIABETES

Diabetes as a Risk Factor for Peripheral Arterial Disease

Peripheral arterial disease is a manifestation of atherosclerosis characterized by occlusive disease of the lower extremities that may or may not have symptoms, and is a marker for atherothrombotic disease in other vascular beds (coronary and cerebral). PAD affects approximately 12 million people in the United States. It is uncertain how many of these have diabetes. Framingham data revealed that 20% of symptomatic patients with PAD had diabetes (7), but this probably greatly underestimates the prevalence, given that many more people with PAD are asymptomatic than are symptomatic. Estimates

are that diabetics may in fact comprise as many as 30% to 40% of patients with PAD. In the PARTNERS study, greater than 40% of patients diagnosed with PAD had diabetes, but this probably represents the bias of the selection criteria (8).

Although there are other well-known risk factors, such as advanced age, hypertension, and hyperlipidemia, diabetes and smoking are the strongest risk factors for PAD (9). Moreover, in at least one analysis, diabetes was the most strongly associated risk factor for PAD, with a relative risk of 4.06 (10). It has also become clear that the risk of PAD may precede the development of overt diabetes and hyperglycemia. The Framingham Heart Study showed a twofold excess of signs of PAD in 924 patients with impaired glucose intolerance (11). This underscores the cardiovascular impact of the metabolic syndrome of glucose intolerance, insulin resistance, and endothelial dysfunction, and lends weight to the new ADA classification of glucose intolerance as "pre-diabetes."

Other potential risk factors are also clustered within the diabetic population, and include elevated levels of fibrinogen, homocysteine, apolipoprotein B, and lipoprotein(a), and increased plasma viscosity. C-reactive protein has also been strongly associated with PAD (12). Hypertension and hypertriglyceridemia are two risk factors that cluster with diabetes and may also explain part of the excess PAD seen in diabetes (13). As for protective factors, an inverse relationship has been suggested between PAD and alcohol consumption.

For people with diabetes, the risk of PAD is further increased by age and the duration of diabetes (14). What has been described clinically is also found epidemiologically. There is a strong association of PAD with diabetic peripheral neuropathy (15). As will be discussed, this association and the coincidence of PAD and neuropathy have implications for the clinical presentation and for the progression of disease. In patients with diabetes, race is also significantly associated factor for PAD. African Americans and Hispanics with diabetes have a higher prevalence of PAD than non-Hispanic whites, even after adjustment for other known risk factors and the excess prevalence of diabetes. The relative risk for African Americans is 2.5 times, and that for Hispanics is 1.5 times, that of their white counterparts (M. Criqui, personal communication). Amputation incidence is also increased in African Americans and Hispanics, although this may also reflect less access to medical care (16).

It is important to note that diabetes as a PAD risk factor is unique in its pattern of disease expression: diabetes is most strongly associated with femoral–popliteal and tibial (below-the-knee) PAD, whereas other risk factors (e.g., smoking and hypertension) are associated with more proximal disease in the aortoiliofemoral vessels (17). Thus as a risk factor for PAD, diabetes stands alone: not only is it the most powerfully associated risk factor, but it uniquely involves the distal territories of the peripheral vasculature, a characteristic that proves crucial in understanding its clinical manifestations.

Prevalence and Impact of Peripheral Arterial Disease in Diabetes

The true prevalence of PAD in persons with diabetes has been difficult to determine because most patients are asymptomatic, or the symptoms are atypical and many persons do not report them. Furthermore, pain perception may be blunted by the frequent presence of peripheral neuropathy. In addition, screening modalities have not been uniformly agreed on or validated. Whereas amputation has been used by some as a measure for PAD prevalence, medical care and local indications for amputation versus revascularization of the patient with critical limb ischemia vary widely. The nationwide age-adjusted amputation rate in diabetes is approximately 8 per 1,000 patient-years, with a prevalence of approximately 3%. However, there is great variability because of the nonuniformity of care. In a study of amputations in Medicare beneficiaries with diabetes, there was nearly a ninefold variation of amputation incidence in the 306 Medicare regions across the United States. Therefore, the incidence and prevalence of amputation may be an imprecise reflection of PAD in diabetes, tainted by bias and randomness of care.

The reported prevalence of PAD is also affected by the methods by which the diagnosis is sought. The most common assessments are the absence of peripheral pulses and a history of claudication. Both, however, suffer from gross insensitivity. A more accurate estimation of the prevalence of PAD in diabetes should rely on the ankle–brachial index (ABI), a validated and reproducible test, which involves measuring the systolic blood pressure in the ankles (dorsalis pedis and posterior tibial arteries) and arms (brachial artery) using a handheld Doppler probe and then calculating a ratio. Simple to perform, it is a noninvasive, quantitative measurement of the patency of the lower extremity arterial system. It has been validated against angiographically confirmed disease, and found to be 95% sensitive and almost 100% specific (19). There are some limitations, however, in using the ABI. Medial arterial calcinosis (MAC) with poorly compressible vessels in the elderly and some patients with diabetes may artificially elevate values. The ABI may also be falsely normal in symptomatic patients with moderate aortoiliac stenoses.

Although these issues complicate the evaluation of an individual patient, they are not prevalent enough to detract from the usefulness of the ABI as an effective epidemiologic test to screen for and diagnose PAD in patients with diabetes. Using ABI, one recent survey in Scotland found a prevalence of PAD in people with type 1 and type 2 diabetes greater than 40 years of age to be greater than 20%, a prevalence greater than anticipated using less reliable measures such as symptoms or absent pulses (20). Moreover, in the PARTNERS study, another survey of patients with diabetes age greater than 50 years of age by general practitioners using the ABI, the prevalence of PAD was 29% (8). It is important to note that most of the patients with PAD were newly diagnosed, and only a small percentage had classic claudication. Thus, the true prevalence of PAD in diabetes, which is largely silent and undetected, appears much higher than previously estimated.

The clinical impact of PAD can be assessed by from two perspectives: first, its progression and the onset or worsening of symptoms, and, second, the excess risk of cardiovascular events associated with systemic atherosclerosis. With regard to disease progression, most patients with PAD remain stable in their symptoms. Over a 5-year period, about 27% of patients with PAD demonstrate progression of symptoms, with limb loss occurring in about 4%. However, whereas the majority of patients remain stable in their lower limb symptomatology, there is systemic atherosclerosis with a striking excess in cardiovascular event rates over the same 5-year time period: 20% of PAD patients sustain nonfatal events (myocardial infarction, stroke) and a 30% die (21). The outcomes and prognosis for more diseased patients with critical limb ischemia (CLI) are predictably worse. Within 6 months of presentation, 30% will have amputations and 20% will die (22). The natural history of PAD in patients with diabetes in particular has not specifically been studied longitudinally; however, it is known from prospective clinical trials of risk interventions that the cardiovascular event rates in patients with PAD and diabetes are higher than those of their nondiabetic counterparts. Thus it is firmly believed that the 5-year natural history for those with diabetes and PAD is worse than that described for PAD alone.

As previously mentioned, the frequent presence of neuropathy strongly influences the clinical presentation. The presence of neuropathy blunts pain perception and makes symptoms such as claudication less common, allowing a later presentation with more severe lesions than in the nondiabetic patient. In a vicious cycle, the presence of PAD increases nerve ischemia and hypoxia, resulting in worsened sensory neuropathy (23). In addition, such arterial lesions may progress undetected for long intervals due to the distal distribution, also making the severity of the underlying PAD often underestimated. This helps explain the unanticipated high prevalence of PAD in diabetes, which has been largely undetected by methods that rely on historical or physical clues. When the patient finally develops symptoms, it is often a late manifestation of severe underlying disease. Accordingly, diabetic patients with PAD are more likely to present with advanced disease compared to nondiabetic patients, often with an ulcer and critical limb ischemia as a presenting symptom (24).

THE PATHOPHYSIOLOGY AND BIOLOGY OF PERIPHERAL ARTERIAL DISEASE IN DIABETES

The proatherogenic changes associated with diabetes are extensive and complex, and have been reviewed more thoroughly than can be allowed in this chapter (25). The genesis of atheroscerosis may pre-date the diagnosis of diabetes. Factors involved include derangements in the regulation of blood flow, abnormalities in the components of blood vessels, and alterations in coagulation and rheology. Thus, atherogenic factors in diabetes can be viewed as Virchow's triad fulfilled (I. Jialal, personal communication). In addition, the changes result in activation of inflammatory pathways, which increase activity of the disease. These changes are associated with an increased risk for accelerated atherogenesis as well as poor outcomes. Given the large size of the peripheral vascular bed, the potential impact of these abnormalities is great.

DIABETES AND ENDOTHELIAL CELL DYSFUNCTION

The endothelial cell lining of the arterial vasculature is a biologically active organ. It modulates the relationship between the cellular elements of the blood and the vascular wall, which mediates the normal balance between thrombosis and fibrinolysis and plays an integral role in leukocyte/cell wall interactions. Abnormalities of endothelial function can render the arterial system susceptible to atherosclerosis and its associated adverse outcomes.

Most patients with diabetes, including those with PAD, demonstrate abnormalities of endothelial function and vascular regulation (26). The mediators of endothelial cell dysfunction in diabetes are numerous, but an important final common pathway is derangement of nitric oxide (NO) bioavailability. Nitric oxide is a potent stimulus for vasodilation and limits inflammation via its modulation of leukocyte–vascular wall interaction. Furthermore, NO inhibits vascular smooth muscle cell migration and proliferation and limits platelet activation. Therefore, the loss of normal NO homeostasis can result in the risk of a cascade of events in the vasculature, leading to atherosclerosis and its consequent complications (27).

Several mechanisms contribute to endothelial dysfunction, including hyperglycemia, insulin resistance, and free fatty acid production. Hyperglycemia blocks the function of endothelial nitric oxide synthase (eNOS), and boosts production of reactive oxygen species, which impairs the vasodilator homeostasis fostered by endothelium. This oxidative stress is amplified because, in endothelial cells, glucose transport is not downregulated by hyperglycemia (28).

In addition to hyperglycemia, insulin resistance plays a role in the loss of normal NO homeostasis, and endothelial dysfunction has been described in insulin-resistant states, including those in first-degree relatives of type 2 diabetics, pre-diabetes, and the metabolic syndrome. This suggests the primacy of endothelial dysfunction in the pathogenesis of atherosclerosis, and explains the onset of vascular disease before the advent of hyperglycemia. The impaired vasoreactivity in response to insulin signaling also may explain in part the defects in glucose metabolism in that there is inadequate fuel delivery to muscle capillary beds (29).

Another consequence of insulin resistance is excess liberation of free fatty acids (FFAs). FFAs may have numerous deleterious effects on normal vascular homeostasis and insulin signaling and sensitivity. With hyperglycemia and oxidative stress, there is accumulation of diacylglycerol intracellularly and activation of protein kinase C (30). In addition, FFAs inhibit the insulin receptor substrate-1 (IRS-1) insulin signaling pathway (an eNOS/vasodilatory pathway), and in turn activate the mitogen-activated protein (MAP) kinase pathway, which is proinflammatory and potentially atherogenic (31). The sum effect of all these leads to the loss of NO homeostasis.

Ultimately, the effects of endothelial cell dysfunction, along with activation of the receptor for advanced glycation end products (RAGE), increase the local inflammatory state of the vascular wall, mediated in part by increased production of the transcription factors nuclear factor-κB (NF-κB) and activator protein-1. In addition, there is increased expression of adhesion molecules. Local increases in these proinflammatory factors, together with the loss of normal NO function, are associated with increased leukocyte chemotaxis, adhesion, transmigration, and transformation into foam cells (32). The latter process is further augmented by increased local oxidative stress. Foam cell transformation is the earliest precursor of atheroma formation.

Diabetes, Inflammation, and Risk for Peripheral Arterial Disease

Inflammation has been established as both a risk marker and perhaps a risk factor for atherothrombotic disease states, including PAD (33). As mentioned earlier, elevated levels of C-reactive protein (CRP) are strongly associated with the development of PAD. In addition, levels of CRP are abnormally elevated in patients with insulin-resistant states, including impaired glucose tolerance (IGT) and diabetes. In addition to being a marker of disease presence, elevation of CRP may also be a culprit in the causation or exacerbation of PAD. CRP has been found to bind to endothelial cell receptors promoting apoptosis, and has been shown to colocalize with oxidized low-density lipoprotein in atherosclerotic plaques. CRP also stimulates endothelial production of procoagulant, tissue factor, and leukocyte adhesion and chemotactic substances. It also inhibits eNOS, resulting in abnormalities in the regulation of vascular tone. Finally, CRP may increase the local production of compounds impairing fibrinolysis, such as plasminogen activator inhibitor-1 (PAI-1) (34).

Diabetes and the Vascular Smooth Muscle Cell

The presence of diabetes is also associated with significant abnormalities in vascular smooth muscle cell (VSMC) function. Diabetes stimulates proatherogenic activity in VSMC via mechanisms similar to that in endothelial cells, including reductions in phosphatidylinositol (PI)-3 kinase, as well as local increases in oxidative stress and upregulation of protein kinase C, RAGE, and NF-κB. The sum total of these changes might be expected to promote the formation of atherosclerotic lesions. These effects also may increase VSMC apoptosis and tissue factor production while reducing *de novo* synthesis of plaque-stabilizing compounds such as collagen. Thus, the foregoing events accelerate atherosclerosis, and are also associated with plaque destabilization and precipitation of clinical events (35).

DIABETES AND THE PLATELET

Platelets play an integral role in the connection between vascular function and thrombosis. Abnormalities in platelet biology not only may promote the progression of atherosclerosis, but also may influence the consequence of plaque disruption and atherothrombosis. As in the endothelial cell, platelet uptake of glucose is unchecked in the setting of hyperglycemia, and similar to the endothelial cell, hyperglycemia results in increased oxidative stress. Consequently, platelet aggregation is enhanced in patients with diabetes. Platelets in patients with diabetes also have increased expression of glycoprotein Ib and IIb/IIIa receptors, which are important in thrombosis via their role in adhesion and aggregation.

DIABETES, COAGULATION, AND RHEOLOGY

Diabetes leads to a hypercoagulable state (36). It is associated with the increased production of tissue factor by endothelial cells and VSMC, as well as increased plasma concentrations of factor VII. Hyperglycemia is also associated with a decreased concentration of antithrombin and protein C, impaired fibrinolytic function, and excess production of PAI-1.

Finally, abnormalities in rheology are seen in diabetes patients including elevation in blood viscosity and fibrinogen. Elevated viscosity and fibrinogen are both correlative with abnormalities in ankle–brachial index among patients with PAD, and elevated fibrinogen (or its degradation products) has been associated with the development, presence, and complications of PAD (37).

In summary, diabetes increases the risk for atherogenesis via deleterious effects on the vessel wall and also has effects on blood cells and rheology. The vascular abnormalities leading to atherosclerosis in patients with diabetes may be evident prior to the diagnosis of diabetes, and they increase with duration of diabetes and worsening blood glucose control. Further studies of the diabetes-specific mechanisms responsible for the development of atherosclerosis, as well as the specific pathways responsible for PAD in this population, are needed.

CLINICAL MANIFESTATIONS AND PRESENTATION OF PERIPHERAL ARTERIAL DISEASE IN DIABETES

The most common symptom of PAD is intermittent claudication, classically defined as pain, cramping, or aching in the calves, thighs, or buttocks that appears reproducibly with walking and is relieved by rest. More extreme presentations of PAD include rest pain, tissue loss, and gangrene. These limb-threatening manifestations of PAD are collectively termed critical limb ischemia. Most patients with PAD are asymptomatic. It has been reported that of those with PAD, over half are asymptomatic or have atypical symptoms, about one-third have claudication, and the remainder have more severe forms of the disease (38).

It is important for the clinician to understand that the presentation of people with diabetes and PAD differs distinctly from those with PAD from other risk factors, such as smoking and hypertension. Although diabetes is an important risk factor for claudication, in patients with diabetes, PAD is often more subtle in its presentation than in those without diabetes. This is related to the pattern of disease distribution and the association with neuropathy. In contrast to the focal and proximal atherosclerotic lesions of PAD found typically in other high-risk patients, in patients with diabetes the lesions are more likely to be more diffuse and distal. Importantly, PAD in persons with diabetes is usually accompanied by peripheral neuropathy with impaired sensory feedback, enabling the silent progression of occlusive disease. Thus, although a classic history of claudication may be less common in diabetes, one may elicit more subtle symptoms such as leg fatigue and slow walking velocity, which the patient may attribute to simply getting older. Indeed, despite the paucity of symptoms, it has been reported that patients with diabetes and PAD experience worse lower extremity function than those with PAD alone (39).

Belying the seriousness of their disease, asymptomatic diabetic patients who have been identified with PAD are also more prone to the danger of the sudden ischemia of arterial thrombosis. In one series, the incidence of acute arterial thombosis in PAD was 35%, with a 21% risk of major amputation in patients with diabetes, compared with 19% and 3%, respectively, in those without diabetes (40). A patient with diabetes and asymptomatic PAD could also have a "pivotal event" that leads acutely to an ischemic ulcer and a limb-threatening situation. A typical story would be a man with PAD and neuropathy who wears a tight-fitting dress shoe to a wedding, and develops an ulcer at the day-long affair. In contrast to the plantar location of neuropathic ulcers, ischemic ulcers are commonly seen around the edges of the foot, including the apices of the toes and the back of the heel. Thus, an asymptomatic, usually undiagnosed patient can lapse abruptly into critical limb ischemia. Clearly, by identifying a patient with subclinical disease and instituting preventative measures, it may be possible to avoid acute, limb-threatening ischemia.

As mentioned previously, PAD is also a major risk factor for lower extremity amputation, especially in a patient with diabetes. Moreover, even for the asymptomatic patient, PAD is a marker for systemic vascular disease involving coronary, cerebral, and renal vessels, leading to an elevated risk of events such as myocardial infarction, stroke, and death. In a study that compared patients with PAD with and without diabetes, those with diabetes had more severe disease below the knee, had a fivefold higher amputation rate, and had double the mortality of the nondiabetics despite similar ABI values (41).

Perhaps most importantly, it should be appreciated that PAD in diabetes also adversely affects quality of life, contributing to long-term disability and functional impairment that is often severe. Patients with claudication have a slower walking speed (generally less than 2 miles per hour) and have limited walking distance. The functioning level is comparable to New York State Heart class III (42). In addition, those with diabetes have worse function even in the absence of claudication, as mentioned. This may result in a "cycle of disability" with progressive deconditioning and loss of function. Too often this initiates a downward spiral to an overall affective and social decline for the patient.

EVALUATION AND ASSESSMENT OF PERIPHERAL ARTERIAL DISEASE IN DIABETES

Clinical Evaluation: History and Physical

Diagnosing PAD is of clinical importance for two reasons. The first is to identify a patient who has a high risk of subsequent myocardial infarction or stroke regardless of whether symptoms of PAD are present. Some have even advocated that PAD be considered a "coronary disease equivalent." The second is to elicit and treat symptoms of PAD, which may be associated with functional disability and risk of limb loss, and attempt to prevent progression of disease.

The initial assessment of PAD in patients with diabetes should begin with a thorough medical history and physical examination to help identify those patients with PAD risk factors, symptoms of claudication, rest pain, and/or functional impairment. Alternative causes of leg pain on exercise are many, including spinal stenosis, and should be excluded. PAD patients present along a spectrum of severity ranging from no symptoms, to intermittent claudication, to rest pain, and finally to nonhealing wounds and gangrene.

A thorough walking history may elicit classic claudication symptoms, though more patients may have atypical symptoms, and most are asymptomatic. In the PARTNERS study, only 5.5% of patients had classic claudication, and almost half had atypical symptoms. Interestingly, a substantial portion of patients may present with PAD and unrelated leg pain resulting from musculoskeletal or neuropathic causes. In a study of patients with PAD as identified by a vascular laboratory, 56% had exertional leg symptoms other than claudication (8). Diabetes, male sex, and older age were associated independently with an absence of exertional symptoms (43). Because most symptoms are often not volunteered, patients should be asked specifically about them.

Two important components of the physical examination are visual inspection of the foot and palpation of peripheral pulses. Dependent rubor, pallor on elevation, absence of hair growth, dystrophic toenails, and cool, dry, fissured skin are signs of vascular insufficiency and should be noted. The interdigital spaces should be inspected for fissures, ulcerations, and infections (44). These signs are extremely useful in distinguishing rest pain from neuropathic pain, as both often have nocturnal exacerbation—rest pain because of recumbancy, neurpathic pain with inactivity. A history of dangling the extremities also supports the diagnosis of rest pain.

Palpation of peripheral pulses should be a routine component of the physical exam and should include assessment of the femoral, popliteal, and pedal vessels. It should be noted that pulse assessment is a learned skill and has a high degree of interobserver variability, with high false-positive and false-negative rates. The dorsalis pedis pulse is reported to be absent in 8.1% of healthy individuals and the posterior tibial pulse is absent in 0.2% (45). In a study of patients with foot and leg ulcers, 15.4% of patients with absent pulses had an ABI within normal limits; conversely, and more striking, 38.8% of patients with palpable pulses had an ABI less than 0.9 (46). Nevertheless, the absence of both pedal pulses, when assessed by a person experienced in this technique, strongly suggests the presence of vascular disease.

Noninvasive Evaluation for Peripheral Arterial Disease: Ankle–Brachial Index

In contrast to the variability of pulse assessment and the often nonspecific nature of information obtained via history and other components of the physical exam, the ABI is a reproducible and reasonably accurate, noninvasive measurement for the detection of PAD and the determination of disease severity (47). The ABI is defined, as noted previously, as the ratio of the highest systolic blood pressure in the ankle divided by the highest systolic blood pressure at the arm. The only tools required to perform the ABI measurement include a handheld 5- to 10-MHz Doppler probe and a blood pressure cuff. An ABI of less than or equal to 0.90 is diagnostic of PAD. An ABI value of greater than 1.3 suggests poorly compressible arteries at the ankle level due to the presence of medial arterial calcification, an issue not uncommon in the diabetic population. This renders the diagnosis of PAD by ABI alone less reliable, and further noninvasive evaluation is necessary. It should be noted that in the evaluation of the individual patient with any test there may be errors, and that the reliability of any diagnostic test is dependent on the prior probability of disease (Bayes's theorem).

Because of the high estimated prevalence of PAD in patients with diabetes, and because most patients are asymptomatic, the American Diabetes Association has recommended that a screening ABI should be performed in patients over 50 years of age who have diabetes (5). If normal, the test should be repeated every 5 years. A screening ABI should be considered in diabetic patients less than 50 years of age who have other PAD risk factors (e.g., smoking, hypertension, hyperlipidemia, or duration of diabetes greater than

10 years). Certainly, a diagnostic ABI should be performed in any patient with symptoms of PAD.

Additional Evaluation

Because the ABI may be unreliable in patients with diabetes and calcified blood vessels, evaluation of a toe pressure is the next appropriate test. A toe/brachial index of less than 0.7 is diagnostic of PAD. In patients with possible critical limb ischemia, a systolic toe pressure may help with clinical decision making regarding revascularization. A toe pressure of less than 40 mm Hg or a toe waveform of less than 4 mm may predict impaired wound healing, and is often used in the evaluation of ischemic ulcer (48). Another method of predicting healing is the measurement of the transcutaneous partial pressure of oxygen ($TcPO_2$). A value less than 30 mm Hg is associated with poor healing of wounds or amputations. Conversely, an initial or postinterventional $TcPO_2$ of greater than 30 mm Hg is almost 90% predictive of healing, and is more accurate than a palpable pedal pulse (49).

Vascular Lab Evaluation: Segmental Pressures and Pulse Volume Recordings

In the patient with a confirmed diagnosis of PAD in whom assessment of the location and severity is desired, the next step is a vascular laboratory evaluation for segmental pressures and pulse volume recordings (PVR). These tests should also be considered for patients with poorly compressible vessels or those with a normal ABI where there is high suspicion of PAD. Segmental pressures and PVRs are determined at the toe, ankle, calf, low thigh, and high thigh. Segmental pressures help with localization of the stenosis or occlusion, and PVRs provide segmental plethysmographic wave form analysis, a qualitative assessment of blood flow.

Treadmill Functional Testing

For patients with atypical symptoms, or a normal ABI with typical symptoms of claudication, functional testing with a graded treadmill may help with diagnosis. The best example is the patient with an ileofemoral stenosis. Patients with claudication typically exhibit a greater than 20-mm Hg drop in the ABI after exercise, allowing a diagnosis to be made. Treadmill testing may also be used as an evaluation of treatment efficacy and as an assessment of physical function, usually at a safe, low work load at 2 miles per hour with small uphill grade.

Anatomic Studies: Duplex Sonography, Magnetic Resonance Angiogram, Contrast Angiography

For those patients in whom revascularization is considered and anatomic localization of stenoses or occlusions is important, an evaluation with a duplex ultrasound or a magnetic resonance angiogram (MRA) may be valuable. Duplex ultrasound can directly visualize vessels, and is also useful in the surveillance of postprocedure patients for graft or stent patency. MRA is noninvasive with minimal risk of renal insult. It may give images that are comparable to conventional x-ray angiography especially in occult pedal vessels, and may be used for anatomic diagnosis. This is especially important in patients with diabetes and tibial disease, where identifying a suitable pedal target vessel is crucial for the success of bypass surgery (50). MRA is rapidly gaining utility in preoperative assessment, especially in the patient with diabetes and difficult-to-visualize pedal vessels. Most centers utilize both contrast-enhanced and time-of-flight images.

Although MRA is a safe and promising new technology, the gold standard for vascular imaging remains x-ray angiography, and it is indicated primarily for the anatomic evaluation of only the patient in whom a revascularization procedure is intended. Because it is an invasive test with a small risk of contrast-induced nephrotoxicity, "exploratory" angiography should not be performed for diagnosing PAD. For patients with suspected pedal ischemia, the angiography should include an aortogram with selective unilateral runoff and a magnified lateral view of the foot to identify candidate target vessels. It should be noted that the decision to perform an angiogram can be made on a clinical basis by an experienced clinician on the need for revascularization, sometimes independent of any prior noninvasive tests.

TREATMENT OF PERIPHERAL ARTERIAL DISEASE IN PATIENTS WITH DIABETES

Treatment of Systemic Atherosclerosis Associated with Peripheral Arterial Disease

Diabetes is now recognized as a cardiovascular equivalent, and thus the clinician is compelled to place the patient with diabetes into primary risk factor interventions. The presence of PAD further increases the risk of cardiovascular events, and suggests considerations for secondary risk interventions. The ADA publishes these clinical practice recommendations annually. The ADA slogan of "know your ABC's" of primary risk interventions refers to A1c (the hemoglobin A1c test), blood pressure, and cholesterol, with target values of A1c less than 7%, blood pressure less than 130/80, and low-density lipoprotein (LDL) cholesterol less than 100 mg%. For people with both PAD and diabetes specifically, there is little prospective data showing that treating these risk factors will improve cardiovascular outcomes; however, expert consensus strongly supports such interventions given that both PAD and diabetes are associated with significantly increased risks of cardiovascular events. Thus, patients with diabetes should be managed by current guidelines; those with PAD as well may benefit from more aggressive interventions.

Cigarette Smoking

Cigarette smoking is the single most important modifiable risk factor for the development and exacerbation of PAD. In patients with PAD, tobacco use is associated with increased progression of atherosclerosis as well as increased risk of amputation (51). Smoking cessation is recommended for all patients with diabetes and/or PAD, with an expectation of improved symptoms and fewer cardiovascular events (52).

Glycemic Control

Hyperglycemia is a contributing cardiovascular risk factor in persons with PAD. Unfortunately, evidence for the benefit of tight glycemic control in ameliorating cardiovascular complications is lacking. In the United Kingdom Prospective Diabetes Study (UKPDS), intensive glycemic control reduced diabetes-related endpoints and diabetes-related deaths compared to conventional treatment (53). However, it was not associated with a significant reduction in the risk of cardiovascular events. In fact, the major reduction in adverse endpoints was due to improved microvascular rather than macrovascular endpoints, with the exception of fewer myocardial infarctions in the subset of the tight control group treated with metformin monotherapy. Although it is likely that many patients with peripheral arterial disease were included in the UKPDS study, the prevalence of PAD was not defined, so that conclusions from this study may not directly relate to patients with diabetes and PAD. Approximately 14% of patients had an absent pedal pulse at entry (54); however, this is not a sensitive or specific criterion for the diagnosis of PAD. Thus, the outcomes of those with PAD are not clear. Despite the fact that there were no differences in amputations between the two groups, one cannot draw conclusions on the effect, or lack thereof, of tight glycemic control on the natural history of PAD. Nevertheless, good glycemic control (hemoglobin A1c less than 7.0%) should be a goal of therapy in patients with PAD and diabetes to prevent microvascular complications.

Hypertension

Hypertension is associated with the development of atherosclerosis and a two- to threefold increased risk of claudication (55). In the UKPDS, diabetic endpoints and risks of strokes were significantly reduced, and risk of myocardial infarction was nonsignificantly reduced, by tight blood pressure control (56). It is noteworthy that this significant improvement in outcomes was related to only a 10-mm Hg lowering of the systolic pressure in the intensely treated group. Risk for amputation due to PAD was not reduced, but once again, the results are limited by the lack of clear diagnostic criteria for PAD in the study.

The benefits of treating hypertension for atherosclerotic disease or for cardiovascular events have not been directly evaluated in patients with both PAD and diabetes specifically. Nevertheless, consensus still strongly supports aggressive blood pressure control (less than 130/80 mm Hg) in patients with PAD and diabetes, to reduce cardiovascular risk (57).

Results of the Heart Outcomes Prevention Evaluation study showed that the use of ramipril, an angiotensin-converting enzyme (ACE) inhibitor, in normotensive high-risk patients, including diabetics, significantly reduced the rate of cardiovascular death, myocardial infarction, and stroke (58).

The benefit was greater in the subgroup of patients with diabetes. Of the greater than 9000 patients in this study, almost half had PAD. Patients with PAD had a similar reduction in the cardiovascular endpoints as those without PAD. Thus ramipril was effective in lowering the risk of fatal and nonfatal ischemic events among all patients, especially those with diabetes, and including those with PAD. Nonetheless, the potential benefit of ACE inhibitors has not been studied in prospective, randomized trials in patients with PAD. Such trials are needed before making definite treatment recommendations regarding the use of an ACE inhibitor as a unique pharmacologic agent in the treatment of PAD.

Finally, a smaller series published recently demonstrated that intensively treating normotensive patients with diabetes and PAD with an ACE inhibitor or a calcium channel blocker resulted in a significant reduction in cardiovascular events (13.6%) compared to placebo controls (38.7%) over a 4-year period (59). If similar results confirm this finding, the impetus for treating normotensive patients with diabetes and PAD will be hastened, and will make the diagnosis of PAD more crucial in guidelines for blood pressure control in patients with diabetes.

Dyslipidemia

Although treating dyslipidemia decreases cardiovascular morbidity and mortality in general, no studies have prospectively studied the treatment of lipid disorders in patients with PAD. In a meta-analysis of randomized trials in patients with PAD and dyslipidemia who were treated by a variety of therapies, Leng et al. reported a nonsignificant reduction in mortality and no change in nonfatal cardiovascular events (60). However, the severity of claudication was reduced by lipid-lowering treatment. Similarly, in a subgroup analysis of the Scandinavian Simvastatin Survival Study, the reduction in cholesterol level by simvastatin was associated with a 38% reduction in the risk of new or worsening symptoms of intermittent claudication (61,62). In the Heart Protection Study, adults with coronary disease, other occlusive arterial disease, or diabetes were randomly allocated to receive simvastatin or placebo. A significant reduction in coronary death rate was observed in people with PAD, but the reduction was similar to and no greater than the effect of the drug on other subgroups (63). Thus, although there are no data showing direct benefits of treating dyslipidemia in persons with *both* PAD and diabetes, dyslipidemia in diabetic patients should be treated according to published guidelines. The American Diabetes Association recommends a target LDL cholesterol level of less than 100 mg per dL (64). Following this guideline, it is believed that lipid-lowering treatment not only may decrease cardiovascular deaths, but also may slow the progression of PAD in diabetes.

Antiplatelet Therapy

The Antiplatelet Trialists' Collaboration reviewed 145 randomized studies in an effort to evaluate the efficacy of prolonged treatment with antiplatelet agents (in most cases, aspirin) (65). This meta-analysis combined data from more than 100,000 patients, including approximately 70,000 high-risk patients with evidence of cardiovascular disease. A 27% reduction in odds ratio in the composite primary endpoint (myocardial infarction, stroke, and vascular death) was found for high-risk patients compared to controls. However, when a subset of greater than 3,000 patients with claudication was analyzed, effects of antiplatelet therapy were not significant. The relative risk reduction of aspirin over placebo was 15%; however, the confidence intervals showed overlap and lack of statistical significance. Thus, the use of aspirin to prevent cardiovascular events and death in patients with PAD specifically is considered equivocal, although, aspirin therapy is recommended by the ADA for people with diabetes (66).

The Clopidogrel versus Aspirin in Patients at Risk of Ischemic Events (CAPRIE) Study evaluated aspirin versus clopidogrel in greater than 19,000 patients with recent stroke, myocardial infarction, or stable PAD (67). The study results showed that 75 mg of clopidogrel per day was associated with a relative risk reduction of 8.7% compared to the benefits of 325 mg of aspirin per day for a composite endpoint (myocardial infarction, ischemic stroke, and vascular death). More striking, in a subgroup analysis of greater than 6,000 patients with PAD, clopidogrel was associated with a risk reduction of 24% compared to aspirin. Clopidogrel was shown to be as well tolerated as aspirin. Based on these results, clopidogrel was approved by the U.S. Food and Drug Administration (FDA) for the reduction of ischemic events in all patients with PAD. Additionally, in the CAPRIE study, about one-third of the patients had diabetes. In those patients, clopidogrel was also superior to aspirin therapy, with a significant absolute risk reduction in total events (68). Because of the higher event rate in the subgroup with diabetes, the relative risk reduction with clopidogrel was comparable to that for the nondiabetics.

In summary, patients with diabetes should be on an antiplatelet agent (e.g., aspirin or clopidogrel) according to current guidelines (28). Those with diabetes and PAD may benefit more by taking clopidogrel.

TREATMENT OF SYMPTOMATIC PERIPHERAL ARTERIAL DISEASE

Intermittent Claudication

Medical therapy for intermittent claudication currently supports exercise rehabilitation as the cornerstone therapy, along with the adjunctive use of pharmacologic agents.

Exercise Rehabilitation

Since 1966, many randomized, controlled trials have demonstrated benefit of supervised exercise training in persons with PAD (69,70). The American Medical Association has recently issued a CPT-4 code to allow reimbursement to facilities conducting exercise programs. These programs call for at least 3 months of intermittent treadmill walking three times per week. Exercise therapy has minimal associated morbidity and is likely to improve the cardiovascular risk factor profile. Of note, however, in nearly all studies, unsupervised exercise regimens have shown lack of efficacy in improving functional capacity (71).

Pharmacologic Therapies

Pentoxifylline, a hemorheologic agent, was approved by the FDA in 1984 for treating claudication. The putative mechanism of action is an increase in red cell deformability. It may also have antiinflammatory effects. The results of postapproval trials, however, suggest that it does not increase walking distance to a clinically meaningful extent. Thus it is given tepid endorsement for the treatment of claudication, in that it is a safe drug that is possibly effective.

Cilostazol was the second drug to gain FDA approval for treating intermittent claudication. It is an oral phosphodiesterase type III inhibitor, and has effects on platelets, thrombosis, and lipids. Its main mechanism of action is probably as a vasodilator acting on vascular smooth muscle. Significant benefit has been demonstrated in increasing maximal walking time in six of eight randomized controlled trials, in addition to improved functional status and health-related quality of life (72). Because of its relatedness to milranone, anther phosphodiesterase III inhibitor, use of this drug is contraindicated if any degree of heart failure is present due to concerns about arrhythmias. In a single trial with a placebo arm, pentoxifyllinewas inferior to treatment with cilostazol (73). Based on these results, cilostazol is the drug of choice if pharmacologic therapy is necessary for the management of PAD in patients with diabetes.

Treatment of the "Neuroischemic Foot"

In contrast to the plantar location of neuropathic ulcers, ischemic ulcers are commonly seen around the edges of the foot, including the apices of the toes and the back of the heel. They are generally associated with a pivotal event: trauma or wearing unsuitable shoes. Important aspects of conservative management include debridement, offloading the ulcer, appropriate dressings, and treatment of infection (74).

Debridement

Debridement should remove all debris and necrotic material to render infection less likely. The preferred method is frequent sharp debridement with a scalpel, normally undertaken at the hospital bedside or in the outpatient setting. Ischemic ulcers are often dry, and have less depth than neuropathic ulcers, so they may also respond to mild enzymatic debriding agents. Urgent indications for surgical debridement include the presence of necrotic tissue, localized fluctuance, drainage of pus, or crepitus with gas in the soft tissues on x-ray examination. Even when ischemia is present, the drainage of contained infection is paramount and should be initiated without delay. Thereafter, plans can be made for revascularization if necessary.

Off-loading

With the neuroischemic foot, the chief aim is to protect the foot from pressure and shear. Ulcers may be prevented from healing if the patient wears ill-fitting or inappropriate shoes. Unlike neuropathic ulcers, which result from elevated plantar pressures, ischemic ulcers more often result from friction and shear (75). It is most important that the shoe does no harm. A shoe that is sufficiently long, broad, and deep and fastens with a lace or strap high on the foot may be all that is needed to protect the margins of the foot and allow healing of the ulcers. It may be necessary, however, to provide special footwear, such as open sandals or short leg-walker braces.

Dressings

Nonadherent dressings should cover diabetic foot ulcers at all times. No single ideal dressing exists, and there is no evidence that any one dressing is better for the diabetic foot than any other. However, the following properties are desirable: ease of removal from the ulcer, nonadherence to healthy tissue, patient comfort, and ability to accommodate pressures of walking. Occlusive dressings may lower the risk of infection. Xeroform dressings are often preferred for their additional stringent and antimicrobial effects. Full-strength antiseptics and iodine solution are discouraged, as they may be toxic to healthy tissue.

Treatment of Infection

Whereas ulcers often become infected, the signs and symptoms of foot infection are diminished in diabetic patients. The early warning signs of infection may be subtle because of an impaired neuroinflammatory response. Furthermore, it may be difficult to differentiate between the erythema of cellulitis and the rubor of ischemia. The redness of ischemia, which is most marked on dependency, will disappear on elevation of the limb, whereas that of cellulitis will remain irrespective of foot position.

Infections in the foot can be classified according to their severity. Non-limb-threatening infections are defined as having less than 2 cm of surrounding cellulites with no evidence of abscess, osteomyeltis, or gangrene. In contrast, limb-threatening infections are characterized by extensive cellulites, or deep space infection with abscess, osteomyelitis, or gangrene. Both wet and dry gangrene can occur in the neuroischemic foot. Wet gangrene is caused by a septic arteritis, secondary to soft-tissue infection or ulceration. Non-limb-threatening (superficial) infections are usually caused by gram-positve bacteria, so an oral cephalosporin, clindamycin, or beta-lactam is appropriate. Recently, a randomized trial showed that linezolid was superior to ampicillin/sulbactam for infected diabetic ulcers (76), and it is now the preferred antibiotic, with an FDA indication. Deep infections in the diabetic foot are often polymicrobial with gram-negative bacteria and anaerobes in addition to gram-positive bacteria. Nearly half of infected ulcers harbor *Staphylococcus aureus*. Broad-spectrum antibiotics are initially indicated. A lactam/lactamase inhibitor, clindamycin with a fluoroquinalone, or ertepenam would be reasonable empiric coverage. If concerns for methicillin-resistant stapholococci exist, then linezolid or vancomycin should be added to the regimen.

Severe infections require intravenous antibiotic therapy and urgent assessment of the need for surgical drainage and debridement. It is important to emphasize that medical treatment of infection with antibiotics alone is insufficient to resolve the majority of diabetic foot infections. In a large retrospective series, patients with foot infections had better outcomes when early surgical drainage and debridement was performed than with antibiotics alone (77).

Limb Salvage Procedures

Incision and drainage is the basic approach to treatment for nearly all infections of the diabetic foot. Sometimes amputation of a toe, toes, or ray(s) may be necessary to establish drainage. Salvage of the diabetic foot is usually possible, but may require aggressive debridement even in the setting of ischemia. Healthy tissue should be left intact. Postoperatively there may be considerable tissue deficit or exposure of bone or tendon. In such circumstances the foot should be revascularized as indicated and soft-tissue deficits may be repaired by reconstructive surgery at a latter stage. Outcomes may be improved when debridement, revascularization, and closure are staged patiently, with appreciation of the distict "angiosomes" or vascular territories of the foot (78). A vacuum-assisted wound-closure device provides topical subatmospheric pressure that is often helpful in staged procedures when wound-bed preparation is crucial.

Dry gangrene is secondary to a severe reduction in arterial perfusion and occurs in chronic critical ischemia. Revascularization should be initially carried out followed by surgical debridement. If revascularization is not possible, surgical debridement or amputation should be considered if the necrotic toe or any other area of necrosis is painful or if the circulation is not severely impaired. Otherwise the necrosis should be allowed to autoamputate, as a surgical procedure may result in further necrosis and a higher level of amputation.

Critical Limb Ischemia and Revascularization

The indications for limb revascularization are disabling claudication or critical limb ischemia—rest pain or tissue loss—refractive to conservative therapy. Disabling claudication is a relative, not absolute indication and requires significant patient consultation.

One must weigh existing symptoms against the risk of the procedure and its expected effect and durability. Although most ischemic limbs can be revascularized, some cannot. Lack of a target vessel, unavailability of autogenous vein, or irreversible gangrene beyond the midfoot may preclude revascularization. In such patients a choice must be made between prolonged medical therapy and primary amputation.

Two general techniques of revascularization exist: open surgical procedures and endovascular interventions. The two approaches are not mutually exclusive and may be combined, such as iliac angioplasty combined with infrainguinal saphenous vein bypass. The risks, expected benefit, and durability of each must be considered. In either approach, meticulous technique, flexibility and resourcefulness of judgment, and contingency plans are important. Appropriate patient preparation, intraprocedure monitoring, and postprocedure care will minimize complications.

Endovascular intervention is more appropriate in patients with focal disease, especially stenosis of larger, more proximal vessels, and when the procedure is performed for claudication. Open procedures have been successfully carried out for all lesions and tend to have greater durability. However, open procedures are associated with a small but consistent morbidity and mortality. The choice between the two modalities in an individual patient is a complex decision and requires team consultation.

Aortoiliac disease istraditionally and effectively treated with prosthetic aortofemoral bypass, but is increasingly amenable to endovascular angioplasty and stenting (79). Although percutaneous angioplasty and stenting have achieved their best results in the aortoiliac vessels, open revascularization probably offers results that are more durable when diffuse aortoiliac disease or occlusion is present.

Stenoses of the superficial femoral artery may be treated with an endovascular approach, but restenosis is common, especially in patients with diabetes and poor runoff (80). More durable results appear obtainable with open bypass to the popliteal artery, particularly using saphenous vein. Whether newer endovascular techniques, such as stents to prevent restenosis, will affect the longer term outcome of endovascular management of superficial femoral artery occlusions remains speculative. Thus far, data are lacking to support widespread use.

Bypass to the tibial or pedal vessels with autogenous vein has a long track record in limb salvage and remains the best and most predictable method of improving blood flow to the threatened limb (81). The procedure is safe, durable, and effective. Below-the-knee bypass accounts for 75% of infrainguinal procedures in patients with diabetes, with the anterior tibial/dorsalis pedis artery the most common target vessel. In the state of the art, surgical bypass with greater saphenous vein has become the procedure of choice for patients with diabetes and tibial disease. The employment of endovascular interventions including stenting for tibial arteries cannot be recommended as an alternative to bypass because of poor long-term patency and durability. Nonetheless, in selected patients, especially high-risk or moribund individuals, tibial angioplasty and stenting may serve as a "buy-time" maneuver to resolve an episode of critical limb ischemia (82). Limb salvage rates in general exceed patency rates in all vascular procedures.

Vascular Surgery in the Patient with Diabetes

There have been several guidelines drafted to assist in the assessment and perioperative management of patients with coronary disease (83), although none specifically addresses the issues of the patient with diabetes. The noncardiac procedures that pose the greatest risk to the patient with coronary disease are emergency procedures and peripheral vascular surgery. In addition to the type of procedure, the preoperative assessment should include identification of potentially serious heart disease. Symptoms of angina may be masked in patients with neuropathy and claudication, with limited work load. Advanced age (greater than 70 years) is per se an added risk factor. When these historical features are considered, along with the general history of comorbid conditions, the physical exam, functional capacity, and the resting electrocardiogram, a fairly accurate assessment of low risk versus high risk can be made (84). This Bayesian approach has been advocated as a simple and reliable method of risk stratification.

Further preoperative testing may be necessary. Echocardiography may identify patients with left ventricular dysfunction. A low ejection fraction (less than 35%) increases the risk of noncardiac surgery (85). Pharmacologic stress testing may assist in the evaluation, especially in stratifying patients of indeterminate or moderate risk. The most useful noninvasive evaluation is perfusion nuclear imaging with thallium. For patients with diabetes, advanced age, resting electrocardiogram abnormalities, and thallium abnormalities were shown to be the most important independent predictors of postoperative death (86). It should be noted that in patients with diabetes who are undergoing peripheral vascular surgery, the prevalence of thallium imaging abnormalities is high. At the Deaconess Hospital in Boston, greater than 90% of vascular surgery patients with clinical evidence of cardiac disease had abnormal dipyridimole thallium scans, whereas greater than 50% of those without clinical disease had abnormalities (87). The clinical caveat is that all patients with diabetes undergoing vascular surgery should be managed with a high index of suspicion for significant coronary artery disease.

A more complex decision tree presents when a patient is identified as high risk, with a consideration of proceeding to invasive testing and coronary angiography This decision generally is based on three probabilities: the prior Bayesian probability of coronary artery disease, the risks of the revascularization procedure, and the risks of the proposed surgery. It is generally felt that with close monitoring, the high-risk patient going directly to vascular surgery will fair better in terms of all outcomes than the same patient subjected to the potential morbidity and mortality of presurgical coronary angiography and revascularization (88). The choice of preoperative coronary artery bypass grafts (CABG) is not encouraged, as the risk of two procedures (CABG and leg bypass) exceeds the risk of leg bypass alone. The decision for CABG should be based on the same indications as for the nonoperative patient.

One study on perioperative beta-blockade in high-risk patients undergoing vascular surgery showed a striking reduction of myocardial infarction and death (89). In a prospective randomized trial, patients with abnormal thallium reperfusion imaging were randomized to bisoprolol or placebo before peripheral vascular surgery. There was a significant reduction of perioperative and in-hospital mortality, which persisted throughout the treatment period of 6 months. Most observers consider the beneficial results are class effects of beta-blockers.

The morbidity and mortality of vascular surgical procedures in patients with diabetes has improved significantly, with outcomes now comparable to those for nondiabetic vascular patients (90). The preoperative evaluation of coronary disease may be simply a Bayesian evaluation of clinical risk and prior probability of disease with or without noninvasive studies. The at-risk patient could then be initiated on beta-blockade, and followed vigilantly during and after surgery. One should realize that even in the best circumstances, the mortality rates of vascular surgery in high-risk patients with diabetes most likely remain a finite 1% to 2%.

Regular postoperative follow-up of peripheral vascular patients is mandatory because most late revascularization failures involve progression of intimal hyperplasia at areas of anastomosis, vein injury, valve sites, or angioplasty. History, clinical exam, and the ABI are simple and effective methods of detecting major restenosis, but may miss silent lesions, which may progress to sudden thromboses if uncorrected. These lesions are best detected by duplex ultrasonography, which should be performed every 3 to 6 months. In addition, around 50% of patients with CLI in one limb will develop threatened limb loss in the contralateral limb (91), underscoring the need for ongoing risk factor reduction and close monitoring of lower limb circulation.

Major amputation in the neuroischemic foot is necessary and indicated only when there is overwhelming infection that threatens the patient's life, when rest pain cannot be controlled, or when extensive necrosis secondary to a major arterial occlusion has destroyed the foot. Based on these criteria, the number of major limb amputations should be limited (92). Most amputations can be prevented and limbs salvaged through a multiarmed treatment of antibiotics, debridement, revascularization, and staged wound closure. On the other hand, amputation may offer an expedient return to a useful quality-of-life, especially if a prolonged course of treatment is anticipated with little likelihood of healing. Decisions should be made on an individual basis with rehabilitative and quality-of-life issues considered highly. Diabetic patients should have full and active rehabilitation following amputation.

SUMMARY AND FINAL COMMENTS

In summary, PAD in diabetes is exceedingly prevalent and largely undetected due to the silent nature of its progression. This is best explained by the diffuse and distal nature of the territory involved, and by its dynamic association with peripheral sensory neuropathy. Because of the lack of symptoms, screening programs are necessary, especially in those with diabetes greater than 50 years of age.

By diagnosing PAD in a patient with diabetes, one may elicit symptoms of poor function, and institute treatment measures to improve quality of life and slow progression of disease. Moreover, diagnosis identifies a patient with high cardiovascular risk of myocardial infarction, stroke, and death, and places emphasis on aggressive risk factor interventions.

Treatment of the patient with diabetes and PAD is more successful when it involves several disciplines. The complexity of the management of the patient with diabetes and PAD is beyond the scope of a single clinician. The treatment is best carried out within an interdisciplinary team that places the patient at the center of focus. It is with the cooperative interaction of the varied specialists that the guidelines for care and prevention will most effectively be implemented.

The clinical burden of PAD in diabetes is large, and the prediction of an enormous wave of patients entering their second decade of diabetes presenting with cardiovascular complications is a clarion call. As a responsible medical community, we must admit our inability to penetrate this problem today, and prepare to work cooperatively for the looming challenges of the diabetes epidemic and its cardiovascular complications.

REFERENCES

1. Mokdad AH, Bowman BA, Ford ES, et al. The continuing epidemics of obesity and diabetes in the United States. *JAMA* 2001;286:1195–2001.
2. American Diabetes Association. *National diabetes fact sheet.* Alexandria, VA: Author, 2003.
3. Zimmet PZ. Kelly West Lecture 1991. Challenges in diabetes epidemiology—from West to the rest. *Diabetes Care* 1992;15:232–252.
4. Mokdad AH, Ford ES, Bowman BA, et al. Prevalence of obesity, diabetes, and obesity-related health risk factors, 2001. *JAMA* 2003;289:76–79.

5. Haffner SM, Lehto S, Ronnemaa T, et al. Mortality from coronary heart disease in subjects with type 2 diabetes and in nondiabetic subjects with and without prior myocardial infarction. *N Engl J Med* 1998;339:229–234.
6. American Diabetes Association. Peripheral arterial disease in people with diabetes (Consensus statement). *Diabetes Care (in press)*.
7. Murabito JM, D'Agostino RB, Silbershatz H, et al. Intermittent claudication. A risk profile from the Framingham Heart Study. *Circulation* 1997;96:44–49.
8. Hirsch AT, Criqui MH, Treat-Jacobson D, et al. Peripheral arterial disease detection, awareness, and treatment in primary care. *JAMA* 2001;286:1317–1324.
9. Criqui MH. Peripheral arterial disease—epidemiological aspects. *Vasc Med* 2001;6[Suppl 1]:3–7.
10. Newman AB, Siscovick DS, Manolio TA, et al. Ankle–arm index as a marker of atherosclerosis in the Cardiovascular Health Study. Cardiovascular Heart Study (CHS) Collaborative Research Group. *Circulation* 1993;88:837–845.
11. Brand FN, Kannel WB, Evans J, et al. Glucose intolerance, physical signs of peripheral artery disease, and risk of cardiovascular events: the Framingham Study. *Am Heart J* 1998;136:919–927.
12. Ridker PM, Cushman M, Stampfer MJ, et al. Plasma concentration of C-reactive protein and risk of developing peripheral vascular disease. *Circulation* 1998;97:425–428.
13. Lee AJ, MacGregor AS, Hau CM, et al. The role of haematological factors in diabetic peripheral arterial disease: the Edinburgh artery study. *Br J Haematol* 1999;5:648–654.
14. Katsilambros NL, Tsapogas PC, Arvanitis MP, et al. Risk factors for lower extremity arterial disease in non-insulin-dependent diabetic persons. *Diabet Med* 1996;13:243–246.
15. Asakawa H, Tokunaga K, Kawakami F. Comparison of risk factors of macrovascular complications. Peripheral vascular disease, cerebral vascular disease, and coronary heart disease in Japanese type 2 diabetes mellitus patients. *J Diabetes Complications* 2000;14:307–313.
16. Collins TC, Johnson M, Henderson W, et al. Lower extremity nontraumatic amputation among veterans with peripheral arterial disease: is race an independent factor? *Med Care* 2002;40[1 Suppl]:106–116.
17. Haltmayer M, Mueller T, Horvath W, et al. Impact of atherosclerotic risk factors on the anatomical distribution of peripheral arterial disease. *Int Angiol* 2001;20:200–207.
18. Wrobel JS, Mayfield JA, Reiber GE. Geographic variation of lower-extremity major amputation in individuals with and without diabetes in the Medicare population. *Diabetes Care* 2001;24:860–864.
19. Bernstein EF, Fronek A. Current status of non-invasive tests in the diagnosis of peripheral arterial disease. *Surg Clin North Am* 1982;62:473–487.
20. Elhadd TA, Robb R, Jung RT, et al. Pilot study of prevalence of asymptomatic peripheral arterial occlusive disease in patients with diabetes attending a hospital clinic. *Practical Diabetes Int* 1999;16:163–166.
21. Weitz JI, Byrne J, Byrne J, Clagett GP, et al. Diagnosis and treatment of chronic arterial insufficiency of the lower extremities: a critical review. *Circulation* 1996;94:3026–3049.
22. Dormandy JA, Rutherford RB. Management of peripheral arterial disease (PAD). TASC Working Group. TransAtlantic Inter-Society Consensus (TASC). *J Vasc Surg* 2000;31[1 Pt 2]:S1–S296.
23. Ram Z, Sadeh M, Walden R, et al. Vascular insufficiency quantitatively aggravates diabetic neuropathy. *Arch Neurol* 1991;48:1239–1242.
24. Kannel WB. Risk factors for atherosclerotic cardiovascular outcomes in different arterial territories. *J Cardiovasc Risk* 1994;1:3333–3339.
25. Eckel RH, Wassef M, Chait A, et al. Prevention conference VI: Diabetes and cardiovascular disease: Writing group II: pathogenesis of atherosclerosis in diabetes. *Circulation* 2002;7:105:e138–e143.
26. Veves A, Akbari CM, Primavera J, et al. Endothelial dysfunction and the expression of endothelial nitric oxide synthetase in diabetic neuropathy, vascular disease, and foot ulceration. *Diabetes* 1998;47:457–463.
27. Beckman JA, Creager MA, Libby P. Diabetes and atherosclerosis: epidemiology, pathophysiology, and management. *JAMA* 2002;15:2570–2581.
28. Kaiser N, Sasson S, Feener EP, et al. Differential regulation of glucose transport and transporters by glucose in vascular endothelial and smooth muscle cells. *Diabetes* 1993;42:80–89.
29. Steinberg HO, Baron AD. Vascular function, insulin resistance and fatty acids. *Diabetologia* 2002;45:623–634.
30. Way KJ, Katai N, King GL. Protein kinase C and the development of diabetic vascular complications. *Diabet Med* 2001;18:945–959.
31. Montagnani M, Golovchenko I, Kim I, et al. Inhibition of phosphatidylinositol 3-kinase enhances mitogenic actions of insulin in endothelial cells. *J Biol Chem* 2002;277:1794–1799.
32. Tsao PS, Wang B, Buitrago R, et al. Nitric oxide regulates monocyte chemotactic protein-1. *Circulation* 1997;96:934–940.
33. Libby P. Inflammation in atherosclerosis. *Nature* 2002;420:868–874.
34. Jialal I, Devaraj S, Venugopal SK. Oxidative stress, inflammation, and diabetic vasculopathies: the role of alpha tocopherol therapy. *Free Radic Res* 2002;36:1331–1336.
35. Geng YJ, Libby P. Progression of atheroma: a struggle between death and procreation. *Arterioscler Thromb Vasc Biol* 2002;22:1370–1380.
36. Schneider DL, Sobel BE. Diabetes and thrombosis. In: Johnstone MT, Veves A, eds. *Diabetes and cardiovascular disease.* Totowa, NJ: Humana Press, 2001.
37. McDermott MM, Green D, Greenland P, et al. Relation of levels of hemostatic factors and inflammatory markers to the ankle–brachial index. *Am J Cardiol* 2003;92:194–199.
38. Hiatt WR. Medical treatment of peripheral arterial disease and claudication. *N Engl J Med* 2001;344:1608–1621.
39. Dolan NC, Liu K, Criqui MH, et al. Peripheral artery disease, diabetes, and reduced lower extremity functioning. *Diabetes Care* 2002;25:113–120.
40. McDaniel MD, Cronenwett JL. Basic data related to the natural history of intermittent claudication. *Ann Vasc Surg* 1989;3:273–277.
41. Jude EB, Oyibo SO, Chalmers N, et al. Peripheral arterial disease in diabetic and nondiabetic patients: a comparison of severity and outcome. *Diabetes Care* 2001;24:1433–1437.
42. Bruce RA, Kusumi F, Hosmer D. Maximal oxygen intake and nomographic assessment of functional aerobic impairment in cardiovascular disease. *Am Heart J* 1973;85:546–562.
43. McDermott MM, Mehta S, Greenland P. Exertional leg symptoms other than intermittent claudication are common in peripheral arterial disease. *Arch Intern Med* 1999;159:387–392.
44. American Diabetes Association. Preventive foot-care in people with diabetes (Position statement). *Diabetes Care* 2003;26[Suppl 1]:S78–S79.
45. Lundbrook J, Clark AM, McKensie JK. Significance of absent ankle pulse. *Br Med J* 1962;1:1724–1726.
46. Bjellerup M. Does dorsal pedal pulse palpation predict hand-held Doppler measurement of ankle brachial index in leg ulcer patients? *Wounds* 2003;15:237–240.
47. Strandness Jr DE, Bell JW. Peripheral vascular disease: diagnosis and evaluation using a mercury strain gauge. *Ann Surg* 1965;161[Suppl 4]:1.
48. Carter SA, Tate RB. The value of toe pulse waves in determination of risks for limb amputation and death in patients with peripheral arterial disease and skin ulcers or gangrene. *J Vasc Surg* 2001;33:708–714.
49. Ballard JL, Eke CC, Bunt TJ. A prospective evaluation of transcutaneous oxygen measurements in the management of diabetic foot problems. *J Vasc Surg* 1995;22:485–490, discussion 490–492.
50. LoGerfo FW, Coffman JD. Current concepts. Vascular and microvascular disease of the foot in diabetes. Implications for foot care. *N Engl J Med* 1984;311:1615–1619.
51. Lassila R, Lepantalo M. Cigarette smoking and the outcome after lower limb arterial surgery. *Acta Chir Scand* 1988;154:635–640.
52. American Diabetes Association. Smoking and diabetes (Position statement). *Diabetes Care* 2003;26:S89–S91.
53. UK Prospective Diabetes Study (UKPDS) Group. Intensive blood-glucose control with sulphonylureas or insulin compared with conventional treatment and risk of complications in patients with type 2 diabetes (UKPDS 33). *Lancet* 1998;352:837–853.
54. Holman RR. Consultant. 1997;37[Suppl]:S30–S36.
55. Stokes J, Kannel WB, Wolf PA, et al. The relative importance of selected risk factors for various manifestations of cardiovascular disease among men and women from 35 to 64 years old: 30 years of follow-up in the Framingham Study. *Circulation* 1987;75:V65–V73.
56. UK Prospective Diabetes Study (UKPDS) Group. Tight blood pressure control and risk of macrovascular and microvascular complications in type 2 diabetes (UKPDS 38). *BMJ* 1998;317:703–713.
57. American Diabetes Association. Treatment of hypertension in adults with diabetes (Position statement). *Diabetes Care* 2003;26:S80–S82.

58. Yusuf S, Sleight P, Pogue J, et al. Effects of an angiotensin-converting-enzyme inhibitor, ramipril, on cardiovascular events in high-risk patients. The Heart Outcomes Prevention Evaluation Study Investigators. *N Engl J Med* 2000;342:145–153.

59. Mehler PS, Coll JR, Estacio R, et al. Intensive blood pressure control reduces the risk of cardiovascular events in patients with peripheral arterial disease and type 2 diabetes. *Circulation* 2003;107:753–756.

60. Leng GC, Price JF, Jepson RG. Lipid-lowering for lower limb atherosclerosis (Cochrane Review). *Cochrane Database Syst Rev* 2000;2: CD000123.

61. Randomized trial of cholesterol lowering in 4444 patients with coronary heart disease: the Scandinavian Simvastatin Survival Study (4S). *Lancet* 1994;344:1383–1389.

62. Kjekshus J, Pedersen TR. Reducing the risk of coronary events: evidence from the Scandinavian Simvastatin Survival Study (4S). *Am J Cardiol* 1995;76:64C–68C.

63. MRC/BHF Heart Protection Study of cholesterol lowering with simvastatin in 20,536 high-risk individuals: a randomized placebo-controlled trial. *Lancet* 2002;360:7–22.

64. American Diabetes Association. Management of dyslipidemia in adults with diabetes (Position statement). *Diabetes Care* 2003;26:S83–S86.

65. Antiplatelet Trialists' Collaboration. Collaborative overview of randomised trials of antiplatelet therapy—I. Prevention of death, myocardial infarction, and stroke by prolonged antiplatelet therapy in various categories of patients. *BMJ* 1994;308:81–106.

66. American Diabetes Association. Aspirin therapy in diabetes (Position statement). *Diabetes Care* 2003;26[Suppl. 1]:S87–S88.

67. CAPRIE Steering Committee. A randomized, blinded, trial of clopidogrel versus aspirin in patients at risk of ischaemic events (CAPRIE). *Lancet* 1996;348:1329–1339.

68. Bhatt DL, Marso SP, Hirsch AT, et al. Amplified benefit of clopidogrel versus aspirin in patients with diabetes mellitus. *Am J Cardiol* 2002;90:625–628.

69. Larsen OA, Lassen NA. Effect of daily muscular exercise in patients with intermittent claudication. *Lancet* 1966;2:1093–1096.

70. Regensteiner JG, Ware Jr JE, McCarthy WJ, et al. Effect of cilostazol on treadmill walking, community-based walking ability, and health-related quality of life in patients with intermittent claudication due to peripheral arterial disease: meta-analysis of six randomized controlled trials. *J Am Geriatr Soc* 2002;50:1939–1946.

71. Stewart KJ, Hiatt WR, Regensteiner JG, et al. Exercise training for claudication. *N Engl J Med* 2002;347:1941–1951.

72. Packer M, Chair. Cardiovascular and Renal Drugs Advisory Committee, 85th Meeting. Bethesda, MD: U.S. Department of Health and Human Services, Food and Drug Administration, 1998.

73. Dawson DL, Cutler BS, Hiatt WR, et al. A comparison of cilostazol and pentoxifylline for treating intermittent claudication. *Am J Med* 2000;109:523–530.

74. American Diabetes Association. Diabetic foot wound care (Consensus statement). *Diabetes Care* 1999;21:1354–1360.

75. Pitei DL, Lord M, Foster A, et al. Plantar pressures are elevated in the neuroischemic and the neuropathic diabetic foot. *Diabetes Care* 1999;22:1966–1970.

76. Lipsky BA, Armstrong DG, Acin F, et al. Treating diabetic foot infections with linezolid versus aminopenicillins: a randomized international multicenter trial. *Clin Infect Dis (in press).*

77. Tan JS, Friedman NM, Hazelton-Miller C, et al. Can aggressive treatment of diabetic foot infections reduce the need for above-ankle amputation? *Clin Infect Dis* 1996;23:286–291.

78. Attinger CE, Ducic I, Cooper P, et al. The role of intrinsic muscle flaps of the foot for bone coverage in foot and ankle defects in diabetic and nondiabetic patients. *Plast Reconstr Surg* 2002;110:1047–1054.

79. Dormandy JA, Rutherford RB. Management of peripheral arterial disease (PAD). TASC Working Group. TransAtlantic Inter-Society Consensus (TASC). *J Vasc Surg* 2000;31:S1–S296.

80. Stokes J, Kannel WB, Wolf PA, et al. The relative importance of selected risk factors for various manifestations of cardiovascular disease among men and women from 35 to 64 years old: 30 years of follow-up in the Framingham Study. *Circulation* 1987;75:V65–V73.

81. Pomposelli FB, Kansal N, Hamdan AD, et al. A decade of experience with dorsalis pedis artery bypass: analysis of outcome in more than 1000 cases. *J Vasc Surg* 2003;37:307–315.

82. Dorros G, Jaff MR, Dorros AM, et al. Tibioperoneal (outflow lesion) angioplasty can be used as primary treatment in 235 patients with critical limb ischemia: five-year follow-up. *Circulation* 2001;104:2057–2062.

83. Froehlich JB, Karavite D, Russman PL, et al. American College of Cardiology/American Heart Association preoperative assessment guidelines reduce resource ultilization before aortic surgery. *J Vasc Surg* 2002;36:758–763.

84. Fleisher LA, Eagle KA. Screening for cardiac disease in patients having noncardiac surgery. *Ann Intern Med* 1996;124:767–772.

85. Eagle KA, Brundage BH, Chaitman BR, et al. Guidelines for perioperative cardiovascular evaluation for noncardiac surgery: an abridged version of the report of the American College of Cardiology/American Heart Association Task Force on Practice Guidelines. *Mayo Clin Proc* 1997;72:524–531.

86. Cohen MC, Curran PF, L'Italien GJ, et al. Long-term prognostic value of preoperative dipyridamole thallium imaging and clinical indexes in patients with diabetes mellitus undergoing peripheral vascular surgery. *Am J Cardiol* 1999;83:1038–1042.

87. Zarich SW, Cohen MC, Lane SE, et al. Routine perioperative dipyridamole 201T1 imaging in diabetic patients undergoing vascular surgery. *Diabetes Care* 1996;19:355–360.

88. Mangano DT. Assessment of the patient with cardiac disease: an anethesiologist's paradigm. *Anesthesiology* 1999;91:1521.

89. Poldermans D, Boersma E, Bax JJ, et al. The effect of bisoprolol on perioperative mortality and myocardial infarction in high-risk patients undergoing vascular surgery. Dutch Echocardiographic Cardiac Risk Evaluation Applying Stress Echocardiography Study Group. *N Engl J Med* 1999;341:1789–1794.

90. Hamdan AD, Saltzberg SS, Sheahan M, et al. Lack of association of diabetes with increased postoperative mortality and cardiac morbidity: results of 6565 major vascular operations. *Arch Surg* 2002;137:417–421.

91. Dormandy J, Heeck L, Vig S. Major amputations: clinical patterns and predictors. *Semin Vasc Surg* 1999;12:154–161.

92. Eneroth M, Larsson J, Apelqvist J. Deep foot infections in patients with diabetes and foot ulcer: an entity with different characteristics, treatments, and prognosis, *J Diabetes Complications* 1999;13:254–263.

CHAPTER 6

Insulin Resistance and the Metabolic Syndrome

Charles A. Reasner, II

Key Points

- Components of the insulin resistance/metabolic syndrome include obesity, hypertension, hyperglycemia, and dyslipidemia.
- The insulin resistance/metabolic syndrome identifies individuals at increased risk for developing cardiovascular disease as well as diabetes.
- Maintenance of ideal body weight and daily physical exercise should be goals of every individual with this condition.
- Aggressive treatment of hypertension with angiotensin inhibitors has been shown to prevent cardiovascular complications and delay the onset of diabetes.
- Aggressive lipid management has been shown to provide the greatest reduction in cardiovascular mortality.
- The use of insulin sensitizers may prevent cardiovascular disease and holds the promise of delaying or even preventing beta cell failure and the development of diabetes.

DEFINITION

The association of insulin resistance with a clustering of cardiovascular risk factors including hyperinsulinemia, hypertension, abdominal obesity, dyslipidemia, and coagulation abnormalities has been referred to by a variety of names including the insulin resistance syndrome, the metabolic syndrome, the dysmetabolic syndrome, and the deadly quartet, to name a few. Since the description of the insulin resistance syndrome by Reaven in 1988 (1), the number of associated factors has continued to grow.

The most widely used criteria to define this syndrome were published as part of the National Cholesterol Education Program (NCEP) Adult Treatment Panel (ATP) III guidelines for the treatment of hypercholesterolemia (2). The NCEP components of the metabolic syndrome are outlined in Table 6.1. The ATP III guidelines establish a diagnosis of the metabolic syndrome when at least three of the five criteria are present. The metabolic syndrome has been assigned the diagnostic code 277.7 by the *International Classification of Diseases, ninth revision* (3); which enables physicians to be reimbursed for treating patients with this condition. The standards for the individual risk factors vary between ATP III and other expert panels including the World Health

Organization and the American College of Endocrinology. For example, ATP uses waist circumference to define obesity, whereas other expert committees use the body mass index (BMI). The ATP guidelines base glucose intolerance on a fasting glucose, whereas others prefer the results of an oral glucose tolerance test (OGTT). As we become better able to quantify the relationship between these factors and the development of cardiovascular disease, the definition of the syndromes and the individual component values will no doubt continue to be refined.

PREVALENCE

The insulin resistance syndrome (IRS) is common in the United States. Ford et al. analyzed the data from the third National Health and Nutrition Evaluation Survey, carried out in 1988 through 1994 (4). The sample included 20,050 persons aged greater than or equal to 17 years, with glucose tolerance testing performed in 3,302 persons aged 40 to 74 years. Of this population, the triglyceride criterion was positive in 34%, low high-density lipoprotein (HDL) was present in 37%, 40% were hypertensive, and 24% met the glucose tolerance test (GTT) criterion for hyperglycemia. Twenty-five percent of

TABLE 6.1. *The five components of the metabolic syndrome[a]*

Risk factor	Defining level
Abdominal obesity: (waist circumference)	
Men	>102 cm (>40 in.)
Women	>88 cm (>35 in.)
Triglycerides	≥150 mg/dL
High-density lipoprotein C	
Men	<40 mg/dL
Women	<50 mg/dL
Blood pressure	≥130/≥85 mm Hg
Fasting glucose	≥110 mg/dL

[a]Individuals who have at least three components meet the criteria for diagnosis.

From Expert Panel on Detection, Evaluation, and Treatment of High Blood Cholesterol in Adults. Executive summary of the third report of the National Cholesterol Education Program (NCEP) Expert Panel on Detection, Evaluation, and Treatment of High Blood Cholesterol in Adults (Adult Treatment Panel III). *JAMA* 2001;285:2486–2496, with permission.

men and 34% of women met none of the criteria, and about 30% of men and women had one abnormality. When the ATP III standard of three or more metabolic abnormalities was applied to the same population, 26% of the population met the criteria for the metabolic syndrome. The prevalence of the IRS increases with age, with 33% affected at age 40, 40% at age 50, and 50% by 60 years of age. The prevalence of the IRS also differs in various ethnic groups, with 52% of Mexican Americans affected compared to 36% of African Americans and 40% of whites. Although the prevalence of the metabolic syndrome in this survey is staggering, the data are now 10 to 16 years old and the prevalence has almost certainly increased as the population has aged and become more obese.

PATHOGENESIS

Normal Insulin Action

To better understand the insulin-resistant state, we first review normal insulin action. In the fasting state, 75% of total body glucose disposal takes place in the brain and splanchnic tissues (liver and gastrointestinal tissues), which are not dependent on insulin (5). The remaining 25% of glucose metabolism takes place in muscle, which is an insulin-dependent tissue (6,7). In the fasting state, approximately 85% of glucose production is derived from the liver, and the remaining amount is produced by the kidney (5,8,9). In the fed state, carbohydrate ingestion increases the plasma glucose concentration and stimulates insulin release from the pancreatic beta cells. The resultant hyperinsulinemia suppresses hepatic glucose production and stimulates glucose uptake by peripheral tissues (5–7,10–14). The majority (~80% to 85%) of glucose that is taken up by peripheral tissues is disposed of in muscle (5–7,11–14), with only a small amount (~4% to 5%) being metabolized by adipocytes (15).

Although fat tissue is responsible for only a small amount of total body glucose disposal, it plays a very important role in the maintenance of total body glucose homeostasis. Small increments in the plasma insulin concentration exert a potent antilipolytic effect, leading to a marked reduction in the plasma free fatty acid (FFA) level (16). The decline in plasma FFA concentration results in increased glucose uptake in muscle (17) and reduces hepatic glucose production (18). Thus, a decrease in the plasma FFA concentration lowers plasma glucose by both decreasing glucose production and enhancing glucose uptake in muscle (19,20).

Insulin in Type 2 Diabetes Mellitus

Type 2 diabetic individuals are characterized by defects in insulin secretion and insulin resistance involving muscle, liver, and the adipocyte.

Impaired Insulin Secretion

The pancreas in people with a normal-functioning beta cell is able to "read" the severity of insulin resistance and adjust its secretion of insulin to maintain normal glucose tolerance (21). Thus, in nondiabetic individuals, insulin is increased in proportion to the severity of the insulin resistance and glucose tolerance remains normal. Impaired insulin secretion is a uniform finding in type 2 diabetic patients, and the evolution of beta cell dysfunction has been well characterized in diverse ethnic populations.

DeFronzo et al. (22) measured the fasting plasma insulin concentration and performed oral glucose tolerance tests in 77 normal-weight type 2 diabetic patients and greater than 100 lean individuals with normal or impaired glucose tolerance (Fig. 6.1). The relationship between the fasting plasma glucose concentration and the fasting plasma insulin concentration resembles an inverted U or horseshoe (6). As the fasting plasma glucose concentration rises from 80 to 140 mg per dL, the fasting plasma insulin concentration increases progressively, peaking at a value that is 2- to 2.5-fold greater than in normal-weight, nondiabetic controls. When the fasting plasma glucose concentration exceeds 140 mg per dL, the beta cell is unable to maintain its elevated rate of insulin secretion and the fasting insulin concentration declines precipitously. This decrease in fasting insulin is directly related to the increase in hepatic glucose production, which results in an elevated fasting plasma glucose concentration (22).

A type 2 diabetic patient with a fasting plasma glucose concentration of 150 to 160 mg per dL secretes an amount of insulin that is similar to that in a healthy, nondiabetic individual. However, a "normal" amount of insulin in absolute terms in the presence of this degree of hyperglycemia is markedly abnormal. When the fasting glucose exceeds 200 to 220 mg per dL, the plasma insulin response to a glucose challenge is markedly blunted.

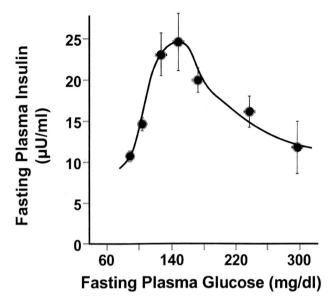

FIG. 6.1. The relationship between fasting plasma insulin and fasting plasma glucose in 177 normal-weight individuals. Plasma insulin and glucose increase together up to a fasting glucose of 140 mg/dL. When the fasting glucose exceeds 140 mg/dL, the beta cell makes progressively less insulin, which leads to an overproduction of glucose by the liver and results in a progressive increase in fasting glucose.

The natural history of type 2 diabetes, starting with normal glucose tolerance and progressing to impaired glucose tolerance (IGT) and overt diabetes mellitus has been observed in a variety of populations including whites, Native Americans, Mexican Americans, and Pacific Islanders (6,23–34). In all of these population studies, the development of type 2 diabetes is strongly associated with the presence of obesity. In populations at high risk to develop type 2 diabetes mellitus, the progression from IGT to type 2 diabetes with mild fasting hyperglycemia (120 to 140 mg per dL, 6.7 to 7.8 mmol per L) is heralded by an inability of the beta cell to maintain its previously high rate of insulin secretion in response to a glucose challenge (6,24,25,30,35) without any further or minimal deterioration in tissue sensitivity to insulin.

Insulin Resistance

Himsworth and Kerr (36), using a combined oral glucose and intravenous insulin tolerance test, were the first to demonstrate that tissue sensitivity to insulin was diminished in diabetic patients. In 1975, Ginsberg and colleagues (37), using the insulin suppression test, found that the ability of insulin to promote tissue glucose uptake in type 2 diabetes was severely reduced. DeFronzo et al., using the more physiological euglycemic insulin clamp technique (38), demonstrated that insulin resistance is similar in type 2 diabetic and obese nondiabetic individuals (Fig. 6.2) (5,6,16,39,40). Obese diabetics with mild to modest elevations in the fasting plasma glucose concentration (mean=150 ± 8 mg per dL, 8.3 ± 0.4 mmol per L) displayed a 40% to 50% reduction in insulin-mediated whole-body glucose disposal. Lean type 2 diabetics with more severe fasting hyperglycemia (198 ± 10 mg per dL) have a similar degree of insulin resistance (Fig. 6.2) (5,6,41,42).

SITES OF INSULIN RESISTANCE IN TYPE 2 DIABETES

Liver

In the overnight fasted state, the liver of healthy individuals produces glucose at the rate of approximately 2.0 mg per kg per min (5,6,16,22). This glucose production is essential to meet the needs of the brain and other neural tissues, which utilize glucose at a constant rate of 1 to 1.2 mg per kg per min (43). Brain glucose uptake accounts for ~50% to 60% of glucose disposal during the fasting state, and this uptake is insulin independent. Therefore, brain glucose uptake occurs at the same rate during fed and fasting periods and is not altered in type 2 diabetes (44). In type 2 diabetic subjects with mild to moderate fasting hyperglycemia (140 to 200 mg per dL, 7.8 to 11.1 mmol per L), basal hepatic glucose production is increased by ~0.5 mg per kg per min. Consequently, during the overnight sleeping hours, the liver of a 80-kg diabetic individual with modest fasting hyperglycemia adds an additional 35 g of glucose to the

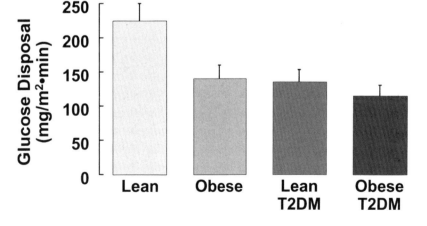

FIG. 6.2. Effect of obesity and type 2 diabetes mellitus on tissue sensitivity to insulin. Whole-body glucose disposal, a measure of insulin resistance, is reduced 40% to 50% in obese nondiabetic and lean type 2 diabetic individuals. Obese diabetic individuals are slightly more resistant than lean diabetic patients. (From DeFronzo RM. Pathogenesis of type 2 diabetes: metabolic and molecular implications for identifying diabetes genes. *Diabetes Rev* 1997;5:177–269, with permission.)

systemic circulation. This increase in fasting hepatic glucose production is the cause of fasting hyperglycemia (5,6,16, 39–41).

Following glucose ingestion, insulin is secreted into the portal vein and carried to the liver, where it suppresses hepatic glucose output. If the liver is resistant to insulin and continues to produce glucose, there will be two inputs of glucose into the body, one from the liver and another from the diet, and marked hyperglycemia will ensue. The glucose released by the liver can be derived from either glycogenolysis or gluconeogenesis (45). Studies employing the hepatic vein catheter technique have shown that the uptake of gluconeogenic precursors, especially lactate, is increased in type 2 diabetic individuals (46). Consistent with this observation, radioisotope turnover studies, using lactate, alanine, and glycerol, have shown that ~90% of the increase in hepatic glucose production (HGP) above baseline can be accounted for by accelerated gluconeogenesis (47,48).

Peripheral (Muscle)

Muscle is the major site of glucose disposal in humans (5–7,14). Under euglycemic hyperinsulinemic conditions, approximately 80% of total body glucose uptake occurs in skeletal muscle (5–7). Studies employing the euglycemic insulin clamp in combination with femoral artery/vein catheterization have examined the effect of insulin on leg glucose uptake in type 2 diabetic and control individuals. Because bone is metabolically inert and adipose tissue takes up less than 5% of an infused glucose load (15,49,50), muscle represents the major tissue responsible for leg glucose uptake. In response to a physiological increase in plasma insulin concentration (~80 to 100 μU per mL), leg (muscle) glucose uptake increases linearly, reaching a plateau value of 10 mg per kg leg weight per min (51). In contrast, in lean type 2 diabetic individuals, the onset of insulin action is delayed for ~40 min and the ability of the hormone to stimulate leg glucose uptake is markedly blunted (51). During the last hour of the insulin clamp study, when the effect of insulin is at its peak, the rate of glucose uptake in muscle was reduced by 50% in the diabetic group (51). These results provide conclusive evidence that the primary site of insulin resistance in type 2 diabetic patients is muscle tissue.

In summary, insulin resistance involving both muscle and liver are characteristic features of the glucose intolerance in type 2 diabetic individuals. In the basal state, the liver represents a major site of insulin resistance, and this is reflected by overproduction of glucose. This accelerated rate of hepatic glucose output is the primary determinant of the elevated fasting plasma glucose concentration in type 2 diabetic individuals. In the fed state, both decreased muscle glucose uptake and impaired suppression of HGP contribute to the hyperglycemia. Following glucose ingestion, the defects in insulin-mediated glucose uptake by muscle and the lack of suppression of HGP by insulin contribute approx-

imately equally to the disturbance in whole-body glucose homeostasis in type 2 diabetes.

Peripheral (Adipocyte)

A similar degree of insulin resistance is seen in obese nondiabetic and lean type 2 diabetic individuals (Fig. 6.2) (52–54). However, lean diabetic individuals manifest marked glucose intolerance, whereas the obese nondiabetic individuals have normal plasma glucose (6). This difference is explained by the plasma insulin response to a glucose challenge. Obese nondiabetic individuals secrete more than twice as much insulin as lean nondiabetic controls and compensate for the insulin resistance. In contrast, normal-weight diabetic patients are unable to augment the secretion of insulin sufficiently to compensate for the insulin resistance. When obesity and diabetes coexist in the same individual, the severity of insulin resistance is only slightly greater than that in either the normal-weight diabetic or nondiabetic obese groups (Fig. 6.2) (6).

Felber and co-workers (35,40,41,55,56) were among the first to demonstrate that in obese nondiabetic and diabetic humans, basal plasma FFA levels are increased and fail to suppress normally after glucose ingestion. FFAs are stored as triglycerides in adipocytes and serve as an important energy source during conditions of fasting. Insulin is a potent inhibitor of lipolysis, and restrains the release of FFA from the adipocyte by inhibiting the enzyme hormone-sensitive lipase. It is now recognized that chronically elevated plasma FFA concentrations can lead to insulin resistance in muscle and liver (5,6,17,19,20,41,57,58) and impair insulin secretion (19,59,60). In addition to FFAs that circulate in plasma in increased amounts, type 2 diabetic and obese nondiabetic individuals have increased stores of triglycerides in muscle (61,62) and liver (63,64), and the increased fat content correlates closely with the presence of insulin resistance in these tissues. The sequence of events via which elevated FFAs inhibit muscle glucose transport, glucose oxidation, and glycogen synthesis is referred to as the Randle cycle (65).

Insulin is a vasodilatory hormone. The vasodilatory effect of insulin is mediated via the release of nitric oxide from the vascular endothelium (66). In insulin-resistant conditions, such as obesity and type 2 diabetes, some investigators have suggested that as much as half of the impairment in insulin-mediated whole-body and leg-muscle glucose uptake is related to a defect in insulin's vasodilatory action (67,68). Because type 2 diabetes and obesity are insulin-resistant states characterized by day-long elevation in the plasma FFA concentration (69) and impaired endothelium-dependent vasodilation (67), investigators have examined the effect of increased plasma FFA levels on limb blood flow and muscle glucose uptake (70,71). In healthy, nondiabetic subjects an acute physiological increase in plasma FFA concentration inhibited methacholine (endothelium-dependent), but not nitroprusside (endothelium-independent) stimulated blood flow in association with an impairment in insulin-stimulated muscle glucose disposal. In subsequent studies, the inhibitory effect of FFA on insulin-stimulated leg blood flow was shown to be associated with decreased nitric oxide production (72).

In summary, in obese individuals and in the majority (greater than 80%) of type 2 diabetic individuals, there is an expanded fat cell mass and the adipocytes are resistant to the antilipolytic effects of insulin (16). Most obese and diabetic individuals are characterized by visceral adiposity (73), and visceral fat cells have a high lipolytic rate, which is especially refractory to insulin (74). Not surprisingly, both type 2 diabetes and obesity are characterized by an elevation in the mean day-long plasma FFA concentration. Elevated plasma FFA levels, as well as increased triglyceride/fatty acyl coenzyme A content in muscle, liver, and the beta cell, lead to the development of muscle/hepatic insulin resistance and impaired insulin secretion.

CELLULAR MECHANISMS OF INSULIN RESISTANCE

The stimulation of glucose metabolism by insulin requires that the hormone must first bind to specific receptors that are present on the cell surface (Fig. 6.3) (5,75–78). After insulin has bound to and activated its receptor, second messengers initiate a series of events involving a cascade of phosphorylation–dephosphorylation reactions (5,75–81) that result in the stimulation of intracellular glucose metabolism. The initial step in glucose metabolism involves activation of the glucose transport system, leading to influx of glucose into insulin target tissues, primarily muscle (5,82,83). The free glucose is metabolized by a series of enzymatic steps that are under the control of insulin.

The insulin receptor is a glycoprotein consisting of two α-subunits and two β-subunits linked by disulfide bonds (5,75–78) (Fig. 6.3). The α-subunit of the insulin receptor is entirely extracellular and contains the insulin-binding domain.

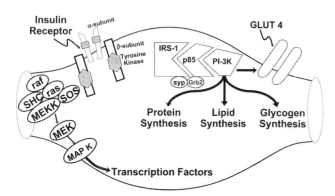

FIG. 6.3. The two insulin-sensitive pathways in muscle. Binding of insulin and activation of the insulin receptor substrate (IRS) leads to the anabolic actins of insulin. Activation of mitogen-activated protein kinase (MAP K) results in the production of transcription factors that promote cell growth, proliferation, and differentiation.

The β-subunit has an extracellular domain, a transmembrane domain, and an intracellular domain that expresses insulin-stimulated kinase activity directed toward its own tyrosine residues. Insulin receptor phosphorylation of the β-subunit, with subsequent activation of insulin receptor tyrosine kinase, represents the first step in the action of insulin on glucose metabolism (75–78).

The binding of insulin to tyrosine kinase stimulates two distinct pathways: the glycogen synthesis pathway and the mitogenic pathway (Fig. 6.3). Once activated, tyrosine kinase phosphorylates specific intracellular proteins, of which at least nine have been identified (83). Four of these belong to the family of insulin-receptor substrate proteins: IRS-1, IRS-2, IRS-3, and IRS-4 (the others include Shc, Cbl, Gab-1, p60[dok], and APS). In muscle, IRS-1 serves as the major docking protein, which interacts with the insulin receptor tyrosine kinase and undergoes tyrosine phosphorylation. This leads to the activation of the enzyme phosphatidylinositol (PI)-3 kinase (75–87). PI-3 kinase activation stimulates glucose transport (75–78) and glycogen synthesis (75,76). Inhibitors of PI-3 kinase impair glucose transport (88) by interfering with the translocation of GLUT 4 transporters from their intracellular location (82,83) and block the activation of glycogen synthase (89). The action of insulin to increase protein synthesis and inhibit protein degradation also is mediated by PI-3 kinase (90,91). Insulin also promotes hepatic triglyceride synthesis, and this lipogenic effect of insulin also appears to be mediated via the PI-3 kinase pathway (75). Thus all of the anabolic effects of insulin are mediated through the IRS/PI-3 kinase pathway. In liver, IRS-2 serves as the primary docking protein, which undergoes tyrosine phosphorylation and mediates the effect of insulin on hepatic glucose production, gluconeogenesis, and glycogen formation (92). In adipocytes, Casitas B-lineage lymphoma protein (Cbl) represents another substrate, which is phosphorylated following its interaction with the insulin receptor tyrosine kinase and is required for stimulation of GLUT 4 translocation (93).

In muscle, insulin stimulates a second pathway, the mitogen-activated protein (MAP) signaling pathway (Fig. 6.3). Activation of this pathway plays an important role in the production of mitogens, which promote cell growth, proliferation, and differentiation. Blockade of the MAP kinase pathway prevents the stimulation of cell growth by insulin, but has no effect on the anabolic actions of the hormone (94–96).

Insulin Signal Transduction Defects in Insulin Resistance

Insulin Receptor Number and Affinity

Muscle and liver represent the major tissues responsible for the regulation of glucose homeostasis *in vivo*, and insulin binding to solubilized receptors obtained from skeletal muscle and liver biopsies has been shown to be normal in both obese and lean diabetic individuals (97–101). The insulin receptor gene has been sequenced in a large number of type 2 diabetic patients from diverse ethnic populations using denaturing-gradient gel electrophoresis or single-stranded conformational polymorphism analysis, and, with very rare exceptions (102), physiologically significant mutations in the insulin receptor gene have not been observed (103,104). Therefore, a structural gene abnormality in the insulin receptor is unlikely to be a common cause of insulin resistance.

Insulin Receptor Tyrosine Kinase Activity

Insulin receptor tyrosine kinase activity has been examined in skeletal muscle and hepatocytes from normal-weight and obese diabetic patients. Most investigators (79,97,98,105–107) have found reduced tyrosine kinase activity. Interestingly, weight loss with normalization of blood glucose levels has been shown to correct the defect in insulin receptor tyrosine kinase activity (108). This observation suggests that the defect in tyrosine kinase may be acquired and results from some combination of hyperglycemia and/or insulin resistance, which are reversed with weight loss.

Insulin Signaling (IRS-1 and PI-3 Kinase) Defects

A physiological increase in the plasma insulin concentration stimulates tyrosine phosphorylation of the insulin receptor and IRS-1 in lean, healthy individuals to 150% to 200% of basal values (81,107,109,110). In obese nondiabetic individuals, the ability of insulin to activate these two early insulin

receptor signaling events in muscle is reduced, whereas in type 2 diabetics, insulin has no significant stimulatory effect on either insulin receptor or IRS-1 tyrosine phosphorylation. The association of p85 protein and PI-3 kinase activity with IRS-1 also is greatly reduced in obese nondiabetic and type 2 diabetic individuals compared to lean healthy individuals (107–111). In the insulin-resistant, normal, glucose-tolerant offspring of two type 2 diabetic parents, IRS-1 tyrosine phosphorylation and the association of p85 protein/PI-3 kinase activity with IRS-1 were also markedly decreased (109). These insulin signaling defects are correlated closely with the severity of insulin resistance (109). In summary, a defect in the association of PI-3 kinase with IRS-1 and its subsequent activation appear to be a characteristic abnormality in type 2 diabetics and is closely correlated with *in vivo* muscle insulin resistance.

The profound defect of the PI-3 kinase signaling pathway in insulin-resistant individuals contrasts markedly with the ability of insulin to stimulate MAP kinase pathway activity (107) (Fig. 6.4). Hyperinsulinemia increases meiosis-specific serine/threonine-protein kinase (MEK1) activity and extracellular signal-related kinase 1/2 (ERK1/2) phosphorylation and activity to the same extent in lean healthy and in insulin-resistant obese nondiabetic and type 2 diabetic patients (107).

Maintenance of insulin stimulation of the MAP kinase pathway in the presence of insulin resistance in the PI-3 kinase pathway may be important in the development of atherosclerosis (Fig. 6.4). Insulin resistance in the anabolic (IRS/PI-3 kinase) pathway, with its compensatory hyperinsulinemia, would lead to excessive stimulation of the MAP

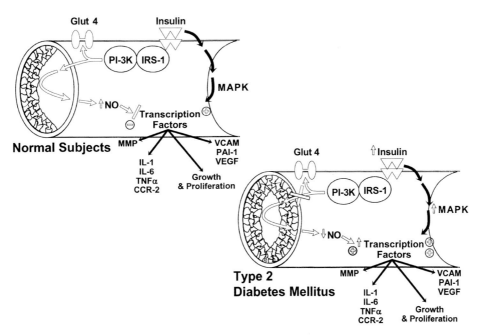

FIG. 6.4. The two insulin-signaling pathways in the vasculature. In the insulin-resistant individual, a block in the anabolic pathway results in compensatory hyperinsulinemia. Because the kinase mitogen-activated protein kinase (MAP K) pathway is intact, an increase in growth factors and inflammatory cytokines may lead to an accelerated rate of atherosclerosis.

kinase pathway in vascular tissue. This would result in the proliferation of vascular smooth muscle cells, increased collagen formation, and increased production of growth factors and inflammatory cytokines, possibly explaining the accelerated rate of atherosclerosis in type 2 diabetic individuals.

Insulin Resistance and the Components of the Insulin Resistance Syndrome

Obesity and Insulin Resistance

The relationship between insulin resistance and weight gain was evaluated in the San Antonio Heart Study (112). Approximately 1,500 Mexican Americans and non-Hispanic whites were divided into two groups: those whose weight increased or decreased during 8 years of follow-up. Fasting insulin was the only independent metabolic predictor of weight change. Those persons who had higher baseline levels of fasting insulin were less likely to gain weight. Similarly, in 97 Pima Indians followed for 3 years, insulin secretion was negatively associated with weight gain (113). When insulin sensitivity was measured in 192 obese Pima Indians, those who were insulin sensitive gained twice as much weight (7.6 kg) as those who were resistant to insulin (3.1-kg weight gain) over 3.5 years (114). In a study of 31 insulin-resistant versus insulin-sensitive persons with BMI between 28 and 35 kg per m^2 who were placed on a hypocaloric liquid diet, there was no correlation of either steady-state plasma glucose (SSPG) or insulin response to meals with weight loss (115). Therefore, the literature does not support the concept that hyperinsulinemia or insulin resistance leads to weight gain in adults.

Whereas insulin resistance does not necessarily result in obesity, weight gain does cause insulin resistance. DeFronzo, utilizing the hyperinsulinemic, euglycemic clamp, demonstrated that obese nondiabetic individuals have the same degree of insulin resistance as lean type 2 diabetic patients (Fig. 6.2) (5). Using the same technique in 1,146 nondiabetic, normotensive individuals, Ferrannini et al. showed a progressive loss of insulin sensitivity when the BMI increased from 18 to 38 kg per m^2 (116). The increase in insulin resistance with weight gain is directly related to the amount of visceral adipose tissue (117,118).

The term visceral adipose tissue (VAT) refers to fat cells located within the abdominal cavity and includes omental, mesenteric, retroperitoneal, and perinephric adipose tissue. VAT has been shown to correlate with insulin resistance and explain much of the variation in insulin resistance seen in a population of African Americans (119). Visceral adipose tissue represents 20% of fat in men and 6% of fat in women. This fat tissue has been shown to have a higher rate of lipolysis than subcutaneous fat, resulting in an increase in free fatty acid production. These fatty acids are released into the portal circulation and drain into the liver, where they stimulate the production of very low density lipoproteins and decrease insulin sensitivity in peripheral tissues (117). VAT also produces a number of cytokines, which cause insulin resistance. These

factors drain into the portal circulation and reduce insulin sensitivity in peripheral tissues (120). Visceral adipose tissue may also lead to elevated levels of cortisol, which would increase insulin resistance. Intraabdominal fat has a high activity of the enzyme 11-beta-hydroxysteroid dehydrogenase. This enzyme converts inactive cortisone to active cortisol. In a weight loss intervention trial carried out in obese, nondiabetic individuals, the best predictor of improvement in insulin sensitivity was a decrease in visceral adiposity (121).

Fat cell size is an important predictor of the development of diabetes (122). Small, newly differentiated adipocytes are more insulin sensitive than large, lipid-laden fat cells. The smaller cells are able to take up glucose and store lipid. In contrast, the larger cells have low rates of insulin-stimulated glucose uptake, less suppression of lipolysis, and a higher rate of cytokine production. This leads to increased amounts of free fatty acids, tumor necrosis factor, and interleukin-6 being transported to the liver, which increases insulin resistance (123,124).

A major health concern in obese diabetics is fatty liver or nonalcoholic steatohepatitis. The prevalence of this condition may be as high as 75% in diabetics with a BMI greater than 30 kg per m^2 (125). The lipid content of the liver is directly correlated with the insulin sensitivity of this tissue in diabetic and nondiabetic individuals (63,126). Fatty liver is also correlated with the increased production of very low density lipoproteins.

The fat cell also has the capability of producing at least one hormone that improves insulin sensitivity—adiponectin. This factor is made in decreasing amounts as an individual becomes more obese (127,128). In animal models, adiponectin decreases hepatic glucose production and increases fatty acid oxidation in muscle (129,130).

Hypertension and Insulin Resistance

The relationship between insulin resistance and hypertension is due in part to increased sympathetic activity caused by increased levels of insulin in obese individuals. Norepinephrine levels increase with increasing BMI and waist-to-hip ratio. Muscle sympathetic nerve activity also increases (131). During fasting, the small fall in glucose and the greater fall in insulin decrease metabolism, leading to a decrease in sympathetic activity, whereas overfeeding increases sympathetic activity. This increase in sympathetic activity in obesity may be an adaptive response to compensate for increase in caloric intake; however, it may lead to an increase in blood pressure.

The classic target tissues of insulin are muscle, fat, and liver. Insulin also has actions in nonclassic tissues, including vascular endothelium (Fig. 6.4). Insulin stimulates the synthesis of the vasodilator nitric oxide (NO) via the IRS pathway. Mice who cannot express endothelial NO synthase (eNOS) have insulin resistance as well as hypertension. The degree of vasodilation with insulin is strongly associated with the degree of insulin sensitivity. FFAs may link the metabolic and hemodynamic abnormalities, causing both insulin resistance and endothelial dysfunction. In classic insulin target tissues, insulin signaling increases phosphorylation of IRS-1 through 4, activating PI-3 kinase, leading to 3′-phosphoinositide-dependent kinase 1 (PDK1) phosphorylation, which leads to phosphorylation of Akt (protein kinase B), causing GLUT4 translocation to the cell membrane (Fig. 6.2). In the endothelial cell, a similar pathway of insulin action increases Akt, leading to eNOS phosphorylation and activation (Fig. 6.4). The common pathway suggests that insulin resistance might have both metabolic and hemodynamic consequences via NO. In a non-insulin-resistant person, insulin has no net effect on blood pressure. However, in the presence of insulin resistance, the compensatory hyperinsulinemia can cause hypertension via the vasoconstrictive pathways of intracellular insulin action on endothelial tissue (132).

Dyslipidemia and Insulin Resistance

Insulin resistance is associated with a dyslipidemia characterized by high triglyceride levels, low HDL-cholesterol levels, and small, dense low-density lipoprotein (LDL)-cholesterol levels (Fig. 6.5) (133).

This atherogenic lipid profile typically precedes the development of type 2 diabetes (134). In addition, hyperglycemia itself may play an etiological role in atherosclerosis through the production of atherogenic glycosylated proteins in vascular walls (135).

Elevated Triglycerides

Insulin resistance results in an enhancement of lipolysis in adipose tissue, fatty acid flux to the liver, and hepatic reesterification of fatty acids into triglycerides (TGs) for their incorporation into very low density lipoprotein (VLDL) (Fig. 6.5) (136). Triglyceride availability is a major factor underlying hepatocellular secretion and transport of apolipoprotein B (apo B). Apo B is present on the surface of VLDL particles and functions as a ligand for the native lipoprotein

lipase receptor (137,138). Elevated free fatty acid levels can also act to enhance insulin resistance (139), which exacerbates the problem. VLDL is removed from the circulation by several high-affinity receptors that recognize surface apoproteins B and E. Glycation of these proteins may reduce their affinity for hepatic receptor-mediated clearance and augment their uptake by vascular macrophages (140,141). Overall, diabetes results in overproduction of and reduced catabolism of TG-rich VLDL, which affects the other components of the dyslipidemic profile.

Low High-density Lipoprotein

High-density lipoprotein promotes reverse cholesterol transport, the primary mechanism of lipid efflux from peripheral tissues (142) (see Chapter 12). Insulin resistance is associated with low serum levels of circulating HDL particles, principally due to a decrease in the antiatherogenic HDL_2 subfraction (143). Under the influence of cholesterol ester transfer protein (CETP), HDL particles take part in a "lipid and protein shuttle" with VLDL and LDL particles, transferring esterified cholesterol in exchange for TG. Enriched with TG, the HDL particles enlarge, are classified progressively as HDL_3, then HDL_2 (Fig. 6.5). Elevated TG levels act to stimulate CETP activity, enriching HDL particles with TG and apo E. More apo E molecules per particle may promote greater HDL catabolism through receptor-mediated clearance.

Small, Dense Low-density Lipoprotein

LDL particles are an end product of lipid and apoprotein transfer and the progressive lipolysis seen during VLDL catabolism (see Chapter 12). Although total LDL concentrations are not appreciably different in diabetic and nondiabetic individuals, there is a qualitative difference related to particle size and density. Elevated serum TG levels stimulate CETP activity, transferring TG from VLDL to LDL in exchange for cholesterol (Fig. 6.5). Subsequent exposure to hepatic lipases

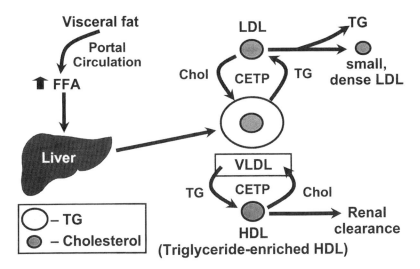

FIG. 6.5. Dyslipidemia in insulin resistance: atherogenic lipid profile. Visceral adipose tissue (VAT) releases free fatty acids (FFAs) into the portal circulation. The FFAs stimulate the assembly and secretion of very low density lipoproteins (VLDL) in the liver. VLDL particles transport triglycerides (TGs) and cholesterol (Chol) in a ratio of 4 or 5 to 1. Cholesterol ester transport protein (CETP) stimulates the exchange of cholesteryl esters from high-density lipoprotein (HDL) and low-density lipoprotein (LDL) for TG carried by VLDL. TG-enriched LDL undergoes lipolysis and become smaller and denser.

removes triglycerides from LDL particles, leaving a population of the smaller, denser, cholesterol-rich particles. This altered LDL species has a reduced affinity for the normal apo B clearance receptor, leading to a greater opportunity for oxidation by free radicals and preferential uptake by the scavenger receptors found on tissue macrophages. The atherosclerotic potential of small, dense LDL particles also derives in part from their greater ease of penetration into vascular tissue (144,145).

TREATMENT OF THE INSULIN RESISTANCE SYNDROME

Insulin Resistance and Hyperinsulinemia

The biguanides and the thiazolidenediones are used to improve insulin sensitivity in target tissues. The biguanides primarily target hepatic tissue, and the thiazolidenediones are more potent insulin sensitizers and interact with peroxisome proliferator-activated receptor gamma receptors found in fat and muscle tissue. Metformin was used in a substudy of overweight individuals in the United Kingdom Prospective Diabetes Study (146). Patients were randomized to treatment with diet and exercise alone or diet and exercise plus drug therapy. Pharmacologic interventions included insulin, chlorpropamide, glibenclamide, or metformin. Patients in the drug treatment group had a 1% lower mean hemoglobin A1c than patients treated with diet and exercise alone. There was no difference in glycemic control between any of the groups receiving pharmacologic therapy. Although all drug-treated patients showed similar reductions in microvascular complications, only the metformin-treated patients had a reduction in macrovascular events. There was a 50% reduction in fatal myocardial infarctions, a 41% reduction in stroke, and a 36% reduction in all-cause mortality in patients treated with metformin compared to patients treated with diet and exercise alone (146).

The thiazolidenediones are the most potent insulin sensitizers and have demonstrated a number of antiatherogenic properties. In a study of 154 type 2 diabetic patients, troglitazone lowered diastolic blood pressure 7 mm Hg (147). Thiazolidenediones provide a consistent increase in HDL cholesterol of 20%. In addition, there is a favorable effect on LDL composition. In a study of type 2 diabetic patients treated with 8 mg of rosiglitazone daily, LDL particle size increased in 71% of patients with a predominance of small, dense LDL (148). Several studies have shown thiazolidenedione treatment favorably alters fat distribution. In a study of 24 type 2 diabetics treated with rosiglitazone ($N = 10$) or placebo ($N = 14$) for 16 weeks, subcutaneous fat increased and hepatic fat content decreased with rosiglitazone therapy (149). Pioglitazone was shown to decrease intraabdominal fat and increase subcutaneous fat in 13 type 2 diabetics treated with 45 mg daily for 16 weeks (150). Thiazolidenediones have also been shown to reduce plasminogen activator inhibitor-1 levels and activity (151,152).

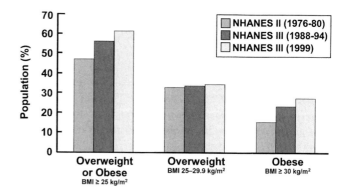

FIG. 6.6. Age-adjusted prevalence of overweight and obesity in the United States between 1975 and 1999. BMI, body mass index. NHANES, National Health and Nutrition Examination Survey. (From National Center for Health Statistics, available at www.cdc.gov/nchs/products/pubs/pubd/hestats/obese/obese99.htm, with permission.)

Insulin Resistance and Obesity

Chapter 9 provides an in-depth discussion of the available treatments for obesity. The impact of obesity on the insulin resistance syndrome cannot be overstated. Obesity is the most prevalent component of the metabolic syndrome, and the prevalence of obesity has increased dramatically over the last 25 years (Fig. 6.6). Indeed, the 33% increase in the prevalence of diabetes mirrors the increased body weight in the United States (153) (Fig. 6.7). Colditz et al. showed there was a continuous increase in the risk of developing diabetes as one gained weight (154) (Fig. 6.8). Individuals who gained more than 20 kg since age 18 years were ten times more likely to develop diabetes than individuals who maintained their weight (154).

Weight loss results in improved insulin sensitivity. In overweight diabetic individuals, a 2.5-kg weight loss resulted in improved glycemic control with lower insulin levels (155). Greater weight loss resulted in progressive reduction in glucose and insulin (155). Clearly, we must use every tool at

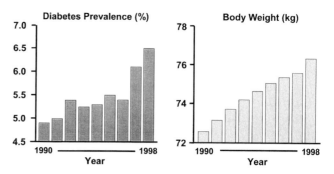

FIG. 6.7. Relationship between prevalence of diabetes and body weight between 1990 and 1998. Data from the Behavioral Risk Factor Surveillance System. (From Mokada A, Ford ES, Bowman BA, et al. Diabetes trends in the U.S.: 1990–1998. *Diabetes Care* 2000;23:1278–1283, with permission.)

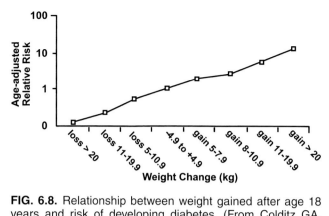

FIG. 6.8. Relationship between weight gained after age 18 years and risk of developing diabetes. (From Colditz GA, Willett WC, Rotnitzky A, et al. Weight gain as a risk factor for clinical diabetes mellitus in women. *Ann Intern Med* 1995;122:481–486, with permission.)

TABLE 6.2. *Effects of lipid-lowering agents in diabetic patients*

	Triglycerides	High-density lipoproteins	Triglycerides
Statins	↓↓↓	↑↔	↓
Fibrates	↔	↑↑	↓↓
Niacin	↓	↑↑↑	↓↓
Resins	↓	↔	↑
Zetia	↓↓	↔	↔

From Lipids Online, available at http://www.lipidsonline. org/, with permission.

our disposal to reverse the progressive weight gain seen in Western cultures.

Insulin Resistance and Hypertension

Reduction in cardiovascular disease and in some cases a reduction in the development of diabetes have been demonstrated with angiotensin-converting enzyme (ACE) inhibitors and angiotensin receptor blockers (ARBs). Cardioprotection with ACE inhibitors has been shown in the Heart Outcomes Prevention Evaluation (HOPE) (156), the Captopril Prevention Project (CAPPP) (157), the Fosinopril vs. Amlodipine (FACET) (158), and the Swedish Trial in Old Patients with Hypertension (STOP-2) (159) trials. In the HOPE study (156), the largest of these trials, 3,577 normotensive diabetic patients were randomized to treatment with ramipril 10 mg per day versus placebo. At the end of the 4-year study period, diabetics in the active treatment group showed a 37% reduction in cardiovascular mortality and a 24% reduction in overall mortality (156). Interestingly, a post hoc analysis of the nondiabetic individuals in the study showed a 30% reduction in the risk of developing diabetes in patients treated with ramipril versus placebo (160). In the LIFE study (161), losartan reduced cardiovascular events more than atenolol in diabetic patients. In addition, nondiabetic individuals who were randomized to this angiotensin receptor blocker were 25% less likely to develop diabetes (162). Drugs that block the angiotensin system should be considered first-line therapy for hypertension in insulin-resistant individuals because of their proven ability to reduce both cardiovascular complications and the progression to diabetes.

Dyslipidemia and Insulin Resistance

Glycemic control may itself have positive effects on serum lipids and lipoproteins. Weight loss and exercise can decrease TG levels and increase HDL-C. In addition, LDL-C

levels may be lowered by 15 to 25 mg per dL (162). Triglyceride levels are significantly reduced by diabetes management that includes oral hypoglycemic agents, and may be reduced by as much as 50% in patients receiving insulin treatment (162). The effects of glycemic control on LDL-C and HDL-C levels are generally more modest. Interestingly, type 2 diabetics requiring treatment with insulin have shown an antiatherogenic redistribution within HDL particles, producing increased HDL₂ and decreased HDL₃ (163).

Patients with atherogenic dyslipidemia will usually require specific lipid-lowering therapy. The various classes of drugs used in the treatment of adult dyslipidemias provide a range of lipid alterations (Table 6.2) (164), and clinical trials have established the value of these agents as monotherapy and in combinations.

Monotherapy

Statins

Statins (3-hydroxy-3-methylglutaryl coenzyme A reductase inhibitors), the most powerful LDL-cholesterol (LDL-C)-lowering class, are usually the initial treatment step in insulin-resistant individuals with elevated LDL-C levels (see Chapters 12 and 13). Although no clinical outcome trials with statins have been performed that specifically target the diabetic patient, post hoc subgroup analyses of the major primary and secondary prevention trials included sufficient type 2 diabetes patients to show at least equivalent benefits of various statins as in the nondiabetic cohort (Table 6.3). A total of 4,619 diabetic patients participated in four trials (4S, CARE/LIPID, HPS, and VA-HIT; see Table 6.3). In these studies of (165–169), there was an 8% prevalence rate of diabetes, similar to the prevalence of diabetes in the general population (170). Because each trial had its own entry criteria, the baseline levels of LDL-C varied from 136 to 186 mg per dL, or 36% to 86% above the current recommended target level for diabetics. Significant LDL-C lowering occurred in all trials, ranging from 25% to 36%. Over the course of the 5- to 6-year average follow-up period, major coronary events were found to be reduced at least as much in diabetic patients (19% to 45%) as in nondiabetic patients (23% to 37%).

The largest placebo-controlled coronary heart disease (CHD) prevention trial of statin therapy, the Heart Protection Study, randomized greater than 20,000 patients considered to be at clinical risk of experiencing a new CHD event by virtue of prior CHD, other atherosclerotic disease, diabetes, or hypertension (171). This high-risk population included 5,963 men and women with diabetes, 3,982 of whom had no prior evidence of CHD. After an average follow-up of 5 years, there was 24% relative risk reduction in major vascular events (CHD death, myocardial infarction, stroke, or revascularization) with simvastatin treatment ($p < 0.0001$) in the total population. Notably, patients with LDL-C less than 116 mg per dL at baseline had similar reductions in events compared to patients with LDL-C greater than 136 mg per dL. In patients with diabetes, there was a similar 25% risk reduction ($p < 0.0001$). The consistent reduction in CHD risk demonstrated in these randomized clinical trials involving over 8,000 diabetics suggests that statins be used in all patients with CHD or CHD equivalent independent of LDL-C level. A moderate effect on lowering TG levels is seen with statin therapy; however, statins have only modest effects on HDL-cholesterol (HDL-C) levels.

Fibrates

A second major class of lipid-modifying drugs used for the reduction of CHD risk is derivatives of fibric acid (including gemfibrozil, fenofibrate, and bezafibrate). A number of clinical trials in diabetic patients have demonstrated lipid-altering effects and CHD risk reduction associated with this class of agents (172–174). The Veterans Administration HDL Intervention Trial (VA-HIT) enrolled 2,531 men with known CHD, low HDL-C, and normal LDL-C levels; approximately 25% of the men who fit these entry criteria had diabetes, whereas 50% had either type 2 diabetes or hyperinsulinemia (174) In the total population, major coronary events were reduced 22% more with gemfibrozil treatment than with placebo over a 7-year period (175). Virtually all the benefit of gemfibrozil was observed in the subgroups of patients with diabetes, hyperinsulinemia, or both (relative risk reductions 30.5%, 27.3%, and 25.2%, respectively; $p \leq 0.02$), whereas little benefit was seen in patients without these conditions (174). Fibrates effectively reduce elevated TG values by 20% to 50% and raise HDL-C levels by approximately 10% (178). These drugs have little effect on LDL-C levels (2). In diabetic patients without elevated LDL-C levels, non-HDL-C control should become the therapeutic target.

Niacin

Niacin is the most effective pharmacologic agent available for increasing HDL-C levels (164). Niacin has been relatively contraindicated in the diabetic population, however, due to early reports of diminished glycemic control and an increase in insulin resistance (176). There is a modest hyperglycemic response to niacin, perhaps due to a secondary

TABLE 6.3. *Secondary coronary heart disease prevention studies: analysis of benefit in the entire cohort (A) and the diabetic patient subgroup (B)[a,b]*

A. Entire cohort

Trial	Drug	Baseline lipids		CHD event rates (%)		Absolute RR (%)	NNT
		LDL-C (mg/dL)	HDL-C (mg/dL)	Placebo	Drug		
4S	Simvastatin	189	46	28	19.4	8.6	12
CARE	Pravastatin	139	39	13.2	10.2	3.0	33
LIPID	Pravastatin	150	37	15.9	12.3	3.6	28
HPS	Simvastatin	131	41	11.8	8.7	3.1	32
VA-HIT	Gemfibrozil	111	32	21.7	17.3	4.4	23

B. Diabetes subanalysis

Trial	n	First major CHD event		Relative RR (95% CI)	Absolute RR (%)	NNT
		Placebo (%)	Drug (%)			
4S	483	37.5	23.5	42 (59 to 20)	14	7
CARE/LIPID	1386	22.1	18.6	17 (35 to 5)	3.5	29
HPS	1981	21.0	17.4	17 (35 to 2)	3.6	28
VA-HIT	769	29.4	21.2	31 (48 to 8)	8.2	12

[a]See text for details.
[b]CHD, coronary heart disease; LDL-C, low-density lipoprotein cholesterol; HDL-C, high-density lipoprotein cholesterol; RR, risk ratio; NNT, number needed to treat; 4S, Scandinavian Simvastatin Survival trial; CARE, Cholesterol and Recurrent Events trial; LIPID, long-term Intervention with Pravastatin in Ischaemic Disease (LIPID) study; HPS, Heart Protection Study; VA-HIT, Veterans Administration HDL Intervention Trial; CI, confidence interval.

rebound in circulating oxidized free fatty acids, leading to reduced insulin-stimulated glucose uptake and increased hepatic glucose output. However, the actions of niacin effectively target the various lipid components of the atherogenic triad, making it particularly attractive for use in type 2 diabetic patients (164) Consequently, several recent studies have reexamined the efficacy and safety of niacin in patients with controlled type 2 diabetes.

The Arterial Disease Multiple Interventions Trial evaluated niacin therapy in 486 patients with peripheral vascular disease, including 125 patients with diabetes, for a period of 1 year. Niacin (average dose of 2.5 gm per day) increased glucose levels by 8.1 mg per dL in the diabetic patients compared with an increase of 6.3 mg per dL in the nondiabetic subjects, and HbA$_{1C}$ levels were not significantly changed from baseline (177). Similarly, the Assessment of Diabetes Control and Evaluation of the Efficacy of Niaspan Trial randomized 148 type 2 diabetic patients to placebo or extended-release niacin (niacin ER). Dose-dependent increases in HDL-C and decreases in TG occurred with niacin ER, 1,000 mg and 1,500 mg, and these changes were accompanied by negligible increases in hemoglobin A1c (178).

Clinically, niacin's ability to decrease cardiovascular events was shown in the Coronary Drug Project, where CHD patients with hypercholesterolemia experienced a 27% relative reduction in nonfatal myocardial infarction rates and an 11% reduction in long-term mortality (179,180). Recently, these results were analyzed by baseline fasting and 1-hour blood glucose (186). In the post-hoc analysis, niacin reduced nonfatal myocardial infarction and total mortality to a similar extent across all baseline glucose levels, even in patients with fasting blood glucose greater than or equal to 126 mg per dL.

Statins Plus Fibrates

Use of this drug combination has been limited following reports in the literature of rhabdomyolysis and renal failure (182–185). However, in controlled clinical trials where study design minimized other drug interactions, only 1% of nearly 600 patients treated with this combination were withdrawn because of myalgias (164). Athyros and colleagues compared atorvastatin plus fenofibrate to either drug alone for 24 weeks in 120 patients with type 2 diabetes (186). The combination reduced LDL-C levels by 46% and TG values by 50%; HDL-C levels increased by 22%. This study shows that a statin–fibrate combination is attractive for diabetic patients with elevated LDL-C and TG levels and for those who continue to have elevated TG after reaching their LDL-C goal with statin monotherapy. Careful monitoring for symptoms of myopathy is recommended (164).

Statins Plus Niacin

Statins and niacin have complementary actions on the atherogenic lipid profile. A study of high-dose atorvastatin–niacin

ER (80 mg–3 g per day) combination therapy was compared with each drug given as monotherapy in 53 diabetic patients with atherogenic dyslipidemia defined by small LDL particle size and/or low HDL$_2$ levels (less than 40% of total HDL) (187). Among patients with small LDL size, atorvastatin and niacin ER monotherapies had different effects on LDL. Reductions in LDL-C concentrations from baseline were significantly greater with atorvastatin (49%) and combination therapy (55%) than with niacin ER monotherapy (20%; $p<0.0002$), whereas increases in LDL particle size were significantly greater with niacin ER and combination therapy (4% each) than with atorvastatin monotherapy (2%; $p<0.05$). Among patients with low HDL$_2$, increases in HDL-C concentrations from baseline were significantly greater with niacin ER and combination therapy (42% each) than with atorvastatin monotherapy (2%; $p<0.005$). Similarly, HDL$_2$ concentrations increased significantly more with niacin ER (100%) and combination therapy (93%) than with atorvastatin monotherapy (50%; $p<0.03$). Overall, combination therapy lowered TG levels more than either drug alone. In the two groups of diabetic patients studied, combined therapy normalized lipoprotein levels and improved particle sizes.

The combination of a statin and niacin was associated with substantial clinical benefits in the HDL-Atherosclerosis Treatment Study (188), which enrolled 160 patients with CHD, including 34 patients with diabetes or impaired fasting glucose levels (189). All patients had low HDL-C, high TG, and mildly elevated LDL-C levels and were randomized to treatment with antioxidants, simvastatin plus niacin, simvastatin plus niacin plus antioxidants, or placebo (188). After 3 years, patients treated with simvastatin–niacin regimens experienced a 60% to 90% reduction in the composite primary endpoint (CHD death, myocardial infarction, stroke, or revascularization) compared with those treated with placebo or antioxidants alone ($p=0.03$). Substantial improvements were also seen in the subgroup of patients with diabetes or impaired fasting glucose; simvastatin–niacin treatment was associated with a 31% decrease in LDL-C, a 40% decrease in TG, and a 30% increase in HDL-C, whereas placebo or antioxidant treatments alone had little effect (189).

In summary, the lipoprotein abnormalities associated with the insulin resistance syndrome are integrally related to the development and progression of atherosclerosis, and there is abundant evidence from clinical trials that type 2 diabetic patients receive benefit from aggressive lipid management. Statins, fibrates, and niacin each improve different aspects of the lipid profile and should be used selectively, based on individual patient characteristics. Combination therapies may provide the best therapeutic option for treating the atherogenic dyslipidemia of type 2 diabetes.

Insulin Resistance and the Prevention of Hyperglycemia

It should be clear from the foregoing discussion that improvements in insulin sensitivity can be achieved by decreasing abdominal fat with diet and exercise. In addition, recent clinical trials have documented the ability of insulin-sensitizing drugs to delay the onset of hyperglycemia in insulin-resistant individuals.

Diet and Exercise

The Diabetes Prevention Program (190) confirmed that modest weight loss in association with exercise can have a dramatic impact on insulin sensitivity and the progression to diabetes. In this study, approximately 2,000 individuals with impaired glucose tolerance were randomized to lifestyle changes versus usual care. The study, which was originally planned to be ongoing for 5 years, was stopped after 2.8 years because the results were so conclusive. The usual-care group developed diabetes at the rate of 11% each year. In the lifestyle arm, diabetes developed at a rate of 5% per year— a 58% reduction in the risk of developing diabetes with diet and exercise (190). Surprisingly, a modest amount of diet and exercise yielded impressive results. The exercise program in the lifestyle group was walking 30 min for 5 days each week. The mean weight loss over the 2.8-year study period was only 8 pounds. Similar results were seen in the Finnish Diabetes Study (191).

Pharmacologic Agents

In the Diabetes Prevention Program (190) just discussed approximately 1,000 of the study patients were randomized to metformin therapy. The metformin-treated patients showed a 4-pound weight loss on average and a reduction in the risk of developing diabetes of 31% compared to placebo (190). Interestingly, young and overweight individuals had a greater reduction in the risk of developing diabetes than normal-weight and older study patients (190).

The TRIPOD study (192) evaluated the ability of troglitazone to prevent the development of diabetes in women with a history of gestational diabetes. The rate of development of diabetes in the placebo arm of the study was approximately 12% per year compared to about 5% in the treatment group. Surprisingly, Buchanan et al. were able to demonstrate total preservation of beta cell function over a 5-year period in women who had near normal beta cell function at baseline and initially responded to the drug (192). The preservation in beta cell function continued 8 months after the drug was discontinued.

REFERENCES

1. Reaven GM. Role of insulin resistance in human disease. *Diabetes* 1988;37:1595–1607.
2. Expert Panel on Detection, Evaluation, and Treatment of High Blood Cholesterol in Adults. Executive summary of the third report of the National Cholesterol Education Program (NCEP) Expert Panel on Detection, Evaluation, and Treatment of High Blood Cholesterol in Adults (Adult Treatment Panel III). *JAMA* 2001;285:2486–2496.
3. Park YW, Zhu S, Palaniappan L, et al. The metabolic syndrome: prevalence and associated risk factor findings in the US population from the Third National Health and Nutrition Examination Survey, 1988–1994. *Arch Intern Med* 2003;163:427–436.
4. Ford ES, Giles WH, Dietz WH. Prevalence of the metabolic syndrome among US adults: findings from the third National Health and Nutrition Examination Survey. *JAMA* 2002;287:356–359.
5. DeFronzo RA. Pathogenesis of type 2 diabetes mellitus: metabolic and molecular implications for identifying diabetes genes. *Diabetes Rev* 1997;5:177–269.
6. DeFronzo RA. Lilly Lecture. The triumvirate: beta cell, muscle, liver. A collusion responsible for NIDDM. *Diabetes* 1988;37:667–687.
7. DeFronzo RA, Jacot E, Jequier E, et al. The effect of insulin on the disposal of intravenous glucose: results from indirect calorimetry. *Diabetes* 1981;30:1000–1007.
8. Gerich JE, Meyer C, Woerle HJ, et al. Renal gluconeogenesis. Its importance in human glucose homeostasis. *Diabetes Care* 2001;24:382–391.
9. Ekberg K, Landau BR, Wajngot A, et al. Contributions by kidney and liver to glucose production in the postabsorptive state and after 60 h of fasting. *Diabetes* 1999;48:292–298.
10. DeFronzo RA. Pathogenesis of type 2 (non-insulin dependent) diabetes mellitus: a balanced overview. *Diabetologia* 1992;35:389–397.
11. Katz LD, Glickman MG, Rapoport S, et al. Splanchnic and peripheral disposal of oral glucose in man. *Diabetes* 1983;32:675–679.
12. Ferrannini E, Bjorkman O, Reichard Jr GA, et al. The disposal of an oral glucose load in healthy subjects. *Diabetes* 1985;34:580–588.
13. Mitrakou A, Kelley D, Veneman T, et al. Contribution of abnormal muscle and liver glucose metabolism to postprandial hyperglycemia in NIDDM. *Diabetes* 1990;39:1381–1390.
14. Mandarino L, Bonadonna R, McGuinness O, et al. Regulation of muscle glucose uptake *in vivo*. In: Jefferson LS, Cherrington AD, eds. *Handbook of physiology, Section 7, The endocrine system,* Vol. II, *The endocrine pancreas and regulation of metabolism.* Oxford: Oxford University Press, 2001:803–848.
15. Jansson PA, Larsson A, Smith U, et al. Lactate release from the subcutaneous tissue in lean and obese men. *J Clin Invest* 1994;93:240–246.
16. Groop LC, Bonadonna RC, Del Prato S, et al. Glucose and free fatty acid metabolism in non-insulin dependent diabetes mellitus. Evidence for multiple sites of insulin resistance. *J Clin Invest* 1989;84:205–215.
17. Santomauro A, Boden G, Silva M, et al. Overnight lowering of free fatty acids with acipimox improves insulin resistance and glucose tolerance in obese diabetic and non-diabetic subjects. *Diabetes* 1999;48:1836–1841.
18. Bergman RN. Non-esterified fatty acids and the liver: why is insulin secreted into the portal vein?. *Diabetologia* 2000;43:946–952.
19. Boden G. Role of fatty acids in the pathogenesis of insulin resistance and NIDDM. *Diabetes* 1997;46:3–10.
20. McGarry JD. Banting Lecture 2001: dysregulation of fatty acid metabolism in the etiology of type 2 diabetes. *Diabetes* 2002;51:7–18.
21. Diamond MP, Thornton K, Connolly-Diamond M, et al. Reciprocal variations in insulin-stimulated glucose uptake and pancreatic insulin secretion in women with normal glucose tolerance. *J Soc Gynecol Invest* 1995;2:708–715.
22. DeFronzo RA, Ferrannini E, Simonson DC. Fasting hyperglycemia in non-insulin-dependent diabetes mellitus: contributions of excessive hepatic glucose production and impaired tissue glucose uptake. *Metabolism* 1989;38:387–395.
23. Sicree RA, Zimmet P, King HO, et al. Plasma insulin response among Nauruans. Prediction of deterioration in glucose tolerance over 6 years. *Diabetes* 1987;36:179–186.
24. Saad MF, Knowler WC, Pettitt DJ, et al. Sequential changes in serum insulin concentration during development of non-insulin-dependent diabetes. *Lancet* 1989;i:1356–1359.
25. Saad MF, Knowler WC, Pettitt DJ, et al. The natural history of impaired glucose tolerance in the Pima Indians. *N Engl J Med* 1988;319:1500–1505.
26. Haffner SM, Miettinen H, Gaskill SP, et al. Decreased insulin secretion and increased insulin resistance are independently related to the 7-year risk of NIDDM in Mexican-Americans. *Diabetes* 1995;44:1386–1391.

27. Weyer C, Hanson RL, Tataranni PA, et al. A high fasting plasma insulin concentration predicts type 2 diabetes independent of insulin resistance. Evidence for a pathogenic role of relative hyperinsulinemia. *Diabetes* 2000;49:2094–2101.

28. Weyer C, Bogardus C, Pratley RE. Metabolic characteristics of individuals with impaired fasting glucose and/or impaired glucose tolerance. *Diabetes* 1999;48:2197–2203.

29. Weyer C, Tataranni PA, Bogardus C, et al. Insulin resistance and insulin secretory dysfunction are independent predictors of worsening of glucose tolerance during each stage of type 2 diabetes development. *Diabetes Care* 2000;24:89–94.

30. Martin BC, Warram JH, Krolewski AS, et al. Role of glucose and insulin resistance in development of type 2 diabetes mellitus: results of a 25-year follow-up study. *Lancet* 1992;340:925–929.

31. Lillioja S, Mott DM, Zawadzki JK, et al. *In vivo* insulin action is a familial characteristic in nondiabetic Pima Indians. *Diabetes* 1987;36:1329–1335.

32. Kahn SE. Clinical review 135. The importance of β-cell failure in the development and progression of type 2 diabetes. *J Clin Endocrinol Metab* 2001;86:4047–4058.

33. Bergman RN, Finegood DT, Kahn SE. The evolution of β-cell dysfunction and insulin resistance in type 2 diabetes. *Eur J Clin Invest* 2002;32:35–45.

34. Lillioja S, Mott DM, Howard BV, et al. Impaired glucose tolerance as a disorder of insulin action. Longitudinal and cross-sectional studies in Pima Indians. *N Engl J Med* 1988;318:1217–1225.

35. Jallut D, Golay A, Munger R, et al. Impaired glucose tolerance and diabetes in obesity: a 6 year follow-up study of glucose metabolism. *Metabolism* 1990;39:1068–1075.

36. Himsworth HP, Kerr RB. Insulin-sensitive and insulin-insensitive types of diabetes mellitus. *Clin Sci* 1939;4:120–152.

37. Ginsberg H, Kimmerling G, Olefsky JM, et al. Demonstration of insulin resistance in untreated adult-onset diabetic subjects with fasting hyperglycemia. *J Clin Invest* 1975;55:454–461.

38. DeFronzo RA, Tobin JD, Andres R. Glucose clamp technique: a method for quantifying insulin secretion and resistance. *Am J Physiol* 1979;6:E214–E223.

39. DeFronzo RA, Simonson D, Ferrannini E. Hepatic and peripheral insulin resistance: a common feature in non-insulin-dependent and insulin-dependent diabetes. *Diabetologia* 1982;23:313–319.

40. Golay A, DeFronzo RA, Ferrannini E, et al. Oxidative and non-oxidative glucose metabolism in non-obese type 2 (non-insulin dependent) diabetic patients. *Diabetologia* 1988;31:585–591.

41. Golay A, Felber JP, Jequier E, et al. Metabolic basis of obesity and noninsulin-dependent diabetes mellitus. *Diabetes Metab Rev* 1988;4:727–747.

42. DeFronzo RA, Sherwin RS, Hendler R, et al. Insulin binding to monocytes and insulin action in human obesity, starvation, and refeeding. *J Clin Invest* 1978;62:204–213.

43. Huang SC, Phelps ME, Hoffman EJ, et al. Non-invasive determination of local cerebral metabolic rate of glucose in man. *Am J Physiol* 1980;238:E69–E82.

44. Reaven GM, Brand RJ, Ida Chen YD, et al. Insulin resistance and insulin secretion are determinants of oral glucose tolerance in normal individuals. *Diabetes* 1993;42:1324–1332.

45. Cherrington AD, Stevenson RW, Steiner KE, et al. Insulin, glucagon, and glucose as regulators of hepatic glucose uptake and production *in vivo*. *Diabetes Metab Rev* 1987;3:307–332.

46. Waldhausl W, Bratusch-Marrain P, Gasic S, et al. Insulin production rate, hepatic insulin retention, and splanchnic carbohydrate metabolism after oral glucose ingestion in hyperinsulinemic type II (non-insulin dependent) diabetes mellitus. *Diabetologia* 1982;23:6–15.

47. Consoli A, Nurjahn N, Capani F, et al. Predominant role of gluconeogenesis in increased hepatic glucose production in NIDDM. *Diabetes* 1989;38:550–556.

48. Nurjhan N, Consoli A, Gerich J. Increased lipolysis and its consequences on gluconeogenesis in noninsulin-dependent diabetes mellitus. *J Clin Invest* 1992;89:169–175.

49. Bjorntorp P, Berchtold P, Holm J. The glucose uptake of human adipose tissue in obesity. *Eur J Clin Invest* 1971;1:480–485.

50. Frayn KN, Coppack SW, Humphreys SM, et al. Metabolic characteristics of human adipose tissue *in vivo*. *Clin Sci* 1989;76:509–516.

51. DeFronzo RA, Gunnarsson R, Bjorkman O, et al. Effects of insulin on peripheral and splanchnic glucose metabolism in non-insulin-dependent (type II) diabetes mellitus. *J Clin Invest* 1985;76:149–155.

52. Bonadonna RC, Bonora E. Glucose and free fatty acid metabolism in human obesity: relationships to insulin resistance. *Diabetes Rev* 1997;5:21–51.

53. Reaven GM, Chen YDI, Donner CC, et al. How insulin resistant are patients with non-insulin-dependent diabetes mellitus? *J Clin Endocrinol Metab* 1985;61:32–36.

54. Lillioja A, Mott DM, Zawadzki JK, et al. Glucose storage is a major determinant of *in vivo* 'insulin resistance' in subjects with normal glucose tolerance. *J Clin Endocrinol Metab* 1986;62:922–927.

55. Hales CN. The pathogenesis of NIDDM. *Diabetologia* 1994;37:S162–S168.

56. Reaven GM, Hollenbeck C, Jeng CY, et al. Measurement of plasma glucose, free fatty acid, lactate, and insulin for 24 hours in patients with NIDDM. *Diabetes* 1988;37:1020–1024.

57. Thiebaud D, DeFronzo RA, Jacot E, et al. Effect of long-chain triglyceride infusion on glucose metabolism in man. *Metabolism* 1982;31:1128–1136.

58. Kelley DE, Mandarino LJ. Fuel selection in human skeletal muscle in insulin resistance. A reexamination. *Diabetes* 2000;49:677–683.

59. Kashyap S, Belfort R, Pratipanawatr T, et al. Chronic elevation in plasma free fatty acids impairs insulin secretion in non-diabetic offspring with a strong family history of T2DM. *Diabetes* 2002;51[Suppl 2]:A12.

60. Carpentier A, Mittelman SD, Bergman RN, et al. Prolonged elevation of plasma free fatty acids impairs pancreatic beta-cell function in obese nondiabetic humans but not in individuals with type 2 diabetes. *Diabetes* 2000;49:399–408.

61. Goodpaster BH, Thaete FL, Kelley BE. Thigh adipose tissue distribution is associated with insulin resistance in obesity and in type 2 diabetes mellitus. *Am J Clin Nutr* 2000;71:885–892.

62. Greco AV, Mingrone G, Giancaterini A, et al. Insulin resistance in morbid obesity. Reversal with intramyocellular fat depletion. *Diabetes* 2002;51:144–151.

63. Ryysy L, Hakkinen AM, Goto T, et al. Hepatic fat content and insulin action on free fatty acids and glucose metabolism rather than insulin absorption are associated with insulin requirements during insulin therapy in type 2 diabetic patients. *Diabetes* 2000;49:749–758.

64. Miyazaki Y, Mahankali A, Matsuda M, et al. Effect of pioglitazone on abdominal fat distribution and insulin sensitivity in type 2 diabetic patients. *J Clin Endocrinol Metab* 2002;87:2784–2791.

65. Randle PJ, Garland PB, Hales CN, et al. The glucose fatty acid cycle. Its role in insulin sensitivity and the metabolic disturbances of diabetes mellitus. *Lancet* 1963;281:785–789.

66. Steinberg HO, Brechtel G, Johnson A, et al. Insulin-mediated skeletal muscle vasodilation is nitric oxide dependent. A novel action of insulin to increase nitric oxide release. *J Clin Invest* 1994;94:1172–1179.

67. Baron AD. Hemodynamic actions of insulin. *Am J Physiol* 1994;267:E187–E202.

68. Mather K, Laakso M, Edelman S, et al. Evidence for physiological coupling of insulin-mediated glucose metabolism and limb blood flow. *Am J Physiol Endocrinol Metab* 2000;279:E1264–E1270.

69. Reaven GM, Hollenbeck C, Jeng CY, et al. Measurement of plasma glucose, free fatty acid, lactate, and insulin for 24 hours in patients with NIDDM. *Diabetes* 1988;37:1020–1024.

70. Steinberg HO, Paradisi G, Hook G, et al. Free fatty acid elevation impairs insulin-mediated vasodilation and nitric oxide production. *Diabetes* 2000;49:1231–1238.

71. Kreutzenberg SV, Crepaldi C, Marchetto S, et al. Plasma free fatty acids and endothelium-dependent vasodilation: effect of chain-length and cyclooxygenase inhibition. *J Clin Endocrinol Metab* 2000;85:793–798.

72. Davda RK, Chandler LJ, Guzman NJ. Protein kinase C modulates receptor-independent activation of endothelial nitric oxide synthase. *Eur J Pharmacol* 1994;266:237–244.

73. Bjorntorp P. Metabolic implications of body fat distribution. *Diabetes Care* 1991;14:1132–1143.

74. Arner P. Regional adiposity in man. *J Endocrinol* 1997;155:191–192.

75. Saltiel AR, Kahn CR. Insulin signaling and the regulation of glucose and lipid metabolism. *Nature* 2001;414:799–806.

76. Virkamaki A, Ueki K, Kahn CR. Protein–protein interaction in insulin signaling and the molecular mechanisms of insulin resistance. *J Clin Invest* 1999;103:931–943.

77. Pessin JE, Saltiel AR. Signaling pathways in insulin action: molecular targets of insulin resistance. *J Clin Invest* 2000;106:165–169.

78. Whitehead JP, Clark SF, Urso B, et al. Signalling through the insulin receptor. *CurrOpin Cell Biol* 2000;12:222–228.

79. Wilden PA, Kahn CR. The level of insulin receptor tyrosine kinase activity modulates the activities of phosphatidylinositol 3-kinase, microtubule-associated protein, and S6 kinases. *Mol Endocrinol* 1994;8:558–567.

80. Haring HU, Mehnert H. Pathogenesis of type 2 (non-insulin-dependent) diabetes mellitus: candidates for a signal transmitter defect causing insulin resistance of the skeletal muscle. *Diabetologia* 1993;36:176–182.

81. Wajtaszewski JFP, Hansen BF, Kiens B, et al. Insulin signaling in human skeletal muscle. Time course and effect of exercise. *Diabetes* 1997;46:1775–1781.

82. Shepherd PR, Kahn BB. Glucose transporters and insulin action. Implications for insulin resistance and diabetes mellitus. *N Engl J Med* 1999;341:248–257.

83. Garvey WT. Insulin action and insulin resistance: diseases involving defects in insulin receptors, signal transduction, and the glucose transport effector system. *Am J Med* 1998;105:331–345.

84. Chou DK, Dull TJ, Russell DS, et al. Human insulin receptors mutated at the ATP-binding site lack protein tyrosine kinase activity and fail to mediate postreceptor effects of insulin. *J Biol Chem* 1987;262:1842–1847.

85. Ebina Y, Araki E, Tiara F, et al. Replacement of lysine residue 1030 in the putative ATP-binding region of the insulin receptor abolishes insulin and antibody-stimulated glucose uptake and receptor kinase activity. *Proc Natl Acad Sci USA* 1987;84:704–708.

86. Backer JM, Myers MG Jr, Shoelson SE, et al. The phosphatidylinositol 3' kinase is activated by association with IRS-1 during insulin stimulation. *EMBO J* 1992;11:3469–3479.

87. Sun XJ, Miralpeix M, Myers Jr MG, et al. The expression and function of IRS-1 in insulin signal transmission. *J Biol Chem* 1992;267:22662–22672.

88. Okada T, Sakuma L, Fukui Y, et al. Essential role of phosphatidylinositol 3-kinase in insulin-induced glucose transport and antilipolysis in rat adipocytes. *J Biol Chem* 1994;269:3568–3573.

89. Cross D, Alessi D, Vandenheed J, et al. The inhibition of glycogen synthase kinase-3 by insulin-like growth factor 1 in the rat skeletal muscle cell line L6 is blocked by wortmannin but not rapamycin. *Biochem J* 1994;303:21–26.

90. Thomas G, Hall MN. TOR signalling and control of cell growth. *Curr Opin Cell Biol* 1997;9:782–787.

91. Nave BT, Ouwens M, Withers DJ, et al. Mammalian target of rapamycin is a direct target for protein kinase B: identification of a convergence point for opposing effects of insulin and amino-acid deficiency on protein translation. *Biochem J* 1999;344[Pt 2]:427–431.

92. Kerouz NJ, Horsch D, Pons S, et al. Differential regulation of insulin receptor substrates-1 and -2 (IRS-1 and IRS-2) and phosphatidylinositol 3-kinase isoforms in liver and muscle of the obese diabetic (ob/ob) mouse. *J Clin Invest* 1997;100:3164–3172.

93. Chiang SH, Baumann CA, Kanzaki M, et al. Insulin-stimulated GLUT4 translocation requires the CAP-dependent activation of TC10. *Nature* 2001;410:944–948.

94. Boulton TG, Nye SH, Robbins DJ, et al. ERKs: a family of protein–serine/threonine kinases that are activated and tyrosine phosphorylated in response to insulin and NGF. *Cell* 1991;65:663–675.

95. Lazar DF, Wiese RJ, Brady MJ, et al. Mitogen-activated protein kinase kinase inhibition does not block the stimulation of glucose utilization by insulin. *J Biol Chem* 1995;270:20801–20807.

96. Dorrestijn J, Ouwens DM, Van den Berghe N, et al. Expression of dominant-negative Ras mutant does not affect stimulation of glucose uptake and glycogen synthesis by insulin. *Diabetologia* 1996;39:558–563.

97. Caro JF, Sinha MK, Raju SM, et al. Insulin receptor kinase in human skeletal muscle from obese subjects with and without non-insulin dependent diabetes. *J Clin Invest* 1987;79:1330–1337.

98. Caro JF, Ittoop O, Pories WJ, et al. Studies on the mechanism of insulin resistance in the liver from humans with non-insulin-dependent diabetes. Insulin action and binding in isolated hepatocytes, insulin receptor structure, and kinase activity. *J Clin Invest* 1986;78:249–258.

99. Comi RJ, Grunberger G, Gorden P. Relationship of insulin binding and insulin-stimulated tyrosine kinase activity is altered in type II diabetes. *J Clin Invest* 1987;79:453–462.

100. Klein HH, Vestergaard H, Kotzke G, et al. Elevation of serum insulin concentration during euglycemic hyperinsulinemic clamp studies leads to similar activation of insulin receptor kinase in skeletal muscle of subjects with and without NIDDM. *Diabetes* 1995;344:1310–1317.

101. Obermaier-Kusser B, White MF, Pongratz DE, et al. A defective intramolecular autoactivation cascade may cause the reduced kinase activity of the skeletal muscle insulin receptor from patients with non-insulin-dependent diabetes mellitus. *J Biol Chem* 1989;264:9497–9503.

102. Cocozza S, Procellini A, Riccardi G, et al. NIDDM associated with mutation in tyrosine kinase domain of insulin receptor gene. *Diabetes* 1992;41:521–526.

103. Moller DE, Yakota A, Flier JS. Normal insulin receptor cDNA sequence in Pima Indians with non-insulin-dependent diabetes mellitus. *Diabetes* 1989;38:1496–1500.

104. Kusari J, Verma US, Buse JB, et al. Analysis of the gene sequences of the insulin receptor and the insulin-sensitive glucose transporter (GLUT4) in patients with common-type non-insulin-dependent diabetes mellitus. *J Clin Invest* 1991;88:1323–1330.

105. Nyomba BL, Ossowski VM, Bogardus C, et al. Insulin-sensitive tyrosine kinase relationship with *in vivo* insulin action in humans. *Am J Physiol* 1990;258:E964–E974.

106. Nolan JJ, Friedenberg G, Henry R, et al. Role of human skeletal muscle insulin receptor kinase in the *in vivo* insulin resistance of noninsulin-dependent diabetes and obesity. *J Clin Endocrinol Metab* 1994;78:471–477.

107. Krook A, Bjornholm M, Galuska D, et al. Characterization of signal transduction and glucose transport in skeletal muscle from type 2 diabetic patients. *Diabetes* 2000;49:284–292.

108. Freidenberg GR, Reichart D, Olefsky JM, et al. Reversibility of defective adipocyte insulin receptor kinase activity in non-insulin dependent diabetes mellitus. Effect of weight loss. *J Clin Invest* 1988;82:1398–1406.

109. Pratipanawatr W, Pratipanawatr T, Cusi K, et al. Skeletal muscle insulin resistance in normoglycemic subjects with a strong family history of type 2 diabetes is associated with decreased insulin-stimulated insulin receptor substrate-1 tyrosine phosphorylation. *Diabetes* 2001;50:2572–2578.

110. Laville M, Auboeuf D, Khalfallah Y, et al. Acute regulation by insulin of phosphatidylinositol-3-kinase, Rad, Glut 4, and lipoprotein lipase in mRNA levels in human muscle. *J Clin Invest* 1996;98:43–49.

111. Kim YB, Nikoulina S, Ciaraldi TP, et al. Normal insulin-dependent activation of Akt/protein kinase B, with diminished activation of phosphoinositide 3-kinase, in muscle in type 2 diabetes. *J Clin Invest* 1999;104:733–741.

112. Valdez R, Mitchell BD, Haffner SM, et al. Predictors of weight change in a bi-ethnic population: the San Antonio Heart Study. *Int J Obes Relat Metab Disord* 1994;18:85–91.

113. Schwartz MW, Boyko EJ, Kahn SE, et al. Reduced insulin secretion: an independent predictor of body weight gain. *J Clin Endocrinol Metab* 1995;80:1571–1576.

114. Swinburn BA, Nyomba BL, Saad MF, et al. Insulin resistance associated with lower rates of weight gain in Pima Indians. *J Clin Invest* 1991;88:168–173.

115. McLaughlin T, Abbasi F, Carantoni M, et al. Differences in insulin resistance do not predict weight loss in response to hypocaloric diets in healthy obese women. *J Clin Endocrinol Metab* 1999;84:578–581.

116. Ferrannini E, Natali A, Bell P, et al. Insulin resistance and hypersecretion in obesity. *J Clin Invest* 1997;100:1166–1173.

117. Montague CT, O'Rahilly S. The perils of portliness: Causes and consequences of visceral adiposity. *Diabetes* 2000;49:883–888.

118. Kelley DE, Williams KV, Price JC, et al. Plasma fatty acids, adiposity and variance of skeletal muscle insulin resistance in type 2 diabetes mellitus. *J Clin Endocrinol Metab* 2001;86:5412–5419.

119. Banerji MA, Lebowitz J, Chaiken RL, et al. Relationship of visceral adipose tissue and glucose disposal is independent of sex in black NIDDM subjects. *Am J Physiol* 1997;273:E425–E432.

120. Kelley DE. The impact of obesity, regional adiposity and ectopic fat on the pathophysiology of type 2 diabetes; Council on Obesity Diabetes Education. 2003;12–20.

121. Goodpaster BH, Kelley DE, Wing RR, et al. Effects of weight loss on insulin sensitivity in obesity: influence of regional adiposity. *Diabetes* 1999;48:839–847.
122. Weyer C, Foley JE, Bogardus C, et al. Enlarged subcutaneous abdominal adipocyte size, but not obesity itself, predicts type 2 diabetes independent of insulin resistance. *Diabetologia* 2000;43:1498–1506.
123. Hotamisligil GS, Arner S, Caro P, et al. Increased adipose tissue expression of tumor necrosis factor-alpha in human obesity and insulin resistance. *J Clin Invest* 1995;95:2409–2415.
124. Kern PA, Saghizadeh, M, Ong JM, et al. The expression of tumor necrosis factor in human adipose tissue: regulation by obesity, weight losss, and relationship to lipoprotein lipase. *J Clin Invest* 1995;95;2111–2119.
125. Chitturi S, Farrell GC. Etiopathogenesis of nonalcolholic steatohepatits. *Semin Liver Dis* 2001;21:27–41.
126. Seppala-Lindroos A, Vehkavaara S, Häkkinen AM, et al. Fat accumulation in the liver is associated with defects in insulin suppression of glucose production and serum fatty acids independent of obesity in normal men. *J Clin Endocrinol Metab* 2002;87:3023–3028.
127. Weyer C, Funahashi T, Tanaka S, et al. Hypoadiponectinemia in obesity and type 2 diabetes: close association with insulin resistance and hyperinsulinemia. *J Clin Endocrinol Metab* 2000;86;1930–1935.
128. Arita Y, Kihara S, Ouchi N, et al. Paradoxical decrease of an adipose-specific protein, adiponectin, in obesity. *Biochem Biophys Res Commun* 1999;257;79–83.
129. Berg AH, Combs TP, Du X, et al. The adipocyte-secreted protein Acrp30 enhances hepatic insulin action. *Nat Med* 2001;7:947–953.
130. Yamauchi T, Kamon J, Waki H, et al. The fat-derived hormone adiponectin reverses insulin resistance associated with both lipatrophy and obesity. *Nat Med* 2001;7:941–946.
131. Grassi G, Seravalle G, Cattaneo BM, et al. Sympathetic activation in obese normotensive subjects. *Hypertension* 1995;25:560–563.
132. Montagnani M, Golovchenko I, Kim I, et al. Inhibition of phosphatidylinositol 3-kinase enhances mitogenic actions of insulin in endothelial cells. *J Biol Chem* 2002;277:1794–1799.
133. Austin MA, King MC, Vranizan KM, et al. Atherogenic lipoprotein phenotype. A proposed genetic marker for coronary heart disease risk. *Circulation* 1990;82:495–506.
134. Haffner SM. Management of dyslipidemia in adults with diabetes. *Diabetes Care* 1998;21:160–178.
135. Nakamura Y, Horii Y, Nishino T, et al. Immunohistochemical localization of advanced glycosylation end products in coronary atheroma and cardiac tissue in diabetes mellitus. *Am J Pathol* 1993;143:1649–1656.
136. Sztalryd C, Kraemer FB. Regulation of hormone-sensitive lipase in streptozotocin-induced diabetic rats. *Metabolism* 1995;44:1391–1396.
137. Ginsberg HN. Diabetic dyslipidemia: basic mechanisms underlying the common hypertriglyceridemia and low HDL cholesterol levels. *Diabetes* 1996;45[Suppl 3]:S27–S30.
138. Brown MS, Kovanen PT, Goldstein JL. Regulation of plasma cholesterol by lipoprotein receptors. *Science* 1981;212:628–635.
139. Boden G, Chen X, Ruiz J, et al. Mechanisms of fatty acid-induced inhibition of glucose uptake. *J Clin Invest* 1994;93:2438–2446.
140. Bucala R, Makita Z, Vega G, et al. Modification of low density lipoprotein by advanced glycation end products contributes to the dyslipidemia of diabetes and renal insufficiency. *Proc Natl Acad Sci USA* 1994;91:9441–9445.
141. Verges BL. Dyslipidaemia in diabetes mellitus. Review of the main lipoprotein abnormalities and their consequences on the development of atherogenesis. *Diabetes Metab* 1999;25[Suppl 3]:32–40.
142. Tall AR. An overview of reverse cholesterol transport. *Eur Heart J* 1998;19[Suppl A]:A31–A35.
143. Howard BV. Insulin resistance and lipid metabolism. *Am J Cardiol* 1999;84[1 Suppl 1]:28–32.
144. Ginsberg HN. Insulin resistance and cardiovascular disease. *J Clin Invest* 2000;106:453–458.
145. Schwartz CJ, Valente AJ, Sprague EA. A modern view of atherogenesis. *Am J Cardiol* 1993;71:9B–14B.
146. UK Prospective Diabetes Study (UKPDS) Group. Effect of intensive blood-glucose control with metformin on complications in overweight patients with type 2 diabetes (UKPDS 34). *Lancet* 1998;352:854–865.
147. Ghazzi MN, Perez JE, Antonucci TK, et al. Cardiac and glycemic benefits of troglitazone treatment in NIDDM. The Troglitazone Study Group. *Diabetes* 1997;46:433–439.
148. Brunzell J, Cohen B, Kreider M, et al. Rosiglitazone favorably affects LDL-C, and HDL-C heterogeneity in type 2 diabetes [Abstract 567-P]. *Diabetes* 2001;50[suppl 2];A141.
149. Carey DG, Galloway G, Dodrell D, et al. *Rosiglitazone reduces hepatic fat and increases subcutaneous but not intrabdominal fat depots* [Abstract 271]. Presented at the 36th Annual Meeting of the European Association for the Study on Diabetes, September 17–21, 2000, Jerusalem.
150. Miyazaki Y, Mahankali A, Matsuda M, et al. Relationship between visceral fat and enhanced peripheral/hepatic insulin sensitivity after pioglitazone in type 2 diabetes [Abstract 506-P]. *Diabetes* 2001;50[Suppl 2]:A126.
151. Freed M, Fuell D, Menci L, et al. Effect of combination therapy with rosiglitazone and glibenclamide on PAI-1 antigen, PAI-1 activity, and tPA in patients with type 2 diabetes [Abstract 1024]. *Diabetologia* 2000;43[Suppl 1]:A267.
152. Fonseca VA, Reynolds T, Hemphill D, et al. Effect of troglitazone on fibrinolysis and activated coagulation in patients with non-insulin-dependent diabetes mellitus. *J Diabetes Complications* 1998;12:181–186.
153. Mokdad AH, Ford ES, Bowman BA, et al. Diabetes trends in the U.S.: 1990–1998. *Diabetes Care* 2000;23;1278–1283.
154. Colditz GA, Willett WC, Rotnitzky A, et al. Weight gain as a risk factor for clinical diabetes mellitus in women. *Ann Intern Med* 1995;122;481–486.
155. Wing RR, Koeske R, Epstein LH, et al. Long-term effects of modest weight loss in type II diabetic patients. *Arch Intern Med* 1987;147:1749–1753.
156. Effects of ramipril on cardiovascular and microvascular outcomes in people with diabetes mellitus: results of the HOPE study and MICRO-HOPE substudy. *Lancet* 2000A;355:253–259.
157. Hansson L, Lindholm LH, Niskanen L, et al. Effect of angiotensin-converting enzyme inhibition compared with conventional therapy on cardiovascular morbidity and mortality in hypertension: the Captopril Prevention Project (CAPPP) randomized trial. *Lancet* 1999;353:611–616.
158. Tatti P, Pahor M, Byington RP, et al. Outcome results of the Fosinopril Versus Amlodipine Cardiovascular Events Randomized Trial (FACET) in patients with hypertension and NIDDM. *Diabetes Care* 1998;21:597–603.
159. Hansson L, Lindholm L, Ekbom T, et al. Randomized trial of old and new anti-hypertensive drugs in elderly patients: Cardiovascular mortality and morbidity. The Swedish Trial in Old Patients with Hypertension-2 Study. *Lancet* 1999;354:1751–1756.
160. Yusuf S, Gerstein H, Hoogwerf B, et al. Ramipril and the development of diabetes. *JAMA* 2001;286:1882–1885.
161. Tatti P, Pahor M, Byington RP, et al. Outcome results of the Fosinopril Versus Amlodipine Cardiovascular Events Randomized Trial (FACET) in patients with hypertension and NIDDM. *Diabetes Care* 1998;21:597–603.
162. American Diabetes Association. Management of dyslipidemia in adults with diabetes. *Diabetes Care* 2002;25[Suppl 1]:S74–S77.
163. Taskinen MR, Kuusi T, Helve E, et al. Insulin therapy induces antiatherogenic changes of serum lipoproteins in noninsulin-dependent diabetes. *Arteriosclerosis* 1988;8:168–177.
164. Expert Panel on Detection, Evaluation, and Treatment of High Blood Cholesterol in Adults. *National Cholesterol Education Program: Adult Treatment Panel III report executive summary.* Bethesda, MD: National Heart, Lung, and Blood Institute, 2001.
165. The Long-Term Intervention with Pravastatin in Ischaemic Disease (LIPID) Study Group. Prevention of cardiovascular events and death with pravastatin in patients with coronary heart disease and a broad range of initial cholesterol levels. *N Engl J Med* 1998;339:1349–1357.
166. Downs JR, Clearfield M, Weis S, et al. Primary prevention of acute coronary events with lovastatin in men and women with average cholesterol levels: results of AFCAPS/TexCAPS. *JAMA* 1998;279:1615–1622.
167. Goldberg RB, Mellies MJ, Sacks FM, et al. Cardiovascular events and their reduction with pravastatin in diabetic and glucose-intolerant myocardial infarction survivors with average cholesterol levels: subgroup

analyses in the cholesterol and recurrent events (CARE) trial. The Care Investigators. *Circulation* 1998;98:2513–2519.

168. Keech A, Colquhoun D, Baker J, et al. Benefits of long term cholesterol lowering therapy using pravastatin among patients with diabetes in the lipid study [Abstract]. *Aust N Z J Med* 2000;30:172.

169. Haffner SM, Alexander CM, Cook TJ, et al. Reduced coronary events in simvastatin-treated patients with coronary heart disease and diabetes or impaired fasting glucose levels: subgroup analyses in the Scandinavian Simvastatin Survival Study. *Arch Intern Med* 1999;159:2661–2667.

170. Centers for Disease Control and Prevention. *National diabetes fact sheet.* Accessed December 18, 2002, at http://www.cdc.gov/diabetes/pubs/general.htm

171. Heart Protection Study Collaborative Group. MRC/BHF Heart Protection Study of cholesterol lowering with simvastatin in 20536 high-risk individuals: a randomised placebo-controlled trial. *Lancet* 2002;360:7–22.

172. Koskinen P, Mänttäri M, Manninen V, et al. Coronary heart disease incidence in NIDDM patients in the Helsinki Heart Study. *Diabetes Care* 1992;15:820–825.

173. Effect of fenofibrate on progression of coronary-artery disease in type 2 diabetes: the Diabetes Atherosclerosis Intervention Study, a randomised study. *Lancet* 2001;357:905–910.

174. Robins SJ, Collins D, Rubins HB. Diabetes, hyperinsulinemia and recurrent coronary events in the VA-High Density Lipoprotein Intervention Trial (VA-HIT) [Abstract 4069]. *Circulation* 2002;102:II–847.

175. Rubins HB, Robins SJ, Collins D, et al. Gemfibrozil for the secondary prevention of coronary heart disease in men with low levels of high-density lipoprotein cholesterol. *N Engl J Med* 1999;341:410–418.

176. Garg A, Grundy SM. Nicotinic acid as therapy for dyslipidemia in non–insulin-dependent diabetes mellitus. *JAMA* 1990;264:723–726.

177. Elam MB, Hunninghake DB, Davis KB, et al. Effect of niacin on lipid and lipoprotein levels and glycemic control in patients with diabetes and peripheral arterial disease. The ADMIT study: a randomized trial. *JAMA* 2000;284:1263–1270.

178. Grundy SM, Vega GL, McGovern ME, et al. Efficacy, safety, and tolerability of once-daily niacin for the treatment of dyslipidemia associated with type 2 diabetes: results of the assessment of diabetes control and evaluation of the efficacy of Niaspan trial. *Arch Intern Med* 2002;162:1568–1576.

179. The Coronary Drug Project Research Group. Clofibrate and niacin in coronary heart disease. *JAMA* 1975;231:360–381.

180. Canner PL, Berge KG, Wenger NK, et al. Fifteen year mortality in Coronary Drug Project patients: long-term benefit with niacin. *J Am Coll Cardiol* 1986;8:1245–1255.

181. Canner PL, Furberg CD, McGovern ME. Niacin decreases myocardial infarction and total mortality in patients with impaired fasting glucose or glucose intolerance: results from the coronary drug project [Abstract]. *Circulation* 2002;106[Suppl II]:II–636.

182. Omar MA, Wilson JP. FDA adverse event reports on statin-associated rhabdomyolysis. *Ann Pharmacother* 2002;36:288–295.

183. Marais GE, Larson KK. Rhabdomyolysis and acute renal failure induced by combination lovastatin and gemfibrozil therapy. *Ann Intern Med* 1990;112:228–230.

184. Pierce LR, Wysowski DK, Gross TP. Myopathy and rhabdomyolysis associated with lovastatin–gemfibrozil combination therapy. *JAMA* 1990;264:71–75.

185. Illingworth DR, Bacon S. Influence of lovastatin plus gemfibrozil on plasma lipids and lipoproteins in patients with heterozygous familial hypercholesterolemia. *Circulation* 1989;79:590–596.

186. Athyros VG, Papageorgiou AA, Athyrou VV, et al. Atorvastatin and micronized fenofibrate alone and in combination in type 2 diabetes with combined hyperlipidemia. *Diabetes Care* 2002;25:1198–1202.

187. Van JT, Pan J, Wasty T, et al. Comparison of extended-release *niacin* and *atorvastatin* monotherapies and combination treatment of the atherogenic lipid profile in diabetes mellitus. *Am J Cardiol* 2002;89:1306–1308.

188. Brown BG, Zhao XQ, Chait A, et al. Simvastatin and niacin, antioxidant vitamins, or the combination for the prevention of coronary disease. *N Engl J Med* 2001;345:1583–1592.

189. Morse JS, Brown BG, Zhao XQ, et al. Niacin plus simvastatin protect against atherosclerosis progression and clinical events in CAD patients with low HDLc and diabetes mellitus or impaired fasting glucose [Abstract 842-3]. *J Am Coll Cardiol* 2001;37[Suppl A]:262A.

190. Diabetes Prevention Program Research Group. Reduction in the incidence of type 2 diabetes with lifestyle intervention or metformin. *N Engl J Med* 2002;346:393–403.

191. Tuomilehto J, Lindstrom J, Eriksson JG, et al. Prevention of type 2 diabetes mellitus by changes in lifestyle among subjects with impaired glucose tolerance. *N Engl J Med* 2001;344:1343–1350.

192. Buchanan TA, Xiang AH, Peters RK, et al. Preservation of pancreatic β-cell function and prevention of type 2 diabetes by pharmacological treatment of insulin resistance in high-risk Hispanic women. *Diabetes* 2002;51:2796–2803.

CHAPTER 7

Uncommon Types of Occlusive Arterial Disease

Peter C. Spittell

Key Points

- An important late complication of giant-cell arteritis is thoracic aortic aneurysm, which is 17 times more likely in individuals with such a condition than in normal patients.
- Angiography is the gold standard for diagnosis of distal occlusion of the hand, thromboangiitis obliterans, trauma, Takayasu's disease, severe ergotism, primary arterial dissection, and fibromuscular dysplasia.
- Fibromuscular dysplasia, Takayasu's disease, and giant-cell arteritis are more common in women than in men.
- Primary arterial dissection of the peripheral vessels without involvement of the aorta is a rare condition.
- Corticosteroids are the primary treatment for Takayusu's disease and giant-cell arteritis, and in the case of giant-cell arteritis, may require low-dose treatment for several years.

Familiarity with the less common types of occlusive peripheral arterial disease offers the informed clinician diagnostic and therapeutic opportunities that are too important to neglect. In the broadest sense, the uncommon types of occlusive peripheral arterial disease include thromboangiitis obliterans (Buerger's disease), giant-cell arteritis (cranial and Takayasu's disease), and occlusive arterial disease due to blunt trauma or arterial entrapment. Other disorders worthy of attention include cystic adventitial disease, fibromuscular dysplasia, ergotism, and acute aortic dissection.

In general, an uncommon type of occlusive peripheral arterial disease is suggested by the youth of the patient, involvement of only the upper extremity or digits, or the presentation of acute ischemia without a prior history of occlusive arterial disease. The uncommon types of peripheral arterial occlusive disease have distinctive clinical features and if recognized early and managed properly, their progression to complications can be prevented.

THROMBOANGIITIS OBLITERANS (BUERGER'S DISEASE)

Thromboangiitis obliterans (TAO, Buerger's disease) is an idiopathic inflammatory arteriopathy that involves small and medium-size arteries and veins of both the upper and lower extremities. Typically, persons with thromboangiitis obliterans are heavy smokers, more often men than women, whose symptoms often appear before age 30 years. TAO has been demonstrated to have a strong positive association with the HLA antigens (HLA-DrB1*1501), suggesting an important role of HLA-linked factors in governing susceptibility to the disorder (1). The diagnostic clinical criteria for thromboangiitis obliterans (Buerger's disease) are listed in Table 7.1 (2). A definitive diagnosis of thromboangiitis obliterans requires angiography, which usually reveals multiple, bilateral focal segments of arterial stenosis or occlusion, normal proximal vessels, and collateral vessels that have a corkscrew appearance (Fig. 7.1). The anterior or posterior tibial arteries are the most commonly affected, but approximately 25% of patients have upper extremity artery (most commonly ulnar artery) involvement.

Treatment of thromboangiitis obliterans is the same as for other types of occlusive peripheral arterial disease, with particular emphasis on the need for permanent abstinence from all forms of tobacco. Smoking cessation ameliorates the course of the disease, but does not invariably stop further exacerbations. Abstinence from tobacco significantly reduces the risk of ulcer formation and amputation, thus

TABLE 7.1. *Clinical criteria for the diagnosis of buerger's disease[a]*

Age	<50 years (often <30 years)
Gender	Men most often
Habits	Tobacco, cannabis use
History	Superficial phlebitis
	Claudication, arch or calf
	Raynaud's phenomenon
	Absence of atherosclerotic risk factors other than smoking
Examination	Small arteries involved
	Infrapopliteal arterial disease
	Upper extremity involved (positive Allen test)
Laboratory	Normal glucose, blood counts, sedimentation rate, lipids, and screening tests for connective tissue disease
X-ray	No arterial calcification

[a] See Shinoya (2).

improving quality of life in patients with thromboangiitis obliterans (3). Because the arteries involved are small, arterial reconstructions for ischemia in patients with Buerger's disease are technically challenging. Distal arterial reconstruction, if necessary, is indicated to prevent ischemic limb loss. Collateral artery bypass is an option when the main arteries are affected by the disease. A patent but diseased artery should be avoided as a target for reconstruction (4). Sympa-

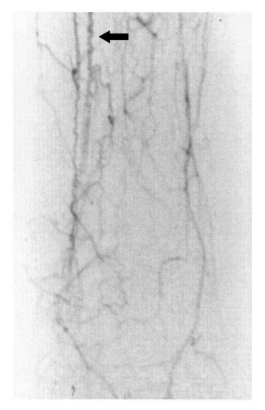

FIG. 7.1. Classic angiographic features of thromboangiitis obliterans with multiple focal segments of arterial stenosis or occlusion of the tibioperoneal arteries, with collateral vessels that have a corkscrew appearance (*arrow*).

thectomy may be useful in severe digital ischemia with ulceration to control pain and to improve cutaneous blood flow. Intravenous cyclophosphamide has been shown to increase initial claudication distance, relieve ischemic rest pain, and improve ulcer healing in a small retrospective treatment trial (5). Therapeutic angiogenesis with phVEGF165 gene transfer may be beneficial in patients with advanced Buerger's disease that is unresponsive to standard medical or surgical treatment methods (6).

ARTERITIS

Giant-Cell Arteritis

Giant-cell arteritis (formerly called temporal arteritis or cranial arteritis) is a subacute and chronic vasculitis of large and medium-size vessels with local and systemic manifestations. Although arterial involvement may be widespread, the extracranial branches of the arteries originating from the aortic arch are the most commonly involved. Involvement of the thoracic aorta and its branches may be minimal and asymptomatic, or it can result in occlusion of one or more branches of the aortic arch, fusiform or saccular aneurysm of the aorta, or even aortic dissection.

The average annual incidence of giant-cell arteritis is reported to be 17.8 cases per 100,000 persons greater than or equal to 50 years of age, and the incidence appears to be increasing (7). Women are affected twice as often as men. Morbidity of giant-cell arteritis is primarily attributed to either luminal stenosis or occlusion of the involved arteries or weakening of the inflamed arterial wall, resulting in aneurysm formation (8). The mortality rate of giant-cell arteritis is similar to that expected in the general population, although thoracic aortic aneurysms and dissection of the aorta are important late complications.

The cause of giant-cell arteritis is unknown, although it is probably a polygenic disease in which multiple environmental and genetic factors influence susceptibility and severity. Pathologically, arteries originating from the aortic arch are usually affected by a focal and segmental inflammatory infiltrate with marked disruption of the internal elastic lamina. "Skip" lesions between areas of involvement are characteristic; therefore, a negative temporal artery biopsy does not necessarily exclude the diagnosis of giant-cell arteritis. The classic histological picture of giant-cell arteritis is one of granulomatous inflammation in which giant cells are usually located between the intima and media. Atypical or nongranulomatous arteritis and predominantly intimal hyperplasia with little active inflammation are other types of vascular injury which may occur.

The onset of symptoms of giant-cell arteritis may be gradual or abrupt, and systemic symptoms (malaise, fatigue, weight loss, anorexia, low-grade fever) are present in about half of patients. Musculoskeletal manifestations, including polymyalgia rheumatica, are common early symptoms. A headache localized over the temporal or occipital areas is probably the most frequent symptom and occurs in two-thirds of patients. On physical examination, the frontal or parietal branches of the superficial temporal arteries may be thickened, nodular, tender, or occasionally erythematous. Nearly half of patients suffer from jaw claudication. Occasionally, intermittent claudication may occur in the muscles of the tongue or those involved in swallowing. In rare cases, more marked vascular narrowing may lead to infarction of the scalp or the tongue. Permanent partial or complete loss of vision in one or both eyes occurs in up to 20% of patients and is often preceded by amaurosis fugax (9). Fundoscopic findings can include ischemic optic neuritis with a slight pallor and edema of the optic disk and scattered cotton-wool patches and small hemorrhages. Other neurological manifestations (mononeuropathies or peripheral polyneuropathies of the upper or lower extremities, and less commonly, transient ischemic attacks or stroke) occur in one-third of patients.

In approximately 10% to 15% of patients, intermittent claudication of the upper extremities develops due to stenosis of branches of the aortic arch—in particular, the subclavian and axillary arteries—and may provide an important clue to the diagnosis of giant-cell arteritis (10). Examination will usually reveal diminished or absent pulses in the upper extremities and/or neck. Bruits may be heard on auscultation over the carotid, subclavian, axillary, and brachial arteries. Simultaneous palpation of the radial pulses will demonstrate a delay of the radial pulse ipsilateral to a significant upper extremity artery stenosis. The brachial systolic pressure will usually be reduced on the side of significant subclavian artery stenosis.

An important late complication of giant-cell arteritis is thoracic aortic aneurysm, which is 17 times as likely in patients with giant-cell arteritis as in those without the disease (8). Thoracic aortic aneurysm usually occurs several years after the diagnosis and when other symptoms have subsided. An annual chest radiograph is indicated to screen for thoracic aortic aneurysm.

Laboratory findings in giant-cell arteritis include a mild to moderate anemia of chronic disease and often mildly abnormal liver function tests. Laboratory criteria of the American College of Rheumatology include an erythrocyte sedimentation rate (ESR) of at least 50 mm per hour; however, this test is normal in more than 20% of patients. Therefore, a normal ESR rate does not exclude a diagnosis of giant-cell arteritis. The C-reactive protein level is a more sensitive indicator of disease activity than the ESR both at diagnosis and during relapse.

When extracranial giant-cell arteritis is clinically suspected, angiography, computed tomography (CT), and/or magnetic resonance imaging (MRI) are often indicated, the choice of test depending on the patient's clinical presentation. When arterial stenosis(es) are suspected based on the physical examination, angiography (standard contrast angiography or magnetic resonance angiography [MRA] with gadolinium enhancement) is the test of choice. The typical angiographic findings in giant-cell arteritis are dilation of the ascending aorta and possible thickening of its wall; and involvement of branches of the aortic arch, which, when present, is often bi-

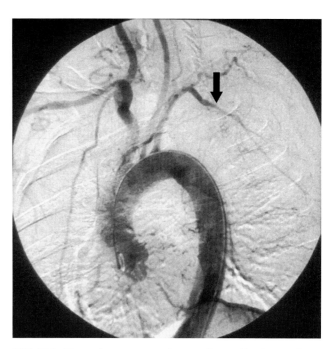

FIG. 7.2. Thoracic aortagram in a patient with giant cell arteritis, demonstrating a tapered arterial stenosis involving the distal left subclavian artery.

lateral, with segmental areas of smooth, tapered arterial stenosis and/or occlusion in the absence of atherosclerotic changes (Fig. 7.2). The femoral arteries are less commonly involved. If a chest radiograph suggests thoracic aortic aneurysm, CT or MRI/MRA is indicated to determine aneurysm size, location, and extent. The finding of a thickened aortic wall on CT or MRI is a direct indication of inflammation of the aortic wall and thus of active disease (11,12). The role of fluorine-18 fluorodeoxyglucose positron emission tomography (FDG PET) in the diagnosis of giant-cell arteritis is still evolving, but preliminary reports suggest it is more reliable than MRI in monitoring disease activity during immunosuppressive therapy (13,14).

The diagnosis of giant-cell arteritis is typically confirmed by biopsy of the superficial temporal artery. However, angiography is useful in confirming the diagnosis of aortic and branch vessel involvement and in differentiating this disorder from atherosclerotic occlusion. Of note, the histopathologic and radiographic findings of giant-cell arteritis may sometimes be indistinguishable from those observed in Takayasu's arteritis. The age at onset and the distribution of lesions usually allow the proper diagnosis to be made (15).

Corticosteroids are the drugs of choice to treat giant-cell arteritis. The initial dose of prednisone is at least 40 to 60 mg as a single or divided dose. Initial pulsed intravenous doses of methylprednisolone (1,000 mg every day for 3 days) may be given to patients with recent or impending visual loss. Corticosteroids may prevent, but usually do not reverse visual loss. The response to corticosteroids is usually rapid, with resolution of many symptoms after a few days of therapy. The initial dose of corticosteroids is usually given for 2 to 4 weeks;

then, it can be gradually reduced each week by a maximum of 10% of the total daily dose. When the corticosteroid dose is reduced too quickly, a relapse usually occurs, although spontaneous exacerbations of the disease, independent of the corticosteroid dose, are not uncommon in the first 2 years.

Regular assessment of clinical symptoms and laboratory markers (ESR and/or C-reactive protein) is indicated, although an elevated ESR or C-reactive protein during treatment in the absence of symptoms is not a valid reason to increase the dose of corticosteroids (16). One to 2 years of treatment is usually required, although some patients have a more chronic, relapsing course and may require low doses of corticosteroid for several years. Corticosteroid-related adverse events are common and should be carefully looked for during follow-up. Calcium and vitamin D supplementation (bisphosphonates in patients with reduced bone mineral density) should be given with corticosteroid therapy in all patients with giant-cell arteritis. Methotrexate, when used as a steroid-sparing drug in patients with giant-cell arteritis, has given conflicting results; however, it should be considered in patients who need high doses of corticosteroids to control active disease and who have serious side effects. Arterial changes are reversible with adequate therapy, but when corticosteroid therapy has been insufficient to suppress the arteritis, there may be progressive involvement of the aorta and resultant dissection or rupture (17). As with any rare disorder, randomized controlled treatment trials are lacking or based on small patient numbers, making management decisions difficult.

Takayasu's Disease

Takayasu's disease (pulseless disease, occlusive thromboaortopathy, idiopathic medial aortopathy, and arteriopathy) is a chronic inflammatory fibrosing arteritis affecting primarily the aorta and its major branches. Takayasu's disease is rare, with an incidence of approximately 2.6 per million per year in North America (18). In contrast to patients with giant-cell arteritis, most patients with Takayasu's disease are less than 40 years old, although it also occurs more commonly in women (greater than 80% of cases).

Pathologically, the aorta is thickened secondary to fibrosis of all three arterial layers, in particular the adventitia and the intima. Often, the thick intima may reveal longitudinal wrinkling and ridging, giving the gross appearance of tree bark, a gross morphological feature characteristic of many types of aortitis. Extension of the adventitial fibrosis and round cell infiltration to the adjacent structures may imitate retroperitoneal fibrosis and also induce a fibrosing pericarditis. Microscopically, the vasculitis may be divided into an acute florid inflammatory phase and a healed fibrotic phase (19).

Clinical manifestations range from asymptomatic disease found as a result of impalpable pulses or bruits to catastrophic neurological impairment. A two-stage process has been suggested, with a "pre-pulseless" phase characterized by nonspecific inflammatory features (fever, night sweats, anorexia, malaise, weight loss, arthralgia, myalgia, and fa-

tigue), followed by a chronic phase with the development of vascular insufficiency. The early subacute phase often goes unrecognized, with the diagnosis first being suspected when symptoms and signs of the occlusive phase develop.

The clinical manifestations of the chronic or "pulseless" phase can include hypertension, cerebrovascular insufficiency, arterial insufficiency of the upper or lower extremities, and less commonly mesenteric insufficiency, depending on the location of the aortitis and arteritis. Systemic hypertension is present in 33% to 83% of patients, generally reflecting renal artery stenosis, and less commonly stenosis of the descending thoracic aorta, causing a form of acquired aortic coarctation (20). Stenotic lesions predominate and tend to be multiple and bilateral. The aortic lumen becomes narrowed in a "skip" lesion fashion, alternating with regions of fusiform or saccular aneurysm formation. Nearly all patients with aneurysms also have stenoses and most have extensive vascular lesions. Characteristic clinical features in the chronic phase include diminished or absent pulses (84% to 96% of patients), often with limb claudication and blood pressure discrepancies (21). Arterial bruits are present in the majority of patients, are often multiple, and are usually located over involved segments of the carotid, subclavian, and abdominal vessels. Congestive heart failure can result from aortic regurgitation, systemic hypertension, myocardial ischemia, and/or dilated cardiomyopathy (20). Pulmonary artery involvement is not uncommon and can be useful in the differential diagnosis of aortitis. Other features include neurological symptoms secondary to hypertension and/or ischemia, Takayasu retinopathy, dyspnea, headache, carotodynia, chest wall pain, and erythema nodosum.

Specific diagnostic criteria for Takayasu's disease have been formulated by the American College of Rheumatology (ACR) incorporating the more typical clinical features of the disorder (Table 7.2) (22).

Angiography remains the gold standard for diagnosis. Segmental narrowing of a variable length of descending or abdominal aorta or narrowing of the origin of major branches of the aorta occur as a result of thickening of the aorta or arterial wall (Fig. 7.3). This usually allows distinction of Takayasu's disease from other causes of the aortic arch syndrome. Aneurysmal dilation of the thoracic aorta can occur in Takayasu's disease, but it is not common or distinctive in this disorder. No single laboratory assay or imaging modality establishes disease activity, although T2-weighted MRI, MRA, spiral CT angiography, and fluorine-18 FDG PET have shown potential in identifying acute inflammatory changes within the vessel wall (12,14,23).

The natural history of Takayasu's disease is notable for the complications of Takayasu retinopathy, secondary hypertension, aortic regurgitation, and aneurysm formation. The overall 5-year survival rate after diagnosis is greater than 80%, with mortality attributed primarily to cerebrovascular disease and congestive heart failure (24).

Corticosteroids are the mainstay of treatment for Takayasu's disease, but reports of efficacy vary. This may relate to the stage of disease at which treatment is introduced

TABLE 7.2. *1990 American college of rheumatology criteria for the classification of Takayasu arteritis*[a]

Criterion	Definition
Age at disease onset ≤40 years	Development of symptoms or findings related to Takayasu arteritis at age ≤40 years
Claudication of extremities	Development and worsening of fatigue and discomfort in muscles of one or more extremities while in use, especially the upper extremities
Decreased brachial artery pulse	Decreased pulsation of one or both brachial arteries
Blood pressure difference >10 mm Hg	Difference of >10 mm Hg in systolic blood pressure between arms
Bruit over subclavian arteries or aorta	Bruit audible on auscultation over one or both subclavian arteries or abdominal aorta
Angiogram abnormality	Angiographic narrowing or occlusion of the entire aorta, its primary branches, or large arteries in the proximal upper or lower extremities, not caused by atherosclerosis, fibromuscular dysplasia, or similar causes; changes usually focal or segmental

[a]A diagnosis of Takayasu's disease requires that at least three of the six criteria are met.

in addition to disease extent. Currently, the best evidence-based treatments include steroids, to which 50% respond, and methotrexate, to which a further 50% respond (25,26). The other important medical issues relate to the management of hypertension, which can be worsened by the use of corticosteroids with their fluid-retaining side effects. The use of angiotensin-converting enzyme inhibitors requires careful monitoring in view of the frequency of renal artery stenosis.

Indications for surgery include systemic hypertension due to critical renal artery stenosis or acquired coarctation of the aorta, lifestyle-limiting extremity claudication, cerebrovascular ischemia or critical stenoses of three or more cerebral vessels, significant aortic regurgitation, and cardiac

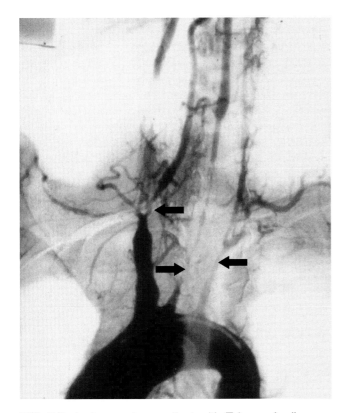

FIG. 7.3. Aortagram in a patient with Takayasu's disease, demonstrating the characteristic tapered narrowings (*arrow*) of the origin of major branches of the aorta.

ischemia with confirmed coronary artery involvement. In general, surgery is recommended at a time of quiescent disease to avoid the complications of restenosis, thrombosis, hemorrhage, infection, and anastamotic failure (21).

Long-term follow-up is recommended and generally utilizes noninvasive cardiovascular imaging techniques such as Doppler ultrasound, MRA, and/or CT angiography.

TRAUMA

Acute injury to arteries from penetrating or crushing injuries, fractures, dislocations, sudden deceleration, and iatrogenic causes can have various results. Arterial laceration, local thrombosis, secondary hemorrhage, embolism, delayed traumatic aneurysm, arteriovenous fistula, and/or complete severance are all possible outcomes. Traumatic pseudoaneurysms may result from seemingly minor trauma and are treated surgically.

Incomplete rupture of the thoracic aorta (in the region of the aortic isthmus) results from a sudden deceleration injury. It is seen most often in motor vehicle accident victims and should be suspected when there is evidence of chest wall trauma, decreased or absent leg pulses, left-sided hemothorax, and/or widening of the superior mediastinum on chest radiography. These patients are usually hypertensive at initial presentation. The diagnosis can be confirmed by transesophageal echocardiography, CT, MRI, or angiography. Treatment is emergent surgical repair in patients who are suitable surgical candidates. At initial presentation, the condition of 40% to 50% of the patients is unstable; furthermore, there are no clinical or imaging criteria that accurately predict future complete rupture. Therefore, even if a patient presents with a chronic incomplete rupture, surgery is indicated. Most of the patients are young, and the risk of elective surgical repair is low, with an otherwise good prognosis for long-term survival if aortic repair is successful.

Chronic occlusive arterial disease may result from repetitive blunt trauma, chronic compression of an artery by musculotendinous structures, and chronic and repetitive impingement on an artery by bony structures.

In the upper extremity, the usual types of occlusive arterial disease due to trauma are seen in two locations, the arteries of the hand (chronic occupational trauma) and the subclavian artery (thoracic outlet compression). In the lower extremity, chronic occlusive disease of the popliteal artery can result from compression of the popliteal artery by muscle or tendon (popliteal artery entrapment). In addition, compression of the superficial femoral artery by the tendinous band at the outlet of Hunter's canal in the thigh can produce atherosclerotic lesions at this location.

Chronic Occupational Occlusive Arterial Disease of the Hand

The superficial location and close approximation to bone of many of the arteries of the hands and fingers, combined with frequent exposure of the hands to repetitive blunt or compressive trauma in many occupations, activities, and hobbies, make occlusive arterial disease of the hand due to blunt trauma more common than is generally accepted (27). The majority of patients are current or former smokers. A history of repetitive blunt trauma, even if apparently minor, to the hands and digits should suggest the diagnosis in a person presenting with signs and symptoms of ischemia in the hands and fingers. The dominant hand is usually the one involved, although in an occasional person, the nondominant hand may be affected. Patients often describe a sudden onset of pain in the traumatized hand or fingers, followed by a latent period from a day to several weeks before ischemic symptoms appear. Symptoms can range from cold sensitivity, intermittent coldness, paresthesia, numbness, and/or Raynaud's phenomenon of the involved digits to hand claudication and/or ischemic pain or ulceration of one or more digits, depending on the severity of the ischemia.

Examination may reveal decreased skin temperature, pallor, cyanosis, cutaneous infarction, ischemic ulceration, and, rarely, gangrene of one or more digits. Careful evaluation of the pulsations of the radial and ulnar arteries in every patient and performance of the Allen test (see Chapter 3) to confirm their patency, as well as to evaluate the circulation of the hand, will identify even asymptomatic patients, who can be instructed in protection of the hand from further blunt and other types of trauma. The presence or absence of ischemic symptoms, especially in ulnar artery occlusion, depends on the completeness of the superficial palmar arch. The superficial palmar arch is complete in 80% of cases, and a complete deep palmar arch exists in greater than 97% of cases. In general, the superficial palmar arch and deep palmar arch provide arterial blood supply to the second through fifth digits and first digits, respectively (28). Because thoracic outlet compression can lead to localized injury of the subclavian artery and/or poststenotic dilation with thrombus formation and distal embolization to the hands or fingers, careful evaluation of the subclavian artery in the supraclavicular space and performance of the thoracic outlet maneuvers are essential parts of the examination as well. Additional studies that are useful in supporting the diagnosis include a complete blood count, fasting blood glucose, and erythrocyte sedimentation rate; radiography of the chest and cervical spine should be per-

formed to exclude cervical or abnormal first ribs, as these are not always evident on physical examination. An electrocardiogram is useful for identifying rhythm disturbances or myocardial disease or infarction that could account for embolic arterial occlusion. Other tests often indicated in the evaluation of patients with occlusive arterial disease of the hands and digits include serum protein electrophoresis, rheumatoid factor, serological test for syphilis, antinuclear antibody, hepatitis serology, serum cryoglobulins, and cryofibrinogen and antiphospholipid antibodies. Thromboangiitis obliterans presents a diagnostic challenge in a person who smokes, but is unlikely in the absence of a history of Raynaud's phenomenon, superficial thrombophlebitis, or intermittent claudication or evidence of occlusive arterial disease in more than just one hand.

Although occlusive arterial disease of the hand and/or digits can be confirmed by noninvasive testing (digital systolic blood pressures, pulse volume records, and digital skin temperatures), angiography remains the standard for the diagnosis, revealing occlusion of the distal ulnar or radial artery, the palmar arch, and/or the digital arteries (Fig. 7.4). Furthermore, arteriography is useful for excluding proximal arterial causes of distal embolic occlusive arterial disease.

Treatment is guided by both the severity of the clinical manifestations and angiographic findings. The majority of patients with occlusive arterial disease of the hand can be treated conservatively. For milder cases of ischemia, avoidance of any occupational trauma that induced the lesion is of paramount importance. Additional measures include hand protection from all types of mechanical and thermal trauma, use of padded gloves or tools prescribed to perform tasks that require impact or pounding rather than using the hand for such purposes, and discontinuation of tobacco. Various orally administered vasodilators, including prazosin, terazosin, doxazosin, nifedipine, and diltiazem, have been used to alleviate episodic digital vasospasm often seen in association with occlusive arterial disease of the hand. In some persons, vasodilator therapy is required only during cold weather or periods of occupational exposure to cold. More severe ischemia may require surgical therapy to hasten healing of ischemic ulceration. Thoracoscopic sympathectomy in patients with severe ischemia can provide effective symptom control and maximum tissue salvage (29). Periarterial microsympathectomy (stripping of the adventitia) and/or direct revascularization by interposition vein grafting or end-to-end anastomosis using microvascular techniques have been reported with increasing success (30).

ARTERIAL ENTRAPMENT

Thoracic Outlet Compression

Compression of the subclavian artery in the thoracic outlet (thoracic outlet compression syndrome) may result in intimal trauma and subsequent stenosis, thrombosis within the lumen of the subclavian artery, and/or embolization to the

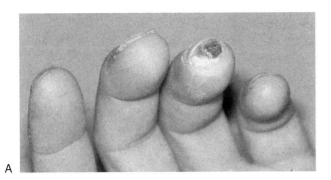

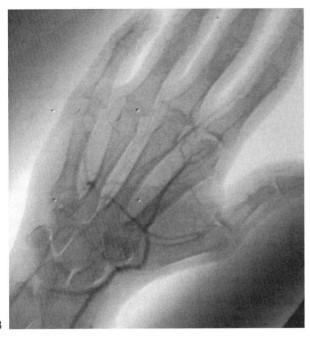

FIG. 7.4. (See Color Fig. 7.4A.) **A:** Ischemic digital ulceration in a left-hand-dominant automotive mechanic from repetitive blunt trauma to the hand. **B:** Angiography demonstrating occlusion of the left ulnar artery (*arrow*) and multiple digital arteries.

more distal arteries in the upper extremity. Subclavian artery compression can occur at several points, most commonly in the costoclavicular space between the uppermost rib (cervical or first thoracic) and the clavicle (31,32). Other, less common anatomic and/or developmental anomalies described in association with thoracic outlet compression include scalene muscle segmentation or insertion abnormalities and hypertrophy of the subclavius muscle or tendon (31,32).

The clinical presentation of thoracic outlet syndrome with arterial compression can vary depending on the location and extent of the arterial occlusion. Symptoms range from none to severe ischemia, cold sensitivity of the hand, Raynaud's phenomenon in one or more fingers of the ipsilateral hand, digital cyanosis or ulceration, upper extremity emboli, and claudication of the arm or forearm.

Arterial examination in the upper extremity with the patient's arms in a neutral position may be normal. Both the radial and ulnar artery pulsations should be carefully evalu-

ated and the Allen test used to confirm and localize occlusive arterial disease in the hand. When a cervical rib or abnormal first rib is the basis of the compression of the subclavian artery, it is often palpated as a mass in the supraclavicular area. Compression of the subclavian artery in the thoracic outlet can be demonstrated by changing the position of the arm or shoulder, listening for a bruit over the subclavian artery, and/or noting a decrease in amplitude of pulsation of the corresponding radial artery. The clinical tests most often used to demonstrate thoracic outlet compression at the bedside include the costoclavicular maneuver, both active and passive, the hyperabduction maneuver, and the Adson maneuver (see Chapter 3). It is important to remember, however, that many persons in whom one or more of the maneuvers are positive do not have symptomatic thoracic outlet compression.

Subclavian artery compression in the thoracic outlet can be confirmed noninvasively by measuring pulse volume recordings of the radial artery while the various maneuvers are performed. Duplex ultrasonography, helical computed tomography, and MRI/MRA are additional noninvasive tests that can be used to diagnose thoracic outlet compression and have the advantage of providing more precise information regarding severity of arterial compression (ultrasound, CT, and MRI) as well as the exact mechanism of arterial compression (CT and MRI) (33,34). All of these methods rely on demonstrating subclavian artery compression with reduced or abolished subclavian artery blood flow occurring with the arm in the hyperabducted position (see Chapter 3). Contrast angiography is required before surgical therapy to define the arterial circulation proximal and distal to the compressed arterial segment.

Over time, compression of the subclavian artery in the thoracic outlet can result in poststenotic dilation, aneurysm formation, or intimal thickening with superimposed thrombus at the site of arterial injury. With any of these changes, the complications of thrombosis of the subclavian artery and/or embolization of more distal arteries in the upper extremity, sometimes leading to loss of digits, can result.

The optimal therapy for thoracic outlet compression is a subject of controversy. In general, treatment depends on the severity of the patient's symptoms. In minimally symptomatic patients, physical therapy and education regarding the relationship of arm and body position to arterial compression may be all that is required. In patients who have more severe symptoms, aneurysm formation, distal embolization, or digital ischemia, surgical treatment should be considered. Surgical resection of the first thoracic or cervical rib is the most effective way to relieve the arterial compression. In some cases, thrombectomy and reconstruction of the subclavian artery in patients with subclavian artery stenosis, thrombosis, and/or occlusion are also indicated (35). Sympathectomy may also be utilized as an adjunctive surgical procedure when there is significant digital or hand ischemia. Stent placement in residual subclavian artery stenoses has been successful, but needs to be performed after surgical decompression of the costoclavicular space to decrease the likelihood of recurrence and/or stent damage.

External Iliac Arteriopathy

Obstruction of the external iliac arteries may occur in avid or competition bicyclists and is thought to be the result of hemodynamic injury secondary to the shear stresses of very high blood flow coupled with the mechanical stress to the artery from the cyclist's body position (36–38). Patients usually present with intermittent claudication of one lower limb, most commonly the left, occurring during maximal exertion on the cycle. Progression to acute or subacute arterial occlusion is uncommon. Although the ratio of resting ankle to brachial systolic blood pressures (ankle–brachial index, ABI) is usually normal, ergometric bicycle stress testing will usually reveal a transient decrease of the ABI of the affected limb (38). Duplex ultrasound is also accurate in diagnosing external iliac arteriopathy and for postoperative surveillance (39). Angiographic evaluation is warranted in patients with lifestyle-limiting symptoms or in those with critical limb ischemia, and characteristically demonstrates a moderate stenosis of the external iliac artery (Fig. 7.5) (38). In patients who are severely compromised and in those with critical limb ischemia, surgical revascularization has shown benefit (40).

Popliteal Artery Entrapment

Popliteal artery entrapment is an uncommon congenital abnormality that is often overlooked clinically. It is an important syndrome because repeated compression of the popliteal artery can lead to localized atherosclerosis, poststenotic dilation, and/or thrombosis, resulting in significant ischemia in

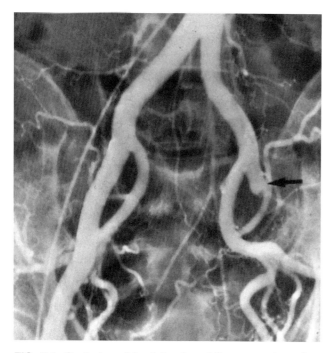

FIG. 7.5. Occlusion of the left external iliac artery (*arrow*) in a competitive cyclist.

the distal leg or foot. This anomaly occurs most often in young men, who may present with a complaint of intermittent claudication in the arch of the foot or calf. An observant patient may note intermittent claudication with walking and not with running. If the popliteal artery is not already occluded, the finding of reduced pedal pulses with sustained active plantar flexion should increase suspicion of the disorder.

Popliteal artery entrapment can occur by several mechanisms. The artery can be compressed because of its anomalous relationship to the medial head of the gastrocnemius (looping around and under or through the gastrocnemius), by its displacement by an anomalous insertion of the plantaris muscle, or by passing beneath rather than behind the popliteus muscle.

The diagnosis of popliteal artery entrapment can be made noninvasively with duplex ultrasound, CT, and MRI (41–43). MRI has been demonstrated to be superior to ultrasonography and CT in defining the exact abnormality in popliteal artery entrapment, with results similar to those seen with digital subtraction angiography (43). The combined morphological and functional evaluation of the popliteal fossa makes MRI the investigation of choice in the management of young adults with intermittent claudication. MRI is the ideal screening test before angiography or surgery and is particularly useful when the popliteal artery is occluded, in which situation ultrasonography and angiography are of limited value.

Angiographic assessment in popliteal artery entrapment demonstrates irregularity of the wall of the popliteal artery in an otherwise normal arterial tree, often associated with prestenotic or poststenotic dilatation. If the artery is still patent, medial displacement of the popliteal artery from its normal position in the popliteal space, and/or popliteal artery compression with extension of the knee and dorsiflexion of the foot, are diagnostic angiographic findings. If the mechanism of compression is by the plantaris or popliteus muscle, the position of the artery may appear normal on the arteriogram. If popliteal artery entrapment has been diagnosed in one limb, the contralateral limb should be screened, as bilateral disease occurs in more than 25% of patients (44).

The management of popliteal artery entrapment depends on the clinical presentation and anatomic findings. Although the natural history of popliteal artery entrapment is not well defined, surgery has been advocated to prevent progression of the disease from repetitive arterial trauma. Detection and treatment of popliteal artery entrapment at an early stage permits better long-term results. If the artery is undamaged, simple release of the popliteal artery by division of the medial head of the gastrocnemius muscle or other abnormal slips of muscle and tendon may be all that is required (44). If the popliteal artery is damaged or occluded, autologous saphenous vein interposition grafting seems to give the best results (45).

ADDUCTOR CANAL OUTLET SYNDROME

Compression of the superficial femoral artery by the tendinous band at the outlet of Hunter's canal in the distal thigh has been implicated as the cause of atherosclerotic lesions so often seen at this location (46). Mechanical trauma occurs at the point where the femoral artery crosses the adductor magnus tendon (47). In addition, certain types of aerobic exercise, such as jogging and cross-country skiing, can exaggerate any compression of the superficial femoral artery and may cause acute arterial injury and thrombosis at this location (47). An awareness of the relationship of these activities to acute intimal injury and thrombosis is key to providing effective treatment.

CYSTIC ADVENTITIAL DISEASE

Cystic adventitial disease of the popliteal artery is an uncommon arteriopathy in which a mucin-containing cystic structure arises in the outer tunica media or subadventitial layer of the popliteal artery wall. As the cyst grows, intracystic pressure eventually exceeds that in the lumen of the artery, causing arterial stenosis and resultant intermittent claudication. Possible etiologies include repeated minor trauma causing recurrent intramural bleeding, synovium tracking along small vessels to the popliteal artery from the knee, and incorporation of synovial precursor cells into the arterial wall during development (48).

The estimated prevalence of popliteal artery cystic adventitial disease is 1 for every 1,200 cases of calf claudication (49). Most affected persons are men between 20 and 50 years of age without risk factors for atherosclerotic disease. The clinical presentation is usually intermittent claudication, with normal or reduced popliteal and pedal pulses. Therefore, intermittent claudication in a younger individual in the absence of atherosclerotic risk factors should heighten the clinical suspicion of cystic adventitial disease.

ABIs may be reduced because of arterial stenosis. Angiography typically reveals a smoothly tapered eccentric or concentric narrowing of the mid popliteal artery in an otherwise normal arterial tree. Angiography is not able to distinguish cystic adventitial disease from other causes of external compression. Duplex ultrasonography is able to show the popliteal artery stenosis and can also demonstrate the intramural cyst, which usually lies eccentric to the artery, is hypoechoic, and shows no internal flow (50). CT and MRI are also accurate in the diagnosis of cystic adventitial disease (51–53).

Some patients may have symptoms of intermittent claudication spontaneously resolve because of coalescence of multiple cyst loculi or cyst rupture relieving arterial compression, but symptom recurrence is common. If the diagnosis is made when arterial stenosis is present, cyst decompression may be performed with CT or sonographic guidance. Surgical intervention is required for those patients who develop complete arterial occlusion or thrombosis.

FIBROMUSCULAR DYSPLASIA

Fibromuscular dysplasia (FMD) is an uncommon arteriopathy, which occurs in young to middle-aged individuals, pre-

dominantly women. The presence of FMD has been demonstrated in almost every vascular bed. Renal artery involvement is most common (60% to 75%), followed by the cervicocranial arteries (25% to 30%), visceral arteries (9%), and the arteries of the extremities (5%) (54). There are rare reports of FMD involving the subclavian, axillary, radial, and ulnar arteries. In the lower extremity, the external iliac arteries are most often involved; less commonly, the femoral, popliteal, tibial, and peroneal arteries are involved. Although the pathogenesis of FMD is not completely understood, humoral, mechanical, and genetic factors and mural ischemia may play a role. The natural history of FMD is relatively benign, with progression occurring in only a minority of the patients (55).

The clinical presentation is variable, ranging from asymptomatic bruits to intermittent claudication, cold legs, or evidence of distal embolism (56). Upper extremity arterial involvement is most often in the subclavian artery and can result in weakness, paresthesias, and/or claudication of the involved upper extremity, a difference in brachial systolic blood pressure, and the subclavian steal syndrome. Less commonly, the axillary, brachial, radial, and ulnar arteries are affected by FMD (57).

The diagnosis of FMD is most often made by the characteristic angiographic "string of beads" appearance, where the "bead" diameter is larger than the proximal vessel (Fig. 7.6).

In patients with symptoms, percutaneous transluminal angioplasty has emerged as the treatment of choice (56). Surgical bypass/resection is less often required. Prospective studies are needed to determine the optimal management of FMD in the upper and lower extremity arteries.

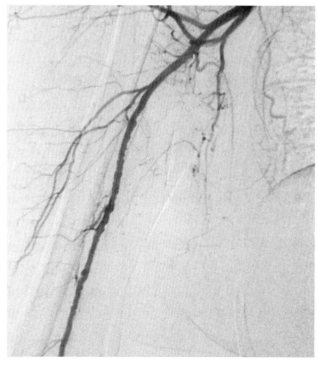

FIG. 7.6. Fibromuscular dysplasia of the brachial artery.

ERGOTISM

Ergotism is most commonly caused by the use of ergotamine preparations for migraine headaches and should be suspected in any patient exhibiting ischemic symptoms while receiving an ergot preparation. Ergot produces intense vasospasm of the digits and large blood vessels by stimulation of α-adrenergic agonist activity and prostaglandin action as well as calcium and serotonin effects. Vasospasm occurs from excess doses of the drugs, usually greater than 10 mg per week. A detailed medication history is important, as several agents can raise ergotamine levels (i.e., erythromycin, tetracycline, clarithromycin, and ritonavir), provoking vascular symptoms in patients chronically taking ergotamine preparations (58).

The diagnosis of ergotism is usually made by a careful history and physical examination. Digital, carotid, axillary, renal, coronary, ophthalmic, splanchnic vessels, and lower extremity arteries may be involved (59). Early symptoms of ergotamine intoxication include coldness of the hands and feet, numbness or a sensation of muscular stiffness, or both. Pallor, cyanosis, or both may be observed, along with a lack of arterial pulsations in the distal parts of the extremities. More rarely, the upper extremities are affected. The manifestations tend to be symmetric, and major arterial pulsations may be absent as a result of ergotism. In cases of severe ischemia, angiography is indicated and usually demonstrates smooth narrowing to complete occlusion of arterial segments of varying lengths. The correct recognition of arterial spasm due to ergotism is basic to avoiding unnecessary arterial surgery. In the milder case, merely discontinuing the ergot-containing preparation will result in a return of pulses and relief of symptoms in 2 to 4 days. When the spasm and resulting ischemia are more intense, intravenous sodium nitroprusside will relieve the spasm in several hours in the vast majority of cases (60,61).

Acute Aortic Dissection

Ischemia of the extremities is an uncommon but important manifestation of acute aortic dissection. Peripheral pulse deficits are noted in up to 40% of patients, and more commonly in patients with proximal aortic dissection, and can provide an important clue to the diagnosis (62–64). Like other arteries arising from the aorta, the iliac and subclavian arteries can be variably occluded by extension of the intramural hematoma into their walls, by constriction of their orifice when the dissection surrounds their origin from the aorta, and even by severance from the aorta by the dissection. Pulse deficits may be transitory due to oscillation of the intimal flap or distal reentry of the hematoma into the true lumen. A difference in blood pressure between the arms is not uncommon. In the iliac artery, occlusion of the lumen by thrombus at the site of reentry of the dissection sometimes also occurs. Acute lower extremity ischemia, with or without chest pain, as a result of dissection extending into the iliac arteries occurs in from 6% to 12% of patients.

In any patient with a catastrophic illness associated with systemic hypertension and physical findings of vascular origin, especially in the presence of chest pain, aortic dissection should always be included in the differential diagnosis. Awareness and recognition of the occasional involvement of the blood supply to the extremities by the dissection may serve the astute clinician well. Correct management is that of aortic dissection. Specific measures to restore pulsatile flow to an ischemic extremity may be necessary if the ischemia is severe and does not improve with treatment of the aortic dissection. Aortic fenestration may be indicated when there is evidence of severe limb ischemia complicating either acute or chronic aortic dissection. Fenestration, either surgical or percutaneous techniques, can effectively relieve the ischemia and can be performed safely in chronic aortic dissection (66,67).

Primary arterial dissection of the peripheral vessels without involvement of the aorta is a rare condition. The dissection occurs most frequently in small to medium-size muscular arteries, close to their origins from the aorta, the regions of marked rheologic change. The dissection generally involves greater than 50% of the circumference of the artery, and the occurrence of symptoms depends largely on the degree of ischemia produced by compression of the arterial lumen. The complications of peripheral arterial dissections include arterial occlusion by obliteration of the lumen or thrombosis and rupture with hemorrhage. Thrombus formation can greatly affect the degree of ischemia and can result in an acute ischemia episode. Primary arterial dissection is more common in men less than 50 years of age and in persons with hypertension or a history of trauma. Primary arterial dissection must always be considered in the differential diagnosis of acute limb ischemia, especially when this occurs in younger patients.

When the subclavian artery is involved, there is commonly a history of trauma, and usually pain in the ipsilateral shoulder region with radiation to the neck and arm. Paresthesia and coolness of the ipsilateral extremity can also occur (68). Examination may reveal a bruit over a pulsatile mass in the supraclavicular fossa, a difference in brachial systolic pressures, and/or a difference in upper extremity peripheral pulses. Primary arterial dissection involving the femoral and/or popliteal arteries is extremely rare and is usually of atherosclerotic origin, but may also occur secondary to blunt or penetrating trauma, connective tissue disorders, or inflammatory arterial diseases (69). The degree of symptoms depends on the severity of limb ischemia secondary to compression of the true lumen by the arterial dissection. Patients may experience pain following trauma, with a picture of acute arterial occlusion, or with intermittent claudication of new onset.

Diagnosis of primary arterial dissection is by angiography, and the optimal treatment depends on the acuteness and the severity of the presenting symptoms. Surgical resection with autogenous vein or prosthetic graft interposition is indicated in symptomatic patients.

Spontaneous dissection of the cervical cephalic arteries is uncommon but important for two reasons. Most patients present with one of two clinical syndromes—either hemicrania with oculosympathetic paresis or hemicrania with delayed focal cerebral ischemic symptoms—and the prognosis is good for recovery and recurrences are rare.

REFERENCES

1. Mehra NK, Jaini R. Immunogenetics of peripheral arteriopathies. *Clin Hemorheol Microcirc* 2000;23:225–232.
2. Shinoya SL. Diagnostic criteria of Buerger's disease. *Int J Cardiol* 1998[Suppl 1]:S243–S245.
3. Sasaki S, Sakuma M, Yasuda K. Current status of thromboangiitis obliterans (Buerger's disease) in Japan. *Int J Cardiol* 2000[75 Suppl 1]:S175–S181.
4. Shindo S, Matsumoto H, Ogata K, et al. Arterial reconstruction in Buerger's disease: by-pass to disease-free collaterals. *Int Angiol* 2002;21:228–232.
5. Saha K, Chabra N, Gulati SM. Treatment of patients with thromboangiitis obliterans with cyclophosphamide. *Angiology* 2001;52:399–407.
6. Isner JM, Baumgartner I, Rauh G, et al. Treatment of thromboangiitis obliterans (Buerger's disease) by intramuscular gene transfer of vascular endothelial growth factor: preliminary clinical results. *J Vasc Surg* 1998;28:964–973.
7. Salvarani C, Gabriel SE, O'Fallon WM, et al. The incidence of giant cell arteritis in Olmsted County, Minnesota: apparent fluctuations in a cyclic pattern. *Ann Intern Med* 1995;123:192–194.
8. Evans JM, O'Fallon WM, Hunder GG. Increased incidence of aortic aneurysm and dissection in giant cell (temporal) arteritis. *Ann Intern Med* 1995;122:502–507.
9. Gonzalez-Gay MA, Blanco R, Rodriguex-Valverde V, et al. Permanent visual loss and cerebrovascular accidents in giant cell arteritis: predictors and response to treatment. *Arthritis Rheum* 1998;41:1497–1504.
10. Klein RG, Hunder GG, Stanson AW, et al. Large artery involvement in giant cell (temporal) arteritis. *Ann Intern Med* 1975;83:806–812.
11. Stanson AW. Imaging findings in extracranial (giant cell) temporal arteritis. *Clin Exp Rheumatol* 2001;18[Suppl 20]:S43–S48.
12. Atalay MK, Bluemke DA. Magnetic resonance imaging of large vessel vasculitis. *Curr Opin Rheumatol* 2001;13:41–47.
13. Turlakow A, Yeung HWD, Pui J, et al. Fludeoxyglucose positron emission tomography in the diagnosis of giant cell arteritis. *Arch Intern Med* 2001;161:1003–1007.
14. Meller J, Strutz F, Siefker U, et al. Early diagnosis and follow-up of aortitis with [(18)F] FDG PET and MRI. *Eur J Nucl Med Mol Imaging* 2003;30:730–736.
15. Salvarani C, Fabrizio C, Boiardi L, et al. Polymyalgia rheumatica and giant-cell arteritis. *N Engl J Med* 2002;347:261–271.
16. Cantini F, Salvarani C, Olivieri I, et al. Erythrocyte sedimentation rate and C-reactive protein in the evaluation of disease activity and severity in polymyalgia rheumatica: a prospective follow-up study. *Semin Arthritis Rheum* 2000;30:17–24.
17. Hunder GG, Ward LE, Burbank MK. Giant-cell arteritis producing an aortic arch syndrome. *Ann Intern Med* 1967;66:578–582.
18. Hall S, Barr W, Lie JT, et al. Takayasu arteritis. A study of 32 North American patients. *Medicine* 1985;64:89–99.
19. Johnston SL, Lock RJ, Gompels MM. Takayasu arteritis: a review. *J Clin Pathol* 2002;55:481–486.
20. Kerr GS, Hallahan CW, Giordano J, et al. Takayasu arteritis. *Ann Intern Med* 1994;120:919–929.
21. Subramanyan R, Joy J, Balakrishnan KG. Natural history of aortoarteritis (Takayasu's disease). *Circulation* 1989;80:429–437.
22. Arend WP, Michel BA, Bloch DA, et al. The American College of Rheumatology 1990 criteria for the classification of Takayasu arteritis. *Arthritis Rheum* 1990;33:1129–1134.
23. Mohan N, Kerr G. Takayasu's arteritis. *Curr Treat Options Cardiovasc Med* 1999;1:35–42.
24. Ishikawa K. Natural history and classification of occlusive thromboaortopathy (Takayasu's disease). *Circulation* 1978;57:27–35.
25. Shelhamer JH, Volkman DJ, Parrillo JE, et al. Takayasu's arteritis and its therapy. *Ann Intern Med* 1985;103:121–126.
26. Hoffmann GS, Leavitt RY, Kerr GS, et al. Treatment of glucocorticoid-resistant or relapsing Takayasu arteritis with methotrexate. *Arthritis Rheum* 1994;37:578–582.
27. Spittell PC, Spittell Jr JA. Occlusive arterial disease of the hand due to repetitive blunt trauma: a review with illustrative cases. *Int J Cardiol* 1993;38:281–292.
28. Coleman SS, Anson BJ. Arterial patterns in the hand based upon a study of 650 specimens. *Surg Gynecol Obstet* 1961;4:409–424.
29. De Giacomo T, Rendina EA, Venuta F, et al. Thoracoscopic sympathectomy for symptomatic arterial obstruction of the upper extremities. *Ann Thorac Surg* 2002;74:885–888.
30. Mehlhoff TL, Wood MB. Ulnar artery thrombosis and the role of interposition vein grafting: patency with microsurgical technique. *J Hand Surg* 1991;16:274–278.
31. Roos DB. Congenital anomalies associated with thoracic outlet syndrome. *Am J Surg* 1976;132:771–778.
32. Makhoul RG, Machleder HI. Developmental anomalies at the thoracic outlet. *J Vasc Surg* 1992;16:534–545.
33. Matsumura JS, Rilling WS, Pearce WH, et al. Helical computed tomography of the normal thoracic outlet. *J Vasc Surg* 1999;26:776–783.
34. Dymarkowski S, Bosmans H, Marchal G, et al. Three-dimensional MR angiography in the evaluation of thoracic outlet syndrome. *Am J Roentgenol* 1999;173:1005–1008.
35. Coletta JM, Murray JD, Reeves TR, et al. Vascular thoracic outlet syndrome: successful outcomes with multimodal therapy. *Cardiovasc Surg* 2001;9:11–15.
36. Mosimann J, Walder J, Van Melle G. Stenotic intimal thickening of the external iliac artery: illness of the competition cyclists?. *Vasc Surg* 1985;19:258–263.
37. Chevalier JM, Enon B, Walder J, et al. Endofibrosis of the external iliac artery in bicycle racers: an unrecognized pathological state. *Ann Vasc Surg* 1986;1:297–303.
38. Rousselet MC, Saint-Andre JM, L'Hoste P, et al. Stenotic intimal thickening of the external iliac artery in competition cyclists. *Hum Pathol* 1990;21:524–529.
39. Ehrsam JE, Spittell PC. Endofibrosis of the external iliac artery in a competitive cyclist: diagnosis and follow-up by duplex ultrasonography. *J Vasc Technol* 1996;20:107–109.
40. Kral CA, Han DC, Edwards WD, et al. Obstructive external iliac arteriopathy in avid bicyclists: new and variable histopathologic features in four women. *J Vasc Surg* 2002;36:565–570.
41. Hoffmann U, Better J, Rainoni L, et al. Popliteal artery compression and force of active plantar flexion in young healthy volunteers. *J Vasc Surg* 1997;26:281–287.
42. Beregi JP, Djabbari M, Desmoucelle F, et al. Popliteal vascular disease: evaluation with spiral CT angiography. *Radiology* 1997;203:477–483.
43. Atilla S, Akpek ET, Yucel C, et al. MR imaging and MR angiography in popliteal artery entrapment syndrome. *Eur J Radiol* 1998;8:1025–1029.
44. Lambert AW, Wilkins DC. Popliteal artery entrapment syndrome. *Br J Surg* 1999;86:1365–1370.
45. Levien LJ, Veller MG. Popliteal artery entrapment syndrome: more common than previously recognized. *J Vasc Surg* 1999;30:587–598.
46. Haimovici H. Patterns of arteriosclerotic lesions of the lower extremity. *Arch Surg* 1967;95:918–933.
47. Balaji MR, DeWeese JA. Adductor canal outlet syndrome. *JAMA* 1981;245:167–170.
48. Levien LJ, Benn CA. Adventitial cystic disease: a unifying hypothesis. *J Vasc Surg* 1998;28:193–205.
49. Flanigan DP, Burnham SJ, Godreau JJ, et al. Summary of cases of adventitial cystic disease of the popliteal artery. *Ann Surg* 1979;189:165–175.
50. Elias DA, White LM, Rubenstein JD, et al. Clinical evaluation and MR imaging features of popliteal artery entrapment and cystic adventitial disease. *Am J Roentgenol* 2003;180:627–632.
51. Jasinski RW, Masselink BA, Partridge RW, et al. Adventitial cystic disease of the popliteal artery. *Radiology* 1987;163:153–155.
52. Ruckert RI, Taupits M. Cystic adventitial disease of the popliteal artery. *Am J Surg* 2000;180:53.
53. Ricci P, Panzetti C, Mastantuono M, et al. Cross-sectional imaging in a case of adventitial cystic disease of the popliteal artery. *Cardiovasc Intervent Radiol* 1999;22:71–74.

54. Gray BH, Young JR, Olin JW. Miscellaneous arterial diseases. In: Young JR, Oliin JW, Bartholomew JR, eds. *Peripheral vascular diseases,* 2nd ed. St. Louis: Mosby–Year Book, 1996:425–440.

55. Luscher TF, Lie JT, Stanson AW, et al. Arterial fibromuscular dysplasia. *Mayo Clin Proc* 1987;62:931–952.

56. Sauer L, Reilly LM, Goldstone J, et al. Clinical spectrum of symptomatic external iliac fibromuscular dysplasia. *J Vasc Surg* 1990;12:488–496.

57. Begelman SM, Olin JW. Fibromuscular dysplasia. *Curr Opin Rheum* 2000;12:41–47.

58. Ausband SC, Goodman PE. An unusual case of clarithromycin associated ergotism. *J Emergency Med* 2001;21:411–413.

59. Greene FL, Ariyan S, Stansel Jr HC. Mesenteric and peripheral vascular ischemia secondary to ergotism. *Surgery* 1977;81:176–179.

60. Wells KE, Steed DL, Zajko AB, et al. Recognition and treatment of arterial insufficiency from cafergot. *J Vasc Surg* 1986;4:8–15.

61. Carliner N, Denune DP, Finch CS, et al. Sodium nitroprusside treatment of ergotamine-induced peripheral ischemia. *JAMA* 1974;227:308–309.

62. Lindsay Jr J, Hurst JW. Clinical features and prognosis in dissecting aneurysm of the aorta: a reappraisal. *Circulation* 1967;35:880–888.

63. Slater EE, Desanctis RW. The clinical recognition of dissecting aortic aneurysm. *Am J Med* 1976;60:625–633.

64. Hagan PG, Nienaber CA, Isselbacher EM, et al. The International Registry of Acute Aortic Dissection (IRAD). New insights into an old disease. *JAMA* 2000;283:897–903.

65. Cambria RP, Brewster DC, Gertler J, et al. Vascular complications associated with spontaneous aortic dissection. *J Vasc Surg* 1988;7:199–209.

66. Pannenton JM, Teh SH, Cherry KJ, et al. Aortic fenestration for acute or chronic aortic dissection: an uncommon but effective procedure. *J Vasc Surg* 2000;32:711–721.

67. Beregi JP, Prat A, Gaxotte V, et al. Endovascular treatment for dissection of the descending aorta. *Lancet* 2000;356:482–483.

68. Wychulis AR, Kincaid OW, Wallace RB. Primary dissecting aneurysm of the peripheral arteries. *Mayo Clin Proc* 1969;44:804–810.

69. Rahmani O, Gallagher JJ. Spontaneous superficial femoral artery dissection with distal embolization. *Ann Vasc Surg* 2002;16:358–362.

CHAPTER 8

Hypertension

Evaluation, Therapy, and Review of Landmark Trials

Mohanram Narayanan, Ralph E. Watson, and Donald J. DiPette

Key Points

- There is a new, simplified classification of hypertension.
- Accurate and thorough evaluation of the hypertensive patient is important.
- There are new treatment guidelines from the Joint National Committee of the National Heart, Lung, and Blood Institute.
- Most patients will need at least two drugs to reach goal blood pressure.
- Summary of the major hypertension clinical trials.

INTRODUCTION

Hypertension is probably the most important public health problem in developed countries (1). The World Health Organization estimates that hypertension causes one in every eight deaths worldwide, making it the third leading killer in the world (2,3). It affects 50 million people in the United States and nearly 1 billion people worldwide (4). Recent data from the Framingham Heart Study indicate that people who are normotensive at age 55 years have a 90% lifetime risk for developing hypertension (5). Hypertension is the most common primary diagnosis in the United States, causing 35 million office visits yearly (6). It is one of the most important and easily remediable risk factors for adverse cardiovascular outcomes, including stroke, myocardial infarction, renal failure, and death. Despite the fact that simple methods of measuring blood pressure (BP) have been available for more than 100 years and despite the overwhelming evidence that the relative risk of having a stroke or a coronary event is clearly associated with a rise in diastolic BP (DBP) or systolic BP (SBP), data from the third National Health and Nutrition Examination Survey (1999 to 2000) show that control rates, although improved at 34%, are still far below the 50% goal in *Healthy People 2010* (4,7–9). Hypertension awareness decreased from 73% to 70%, and treatment rates only increased from 55% to 59% between 1991 and 2000 (Table 8.1)

(4). Thus, despite intensive public awareness and education programs, documented efficacious nonpharmacologic modalities, and the availability of multiple classes of pharmacologic antihypertensive agents, hypertension remains a major public health concern.

Data from the Framingham Study (1950s and 1960s), other epidemiologic surveys, and several large insurance company databases have unequivocally shown that high BP is a powerful predictor of future cardiovascular events, especially stroke, myocardial infarction, and death (10). Controlling hypertension in clinical trials has been associated with a 35% to 40% decrease in the incidence of stroke, a 50% decrease in congestive heart failure, and a 20% to 25% decrease in myocardial infarction (11).

This chapter is organized into two parts: (a) a discussion of the clinical approach to the patient with hypertension, and (b) an overview of landmark hypertension clinical trials.

CLINICAL APPROACH TO THE PATIENT WITH HYPERTENSION

Classification of Blood Pressure

The recently published seventh report of the Joint National Committee on Prevention, Detection, Evaluation, and

TABLE 8.1. *Trends in awareness, treatment, and control of high blood pressure in adults with hypertension aged 18 to 74 years[a]*

	National Health and Nutrition Examination Surveys (weighted %)			
	II (1976–1980)	III (phase 1, 1988–1991)	III (phase 2, 1991–1994)	1999–2000
Awareness	51	73	68	70
Treatment	31	55	54	59
Control[b]	10	29	27	34

[a]Data for 1999–2000 were computed (M. Wolz, unpublished data, 2003) from the National Heart, Lung, and Blood Institute, and data for National Health and Nutrition Examination Surveys II and III (phases 1 and 2) are from The Sixth Report of the Joint National Committee on Prevention, Detection, Evaluation, and Treatment of High Blood Pressure. High Blood Pressure is systolic blood pressure of $\geq$140 mm Hg, diastolic blood pressure of $\geq$90 mm Hg, or taking antihypertensive medication.
[b]Systolic blood pressure of <140 mm Hg and diastolic blood pressure of <90 mm Hg.

Treatment of High Blood Pressure (JNC 7) changed the classification of BP (Table 8.2) (4). The BP is based on the mean of two or more seated BP readings on each of two or more office visits. Compared to JNC 6, JNC 7 combined Stages 2 and 3 and created a new category, prehypertension. Prehypertension is defined as a SBP between 120 and 139 mm Hg and a DBP between 80 and 89 mm Hg. The justification for this new category is based on Framingham data, which indicate that patients in this category are at increased risk for progression to hypertension, with those having 130/80 to 139/89 mm Hg being at twice the risk to develop hypertension compared to those with lower blood pressures (12).

Blood Pressure Measurement in the Office

Auscultation with a calibrated and validated sphygmomanometer should be used (4,13). The proper condition is the patient seated quietly for at least 5 minutes in a chair rather than on an examining table, with feet on the floor and arm supported at heart level. Patients should refrain from smoking or caffeine for 30 minutes before the measurement. The BP should also be determined in the standing position in patients at risk for postural hypotension. The correct-sized cuff is one that has a bladder that encircles at least 80% of the upper arm. At least two measurements should be taken each

TABLE 8.2. *Classification and management of blood pressure for adults aged 18 years or older[a]*

				Management[b]	
				Initial drug therapy	
BP classification	Systolic BP (mm Hg)		Diastolic BP (mm Hg)	Lifestyle modification	Without compelling indication	With compelling indications[c]
Normal	<120	and	<80	Encourage		
Prehypertension	120–139	or	80–89	Yes	No antihypertensive drug indicated	Drug(s) for the compelling indications[d]
Stage 1 hypertension	140–159	or	90–99	Yes	Thiazide-type diuretics for most; may consider ACE inhibitor, ARB, β-blocker, CCB, or combination	Drug(s) for the compelling indications; other antihypertensive drugs (diuretics, ACE inhibitor, ARB, β-blocker, CCB) as needed
Stage 2 hypertension	$\geq$160	or	$\geq$100	Yes	Two-drug combination for most (usually thiazide-type diuretic and ACE inhibitor, or ARB, or β-blocker, or CCB)[e]	Drug(s) for the compelling indications; other antihypertensive drugs (diuretics, ACE inhibitor, ARB, β-blocker, CCB) as needed

[a]ACE, Angiotensin-converting enzyme; ARB, angiotensin-receptor blocker; BP, blood pressure; CCB, calcium channel blocker.
[b] Treatment determined by highest BP category.
[c]See Table 8.4.
[d]Treat patients with chronic kidney disease or diabetes to BP goal of <130/80 mm Hg.
[e]Initial combined therapy should be used cautiously in those at risk for orthostatic hypotension.

time. The SBP is the point at which the first of two or more sounds is heard (Korotkoff phase 1). The DBP is the point before the disappearance of sounds (Korotkoff phase 5). The physician should provide the patient with the BP numbers and the goal BP.

Patient Self-Measurement of BP

Home measurement devices should be checked regularly for accuracy (4). Patient self-measurement of BP can improve compliance, aid in determining the response to therapy, and help in the evaluation for "white coat hypertension," Home BPs of greater than 135/85 mm Hg are generally considered high.

Ambulatory Blood Pressure Monitoring

Ambulatory BP monitoring is warranted for the evaluation of "white coat hypertension" when no target-organ damage is present (4,14). It is also helpful in patients with apparent resistant hypertension, hypotensive symptoms, and episodic hypertension. Ambulatory BP readings are usually lower than office BPs. Elevated ambulatory mean readings are greater than 135/85 mm Hg during the day and greater than 120/75 mm Hg during sleep. Ambulatory BP levels correlate better with target-organ damage than office BP levels (15).

Goals of the Patient Evaluation

There are three objectives: (a) assess lifestyle and identify cardiovascular risk factors or concomitant conditions that could influence treatment decisions, (b) determine the presence of secondary causes of high BP, and (c) determine the presence of target-organ damage (4).

The History

The history should include inquiry about symptoms related to (a) the high BP itself, (b) hypertensive vascular disease, and (c) secondary causes for high BP (4,13). Most patients with hypertension have no symptoms caused by the elevated blood pressure itself. Patients with severe hypertension may have occipital headaches on awakening in the morning. Other symptoms of elevated blood pressure include dizziness, palpitations, easy fatigability, and impotence. Hypertensive vascular disease can cause epistaxis, hematuria, blurred vision, weakness due to transient cerebral ischemia, angina, and dyspnea due to congestive heart failure. Occasionally, pain from a dissecting or leaking aneurysm of the aorta is a presenting symptom.

Examples of symptoms related to secondary causes of hypertension are (a) primary aldosteronism, causing hypokalemia and the resultant polyuria, polydipsia, and muscle weakness; (b) Cushing's syndrome, causing weight gain and emotional lability; (c) pheochromocytoma, presenting with episodic headaches, palpitations, diaphoresis, weight loss, and postural dizziness; (d) the loud snoring of obstructive sleep apnea; (e) the leg claudication of aortic coarctation; (f) the repeated urinary tract infections of chronic pyelonephritis; and (g) the nervousness, increased sweating, heat intolerance, palpitations, dyspnea, fatigue, weight loss, and increased appetite of hyperthyroidism.

The history should inquire about the use of prescription or over-the-counter medications and illicit drugs that can increase BP. These include corticosteroids, nonsteroidal anti-inflammatory agents, oral contraceptives, tricyclic antidepressants, sumatriptan, cyclosporin, appetite suppressants, decongestants, amphetamines, phencyclidine, and cocaine.

A strong family history of hypertension and a history of intermittent blood pressure elevation in the past suggest essential hypertension. Age of onset of BP elevation before 35 years or after 55 years may suggest secondary hypertension. A history suggesting the presence of target-organ damage would include angina pectoris and symptoms of cerebrovascular insufficiency, congestive heart failure, or peripheral vascular disease. The history should also determine whether other risk factors for cardiovascular disease are present, including cigarette smoking, dyslipidemia, diabetes mellitus, leisure-time physical inactivity, and family history of premature cardiovascular disease (men less than 55 years old, women less than 65 years old).

The results and adverse effects of previous BP medications should be determined. The patient's lifestyle, environmental (neighborhood, housing, workplace), and psychosocial factors must also be explored. This should include sodium, alcohol, saturated fat, and caffeine intake. The family and financial situation, employment status, working conditions, and educational level can affect the BP and can influence the treatment and patient education decisions.

The Physical Examination

The physical examination starts with inspection of the general appearance (4,13). "Moon face," truncal obesity, and "Buffalo hump" suggest Cushing's syndrome. Decreased muscular development in the legs compared to the arms suggests aortic coarctation. The next step is accurate measurement of the BP, as described previously. At least initially, the BP should be compared with the contralateral arm. An increase in BP, particularly the DBP, from sitting to standing position is expected in essential hypertension. A decrease, in the absence of BP medications, suggests secondary hypertension. The body mass index should be calculated as the weight in kilograms divided by the square of the height in meters.

Examination of the optic fundi is important because these findings are one of the best indicators of vascular damage and prognosis. Auscultation for carotid, femoral, and renal artery bruits must be included. Other areas of focus are palpation of the thyroid, thorough examination of the heart and lungs, and examination of the abdomen for the bruit of renal artery stenosis, enlarged kidneys of polycystic renal disease, masses, and abnormal aortic pulsations. Palpation of the extremities for edema and pulses and a neurological examination must also be performed. The femoral pulse should be felt and, if it is decreased or delayed compared to the radial pulse, the blood pressure in the legs must be measured to rule out aortic coarctation, especially in young patients.

Laboratory and other Diagnostic Tests

Prior to starting antihypertensive therapy, the recommended routine laboratory tests include hematocrit, potassium, creatinine, blood glucose, calcium, urinalysis, fasting (9 to 12 hours) lipid profile, and electrocardiogram (4,13). Optional tests include measurement of urinary albumin excretion and albumin/creatinine ratio.

More extensive testing is only indicated if BP control is not achieved or the history, physical examination, or routine labs suggest secondary hypertension. The studies to screen for secondary hypertension are as follows:

1. Renovascular disease: magnetic resonance angiography, angiotensin-converting enzyme inhibitor radionuclide renal scan, and renal duplex Doppler flow studies. For more details, see Chapters 18 and 19.
2. Pheochromocytoma: 24-hour urine assay for creatinine, metanephrines, and catecholamines
3. Cushing's syndrome: overnight dexamethasone suppression test or 24-hour urine assay for cortisol and creatinine.
4. Primary aldosteronism: plasma aldosterone–renin activity ratio.

Treatment

The ultimate goal of the treatment of hypertension is a decrease in cardiovascular and renal mortality and morbidity (4). The BP goal in uncomplicated hypertensive patients is less than 140/90 mm Hg. In patients with diabetes (16) or renal disease (17), the goal is less than 130/80 mm Hg (4). In patients with renal insufficiency and proteinuria (greater than 1 g per 24 hours), the BP goal may be lower (less than 125/75 mm Hg) (Fig. 8.1).

Lifestyle Modifications

Healthy lifestyle modifications are essential for prevention of hypertension, and are an important part of the treatment of hypertension (4). Lifestyle modifications that significantly lower blood pressure include (a) weight loss in overweight patients (18,19), (b) dietary sodium reduction (20,21), (c) the Dietary Approaches to Stop Hypertension (DASH) diet, which is high in potassium and calcium (22), (d) physical activity, and (e) moderation of alcohol consumption (Table 8.3).

Drug Therapy

Several classes of medications have been proven to reduce the complications of hypertension, including thiazide-type diuretics, beta-blockers (BBs), angiotensin-converting enzyme inhibitors (ACE-Is), angiotensin-receptor blockers (ARBs),

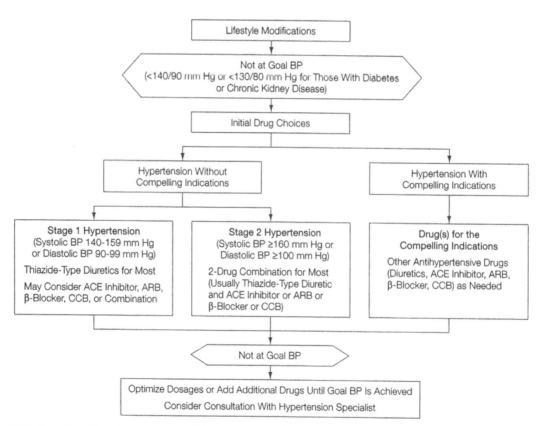

FIG. 8.1. Algorithm for treatment of hypertension. BP, blood pressure; ACE, angiotensin-converting enzyme; ARB, angiotensin-receptor blocker, CCB, calcium channel blocker.

TABLE 8.3. *Lifestyle modifications to manage hypertension*[a,b]

Modification	Recommendation	Approximate systolic BP reduction, range
Weight reduction	Maintain normal body weight (BMI, 18.5–24.9)	5–20 mm Hg/10-kg weight loss (23,24)
Adopt DASH eating plan	Consume a diet rich in fruits, vegetables, and low-fat dairy products with a reduced content of saturated and total fat	8–14 mm Hg (25,26)
Dietary sodium reduction	Reduce dietary sodium intake to ≤100 mEq/L (2.4 g sodium or 6 g sodium chloride)	2–8 mm Hg (25–27)
Physical activity	Engage in regular aerobic physical activity such as brisk walking (≥30 min/d, most days of the week)	4–9 mm Hg (28,29)
Moderation of alcohol consumption	Limit consumption to ≤2 drinks per day (1 oz or 30 mL ethanol, e.g., 24 oz beer, 10 oz wine, or 3 oz of 80-proof whiskey) in most men, and ≤1 drink per day in women and lighter-weight persons	2–4 mm Hg (30)

[a]BMI, Body mass index calculated as weight in kilograms divided by the square of height in meters; BP, blood pressure; DASH, Dietary Approaches to Stop Hypertension.

[b]For overall cardiovascular risk reduction, stop smoking. The effects of implementing these modifications are dose and time dependent, and could be higher for some individuals.

and calcium channel blockers (CCBs) (11,23–29). Many trials have shown that thiazide-type diuretics are as effective at preventing cardiovascular complications as any other class of antihypertensive medications (29). This was confirmed by the recently published Antihypertensive and Lipid-Lowering Treatment to Prevent Heart Attack Trial (ALLHAT) (25). In contrast, the recent Second Australian National Blood Pressure (ANBP2) trial demonstrated that ACE-Is may be more beneficial than diuretics, particularly in elderly men (28). It is important to note that diuretics are inexpensive and enhance the effectiveness of other antihypertensive medications when used in combination (4).

When deciding on drug therapy policy, it is important to consider the ALLHAT study (25,30–32). It is the largest randomized trial of antihypertensive treatment conducted to date (25,30). Over a 5-year period, relatively high-risk hypertensives were randomized to either a thiazide-type diuretic (chlorthalidone), a CCB (amlodipine), an ACE-I (lisinopril), or an alpha-blocker (doxazocin). It included large numbers of previously underrepresented populations in blood pressure trials (47% women, 35% African Americans, 19% Hispanics, 36% diabetics). The alpha-blocker arm of the study was stopped prematurely due to the observation that there was a significantly greater incidence of congestive heart failure and, to a lesser extent, strokes in the hypertensives treated with the alpha blocker than those treated with the diuretic. Among the remaining three groups, there was no difference in the primary outcome of fatal or nonfatal coronary heart disease events and no mortality difference. This was true regardless of sex, race, and the presence or absence of diabetes. The only difference in the major secondary outcomes was that lisinopril was significantly less effective than the diuretic at reducing stroke and combined cardiovascular disease. In addition, congestive heart failure was seen more often in the CCB and ACE-I groups than in the diuretic group. This find-

ing must be viewed with caution because it was not a primary or major secondary endpoint, and diuretics treat the signs and symptoms of congestive heart failure. In addition, the BP in the diuretic group was 2 mm Hg lower than that in the other two groups overall, and 4 mm Hg lower in the African American patients, which can have a major impact on outcomes. In addition, for nondiabetics entering the study, there was a significantly higher 4-year incidence of new-onset diabetes in the diuretic group (18% higher than with amlodipine and 43% higher than with lisinopril). This increase in new-onset diabetes in the diuretic group did not translate into increased cardiovascular events during this relatively short period after the diagnosis. It is also important to note that the diuretic used in this study was chlorthalidone and not hydrochlorothiazide (HCTZ). This may be important due to the greater half-life and potency of chlorthalidone compared to HCTZ.

What can we conclude from ALLHAT (25,30–33)?

1. There were no differences among diuretics, CCBs, and ACE-Is in the primary outcome of fatal or nonfatal coronary heart disease and no mortality difference, regardless of sex, race, or the presence or absence of diabetes (30–33).
2. Lisinopril was significantly less effective than the diuretic at reducing stroke and combined cardiovascular disease, but this may have been affected by the 2- to 4-mm Hg lower blood pressure in the diuretic group (30–32).
3. Heart failure was seen more often in the CCB and ACE-I groups than in the diuretic group, but this finding must be viewed with caution because it was not a primary or major secondary endpoint and may not have been well validated (30–32).
4. Chlorthalidone is at least as effective as a first-line treatment as more expensive alternatives in uncomplicated hypertensives. Diuretics should be an integral part of

TABLE 8.4. *Clinical trial and guideline basis for compelling indications for individual drug classes[a]*

High-risk conditions with compelling indication[b]	Recommended drugs						Clinical trial basis[c]
	Diuretic	β-Blocker	ACE inhibitor	ARB	CCB	Aldosterone antagonist	
Heart failure	•	•	•	•		•	ACC/AHA Heart Failure Guideline (40), MERIT-HF (41), COPERNICUS (42), CIBIS (43), SOLVD (44), AIRE (45), TRACE (46), ValHEFT (47), RALES (48)
Post-myocardial infarction		•	•			•	ACC/AHA post-MI guideline (49), BHAT (50), SAVE (51), Capricom (52), EPHESUS (53)
High coronary disease risk	•	•	•		•		ALLHAT (33), HOPE (34), ANBP2 (35), LIFE (32), CONVINCE (31)
Diabetes	•	•	•	•	•		NKF–ADA guideline (21,22), UKPDS (54), ALLHAT (33)
Chronic kidney disease			•	•			NKF guideline (22), Captopril trial (55), RENAAL (56), IDNT (57), REIN (58), AASK (59)
Recurrent stroke prevention	•		•				PROGRESS (35)

[a]AASK, African American Study of Kidney Disease and Hypertension; ACC/AHA, American College of Cardiology/American Heart Association; ACE, angiotensin-converting enzyme; AIRE, Acute Infarction Ramipril Efficacy; ALLHAT, Antihypertensive and Lipid-Lowering Treatment to Prevent Heart Attack Trial; ANBP2, Second Australian National Blood Pressure Study; ARB, angiotensin-receptor blocker; BHAT, β-Blocker Heart Attack Trial; CCB, calcium channel blocker; CIBIS, Cardiac Insufficiency Bisoprotol Study; CONVINCE, Controlled Onset Verapamil Investigation of Cardiovascular End Points; COPERNICUS, Carvedilol Prospective Randomized Cumulative Survival Study; EPHESUS, Eplerenone Post-Acute Myocardial Infarction Heart Failure Efficacy and Survival Study; HOPE, Heart Outcomes Prevention Evaluation Study; IDNT, Inbesartan Diabetic Nephropathy Trial; LIFE, Losartan Intervention For Endpoint Reduction in Hypertension study; MERIT-HF, Metoprolol CR/XL Randomized Intervention Trial in Congestive Heart Failure; NKF-ADA, National Kidney Foundation–American Diabetes Association; PROGRESS, Perindopril Protection Against Recurrent Stroke Study; RALES, Randomized Aldactone Evaluation Study; REIN, Ramipril Efficacy in Nephropathy Study; RENAAL, Reduction of Endpoints in Non–Insulin-Dependent Diabetes Mellitus with the Angiotensin II Antagonist Losartan Study; SAVE, Survival and Ventricular Enlargement Study; SOLVD, Studies of Left Ventricular Dysfunction; TRACE, Trandolapril Cardiac Evaluation Study; UKPDS, United Kingdom Prospective Diabetes Study; ValHEFT, Valsartan Heart Failure Trial.

[b]Compelling indications for antihypertensive drugs are based on benefits from outcome studies or existing clinical guidelines; the compelling indication is managed in parallel with the blood pressure.

[c]Conditions for which clinical trials demonstrate benefit of specific classes of antihypertensive drugs.

hypertension therapy and should be strongly considered as initial therapy, especially in the elderly and African Americans (30–32).

5. The concerns about the use of thiazide-type diuretics in diabetic patients may be unfounded, at least in the short term (30–32).

6. Most patients (63%) required two or more drugs to control the blood pressure.

7. The most important message is that what matters most in uncomplicated hypertensives is getting the blood pressure controlled, and that this is overwhelmingly more important than the means (30).

JNC 7 recommends that thiazide-type diuretics be used as initial therapy, either alone or in combination with a drug in the other classes of medications that have been proven to reduce complications of hypertension (BBs, ACE-Is, ARBs, and CCBs) (4) (see Fig. 8.1). Initial therapy should start with other drugs if there is a compelling indication (Table 8.4). Other considerations include concurrent medications, BP goal, and side effects encountered. In many cases specialist consultation may be indicated (4).

Compelling Indications

Certain comorbidities require particular drug classes (Table 8.4).

Ischemic Heart Disease

For hypertensive patients with stable angina pectoris, the initial therapy is usually a BB. Alternatively, a long-acting CCB can also be used (4). Patients with unstable angina or acute myocardial infarction (MI) should have their hypertension treated initially with a BB or ACE-I (34). In post-MI patients ACE-Is, BBs, and ARBs are most beneficial (35–37).

Diabetes Mellitus

ACE-Is and ARBs decrease the progression of nephropathy in diabetic hypertensives (38–40). At least two drugs are usually needed to attain the goal of 130/80 mm Hg (16,17). Reductions in cardiovascular disease and stroke incidence have been achieved in these patients with thiazide-type diuretics, BBs, ACE-Is, ARBs, and CCBs (25,41,42).

Congestive Heart Failure

In asymptomatic patients with ventricular dysfunction, ACE-Is and BBs are the preferred initial therapy (36,37). For symptomatic patients and those with end-stage heart failure, loop diuretics in addition to ACE-Is, BBs, ARBs, and aldosterone blockers are recommended (43–49).

Renal Insufficiency

JNC 7 defines chronic kidney disease as either glomerular filtration rate (GFR) less than 60 mL per min per 1.73 m^2 (or serum creatinine greater than 1.5 mg per dL in men, greater than 1.3 mg per dL in women) or albuminuria greater than 300 mg per day (or 200 mg of albumin per gram of creatinine) (4). The goals in these patients are to slow the progression of the renal disease and to prevent cardiovascular disease. They often require at least three drugs to reach their target BP of 130/80 mm Hg (50,51). ACE-Is and ARBs decrease the progression of diabetic and nondiabetic renal disease (38–40,50,51). After starting an ACE-I or ARB, an increase in creatinine of up to 35% can be expected. The drug should not be stopped unless the rise is more than this or hyperkalemia occurs (52). Increasing doses of loop diuretics need to be added to the regimen in advanced renal disease (GFR less than 30 mL per min per 1.73 m^2 or serum creatinine greater than 2.5 mg per dL) (4).

Cerebrovascular Disease

Recurrent strokes are decreased by the combination of an ACE-I and a thiazide-type diuretic (27). There are no clear guidelines for lowering the blood pressure during an acute stroke. However, JNC 7 recommends that the BP be lowered to approximately 160/100 mm Hg until the condition stabilizes or improves (4).

Other Special Considerations

Minority Populations

BP control rates are lowest in Mexican Americans and Native Americans (4). African-American hypertensives have significantly higher rates of cardiovascular mortality, stroke, hypertension-related heart disease, congestive heart failure, hypertensive nephropathy, and end-stage renal disease than whites (53). The prevalence and severity of hypertension are also increased in African Americans (4). As monotherapy,

the blood pressure-lowering efficacy of both thiazide-type diuretics and CCBs are superior to that of ACE-Is, ARBs, and BBs (4,25,53–55). However, most patients will require at least two drugs to reach current BP goals (56,57), and these differences are eliminated by drug combinations that include adequate doses of a diuretic (4). In addition, ACE-I-induced angioedema occurs two to four times as frequently in African-American hypertensives as in other groups (25). However, where compelling indications have been identified for prescribing BBs, ACE-Is, or ARBs in certain groups of patients with hypertension, these indications should be applied equally to African-American patients (53).

Elderly

Hypertension is seen in two-thirds of all people older than age 65 years (4). Two large clinical trials proved the benefits of treating isolated systolic hypertension in older patients (58,59). The treatment recommendations for these patients is the same as for all other hypertensives (4). It may be necessary to start with lower doses in this population to avoid symptoms (4).

Obesity and the Metabolic Syndrome

The metabolic syndrome is defined as the presence of three or more of the following: abdominal obesity [waist circumference greater than 102 cm (40 in.) in men or greater than 89 cm (35 in.) in women], glucose intolerance (fasting glucose at least 110 mg per dL), BP at least 130/85 mm Hg, triglycerides at least 150 mg per dL, or low high-density lipoprotein cholesterol (less than 40 mg per dL in men or less than 50 mg per dL in women) (60). Each component must be treated with appropriate drug therapy, and intensive lifestyle modifications should be pursued with all of these patients (4). See Chapters 6 and 9 on metabolic syndrome and obesity.

Left Ventricular Hypertrophy

Left ventricular hypertrophy is an independent risk factor that increases the risk of subsequent cardiovascular disease. Providing equal BP control, regression is achieved by all classes of antihypertensive medications except direct vasodilators (hydralazine and minoxidil) (4,61).

Peripheral Vascular Disease

Peripheral vasculature disease (PVD) is associated with high cardiovascular morbidity and mortality (62). Intermittent claudication is not only its most common symptom, but also is an important predictor of cardiovascular death, increasing it threefold and increasing all-cause mortality by two- to fivefold (62). Hypertension is an important risk factor for PVD (62). Between 2% and 5% of hypertensives at presentation have intermittent claudication, and 35% to 55% of patients with PVD have hypertension at presentation (62).

Hypertension contributes to the pathogenesis of atherosclerosis and is associated with abnormalities of hemostasis and lipids, causing an increased atherothrombotic state (62). Any class of drugs can be used in most patients with PVD, but hypotension must be avoided (4,63). In the short term, decreasing the BP may worsen intermittent claudication (64). BBs, because they cause peripheral vasoconstriction, may increase symptoms such as claudication and cold extremities in this population. However, the other classes of antihypertensive medications also have not proven to be beneficial to the intermittent claudication in these patients and may also worsen it (63,64). During exercise, they cause vasodilation distal to the sites of significant arterial stenosis, resulting in a fall in perfusion pressure (63).

Orthostatic Hypotension

A decrease in systolic blood pressure on standing of greater than 10 mm Hg is seen more frequently in the elderly with isolated systolic hypertension, in diabetics, and in patients taking diuretics, venous dilators (peripheral alpha blockers, nitrates, and sildenafil), and some psychotropic medications (4). Intravascular depletion should be avoided in these patients, and standing blood pressures must be monitored carefully (4).

Women

Oral contraceptives may cause an increase in BP (4). However, hormone replacement therapy does not increase BP (65). In pregnancy, methyldopa, BBs, combined alpha and BBs such as labetalol, and vasodilators are the treatments of choice (66). ACE-Is and ARBs must be avoided in pregnancy and in patients who are likely to become pregnant, because of the high risk of fetal defects (66). Preeclampsia and eclampsia are beyond the scope of this chapter and are well covered elsewhere (66).

Potential Favorable Effects of BP Medications (4)

Peripheral alpha blockers are often useful in prostatic urethral obstruction. Thiazide-like diuretics decrease the demineralization of osteoporosis. BBs also treat tachyarrhythmias, migraines, essential tremor, thyrotoxicosis, and perioperative hypertension. CCBs are often useful in Raynaud's syndrome and in some arrhythmias.

Potential Unfavorable Effects of BP Medications (1,4)

ACE-Is and ARBs must be avoided in pregnancy and in patients who are likely to become pregnant, because of the high risk of fetal defects. ACE-Is should not be given to patients with any history of angioedema. Aldosterone antagonists and potassium-sparing diuretics can cause hyperkalemia and should be avoided in patients with serum potassium greater than 5 mg per dL. BBs should generally be avoided in patients with reactive airway disease or second- or third-degree heart block. BBs may also cause cold extremities and Raynaud's

phenomenon (63). Because they inhibit the usual sympathetic responses to hypoglycemia and block some of the symptoms of hypoglycemia, BBs must be used with caution in diabetics receiving hypoglycemic medications (1). Verapamil and diltiazem either alone or in combination with BBs can cause significant bradycardia and heart block. Thiazide-type diuretics must be used with caution in patients with gout or a history of hyponatremia, especially in the elderly.

Achieving Blood Pressure Control

Trials have shown that most patients will require two or more drugs to achieve the current BP goals (56,57). A second drug from a different class should be added if the goal is not reached. A meta-analysis found that the systolic blood pressure decreased by 13 and 18 mm Hg during treatment with low- and high-dose thiazide-type diuretics, respectively (67). Therefore it seems reasonable that when the initial BP is greater than 20/10 mm Hg above goal, initiating therapy with two drugs should be considered, either separate pills or a fixed-dose combination (4). This may achieve the goal BP more quickly, but caution is advised in patients at risk for orthostatic hypotension, including the elderly and patients with diabetes or other autonomic dysfunction (4). Fixed-dose combinations and generics often can decrease cost.

Motivation to take the prescribed medication and maintain a healthy lifestyle improves when patients trust and have positive experiences with their physicians. Patient attitudes and behaviors are greatly influenced by cultural differences, health and illness beliefs, and previous experiences with the health care system. These attitudes must be understood if the physician is to build trust and increase communication with patients and families (68). Knowledge of cultural issues can give the physician insight into the patient's world, assist in the development of more effective strategies for clinical care, and encourage greater compliance. Practicing culturally sensitive medicine and responding to the patient's cues on cultural etiquette can help the physician avoid misunderstandings and barriers to communication.

OVERVIEW OF LANDMARK HYPERTENSION CLINICAL TRIALS

Studies of Diastolic Hypertension

Evidence from many placebo-controlled trials of treatment of diastolic hypertension spanning the extremes of severity from the first Veterans Administration study of patients with DBPs between 115 and 129 mm Hg (69,69a) to several studies of young patients with DBPs between 90 and 99 mm Hg (70,71) have shown that treatment decreases cardiovascular risk. Due to the multifactorial nature of atherosclerosis leading to coronary heart disease, it has been easier to demonstrate reduced risk of cerebrovascular events than cardiac events with BP lowering. Recent meta-analyses of clinical trials have shown that the risk of stroke is reduced by 42% compared with placebo (29). Although the beneficial effect of antihypertensive therapy on coronary heart disease (CHD) mortality was difficult to show in earlier trials, (72) more recent trials (73,74), especially in older persons, have demonstrated a significant reduction in CHD endpoints in the group randomized to active antihypertensive drug therapy. Current evidence indicates an improvement of approximately 16% in CHD endpoints.

The progression of hypertension to higher stages and the development of heart failure are substantially prevented by antihypertensive drug therapy (75). A recent meta-analysis indicates that the development of heart failure is reduced by 42% by either a low-dose diuretic or a beta blocker as first-line therapy. In some placebo-controlled trials (76), the group randomized to active antihypertensive therapy had a 94% decreased risk of progression to higher stages of hypertension.

As noted from the data derived from the large Multiple Risk Factor Intervention Trial screenees (77), hypertension is an important risk factor for the development of renal failure and the need for renal replacement therapy. Other recent large trials [the Collaborative Study Group (38), Modification of Diet in Renal Disease (78), and ACE Inhibition in Progressive Renal Insufficiency (79)] also showed that antihypertensive therapy improves prognosis in such patients. The JNC 7 report recommends a lower treatment goal for diabetics and patients with renal impairment (4).

Isolated Systolic Hypertension

Framingham data clearly show that the SBP is a stronger risk marker for coronary heart disease than the DBP (69a,80,81). In the last decade, several large intervention trials have addressed the treatment of isolated systolic hypertension in the elderly (elevated SBP, but DBP below 90 mm Hg). The positive results from intervention have resulted in a positive attitude towards treatment, and today this is an accepted and highly effective medical intervention.

In the *Systolic Hypertension in the Elderly Program* (SHEP) (58), 4,736 patients older than 60 years with SBP greater than 160 mm Hg and DBP greater than 90 mm Hg were randomized to either chlorthalidone 12.5 mg or placebo, with additional treatment (atenolol or reserpine) given until the SBP was reduced to 160 mm Hg or less (if baseline SBP was greater than 180 mm Hg) or by 20 mm Hg (if baseline SBP was 160 to 179 mm Hg). After an average of 4.6 years of treatment, there were 33% fewer fatal or non-fatal strokes, 25% fewer coronary heart disease endpoints, 25% fewer cardiac endpoints, and 32% fewer cardiovascular events in the group randomized to active treatment. All of these differences were statistically significant. The results of SHEP show that antihypertensive drug therapy reduces cardiovascular risk in essentially all patient subgroups (men, women, older, younger, nondiabetic, initial SBP greater than 180 mm Hg. vs 160 to 180 mm Hg, previously treated and never treated), even when only the SBP is elevated.

The *Systolic Hypertension in Europe Study* (Syst-Eur) (59), completed in 1997, confirmed the benefits of antihypertensive therapy for isolated systolic hypertension in older

patients. A total of 4,695 patients aged 60 years and older with SBP 160 to 219 mm Hg and DBP less than 95 mm Hg were randomized to placebo or active treatment beginning with nitrendipine followed by enalapril and HCTZ if needed to reach BP goal. The study was terminated after an average of 2 years follow-up by the Data Safety and Monitoring Committee due to a significant (42% to 44%) reduction in stroke incidence among patients randomized initially to nitrendipine. Active treatment was also associated with a statistically significant 26% reduction in sudden death and a 33% reduction in nonfatal cardiovascular events. In an interesting substudy (82) from Syst-Eur, the investigators also found that when compared to placebo-treated individuals, there was a 50% reduction in incidence of dementia in actively treated participants. They estimated that if 1,000 hypertensive patients were treated for 5 years, 19 cases of dementia could be prevented.

The *Systolic Hypertension in China Study* (Syst-China) (83) followed a protocol identical to Syst-Eur with the exception that the allocation of treatment in the 2,394 patients was by sequential alternate assignment rather than randomization. A comparison of nitrendipine 10 to 40 mg daily versus placebo was carried out in 1,253 versus 1,141 individuals, respectively. If BP was not adequately controlled (less than 150 mm Hg systolic), captopril or HCTZ 12.5 to 25 mg twice daily or both were added. Fatal and nonfatal stroke was the primary trial endpoint. After publication of the SHEP results, 21 of the 31 Syst-China centers decided to stop the trial. The medium overall follow-up was thus only 3 years. There was a significant 39% reduction in all-cause mortality, a 58% reduction in stroke mortality, a 37% reduction in all cardiovascular endpoints, and a 38% reduction in fatal and nonfatal stroke in the group allocated to active antihypertensive therapy. The study augmented data available from SHEP and from Syst-Eur in demonstrating that results from those studies were generalizable to the Chinese population and mimicked the Syst-Eur study in demonstrating the safety and efficacy of a long-acting CCB, nitrendipine, in elderly patients with isolated systolic hypertension.

Studies of Lifestyle Modifications

Various dietary modifications have been shown to be beneficial in the treatment of hypertension, including salt and alcohol restriction, weight reduction, possibly increasing potassium and calcium intake, and ingestion of a vegetarian diet or fish oil supplements (84–88,88a). Nondietary modalities of lifestyle modification should also be considered including cessation of smoking to reduce the overall cardiovascular risk and increased physical activity by institution of an aerobic exercise regimen (4).

Most of the studies on lifestyle modifications evaluated only a single factor to prove its efficacy: for example, weight reduction without sodium restriction. In making recommendations to the individual patient, however, the physician should try to modify all of the factors that may be contributing to the elevation in blood pressure. In JNC 7, lifestyle modifications were recommended in all patients as initial and concurrent therapy (4).

Another approach was utilized in the *DASH trial* (22). Rather than evaluating sodium intake or weight loss, DASH randomized 459 patients with blood pressures of less than 160/80–95 mm Hg to a control diet low in fruits and vegetables; a diet rich in fruits and vegetables; or a combination diet rich in fruits and vegetables that includes low-fat dairy products low in saturated and total fat (the last is called the DASH diet). The following observations were noted, where the BP reductions are expressed in relation to the fall in BP seen with the control diet:

- The fruits and vegetables diet reduced the BP by 2.8/1.1 mm Hg compared to the DASH diet which reduced the BP by 5.5/3.0 mm Hg.
- These effects were more pronounced in hypertensives where the BP fell 11.4/5.5 mm Hg compared to 3.5/2.1 mm Hg in normotensives.
- The antihypertensive effects were maximal by the end of week 2 with any of the diets and were then maintained for 8 weeks.

The low-sodium DASH trial evaluated the effect of varying sodium intake in combination with consuming the DASH diet just described (20). In this study, 412 participants were randomly assigned to a control or a DASH diet and, within each diet, ate foods with three levels of sodium content (3.5, 2.3, and 1.2 g) for 30 days each. The following results were reported:

- Independent of sodium intake, the DASH diet resulted in significantly lower systolic and diastolic BP levels than the control diet. With the high-, intermediate-, and low-sodium intakes, the SBP was 5.9, 5.0, and 2.2 mm Hg lower with the DASH diet than with the control diet, respectively. Comparable values for the DBP were 2.9, 2.5, and 1.0 mm Hg lower with the DASH diet, respectively.
- With either diet, lowering the sodium intake reduced BP levels, an effect observed between those with and without hypertension, and among different races and between genders.
- When different phases of diet were compared, the most significant decrease in BP was observed between the high-sodium control and low-sodium DASH diets, as a comparative overall reduction of 8.9 and 4.5 mm Hg in systolic and diastolic BP, respectively, was noted with the low-sodium DASH diet. This benefit was even more significant among hypertensive individuals.

Compared to those consuming the high-sodium control diet, a mean SBP that was 11.5 and 7.1 mm Hg lower was found among patients with and without hypertension, respectively, who were consuming the low-sodium DASH diet.

Thus, the combination of a low-sodium and a DASH diet resulted in the most significant benefit, with decreases in BP comparable to those observed with antihypertensive agents.

Benefits of this low-sodium and/or prudent diet were observed in most patient subgroups, including older and even nonhypertensive individuals (21).

The best data on combined dietary intervention come from the *Treatment of Mild Hypertension Study* (89), a multicenter study in which 902 patients with mild diastolic hypertension (90 to 100 mm Hg) were started on a program consisting of weight reduction, sodium and alcohol restriction, and increased physical activity. Patients were then randomized to placebo or to one of five antihypertensive drugs (ACE-I, CCB, alpha blocker, diuretic, or BB) for a 4-year treatment period. There were initial improvements with nonpharmacologic therapy, which tended to diminish over time. There was a greater reduction in BPs, despite the fact that baseline BPs were only barely elevated (140/91 mm Hg, on average), among the patients randomized to active drug therapy, over and above the reductions seen in patients treated with only lifestyle modifications (16/12 vs. 8.6/8.6 mm Hg). The study was intended primarily as a pilot to see how well tolerated and effective the medications and lifestyle modifications were over the long term, and did not have the statistical power to compare the ability of individual regimens to protect patients against cardiovascular events. Nevertheless, there was a statistically significant ($p<0.05$) difference favoring the drug therapy group when all endpoints were pooled.

Although the BP response to lifestyle modifications alone is less than that seen if drug therapy is added (18,89), lifestyle modifications have the additional cardiovascular advantage of lowering plasma total and low-density lipoprotein (LDL)-cholesterol and raising high-density lipoprotein (HDL)-cholesterol, thereby lowering cardiovascular risk (19). In comparison, chlorthalidone and atenolol may have an unfavorable effect on plasma lipids (19).

Prevention of Hypertension

Dietary modification has also been evaluated in other studies. One such trial consisted of patients with "prehypertension," which was defined as a diastolic pressure between 85 and 89 mm Hg on two visits or between 80 and 84 mm Hg if the patient was more than 10% overweight (90). The patients were randomized to sodium and alcohol restriction and weight reduction or to a regular diet. The treated group had more weight loss and lower sodium and alcohol intakes. At 5 years, the incidence of progression to hypertension (defined as a DBP at least 90 mm Hg) was 19.2% in the control group, but only 8.8% in the treated group. Similar dietary changes, particularly weight reduction due to decreased caloric intake, can also modestly (2 to 3 mm Hg) and persistently lower the BP in patients who are normotensive (91).

Other studies have evaluated the relative efficacy of different lifestyle modifications in both hypertensive and prehypertensive patients. Weight loss in overweight patients is generally most effective, and salt restriction also may be beneficial (91–94). Furthermore, weight reduction and salt restriction used in combination may produce an additive antihypertensive response (92,95,96). The *Trials of Hypertension Prevention, phase II*, randomized 2,382 men and women (aged 30 to 54 years) with a BP greater than 140/83 to 89 mm Hg who were 110% to 165% of ideal body weight (92). The patients were randomized to usual care, salt restriction, weight reduction, or both. Sodium restriction was associated with a 50- and 40-meq decline in sodium intake and a 4.4- and 2.0-kg weight reduction at 6 and 36 months, respectively. Compared to usual care, the BP fell at 6 months by 3.7/2.7 mm Hg with weight loss, 2.9/1.6 mm Hg with salt restriction, and 4.0/2.0 mm Hg with combined therapy. These effects were attenuated at 36 months, but at 48 months, the likelihood of progressing to hypertension was reduced with the lifestyle modifications (relative risk 0.78 to 0.82).

Similar results were obtained in the *Trial of Nonpharmacologic Interventions in Elderly*, which evaluated 975 older persons (aged 60 to 80 years) who had a BP greater than 145/85 mm Hg on one antihypertensive medication; 585 were obese (96). Salt restriction was associated with a 40-meq per day reduction in sodium intake, and, in those patients who were obese, a regimen of diminished caloric intake and increased physical activity was associated with a persistent weight loss of 4 to 5 kg. These parameters were unchanged in the usual-care group. The reduction in blood pressure compared to usual care was 2.6/1.1 mm Hg with sodium restriction, 3.2/0.3 mm Hg with weight loss, and 4.5/2.6 mm Hg with combined therapy. The likelihood of remaining free of high blood pressure, antihypertensive drugs, and cardiovascular events at 30 months was reduced by salt restriction (38% vs. 24% with usual care), by weight reduction in obese subjects (39% vs. 26%), and by combined salt restriction and weight reduction in obese subjects (44% vs. 16%).

In summary, these observations suggest that diet plays an important role in many susceptible patients in the genesis of hypertension (19,22,85). Weight reduction and salt restriction may both lower the blood pressure and have an additive effect when used in conjunction with antihypertensive medications (20,91–93,95,96). A diet rich in fruits and vegetables and low-fat dairy products may also be beneficial (20,22,85).

What Is the Blood Pressure Goal for Most Patients?

The issue of whether the traditional BP goal (less than 140/90 mm Hg) is low enough for all patients is an important and debatable point (69a). National and international recommendations for the treatment of hypertension have universally included a goal of less than 140/90 mm Hg for the majority of hypertensive patients. These guidelines have been formulated to apply to both young and old patients, even those above the age of 75 or 80 years with isolated systolic hypertension.

The *Hypertension Detection and Follow-up Program* showed a 15% to 28% reduction in 5-year death rates in subgroups randomized to "stepped care" (average DBP 83 mm Hg) compared with those randomized to "referred care" (DBP of 88 mm Hg) (97). Data from several clinical trials suggest that a lower-than-usual BP goal, as recommended by JNC 7, is appropriate for high-risk patients (4).

Subgroups in which more aggressive therapy may be warranted or may be desirable include the following.

Renal Disease

Retrospective analysis of the *MDRD trial* (79) indicated less progression of renal disease in those patients randomized to the lower blood pressure goal of less than 125/75 mm Hg over the 2 years of follow-up. The MDRD study was a success more for the results of its BP intervention than for those obtained with dietary protein restriction. The *African American Study of Kidney Disease and Hypertension trial* (98), one of the largest of the National Institutes of Health-sponsored trials, also suggested that the lower the blood pressure in patients with renal disease, the better was the outcome. This trial included 1,094 African Americans with longstanding hypertension, otherwise unexplained slowly progressive chronic renal failure, and proteinuria (mean about 500 to 600 mg per day). The patients were allocated to one of three drugs—ramipril (436 patients), metoprolol (441 patients), or amlodipine (217 patients)—and to one of two blood pressure goals, 125/75 or 140/90 mm Hg. The primary endpoint was the rate of change in GFR; the secondary clinical composite outcome was the time to first event including a 50% reduction in GFR, an actual decrease in GFR of 25 mL per min per 1.73 m^2, the onset of renal failure, or death. At study end after approximately 4 years, the average blood pressure was 128/78 and 141/85 mm Hg in the lower and usual blood pressure groups, respectively.

Diabetes

In the *United Kingdom Prospective Diabetes Study* (UKPDS) (99), greater than 1,100 diabetic patients were treated with different antihypertensive regimens. Patients who achieved tight blood pressure control (144/82 mm Hg) compared with those who achieved less tight blood pressure control (154/87 mm Hg), a difference of only 10/5 mm Hg, achieved a marked decrease in both diabetic and nondiabetic cardiovascular complications. This study indicates that careful blood pressure control, especially in diabetic patients, is beneficial. Because the mean tight blood pressure control result was 144/82 mm Hg, it is obvious that many of the patients in this group must have achieved blood pressures considerably lower than 140/80 mm Hg. A subset analysis of the patients who achieved SBP levels of less than 140 mm Hg indicated additional benefit as pressure was lowered. Thus, an SBP goal of less than 130 mm Hg in diabetic persons is a reasonable one, if it can be achieved.

The *Hypertension Optimum Treatment* (HOT) (100) study in Sweden attempted to answer the question: Is there a difference in outcome if blood pressure levels are lowered more in one group than in another? In other words, does it matter how blood pressure is lowered, that is, which drug regimen is used? This randomized trial of nearly 19,000 patients from 26 countries showed that DBP could be lowered from an average of 105 mm Hg to an optimal level of 83 mm Hg, and that further lowering was safe, but not associated with further reductions in cardiovascular events. The original design of the trial was to randomize patients to three different DBP goals: 90 mm Hg or less, 85 mm Hg and less, and 80 mm Hg or less. Although there were fewer cardiovascular events than expected during the average 3.8 years of follow-up (only 3.8 cardiovascular deaths/1,000 patient-years compared with 6.5/1,000 in previous meta-analyses), there was a progressive reduction in risk seen with each 5-mm Hg decrement in achieved DBP from 100 to 80 mm Hg, with the "optimum" at 83 mm Hg. The intention-to-treat analysis for 1,501 diabetics in the HOT study also showed a statistically significant benefit of intensified treatment, with the greatest reductions in major cardiovascular events occurring in the group randomized to the lowest BP goal. There was no evidence for a J-shaped curve in the rates of cardiovascular morbidity and mortality for patients with known cardiovascular disease, and all patients appeared to tolerate the lower level of BP. The greatest improvement in quality-of-life scores occurred in those randomized to the lowest BP goal. In short: Lower is better, regardless of how it is achieved (this was one of the studies that led to recommendations that diabetic patients should have their DBP levels lowered to less than 80 mm Hg).

The recently completed major results of *ALLHAT* (25,100a), the largest clinical hypertension trial ever conducted, suggests that blood pressure can be reduced to levels close to recommended goals in a high percentage of patients. Mean age in this trial was 67 years of age, indicating a relatively older population, and yet, with a total enrollment of more than 33,000 patients, greater than 90% achieved DBP goals of less than 90 mm Hg, 60% achieved SBP goals of less than 140 mm Hg, and 66% achieved blood pressure levels of less than 140/90 mm Hg. These results were achieved in an ethnically diverse enrollment, in a widely dispersed North American region, and in private practice or public clinic settings. An important caveat to these results is that greater than 60% of the patients required two or more medications for control. Nevertheless, in a private-practice follow-up study of more than 8 years' duration, almost 80% of patients achieved the stringently defined goal blood pressure levels, even though the choice of medications was limited by trial design at the time of the study.

In summary, there are two important lessons to be learned from these recent clinical trials. (a) There are effective and safe medications, especially if they are employed in the appropriate combinations, which are capable of accomplishing these lower BP goals. It is incumbent on all physicians to utilize these agents in appropriate dosages and combinations so that a greater reduction in cardiovascular events can be achieved. (b) There is little evidence to support the notion that reducing blood pressure to even lower levels than those set in recent recommendations poses any danger.

Benefits of Antihypertensives Beyond Blood Pressure Control

Even though the benefits of decreasing BP are well known, there are certain antihypertensive agents that provide benefits to certain patient groups above and beyond their BP-lowering effects.

Diabetic Retinopathy

ACE-Is may have the same benefit in diabetic retinopathy as they do in nephropathy (100b). A randomized trial by Chaturvedi et al. (101) assessed the efficacy of lisinopril in normotensive patients with type 1 diabetes and retinopathy. Retinopathy, assessed on a five-level scale (none to proliferative), progressed by one level in 21 of 159 patients (13%) receiving lisinopril compared to 39 of 166 patients (23%) receiving placebo. Lisinopril also decreased progression by two or more levels (odds ratio 0.27) and the progression to proliferative retinopathy (odds ratio 0.18). The mechanism by which ACE-Is might inhibit the progression of retinopathy is unclear. In the case of captopril, the benefit may be related to its sulfhydryl group rather than to ACE inhibition. In an *in vitro* study, captopril blocked neovascularization in rat cornea by inhibition of zinc-dependent endothelial cell metalloproteinases (102). The applicability of this observation to humans remains to be determined, particularly since lisinopril also may be effective.

Cardiovascular Disease

There has been concern about the dihydropyridine calcium channel blockers in diabetic patients with hypertension (102a,102b). Two relatively small initial trials suggested increased cardiovascular complications with nisoldipine or amlodipine compared to an ACE-I. The *Appropriate Blood Pressure Control in Diabetes* (ABCD) *trial* (103) was a prospective, randomized, blinded trial comparing the effects of moderate control of blood pressure (target diastolic pressure 80 to 89 mm Hg) with those of intensive control of BP (diastolic pressure 75 mm Hg) on the incidence and progression of complications of diabetes. The study also compared nisoldipine with enalapril as a first-line antihypertensive agent in terms of the prevention and progression of complications of diabetes. Data were also analyzed on a secondary endpoint (the incidence of myocardial infarction) in the subgroup of patients in the ABCD trial who had hypertension. In this analysis, the 470 hypertensive patients (baseline diastolic BP = 90 mm Hg) showed similar control of BP, blood glucose and lipid concentrations, and smoking behavior in the nisoldipine group (237 patients) and the enalapril group (233 patients) throughout 5 years of follow-up. Using a multiple logistic-regression model with adjustment for cardiac risk factors, it was found that nisoldipine was associated with a higher incidence of fatal and nonfatal myocardial infarctions (24) than enalapril (4) (risk ratio = 9.5; 95% confidence interval [CI] = 2.7 to 33.8). It was presumed that this difference represented a benefit from the ACE-I rather than an increase in risk with the dihydropyridine. Whether this difference was due to the greater use of diuretics or beta-blockers in the enalapril group, a worsened prognosis with the CCB, or chance is unclear.

The primary aim of the *Fosinopril Versus Amlodipine Cardiovascular Events Randomized Trial* (FACET) (104) was to compare the effects of fosinopril and amlodipine on serum lipids and diabetic control in non-insulin-dependent diabetes mellitus (NIDDM) patients with hypertension. Prospectively defined cardiovascular events were assessed as secondary outcomes. Inclusion criteria included a diagnosis of NIDDM and hypertension (SBP of greater than 140 mm Hg or DBP of greater than 90 mm Hg). Exclusion criteria included a history of coronary heart disease or stroke, serum creatinine greater than 1.5 mg per dL, albuminuria greater than 40 mg per minute, and use of lipid-lowering drugs, aspirin, or antihypertensive agents other than BBs or diuretics. A total of 380 hypertensive diabetics were randomly assigned to open-label fosinopril (20 mg per day) or amlodipine (10 mg per day) and followed for up to 3.5 years. If blood pressure was not controlled, the other study drug was added. Both treatments were effective in lowering blood pressure. At the end of follow-up, there was no significant difference between the two groups in total serum cholesterol, HDL cholesterol, hemoglobin A1c, fasting serum glucose, or plasma insulin (primary endpoint). However, the patients receiving fosinopril had a significantly lower risk of the combined outcome of acute myocardial infarction, stroke, or hospitalized angina than those receiving amlodipine (14/189 vs. 27/191; $p<0.05$; hazards ratio = 0.49, 95% CI=0.26 to 0.95).

Both the ABCD and FACET trials may show the danger of small (400 patients) trials, one open label, and both reporting secondary endpoints. In the much larger (33,000 patients) ALLHAT (25), there were no differences among the three groups (diuretic, ACE-I, CCB) in the primary outcome of fatal or nonfatal coronary heart disease and there was no mortality difference, as discussed earlier.

The *Heart Outcomes Prevention Evaluation* (HOPE) *trial,* in a substudy named *MICRO-HOPE* (microalbuminuria, cardiovascular, and renal outcomes) (105), randomized 3,577 at-risk patients (greater than 55 years of age) with diabetes (among a total of 9,541 participants) to either ramipril (10 mg per day) or placebo. High risk was defined as diabetes plus a history of previous cardiovascular event or presence of at least one other risk factor for cardiovascular disease: total serum cholesterol greater than 200 mg per dL, low HDL-cholesterol, hypertension (present in 56%), known microalbuminuria, or current smoking. Previous coronary disease was present in 60% and most patients were on other cardioprotective medications including aspirin (55%), beta-blockers (29%), and lipid-lowering agents (23%). The combined primary outcome was MI, stroke, or cardiovascular death. The study was stopped 6 months early by the independent data safety and monitoring board due to consistent benefit with ramipril compared to placebo. At a mean follow-up of 4.5 years, ramipril therapy lowered the risk of the combined primary outcome by 25% and significantly lowered the incidence of myocardial infarction, stroke, and total mortality by 22%, 33%, and 24%, respectively. Additionally it lowered revascularization by 17% and overt nephropathy by 24%. This benefit remained after adjustments for the small decrease in blood pressure (2.4 mm Hg systolic and 1.0 mm Hg diastolic) observed with active therapy, and it was felt that the large improvement in outcomes was most likely attributable to favorable vascular effects of ACE-I.

However, it is possible that the benefits of ramipril therapy in HOPE (16,106) were, to a larger extent than initially reported, due to BP lowering, an effect that was masked by the design of the study. Ramipril was given before bedtime and the office blood pressure was measured about 10 to 18 hours later. In a subset of 38 patients with peripheral vascular disease, ambulatory monitoring was performed at baseline and at 1 year. Although there was no significant reduction in office blood pressure with ramipril therapy, 24-hour ambulatory pressure was significantly reduced, largely due to a more prominent fall in blood pressure during the night (17/8 mm Hg compared to placebo). Based on the results of the HOPE trial, the U.S. Food and Drug Administration has approved the use of ramipril for the reduction of MI, stroke, and cardiovascular and all-cause mortality in high-risk patients, including diabetics, as defined by the trial. However, approval did not include the use of ramipril for the prevention of diabetic complications. In addition, approximately 90% of the patients were white, leaving it unclear whether the observed benefits apply to other groups.

In contrast, the *Losartan Intervention for Endpoint Reduction in Hypertension* (LIFE) *trial* (24), in which the efficacy of an ARB was compared with a BB, reported a significant reduction in cardiovascular morbidity and mortality with losartan in a subset of high-risk patients. Unlike the RENAAL and IDNT studies discussed later, the LIFE trial (which enrolled a total 9,193 patients, of whom 1,105 were diabetic) was sufficiently powered to provide comparative efficacy data. The entry criteria included clinical hypertension (sitting blood pressure 160 to 200/95 to 115 mm Hg) and electrocardiographic evidence of left ventricular hypertrophy. In the LIFE diabetic trial substudy (42), all diabetic patients (most of whom had type 2 diabetes) between the ages of 55 and 80 years who fulfilled the entry criteria were randomly assigned to either losartan- or atenolol-based therapy. The substudy was performed in parallel with and analyzed similarly as the larger LIFE study. The primary endpoint was one of cardiovascular death, myocardial infarction, or stroke, and the composite endpoint was any one of these primary events. The administration of losartan resulted in marked benefits. At a mean follow-up of 4.7 years, the ARB was associated with significant reductions in the primary composite endpoint (18% vs. 23% for atenolol), cardiovascular mortality (6% vs. 10%), and total mortality (11% vs. 17%). These differences were primarily due to a marked reduction in stroke in the losartan-treated group compared to the atenolol-treated group.

There is no evidence that the benefits from ACE-Is or ARBs, as observed in HOPE and LIFE, are seen in diabetics who are not at high risk for adverse cardiovascular outcomes. Data from the UKPDS (99), for example, found that atenolol was as effective as captopril in terms of both blood pressure lowering and protection against macrovascular and microvascular disease among patients with type 2 diabetes who were not selected for being at increased risk for cardiovascular disease.

In the most recently conducted *Second Australian National Blood Pressure Study* (28), ACE-I-based therapy in elderly subjects with hypertension, particularly men, was associated with a significant cardiovascular benefit compared to diuretic therapy, despite equivalent BP control. This was a 4-year prospective, randomized, open-label study with blinded assessment of endpoints in 6,083 subjects (95% white) aged 65 to 84 years with hypertension (greater than 160/90 mm Hg). There was an 11% reduction in the total burden of cardiovascular events or death from any cause in the ACE inhibitor-treated group, comprising a 14% reduction in the rate of first nonfatal cardiovascular events and a 32% decrease in the rate of first nonfatal myocardial infarctions.

Renal Disease

Diabetic nephropathy is a common problem that is most likely to occur in patients who have poor glycemic control, hypertension, and glomerular hyperfiltration, or who are African American, Mexican, or Pima Indian (106a). The risk of nephropathy is roughly equivalent in type 1 and type 2 diabetes. Extensive studies in diabetic animals suggest that intraglomerular hypertension and glomerular hypertrophy play an important role, being present early in the disease (because diabetes induces renal vasodilation and often a rise in glomerular filtration rate) and then being exacerbated by the compensatory response to nephron loss.

Type 1 Diabetes

The benefit of antihypertensive therapy with an ACE-I in type 1 diabetes can be demonstrated early in the course of the disease when microalbuminuria is the only clinical manifestation. The *European Microalbuminuria Captopril Study Group* (107,108) showed that the administration of an ACE inhibitor to normotensive type 1 diabetics with microalbuminuria decreased both albumin excretion and, at 2 years, progression to overt diabetic nephropathy when compared to patients treated with placebo.

However, in the landmark study by Lewis et al. in the *Collaborative Study Group* (38), a more pronounced benefit was demonstrated in type 1 diabetics with overt nephropathy. Patients with overt proteinuria and a plasma creatinine concentration no greater than 2.5 mg per dL (220 μmol per L) were randomized to therapy with either captopril or placebo ($n = 409$). Further antihypertensive drugs were then added as necessary, although CCBs and other ACE inhibitors were excluded. After approximately 4 years of nearly equivalent blood pressure control, patients treated with captopril had a slower rate of increase in the plasma creatinine concentration and a lesser likelihood of progressing to end-stage renal disease or death. This benefit was limited to patients with an initial plasma creatinine concentration of at least 1.5 mg per dL (132 μmol per L), in whom the rate of rise in the plasma creatinine concentration was reduced by over 50% from 1.4 mg per dL per year (123 μmol per L) in the placebo group to 0.6 mg per dL per year (53 μmol per L) with captopril. In comparison, no improvement could be demonstrated in the patients with a lower baseline plasma creatinine concentration because the rate of progression was very slow in this group, with the plasma creatinine concentration rising by only 0.1 to 0.2 mg per dL per year (9 to 18 μmol per L).

The beneficial response to captopril, which was seen in both hypertensive and normotensive subjects (109,110), is consistent with smaller studies, which suggested that antihypertensive therapy, particularly with an ACE inhibitor, slowed the rate of progression in diabetic nephropathy.

Type 2 Diabetes

There has been much less information on the effect of antihypertensive therapy with ACE-Is in patients with nephropathy due to type 2 diabetes, although a similar benefit appears to be present. More data are available on the efficacy of ARBs. Two major trials have demonstrated a clear benefit in terms of renoprotection with ARBs in patients with nephropathy due to type 2 diabetes. A deficiency of these trials is the lack of comparison of ARBs to ACE-Is (111).

In the *Irbesartan Diabetic Nephropathy Trial* (IDNT) (40), 1,715 hypertensive patients with nephropathy due to type 2 diabetes were randomly assigned to irbesartan (300 mg per day), amlodipine (10 mg per day), or placebo. At 2.6 years, irbesartan was associated with a risk of the combined endpoint (doubling of the serum creatinine, development of end-stage renal disease, or death from any cause) that was 23% and 20% lower than with amlodipine and placebo, respectively; the respective values were 37% and 30% lower for doubling of the plasma creatinine. Furthermore, the risk of doubling of the plasma creatinine was increased by 7% in the amlodipine group compared to the ARB group. These benefits were not directly related to differences in the magnitude of blood pressure reduction among the groups.

In the *Reduction of Endpoints in NIDDM with the Angiotensin II Antagonist Losartan* (RENAAL) *trial* (39), 1,513 patients with type 2 diabetes and nephropathy were randomly assigned to losartan (50 to 100 mg per day) or placebo, both in addition to conventional antihypertensive therapy (except ACE-Is). The primary outcome was the composite of a doubling of the baseline serum creatinine, end-stage renal disease, or death. Secondary endpoints included a composite of morbidity and mortality from cardiovascular causes, proteinuria, and the rate of progression of renal disease. Compared to placebo, losartan reduced the incidence of a doubling of the plasma creatinine by 25% and end-stage renal disease by

28%; the mean follow-up was 3.4 years. The level of proteinuria declined by 35% with losartan compared to placebo. These benefits were again not associated with differences in blood pressure levels between the groups.

Although both studies showed the ARB groups had significant reductions in the development of and subsequent hospitalization for heart failure, neither study showed any significant cardiovascular mortality reduction, as these trials were underpowered and of too short duration to detect a possible cardiovascular benefit.

Joint National Committee VII Report

The much anticipated Seventh Report of the Joint National Committee on Prevention, Detection, Evaluation, and Treatment of High Blood Pressure was released recently (4). As mentioned earlier, the key highlights of the report include (a) the importance of systolic hypertension (greater than 140 mm Hg) as a cardiovascular risk factor in addition to DBP, (b) the recognition of "prehypertension" (SBP 120 to 139 mm Hg and DBP of 80 to 89 mm Hg) so that appropriate lifestyle modifications can be initiated to prevent cardiovascular disease, (c) the continuous positive correlation of cardiovascular disease risk with each increment of 20/10 mm Hg, (d) the simplification of classifying BP, (e) the emphasis on use of thiazide-type diuretics alone or in combination for most patients with uncomplicated hypertension, and (f) the almost universal need to use two or more agents in achieving therapeutic goals and to initiate therapy with two drugs if initial BP is greater than 20/10 mm Hg above goal BP.

WHERE ARE WE AND WHERE DO WE GO FROM HERE IN THE TREATMENT AND MANAGEMENT OF HYPERTENSION?

Excellent clinical trial outcome data (evidence-based medicine) prove that lowering BP with several differing classes of pharmacologic antihypertensive agents, including ACE-Is, ARBs, CCBs, and thiazide-type diuretics, will reduce the complications of hypertension. Recommendations for therapy (112) may be summarized as follows:

1. Most patients with hypertension will require two or more antihypertensive medications to achieve the new recommended BP goals (56,57).
2. Thiazide-type diuretics have been the basis of antihypertensive therapy in most outcome trials, including the recent large ALLHAT. In uncomplicated hypertensives, diuretics appear to be as effective in reducing morbidity and mortality as any of the other classes of agents. They enhance the antihypertensive efficacy of multidrug regimens, are useful in achieving BP control, and are more affordable than other antihypertensive agents. They should continue to be recommended as initial therapy for most patients with uncomplicated hypertension, either alone or in combination with one of the other classes.

3. Cardiovascular events, particularly congestive heart failure and stroke, are negatively influenced by the use of alpha-blockers and should not be considered as preferred initial therapy.
4. CCBs should be considered as second-line or third-line therapy except in special situations. Although CCBs are effective in reducing BP and are generally well tolerated, studies on primary or secondary prevention of myocardial infarction have been disappointing (113–115). Only the nondihydropyridines, that is, diltiazem and verapamil, have been shown to reduce reinfarction in patients with previous myocardial infarctions.
5. An ACE-I- or an ARB-based treatment program should be one of the preferred approaches in the management of type 1 or type 2 diabetic patients with nephropathy, respectively.

In summary, despite significant advances in understanding the pathophysiology of hypertension as well as its detection and management, awareness, treatment, and control rates remain very disappointing. Hypertension continues to be a major public health problem. The new guidelines coupled with the understanding of the health care community, patient education programs, and continued basic and clinical investigation should, we hope, increase our treatment and control of this major cardiovascular disease.

ACKNOWLEDGMENTS

The authors would like to express their appreciation to Rebecca McMahon for her assistance in the preparation of this chapter.

REFERENCES

1. Williams GH. Hypertensive vascular disease. In: Braunwald E, Fauci AS, Kasper DL, et al., eds., *Harrison's principles of internal medicine,* Vol. 1, 15th ed. New York: McGraw-Hill, 2001:1414–1430.
2. Kottke TE, Stroebel RJ, Hoffman RS. JNC7—It's more than high blood pressure. *JAMA* 2003;289:2573–2575.
3. World Health Organization. *The world health report 2002. Reducing risks, promoting healthy life.* Geneva: Author, 2002.
4. Chobanian AV, Bakris GL, Black HR, et al. The seventh report of the Joint National Committee on Prevention, Detection, Evaluation, and Treatment of High Blood Pressure: the JNC7 complete version. *Hypertension* 2003;42:1206–1252.
5. Vasan RS, Beiser A, Seshadri S, et al. Residual lifetime risk for developing hypertension in middle-aged women and men: the Framingham Heart Study. *JAMA* 2002;287:1003–1010.
6. Cherry DK, Woodwell DA. National ambulatory medical care survey: 2000 summary. *Advance Data* 2002;328:1–32.
7. Hajjar I, Kotchen TA. Trends in prevalence, awareness, treatment, and control of hypertension in the United States, 1988–2000. *JAMA* 2003;290:199–206.
8. Burt VL, Cutler JA, Higgins M, et al. Trends in the prevalence, awareness, treatment, and control of hypertension in the adult US population. *Hypertension* 1995;26:60–69.
9. U.S. Department of Health and Human Services. *Healthy people 2010: Understanding and improving health,* 2nd ed. Washington, U.S. Government Printing Office, 2000.
10. Kannel WB, Schwartz MJ, McNamara PM. Blood pressure and risk of coronary heart disease: the Framingham Study. *Dis Chest* 1969;56:43–52.

11. Neal B, MacMahon S, Chapman N. Effects of ACE inhibitors, calcium antagonists, and other blood pressure-lowering drugs. *Lancet* 2000;356:1955–1964.

12. Vasan RS, Larson MG, Leip EP, et al. Assessment of frequency of progression to hypertension in non-hypertensive participants in the Framingham Heart Study: a cohort study. *Lancet* 2001;358:1682–1686.

13. Williams GH. Approach to the patient with hypertension. In: Braunwald E, Fauci AS, Kasper DL, et al., eds., *Harrison's principles of internal medicine,* Vol. 1, 15th ed. New York: McGraw-Hill, 2001:211–214.

14. Pickering T. Recommendations for the use of home (self) and ambulatory blood pressure monitoring. *Am J Hypertens* 1996;9:1–11.

15. Verdecchia P. Prognostic value of ambulatory blood pressure. *Hypertension* 2000;35:844–851.

16. American Diabetes Association. Treatment of hypertension in adults with diabetes. *Diabetes Care* 2003;26[Suppl 1]:S80–S82.

17. National Kidney Foundation guideline. K/DOQI clinical practice guidelines for chronic kidney disease: Kidney Disease Outcome Initiative. *Am J Kidney Dis* 2002;39[Suppl 2]:S1–S246.

18. Wassertheil-Smoller S, Blaufox MD, Oberman AS, et al. The Trial of Antihypertensive Interventions and Management (TAIM) study. Adequate weight loss, alone and combined with drug therapy in the treatment of mild hypertension. *Arch Intern Med* 1992;152:131–136.

19. Oberman A, Wassertheil-Smoller S, Langford HG, et al. Pharmacologic and nutritional treatment of mild hypertension: changes in cardiovascular risk status (TAIM). *Ann Intern Med* 1990;112:89–95.

20. Sacks FM, Svetkey LP, Vollmer WM, et al. Effects on blood pressure of reduced dietary sodium and the Dietary Approaches to Stop Hypertension (DASH) diet. DASH–Sodium Collaborative Research Group. *N Engl J Med* 2001;344:3–10.

21. Vollmer WM, Sacks FM, Ard J, et al. Effects of diet and sodium intake on blood pressure: subgroup analysis of the DASH–Sodium Trial. *Ann Intern Med* 2001;135:1019–1028.

22. Appel LJ, Moore TJ, Obarzanek E, et al. A clinical trial of the effects of dietary patterns on blood pressure. DASH Collaborative Research Group. *N Engl J Med* 1997;336:1117–1124.

23. Black HR, Elliott WJ, Grandits G, et al. Principal results of the Controlled Onset Verapamil Investigation of Cardiovascular End Points (CONVINCE) Trial. *JAMA* 2003;289:2073–2082.

24. Dahlof B, Devereux RB, Kjeldsen SE, et al. Cardiovascular morbidity and mortality in the Losartan Intervention For Endpoint reduction in hypertension study (LIFE): a randomized trial against atenolol. *Lancet* 2002;359:995–1003.

25. The ALLHAT Officers and Coordinators for the ALLHAT Collaborative Research Group. Major outcomes in high-risk hypertensive patients randomized to angiotensin-converting enzyme inhibitor or calcium channel blocker vs. diuretic. *JAMA* 2002;288:2981–2997.

26. The Heart Outcomes Prevention Evaluation Study Investigators. Effects of an angiotensin-converting enzyme inhibitor, ramipril, on cardiovascular events in high-risk patients. *N Engl J Med* 2000;342:145–153.

27. PROGRESS Collaborative Group. Randomised trial of a perindopril-based blood pressure-lowering regimen among 6105 individuals with previous stroke or transient ischamic attack. *Lancet* 2001;358:1033–1041.

28. Wing LMH, Reid CM, Ryan P, et al. A comparison of outcomes with angiotensin-converting-enzyme inhibitors and diuretics for hypertension in the elderly. *N Engl J Med* 2003;348:583–592.

29. Psaty BM, Smith NL, Siscovick DS, et al. Health outcomes associated with antihypertensive therapies used as first-line agents: a systematic review and meta-analysis. *JAMA* 1997;277:739–745.

30. Williams B. Drug treatment of hypertension. *BMJ* 2003;326:61–62.

31. Moser M. Results of the ALLHAT trial: is the debate about initial antihypertensive drug therapy over? *J Clin Hypertens* 2003;5:5–8.

32. Weber MA. The ALLHAT report: a case of information and misinformation. *J Clin Hypertens* 2003;5:9–13.

33. Frohlich ED. Treating hypertension—what are we to believe? *N Engl J Med* 2003;348:639–641.

34. Braunwald E, Antman EM, Beasley JW, et al. ACC/AHA 2002 guideline update for the management of patients with unstable angina and non-ST-segment elevation myocardial infarction—summary article: a report of the American College of Cardiology/American Heart Association Task Force on Practice Guidelines (Committee on the Management of Patients With Unstable Angina). *J Am Coll Cardiol* 2002;40:1366–1374.

35. Beta Blocker Heart Attack Trial Research Group. A randomized trial of propranolol in patients with acute myocardial infarction, I: mortality results. *JAMA* 1982;247:1707–1714.

36. The Capricorn Investigators. Effect of carvedilol on outcome after myocardial infarction in patients with left-ventricular dysfunction: the CAPRICORN randomized trial. *Lancet* 2001;357:1385–1390.

37. Pfeffer MA, Braunwald E, Moye LA, et al. Effect of captopril on mortality and morbidity in patients with left ventricular dysfunction after myocardial infarction. Results of the survival and ventricular enlargement trial. The SAVE investigators. *N Engl J Med* 1992;327:669–677.

38. Lewis EJ, Hunsicker LG, Bain RP, et al. The effect of angiotensin-converting-enzyme inhibition on diabetic nephropathy. The Collaborative Study Group. *N Engl J Med* 1993;329:1456–1462.

39. Brenner BM, Cooper ME, de Zeeuw D, et al. Effects of losartan on renal and cardiovascular outcomes in patients with type 2 diabetes and nephropathy. RENAAL study investigators. *N Engl J Med* 2001;345:861–869.

40. Lewis EJ, Hunsicker LG, Clarke WR, et al. Renoprotective effects of the angiotensin-receptor antagonist irbesartan in patients with nephropthy due to type 2 diabetes. *N Engl J Med* 2001;345:851–860.

41. UK Prospective Diabetes Study Group. Efficacy of atenolol and captopril in reducing risk of macrovascular and microvascular complications of type 2 diabetes: UKPDS 39. *BMJ* 1998;317:713–720.

42. Lindholm LH, Ibsen H, Dahlof B, et al. Cardiovascular morbidity and mortality in patients with diabetes in the Losartan Intervention For Endpoint reduction in hypertension study (LIFE): a randomized trial against atenolol. *Lancet* 2002;359:1004–1010.

43. Hunt SA, Baker DW, Chin MH, et al. ACC/AHA guidelines for the evaluation and management of chronic heart failure in the adult: executive summary. *J Am Coll Cardiol* 2001;38:2101–2113.

44. Packer M, Coats AJS, Fowler MB, et al. Effect of carvedilol on survival in severe chronic heart failure. *N Engl J Med* 2001;344:1651–1658.

45. CIBIS Investigators and Committees. A randomized trial of beta-blockade in heart failure: the Cardiac Insufficiency Bisoprolol Study (CIBIS). *Circulation* 1994;90:1765–1773.

46. The SOLVD Investigators. Effect of enalaril on survival in patients with reduced left ventricular ejection fractions and congestive heart failure. *N Engl J Med* 1991;325:293–302.

47. The Acute Infarction Ramipril Efficacy (AIRE) Study Investigators. Effect of ramipril on mortality and morbidity of survivors of acute myocardial infarction with clinical evidence of heart failure. *Lancet* 1993;342:821–828.

48. Cohn JN, Tognoni G. A randomized trial of the angiotensin-receptor blocker valsartan in chronic heart failure. *N Engl J Med* 2001;345:1667–1675.

49. Pitt B, Zannad F, Remme WJ, et al. The effect of spironolactone on morbidity and mortality in patients with severe heart failure. *N Engl J Med* 1999;341:709–717.

50. Wright JT, Agodoa L, Contreras G, et al. Successful blood pressure control in the African American Study of Kidney Disease and Hypertension (AASK). *Arch Intern Med* 2002;162:1636–1643.

51. Bakris GL, Williams M, Dworkin L, et al. Preserving renal function in adults with hypertension and diabetes: a consensus approach. National Kidney Foundation Hypertension and Diabetes Executive Committee Working Group. *Am J Kidney Dis* 2000;36:646–661.

52. Bakris GL, Weir MR. Angiotensin-converting enzyme inhibitor-associated elevations in serum creatinine. *Arch Intern Med* 2000;160:685–693.

53. Douglas JG, Bakris GL, Epstein M, et al. Management of high blood pressure in African Americans: consensus statement of the Hypertension in African Americans Working Group of the Internatonal Society on Hypertension in Blacks. *Arch Intern Med* 2003;163:525–541.

54. Saunders E, Weir MR, Kong BW, et al. A comparison of the efficacy and safety of a beta-blocker, a calcium channel blocker, and a converting enzyme inhibitor in hypertensive blacks. *Arch Intern Med* 1990;150:1707–1713.

55. Materson BJ, Reda DJ, Williams D. Lessons from combination therapy in Veterans Affairs Studies. *Am J Hypertens* 1996;9:187S–191S.

56. Cushman WC, Ford CE, Cutler JA, et al. Success and predictors of blood pressure control in diverse North American settings: the

Antihypertensive and Lipid-Lowering Treatment to Prevent Heart Attack Trial (ALLHAT). *J Clin Hypertens* 2002;4:393–405.

57. Black HR, Elliott WJ, Neaton JD, et al. Baseline characteristics and early blood pressure control in the CONVINCE trial. *Hypertension* 2001;37:12–18.

58. SHEP Cooperative Research Group. Prevention of stroke by antihypertensive drug treatment in older persons with isolated systolic hypertension. Final results of the Systolic Hypertension in the Elderly Program (SHEP). *JAMA* 1991;265:3255–3264.

59. Staessen JA, Fagard R, Thijs L, et al. Randomised double-blind comparison of placebo and active treatment for older patients with isolated systolic hypertension (Syst-Eur). *Lancet* 1997;350:757–764.

60. National Cholesterol Education Program. Third report of the National Cholesterol Education Program (NCEP) Expert Panel on Detection, Evaluation, and Treatment of High Blood Cholesterol in Adults (Adult Treatment Panel III) final report. *Circulation* 2002;106:3143–3421.

61. Kjeldsen SE, Dahlof B, Devereux RB, et al. Effects of losartan on cardiovascular morbidity and mortality in patients with isolated systolic hypertension and left ventricular hypertrophy: a Losartan Intervention For Endpoint Reduction (LIFE) substudy. *JAMA* 2002;288:1491–1498.

62. Makin A, Lip GY, Silverman S, et al. Peripheral vascular disease and hypertension: a forgotten association? *J Hum Hypertens* 2001;15:447–454.

63. Creager MA, Dzau VJ. Vascular diseases of the extremities. In: Braunwald E, Fauci AS, Kasper DL, et al., eds., *Harrison's principles of internal medicine,* Vol. 1, 15th ed. New York: McGraw-Hill, 2001:1434–1442.

64. Burns P, Gough S, Bradbury AW. Management of peripheral arterial disease in primary care. *BMJ* 2003;326:584–588.

65. Writing Group for the Women's Health Initiative Investigators. Risks and benefits of estrogen plus progestin in healthy postmenopausal women. *JAMA* 2002;288:321–333.

66. National High Blood Pressure Education Program. Report of the National High Blood Pressure Education Program Working Group on High Blood Pressure in Pregnancy. *Am J Obstet Gynecol* 2000;183: S1–S22.

67. Ames RP. A comparison of blood lipid and blood pressure responses during the treatment of systemic hypertension with indapamide and with thiazides. *Am J Cardiol* 1996;77:12B–16B.

68. Betancourt JR, Carrillo JE, Green AR. Hypertension in multicultural and minority populations. *Curr Hypertens Rep* 1999;1:482–488.

69. VA Cooperative Study Group on Antihypertensive Agents. Effects of treatment on morbidity in hypertension. Results in patients with diastolic blood pressures averaging 115 through 129 mm Hg. *JAMA* 1967;202:1028–1034.

69a. Elliott WJ, Black HR. Benefits of treating hypertension - lessons from clinical trials. In: Oparil S, Weber MA eds. *Hypertension: a companion to Brenner & Rector's the kidney.* Philadelphia: WB Saunders Co., 2000:331–341.

70. Medical Research Council Working Party. MRC trial of treatment of mild hypertension: principal results. *BMJ* 1985;291:97–104.

71. Management Committee. The Australian therapeutic trial in mild hypertension. *Lancet* 1980;1:1261–1267.

72. Collins R, Peto R, MacMahon S, et al. Blood pressure, stroke, and coronary heart disease. Part 2, short-term reductions in blood pressure: overview of randomised drug trials in their epidemiological context. *Lancet* 1990;335:827–838.

73. Mulrow CD, Cornell JA, Herrera CR, et al. Hypertension in the elderly. Implications and generalizability of randomized trials. *JAMA* 1994;272:1932–1938.

74. Insua JT, Sacks HS, Lau TS, et al. Drug treatment of hypertension in the elderly: a meta-analysis. *Ann Intern Med* 1994;121:355–362.

75. Moser M, Hebert PR. Prevention of disease progression, left ventricular hypertrophy and congestive heart failure in hypertension treatment trials. *J Am Coll Cardiol* 1996;27:1214–1218.

76. Kostis JB, Davis BR, Cutler J, et al. Prevention of heart failure by antihypertensive drug treatment in older persons with isolated systolic hypertension. SHEP Cooperative Research Group. *JAMA* 1997;278:212–216.

77. Klag MJ, Whelton PK, Randall BL, et al. End-stage renal disease in African-Americans and white men. 16-year MRFIT findings. *JAMA* 1997;277:1293–1298.

78. Maschio G, Alberti D, Janin G, et al. Effect of the angiotensin-converting-enzyme inhibitor benazepril on the progression of chronic renal insufficiency. *N Engl J Med* 1996;334:939–945.

79. Klahr S, Levey AS, Beck GJ, et al. The effect of dietary protein restriction and blood-pressure control on the progression of chronic renal disease. *N Engl J Med* 1994;330:877–884.

80. Kannel WB, Gordon T, Schwartz MJ. Systolic versus diastolic blood pressure and risk of coronary heart disease. The Framingham Study. *Am J Cardiol* 1971;27:335–346.

81. Izzo JL, Levy D, Black HR. Importance of systolic blood pressure in older Americans. *Hypertension* 2000;35:1021–1024.

82. Forette F, Seux ML, Staessen JA et al. Prevention of dementia in randomised double-blind placebo-controlled Systolic Hypertension in Europe (Syst-Eur) trial. *Lancet* 1998;352:1347–1351.

83. Liu L, Wang JG, Gong L, et al. Comparison of active treatment and placebo in older Chinese patients with isolated systolic hypertension. Systolic Hypertension in China (Syst-China) Collaborative Group. *J Hypertens* 1998;16:1823–1829.

84. Conlin PR. Dietary modifications and changes in blood pressure. *Curr Opin Nephrol Hypertens* 2001;10:359–363.

85. Kotchen TA, McCarron DA. Dietary electrolytes and blood pressure: a statement for healthcare professionals from the American Heart Association Nutrition Committee. *Circulation* 1998;98:613–616.

86. Duffy SJ, Gokce N, Holbrook M, et al. Treatment of hypertension with ascorbic acid. *Lancet* 1999;354:2048–2049.

87. John JH, Ziebland S, Yudkin P, et al. Effects of fruit and vegetable consumption on plasma antioxidant concentrations and blood pressure: a randomised controlled trial. *Lancet* 2002;359:1968–1974.

88. Stamler J, Liu K, Ruth KJ, et al. Eight-year blood pressure change in middle-aged men: relationship to multiple nutrients. *Hypertension* 2002;39:1000–1006.

88a. Kaplan NM, Rose BD. Diet and hypertension. In: Rose BD ed. *UpToDate.* Wellesley MA, 2003.

89. Neaton JD, Grimm Jr RH, Prineas RJ, et al. Treatment of Mild Hypertension Study. Final results. Treatment of Mild Hypertension Study Research Group. *JAMA* 1993;270:713–724.

90. Stamler R, Stamler J, Gosch FC, et al. Primary prevention of hypertension by nutritional–hygienic means. Final report of a randomized, controlled trial. *JAMA* 1989;262:1801–1807.

91. The effects of nonpharmacologic interventions on blood pressure of persons with normal levels. Results of the Trials of Hypertension Prevention, Phase I. *JAMA* 1992;267:1213–1220.

92. Effects of weight loss and sodium reduction intervention on blood pressure and hypertension incidence in overweight people with high-normal blood pressure. The Trials of Hypertension Prevention, phase II. The Trials of Hypertension Prevention Collaborative Research Group. *Arch Intern Med* 1997;157:657–667.

93. Elliott P, Stamler J, Nichols R, et al. Intersalt revisited: further analyses of 24 hour sodium excretion and blood pressure within and across populations. Intersalt Cooperative Research Group. *BMJ* 1996;312:1249–1253.

94. He J, Whelton PK, Appel LJ, et al. Long-term effects of weight loss and dietary sodium reduction on the incidence of hypertension. *Hypertension* 2000;35:544–549.

95. Dyer AR, Elliott P, Shipley M, et al. Body mass index and associations of sodium and potassium with blood pressure in INTERSALT. *Hypertension* 1994;23:729–736.

96. Whelton PK, Appel LJ, Espeland MA, et al. Sodium reduction and weight loss in the treatment of hypertension in older persons: a randomized controlled trial of nonpharmacologic interventions in the elderly (TONE). *JAMA* 1998;279:839–846.

97. Hypertension Detection and Follow-up Program Cooperative Group. Five-year findings of the hypertension detection and follow-up program. II. Mortality by race, sex and age. Hypertension Detection and Follow-up Program Cooperative Group (HDFP). *JAMA* 1979;242: 2572–2577.

98. Wright JT, Bakris G, Greene T, et al. Effect of blood pressure lowering and antihypertensive drug class on progression of hypertensive kidney disease: results from AASK trial. *JAMA* 2002;288:2421–2431.

99. UK Prospective Diabetes Study Group. Tight blood pressure control and risk of macrovascular and microvascular complications in type 2 diabetes: UKPDS 38. *BMJ* 1998;317:703–713.

100. Hansson L, Zanchetti A, Carruthers SG, et al. Effects of intensive blood pressure lowering and low-dose aspirin in patients with hypertension: principal results of the Hypertension Optimal Treatment

(HOT) randomised trial. HOT Study Group. *Lancet* 1998;351:1755–1762.

100a. Moser MM. Guidelines & goals in the management of hypertension. *Medscape Cardiology* 7(1), 2003.

100b. McCulloch DK. Screening for and treatment of diabetic retinopathy. In: Rose BD ed. *UpToDate*. Wellesley MA, 2003.

101. Chaturvedi N, Sjolie AK, Stephenson JM, et al. Effect of lisinopril on progression of retinpathy in normotensive people with type 1 diabetes. The EUCLID Study Group. EURODIAB Controlled Trial of Lisinopril in Insulin-Dependent Diabetes Mellitus. *Lancet* 1998;351:28–31.

102. Volpert OV, Ward WF, Lingen MW, et al. Captopril inhibits angiogenesis and slows the growth of experimental tumors in rats. *J Clin Invest* 1996;98:671–679.

102a. Reeder GS, Kaplan NM. ACE inhibition or A-II receptor antagonism in patients at high risk for a cardiovascular event. In: Rose BD ed. *UpToDate*. Wellesley MA, 2003.

102b. Kaplan NM, Rose BD. Treatment of hypertension in diabetes mellitus-1. In: Rose BD ed. *UpToDate*. Wellesley MA, 2003.

103. Estacio RO, Jeffers BW, Hiatt WR, et al. The effect of nisoldipine as compared with enalapril on cardiovascular outcomes in patients with non-insulin-dependent diabetes and hypertension (ABCD). *N Engl J Med* 1998;338:645–652.

104. Tatti P, Pahor M, Byington RP, et al. Outcome results of the Fosinopril Versus Amlodipine Cardiovascular Events Randomized Trial (FACET) in patients with hypertension and NIDDM. *Diabetes Care* 1998;21:497–603.

105. Effects of ramipril on cardiovascular and microvascular outcomes in people with diabetes mellitus: results of the HOPE study and MICRO-HOPE substudy. Heart Outcomes Prevention Evaluation Study Investigators. *Lancet* 2000;355:253–259.

106. Dagenais GR, Yusuf S, Bourassa MG, et al. Effects of ramipril on coronary events in high-risk persons: results of the Heart Outcomes Prevention Evaluation Study. *Circulation* 2001;104:522–526.

106a. Rose BD, Bakris GL. Treatment of diabetic nephropathy-1. In: Rose BD ed. *UpToDate*. Wellesley MA, 2003.

107. Viberti G, Mogensen CE, Groop LC, et al. Effect of captopril on progression to clinical proteinuria in patients with insulin-dependent diabetes mellitus and microalbuminuria. European Microalbuminuria Captopril Study. *JAMA* 1994;271:275–279.

108. The Microalbuminuria Captopril Study Group. Captopril reduces the risk of nephropathy in IDDM patients with microalbuminuria. *Diabetologia* 1996;39:587–593.

109. Kasiske BL, Kalil RS, Ma JZ, et al. Effect of antihypertensive therapy on the kidney in patients with diabetes: a meta-regression analysis. *Ann Intern Med* 1993;118:129–138.

110. Parving HH, Hommel E, Jensen BR, et al. Long-term beneficial effect of ACE inhibition on diabetic nephropathy in normotensive type 1 diabetic patients. *Kidney Int* 2001;2001:228–234.

111. Hostetter TH. Prevention of end-stage renal disease due to type 2 diabetes. *N Engl J Med* 2001;345:910–912.

112. Moser M. Current recommendations for the treatment of hypertension: are they still valid? *J Hypertens* 2002;20 [Suppl 1]:S3–S10.

113. Hansson L, Hedner T, Lund-Johansen P, et al. Randomised trial of effects of calcium antagonist compared with diuretics and beta-blockers on cardiovascular morbidity and mortality in hypertension: the Nordic diltiazem (NORDIL) study. *Lancet* 2000;356:359–365.

114. Brown MJ, Palmer CR, Castaigne A, et al. Morbidity and mortality in patients randomised to double-blind treatment with a long-acting calcium-channel blocker or diuretic in the International Nifedipine GITS study: Intervention as a Goal in Hypertension Treatment (INSIGHT). *Lancet* 2000;356:366–372.

115. Zanchetti A, Rosei EA, Dal Palu C, et al. The Verapamil in Hypertension and Atherosclerosis Study (VHAS): results of long-term randomized treatment with either verapamil or chlorthalidone on carotid intima–media thickness. *J Hypertens* 1998;16:1667–1676.

CHAPTER 9

Obesity

An Epidemic

Ved V. Gossain

Key Points

- Obesity is defined as a condition in which an individual has excess body fat.
- By consensus, a body mass index of 25 to 29.9 kg per m^2 defines overweight and a body mass index of 30 kg per m^2 defines obesity.
- Sixty-four percent of the U.S. population is overweight and 30% is obese.
- The cost of obesity and related diseases is estimated to be 238 billion dollars (20% of U.S. health care cost).
- Obesity is associated with insulin resistance and increased risk for developing diabetes, hypertension, cardiovascular disorders, osteoarthritis, hepatobiliary diseases, and certain types of cancers.
- Obesity is a chronic illness, requiring long-term management.
- Treatment options include lifestyle changes (diet and exercise), pharmacology, and surgical treatment.
- Weight loss results in improvement in associated morbidities.
- Although no definite data are available showing that weight loss improves longevity, obese people should be motivated to lose weight.

DEFINITION

Obesity is defined as a condition in which an individual has an excess accumulation of body fat. Although several methods are available for estimating body fat, it is difficult to measure it accurately, and no method is readily available for routine clinical use. In young adults, normal levels of body fat are 12% to 20% of body weight for men and 20% to 30% of body weight for women. Body fat greater than 25% in men and greater than 33% in women has been considered an indication of obesity (1) (Table 9.1).

The most widely used clinical measure for obesity is the body mass index (BMI), which is calculated by the following formula:

$$BMI = \text{weight in kg}/(\text{height in meters})^2$$

By consensus, individuals with a BMI of 25 to 29.9 kg per m^2 are classified as overweight and individuals with a BMI of greater than 30 kg per m^2 are classified as obese (2,3).

PREVALENCE

The prevalence of obesity has been increasing worldwide in recent years (2). The prevalence of obesity increased from 12% in 1991 to 17.9% in 1998 in the United States (4). It further increased to 19.8% in 2000 and to 20.9% in 2001 (5). These estimates are based on self-reported height and weight data. However, based on the National Health and Nutrition Examination Survey (NHANES) data, the prevalence of obesity was 30.5% in 1999 to 2000 (6).

TABLE 9.1. *Criteria for obesity in men and women*

	Body fat %	
Category	Men	Women
Normal	12–20	20–30
Borderline	21–25	31–33
Obese	>25	>33

From Bray GA *Contemporary diagnosis and management of obesity*. Newtown, PA: Handbooks in Health Care, 1998: 9–34, with permission.

The prevalence of persons who were either overweight or obese (BMI greater than or equal to 25) was 55.9% in NHANES III, and increased to 64.5% in 1999–2000 (6).

Not only among adults, but also among children and adolescents the prevalence of obesity has been increasing in recent years. In 1999 to 2000, the prevalence of overweight was 15.5% among 12- to 19-year-olds, 15.3% among 6- to 11-year-olds, and 10.4% among 2- to 5-year-olds (7).

METHODS OF DETERMINING BODY FAT

Table 9.2 lists methods of determining body fat. Only those methods that are available for clinical use are briefly described. Underwater weighing has been the gold standard for measuring body fat, against which other methods are compared, but dual energy x-ray absorptiometery is rapidly becoming the method of choice because of its ease and availability. Both computed tomography scans and magnetic resonance imaging have been used to measure body fat and have

the added advantage that regional fat distribution can also be measured. Ultrasound can also be employed to measure total/regional body fat distributions, but is less often utilized. Bioelectric impedance based on the principle that electric impedance of adipose tissue is different than that of lean body mass is also an easy, readily available, and fairly accurate method of body fat determination. For details of methods employed in estimating body fat, the reader is referred to other reviews (8–11).

CLASSIFICATION OF OBESITY

The primary classification of overweight and obesity is based on assessment of BMI. This classification relates the BMI to the risk of disease. Increasing body weight is associated with an increased risk for mortality (12). Not only the total obesity, but also the regional distribution of fat, that is, increased abdominal obesity, is an independent risk factor for cardiovascular morbidity and mortality (2,3,13,14). Therefore, waist circumference measurements are also included in the assessment of obesity. Although waist circumference and BMI are interrelated, waist circumference provides an independent measure of risk and is particularly useful in individuals with BMI of 25 to 34.9 kg per m^2. A large waist circumference is associated with an increased risk for type 2 diabetes, dyslipidemia, hypertension, and cardiovascular disease (CVD) (14–16). In some populations (e.g., Asian Americans or persons of Asian descent), waist circumference is a better indicator of relative disease risk than BMI (17).

TABLE 9.2. *Methods of estimating body fat and its distribution*

Method	Cost[a]	Ease of use	Accuracy	Measures regional fat
Height and weight	$	Easy	High	No
Skin folds	$	Easy	Low	Yes
Circumferences	$	Easy	Moderate	Yes
Ultrasound	$$	Moderate	Moderate	Yes
Density				
Immersion	$	Moderate	High	No
Plethysmograph	$$$	Difficult	High	No
Heavy water				
Tritiated	$$	Moderate	High	No
Deuterium oxide or heavy oxygen	$$$	Moderate	High	No
Potassium isotope (^{40}K)	$$$$	Difficult	High	No
Total body electrical conductivity	$$$	Moderate	High	No
Bioelectric impedance	$$	Easy	High	No
Fat-soluable gas	$$	Difficult	High	No
Absorptiometry (dual-energy x-ray absorptiometry, dual-photon absorptiometry)	$$$	Easy	High	No
Computed tomography	$$$$	Difficult	High	Yes
Magnetic resonance imaging	$$$$	Difficult	High	Yes
Neutron activation	$$$$	Difficult	High	No

[a]$, Low cost; $$, moderate cost; $$$, high cost; $$$$, very high cost.
From Harsha DW, Bray GA. Body composition and childhood obesity. *Endocrinol Metab Clin North Am* 1996;25:871–885, with permission.

TABLE 9.3. *Classification of overweight and obesity by body mass index (BMI), waist circumference, and associated disease risk*

	BMI (kg/m^2)	Obesity class	Disease risk[a] (Relative normal weight and waist circumference)	
			Men ≤40 in. (≤102 cm), women ≤35 in. (≤88 cm)	Men >40 in. (>102 cm), women >35 in. (>88 cm)
Underweight	<18.5		—	—
Normal[b]	18.5–24.9		—	—
Overweight	25.0–29.9		Increased	High
Obesity	30.0–34.9	I	High	Very high
Obesity	35.0–39.9	II	Very high	Very high
Extreme obesity	≥40	III	Extremely high	Extremely high

[a]Disease risk for type 2 diabetes, hypertension, and cardiovascular disease.
[b]Increased waist circumference can also be a marker for increased risk even in persons of normal weight.
Adapted from World Health Organization. Obesity: *preventing and managing the global epidemic of obesity. Report of the World Health Organization Consultation on Obesity.* Geneva: Author, 1998, with permission.

The classification of obesity recommended by the World Health Organization and National Institute of Health is given in Table 9.3. A BMI chart, which should be available in every physician's office, is given in Fig. 9.1. It provides an easy measure of overweight/obesity. Although BMI correlates well with total body fat, there are ethnic variations (18,19). Deurenberg et al demonstrated that among Asians, for the same BMI their percentage body fat was 3% to 5% higher than that of whites (19). For these reasons, it has been recommended that lower cutoff limits for overweight (greater than or equal to 23.0 kg per m^2) and obesity (greater than or equal to 25.0 kg per m^2) be used for Asians (20).

ETIOLOGY OF OBESITY

The etiology of human obesity is multifactorial, and both nature (genetics) and nurture (environmental factors) play a role. The genetic predisposition to obesity was confirmed by

Overweight   Obese

BMI	19	20	21	22	23	24	25	26	27	28	29	30	31	32	33	34	35	36	37	38	39	40

WEIGHT (in pounds)

HEIGHT																						
4'10"	91	96	100	105	110	115	119	124	129	134	138	143	148	153	158	162	167	172	177	181	186	191
4'11"	94	99	104	109	114	119	124	128	133	138	143	148	153	158	163	168	173	178	183	188	193	198
5'	97	102	107	112	118	123	128	133	138	143	148	153	158	163	168	174	179	184	189	194	199	204
5'1"	100	106	111	116	122	127	132	137	143	148	153	158	164	169	174	180	185	190	195	201	206	211
5'2"	104	109	115	120	126	131	136	142	147	153	158	164	169	175	180	186	191	196	202	207	213	218
5'3"	107	113	118	124	130	135	141	146	152	158	163	169	175	180	186	191	197	203	208	214	220	225
5'4"	110	116	122	128	134	140	145	151	157	163	169	174	180	186	192	197	204	209	215	221	227	232
5'5"	114	120	126	132	138	144	150	156	162	168	174	180	185	192	198	204	210	216	222	228	234	240
5'6"	118	124	130	136	142	148	155	161	167	173	179	186	192	198	204	210	216	223	229	235	241	247
5'7"	121	127	134	140	146	153	159	166	172	178	185	191	198	204	211	217	223	230	236	242	249	255
5'8"	125	131	138	144	151	158	164	171	177	184	190	197	203	210	216	223	230	236	243	249	256	262
5'9"	128	135	142	149	155	162	169	176	182	189	196	203	209	216	223	230	236	243	250	257	263	270
5'10"	132	139	146	153	160	167	174	181	188	195	202	209	216	222	229	236	243	250	257	264	271	278
5'11"	136	143	150	157	165	172	179	186	193	200	208	215	222	229	236	243	250	257	265	272	279	286
6'	140	147	154	162	169	177	184	191	199	206	213	221	228	235	242	250	258	265	272	279	287	294
6'1"	144	151	159	166	174	182	189	197	204	212	219	227	235	242	250	257	265	272	280	288	295	302
6'2"	148	155	163	171	179	186	194	202	210	218	225	233	241	249	256	264	272	280	287	295	303	311
6'3"	152	160	168	176	184	192	200	208	216	224	232	240	248	256	264	272	279	287	295	303	311	319
6'4"	156	164	172	180	189	197	205	213	221	230	238	246	254	263	271	279	287	295	304	312	320	328

FIG. 9.1. Values of body mass index (kg per m^2).

the discovery of obese (*ob*) gene, which linked mutations of this gene to extreme obesity of *ob/ob* mice (21). In humans and animals, this gene codes for leptin. The gene has been identified and cloned (21). Leptin is secreted by the adipose tissue, acts on the central nervous system, and has profound effects on appetite and regulation of body fat (22,23). Leptin-deficient mice are hyperphagic, hyperinsulinemic, insulin resistant, and infertile. Leptin administration reverses all the features of this syndrome (22). The levels of leptin increase as the body fat increases (24). Obese individuals have very high levels, indicating that they are resistant to the action of leptin on food intake and energy expenditure. Therefore, although a deficiency of leptin may not be a common cause of obesity, extreme obesity due to leptin deficiency has been described in humans, which improves with administration of leptin (25,26).

To evaluate the genetic contribution to obesity, Stunkard et al. studied 93 pairs of identical twins reared apart or together (27). They observed that there was a correlation in the body mass index of twins reared apart (27). Additionally, identical twins respond similarly to long-term excess caloric intake (28). Although it is difficult to estimate accurately the genetic contribution to obesity, it has been estimated that it may range between 25% and 70% (29). The recent trend of increasing obesity in industrialized populations is almost certainly due to a tendency of increasingly sedentary lifestyle along with an increased energy intake.

HORMONAL ABNORMALITIES ASSOCIATED WITH OBESITY

There are a number of endocrine abnormalities seen in obesity. In general, these abnormalities are more common in central (visceral) obesity than peripheral obesity. With weight loss, many of these abnormalities revert toward normal, suggesting that they may be secondary to obesity. These abnormalities are summarized in Table 9.4.

Insulin resistance, defined as a subnormal response to a given concentration of insulin, is one of the most common abnormalities associated with obesity (30,31). Although insulin resistance is present in several tissues, this term is commonly used to define an impairment of insulin stimulated glucose disposal. Insulin resistance leads to a compensatory increase in insulin secretion (32,33). In nondiabetic subjects, increased insulin concentrations reflect insulin resistance, and in patients with type 2 diabetes, the fasting insulin level may be a reasonable surrogate for insulin resistance (34). The compensatory increase in insulin secretion can maintain the fasting plasma glucose levels in a normal range for years, but eventually the failure of beta cells leads to the development of diabetes mellitus in susceptible individuals (35).

The insulin resistance of obesity may result from a decrease in the number of insulin receptors, whereas both receptor and postreceptor defects are implicated in the pathogenesis of type 2 diabetes (36,37). Insulin resistance is associated not only with abnormalities of carbohydrate metabolism, but also with hypertension and dyslipidemia. The combination of insulin resistance, hypertension, and dyslipidemia was originally called Syndrome X by Reaven (33). It is now commonly referred to as the metabolic syndrome. Subsequently, other metabolic abnormalities have been associated with this syndrome, including obesity, microalbuminuria, and abnormalities of fibrinolysis and coagulation (38,39). Although the spectrum of metabolic syndrome appears to be ever expanding, for clinical purposes the National Cholesterol Education Program Expert Panel on Detection, Evaluation, and Treatment of High Cholesterol in Adults has defined the "metabolic syndrome" according to the criteria given in Table 9.5 (40). The World Health Organization uses a slightly different definition (41). The presence of metabolic syndrome

TABLE 9.4. *Hormonal abnormalities associated with obesity*[a]

		Ref.
Pancreas		
Insulin	Insulin resistance and hyperinsulinemia	30–34
	Metabolic syndrome	40,41
Glucagon	Normal or increased	44–46
Pituitary/gonadal axis		
Men	Low levels of testosterone	47,48
Women	Menarche at a younger age	49
	Total testosterone normal	50
	Sex hormone-binding globulin decreased	50
	Free testosterone increased	50
	Polycystic ovarian syndrome	51
Pituitary/adrenal axis	Increased cortisol secretion rate	52
	Normal circadian rhythm of cortisol	49
	Normal response to dexamethasone suppression	49
Pituitary/growth hormone axis	Decreased secretion of growth hormone	53,54
	Insulin-like growth factor 1 levels variable	55
Pituitary/thyroid axis	Normal	55

[a]Other reviews (49,52,55) may be consulted for more details.

TABLE 9.5. *Clinical identification of the metabolic syndrome*

Risk factor	Defining level
Abdominal obesity (waist circumference)[a]	
Men[b]	>102 cm (>40 in.)
Women	>88 cm (>35 in.)
Triglycerides	≥150 mg/dL
High-density lipoprotein cholesterol	
Men	<40 mg/dL
Women	<50 mg/dL
Blood pressure	≥130/≥85 mm Hg
Fasting glucose	≥110 mg/dL

[a]Overweight and obesity are associated with insulin resistance and the metabolic syndrome. However, the presence of abdominal obesity is more highly correlated with the metabolic risk factors than is an elevated body mass index. Therefore, the simple measure of waist circumference is recommended to identify the body weight component of the metabolic syndrome.

[b]Some male patients can develop multiple metabolic risk factors when the waist circumference is only marginally increased, e.g., 94–102 cm (37–40 in.). Such patients may have a strong genetic contribution to insulin resistance, and they should benefit from changes in life habits, similarly to men with categorical increases in waist circumference.

From Executive summary of the third report of the National Cholesterol Education Program (NCEP) Expert Panel on Detection, Evaluation, and Treatment of High Blood Cholesterol in Adults (Adult Treatment Panel III). *JAMA* 2001;285:2486–2497, with permission.

is associated with increased cardiovascular morbidity and mortality. The risk for coronary heart disease and stroke is increased threefold, and the cardiovascular mortality is two to three times higher in those with the metabolic syndrome than in those without it (42,43).

ADIPOSE TISSUE AS AN ENDOCRINE ORGAN

Traditionally, adipose tissue has been viewed as an organ of energy storage. However, adipose tissue is now known to produce several bioactive proteins including leptin, resistin, tumor necrosis factor-α (TNF-α), interleukin-6, and adiponectin (56,57). The exact role of these hormones is not well understood, but they could be important as part of the link between obesity and health complications, for example, insulin resistance and atherosclerosis (57,58).

LIPID ABNORMALITIES

Obesity is associated with various lipid abnormalities. Many patients with obesity, particularly those with central obesity, have metabolic syndrome and the accompanying lipid abnormalities, that is, high triglycerides, low high-density lipoprotein cholesterol (HDL-C) levels, and small, dense low-density lipoprotein (LDL) particles (40). According to NHANES III (1988 to 1994), the prevalence of high cholesterol and mean levels of cholesterol were higher in people with BMI of greater than 25 kg per m^2 than in people with a BMI of less than 25 kg per m^2, but did not consistently increase

with increasing BMI of greater than 25 kg per m^2. Mean levels of HDL-C were higher in women than in men, and they decreased with increasing BMI in both sexes. When dyslipidemia was defined as the ratio of total cholesterol to HDL-C of greater than or equal to 4.5, the prevalence of this condition increased with increasing BMI levels in both sexes and among all race/ethnic groups (59). Martins et al. (60) observed that the prevalence of dyslipidemia was 46% among overweight or obese women, but serum cholesterol concentrations were not significantly related to anthropometeric indexes. On the other hand, positive correlation between BMI and waist circumference with total cholesterol, triglycerides, and LDL-C in both sexes have been described by others (61).

Plasma free fatty acid levels are increased in obese subjects compared to nonobese individuals (62). It has been suggested that increased free fatty acid delivery to the liver leads to increased triglyceride synthesis and subsequently increased secretion of very low density lipoprotein (VLDL)-apolipoprotein B (apoB). Low HDL and the increase in small, dense LDL particles are the indirect consequences of elevated triglyceride-rich VLDL via increased cholesterol ester transfer protein and hepatic lipase activity (62) (see Chapter 12).

Increased levels of apoB (63–66) have been described in obesity. The effect of weight loss on apoB levels has been somewhat controversial. In our studies (66), apoB levels were reduced after weight loss, whereas Manzato et al. (63) did not observe a change in apoB levels with weight loss. It may be important to evaluate the apolipoprotein levels in obesity because some studies have suggested that apoproteins may be better predictors of coronary heart disease risk than levels of LDL and HDL cholesterol (67,68).

COST OF OBESITY

Obesity is associated with several other medical conditions, which increase morbidity and mortality. Obesity accounts for greater than 280,000 deaths annually in the United States and will soon overtake smoking as the primary preventable cause of death if the current trends continue (69). Using data from U.S. life tables and the NHANES I, NHANES II, NHANES III studies, Fontaine et al. estimated the years of life lost due to obesity (70). A J-shaped or U-shaped association between BMI and years of life lost was observed at all ages. The optimal BMI (i.e., BMI associated with the greatest longevity) for adults is 23 to 25 kg per m^2 for whites and 23 to 30 kg per m^2 for blacks. Figure 9.2 demonstrates the relationship between obesity and mortality.

The total cost attributable to obesity has been estimated to be 99.2 billion dollars (1995 dollars), of which 51.64 billion dollars is in direct medical costs (71). Gorsky et al. estimated that an estimated 16 billion dollars will be spent during the next 25 years in treating health outcomes associated with overweight among middle-aged women in the United States (72). According to more recent estimates, the cost of treating obesity-related diseases in the United States is $238 billion, or approximately 20% of the total U.S. health care bill (73).

Men

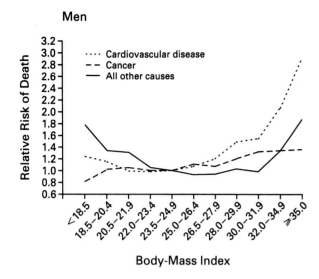

Women

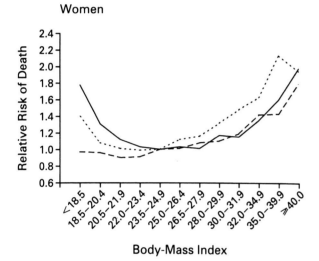

FIG. 9.2. Multivariate relative risk of death from cardiovascular disease, cancer, and all other causes among men and women who had never smoked and who had no history of disease at enrolment, according to body mass index. From Calle EE, Thun MJ, Petrelli JM, et al. Body-mass index and mortality in a prospective cohort of U.S. adults. *N Engl J med* 1999;341:1097–1105, with permission.

HEALTH RISKS OF OBESITY

Obesity affects every organ system in the body. The health consequences of clinically severe obesity are summarized in Table 9.6.

CARDIOVASCULAR SYSTEM

Hypertension

The prevalence of hypertension among the obese is increasing (59,74). According the NHANES III, the age-adjusted prevalence of hypertension (defined as blood pressure [BP] greater than or equal to 140/90 mm Hg or the need for antihypertensive medication) in obese men and women is 42% and 38%, respectively. These prevalence rates are more than

TABLE 9.6. *Health risks of obesity*

Cardiovascular system
  Hypertension
  Coronary artery disease
  Congestive heart failure
  Stroke
  Electrocardiographic changes
  C-reactive protein
  Endothelial dysfunction
Respiratory system
  Hypoventilation
  Sleep apnea
Endocrine and metabolic system
  Insulin resistance
  Diabetes mellitus
  Dyslipidemia
Gastrointestinal system
  Gallstones
  Nonalcoholic fatty liver disease
Musculoskeletal system
  Osteoarthritis
  Hyperuricemia/gout
  Carpal tunnel syndrome
Prothrombotic state
  Venous thrombosis/pulmonary embolism
  Poor wound healing
Cancer
  Increased risk of breast, endometrium, and ovary cancers
  Increased risk of prostate, colorectal, liver, and kidney cancers
Psychosocial
  Work disability
  Social discrimination
  Depression

twice the prevalence among nonobese individuals (15% for subjects with BMI of less than 25 kg per m^2) (59). The relationship of BMI and BP is linear (75,76). The exact cause(s) of obesity leading to hypertension are not clear, but may include increased sodium reabsorption by the kidney because of hyperinsulinemia and increased sympathetic tone (77,78).

Coronary Heart Disease

The risk of coronary artery disease among obese subjects is increased because of associated risk factors for cardiovascular disease such as hypertension, dyslipidemia, impaired glucose tolerance, or type 2 diabetes (79). Long-term studies have demonstrated that being overweight is also a predictor of CVD, independent of its effect on the traditional risk factors (80,81). In women 30 to 55 years of age, higher levels of body weight within the normal range and a modest weight gain after 18 years of age are associated with increased risk of coronary heart disease (82).

Congestive Heart Failure

The cellular metabolism of cations may be altered in obesity and may lead to changes in vascular responsiveness and increased vascular resistance. These changes can lead to structural adaptations, characterized by concentric–eccentric left ventricular hypertrophy. The hypertrophic condition provides the basis for the development of congestive heart failure and cardiac arrhythmias, which may explain the higher rates of sudden cardiac death in these patients. Congestive heart failure has also been documented as a common complication of morbid obesity, regardless of the presence of hypertension (83). However, in patients with advanced heart failure of multiple etiologies, obesity is not associated with increased mortality (84).

Stroke

The risk of fatal and nonfatal ischemic stroke is increased among obese compared to nonobese persons (85,86) and increases progressively with increasing BMI.

Electrocardiographic Changes

Prolonged QT interval on the electrocardiogram has been described in patients with obesity (87). In our studies, approximately 10% to 24% of patients had prolonged QT intervals (greater than 0.445). The alterations in the QT changes improved with weight loss (88). The prolongation of QT intervals was present even in those patients who were free of other cardiovascular risk factors. It is possible, therefore, that these electrocardiographic changes may be responsible for some sudden deaths in obese patients.

Obesity, Coronary Heart Disease, and Inflammation

The role of inflammation in the pathogenesis of atherosclerosis is now well recognized (89). Acute-phase C-reactive protein (CRP) is a sensitive marker for systemic inflammation. In a meta-analysis of seven prospective studies, elevated CRP concentration was shown to predict future risk of coronary heart disease (90). In a prospective study of 27,939 apparently healthy women who were followed for a mean of 8 years, CRP was a stronger predictor of cardiovascular events than LDL cholesterol (91). Higher BMI is associated with higher CRP concentrations, suggesting that a state of low-grade systemic inflammation exists in overweight and obese persons (92). It is now generally believed that injury to endothelium plays a critical role in the development of atherosclerosis (93). Obesity/insulin resistance is also associated with endothelial dysfunction (94), thus predisposing obese individuals to the development of atherosclerosis (see Chapter 2).

Endocrine System

Diabetes

The risk of developing diabetes (type 2) increases as the body weight increases. The prevalence of diabetes has increased in parallel with the increased prevalence of obesity. Based on the American Diabetes Association criteria, the prevalence of diabetes (diagnosed plus undiagnosed) in the total population of people who were 40 to 74 years of age increased from 8.9% in the period 1976 to 1980 to 12.3% by 1988 to 1994 (95). In 2000, the prevalence of obesity (BMI of greater than or equal to 30 kg per m^2) was 19.8% and the prevalence of self-reported diabetes was 7.3% (96). In 2001, the prevalence of obesity rose to 20.9% (an increase of 5.6%), and the prevalence of diabetes rose from 7.3% to 7.9% (an increase of 8.2%) (5). In the Nurse's Health Study, overweight and obesity was the single most important predictor of development of diabetes (97).

As previously mentioned, insulin resistance associated with obesity leads to a compensatory increase in insulin secretion; eventually the beta cells of pancreas are unable to compensate for the insulin resistance, resulting in the development of diabetes (32,33,35,36). Development of diabetes is associated with an increased risk for the development of macrovascular complications (98,99). Although diabetes mellitus is associated with other cardiovascular risk factors (hypertension, dyslipidemia, obesity), there is evidence that diabetes is an independent risk factor for CVD in both men and women (100–102). Women with diabetes seem to lose most of their inherent protection against development of CVD (100,103). The cardiovascular mortality in patients with diabetes is increased two- to fourfold (102–104), and the impact of diabetes on the risk of coronary death is significantly greater for women than men (105). The incidence of myocardial infarction in patients with diabetes, but without previous myocardial infarction, is 20% over 7 years, similar to that in nondiabetic patients with previous myocardial infarction (18.8%) (106). Nearly 80% of all patients die of CVD (107,108). For these reasons, it has been proposed that "Diabetes is a cardiovascular disease" (109). Although there is clear evidence that control of hyperglycemia reduces the risk of development of microvascular complications, the evidence for reduction of macrovascular complication is less strong (110). The risk of myocardial infarction in the United Kingdom Prospective Diabetes Study was reduced by 16% in the group with strict control of glycemia compared to the control group, but this difference was not statistically significant (110). However, when the relationship of hemoglobin A1c and myocardial infarction was further examined, each 1% reduction of hemoglobin A1c was associated with 21% reduction of risk of myocardial infarction (111).

Respiratory System

Other cardiopulmonary dysfunctions associated with obesity include sleep apnea syndrome, hypoventilation syndrome, pulmonary hypertension, and heart failure, which can occur alone or in combination (112). Obesity is a major correlate of sleep apnea in men and women, with those having a BMI of at least 30 kg per m^2 being at greatest risk (113,114). Because of increased weight on the chest, obesity results in decreased respiratory compliance, increased work of breathing, decreased total lung capacity, and limited ventilation of lung bases (114). The nocturnal disruption of sleep is associated with daytime somnolence, hypercapnia morning headaches, pulmonary hypertension, and eventually right heart failure (114–116).

Gastrointestinal System

Gallbladder Disease

The risk of developing gallstones increases linearly with increasing weight (117–119) The relative risk of developing symptomatic gallstones in obese individuals (BMI greater than 30 kg per m^2) is 3.7 compared to nonobese individuals (120).

Liver Disease

Obesity is associated with nonalcoholic fatty liver disease (NAFLD) (121). The spectrum of NAFLD is broad, ranging from steatosis and nonalcoholic hepatitis to cirrhosis and liver failure (121,122). NAFLD has been associated with the metabolic syndrome (123). It has been suggested that insulin resistance and NAFLD may result from increased levels of inflammatory cytokines including TNF-α (124).

Musculoskeletal System

Obesity is associated with an increased risk for osteoarthritis (125,126). Osteoarthritis of the knees and ankles may be directly related to trauma associated with degree of excess body weight (127), although dietary and metabolic factors have been implicated (126). Obesity has also been associated with increased risk for hyperuricemia, gout (128), and carpal tunnel syndrome (129).

Cancer

There is an increased risk of endometrium, ovary, breast, prostate, colorectal, liver, kidney, and gallbladder cancers (2,130,131). In the Nurses Health Study, increased BMI was associated with an increased risk of breast cancer in postmenopausal, but not in premenopausal, women (132). Increased body weight is also associated with increased death rates for all cancers combined and for cancers at multiple specific sites (133).

Other Health Conditions

Obesity is a prothrombotic state (134) and is also associated with an increased risk for venous insufficiency, deep vein thrombosis (135,136), and poor wound healing (137).

Psychosocial Functions

The relationship between obesity and psychosocial functioning is complex (138). Prior to the 1960s, it was believed that obesity was in part caused by certain psychological abnormalities, but that has not been established. It is also a common perception that obese individuals have a lower self-esteem compared to average people, but this perception may not be correct. An obese person's self-esteem may be affected by negative stereotypes. Obesity is often seen as a sign of laziness and lack of self-control. Obese individuals are often discriminated against with regard to employment, educational opportunities, and even treatment by health care professionals (138).

TREATMENT OF OBESITY

The principles of treatment of obesity are simple, but have been difficult to implement with success. At any one time, about 45% of women and 30% of men in the United States are actively seeking to lose weight, in most cases without success (139). Obesity should be approached as a chronic illness that requires long-term ongoing management. Prior to initiation of a therapeutic program for obese individuals, as in any other chronic illness, a thorough evaluation should be completed. It is recommended that this evaluation should include a thorough medical, behavioral, psychological, and psychiatric (binge eating disorder, bulimia, body image disturbance) history and history of previous attempts at weight loss and their results. The patient's readiness to undertake the weight loss program, and also the patient's expectation from the weight loss program, should be assessed (3,140). Physical exam should include height, weight (to calculate BMI), and blood pressure measurement with an appropriate sized cuff. An assessment of health risks associated with obesity (Table 9.6) should be completed and appropriate laboratory tests ordered. At a minimum, the laboratory tests should include a fasting plasma glucose and a lipid profile (total cholesterol, triglycerides, HDL and LDL cholesterol). Obtaining other laboratory tests will be dictated by presence of associated conditions such as coronary artery disease, gallbladder/liver disease, sleep apnea, and so on.

Available therapeutic options for treatment of obesity are as follows:

1. Lifestyle management, which includes (a) dietary therapy; (b) increased physical activity, and (c) behavior therapy.
2. Pharmacotherapy
3. Surgery.

Table 9.7 provides a guide to selecting these therapeutic options.

Goals of Therapy

Goals of therapy are to reduce body weight and maintain a lower body weight over the long term. An initial weight loss of 10% body weight achieved over a 6-month period is a recommended target (3).

Lifestyle Management

Patients beginning a weight loss program need to understand how body weight is regulated. Simplistically speaking,

TABLE 9.7. *A guide to selecting treatment for obesity*

Treatment	Body mass index category				
	25–26.9	27–29.9	30–34.9	35–39.9	≥40
Diet, physical activity, and behavior therapy	With comorbidities	With comorbidities	+	+	+
Pharmacotherapy		With comorbidities	+	+	+
Surgery			With comorbidities	With comorbidities	With comorbidities

From National Institutes of Health. *The practical guide. Identification, evaluation, and treatment of overweight and obesity in adults.* Bethesda, MD: Author, 2000, with permission.

weight gain or weight loss is a matter of energy balance. If the intake of energy (calories ingested) exceeds the energy utilized, weight gain will result, and weight loss will occur if the reverse is the case. A referral to a registered dietitian should be made for better understanding of the nutritional principles and development of an individualized meal plan. Many patients find it helpful to join a self-help group or enroll in a commercial weight loss program because they provide encouragement, accountability, and social support needed for success (140).

Dietary Therapy

Dietary therapy may consist of a low-calorie diet (LCD) or a very low calorie diet (VLCD). The National Heart, Lung, and Blood Institute guidelines recommend that the intake should be reduced by 500 to 1,000 Kcal per day (3). In general, diets containing 1,000 to 1,200 Kcal per day should be selected for most women. For men, a diet containing between 1,200 and 1,600 cal per day may be chosen and may also be more appropriate for women who weigh 165 lb or more. There is evidence that diets consisting of 1,000 to 1,500 cal per day induce about an 8% weight loss in 16 to 26 weeks (113). The conventional dietary approach to weight management recommended by leading research and medical societies is a high-carbohydrate, low-fat, and energy-deficient diet (3,141,142). A typical recommended weight-reduction diet consists of the following:

Calories: 1,000 to 1,500 per day
Carbohydrates: 55% to 65% of total calories
Fat: 20% to 30% of total calories
Protein: 15% to 20% of total calories
Cholesterol: less than 300 mg per day
Alcohol: limit to one drink per day for women and two drinks per day for men
Fiber content: 20 to 30 g per day

A review of the literature suggests that weight loss is independent of diet composition (143). Altering the macronutrient composition does not induce weight loss unless the calorie intake is also reduced. Low-carbohydrate diets have become increasingly popular and have been promoted by best-selling diet books (144,145). However, the safety and effectiveness of these diets have not been established (146). Two recent studies have demonstrated that low-carbohydrate diets produced a greater weight loss than did the conventional diets for the first 6 months (147,148). However, this difference was not maintained at 1 year, and weight loss was small relative to the excess weight carried by these obese individuals. In both studies, there was a significant dropout rate. More studies will be needed before this issue can be completely resolved.

Very Low Calorie Diets

VLCD are diets containing 800 calories or less per day. They have been utilized successfully in the treatment of obesity (66,88,149–151). These diets are generally prescribed to patients who are moderately to severely (60% to 90% overweight) obese and should be carried out under careful medical supervision. VLCD result in weight loss of 1.5 to 2 kg per week with a total loss of approximately 20 kg over 12 to 16 weeks (152). To preserve the lean body mass, protein content of the diet should be at least 1 g per kg of ideal body weight. It is important to emphasize that VLCD should be part of a comprehensive weight management program. Although VLCD have been shown to result in a greater weight loss compared to LCD, this advantage is not maintained in long-term studies (151–153).

Increasing Physical Activity

Increasing physical activity should be an integral part of every weight loss program. Increasing physical activity helps establish the negative energy balance required for weight loss. Exercise training even without weight loss improves insulin sensitivity (154). Increasing physical activity is also beneficial for its cardiovascular benefits (155,156). In a study by Leermakers et al., physically fit men had lower cardiovascular disease and all-cause mortality than unfit men with the same level of body fat (157). Physicians can play an important role in motivating patients to increase their physical activity (158). Obese patients should be advised to begin exercise slowly, and to increase the intensity of exercise slowly. Simple ways to increase physical activity such as parking farther away from place of work and/or taking stairs instead of elevators should be emphasized. Patients can start walking 10 minutes three times a week and increase gradually to 30 to 45 minutes of intense walking at least three times a week and increase to most if not all days (3,159,160). In addition to being an adjunct for weight loss, sustained physical activity is very helpful in the prevention of weight regain (113,157).

Behavior Therapy

The goal of behavior therapy is to help obese patients identify and modify habits that contribute to their excess weight (161). Behavioral approaches attempt to identify and disconnect the triggers that lead to overeating. Behavioral treatment usually includes multiple components such as self-monitoring (keeping a journal of food intake and physical activity, weighing foods), stimulus control (e.g., not eating in front of the TV, not eating in the car, using smaller plates), social support, and cognitive restructuring (161,162). Data from the National Weight Control Registry suggest that the strategies for successful weight maintainers (average weight loss 30 kg for an average of 5.5 years) include eating a diet low in fat, frequently self-monitoring body weight and food intake, and engaging in high levels of regular physical activity (163).

Pharmacotherapy

Pharmacologic therapy for weight loss should be considered for individuals with a BMI of 30 kg per m² and for those who have a BMI of 27 to 29.9 kg per m² and also have obesity-related risk factors or diseases. Drug therapy should be given as part of a comprehensive weight management program, which includes dietary, physical exercise, and behavior therapy (164). Although many drugs may contribute to weight loss, only a few are available for clinical use.

Drugs available for use in the treatment of obesity can be classified as centrally acting or peripherally acting anorexiants; they have recently been reviewed (165) (Table 9.8).

Anorexiants act centrally in the hypothalamus and thereby promote satiety. Sibutramine functions as a serotonin and norepinephrine reuptake inhibitor, whereas the other anorexiants act by either stimulating norepinephrine release or blocking its reuptake. In the last few years, three anorexiants were withdrawn from the market—fenfluramine and dexfenfluramine, due to their cardiac effects, and phenylpropanolamine, for increased risk of hemorrhagic stroke associated with its use (166,167).

Both sibutramine and orlistat have been found to be more effective than placebo in randomized controlled trials of up to 2 years duration (168,169). Only these two drugs are currently approved for long-term use in the treatment of obesity.

Surgical Treatment of Obesity

Gastrointestinal surgery is the most effective way to achieve major weight loss in severely obese individuals. This type of surgery is indicated for subjects with a BMI of 40 kg per m²

TABLE 9.8. *Weight loss drugs*

Generic name	Trade names	Mechanism of action	Dosage	Contraindications
Benzphetamine	Didrex	Noradrenergic	25–50 mg 1–3 times/d	Hypertension, advanced cardiovascular disease, hyperthyroidism, glaucoma, agitated states, history of drug abuse
Phendimetrazine	Bontril, Plegine, Prelu-2, X-Trozine	Noradrenergic	17.5–70 mg 2–3 times/d, or 105 mg sustained-release/d	Same as benzphetamine
Phentermine	Adipex-P, Fastin, Oby-Cap, others	Noradrenergic	18.75–37.5 mg/d	Same as benzphetamine
Phentermine resin	Ionamin	Noradrenergic	15–30 mg/d	Same as benzphetamine
Diethylpropion	Tenuate, Dospan, Tepanil	Noradrenergic	25 mg 3 times/d or 75 mg sustained-release/d	Same as benzphetamine
Sibutramine	Meridia	Mixed noradrenergic and serotonergic	5–15 mg/d	Uncontrolled hypertension, severe renal impairment, severe hepatic dysfunction, narrow-angle glaucoma, or history of substance abuse, coronary artery disease, congestive heart failure, arrhythmias, or stroke
Orlistat	Xenical	Lipase inhibitor	120 mg 3 times/d with or within 1 h after fat-containing meals, plus a daily multivitamin	Chronic malabsorption syndromes, cholestasis

Adapted from Yanovski SZ, Yanovski JA. Drug therapy—obesity. *N Engl J Med* 2002;346:591–602, with permission.

or a BMI of 35 kg per m^2 with comorbidities and who have not responded to the other therapeutic modalities (3,170). For best results, patients need to be carefully selected by a multidisciplinary team, operated on by experienced surgeons, and remain under lifelong medical surveillance after surgery. Successful weight loss surgery can lead to sustained weight loss for more than five years in most patients. Several surgical procedures have been performed to induce weight loss (171).

Gastroplasty or gastric restriction procedures involve creating a small upper part or pouch (approximately 30 mL in volume) that communicates with the remainder of the stomach through a narrow channel. This can be done by surgical stapling devices (stomach stapling). The currently accepted gastroplasty of choice is the vertical band (or ring) gastroplasty. The newest gastric restrictive procedure is gastroplasty by adjustable gastric banding (171,172). The complications associated with gastroplasty include staple line disruption, stomal stenosis, and gastroesophageal reflux (56).

Gastric bypass, also known as Roux-en-Y gastric bypass, consists of an operation in which the proximal small gastric pouch (approximately 10 mL in volume) is anastamosed to a segment of jejunum, bypassing most of the stomach. Gastric bypass appears to be a more effective procedure than gastroplasty in inducing and maintaining weight loss (173,174).

Partial biliopancreatic bypass involves a partial gastrectomy and bypass of a considerable portion of small intestine from biliary and pancreatic secretions (175). A modification of this procedure, partial biliopancreatic bypass with a duodenal switch, results in an equal amount of weight loss, but with fewer side effects (176). Both procedures induce malabsorption of protein, fat, fat-soluble vitamins, iron, calcium, and vitamin B12 (56,171,177). Jejunoileal bypass, in which a major portion of small intestine is bypassed, is of historical interest only. Originally introduced in 1969 (178), the procedure is no longer performed because of associated side effects (171).

BENEFITS OF INTENTIONAL WEIGHT LOSS

Although there are no long-term convincing data that intentional weight loss reduces the mortality associated with obesity, intentional weight loss improves many of the medical conditions associated with obesity. A 10% reduction in body weight reduces disease risk factors (3).

Effect on Morbidity

It is now well documented that intentional weight loss over the short term is accompanied by reduction of risk factors associated with obesity (137,180,181).

Insulin Resistance and Diabetes

Successful weight loss improves insulin sensitivity and reduces the risk of development of diabetes. The greatest improvement in insulin sensitivity occurs in those who are insulin resistant at baseline. McLaughlin et al. (181) demonstrated that a short-term weight loss of approximately 10% was associated with improvements in insulin sensitivity in individuals who were insulin resistant at baseline, but not in those who were insulin sensitive.

In a recent analysis, a Swedish study of obese subjects randomized to either obesity surgery or conventional obesity treatment found that at 2 years an average weight loss of 28 kg was accompanied by reduced incidence of diabetes and hypertension (182). Data from the Finnish diabetes prevention study suggests that lifestyle modification (i.e., change in diet and increased physical activity) that produced modest weight loss reduces the risk of type 2 diabetes (183). These findings were recently confirmed by the data from the Diabetes Prevention Program, where a weight loss of 7% was associated with a 58% reduction in progression to diabetes in patients with impaired glucose tolerance (184). In obese type 2 diabetes patients, both dietary restriction and weight loss are associated with improved insulin action and glycemic control (185,186).

Hypertension

Reduction in blood pressure with weight loss has also been reported by many studies (187–190). A 6% reduction in the risk of coronary heart disease and a 15% reduction in risk of stroke and transient ischemic attacks has been reported with as little as a 2-mm Hg reduction in diastolic blood pressure (191).

Lipids

The effects of weight loss on lipids are complex and inconsistent (192). Acute weight loss has been reported to reduce total cholesterol, LDL cholesterol, and triglyceride concentration (190,193–195). The changes in HDL cholesterol are more variable (194,195). Wadden et al. (194) observed that HDL cholesterol declined significantly at 8 weeks, but returned to baseline by week 24. No significant change in HDL cholesterol was observed in the European trial (195), whereas a small but nonsignificant fall was noted by Krebs et al. (190).

Modest weight loss may reduce the entire cluster of risk factors. In the Framingham Heart Study, a weight gain of 2.25 kg (5 lb) over 16 years was associated with an increased risk factor sum in men and women. A 2.25-kg (5-lb) weight loss was associated with a 48% decrease in risk factor sum in men and a 40% decrease in women. Clusters of three or more risk factors were associated with a 2.39 and a 5.9 times greater risk of coronary heart disease in men and women, respectively (196).

Pulmonary Disease

Weight loss results in improvement in sleep apnea, improved sleep pattern, and decreased daytime somnolence (197).

More marked weight loss with bariatric surgery is accompanied by improvements in resting room air arterial blood gases, lung volumes, and cardiac filling pressure (198). We have demonstrated an increase in lung volumes and modest improvement in maximum aerobic capacity in patients who lost an average of 23 kg with VLCD treatment (199).

Despite these short-term benefits, the evidence that intentional weight loss improves long-term health status as measured by disability, morbidity, longevity, and quality of life is limited. There is a need to understand the long-term health effects of intentional weight loss, which may be provided by a well-designed randomized controlled trial (200).

Effect on Mortality

Although it is well known that obesity is associated with increased mortality (12), there is no convincing evidence that intentional weight loss in obese persons reduces mortality. As a matter of fact, conflicting opinions regarding the relationship of weight loss and mortality have been expressed (201,202). A detailed discussion of the relationship of obesity and mortality is provided by Sorensen and Yang et al. (201,202). On the whole, epidemiologic studies, even after adjusting for confounding factors (i.e., intentional vs. unintentional weight loss excluding unhealthy subjects), indicate that intentional weight loss appears to neither increase nor decrease mortality rate. Yang et al. (202) concluded (and we agree) that it seems more likely than not that intentional weight loss achieved by medically recommended methods does not increase and probably decreases mortality rate. Therefore, despite the limited success of long-term weight reduction programs, it seems worthwhile to motivate overweight people to attempt a modest weight loss because it reduces cardiovascular risk factors and may reduce mortality over the long term.

SUMMARY AND CONCLUSION

Obesity is defined as a condition in which individuals have excess body fat. By consensus, a BMI of 25 kg per m^2 is defined as overweight, and a BMI of 30 kg per m^2 as obese. Prevalence of obesity has been increasing in recent years and has reached epidemic proportions. Obesity, particularly central obesity, is associated with insulin resistance, type 2 diabetes, dyslipidemia, hypertension, osteoarthritis, gallbladder disease, increased tendency toward thrombosis, and certain types of cancers. These associated diseases increase obesity-related morbidity and mortality. Obesity should be approached as a chronic illness requiring long-term medical management. The therapeutic principles include lifestyle modification, that is, decreased caloric intake, increased physical activity, and behavior therapy. Patients with severe obesity, particularly those with comorbidities, may also require pharmacologic or surgical therapy. Over the short term, weight loss is achieved with these approaches, but maintenance of lower weight over a prolonged period is difficult. Short-term studies indicate

that intentional weight loss is accompanied by reduction in cardiovascular disease and other benefits. However, long-term data on the benefits of intentional weight loss are limited. There are no definitive data to indicate whether intentional weight loss is associated with an increase or a decrease in the mortality rate. Despite the limited data, it is recommended that overweight and obese people should be motivated to lose weight. Weight loss is associated with lowering of cardiovascular risk factors over the short term and may reduce mortality over the long term.

REFERENCES

1. Bray GA. *Contemporary diagnosis and management of obesity.* Newtown, PA: Handbooks in Health Care, 1998:9–34.
2. World Health Organization. *Obesity: preventing and managing the global epidemic of obesity. Report of the WHO Consultation on Obesity.* Geneva: Author, 1998.
3. National Institutes of Health. *The practical guide. Identification, evaluation; and treatment of overweight and obesity in adults.* Bethesda, MD: Author, 2000.
4. Mokdad AH, Serdula MK, Dietz WH, et al. The spread of the obesity epidemic in the United States, 1991–1998. *JAMA* 1999;282:1519–1522.
5. Mokdad AH, Ford ES, Bowman BA, et al. Prevalence of obesity, diabetes, and obesity-related health risk factors, 2001. *JAMA* 2003;289:76–79.
6. Flegal KM, Carroll MD, Ogden CL, et al. Prevalence and trends in obesity among US adults, 1999–2000. *JAMA* 2002;288:1723–1727.
7. Ogden CL, Flegal KM, Caroll MD, et al. Prevalence and trends in overweight among US children and adolescents, 1999–2000. *JAMA* 2002;288:1728–1732.
8. Harsha DW, Bray GA. Body composition and childhood obesity. *Endocrinol Metab Clin North Am* 1996;25:871–885.
9. Brodie DA. Techniques of measurement of body composition. Part I. *Sports Med* 1988;5:11–40.
10. Brodie DA. Techniques of measurement of body composition. Part II. *Sports Med* 1988;5:74–98.
11. Goodpaster BH. Measuring body fat content in humans. *Curr Opin Clin Nutr Metab Care* 2002;5:481–487.
12. Calle EE, Thun MJ, Petrelli JM, et al. Body mass index and mortality in a prospective cohort of US adults. *N Engl J Med* 1999;341:1097–1105.
13. Lapidus L, Bengtsson C, Larsson B, et al. Distribution of adipose tissue and risk of cardiovascular disease and death: a 12 year follow up of participants in the population study of women in Gothenburg, Sweden. *Br Med J* 1984;289:1257–1261.
14. Despres JP, Moorjani S, Lupien PJ, et al. Regional distribution of body fat, plasma lipoproteins and cardiovascular disease. *Arteriosclerosis* 1990;10:497–511.
15. Chan JM, Rimm EB, Colditz GA, et al. Obesity, fat distribution, and weight gain as risk factors for clinical diabetes in men. *Diabetes Care* 1994;17:961–969.
16. Depres JP. Health consequences of visceral obesity. *Ann Med* 2001;33:534–541.
17. Fujimoto WY, Newell-Morris LL, Grote M, et al. Visceral fat obesity and morbidity: NIDDM and atherogenic risk in Japanese American men and women. *Int J Obes* 1991;15[Suppl 2]:41–44.
18. Deurenberg-Yap M, Schmidt G, Staveren WA, et al. The paradox of low body mass index and high body fat percentage among Chinese, Malays and Indians in Singapore. *Int J Obes Relat Metab Disord* 2000;24:1011–1017.
19. Deurenberg P, Deurenberg-Yap M, Guricci S. Asians are different from Caucasians and from each other in their body mass index/body fat percent relationship. *Obes Rev* 2002;3:141–146.
20. Regional Office for the Western Pacific, World Health Organization, the International Association for the Study of Obesity, and the International Obesity Task Force. *The Asia–Pacific perspective: redefining obesity and its treatment.* Sydney, Australia: Health Communications Australia, 2000.

21. Zhang YY, Proenca R, Maffei M, et al. Positional cloning of the mouse gene and its human homologue. *Nature* 1994;372:425–432.
22. Bray GA, York DA. Clinical review 90: Leptin and clinical medicine: a new piece in the puzzle of obesity. *J Clin Endocrinol Metab* 1997;82:2771–2776.
23. Rosenbaum M, Nicolson M, Hirsch J, et al. Effects of gender, body composition, and menopause on plasma concentrations of leptin. *J Clin Endocrinol Metab* 1996;81:3424–3427.
24. Rosenbaum M, Nicolson M, Hirsch J, et al. Effects of weight change on plasma leptin concentration and energy expenditure. *J Clin Endocrinol Metab* 1997;82:3647–3654.
25. Montague CT, Farooqi IS, Whitehead JP, et al. Congenital leptin deficiency is associated with severe early-onset obesity in humans. *Nature* 1997;387:903–908.
26. Farooqi IS, Jebb SA, Langmack G, et al. Effects of recombinant leptin therapy in a child with congenital leptin deficiency. *N Engl J Med* 1999;341:879–884.
27. Stunkard AJ, Harris JR, Pedersen NL, et al. The body-mass index of twins who have been reared apart. *N Engl J Med* 1990;322:1483–1487.
28. Bouchard C, Tremblay A, Despres JP, et al. The response to long-term overfeeding in identical twins. *N Engl J Med* 1990;322:1477–1482.
29. Hill JO, Wyatt HR, Melanson EL. Genetic and environmental contributions to obesity. *Med Clin North Am* 2000;84:333–346.
30. Moller DE, Flier JS. Insulin resistance—mechanisms, syndromes, and implications. *N Engl J Med* 1991;325:938–948.
31. Campbell PJ, Gerich JE. Impact of obesity on insulin action in volunteers with normal glucose tolerance: demonstration of a threshold for the adverse effects of obesity. *J Clin Endocrinol Metab* 1990;70:1114–1118.
32. Reaven GM, Hollenbeck CB, Chen YD. Relationship between glucose tolerance, insulin secretion, and insulin action in non-obese individuals with varying degrees of glucose tolerance. *Diabetologia* 1989;32:52–55.
33. Reaven GM. Banting Lecture 1988. Role of insulin resistance in human disease. *Diabetes* 1988;37:1595–1607.
34. Laasko M. How good a marker is insulin level for insulin resistance? *Am J Epidemiol* 1993;137:959–965.
35. Kruszynska Y, Olefsky JM. Cellular and molecular mechanism of non-insulin dependent diabetes mellitus. *J Invest Med* 1996;44:413–428.
36. Olefsky JM. Insulin resistance and insulin action in obesity and noninsulin-dependent (type II) diabetes mellitus. In: Brodoff BN, Bleicher SJ, eds. *Diabetes mellitus and obesity.* Baltimore: Williams & Wilkins, 1982:250–260.
37. Olefsky JM. The insulin receptor: its role in insulin resistance in obesity and diabetes. *Diabetes* 1976;25:1154–1162.
38. Bjorntorp P. Abdominal obesity and the metabolic syndrome. *Ann Med* 1992;24:465–468.
39. Groop L. Ekstrand A, Forsblom C, et al. Insulin resistance, hypertension, and microalbuminuria in patients with type 2 (non-insulin-dependent) diabetes mellitus. *Diabetologia* 1993;36:642–647.
40. Executive summary of the third report of the National Cholesterol Education Program (NCEP) Expert Panel on Detection, Evaluation, and Treatment of High Blood Cholesterol in Adults (Adult Treatment Panel III). *JAMA* 2001;285:2486–2497.
41. Alberti KG, Zimmett PZ. Definition, diagnosis and classification of diabetes mellitus and its complications. Part 1: diagnosis and classification of diabetes mellitus provisional report of a WHO consultation. *Diabetes Med* 1998;15:539–553.
42. Isomaa B, Almgren P, Tuomi T, et al. Cardiovascular morbidity and mortality associated with the metabolic syndrome. *Diabetes Care* 2001;24:683–689.
43. Lakka HM, Laaksonen DE, Lakka TA, et al. The metabolic syndrome and total cardiovascular disease mortality in middle-aged men. *JAMA* 2002;288:2709–2716.
44. Gossain VV, Srivastava L, Rovner DR et al. Plasma glucagon in simple obesity: effect of exercise. *Am J Med Sci* 1983;286:4–10.
45. Kalkhoff RK, Gossain VV, Matute ML. Plasma glucagon in obesity. Response to arginine, glucose and protein administration. *N Engl J Med* 1973;289:465–467.
46. Hill P, Garbaczewski L, Koppeschaar H, et al. Glucagon and insulin response to meals in non-obese and obese Dutch women. *Clin Chim Acta* 1987;165:253–261.
47. Strain GW, Zumoff B, Kream J. Mild hypogonadotropic hypogonadism in obese men. *Metabolism* 1982;31:871–875.
48. Barrett-Connor E, Khaw KT. Endogenous sex hormones and cardiovascular disease in men. A prospective population-based study. *Circulation* 1988;78:539–545.
49. Bray GA. Obesity: an endocrine perspective. In DeGroot L., ed. *Endocrinology.* Philadelphia: WB Saunders, 1989:2303–2337.
50. Zumoff B. Hormonal abnormalities in obesity. *Acta Med Scand Suppl* 1988;723:153–160.
51. Franks S. Polycystic ovary syndrome. *N Engl J Med* 1995;333:853–861.
52. Bjorntorp P. Endocrine abnormalities in obesity. *Diabetes Rev* 1997;5:52–68.
53. Strobl JS, Thomas MJ. Human growth hormone. *Pharmacol Rev* 1994;46:1–34.
54. Weltman A, Weltman JY, Hartman ML, et al. Relationship between age, percentage body fat, fitness, and 24-hour growth hormone release in healthy young adults: effects of gender. *J Clin Endocrinol Metab* 1994;78:543–548.
55. Smith SR. The endocrinology of obesity. *Endocrinol Metab Clin North Am* 1996;25:921–942.
56. Klein S, Romijn JA. Obesity. In Larsen PR, Kronenberg HM, Melmed S, et al., eds. *Williams textbook of endocrinology.* Philadelphia: WB Saunders, 2003:1619–1641.
57. Arner P. The adipocyte in insulin resistance: key molecules and the impact of thiazolidinediones. *Trends Endocrinol Metab* 2003;14:137–145.
58. Bruun JM, Lihn AS, Verdich C, et al. Regulation of adiponectin by adipose tissue-derived cytokines: *in vivo* and *in vitro* investigations in humans. *Am J Physiol Endocrinol Metab* 2003;285:E527–E533.
59. Brown CD, Higgins M, Donato KA, et al. Body mass index and the prevalence of hypertension and dyslipidemia. *Obes Res* 2000;8:605–619.
60. Martins JM, Carreiras F, Falcao J, et al. Dyslipidaemia in female overweight and obese patients. Relation to anthropometric and endocrine factors. *Int J Obes Relat Metab Disord* 1998;22:164–170.
61. Njelekela MA, Negishi H, Nara T, et al. Obesity and lipid profiles in middle aged men and women in Tanzania. *East Afr Med J* 2002;79:58–64.
62. Sheehan MT, Jensen MD. Metabolic complications of obesity. Pathophysiologic considerations. *Med Clin North Am* 2000;84:363–385.
63. Manzato E, Zambon S, Zambon A, et al. Lipoprotein sub-fraction levels and composition in obese subjects before and after gastroplasty. *Int J Obes Relat Metab Disord* 1992;16:573–578.
64. Marsh JB, Welty FK, Lichtenstein AH, et al. Apolipoprotein B metabolism in humans: studies with stable isotope-labeled precursors. *Atherosclerosis* 2002;162:227–244.
65. Chan DC, Watts GF, Redgrave TG, et al. Apolipoprotein B-100 kinetics in visceral obesity: associations with plasma apolipoprotein C-III concentration. *Metabolism* 2002;51:1041–1046.
66. Gossain VV, Gunaga KP, Carella MJ, et al. Apolipoproteins in obesity. *J Med* 1997;28:251–263.
67. Walldius G, Jungner I, Holme I, et al. High apoprotein B, low apolipoprotein A-I, and improvement in the prediction of fatal myocardial infarction (AMORIS study): a prospective study. *Lancet* 2001;358:2026–2033.
68. Talmud PJ, Hawe E, Miller GJ, et al. Nonfasting apolipoprotein B and triglyceride levels as a useful predictor of coronary heart disease risk in middle-aged UK men. *Arterioscler Thromb Vasc Biol* 2002;22:1918–1923.
69. Allison DB, Fontaine KR, Manson JE, et al. Annual deaths attributable to obesity in the United States. *JAMA* 1999;282:1530–1538.
70. Fontaine KR, Redden DT, Wang C, et al. Years of life lost due to obesity. *JAMA* 2003;289:187–193.
71. Wolf AM, Colditz GA. Current estimates of the economic cost of obesity in the United States. *Obes Res* 1998;6:97–106.
72. Gorsky RD, Pamuk E, Williamson DF, et al. The 25-year health care costs of women who remain overweight after 40 years of age. *Am J Prev Med* 1996;12:388–394.
73. Rubin R. Treating obese patients accounts for one-fifth of nation's health care costs. Accessed April 2003 from http://my.webmd.com/content/article/1728.50064
74. Must A, Spadano J, Coakley EH, et al. The disease burden associated with overweight and obesity. *JAMA* 1999;282:1523–1529.
75. Hubert HB, Feinleib M, McNamara PM, et al. Obesity as an independent risk factor for cardiovascular disease: a 26-year follow-up of

participants in the Framingham Heart Study. *Circulation* 1983;67:968–977.

76. Stamler R, Stamler J, Riedlinger WF, et al. Weight and blood pressure. Findings in hypertension screening of 1 million Americans. *JAMA* 1978;240:1607–1610.

77. Sechi LA, Bartoli E. Mechanisms of insulin resistance leading to hypertension: what can we learn from experimental models. *J Invest Med* 1997;45:238–251.

78. Reaven GM, Hoffman BB. Role for insulin in the aetiology and course of hypertension? *Lancet* 1987;2:435–437.

79. Eckel RH. Obesity and heart disease:a statement for healthcare professionals from the Nutrition Committee, American Heart Association. *Circulation* 1997;96:3248–3250.

80. Manson JE, Willett WC, Stampfler MJ, et al. Body weight and mortality among women. *N Engl J Med* 1995;333:677–685.

81. Garrison RJ, Castelli WP. Weight and thirty-year mortality of men in the Framingham Study. *Ann Intern Med* 1985;103:1006–1009.

82. Willett WC, Manson JE, Stampfer MJ, et al. Weight, weight change and coronary heart disease in women. Risk within 'normal' weight range. *JAMA* 1995;273:461–465.

83. Zhang R, Reisin E. Obesity-hypertension: the effects on cardiovascular and renal systems. *Am J Hypertens* 2000;13:1308–1314.

84. Horwich TB, Fonarow GC, Hamilton MA, et al. The relationship between obesity and mortality in patients with heart failure. *J Am Coll Cardiol* 2001;38:789–795.

85. Walker SP, Rimm EB, Ascherio A, et al. Body size and fat distribution as predictors of stroke among US men. *Am J Epidemiol* 1996;144:1143–1150.

86. Rexrode KM, Hennekens CH, Willett WC, et al. A prospective study of body mass index, weight change, and risk of stroke in women. *JAMA* 1997;277:1539–1545.

87. Frank S, Colliver JA, Frank A. The electrocardiogram in obesity: statistical analysis of 1,029 patients. *J Am Coll Cardiol* 1986;7;295–299.

88. Carella MJ, Mantz SL, Rovner DR, et. al. Obesity, adiposity, and lengthening of the QT interval: improvement after weight loss. *Int J Obes Relat Metab Disord* 1996;20:938–942.

89. Ross R. Atherosclerosis—an inflammatory disease. *N Engl J Med* 1999;340:115–126.

90. Danesh J, Collins R, Appleby P, et al. Association of fibrinogen, C-reactive protein, albumin or leukocyte count with coronary heart disease. *JAMA* 1998;279:1477–1482.

91. Ridker PM, Rifai N, Rose L, et al. Comparison of C-reactive protein and low-density lipoprotein cholesterol levels in the prediction of first cardiovascular events. *N Engl J Med* 1998;347:1557–1565.

92. Visser M, Bouter LM, McQuillan GM, et al. Elevated C-reactive protein levels in overweight and obese adults. *JAMA* 1999;282:2131–2135.

93. Quyyumi AA. Endothelial function in health and disease: new insights into the genesis of cardiovascular disease. *Am J Med* 1998;105:S32–S39.

94. Steinberg HO, Chaker H, Leaming R, et al. Obesity/insulin resistance is associated with endothelial dysfunction. Implications for the syndrome of insulin resistance. *J Clin Invest* 1996;97:2601–2610.

95. Harris MI, Flegal KM, Cowie CC, et al. Prevalence of diabetes, impaired fasting glucose, and impaired glucose tolerance in U.S. adults. The Third National Health and Nutrition Examination Survey, 1988–1994. *Diabetes Care* 1998;21:518–524.

96. Mokdad AH, Bowman BA, Ford ES, et. al. The continuing epidemics of obesity and diabetes in the United States. *JAMA* 2001;286:1195–1200.

97. Hu FB, Manson JE, Stampfer MJ, et al. Diet, lifestyle, and the risk of type 2 diabetes mellitus in women. *N Engl J Med* 2001;345:790–797.

98. Harris MI. Classification, diagnostic criteria, and screening for diabetes. In: Harris MI, Cowie CC, Stern MP, et al., eds. *Diabetes in America*, 2nd ed. Bethesda, MD: National Institutes of Health, 1995:15–32.

99. Kannel WB, McGee DL. Diabetes and cardiovascular disease. The Framingham Study. *JAMA* 1979;241:2035–2038.

100. Wilson PW, D'Agostino RB, Levy D, et al. Prediction of coronary heart disease using risk factor categories. *Circulation* 1998;97:1837–1847.

101. Wilson PW. Diabetes mellitus and coronary heart disease. *Am J Kidney Dis* 1998;32[5 Suppl 3]:S89–S100.

102. American Diabetes Association. Consensus development conference on the diagnosis of coronary heart disease in people with diabetes. *Diabetes Care* 1998;21:1551–1559.

103. Wingard DL, Barrett-Connor E. Heart disease and diabetes. In: Harris

MI, Cowie CC, Stern MP, et al., eds. *Diabetes in America*, 2nd ed. Bethesda MD: National Institute of Health, 1995:429–448.

104. Stamler J, Vaccaro O, Neaton JD, et. al. Diabetes, other risk factors, and 12-yr cardiovascular mortality of men screened in the Multiple Risk Factor Intervention Trial. *Diabetes Care* 1993;16:434–444.

105. Lee WL, Cheung AM, Cape D, et al. Impact of diabetes on coronary artery disease in women. *Diabetes Care* 2000;23:962–968.

106. Haffner SM, Lehto S, Ronnemaa T, et. al. Mortality from coronary heart disease in subjects with type 2 diabetes and in nondiabetic subjects with and without prior myocardial infarction. *N Engl J Med* 1998;339:229–234.

107. O'Keefe JH, Miles JM, Harris WH, et al. Improving the adverse cardiovascular prognosis of type 2 diabetes. *Mayo Clin Proc* 1999;74:171–180.

108. American Diabetes Association. Role of cardiovascular risk factors in prevention and treatment of macrovascular disease in diabetes. *Diabetes Care* 1993;16[Suppl 2]:72–78.

109. Grundy SM, Benjamin IJ, Burke GL, et. al. Diabetes and cardiovascular disease: a statement for healthcare professionals from the American Heart Association. *Circulation* 1999;100:1134–1146.

110. UK Prospective Diabetes Study Group (UKPDS). Intensive blood-glucose control with sulphonylureas or insulin compared with conventional treatment and risk of complications in patients with type 2 diabetes (UKPDS 33). *Lancet* 1998;352:837–852.

111. Stratton IM, Adler AI, Neil AW, et al. Association of glycaemic with macrovascular and microvascular complications of type 2 diabetes (UKPDS 35): prospective observational study. *BMJ* 2000;321:405–412.

112. Lopata M, Onal E. Mass loading, sleep apnea, and the pathogenesis of obesity hypoventilation. *Am Rev Respir Dis* 1982;126:640–645.

113. National Institutes of Health. *Clinical guidelines on the identification, evaluation, and treatment of overweight and obesity in adults—the evidence report*. Bethesda, MD: Author, 1998.

114. Strohl KP, Strobel RJ, Parisi RA. Obesity and pulmonary function. In: Bray GA, Bouchard C, James WPT, eds. *Handbook of obesity*. New York: Marcell Dekker, 1998:725–739.

115. Vgontzas AN, Tan TL, Bixler EO, et al. Sleep apnea and sleep disruption in obese patients. *Arch Intern Med* 1994;154:1705–1711.

116. Strollo Jr PJ, Rogers RM. Obstructive sleep apnea. *N Engl J Med* 1996;334:99–104.

117. Maclure KM, Hayes KC, Colditz GA, et al. Weight, diet, and risk of symptomatic gallstones in middle-aged women. *N Engl J Med* 1989;321:563–569.

118. Stampfer MJ, Maclure KM, Colditz GA. Risk of symptomatic gallstones in women with severe obesity. *Am J Clin Nutr* 1992;55:652–658.

119. Field AE, Coakley EH, Must A, et al. Impact of overweight on the risk of developing common chronic diseases during a 10-year period. *Arch Intern Med* 2001;161:1581–1586.

120. Nakeeb A, Comuzzie AG, Martin L, et al. Gallstones: genetics versus environment. *Ann Surg* 2002;235:842–849.

121. Scheen AJ, Luyckx FH. Obesity and liver disease. *Best Pract Res Clin Gastroenterol* 2002;16:703–716.

122. McCullough AJ. Update on nonalcoholic fatty liver disease. *J Clin Gastroenterol* 2002;34:255–262.

123. Marchesini G, Bugianesi E, Forlani G, et al. Nonalcoholic fatty liver, steatohepatitis, and the metabolic syndrome. *Hepatology* 2003;37:917–923.

124. Li Z, Clark J, Diehl AM. The liver in obesity and type 2 diabetes mellitus. *Clin Liver Dis* 2002;6:867–877.

125. Hochberg MC, Lethbridge-Cejku M, Scott Jr WW, et al. The association of body weight, body fatness and body fat distribution with osteoarthritis of the knee: data from the Baltimore Longitudinal Study of Aging. *J Rheumatol* 1995;22:488–493.

126. Felson DT. Does excess weight cause osteoarthritis and, if so, why? *Ann Rheum Dis* 1996;55:668–670.

127. Felson DT, Anderson JJ, Naimark A, et al. Obesity and knee osteoarthritis. The Framingham Study. *Ann Intern Med* 1988;109:18–24.

128. Roubenoff R, Klag MJ, Mead LA, et al. Incidence and risk factors for gout in white men. *JAMA* 1991;266:3004–3007.

129. Werner RA, Albers JW, Franzblau A, et al. The relationship between body mass index and the diagnosis of carpal tunnel syndrome. *Muscle Nerve* 1994;17:632–637.

130. Carroll KK. Obesity as a risk factors for certain types of cancer. *Lipids* 1998;33:1055–1059.
131. Bergstrom A, Pisani P, Tenet V, et al. Overweight as an avoidable cause of cancer in Europe. *Int J Cancer* 2001;91:421–430.
132. Huang Z, Hankinson SE, Colditz GA, et al. Dual effects of weight and weight gain on breast cancer risk. *JAMA* 1997;278:1407–1411.
133. Calle EE, Rodriguez C, Walker-Thurmond K, et al. Overweight, obesity, and mortality from cancer in a prospectively studied cohort of U.S. adults. *N Engl J Med* 2003;348:1625–1638.
134. Grundy SM. Metabolic complications of obesity. *Endocrine* 2000;13:155–165.
135. Scott TE, LaMorte WW, Gorin DR, et al. Risk factors for chronic venous insufficiency: a dual case–control study. *J Vasc Surg* 1995;22:622–628.
136. Persson AV, Davis RJ, Villavicencio JL. Deep venous thrombosis and pulmonary embolism. *Surg Clin North Am* 1991;71:1195–1199.
137. National Task Force on the Prevention and Treatment of Obesity. Overweight, obesity, and health risk. *Arch Intern Med* 2000;160:898–904.
138. Allison DB, Saunders SE. Obesity in North America. An overview. *Med Clin North Am* 2000;84:305–332.
139. Serdula MK, Mokdad AH, Williamson DF, et al. Prevalence of attempting weight loss and strategies for controlling weight. *JAMA* 1999;282:1353–1358.
140. Kushner RF, Weinsier RL. Evaluation of the obese patient. Practical considerations. *Med Clin North Am* 2000;84:387–399.
141. Position of the American Dietetic Association: weight management. *J Am Diet Assoc* 1997;97:71–74.
142. Kraus RM, Deckelbaum RJ, Ernst N, et al. Dietary guidelines for healthy American adults: a statement for health professionals from the Nutrition Committee, American Heart Association. *Circulation* 1996;94:1795–1800.
143. Kennedy ET, Bowman SA, Spence JT, et al. Popular diets: correlation to healthy, nutrition and obesity. *J Am Diet Assoc* 2001;101:411–420.
144. Eades MR, Eades MD. *Protein power.* New York: Bantam, 1999.
145. Atkins RC. *Dr. Atkins' new diet revolution,* rev. ed. New York: Avon, 1998.
146. Freedman MR, King J, Kennedy E. Popular diets: A scientific review. *Obes Res* 2001;9[Suppl 1]:1S–40S.
147. Samaha FF, Iqbal N, Seshadri P, et al. A low-carbohydrate as compared with a low-fat diet in severe obesity. *N Engl J Med* 2003;348:2074–2081.
148. Foster GD, Wyatt HR, Hill JO. A randomised trial of low-carbohydrate diet for obesity. *N Engl J Med* 2003;348:2082–2090.
149. Wing RR, Marcus MD, Salata R, et al. Effects of a very-low-calorie diet on long-term glycemic control in obese type 2 diabetic subjects. *Arch Intern Med* 1991;151:1334–1340.
150. Wadden TA, Stunkard AJ, Brownell KD. Very low calorie diets: Their efficacy, safety, and future. *Ann Intern Med* 1983;99:675–684.
151. Togerson JS, Lissner L, Lindroos AK, et al. VLCD plus dietary and behavioral support versus support alone in the treatment of severe obesity. A randomised two-year clinical trial. *Int J Obes Relat Metab Disord* 1997;21:987–994.
152. National Task Force on the Prevention and Treatment of Obesity. Very low-calorie diets. *JAMA* 1993;270:967–974.
153. Wadden TA, Foster GD, Letizia KA. One-year behavioral treatment of obesity: comparison of moderate and severe caloric restriction and the effects of weight maintenance therapy. *J Consult Clin Psychol* 1994;62:165–171.
154. Duncan GE, Perri MG, Theriaque DW, et al. Exercise training, without weight loss, increases insulin sensitivity and postheparin plasma lipase activity in previously sedentary adults. *Diabetes Care* 2003;26:557–562.
155. Morris JN, Clayton DG, Everitt MG, et al. Exercise in leisure time: coronary attack and death rates. *Br Heart J* 1990;63:325–334.
156. Lee CD, Blair SN, Jackson AS. Cardiorespiratory fitness, body composition, and all-cause and cardiovascular disease mortality in men. *Am J Clin Nutr* 1999;69:373–380.
157. Leermakers EA, Dunn AL, Blair SN. Exercise management of obesity. *Med Clin North Am* 2000;84:419–440.
158. Calfas KJ, Long BJ, Sallis JF, et al. A controlled trial of physician counseling to promote the adoption of physical activity. *Prev Med* 1996;25:225–233.
159. NIH consensus development panel on physical activity and cardio-

vascular health. Physical activity and cardiovascular health. *JAMA* 1996;276:241–246.
160. Pate RR, Pratt M, Blair SN, et al. Physical activity and public health. A recommendation from the Centers for Disease Control and Prevention and the American College of Sports Medicine. *JAMA* 1995;273:402–407.
161. Wadden TA, Foster GD. Behavioral treatment of obesity. *Med Clin North Am* 2000;84:441–461.
162. Kushner RF. Medical management of obesity. *Semin Gastrointestinal Dis* 2002;13:123–132.
163. Wing RR, Hill JO. Successful weight loss maintenance. *Annu Rev Nutr* 2001;21:323–241.
164. Wadden TA, Berkowitz RI, Sarwer DB, et al. Benefits of lifestyle modification in the pharmacologic treatment of obesity. *Arch Int Med* 2001;161:218–227.
165. Yanovski SZ, Yanovski JA. Drug therapy—obesity. *N Engl J Med* 2002;346:591–602.
166. Khan MA, Herzog CA, St. Peter JV, et al. The prevalence of cardiac valvular insufficiency assessed by transthoracic echocardiography in obese patients treated with appetite-suppressant drugs. *N Engl J Med* 1998;339:713–718.
167. Kernan WN, Viscoli CM, Brass LM, et al. Phenylpropanolamine and the risk of hemorrhagic stroke. *N Engl J Med* 2000;343:1826–1832.
168. James WP, Astrup A, Finer N, et al. Effect of sibutramine on weight maintenance after weight loss: a randomized trial. STORM Study Group. Sibutramine Trial of Obesity Reduction and Maintenance. *Lancet* 2000;356:2119–2125.
169. Davidson MH, Hauptman J, DiGirolamo M, et al. Weight control and risk factor reduction in obese subjects treated for 2 years with orlistat: a randomized controlled trial. *JAMA* 1999;281:235–242; Erratum, *JAMA* 1999;281:1174.
170. Gastrointestinal surgery for severe obesity: National Institutes of Health Consensus Development Conference Statement. *Am J Clin Nutr* 1992;55:615s–619s.
171. Balsiger BM, Murr MM, Poggio JL, et al. Bariatric surgery. Surgery for weight control in patients with morbid obesity. *Med Clin North Am* 2000;84:477–489.
172. O'Brien PE, Brown WA, Smith A, et al. Prospective study of a laparoscopically placed, adjustable gastric band in the treatment of morbid obesity. *Br J Surg* 1999;86:113–118.
173. MacLean LD, Rhode BM, Sampalis J, et al. Results of the surgical treatment of obesity. *Am J Surg* 1993;165:155–162.
174. Howard L, Malone M, Michalek A, et al. Gastric bypass and vertical banded gastroplasty—a prospective randomized comparison and 5-year follow-up. *Obes Surg* 1995;5:55–60.
175. Scopinaro N, Gianetta E, Adami GF, et al. Biliopancreatic diversion for obesity at eighteen years. *Surgery* 1996;119:261–268.
176. Marceau P, Hould FS, Simard S, et al. Biliopancreatic diversion with duodenal switch. *World J Surg* 1998;22:947–954.
177. Murr MM, Balsiger BM, Kennedy FP, et al. Malabsorptive procedures for severe obesity: comparison of pancreaticobiliary bypass and very very long limb Roux-en-Y gastric bypass. *J Gastrointest Surg* 1999;3:607–612.
178. Payne JH, Dewind LT. Surgical treatment of obesity. *Am J Surg* 1969;118:141–147.
179. Vidal J. Updated review on the benefits of weight loss. *Int J Obes Relat Metab Disord* 2002;26 [Suppl 4]:S25–S28.
180. Van Gaal LF, Wauters MA, De Leeuw IH. The beneficial effects of modest weight loss on cardiovascular risk factors. *Int J Obes Relat Metab Disord* 1997;21[Suppl 1]:S5–S9.
181. McLaughlin T, Abbasi F, Kim HS, et al. Relationship between insulin resistance, weight loss, and coronary heart disease risk in healthy, obese women. *Metabolism* 2001;50:795–800.
182. Torgerson JS, Sjostrom L. The Swedish Obese Subjects (SOS) study: rationale and results. *Int J Obes Relat Metab Disord* 2001;25:S2–S4.
183. Tuomilehto J, Lindstrom J, Eriksson JG, et al. Prevention of type 2 diabetes mellitus by changes in lifestyle among subjects with impaired glucose tolerance. *N Engl J Med* 2001;344:1343–1350.
184. Diabetes Prevention Program Research Group. Reduction in the incidence of type 2 diabetes with lifestyle intervention or metformin. *N Engl J Med* 2002;346:393–403.
185. Wing RR, Koeske R, Espstein LH, et al. Long-term effects of modest weight loss in type II diabetic patients. *Arch Intern Med* 1987;147:1749–1753.

186. Markovic TP, Jenkins AB, Campbell LV, et al. The determinants of glycemic responses to diet restriction and weight loss in obesity and NIDDM. *Diabetes Care* 1998;21:687–694.

187. Stevens VJ, Obarzanek E, Cook NR, et al. Long-term weight loss and changes in blood pressure: results of the Trials of Hypertension Prevention, phase II. *Ann Intern Med* 2001;134:1–11.

188. The Trials of Hypertension Prevention, phase II. The Trials of Hypertension Prevention Collaborative Research Group. Effects of weight loss and sodium reduction intervention on blood pressure and hypertension incidence in overweight people with high-normal blood pressure. *Arch Intern Med* 1997;157:657–667.

189. Whelton PK, Appel LJ, Espeland MA, et al. Sodium reduction and weight loss in the treatment of hypertension in older persons: a randomised controlled trial of nonpharmacologic interventions in the elderly (TONE). *JAMA* 1998;279:839–846.

190. Krebs JD, Evans S, Cooney L, et al. Changes in risk factors for cardiovascular disease with body fat loss in obese women. *Diabetes Obes Metab* 2002;4:379–387.

191. Cook NR, Cohen J, Hebert PR, et al. Implications of small reductions in diastolic blood pressure for primary prevention. *Arch Intern Med* 1995;155:701–709.

192. Eckel RH. The importance of timing and acute interpretation of the benefits of weight reduction on plasma lipids [Editorial]. *Obes Res* 1999;7:227–228.

193. Ditschuneit HH, Flechtner-Mors M, Johnson TD, et al. Metabolic and weight-loss effects of a long-term dietary intervention in obese patients. *Am J Clin Nutr* 1999;69:198–204.

194. Wadden TA, Anderson DA, Foster GD. Two year changes in lipids and lipoproteins associated with the maintenance of a 5% to 10% reduction in initial weight. Some findings and some questions. *Obes Res* 1999;7:170–178.

195. Sjostrom L, Rissanen A, Andersen T, et al. Randomised placebo-controlled trial of orlistat for weight loss and prevention of weight regain in obese patients. European Multicentre Orlistat Study Group. *Lancet* 1998;352:167–172.

196. Wilson PW, Kannel WB, Silbershatz H, et al. Clustering of metabolic factors and coronary heart disease. *Arch Intern Med* 1999:159:1104–1109.

197. Smith PL, Gold AR, Meyers DA, et al. Weight loss in mildly to moderately obese patients with obstructive sleep apnea. *Ann Intern Med* 1985;103:850–855.

198. Sugerman HJ, Baron PL, Fairman RP et al. Hemodynamic dysfunction in obesity hypoventilation syndrome and the effects of treatment with surgically induced weight loss. *Ann Surg* 1988;207:604–613.

199. Carella MJ, Blonshine C, Mohan G, et al. Improvement in pulmonary and exercise performance in obese patients after weight loss. *Respir Care* 1999;44:1458–1464.

200. Yanovski SZ, Bain RP, Williamson DF. Report of a National Institutes of Health–Centers for Disease Control and Prevention workshop on the feasibility of conducting a randomized clinical trial to estimate the long-term health effects of intentional weight loss in obese persons. *Am J Clin Nutr* 1999;69:366–372.

201. Sorensen TIA. Weight loss causes increased mortality: pros. *Obes Rev* 2003;4:3–7.

202. Yang D, Fontaine KR, Wang C, et al. Weight loss causes increased mortality: cons. *Obes Rev* 2003;4:9–16.

CHAPTER 10

Peripheral Neuropathy

Cardiovascular Implications

Martin J. Stevens

Key Points

- Diabetic peripheral neuropathy comprises three distinct syndromes, peripheral somatic polyneuropathy, focal neuropathy, and autonomic neuropathy, which frequently overlap.
- Diabetic peripheral neuropathy can affect greater than 50% of diabetic patients.
- Damage to the peripheral autonomic nerves may be a prerequisite for the development of foot ulceration.
- Cardiovascular denervation can result in abnormal exercise-induced cardiovascular performance, orthostatic hypotension, cardiac denervation syndrome, and peripheral autonomic denervation.
- Positron emission tomography using sympathetic neurotransmitter analogues has shown that sympathetic denervation of the heart begins in the distal inferolateral walls and spreads proximally and circumferentially.
- Cardiac sympathetic hyperinnervation and denervation supersensitivity may predispose to life-threatening arhythmogenesis.

In diabetes, several distinct syndromes can affect the peripheral nervous system. The classic "glove-and-stocking" diabetic polyneuropathy (DPN), which represents the most frequently diagnosed neuropathy in the Western world (1–3), results from damage to sensory and motor nerves in a distal-to-proximal pattern. A number of other manifestations of diabetic neuropathy are less commonly seen, but can be equally disabling. For example, nerve roots and the lumbosacral plexus are also targets of diabetes-mediated injury leading to diabetic polyradiculopathy, also known as diabetic amotrophy (4) (Table 10.1). Diabetes can also impair cranial nerve function, particularly cranial nerves III and IV, as well as multiple individual peripheral nerves, such as the median, ulnar, and peroneal, leading to the syndrome of diabetic mononeuritis multiplex (4). Additionally, diabetes can have profound effects on the autonomic nervous system, leading to diabetic autonomic neuropathy (DAN) (4–6), which may

result in a broad spectrum of clinical manifestations, from impaired peripheral sweating to sudden cardiac death. This chapter focuses on the two most common manifestations of neuropathy, DPN and DAN, particularly with regard to the cardiovascular consequences of these syndromes. The pathogenesis, diagnosis, epidemiology, and treatment of DPN and DAN are discussed.

DIABETIC POLYNEUROPATHY AND DIABETIC AUTONOMIC NEUROPATHY: PATHOGENESIS

The contribution of hyperglycemia to the pathogenesis of microvascular complications including diabetic neuropathy both in type 1 diabetes (7) and most recently in type 2 diabetes (8) is now beyond dispute. However, the mechanisms contributing to glucose toxicity appear complex and multifactorial. The most commonly invoked metabolic defects

TABLE 10.1. *Diabetes mellitus: peripheral nervous system manifestations*

Mononeuropathy or mononeuritis multiplex
  Cranial or peripheral nerve lesions (e.g., cranial nerves III and IV, ulnar, median, femoral, or peroneal nerves)
Radiculopathy, polyradiculopathy, or plexopathy
  Thoracic/lumbosacral
  Diabetic amyotrophy
Autonomic neuropathy
  Cardiac denervation syndromes
  Peripheral autonomic denervation
  Other (gastrointestinal/genitorurinary, etc.)
Sensorimotor polyneuropathy
  Diffuse
  Painful

include activation of the polyol or sorbitol pathway, accelerated advanced glycosylated end (AGE) product formation, and increased oxidative damage (9,10). These metabolic defects may directly damage specific critical cellular components of complication-prone tissue or they may contribute to end-organ dysfunction and damage indirectly through functional and/or structural defects involving the extracellular matrix or microvasculature. Alternatively, metabolic defects could induce systemic or localized blood flow abnormalities or defects in vasoactive or growth-promoting agents that in turn alter target-organ structure and/or function. Recently, increased oxidative stress has emerged as the leading candidate responsible for the development of diabetic microvascular complications, a concept that is supported by both clinical (10–12) and preclinical (9,13) studies. Oxidative stress can be regarded as a balancing act, which depends both on systemic oxidative stress buffering capacity and reactive oxygen species (ROS) generation (Fig. 10.1). For example, oxidative

stress buffering capacity, when measured as total radical-trapping antioxidant parameter (TRAP), is reduced in type 1 (11) and type 2 diabetes (14), which, when coupled with diabetes-induced increased ROS production, results in tissue-damaging oxidative stress. This can be measured clinically as elevated levels of plasma protein carbonyls (15) and increased urine 8-epi prostaglandin F2as (12). In experimental animal models of diabetes, evidence of increased oxidative stress and impaired antioxidant defense enzymes occur in complication-prone tissues of diabetes, including the nerve (13,16). Support for a central role of oxidative stress in the development of diabetic neuropathy has been provided by the demonstration that potent antioxidants are able to prevent or correct many functional and metabolic defects in diabetic rodents. For example, antioxidants can correct nerve blood flow (9,16) and nerve functional deficits (9,13,16) in diabetic rodents.

Although there have been fewer studies exploring the pathogenesis of DAN mechanistically, many of the same pathological pathways implicated in DPN are thought to contribute to DAN (17). Risk factors for the development of DAN include age, glycemic control, duration of diabetes, hypertension, hyperinsulinemia, and hyperlipidema (18) and the presence of microvascular and macrovascular complications. Autoimmunity has also been implicated in the development of DAN complicating type 1 diabetes. A weak correlation has been found between the presence of autoantibodies against the sympathetic nervous system and scintigraphically detected deficits of cardiac sympathetic innervation in type 1 diabetics (19). Complement-fixing autoantibodies to the vagus, sympathetic ganglia, and adrenal medulla have been identified in up to 30% of type 1 diabetic patients (20). However, the relationship of autoimmunity to DAN remains controversial because antibodies against autonomic nervous system antigens have been inconsistently found in diabetes and may be associated with coincidental autoimmunity against other organs (21). In general, autonomic ganglia autoantibodies appear to be common in type 1 diabetes, but their role in the pathogenesis of DAN is uncertain (22).

Diabetic Polyneuropathy: Epidemiology

Diabetic peripheral neuropathy commonly complicates diabetes and may be present in up to half of all diabetic patients, and the prevalence rates rise in concert with age. The reported prevalence of diabetic neuropathy varies, however, which reflects differences in terminology, diagnostic criteria, and study populations. In a frequently quoted landmark study, Pirart reported an overall 12% prevalence rate of diabetic neuropathy in patients newly diagnosed with diabetes (23). In this study, the incidence of neuropathy increased with the duration of diabetes, and, after 25 years of diabetes, affected over 50% of diabetic patients. More recently, similar results were obtained in cross-sectional multicenter studies of type 1 and 2 diabetic patients. For example, in a study of over 6,000 diabetic patients in the United Kingdom, assessment using ankle reflexes, vibration perception thresholds, pin prick, and temperature sensation together with a nine-point symptom score

Oxidative Stress
F2 Isoprostanes
C-reactive Protein

Antioxidant Capacity
  TRAP

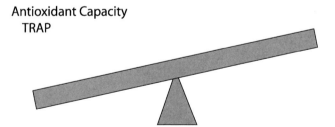

FIG. 10.1. *The oxidative stress balance in diabetes.* Oxidative stress can be regarded as a balancing act, which depends both on systemic oxidative stress buffering capacity and reactive oxygen species (ROS) generation. In diabetes, reduced oxidative stress buffering capacity, which can be measured as total radical-trapping antioxidant parameter (TRAP), decreases the neutralization of ROS, resulting in tissue-damaging oxidative stress. In turn, increased oxidative stress can lead to a number of downstream consequences, including elevations of C-reactive protein.

identified neuropathy in 5% of patients aged between 20 and 29 years old and in 44% in patients in the eighth decade (24). In another study, assessment of ankle reflexes and great toe sensation in over 8,000 diabetic patients identified 32% of patients with peripheral neuropathy (25). In the Rochester Diabetic Neuropathy Study, 54% of type 1 and 45% of type 2 diabetic patients had polyneuropathy (26).

In the Diabetes Control and Complication Trial (DCCT), which comprised a cohort of 278 healthy type 1 diabetic patients, neuropathy was identified in 39% (defined as an abnormal neurological examination plus either abnormal nerve conduction studies in two nerves or abnormal autonomic function testing) (27). Similarly, in the Pittsburgh Epidemiology of Diabetes Complications Study, neuropathy was identified in 18% of type 1 patients 18 to 29 years of age and in 58% of patients greater than 30 years of age (28). In the EURODIAB complications study, which comprised 3,250 type 1 diabetic patients from 16 European countries, diabetic neuropathy was identified in 28% of patients (29). A significant correlation was identified with age, diabetes duration, and glycemic control (29). Similar prevalance rates have been found in patients with type 2 diabetes. For example, in one longitudinal study, neuropathy was diagnosed in 8% of newly diagnosed type 2 patients, and its prevalence increased to 42% after 10 years of diabetes (30). Other studies in type 2 patients reported that 22% and 49% demonstrated neuropathy 4 years and 12 years, respectively, after diagnosis (31,32). Therefore these studies demonstrate the high prevalence of diabetic neuropathy in both type 1 and type 2 diabetes, which rises with age, diabetes duration, and impaired quality of metabolic control.

Diabetic Autonomic Neuropathy: Epidemiology

Diabetic autonomic neuropathy also commonly complicates diabetes and is usually found in association with distal symmetrical polyneuropathy. Traditionally, it can be detected using indirect cardiovascular reflex tests, which assess the integrity of complex reflex arcs, or by more direct tests of peripheral sympathetic function. Abnormalities of cardiovascular reflex testing can be identified in approximately 16% to 20% of diabetic patients (33–39). For example, in the EURODIAB IDDM Complications Study and an earlier report (38), abnormalities of heart rate variability were detected in approximately 19% and 25%, respectively, of patients. Other studies have estimated the prevalence of abnormalities of both heart rate variabilty (HRV) and the Valsalva ratio to be approximately 17% (37). In the DCCT, in type 1 diabetes, in the primary prevention cohort, deficits of HRV were found in less than 2% of patients (27). In patients with baseline complications, this prevalence was increased to approximately 6% (40,41). Much debate has centered on the observation that young women with type 1 diabetes appear to be particularly susceptible to the development of aggressive, early-onset autonomic failure, which may develop in the absence of other chronic complications. This risk appears to be particularly great in the presence of an eating disorder. In type 2 diabetes,

the frequency of parasympathetic DAN has been reported to be 20% at 5 years and 65% at 10 years (42), and that of sympathetic DAN to be 7% at 5 years and 24% at 10 years.

Direct assessment of cardiovascular sympathetic deficits has become possible by the recent introduction of radiolabeled analogues of norepinephrine (NE), which are actively taken up by the sympathetic nerve terminals of the heart (43–52). Quantitative scintigraphic assessment of the pattern of sympathetic innervation of the human heart is possible with either (^{131}I)metaiodobenzylguanidine (MIBG) or (^{11}C)hydroxyephedrine (HED). HED undergoes highly specific and rapid uptake into sympathetic nerve varicosities via NE transporters (NET; "uptake-1"). HED is metabolically stable and its neuronal retention requires intact vesicular storage (Fig. 10.2). HED retention is significantly correlated with myocardial NE content and NET density (53,54). In the transplanted human heart, studies using (^{11}C)HED have demonstrated increased tracer retention in the proximal anterior

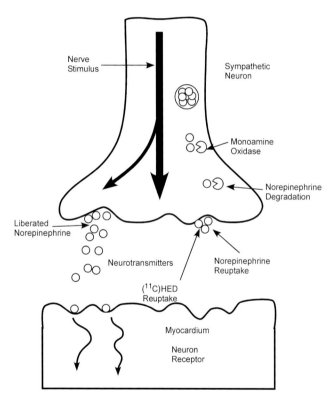

FIG. 10.2. *Visualization of the cardiac sympathetic nerve terminal using positron emission tomography and (^{11}C) hydroxyephedrine [(^{11}C)HED].* Activation of the sympathetic nerve terminal stimulates the release of norepinephrine into the synaptic cleft. This can activate adrenergic receptors on the myocardium and vasculature and/or reuptake ("uptake-1") into the sympathetic neuron. Within the sympathetic nerve terminal, norepinephrine can be broken down by monoamine oxidase or stored within vesicles. (^{11}C)Hydroxyephedrine competes with norepinephrine for neuronal uptake and is not a substrate for monoamine oxidase, and so its retention marks the position of functioning sympathetic terminals. Hydroxyephedrine retention is significantly correlated with myocardial norepinephrine content and norepinephrine transporter density.

wall, which correlated with the presence of axons on histological assessment (53) and with increased myocardial perfusion on sympathetic activation (55), thus confirming the neuronal specificity of HED positron emission tomography (PET) and its ability to assess presynaptic sympathetic nerve integrity. In cross-sectional studies, for example, deficits of left ventricle (^{123}I)MIBG and (^{11}C)HED retention have been identified in type 1 and type 2 diabetic patients with and without abnormalities on cardiovascular reflex testing (43–53) and have been reported even in newly diagnosed diabetic patients (49). In type 1 diabetic patients, for example, abnormalities of (^{11}C)HED retention affecting up to 8% of the left ventricle have been identified in 40% of otherwise healthy subjects without deficits on cardiovascular reflex testing (50). In the mild DAN patients, defects were observed only in the distal inferior wall of the left ventricle, whereas in the severe DAN patients, defects extended to involve the distal and the proximal anterolateral and inferior walls (Fig. 10.3). The presence of an abnormal Valsalva ratio or the presence of symptomatic orthostasis (47,50) predicted a deficit of left ventricular tracer retention of greater than 40%. Deficits of autonomic innervation have been more widely characterized using MIBG single-photon computed tomography (44–46,48,49,51). This technique has demonstrated widespread abnormalities of myocardial tracer retention, which are at least partially correctable by intensive insulin therapy (49). These deficits therefore most likely reflect hyperglycemia-induced neuronal dysfunction, which is sensitive to rapidly improved metabolic control and not more advanced neuronal loss. Unfortunately,

a clinically useful tracer for the quantitative direct assessment of parasympathetic integrity has not been developed and so the evaluation of this component of autonomic integrity remains dependent on heart rate variability assessments.

Diabetic Peripheral Neuropathy: Clinical Manifestations

Diabetic peripheral neuropathy can present with a vast spectrum of clinical manifestations, which reflects the heterogeneity of nerves affected and the widespread consequences of their dysfunction (Table 10.1). Manifestations can range from an imperceptible reduction in temperature perception in the feet to sudden cardiac death. Focal neuropathy is important to recognize because it may be amenable to surgical approaches and have a self-limiting course. Diabetic autonomic neuropathy can result in complex dysfunction of the eye, stomach, bowel, and genitourinary tract. The reader is referred to texts that deal specifically with these syndromes (5,6); this chapter describes the peripheral and cardiovascular manifestations.

Diabetic neuropathy can be either subclinical and symptomatic or clinically apparent and dominate the clinical picture. Subclinical diabetic neuropathy may only be perceptible utilizing electrophysiologic testing or by detailed quantitative sensory testing, and may occur in the complete absence of clinical signs or symptoms. On the other hand, clinical diabetic neuropathy can be diagnosed when symptoms accompany clinically detectable neurological deficits. As described

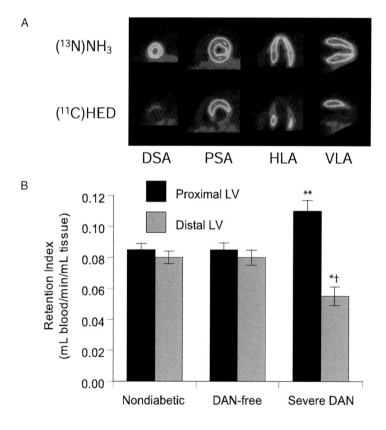

FIG. 10.3. (See Color Fig. 10.3A.) *High-risk cardiac sympathetic dysinnervation complicating diabetes.* **A:** Position emission tomography with (^{11}C)hydroxyephedrine [(^{11}C)HED] was used to quantitate regions of cardiac sympathetic denervation in a 24-year-old patient with type 1 diabetes and symptomatic autonomic and peripheral neuropathy. All cardiovascular reflex tests were abnormal, and the patient suffered from orthostatic hypotension and painful diabetic neuropathy. Blood flow images of the left ventricle appear normal (infact resting perfusion is increased in subjects with cardiovascular autonomic neuropathy, secondary to tachycardia), but abnormalities of tracer retention are extensive, with only the proximal myocardial segments being visualized. DSA, Distal short axis; PSA, proximal short axis; HLA, horizontal long axis; VLA, vertical long axis. **B:** Uptake of tracer is increased above nondiabetic values in the proximal myocardial segments, consistent with "hyperinnervation." Values are decreased distally, consistent with extensive denervation. LV, left ventricle; DAN, diabetic autonomic neuropathy. * $p<0.05$ versus other groups; ** $p<0.01$ versus other groups; $^{+}p<0.01$ versus proximal segments.

in the foregoing, diabetic neuropathy is usually apparent as a variety of clinical syndromes, which may be diffuse or more focal.

Distal symmetrical sensorimotor polyneuropathy is the most common manifestation of diffuse diabetic neuropathy and is characterized by sensory deficits and symptoms with, at least initially, minor motor deficits (56,57). Sensory deficits begin distally in the extremities and progress proximally resulting in the classic stocking-in-glove distribution (56,57). The symptoms and signs of distal symmetrical polyneuropathy are highly dependent on the type of nerve fiber affected. Initially, imperceptible loss of small nerve fibers can result in altered temperature perception (often manifested as an inability to feel water temperature, and which can result in burns), paresthesias, dysesthesias, and/or neuropathic pain. With progression of neuropathy, large nerve fibers also become damaged, which can result in decreased light touch sensation and altered proprioception and ultimately muscle weakness. The earliest manifestations of peripheral autonomic neuropathy are likewise difficult to detect clinically because they may be manifest solely as impaired peripheral vasomotor control or decreased sudomotor function, which may progress to increased arteriovenous shunting (detectable by the presence of distended veins on the lower legs), severe edema, neuroarthropathy (Charcot joints), and neuropathic ulceration. Clinically, early small fiber neuropathy can be difficult to diagnose because reliable tests of vasomotor or temperature perception are not widely available. However, simply inquiring as to whether the feet still sweat can be helpful. Instead, diagnosis usually relies on the detection of more advanced large fiber deficits such as reduced or absent deep-tendon reflexes, especially the Achilles tendon reflex, impaired vibration perception thresholds, and decreased light touch perception (utilizing the 10-g monofilament) (Table 10.2).

Focal neuropathies are importance to recognize because unlike the diffuse neuropathy syndromes, they are usually reversible and many are thought to have an acute vascular etiology (i.e., nerve infarct). These neuropathies may correspond to the distribution of a single peripheral nerve (mononeuropathy) or multiple peripheral nerves (mononeuropathy multiplex). Nerve, areas that can be affected include cranial nerves, regions of the brachial or lumbosacral plexuses (plexopathy), or the nerve roots (radiculopathy). With regard to the manifestations of focal neuropathies affecting the limbs, a relatively common presentation in middle-aged type 2 diabetic men is a unilateral "femoral neuropathy," which may be manifest as an acute onset of pain, weakness, and sensory deficits in the quadriceps muscle, which may become bilateral. These symptoms usually resolve in 1 to 2 years, but some sensory deficits may be persistent. The most common mononeuropathies involve the median or ulnar nerves and may require splinting or surgical intervention. In summary, distal symmetrical polyneuropathy and autonomic neuropathy are common, diffuse, and usually progressive, whereas the focal neuropathies are much rarer, usually sudden in onset, and occur more often in older diabetic patients.

TABLE 10.2. *Testing for diabetic peripheral neuropathy*

Clinical examination findings
  Diffuse neuropathy
    Distal symmetric sensorimotor polyneuropathy
    Autonomic neuropathy
  Focal neuropathy
Abnormal electrophysiologic tests
Abnormal quantitative sensory testing
  Vibration/thermal/light touch perception
Abnormal autonomic function tests
  Parasympathetic
    Heart rate variability studies: Spectral analysis, mid-frequency (0.05–0.15 Hz) and high-frequency (0.15–0.5 Hz) fluctuations
    Maximum/minimum 30:15 ratio
  Sympathetic
    Spectral analysis, low-frequency (0.01–0.05 Hz) fluctuations on standing
    Valsalva ratio
    Postural systolic blood pressure fall
    Pupillary responses
    Blood pressure response to sustained handgrip
    Quantitative sudomotor axon reflex testing
    Plasma norepinephrine (supine and standing)
    Scintigraphic techniques

CARDIOVASCULAR AUTONOMIC NEUROPATHY: CLINICAL MANIFESTATIONS

In general, cardiovascular autonomic neuropathy (CAN) can be divided into four main syndromes: abnormal exercise-induced cardiovascular performance, orthostatic hypotension, cardiac denervation syndrome, and peripheral autonomic denervation (Table 10.3).

Abnormal Cardiovascular Exercise Performance

Advanced CAN may result in reduced cardiovascular performance during exercise, which may be subclinical (17,58). Advanced CAN is accompanied by impaired cardiac ejection fraction, together with abnormal systolic function and decreased diastolic filling (59–61). In diabetes complicated

TABLE 10.3. *Clinical manifestations of cardiovascular autonomic neuropathy*

Cardiovascular	Resting and fixed tachycardia
	Exercise intolerance
	Orthostatic and postprandial hypotension
	Severe hypoglycemia
	Silent myocardial ischemia
	Sudden cardiac death in patients with myocardial ischemia
	Peripheral edema, neuropathic foot ulceration
	Charcot neuroarthropathy, callus formation
Sudomotor	Distal anhidrosis and gustatory sweating (over face, upper chest in response to food)

by autonomic dysfunction, resting heart rate is increased (and may reach 120 beats per min), which reflects decreased parasympathetic tone accompanied by augmented sympathetic activity. With progression of neuropathy, resting heart rate tends to decrease and may become fixed at approximately 90 beats per min. This resting tachycardia is typically unresponsive to mild exercise, and any exercise-induced rise in cardiac output is proportional to the resting vagal tone as measured by resting beat-to-beat heart rate variability. In CAN patients, the resting tachycardia is accompanied by increased myocardial perfusion but impaired vasodilatory reserve in response to stress (43). Consideration needs to be given to the impairment of exercise capacity and silent myocardial ischemia when prescribing exercise regimens in these patients.

Orthostatic Hypotension

Orthostatic hypotension (defined as a fall in systolic blood pressure in excess of 30 mm Hg) is a consequence of cardiovascular denervation and may reflect the consequences of a fixed resting heart rate and impaired visceral as well as lower limb vascular tone. Symptoms can vary from intermittent dizziness, to visual impairment, to syncope, which renders a patient unable to stand. The differential diagnosis includes hypoglycemia or vertigo. The diurnal variation of blood pressure is decreased in subjects with DAN, and may result in nocturnal supine hypertension (which increases the risk for the development of diabetic nephropathy) (62). Profoundly disabling orthostatic hypotension is rare, but highly resistant to treatment. In these patients, there can be a great day-to-day variability of orthostatic symptoms, which may be aggravated by insulin therapy (63,64) and food (65). Anemia secondary to renal denervation can greatly exacerbate orthostatic symptoms and should be actively managed.

Cardiac Denervation Syndrome

The precise metabolic, physiological, and functional consequences of advanced cardiac denervation are the subject of considerable research interest. Potential consequences of cardiac denervation complicating diabetes include abnormal myocardial blood flow regulation, cardiovascular instability during anesthesia, and increased susceptibility to cardiac arrhythmias and sudden death. Because afferent autonomic pathways are also involved in the cardiovascular denervation syndrome, the risk for painless ischemic heart disease is increased.

Implications for Enhanced Cardiac Risk

Cardiovascular autonomic neuropathy is invoked as a cause of sudden cardiac death in diabetes (50,66). Diabetic patients have increased mortality post-myocardial infarction (67–73), which may reflect increased susceptibility to triggering factors, including autonomic imbalance. In diabetes

complicated by myocardial infarction, CAN is predictive of both increased mortality and left ventricle failure (74). A recent meta-analysis of diabetic patients concluded that the mortality of DAN-free patients over 5.5 years was approximately 5%, and this increased to 27% with the development of abnormal cardiovascular reflex tests (75). Mortality increases in proportion to the severity of CAN. For example, in patients with moderately advanced CAN, 5-year mortality approached 30% (36). At the most extreme, longitudinal studies of advanced CAN patients have shown 5-year mortality rates of up to 53%, with the highest mortality associated with advanced cardiovascular sympathetic denervation (16). In contrast, regional cardiac sympathetic hyperactivity is associated with malignant arrhythmogenesis and cardiac death in nondiabetic humans and animals, particularly when accompanied by reduced parasympathetic tone and myocardial ischemia (76–78). The association of increased cardiovascular mortality with decreased cardiac sympathetic innervation in severe CAN therefore appears paradoxical, as does the enhanced protective effects of β-adrenoreceptor blockade in these patients (72,73).

In comparison to nondiabetic individuals, patients with type 1 diabetes have an altered pattern of myocardial ischemia, with the incidence of myocardial infarction decreased in the morning, but increased in the evening. This may reflect decreased sympathetic activation in the morning and impaired evening parasympathetic tone and decreased fibrinolytic activity (79,80). Considerable interest has centered on the role of abnormal myocardial electrical activity in arythmogenesis, including, for example, QT prolongation and altered ventricular repolarization (81). In the EURODIAB Complications Study, the prevalence of QT prolongation in type 1 patients was 16% overall (11% in men, 21% in women (82). The potential mechanisms whereby cardiac denervation increases the risks of myocardial instability have begun to be addressed using scintigraphic techniques. The radiotracer (^{123}I)MIBG has been extensively utilized to explore the contribution of the sympathetic nervous system to enhanced cardiac risk. Decreased inferior and posterior left ventricular (^{123}I)MIBG retention occurs in subjects with silent (83,84) or symptomatic (84) myocardial ischemia. Abnormal myocardial (^{123}I)MIBG uptake correlates with altered left ventricle diastolic filling (60,61) and electrophysiologic defects involving the QT interval (85) and QT dispersion (86). Impaired retention of left ventricle (^{123}I)MIBG in diabetic patients is also predictive of sudden death (87).

In diabetes, quantitative cardiac studies using the sympathetic tracer (^{11}C)HED have shown that abnormalities of left ventricular sympathetic innervation begin distally in the left ventricle and spread circumferentially and proximally, involving anterior, inferior, and lateral ventricular walls, reflecting a proximal–distal progression in the severity of neuropathy (50). Interestingly, despite extensive cardiac denervation, "islands" of proximal myocardial persist, which demonstrate a 30% increase of (^{11}C)HED retention above the same regions in the CAN-free individuals (Fig. 10.3) (50). Despite this increase of tracer retention, no appreciable washout of tracer is observed in the proximal segments, consistent with normal regional tone, but regional sympathetic hyperinnervation. Distally, (^{11}C)HED retention is decreased in severe diabetic CAN by ~30%, and so a dramatic gradient of sympathetic innervation is observed in advanced CAN, which may enhance electrical and chemical instability (50).

Effect of Cardiovascular Autonomic Neuropathy on Myocardial Blood Flow Regulation in Diabetes

PET has been used to explore myocardial blood flow–innervation relationships in type 1 diabetic patients. Maximal impairment in vasodilatory capacity is found in the "hyperinnervated" proximal myocardial segments (43). Other reports have confirmed that DAN is associated with impaired vasodilation of coronary resistance vessels to sympathetic stimulation, which is related to the severity of the sympathetic nerve dysfunction (88). These regions also demonstrate paradoxical reductions of myocardial perfusion on sympathetic stimulation (89) (Fig. 10.4), suggesting that this region of the heart may be the focus of instability.

Adrenergic Responsiveness and Sensitivity Are Altered in Diabetes

Effects of Diabetes on Sympathetic Nervous System Activity

Adrenergic activity is a major determinant of vascular tone, and alterations of adrenergic activity may contribute to abnormalities of regional blood flow regulation and myocardial stability complicating diabetes. Sympathetic nervous system activity is typically studied by measuring plasma levels of norepinephrine and rates of norepinephrine spillover into the circulation. In general, most studies have not found a change in basal sympathetic nervous system activity in diabetes prior to the development of CAN. For example, in diabetes, systemic sympathetic nervous system activity has been reported to be unchanged (90–92), increased (93), or decreased (94–96) compared to nondiabetic controls. Studies in type 1 diabetes with CAN have been more consistent and have demonstrated that plasma norepinephrine levels and norepinephrine spillover into the circulation are decreased, consistent with peripheral sympathetic nerve dysfunction (97). However, the effect of CAN on cardiac norepinephrine spillover is unknown. Because CAN is characterized by a compensatory increase in sympathetic nervous system activity in response to peripheral denervation (5,6), it is interesting to speculate that cardiac sympathetic nervous system activity is increased and may account for the paradoxical association of peripheral denervation with advanced cardiac risk.

Sympathetic nervous system responsiveness can also be explored by evaluating heart rate frequency responses on head-up tilt-table testing (HUTT). Power spectral analysis can indirectly quantify defects in sympathetic and vagal innervation of the heart. The power spectral density of the R–R interval time series can be measured by a 256-point fast-Fourier transformation and can be determined in low-frequency (0.01 to 0.05 Hz), mid-frequency (0.05 to 0.15 Hz), and high-frequency (0.15 to 0.5 Hz) ranges. Abnormality is usually defined as results that are below the 2.3rd percentile for age (39). The low- and high-frequency components are thought to reflect primarily sympathetic and parasympathetic integrity, respectively. The postural response of each measure can be determined during HUTT by evaluating the difference between measurements made in the supine and the tilt positions (value during tilt − value during supine) (98). With this methodology, HRV during standardized HUTT under paced breathing has demonstrated that increased postural change

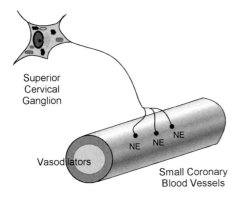
Normal: Vasodilation

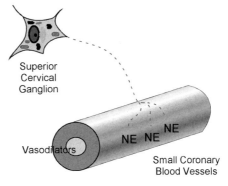
Diabetes: Vasoconstriction

FIG. 10.4. *Model demonstrating alteration of sympathetically mediated myocardial blood flow regulation in diabetes.* The predominant response to sympathetic activation in nondiabetic subjects is vasodilation, which is mediated by a moderate increase in the release of the vasoconstrictor norepinphrine (NE), which is offset by the release of vasodilatory agents such as nitric oxide and prostacyclin. In diabetes, sympathetic hyperresponsiveness or hyperinnervation may result in excess norepinephrine release, which, with a deficiency of vasodilators, may result in paradoxical vasoconstriction.

(supine to upright) in the low-frequency component of the power predicted an increased risk for cardiac death (98), consistent with an augmented sympathetic nervous system reactivity being a risk factor for sudden cardiac death.

In diabetes, myocardial hypertrophy, interstitial and perivascular fibrosis (99,100), and apoptosis (101) characteristically complicate high-risk CAN. Arrhythmogenic right ventricular cardiomyopathy (ARVC) is a recently recognized syndrome, which has some parallels to the myocardial effects of CAN complicating diabetes. It is characterized pathologically by fibrotic and fatty replacement of the right ventricular free wall and progression of myocardial atrophy mediated by apoptotic cell death (102,103). ARVC is characterized by increased cardiac, but not systemic sympathetic nervous system activity, and clinically by ventricular tachycardia, sudden death, and cardioprotection from β-adrenoceptor blockade (102–104), implicating increased cardiac sympathetic nervous system activity in arrhythmogenesis. Therefore, increased sympathetic nerve fiber density (in CAN), increased cardiac sympathetic nervous system activity, and elevated cardiac synaptic norepinephrine (105,106), or enhanced myocardial norepinephrine sensitivity, may augment myocardial norepinephrine-mediated toxicity, predisposing to enhanced cardiac risk in ARVC and diabetic CAN patients.

Enhanced Sympathetic Nervous System Responsiveness May Reflect Nitric Oxide Depletion or Subclinical Denervation

In contrast to the discrepant results regarding alterations in resting sympathetic nervous system activity, recent studies in humans have indicated that responsiveness to infused norepinephrine is increased in diabetes (94,95,107). In response to exercise, increments of norepinephrine are more pronounced in diabetic patients irrespective of complications, although the systolic blood pressure response has been reported to be higher in diabetic microangiopathic patients (93). Exaggerated catecholamine responses to stress are related to suboptimal glycemic control (92,108). In patients with CAN, the epinephrine and norepinephrine responses are blunted (109). Diabetic patients with early microvascular complications exhibit increased systemic sympathetic nervous system responsiveness, contrasting with diabetic CAN patients, in whom norepinephrine responses are blunted. Although the mechanisms of increased norepinephrine responses are unknown, alterations of nitric oxide metabolism [in sympathetic ganglia (110) and/or vascular endothelium (111–114)] and subclinical vascular denervation (91) have been proposed.

Effects of Diabetes and Denervation on Myocardial β-Adrenoreceptor Density and Sensitivity

Diabetes Decreases Myocardial β₁-Adrenoreceptor Density

Understanding the effects of diabetes and cardiovascular denervation on myocardial β-adrenoreceptor density and sensitivity has important implications for myocardial stabil-

ity. In experimental diabetes in rodents, a decrease in β_1-adrenoreceptor density (115–119) and no change or an increased in β_2- and β_3-adrenoreceptor density have been observed, which are associated with acutely (14-day) enhanced β-adrenoreceptor-mediated functional responses to stimulation (115,117). However, in animal models of longer durations of diabetes, the β-adrenoreceptor responses become suppressed (117,120) and the number of voltage-gated Ca^{2+} channels increased (121). In chronic diabetic rodents, decreased myocardial norepinephrine levels (122,123), downregulated myocardial β-adrenoreceptors (117) and α1-adrenoreceptors (124), decreased epinephrine-stimulated adenylyl cyclase activity (125), and defective adrenergic receptor–adenylate cyclase coupling (126) may contribute to the eventual decline in myocardial nerve growth factor protein (122,123) and distal left ventricular denervation. The effects of diabetes on β-adrenoreceptors in humans are, however, unknown.

Denervation Upregulates β₂ Myocardial β-Adrenergic Receptor Density and Sensitivity

The effects of myocardial denervation on β-adrenergic density and subtype have been evaluated in animal models and in human transplanted hearts. In model systems, surgical denervation typically results in both presynaptic and postsynaptic supersensitivity in β-adrenergic receptor pathways and alteration in G protein-mediated signal transduction (127). PET has been serially used in dogs to assess changes in ventricular muscarinic and β-adrenergic receptor densities following chemical or surgical denervation. Denervation has been reported not to effect muscarinic receptor density, but to result in a prolonged upregulation of β-adrenoreceptor (128). Denervation maximally upregulates the β2-adrenoreceptor, which is principally coupled to adenylyl cyclase through Gs. In the denervated myocardium of canine heart, a significant shift from β_1- to β_2-adrenoceptor subtype is observed, whereas the total β-adrenoreceptor density remains unaffected (129). In the denervated transplanted human heart, ventricular β_1-adrenoreceptor density is not changed. By contrast, β_2-adrenoreceptor density is higher in transplant left and right ventricles relative to the respective values in donor ventricles by 33% and 97%, repectively (127). Furthermore, continuous β-adrenoreceptor activation using isoproterenol infusion results in β_2-adrenoreceptor downregulation (130).

Basal adenylyl cyclase activity has been reported to be 40% reduced in sympathectomized membranes as compared with control membranes, which may reflect increased Gi (131). Furthermore, relative stimulation of adenylyl cyclase by isoproterenol has been reported to be twofold greater in sympathectomized heart membranes (132), which is consistent with denervation hypersensitivity. An alteration in Gs interaction with adenylyl cyclase has been implicated in the reduction in basal adenylyl cyclase activity and the increased relative responsiveness of adenylyl cyclase to isoproterenol in chronically sympathectomized ventricular membranes. In denervated pigs, denervation supersensitivity depends on postreceptor elements in the β-adrenoreceptor-responsive pathway, which may be independent of Gs-activated adenylyl cyclase activity. In this model of adrenergic denervation supersensitivity, β-adrenoreceptors, through Gs, may be linked to an alternative effector that drives heart rate responsiveness (133). Therefore, in advanced CAN patients, in the distal denervated myocardium, β-adrenoreceptor subtype may be shifted from β_1 to β_2, which may predispose to denervation supersensitivity and arrhythmogenesis, reflecting the increased coupling of the β_2 subtype to adenyl cyclase or altered interactions of Gs with adenylyl cyclase.

Cardiac sympathetic dysinnervation may therefore contribute to excess mortality in diabetes by a number of different mechanisms and explain the paradoxical association of CAN with increased cardiac risk. In diabetes, left ventricular sympathetic dysinnervation may promote myocardial instability by vascular, chemical, and electrical mechanisms (Fig. 10.5). Proximal myocardial sympathetic hyperinnervation may decrease myocardial vascularity (134), stimulate vascular hyperreactivity (135), and exacerbate paradoxical coronary vasoconstriction (89,136). In the proximal myocardial segments, resting sympathetic nervous system activity may be increased secondary to distal cardiovascular denervation (5,6) and sympathetic ganglionic dysinhibition (110) and further augmented by exercise, hypoglycemia, or ischemia. Accumulation of norepinephrine in the synaptic cleft in the proximal myocardium may perturb intracellular signaling (137) and affect the spatial heterogeneity of calcium transients and increase the dispersion of repolarization (138), thereby enhancing the propensity for ventricular tachyarrhythmias. Additionally, regional accumulation of norepinephrine may precipitate myocardial apoptosis (139,140) and necrosis (141) secondary to increased intracellular calcium and free radical injury (142). Therefore, the islands of persistent proximal innervation in CAN may be the focus of electrical, chemical, and vascular instability, particularly if denervation hypersensitivity is also present (Fig. 10.5).

PERIPHERAL AUTONOMIC DENERVATION

Peripheral autonomic denervation can have many clinical manifestations, and contributes to changes to the skin texture, edema, venous prominence, callus formation, loss of nails, and sweating abnormalities of the feet. Diabetic patients with neuropathic foot ulceration have been shown to have greater

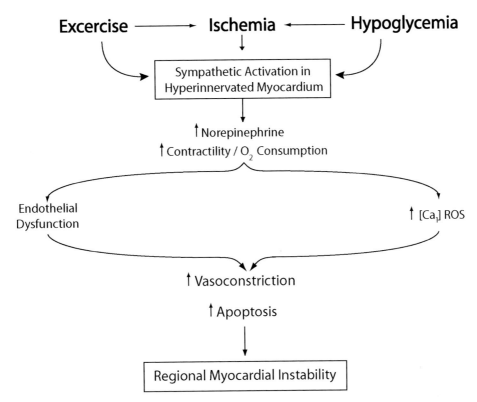

FIG. 10.5. *Hypothetical scheme delineating the potential links between regional hyperinnervation and myocardial instability complicating diabetes.* Sympathetic activation is critically implicated in the development of myocardial instability complicating diabetes. Activation of the sympathetic nervous system in response to exercise, myocardial ischemia, or hypoglycemia may result in excessive release of norepinephrine in the hyperinnervated proximal myocardial segments. This may provoke myocardial oxidative stress and apoptosis, and, in the presence of endothelial dysfunction and vascular smooth muscle hypersensitivity, regional perfusion defects. This, in turn, may lead to regional chemical and electrical instability. ROS, Reactive oxygen species.

impairment in power spectral analysis of heart rate variation than subjects with neuropathy without a history of foot ulcers, despite no differences being found for nerve conduction velocities (143). Diabetic autonomic sudomotor dysfunction is commonly manifested by asymptomatic distal anhidrosis of the lower extremities, which decreases thermal-regulatory capacity (144,145). This may produce a symptomatic compensatory increase in truncal and facial sweating. Gustatory sweating (144) is an abnormal profuse sweating that accompanies the ingestion of certain foods, particularly cheeses. This abnormality of sudomotor function can be quite irritating, and will often be volunteered by the patient. It is highly specific for DAN. Other clinical manifestation of peripheral autonomic denervation include prominent veins in the lower extremities secondary to arteriovenous shunting (146,147), which may impair nutritive skin blood flow. Loss of peripheral vascular sympathetic tone and resultant vasodilation predispose to increased peripheral edema, which, at its worst, can result in cutaneous blistering and infection. Deficits of skin blood flow in the small capillary circulation are found in association with impaired responsiveness to mental arithmetic, cold pressor testing, handgrip, and local heating. In response to local heating, for example, paradoxical vasoconstriction responses have been observed, which may further aggrevate deficits in skin perfusion around a site of active ulceration. The reduction in the amplitude of vasomotion reproduces changes found in premature aging. High peripheral blood flow may play an important role in the development of Charcot arthropathy (neuroarthropathy) by weakening bones in the foot, thereby predisposing to fractures (Fig. 10.6) (See Chapter 30).

Beside clinical inspection, few techniques are available for the assessment of limb peripheral sympathetic nerve activity. Direct recording of sympathetic nervous activity in postganglionic C fibers using microelectrodes is a highly specialized procedure and is not useful in the routine diagnosis of autonomic neuropathy. Galvanic skin responses are easily measured on the skin of the foot and correlate well with the preservation of sympathetic innervation. This technique does not allow gradation of the neuropathy and therefore lacks sensitivity in milder cases. More recently, quantitative sudomotor axon reflex testing has been developed to more accurately quantitate defects on upper and lower limb

autonomic function (148). Peripheral sympathetic denervation can be detected by the finding of abnormal vascular responses in the diabetic foot. Reduced peak skin blood flow after local thermal stimulation and, in particular, paradoxical vasoconstriction responses are detectable before the characteristic finding of biphasic ankle sonograms reflecting reduced peripheral vascular tone. Peripheral autonomic neuropathy usually is found in association with evidence of other small fiber damage, for example, thermal insensitivity, and this may afford an indirect method of assessment.

TREATMENT OF PERIPHERAL NEUROPATHIES

In the absence of an effective treatment to reverse established diabetic neuropathy, therapeutic strategies in diabetic patients can be broadly classified as preventive, for example, recognition of the insensate foot, education about performing regular examination of the feet and foot hygiene, appropriate footware, and instructions regarding when to seek professional help when problems occur. In general, most therapeutic regimens are targeted to the alleviation of symptoms, for example, neuropathic pain, or the diverse manifestations of cardiovascular autonomic dysfunction. The only effective therapeutic modality is intensified metabolic control, which reduces the incidence and slows the progression of diabetic neuropathy (40,41). However, there are no data from large, randomized trials to establish that diabetic polyneuropathy can be reversed by near euglycemia. Rendering the patient euglycemic after a successful pancreas transplant does eventually reverse diabetic neuropathy, but significant improvement may take up to 10 years to become manifest. Understanding the pathophysiology of diabetic neuropathy will facilitate the development of targeted pharmacologic strategies, which should supplement the benefits of intensified metabolic control.

Effects of Metabolic Control

In the DCCT study, 1,441 patients with type 1 diabetes were randomly assigned to intensive therapy or to conventional therapy and followed for a mean of 6.5 years; a hemoglobin A1c difference of 1.9% (9.0% vs. 7.1%, a 20% reduction) was achieved (7,40,41). This trial compared the prevalence

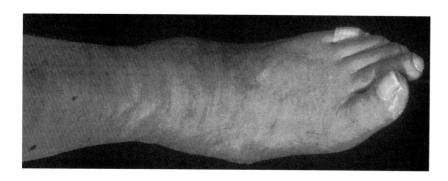

FIG. 10.6. *The diabetic Charcot foot.*

of clinical diabetic neuropathy confirmed by abnormal nerve conduction or autonomic testing in these two groups of type 1 diabetic patients over a 5-year period. Intensive therapy decreased the risk of development of confirmed clinical neuropathy (diagnosed by neurological history and physical examination and confirmed by nerve conduction or autonomic function studies) at year 5 by 69% from 9.8% to 3.1% in the primary prevention cohort, and by 57% from 16.1% to 7.0% in the secondary intervention cohort, with an overall risk reduction of 60% (7,40,41). The DCCT was not designed to test the efficacy of intensive therapy in the treatment of diabetic neuropathy, and patients with clinically significant diabetic neuropathy were excluded from the study. However, 450 patients at baseline had at least one abnormality on clinical examination and were defined as having "possible or definite" clinical neuropathy. The frequency of abnormal nerve conduction was roughly twice as great in patients with possible or definite neuropathy than in those without neuropathy. The likelihood of having abnormal nerve conduction was significantly reduced in patients with possible or definite neuropathy treated with intensive (37%) versus conventional (56%) therapy at 5 years ($p<0.001$). Thus, although not designed to examine the question directly, the DCCT is consistent with the belief that intensive diabetes treatment may benefit patients with existing diabetic neuropathy, at least in it very earliest stage.

More recently, scintigraphic studies have demonstrated widespread abnormalities of myocardial left ventricular MIBG uptake in metabolically compromised, newly diagnosed type 1 diabetic patients, which are partially correctable by intensive insulin therapy (49) and appear to be indicative of a hyperglycemia or insulin deficiency-induced acute neuronal dysfunction. Other scintigraphic studies have shown that poor glycemic control can result in progression of left ventricular sympathetic dysinnervation, which can be prevented (149) or reversed (150) by the institution of near-euglycemia.

In the U.K. Prospective Diabetes Study, the effects of intensive blood-glucose control with either sulfonylurea or insulin (goal fasting plasma glucose [FPG] less than 6 mmol per L) and conventional treatment with diet (best-achievable FPG) on the risk of microvascular and macrovascular complications were evaluated in 3,867 newly diagnosed patients with type 2 diabetes in a randomized controlled trial (8). The microvascular endpoints included vitreous hemorrhage, retinopathy requiring photocoagulation, blindness in one eye, cataract extraction, renal disease, and neuropathy. Over 10 years, hemoglobin A1c was 7.0% (6.2% to 8.2%) in the intensive group and 7.9% (6.9% to 8.8%) in the conventional group, an 11% reduction. Although not as definitive as the DCCT, in this study, a reduction of relative risk for lower limb sensory loss was also beginning to emerge after 15 years.

In DAN, delayed gastric emptying can lead to marked instability of glycemic control. In patients with type 1 diabetes, DAN decreases counterregulatory catecholamine responses, but not symptom awareness, and may increase the risk for severe hypoglycemia (151). In the EURODIAB IDDM Complications Study, the risk of severe hypoglycemia was studied in DAN patients (152). Compared to patients who had not experienced a severe hypoglycemic episode in the previous year, patients who had experienced hypoglycemia were older, had a longer duration of diabetes, had better glycemic control, and had abnormal heart rate variability and postural orthostasis. The odds ratio for severe hypoglycemia was 1.7 for DAN after controlling for other factors. Thus the risk of severe hypoglycemia appears to be increased in DAN patients and may be a precipitating factor contributing to sudden cardiac death. Interestingly, pancreas transplantation improves epinephrine response and normalizes hypoglycemia symptom recognition in patients with DAN (153), implicating a reversible component in some patients. Therefore particular care should be taken in patients with type 1 diabetes complicated by DAN to avoid hypoglycemia, which may result in the rather unsatisfying result of less strict metabolic control.

A number of drugs commonly used to treat painful diabetic neuropathy, including tricyclic antidepressants (154) and clonidine (155), may decrease heart rate variability and prolong the QTc interval and may thus have prognostic implications. They should be used with caution, particularly in subjects with myocardial ischemia. Conversely, heart rate variability has been reported to be increased by the angiotensin-converting enzyme inhibitor quinipril (156), which may contribute to their beneficial effects (157). Considering the enhanced benefits of beta blockade in diabetes, subjects with resting tachycardia may benefit from beta blockade, although outcome studies are lacking demonstrating that this improves mortality in diabetic CAN patients without myocardial ischemia or hypertension. Finally, type 1 patients with CAN may be particularly susceptible to abnormal ventilatory responses to hypoxia and hypercapnia and obstructive sleep apnea (158,159). This may increase the risk of nocturnal hypoxia and respiratory arrests. Nocturnal sleep studies are important in these patients, as is a trial of continuous positive airway pressure (160).

Orthostatic Hypotension

The first step in the management of orthostatic hypotension is the discontinuation, where possible, of therapeutic agents that may be contributing to the problem. Many patients with orthostasis secondary to DAN also have a number of other chronic diabetic complications that require treatment with drugs (e.g., tranquilizers, antidepressants, angiotensin-converting enzyme inhibitors, and diuretics), which can exacerbate postural blood pressure fluctuations. The timing and dosage of these agents may need to be modified to minimize their ability to provoke orthostasis. Occasionally, the patient can be switched to a shorter-acting agent (e.g., captopril) and the timing of the dose altered to minimized daytime orthostatic changes. Other nonneuropathic etiologies such as volume depletion, adrenal insufficiency, anemia, and hypothyroidism should be addressed. Typical initial approaches to the problem include elevating the head of the bed by 30 degrees during the night and instructing the patient to make changes in posture slowly, that is, to "stand in stages." Support stockings are usually prescribed, but may prove ineffective (65), because significant blood pooling probably occurs in the large splanchnic vascular bed. Plasma volume expanders such as a high-salt diet or fludrocortisone (up to 0.4 mg per day), which also increases catecholamine sensitivity, can be used. The sympathomimetic agent midodrine is useful in the treatment of orthostatic hypotension in nondiabetic patients in doses up to 40 mg per day (161). However, midodrine may be less effective in subjects with severe neuropathy. Care has to be taken because of the risk of increasing nocturnal supine hypertension. In the rare severe symptomatic cases, standard therapeutic maneuvers together with atrial tachypacing, the beta-blocker pindolol, or intranasal desmopressin to reduce nocturnal desmopressin often fail. The somatostatin analogue octreotide (50 μg three times daily, subcutaneously) may be helpful, as it acutely increases blood pressure selectively in subjects with autonomic failure (162). Octreotide may, however, be poorly tolerated because it may exacerbate bowel function and fluctuations in glycemic control. Erythropoetin has been shown to improve orthostasis (163), and may work by directly modulating small nerve fiber function in addition to ameliorating anemia. Erythropoetin (5,000 units per week) has been shown to improve orthostasis (164,165) and improve quality of life, particularly in patients who exhibit anemia of autonomic failure and may work in part by directly modulating small nerve fiber function in addition to ameliorating the anemia.

Peripheral Denervation

Peripheral vascular denervation can contribute to decreased skin perfusion and increased bone blood flow and thereby contribute to chronic complications of the diabetic foot. Altered vascular responses, which occur in the feet during the development of Charcot arthropathy, reflect the underlying bony destruction and altered blood flow distribution (146,147,166). These changes in foot blood flow are potentially amenable to therapy. Sympathomimetic drugs (ephedrine and midodrine) can reduce the high arteriovenous shunt flow seen in diabetic peripheral neuropathy (147). Ephedrine (10 to 30 mg three times daily) is an effective treatment of neuropathic edema (147) and may be helpful in the treatment of pain and discomfort. The mechanism by which ephedrine works is unclear, but it probably involves an increase in peripheral vascular tone and increased sodium excretion. This drug has the disadvantage of central side effects, irritability, and insomnia. It also may cause tachycardia and so should be avoided in patients with a history of cardiac disease. It should be used with great caution in patients with hypertension. Midodrine (10 mg three times daily, a selective alpha-adrenergic agonist), which has been shown to be useful in the management of postural hypotension, may be better tolerated because it causes fewer central side effects. Other approaches to treatment of the Charcot foot include the

use of bisphosphonates, although randomized studies of their efficacy are lacking. However, early intervention by instigating non-weight-bearing and supportive foot wear (preferably a surgical cast) at the earliest stages of the Charcot foot remains the principal mode of therapy.

In summary, cardiovascular denervation can result in a wide-ranging spectrum of morbidity and mortality encompassing deficits extending from increased arteriovenous shunting to sudden cardiac death. Improved understanding of the etiology of diabetic neuropathy will facilitate the development of therapeutic strategies aimed at stabilizing or reversing the disabling consequences of this common clinical problem.

ACKNOWLEDGMENTS

This work was supported in part by grants from the Juvenile Diabetes Research Foundation and the National Institutes of Health (R01-DK52391) and a Veterans Administration Career Development Award.

REFERENCES

1. Currie CJ, Morgan CL, Peters JR. The epidemiology and cost of inpatient care for peripheral vascular disease, infection, neuropathy, and ulceration in diabetes. *Diabetes Care* 1998;21:42–48.
2. Morgan CL, Currie CJ, Stott NC, et al. The prevalence of multiple diabetes-related complications. *Diabet Med* 2000;17:146–151.
3. Martyn CN, Hughes RA. Epidemiology of peripheral neuropathy. *J Neurol Neurosurg Psychiatry* 1997;62:310–318.
4. Windebank AJ, Feldman EL. Diabetes and the nervous system. In: Aminoff MJ, ed. *Neurology and general medicine*. 3rd ed. New York: Churchill Livingstone, 2001:341–364.
5. Feldman EL, Stevens MJ, Greene DA. Diabetic neuropathy. In: Turtle JR, Kaneko T, Osato S, eds. *Diabetes in the new millennium*. Sydney: Endocrinology and Diabetes Research Foundation of the University of Sydney, 1999:387–402.
6. Feldman EL, Stevens MJ, Russell JW, et al. Diabetic neuropathy. In: Becker KL, ed. *Principles and practice of endocrinology and metabolism*, 3rd ed. Philadelphia: Lippincott Williams & Wilkins, 2001:1391–1399.
7. DCCT. The effect of intensive treatment of diabetes on the development and progression of long-term complications in insulin-dependent diabetes mellitus. The Diabetes Control and Complications Trial Research Group. *N Engl J Med* 1993;329:977–986.
8. UKPDS. Intensive blood-glucose control with sulphonylureas or insulin compared with conventional treatment and risk of complications in patients with type 2 diabetes (UKPDS 33). UK Prospective Diabetes Study (UKPDS) Group. *Lancet* 1998;352:837–853.
9. Stevens MJ, Feldman EL, Thomas TP, et al. The pathogenesis of diabetic neuropathy. In: Veves A, Conn PMC, eds. *Clinical management of diabetic neuropathy*. Totowa, NJ: Humana Press, 1997:13–47.
10. Greene DA, Stevens MJ, Obrosova I, et al. Glucose-induced oxidative stress and programmed cell death in diabetic neuropathy. *Eur J Pharmacol* 1999;375:217–223.
11. Ghiselli A, Serafini, M, Maiani, G, et al. A fluorescence-based method for measuring total plasma antioxidant capability. *Free Radic Biol Med* 1995;18:29–36.
12. Mezzetti A, Cipollone F, Cuccurullo F. Oxidative stress and cardiovascular complications in diabetes: isoprostanes as new markers on an old paradigm. *Cardiovasc Res* 2000;47:475–488.
13. Bravenboer B, Kappelle AC, Hamers FP, et al. Potential use of glutathione for the prevention and treatment of diabetic neuropathy in the streptozotocin-induced diabetic rat. *Diabetologia* 1992;35:813–817.

14. Ceriello A, Bortolotti N, Falleti E, et al. Total radical-trapping antioxidant parameter in NIDDM patients. *Diabetes Care* 1997;20:194–197.
15. Telci A, Cakatay U, Salman S, et al. Oxidative protein damage in early stage type 1 diabetic patients. *Diabetes Res Clin Pract* 2000;50,213–223.
16. Stevens MJ, Obrosova I, Cao X, et al. Effects of DL-alipoic acid on peripheral nerve conduction, blood flow, energy metabolism, and oxidative stress in experimental diabetic neuropathy. *Diabetes* 2000;49:1006–1015.
17. Vinik AI, Park TS, Stansberry KB, et al. Diabetic neuropathies. *Diabetologia* 2000;43:957–973.
18. Gottsater A, Ahmed M, Fernlund P, et al. Autonomic neuropathy in type 2 diabetic patients is associated with hyperinsulinemia and hypertrigliceridemia. *Diabet Med* 1999;16:49–54.
19. Schnell O, Muhr D, Dresel S, et al. Autoantibodies against sympathetic ganglia and evidence of cardiac sympathetic dysinnervation in newly diagnosed and long-term IDDM patients. *Diabetologia* 1996;39:970–975.
20. Ejskjaer N, Arift S, Dodds W, et al. Prevalence of autoantibodies to autonomic nervous tissue structures in type 1 diabetes mellitus. *Diabet Med* 1999;16:544–549.
21. Stroud CR, Heller SR, Ward JD, et al. Analysis of antibodies against components of the autonomic nervous system in diabetes mellitus. *Q J Med* 1997;90:577–585.
22. Muhr-Becker D, Zielger AG, Druschky A, et al. Evidence for specific autoimmunity against sympathetic and parasympathetic nervous tissues in type 1 diabetes and the relation to cardiac autonomic dysfunction. *Diabetic Med* 1998;15:467–472.
23. Pirart J. Diabetes mellitus and its degenerative complications; a prospective study of 4,400 patients observed between 1947 and 1973. *Diabetes Care* 1978;1:168–188.
24. Young MJ, Boulton AJM, Macleod AF, et al. A multicentre study of the prevalence of diabetic peripheral neuropathy in the United Kingdom hospital clinic population. *Diabetologia* 1993;36:150–154.
25. Fedele D, Comi G, Coscelli C, et al. A multicenter study on the prevalence of diabetic neuropathy in Italy. *Diabetes Care* 1997;20:836–843.
26. Dyck PJ, Kratz KM, Karnes JL, et al. The prevalence by staged severity of various types of diabetic neuropathy, retinopathy, and nephropathy in a population-based cohort: the Rochester Diabetic Neuropathy Study. *Neurology* 1993;43:817–824.
27. The DCCT Research Group. Factors in the development of diabetic neuropathy: baseline analysis of neuropathy in the feasibility phase of the Diabetes Control and Complications Trial (DCCT). *Diabetes* 1988;37:476–481.
28. Maser RE, Steenkiste AR, Dorman JS, et al. Epidemiological correlates of diabetic neuropathy. Report from Pittsburgh Epidemiology of Diabetes Complications Study. *Diabetes* 1989;38:1456–1461.
29. Toeller M, Buyken AE, Heitkamp G, et al. Prevalence of chronic complications, metabolic control and nutritional intake in type 1 diabetes: comparison between different European regions. EURODIAB Complications Study Group. *Horm Metab Res* 1999;31:680–685.
30. Partanen J, Niskanen L, Lehtinen J, et al. Natural history of peripheral neuropathy in patients with non-insulin-dependent diabetes mellitus. *N Engl J Med* 1995;333:89–94.
31. Sands ML, Shetterly SM, Franklin GM, et al. Incidence of distal symmetric (sensory) neuropathy in NIDDM. The San Luis Valley Diabetes Study. *Diabetes Care* 1997;20:322–329.
32. de Wytt CN, Jackson RV, Hockings GI, et al. Polyneuropathy in Australian outpatients with type II diabetes mellitus. *J Diabetes Complications* 1999;13:74–78.
33. Hilsted J, Jeensen SB. A simple test for autonomic neuropathy in juvenile diabetics. *Acta Med Scand* 1979;205:385–387.
34. Dyberg T, Benn J, Christiansen JS, et al. Prevalence of diabetic autonomic neuropathy measured by simple bedside tests. *Diabetologia* 1981;20:190–194.
35. Ewing DJ, Martyn CN, Young RJ, et al. The value of cardiovascular autonomic function tests: 10 years experience in diabetes. *Diabetes Care* 1985;8:491–498.
36. Kennedy WR, Navarro X, Sakuta M, et al. Physiological and clinical correlates of cardiovascular reflexes in diabetes mellitus. *Diabetes Care* 1989;12:399–408.
37. Neil HAW, Thomson AV, John S, et al. Diabetic autonomic neuropathy: the prevalence of impaired heart rate variability in a geographically defined population. *Diabet Med* 1989;6:20–24.
38. EURODIAB IDDM Complications Group. Microvascular and acute complications in IDDM patients: the EURODIAB IDDM Complications Study. *Diabetologia* 1994;37:278–285.
39. Ziegler D, Dannehl K, Muhlen H, et al. Prevalence of cardiovascular autonomic dysfunction assessed by spectral analysis, vector analysis, and standard tests of heart rate variation and blood pressure responses at various stages of diabetic neuropathy. *Diabet Med* 1992;9:806–814.
40. The Diabetes Control and Complications Trial Research Group. The effect of intensive diabetes therapy on the development and progression of neuropathy. *Ann Intern Med* 1995;122:561–568.
41. The Diabetes Control and Complications Trial Research Group. The effect of intensive diabetes therapy on measures of autonomic nervous system function in the Diabetes Control and Complications Trial (DCCT). *Diabetologia* 1998;41:416–423.
42. Toyry JP, Niskanen LK, Mantysaari MJ, et al. Occurrence, predictors and clinical significance of autonomic neuropathy in NIDDM. *Diabetes* 1996;45:308–315.
43. Stevens MJ, Dayanikli F, Raffel DM, et al. Scintigraphic assessment of regionalized defects in myocardial sympathetic innervation and blood flow regulation in diabetic patients with autonomic neuropathy. *J Am Coll Cardiol* 1998;31:1575–1584.
44. Mantysaari M, Kuikka J, Mustonen J, et al. Noninvasive detection of cardiac sympathetic nervous dysfunction in diabetic patients using (123I) metaiodobenzylguanidine. *Diabetes* 1992;41:1069–1075.
45. Kreiner G, Woltzt M, Fasching P, et al. Myocardial m-(123I) iodobenzylguanidine scintigraphy for the assessment of adrenergic cardiac innervation in patients with IDDM. *Diabetes* 1995;44:543–549.
46. Langer A, Freeman ME, Josse RG, et al. Metaiodobenzylguanidine imaging in diabetes mellitus: assessment of cardiac sympathetic denervation and its relation to autonomic dysfunction and silent myocardial ischemia. *J Am Coll Cardiol* 1995;25:610–618.
47. Allman KC, Stevens MJ, Wieland DM, et al. Noninvasive assessment of cardiac diabetic neuropathy by C-11 hydroxyephedrine and positron emission tomography. *J Am Coll Cardiol* 1993;22:1425–1432.
48. Schnell O, Kirsch CM, Stemplinger J, et al. Scintigraphic evidence for cardiac sympathetic dysinnervation in long-term IDDM patients with and without ECG-based autonomic neuropathy. *Diabetologia* 1995;38:1345–1352.
49. Schnell O, Muhr D, Weiss M, et al. Reduced myocardial ^{123}I-metaiodobenzylguanidine uptake in newly diagnosed IDDM patients. *Diabetes* 1996;45:801–805.
50. Stevens MJ, Raffel DM, Allman KC, et al. Cardiac sympathetic dysinnervation in diabetes—an explanation for enhanced cardiovascular risk? *Circulation* 1998;98:961–968.
51. Ziegler D, Weise F, Langen KJ, et al. Effect of glycemic control on myocardial sympathetic innervation assessed by (123I)metaiodobenzylguanidine scintigraphy: a 4-year prospective study in IDDM patients. *Diabetologia* 1998;41:443–451.
52. Stevens MJ, Raffel DM, Allman KC, et al. Regression and progression of cardiac sympathetic dysinnervation in diabetic patients with autonomic neuropathy. *Metabolism* 1999;48:92–101.
53. Schwaiger M, Hutchins GD, Kalff V, et al. Evidence for regional catecholamine uptake and storage sites in the transplanted human heart by positron emission tomography. *J Clin Invest* 1991;87:1681–1690.
54. Ungerer M, Hartmann F, Karoglan M, et al. Regional *in vivo* and *in vitro* characterization of autonomic innervation in cardiomyopathic human heart. *Circulation* 1998;97:174–180.
55. Di Carli MF, Tobes MC, Mangner T, et al. Effects of cardiac sympathetic innervation on coronary blood flow. *Engl J Med* 1997;336:1208–1215.
56. Boulton AJ, Malik RA. Diabetic neuropathy. *Med Clin North Am* 1998;82:909–929.
57. Dyck PJB, Dyck PJ. Diabetic polyneuropathy. In: Dyck PJ, Thomas PK, eds. *Diabetic neuropathy,* 2nd ed. Philadelphia: WB Saunders, 1999:255–278.
58. Hilsted J. Pathophysiology in diabetic autonomic neuropathy: cardiovascular, hormonal, and metabolic studies. *Diabetes.* 1982;31:730–737.
59. Zola B, Kahn JK, Juni JE, et al. Abnormal cardiac function in diabetic patients with autonomic neuropathy in the absence of ischemic heart disease. *J Clin Endocrinol Metab* 1986;63:208–214.

60. Kreiner G, Wolzt M, Fasching P, et al. Myocardial m-(123I)iodobenzylguanidine scintigraphy for the assessment of adrenergic cardiac innervation in patients with IDDM. Comparison with cardiovascular reflex tests and relationship to left ventricular function. *Diabetes* 1995;44:543–549.

61. Mustonen J, Mantysaari M, Kuikka J, et al. Decreased myocardial 123I-metaiodobenzylguanidine uptake is associated with disturbed left ventricular diastolic filling in diabetes. *Am Heart J* 1992;123:804–805.

62. Hornung RS, Mahler RF, Raftery EB. Ambulatory blood pressure and heart rate in diabetic patients: an assessment of autonomic function. *Diabet Med* 1989;6:579–585.

63. Page M, Watkins PJ. Provocation of postural hypotension by insulin in diabetic autonomic neuropathy. *Diabetes* 1975;25:90–95.

64. Mathias CJ, Da Costa DF, Fosbraey P, et al. Hypotensive and sedative effects of insulin in autonomic failure. *Br Med J* 1987;295:161–163.

65. Stevens MJ, Edmonds ME, Mathias CJ, et al. Disabling postural hypotension complicating diabetic autonomic neuropathy. *Diabet Med* 1991;8:870–874.

66. Ewing DJ, Campbell IW, Clarke BF. Assessment of cardiovascular effects in diabetic autonomic neuropathy and prognostic implications. *Ann Intern Med* 1980;92:308–311.

67. Hjalmarson A, Elmfeldt D, Herlitz J, et al. Effect on mortality of metoprolol in acute myocardial infarction, a double-blind randomized trial. *Lancet* 1981;ii:123–127.

68. Beta-blocker Heart Attack Trial Research Group. A randomized trial of propranolol in patients with acute myocardial infarction. I. Mortality results. *JAMA* 1982;247:1707–1714.

69. Norwegian Multicentre Study Group. Timolol-induced reduction in mortality and reinfarction in patients surviving acute myocardial infarction. *N Engl J Med* 1981;304:801–807.

70. Australian and Swedish Pindolol Study Group. The effect of pindolol on the two year mortality after complicated myocardial infarction. *Eur Heart J* 1983;4:367–375.

71. Jaffe AS, Spadaro JJ, Schectman K, et al. Increased congestive heart failure after myocardial infarction of modest extent in patients with diabetes mellitus. *Am Heart J* 1984;108:31–37.

72. Gundersen T, Kjekshus JT. Timolol treatment after myocardial infarction in diabetic patients. *Diabetes Care* 1983;6:285–290.

73. Smith JW, Marcus FI, Serokman R, et al. Prognosis of patients with diabetes mellitus after acute myocardial infarction. *Am J Cardiol* 1984;54:718–721.

74. Fava S, Azzopardi J, Muscatt HA, et al. Factors that influence outcome in diabetic subjects with myocardial infarction. *Diabetes Care* 1993;16:1615–1618.

75. Ziegler D. Cardiovascular autonomic neuropathy: clinical manifestations and measurement. *Diabetes Rev* 1999;7:342–357.

76. Willich SN, Maclure M, Mittleman M, et al. Sudden cardiac death: support for the role of triggering in causation. *Circulation* 1993;87:1442–1450.

77. Lown B, Verrier RL. Neural activity and ventricular fibrillation. *N Engl J Med* 1976;294:1165–1170.

78. Schwartz PJ, Randall WC, Anderson EA, et al. Task Force 4. Sudden cardiac death: Nonpharmacologic interventions. *Circulation* 1987;76:I215–I219.

79. Morning peak in the incidence of myocardial infarction. Experience in the ISIS-2 trial. ISIS-2 (Second International Study of Infarct Survival) Collaborative Group. *Eur Heart J* 1992;13:594–598.

80. Aronson D, Weinrauch LA, D'Elia JA, et al. Circadian patterns of heart rate variability, fibrinolytic activity, and hemostatic factors in type I diabetes mellitus with cardiac autonomic neuropathy. *Am J Cardiol* 1999;84:449–453.

81. Sawicki PT, Kiwitt S, Bender R, et al. The value of QT interval dispersion for identification of total mortality risk in non-insulin-dependent diabetes mellitus. *J Intern Med* 1998;243:49–56.

82. Veglio M, Borra M, Stevens LK, et al. The relation between QTc interval prolongation and diabetic complications. *Diabetologia* 1999;42:68–75.

83. Matsuo S, Takahashi M, Nakamura Y, et al. Evaluating of cardiac sympathetic innervation with iodine-123-metaiodobenzylguanidine imaging in silent myocardial ischemia. *J Nucl Med* 1996;37:712–717.

84. Koistinen MJ, Airaksinen KEJ, Huikiri HV, et al. No difference in cardiac innervation of diabetic patients with painful and asymptomatic coronary artery disease. *Diabetes Care* 1996;19:231–235.

85. Langen KJ, Ziegler D, Weise F, et al. Evaluation of QT interval length, QT dispersion and myocardial m-iodobenzylguanidine uptake in insulin-dependent diabetic patients with autonomic neuropathy. *Clin Sci* 1997;92:325–333.

86. Shimabukuro M, Chibana T, Yoshida H, et al. Increased QT dispersion and cardiac adrenergic dysinnervation in diabetic patients with autonomic neuropathy. *Am J Cardiol* 1996;78:1057–1059.

87. Kahn JK, Sisson JC, Vinik AI. Prediction of sudden cardiac death in diabetic autonomic neuropathy. *J Nucl Med* 1988;29:1605–1606.

88. Di Carli MF, Bianco-Batlles D, Landa ME, et al. Effects of autonomic neuropathy on coronary blood flow in patients with diabetes mellitus. *Circulation* 1999;100:813–819.

89. Stevens MJ. New imaging techniques for cardiovascular autonomic neuropathy: a window on the heart. *Diabetes Technol Therap* 2001;3:9–22.

90. Weidmann P, Beretta-Piccoli C, Trost BN. Pressor factors and responsiveness in hypertension accompanying diabetes mellitus. *Hypertension* 1985;7:II33–II42.

91. Hogikyan RV, Galecki AT, Halter JB, et al. Heightened norepinephrine-mediated vasoconstriction in type 2 diabetes. *Metabolism* 1999;48:1536–1541.

92. Christensen NJ. Plasma norepinephrine and epinephrine in untreated diabetics, during fasting and after insulin administration. *Diabetes* 1974;23:1–8.

93. Hoogenberg K, Dullaart RP. Abnormal plasma noradrenaline response and exercise induced albuminuria in type 1 (insulin-dependent) diabetes mellitus. *Scand J Clin Lab Invest* 1992;52:803–811.

94. Eckberg DL, Harkins SW, Fritsch JM, et al. Baroreflex control of plasma norepinephrine and heart period in healthy subjects and diabetic patients. *J Clin Invest* 1986;78:366–374.

95. Eichler HG, Blaschke TF, Kraemer FB, et al. Responsiveness of superficial hand veins to alpha-adrenoceptor agonists in insulin-dependent diabetic patients. *Clin Sci (Lond)* 1992;82:163–168.

96. Hoffman RP, Sinkey CA, Kienzle MG, et al. Muscle sympathetic nerve activity is reduced in IDDM before overt autonomic neuropathy. *Diabetes* 1993;42:375–380.

97. Hilsted J. Catecholamines and diabetic autonomic neuropathy. *Diabet Med* 1995;12:296–297.

98. Hayano J, Mukai S, Fukuta H, et al. Postural response of low-frequency component of heart rate variability is an increased risk for mortality in patients with coronary artery disease. *Chest.* 2001;120:1942–1952.

99. Francis GS. Diabetic cardiomyopathy: fact or fiction? *Heart* 2001;85:247–248.

100. Chatham JC, Forder JR, McNeill JH. *The heart in diabetes.* Norwell, MA: Kluwer Academic Publishers, 1996.

101. Frustaci A, Kajstura J, Chimenti C, et al. Myocardial cell death in human diabetes. *Circ Res* 2000;87:1123–1132.

102. Marcus FI, Fontaine GH, Guiraudon G, et al. Right ventricular dysplasia: a report of 24 adult cases. *Circulation* 1982;65:384–398.

103. Thiene G, Nava A, Corrado D, et al. Right ventricular cardiomyopathy and sudden death in young people. *N Engl J Med* 1988;318:129–133.

104. Mallat Z, Tedgui A, Fontaliran F, et al. Evidence of apoptosis in arrhythmogenic right ventricular dysplasia. *N Engl J Med* 1996;335:1190–1196.

105. Paulson DJ, Light KE. Elevation of serum and ventricular norepinephrine content in the diabetic rat. *Res Commun Chem Pathol Pharmacol* 1981;33:559–562.

106. Felten SY, Peterson RG, Shea PA, et al. Effects of streptozotocin diabetes on the noradrenergic innervation of the rat heart: a longitudinal histofluorescence and neurochemical study. *Brain Res Bull* 1982;8:593–607.

107. Weidmann P, Beretta-Piccoli C, Trost BN. Pressor factors and responsiveness in hypertension accompanying diabetes mellitus. *Hypertension* 1985;7:II33–II42.

108. Tamborlane WV, Sherwin RS, Koivisto V, et al. *Diabetes* 1979;28:785–788.

109. Meyer C, Grossmann R, Mitrakou A, et al. Effects of autonomic neuropathy on counterregulation and awareness of hypoglycemia in type 1 diabetic patients. *Diabetes Care* 1998;21:1960–1966.

110. Shindo H, Thomas TP, Larkin DD, et al. Modulation of basal nitric oxide-dependent cyclic-GMP production by ambient glucose, myo-inositol, and protein kinase C in SH-SY5Y human neuroblastoma cells. *J Clin Invest* 1996;97:736–745.

111. Tesfamariam B, Cohen RA. Free radicals mediate endothelial cell dysfunction caused by elevated glucose. *Am J Physiol* 1992;263:H321–H326.

112. Cipolla MJ, Harker CT, Porter JM. Endothelial function and adrenergic reactivity in human type-II diabetic resistance arteries. *J Vasc Surg* 1996;23:940–949.

113. Vanhoutte PM, Miller VM. Alpha 2-adrenoceptors and endothelium-derived relaxing factor. *Am J Med* 1989;87:1S–5S.

114. Haefeli WE, Srivastava N, Kongpatanakul S, et al. Lack of role of endothelium-derived relaxing factor in effects of alpha-adrenergic agonists in cutaneous veins in humans. *Am J Physiol* 1993;264:H364–H369.

115. Sellers DJ, Chess-Williams R. The effect of streptozotocin-induced diabetes on cardiac beta-adrenoceptor subtypes in the rat. *J Auton Pharmacol* 2001;21:15–21.

116. Matsuda N, Hattori Y, Gando S, et al. Diabetes-induced downregulation of beta1-adrenoceptor mRNA expression in rat heart. *Biochem Pharmacol* 1999;58:881–885.

117. Austin CE, Chess-Williams R. Transient elevation of cardiac beta-adrenoceptor responsiveness and receptor number in the streptozotocin-diabetic rat. *J Auton Pharmacol* 1992;12:205–214.

118. Nishio Y, Kashiwagi A, Kida Y, et al. Deficiency of cardiac beta-adrenergic receptor in streptozocin-induced diabetic rats. *Diabetes* 1988;37:1181–1187.

119. Ramanadham S, Tenner Jr TE. Alterations in the myocardial beta-adrenoceptor system of streptozotocin-diabetic rats. *Eur J Pharmacol* 1987;136:377–389.

120. Dincer UD, Bidasee KR, Guner S, et al. . The effect of diabetes on expression of beta1-, beta2-, and beta3-adrenoreceptors in rat hearts. *Diabetes* 2001;50:455–461.

121. Gotzsche LB, Rosenqvist N, Gronbaek H, et al. Increased number of myocardial voltage-gated Ca2+ channels and unchanged total beta-receptor number in long-term streptozotocin-diabetic rats. *Eur J Endocrinol* 1996;134:107–113.

122. Hellweg R, Hartung, HD. Endogenous levels of nerve growth factor (NGF) are altered in experimental diabetes mellitus: a possible role for NGF in the pathogenesis of diabetic neuropathy. *J Neurosci Res* 1990;26:258–267.

123. Schmid H, Forman LA, Cao X, et al. Heterogenous cardiac sympathetic denervation and decreased myocardial nerve growth factor in streptozotocin diabetic rats. *Diabetes* 1999;48:603–608.

124. Tanaka Y, Kasiwagi A, Saeki Y, et al. Abnormalities in cardiac a1-adrenoceptor and its signal transduction in streptozotocin-induced diabetic rats. *Am J Physiol* 1992;263:E425–E429.

125. Dhalla NS, Liu X, Panagia V, et al. Subcellular remodelling and heart dyfunction in chronic diabetes. *J Cardiovasc Res* 1998;40:239–247.

126. Smith CI, Pierce GN, Dhalla, NS. Alterations in adenylate cyclase activity due to streptozotocin-induced diabetic cardiomyopathy. *Life Sci* 1984;34:1223–1230.

127. Farrukh HM, White M, Port JD, et al. Up-regulation of beta 2-adrenergic receptors in previously transplanted, denervated nonfailing human hearts. *J Am Coll Cardiol* 1993;22:1902–1908.

128. Valette H, Deleuze P, Syrota A, et al. Canine myocardial beta-adrenergic, muscarinic receptor densities after denervation: a PET study. *J Nucl Med* 1995;36:140–146.

129. Van der Vusse GJ, Dubelaar ML, Coumans WA, et al. Depletion of endogenous dopamine stores and shift in beta-adrenoceptor subtypes in cardiac tissue following five weeks of chronic denervation. *Mol Cell Biochem* 1998;183:215–219.

130. Kompa AR, Molenaar P, Summers RJ. Effect of chemical sympathectomy on (−)-isoprenaline-induced changes in cardiac beta-adrenoceptor subtypes in the guinea-pig and rat. *J Auton Pharmacol* 1994;14:411–423.

131. Hershberger RE, Feldman AM, Anderson FL, et al. *Mr* 40,000 and *Mr* 39,000 pertussis toxin substrates are increased in surgically denervated dog ventricular myocardium. *J Cardiovasc Pharmacol* 1991;17:568–575.

132. Quist EE, Lee SC, Vasan R, et al. Chronic sympathectomy of canine cardiac ventricles affects Gs-adenylyl cyclase coupling and muscarinic receptor density. *J Cardiovasc Pharmacol* 1994;23:936–943.

133. Hammond HK, Roth DA, Ford CE, et al. Myocardial adrenergic denervation supersensitivity depends on a postreceptor mechanism not linked with increased cAMP production. *Circulation* 1992;85:666–679.

134. Torry RJ, Connell PM, O'Brien DM, et al. Sympathectomy stimulates capillary but not precapillary growth in hypertrophic hearts. *Am J Physiol* 1991;260:H1515–H1521.

135. Whall CW, Myers MM, Halpern W. Norepinephrine sensitivity, tension development and neuronal uptake in resistance arteries from spontaneously hypertensive and normotensive rats. *Blood Vessels* 1980;17:1–15.

136. Koltai M, Jermendy G, Kiss V, et al. The effects of sympathetic nerve stimulation and adenosine on coronary circulation and heart function in diabetes mellitus. *Acta Physiol Hung* 1984;63:119–125.

137. Ungerer M, Böhm M, Elce JS, et al. Altered expression of (beta)-adrenergic receptor kinase and (beta)1-adrenergic receptors in the failing human heart. *Circulation* 1993;87:454–463.

138. Wichter T, Schafers M, Rhodes CG, et al. Abnormalities of cardiac sympathetic innervation in arrhythmogenic right ventricular cardiomyopathy: quantitative assessment of presynaptic norepinephrine reuptake and postsynaptic beta-adrenergic receptor density with positron emission tomography. *Circulation* 2000;101:1552–1558.

139. Communal C, Singh K, Pimentel DR, et al. Norepinephrine stimulates apoptosis in adult rat ventricular myocytes by activation of the beta-adrenergic pathway. *Circulation* 1998;98:1329–1334.

140. Iwai-Kanai E, Hasegawa K, Araki M, et al. (alpha)- and (beta)-Adrenergic pathways differentially regulate cell type-specific apoptosis in rat cardiac myocytes. *Circulation* 1999;100:305–311.

141. Cruickshank JM, Neil-Dwyer G, Degaute J, et al. Reduction of stress/catecholamine-induced cardiac necrosis by beta1-selective blockade. *Lancet* 1987;ii:585–589.

142. Haggendal J, Jonsson L, Johansson, et al. Catecholamine-induced free radicals in myocardial cell necrosis on experimental stress in pigs. *Acta Physiol Scand* 1987;131:447–452.

143. Aso Y, Fujiwara Y, Inukai T, et al. Power spectal analysis of heart rate variation in diabetic patients with neuropathic foot ulceration. *Diabetes Care* 1998;21:1173–1177.

144. Thomas PK, Eliasson S. In: Dyck PJ, Thomas PK, Lambert EM, eds. *Peripheral neuropathy*. Philadelphia: WB Saunders, 1975:956–981.

145. Odel HM, Roth GM, Keating FR. Autonomic neuropathy simulating the effects of sympathectomy as a complication of diabetes mellitus. *Diabetes* 1955;4:92–98.

146. Edmonds ME, Archer AG, Watkins PJ. Ephedrine: a new treatment for diabetic neuropathic oedema. *Lancet* 1983;i:548–551.

147. Edmonds ME, Roberts VC, Watkins PJ. Blood flow in the diabetic neuropathic foot. *Diabetologia* 1982;22:9–15.

148. Low PA. Antonomic neuropathies. Low PA, ed. Clinical Antonomic Disorders Philadelphia: Lippincott-Raven, 1997: 463–486.

149. Ziegler D, Weise F, Langen KJ, et al. Effect of glycemic control on myocardial sympathetic innervation assessed by (123I)meta-iodobenzylguanidine scintigraphy: a 4-year prospective study in IDDM patients. *Diabetologia* 1998;41:443–451.

150. Stevens MJ, Raffel DM, Allman KC, et al. Regression and progression of cardiac sympathetic dysinnervation in diabetic patients with autonomic neuropathy. *Metabolism* 1999;48:92–101.

151. Meyer C, Grossmann R, Mitrakou A, et al. Effects of autonomic neuropathy on counterregulation and awareness of hypoglycemia in type 1 diabetic patients. *Diabetes Care* 1998;21:1960–1966.

152. Stephenson JM, Kempler P, Perin PC, et al. Is autonomic neuropathy a risk factor for severe hypoglycaemia? The EURODIAB IDDM Complications Study. *Diabetologia* 1996;39:1372–1376.

153. Kendall DM, Rooney DP, Smets YF, et al. Pancreas transplantation restores epinephrine response and symptom recognition during hypoglycemia in patients with long-standing type I diabetes and autonomic neuropathy. *Diabetes* 1997;46:249–257.

154. Rechlin T. The effect of amitriptyline, doxepin, fluvoxamine and paroxetine treatment on heart rate variability. *J Clin Psychopharmacol* 1994;14:392–395.

155. Elghozi JL, Laude D, Janvier F. Clonidine reduces blood pressure and heart rate oscillations in hypertensive patients. *J Cardiovasc Pharmacol* 1991;17:935–940.

156. Kontopoulos AG, Athros VG, Didangelos TP, et al. Effect of chronic quinapril administration on heart rate variability in patients with diabetic autonomic neuropathy. *Diabetes Care* 1997;20:355–361.

157. Lewis EJ, Hunsicker LG, Bain RP, et al. The effect of angiotensin-converting-enzyme inhibition on diabetic nephropathy. *N Engl J Med* 1993;329:1456–1462.

158. Sobotka PA, Liss HP, Vinik AI. Impaired hypoxic ventilatory drive in diabetic patients with autonomic neuropathy. *J Clin Endocrinol Metab* 1986;62:658–663.

159. Ficker JH, Dertinger SH, Siegfried W, et al. Obstructive sleep apnoea and diabetes mellitus: the role of cardiovascular autonomic neuropathy. *Eur Respir J* 1998;11:14–19.

160. Veale D, Chailleux E, Hoorelbeke-Ramon A, et al. Mortality of sleep apnoea patients treated by nasal continuous positive airway pressure registered in the ANTADIR observatory. *Eur Respir J* 2000;15:326–331.

161. Kaufmann H, Brannan T, Krakoff L, et al. Treatment of orthostatic hypotension due to autonomic failure with a peripheral alpha adrenergic agonist (midodrine). *Neurology* 1988;38:951–956.

162. Pop-Busui R, Chey W, Stevens MJ. Severe hypertension induced by the long-acting somatostatin analogue Sandostatin LAR in a patient with diabetic autonomic neuropathy. *J Clin Endocrinol Metab* 2000;85:943–946.

163. Hoeldtke RD, Streeten DH. Treatment of orthostatic hypotension with erythropoietin. *N Engl J Med* 1993;329:611–615.

164. Winkler AS, Marsden J, Chaudhuri KR, et al. Erythropoietin depletion and anaemia in diabetes mellitus. *Diabet Med* 1999;16:813–819.

165. Bosman DR, Osborne CA, Marsden JT, et al. Erythropoietin response to hypoxia in patients with diabetic autonomic neuropathy and non-diabetic chronic renal failure. *Diabet Med* 2002;19:65–69.

166. Stevens MJ, Edmonds ME, Foster AVM, et al. Selective neuropathy and preserved vascular responses in the diabetic Charcot foot. *Diabetologia* 1992;35:148–154.

CHAPTER 11

Erectile Dysfunction as an Indicator of Vascular Disease

Dana A. Ohl and Susanne A. Quallich

Key Points

- Erectile dysfunction is highly prevalent in the general population, and much more common in the vascular disease patient.
- Erectile dysfunction may be an early symptom of cardiovascular disease, and many men presenting with erectile dysfunction are found to have cardiovascular disease risk factors.
- The nitric oxide/cyclic guanosine monophosphate (cGMP) system is extremely important in generating the penile smooth muscle relaxation that is responsible for blood trapping during erection.
- Inhibition of the type 5 phosphodiesterase (PDE5) enzyme in penile tissue leads to increased levels of cGMP and prolonged smooth muscle relaxation.
- The PDE5 inhibitors sildenafil, vardenafil, and tadalafil are safe and effective in improving erectile function in men with widely varying etiologies of erectile dysfunction.
- PDE5 inhibitors can be safely used in vascular patients as long as pretreatment evaluation suggests low general cardiac risk.

INTRODUCTION

Male erectile dysfunction (ED) is an extremely common problem (1) and may have far-reaching effects on the self-esteem and relationships of those involved. Despite these facts, the overall incidence of erectile dysfunction is both underrecognized and underreported, as questions regarding sexual health may be overlooked or neglected during a routine examination. A large number of men suffer from erectile dysfunction, estimated by some studies to be 30 million in the United States alone. The worldwide incidence of ED is projected to rise to 322 million by 2025 (2). Because of discomfort on the part of patients to discuss this problem with their physicians due to embarrassment or other reasons, and lack of willingness on the part of physicians to include questions regarding sexual function during the patient encounter, only a small percentage of these men are being diagnosed and treated.

Historically, treatments for erectile dysfunction have been invasive, cumbersome, or ineffective. The search for a highly effective oral agent for the treatment of this condition has been difficult. Although there is a basis in folklore (3) and more recently in medical studies (4) of the aphrodisiac and erectogenic properties of the herbal remedy yohimbine, the real efficacy of this drug in the treatment of ED has been questioned (5,6). Many other oral agents, usually natural supplements, have been professed in the lay literature to be effective, but lack supportive double-blind, placebo-controlled studies. Lack of effective oral agents is also a contributing factor to patient unwillingness to seek treatment for erectile dysfunction.

The development of phosphodiesterase type 5 (PDE5) inhibitors for the treatment of erectile dysfunction heralded a new era for this condition. With effective and noninvasive therapy available, patient acceptance of the condition, and a significant increase in public awareness of the condition, more men are being treated now than in the past.

In this chapter, we review the basic physiology of erection, including the relationship of the nitric oxide/cGMP system and endothelial function to the process of penile tumescence. We then discuss the epidemiology of erectile dysfunction in patients with vascular disease and/or vascular risk factors. Urological treatments are briefly discussed, but most of the treatment explanations are of the newer oral therapies. Finally, cardiac safety of the PDE5 inhibitors and safety of initiating sexual dysfunction treatment in the cardiac patient are reviewed.

NORMAL PHYSIOLOGY OF ERECTION

Penile erection is a complex process, dependent on psychogenic, hormonal, neural, arterial, and penile tissue factors. Coordination of all of these processes is essential for normal erectile function.

The function of the brain in the penile erection process is poorly understood. It appears that the medial preoptic and anterior hypothalamic regions integrate information to initiate this function. Serotonin and noradrenaline inhibit sexual function, whereas dopamine augments both sexual drive and penile erection (7). The central excitatory effects of dopamine are the basis for the development and testing of sublingual apomorphine, a D2 receptor agonist, for the treatment of erectile dysfunction (8).

The peripheral neural input into the erectile process is via pelvic parasympathetics arising from sacral levels two through four and traveling in the pelvic nerve. The cavernous nerves leading to the penis course very close to the prostate before entering the penile tissue, which explains the propensity for injury to these nerves and erectile dysfunction from pelvic surgery (9). Sympathetic fibers responsible for the reversal of penile erection (detumescence) arise from the thoracolumbar junction and also travel to the penis via the cavernous nerves (10). In the penile tissue, the final neurotransmitter control is complex, and may involve acetylcholine, vasoactive intestinal peptide, neuropeptide Y, as well as the most important neurotransmitter, nitric oxide (NO; discussed later) (10).

Under the appropriate neural stimulation, vascular changes result in erection. The minimal baseline arterial flow during the flaccid state due to baseline adrenergic tone (11) markedly increases to allow penile filling. Diseases that limit an increase in arterial flow, such as atherosclerosis in the penile vascular bed, lead to arteriogenic erectile dysfunction (12). Increase in penile size and intrapenile blood trapping, however, are also dependent on proper penile tissue physiology.

The central function leading to normal blood trapping is smooth muscle relaxation in the lacunar spaces of the corpora cavernosa. Such smooth muscle relaxation allows increased size of the penis due to increased capacity to hold blood and blood trapping, which is due to the ability of the expanded tissue mass to compress the venules that drain the penile tissue. Failure of corporal smooth muscle relaxation leads to failure of blood trapping and the syndrome of venoocclusive dysfunction or "venous leak" erectile dysfunction (13).

This central function of smooth muscle relaxation in the corpus cavernosum is dependent on the NO/cyclic guanosine monophosphate (cGMP) pathway.

Nitric Oxide/Cyclic GMP System and Role of Phosphodiesterases

The important role of NO in penile erection was described by several investigators in the early 1990s (14–16). Nitric oxide synthase (NOS) catalyzes the conversion of L-arginine to NO and citrulline (17). Both neuronal nitric oxide synthase (nNOS) in nitrergic neurons and endothelial NOS (eNOS) in endothelial cells of the lacunar spaces appear to be important sources of NO in normal penile tissue (18). In the case of endothelial dysfunction associated with vascular disease or vascular risk factors, production of NO by eNOS may be deficient.

Liberation of NO in the penile tissue activates guanylate cyclase to convert GTP to cGMP. The presence of cGMP leads to calcium flux out of the cell, with the decreased intracellular calcium level ultimately leading to corporal smooth muscle relaxation (19). Other pathways leading to smooth muscle relaxation are present in penile tissue, but their importance appears to be less than the NO/cGMP system.

Cyclic nucleotides are inactivated by phosphodiesterase (PDE) enzymes, which convert them to the noncyclic nucleotide, thus ending their biological activity. There are 11 families of PDE enzymes, characterized by their substrate of action, types of inhibitors, and response to calmodulin. The major PDE present in the penile corporal tissue is type 5, which is cGMP specific and is inhibited by zaprinast and sildenafil. Types 2, 3, and 4 are also present in the penile tissue, but to a much lesser extent.

PDE6 is present in the retina of the eye and has a role in color vision processing. The newly discovered PDE11 enzyme family is present in skeletal muscle, cardiac myocytes, pituitary gland, and testis, including the germ cells. The function of PDE11 and effects of its inhibition are unknown. PDE5 is also found in vascular smooth muscle, platelets, and other smooth muscles in the body (20).

ERECTILE DYSFUNCTION AS AN INDICATOR OF VASCULAR DISEASE

Erectile dysfunction is defined as the inability to attain and/or maintain an erection sufficient for satisfactory sexual activity (21). Two points need to be stressed regarding this statement. First, the term erectile dysfunction should be used instead of the older term impotence because it is more descriptive and less derogatory. Second, patients and their partners presenting with ED will have different expectations about what satisfactory sexual activity is for them. Within medical reason, physicians should try to help their patients/couples achieve their personal goals with treatment, rather than try to define a treatment endpoint that fits all cases.

There are many similarities between vascular smooth muscle and penile tissue physiology. Endothelium, specifically nitric oxide production from endothelium, plays an important role in erectile function. Factors that cause endothelial dysfunction lead to both systemic vascular disease and erectile dysfunction. Furthermore, the cavernosal arteries are subject to the same stressors as the remainder of the cardiovascular system, and suffer the same detrimental effects of hypertension, smoking, hypercholesterolemia, and poorly managed diabetes. Atherosclerotic lesions in the penile arteries causing stenosis and impaired flow can prevent the ability of the penile arteries to fill the tissue, leading to arteriogenic ED. Because the penile arteries are very small and require a marked increase in flow to perform their function, ED may be the first manifestation of developing systemic arterial disease.

Vascular disease is one of the most common causes of organic ED. It is conceivable that a diagnosis of vasculogenic ED can be considered a predictor of increased risk for developing other forms of vascular disease. If this is true, bringing the problem of ED to the forefront in a routine fashion in all medical interactions may, in fact, allow for a diagnosis of a potentially serious generalized vascular condition. In other words, it is conceivable that ED is an early indicator of otherwise subclinical vascular disease. The literature supports this contention.

In one study of 1,276 men presenting to an andrology clinic for evaluation of erectile dysfunction, basic ED testing revealed the presence of ED-associated significant medical conditions in 57% of cases. These included hypertension (12.4%), cardiac disease (9.2%), dyslipidemia (11.9%), and diabetes (15.5%). Many of these risk factors were diagnosed in men previously unaware of their conditions (21).

The risk factors that contribute to an increased incidence of ED are the same factors that contribute to increased incidence of vascular disease and cardiac morbidity and mortality: hypertension, diabetes mellitus, dyslipidemia, smoking, and obesity. Virag et al. showed that as the number of vascular risk factors increased, so did the degree of penile vascular impairment (22). Feldman et al. demonstrated in the longitudinal portion of the Massachusetts Male Aging Study (MMAS) that development of ED during the several-year follow-up was associated with smoking, and obesity, and (to a smaller extent) hypertension and high-fat diet (23). Modification of risk factors may affect the rate of development of ED in those at risk. Derby et al. reported that exercise, even if started in mid-life, may have an important role in decreasing the risk for ED (24).

Monitoring the severity of a patient's ED offers another way to monitor the progression of his vascular disease. In a 2001 study, Burchardt et al. showed that ED in patients with hypertension was a significant marker for cardiovascular complications as well as an indicator for overall psychosocial functioning (25).

In general, establishing a precise cause for a particular patient's ED will have little impact on the course of treatment. The value of a thorough evaluation instead lies in the ability to diagnose cardiovascular risk factors in patients who have not been diligent in receiving care from a primary care physician or cardiologist and only present to the doctor when a troublesome symptom (ED) arises.

We now discuss the relationship of ED to specific vascular risk factors.

Erectile Dysfunction and Hypertension

Many epidemiologic studies have shown that not only does ED coexist with hypertension, but that as the severity of hypertension increases, so do patient reports of ED severity. Traditional thought attributed erectile difficulties to atherosclerotic lesions in the hypogastric bed coupled with decreased flow through the penile arteries. This has changed with the recognition of the role of cavernosal relaxation in the process of erection. Burchardt et al. found an ED prevalence of 70% in a survey mailed to patients with hypertension (26). Interestingly, this study showed that the duration of hypertension did not affect the risk of ED or its severity (26).

There has long existed a debate contrasting the effects of hypertension on erectile function with those of hypertensive medications contributing to ED (27). Many patients report the onset of ED after beginning antihypertensive medications, and this creates a new treatment challenge in compliance with the medical plan. Many older antihypertensives, such as ganglion blockers, could cause ED from a neurogenic source, but with modern medication, the reason for development of symptoms is not clear. This is demonstrated by calcium channel blockers, which have been implicated in ED. Verapamil, when injected directly into the penile tissue, is capable of causing a partial erection (28). Why, then, should systemic verapamil cause ED?

The answer most likely lies in the fact that antihypertensive agents simply lower the perfusion pressure in the penile arteries. Jensen et al. found that men whose ED was suspected to be caused by antihypertensive medication had fewer arteries visible on penile Doppler ultrasound (27). This is theorized to be due to atherosclerotic lesions developed because of hypertension. At hypertensive perfusion pressures, enough blood entered the penis to cause erection, but flow was inadequate at normotensive blood pressures (27). By this reasoning, any antihypertensive medication can "cause" ED simply due to the fact that it lowers blood pressure.

Conversely, lowering of the blood pressure may improve endothelial function, blunting such an adverse event. Guay et al. suggested that lowering of the blood pressure to normotensive range along with reducing other cardiovascular risk factors may result in improved success rates in treating men with oral ED therapy (29).

Erectile Dysfunction and Smoking

The precise cause of erectile dysfunction in men who smoke is not well understood, but appears to involve both long-term structural changes in arteries (atherosclerosis) and functional changes in the smooth muscle relaxation of the vascular endothelium. This may be the result of impaired nitric oxide synthase, and may have resulting long-term effects on the health of the corporal tissue (30). ED can result from either direct smoking or passive exposure to cigarettes (second-hand smoke). Smoking is associated with a twofold increase in the risk of ED (23,30). Possible mechanisms for smoking-induced ED include impairment of endothelial-dependent smooth muscle relaxation, increased sympathetic tone, alteration of fibrinogen levels, increased platelet aggregation, and increasing risk of vasospasm.

In one study, up to 86% of chronic smokers were found to have abnormal penile vascular function (31). Klein et al. reported that as the number of pack-years smoked increased, so did the incidence of ED (32). A synergy exists between smoking and other risk factors for cardiovascular disease that increases the risk of ED. Data from the MMAS support this conclusion, and show that age is a less important correlate of ED than other cardiovascular risk factors (33).

A history of smoking is more common in men reporting ED than in the general population (30) and is likely to be due to the increased incidence of atherosclerotic plaques that have been reported in the internal pudendal and common penile arteries in young smokers with erectile complaints (34). Alterations to lipid metabolism from smoking may be a significant contributing factor in development of vessel disease.

A few studies have shown that there is some degree of reversibility of ED with smoking cessation. The results appear to be confined to younger men with no or few other existing cardiovascular risk factors. In one study, within 1 month of smoking cessation, both penile rigidity and tumescence improved (35). In contrast, subjects in the longitudinal portion of the MMAS were not able to alter their risk of development of ED by smoking cessation. Perhaps the lack of effect is age related, as all men participating in the MMAS were greater than 40 years of age at study beginning (24). This underscores the importance of early identification and intervention with men who evidence lifestyle choices that are known risk factors for both ED and vascular disease. It may be possible to slow or even reverse (in some populations) the progression of erectile dysfunction.

Erectile Dysfunction and Dyslipidemia, Coronary Disease, and Atherosclerosis

It has been shown that there is a clear relationship between the number of occluded coronary vessels and the severity of patient-reported ED (36). Erectile dysfunction often predates a diagnosis of coronary artery disease by a significant period of time. Given the specialized arterial supply of the penis and corpora cavernosa and their small diameters, it is likely that these arteries may manifest atherosclerotic changes early in the natural history of the disease.

Penile vascular studies have shown that patients with a history of myocardial infarction or vascular risk factors (smoking, hypertension) suffer from impairment of the penile vascular system (37). Plaque formation contributes to erectile difficulties through several mechanisms: narrowing pelvic and penile arteries, damaging endothelial and corporal tissues, and causing poor compliance and venous leak. Patients

with atherosclerotic disease also suffer from endothelial dysfunction, which predates the formation of plaques (38) and provides an additional parallel association between cardiovascular disease and ED.

In an animal model, erectile function that has been impaired by atherosclerotic lesions has been improved with dietary modifications or the prescription of lipid-lowering agents (39). These same animal models showed that the extent of the atherosclerotic lesions extended to the cavernosal sinusoids.

Erectile Dysfunction and Diabetes

The incidence of ED in diabetic men has been estimated to be between 35% and 75% (39,40). Diabetic men have a three-fold greater incidence of ED, and it often occurs at an earlier age, in many cases predating the diagnosis of diabetes (33). Sairam et al. investigated a population of 127 men with self-reported ED, and found the prevalence of undiagnosed diabetes mellitus to be 4.7%, with another 12% showing evidence of impaired glucose tolerance (41). This study also showed that the simple urine dipstick test missed 80% of patients with elevated serum glucose (41). This resulted in the conclusion that in men presenting with ED, a fasting blood glucose level should be part of the routine evaluation to investigate their potential for occult diabetes (41).

Studies have shown that there exists a correlation between poor glycemic control and erectile dysfunction (42), with the obvious suggestion that the onset of ED may be delayed or prevented by improved glycemic control. This further underscores the need to identify occult diabetes in men presenting with new-onset ED so that their entire future course may be altered.

Investigators have shown an association between erectile dysfunction in diabetic male patients and age, retinopathy, nephropathy, poor glycemic control, smoking, alcohol intake, peripheral neuropathy, pharmacologic treatment for diabetes, and autonomic neuropathy. ED in diabetes results from multifactorial causes (43), including large vessel disease, diabetic neuropathy, and microscopic changes in the corporal tissue. Diabetic men with ED demonstrate impaired neurogenic- and endothelium-dependent relaxation in the corpus cavernosum (39). As a result, nitric oxide levels are diminished in the cavernosal tissue of diabetic men (39,42).

Erectile Dysfunction and Obesity

Many studies have established that obesity is a clear risk factor for the development of a variety of conditions, including diabetes, hypertension, and atherosclerotic disease. Because obesity commonly coexists with a sedentary lifestyle, obese men may also have a decreased exercise tolerance, creating a higher risk for cardiac events when under any type of physiological stress.

Several authors have reported a direct association between obesity and erectile difficulties. Derby et al. reported that in a follow-up of 593 men in the MMAS with an average 8-year follow-up, obesity at initiation of the study led to a higher incidence of ED at the study's conclusion, and a sedentary lifestyle at the conclusion of the study also indicated a higher prevalence of ED (24).

Obesity, defined as a body mass index (BMI) of greater than 30 kg per m² for men (overweight=BMI ≥28 kg per m²), can contribute to ED by several mechanisms. The obese male, because of his increased percentage of body fat, may suffer decreased erectile function and loss of libido due to the conversion of testosterone to estradiol in fatty tissue (44). In addition, up to 80% of obese adults have one medical condition and 40% have two conditions associated with development of ED, such as hyperlipidemia, diabetes, and hypertension (45).

DIAGNOSIS AND TREATMENT OF ERECTILE DYSFUNCTION

Diagnostic Evaluation

The diagnostic evaluation of erectile dysfunction may lead to the discovery of underlying conditions that put the patient at risk for development of cardiovascular disease. It is the potential discovery of these risk factors that gives the main value to specific evaluation of ED etiology. A patient who has occult vascular disease or vascular risk factors may be helped by specific testing to define a vascular etiology of his ED, as improvement in his general health may result. However, by the time many patients seek treatment for ED, in our current medical environment, such conditions have already been diagnosed and managed by their primary care physicians and/or cardiologists. In this circumstance, rather then carefully diagnosing the condition, we may begin a treatment plan directly when presented with the symptoms. The reason for not pursuing a complete diagnostic battery of tests is that the information is rarely useful in determining a course of action.

For instance, although it is tempting to consider microsurgical penile revascularization when confronted with a patient whose specific testing demonstrates arteriogenic which appear bypassable, this operation is only performed in a rare circumstance. This would be in young men with arterial trauma as the etiology of their ED. In these cases, return of normal erectile function may be seen in 75% of those undergoing microsurgical penile revascularization (46). In young trauma victims with ED, specific testing can be justified.

However, arteriogenic ED is more commonly seen in association with cardiovascular risk factors and in older men. Results of penile revascularization are particularly poor in men over 50 years of age and in those with diabetes mellitus and/or generalized atherosclerosis. Because the results of surgery are so poor, this is not a treatment option for these men. Taking this a step further, if surgery is not going to be performed, then data from an arteriogram or other invasive testing are not necessary, and one has to question the wisdom of performing such tests when the information will not be used for practical purposes.

Available diagnostic testing modalities include the following: *nocturnal penile tumescence (NPT) monitoring,* in which sleep-related erections are monitored, with a normal test indicating absence of vascular disease, and most probably a psychogenic basis for the ED; *duplex ultrasonography of the penile vessels with pharmacologic erection,* which involves examining the changes in flow velocities of the cavernosal arteries after injection of a vasoactive agent known to cause erection in men with normal vascular physiology (prostaglandin E1 or papaverine/phentolamine); one can screen for both arterial inflow disease as well as corporal venocclusive dysfunction with duplex ultrasound; *cavernosometry/cavernosography,* an invasive test to measure the ability of penile tissue to trap blood, by measuring its ability to trap infused saline under pharmacologic stimulation; and phalloarteriography (Fig. 11.1), an arteriogram of the penile vessels; in those men considered candidates for

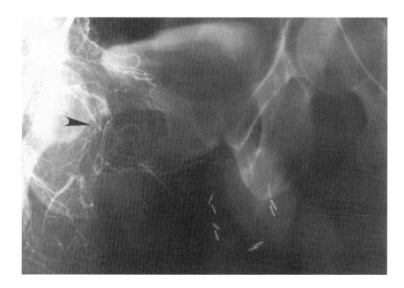

FIG. 11.1. A penile arteriogram in a man with vasculogenic erectile dysfunction. The *arrow* points to an area of narrowing in the blood supply to the penis.

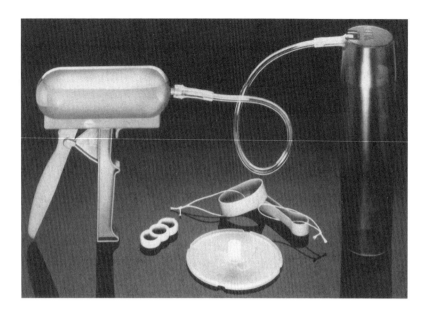

FIG. 11.2. Vacuum constriction device used for erectile dysfunction. The hand pump evacuates air from the cylinder to draw blood into the penis. A variety of bands may be used to keep the blood in the penis.

penile revascularization, an arteriogram is essential to determine a surgical route for bringing more blood into the penis.

To reiterate, although often testing will not be performed, it may be beneficial to perform some or all of the tests just mentioned to allow the treating physician to assess a patient's risk for hitherto undiagnosed vascular disease.

Nonoral Erectile Dysfunction Therapies

Usually patients progress from the least invasive treatments to the more invasive options. Initial attempts at improving erection usually involve the use of oral PDE5 inhibitors, which is discussed in detail in the next section. There are, however, many patients who will not respond to oral agents, and thus become candidates for referral to a urologist. It is important to have a cursory understanding of the other options for treatment of ED that the urologist may offer, for proper preparation and counseling of patients.

Intraurethral administration of prostaglandin E1 (PGE1) can produce an erection following transfer to the corpus cavernosum, by activating the production of cAMP system in penile tissue. An erection is produced in about 40% of subjects attempting this treatment (47). Higher efficacy (80%) is seen by direct *intrapenile injection of PGE1* into the corpus cavernosum (48). With both of these methods, the most common adverse event seen is penile pain (35% to 40% of men). Priapism (prolonged erection) can be seen after penile injection, but is very rare with the intraurethral method. Agents other than PGE1, such as papaverine and phentolamine, have been used alone and in combination for penile injection therapy, but these have not been approved by the U.S. Food and Drug Administration for this use.

For individuals who do not respond to oral or more invasive pharmacologic treatments, mechanical solutions to create an erection are possible. An external vacuum device (Fig. 11.2) placed over the penis can draw blood into the cavernosal bodies, and a constriction band placed at the base of the penis can trap the blood, leading to an erection-like state suitable for intercourse (49). Satisfaction rates from such vacuum-erection devices approximate 50%. Complaints include discoloration of the penis, change in temperature, pain with ejaculation, and loss of erection with time.

The most invasive treatment option for ED is the penile prosthesis (50). These surgically implanted devices vary in design from semirigid rods to fully inflatable models (Fig. 11.3). Satisfaction rates from the inflatable penile prosthesis is greater than 90% for both patients and their partners. The most worrisome adverse event from the implantation surgery is infection, which may lead to loss of the implant.

Phosphodiesterase Inhibitors for Erectile Dysfunction

The ability of type 5 PDE inhibitors to augment penile tissue function is due to their ability to make favorable changes in penile tissue chemistry that promote cavernosal smooth muscle relaxation. As discussed previously, when stimulation of penile erection occurs in a normal man, NO is released by endothelium and nitrergic neurons, leading to production of cGMP, calcium flux, and smooth muscle relaxation, which leads to blood trapping. The effect of cGMP is neutralized by conversion of cGMP to the inactive noncyclic nucleotide by type 5 PDE. In the presence of a PDE5 inhibitor, binding of cGMP to the enzyme is markedly inhibited, and without binding, the cGMP cannot be degraded. This causes increased levels of cGMP in the penile tissue and therefore prolongation of the downstream effects, ultimately leading to augmentation of the smooth muscle relaxation and an increase in blood trapping (20).

In men with ED, one or more of the components of the system may be insufficient, and erection therefore does not

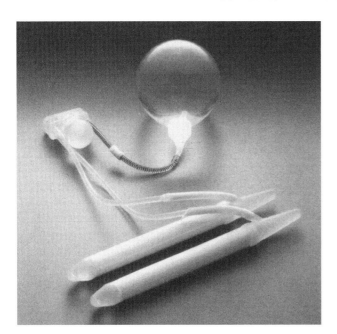

FIG. 11.3. Three-piece inflatable penile prosthesis. There are two cylinders, a pump and a reservoir. The patient activates the scrotal pump to draw fluid from the reservoir to inflate the cylinders and create an erection. The process is then reversed to cause detumescence.

develop. Some men will suffer a lack of production of nitric oxide due to penile tissue endothelial dysfunction or microneuropathy. For these individuals, PDE5 inhibition may specifically address the pathophysiology. However, even those men with the inability to fill the penis with blood, such as in those with arterial inflow disease, PDE5 inhibitors have the ability to increase blood trapping, optimizing the use of whatever blood is able to be delivered, and these inhibitors have demonstrated efficacy in this patient population.

Despite the favorable effects of PDE5 inhibition on the penile tissue, these agents do not *initiate* an erection. Rather, normal mechanisms of activating the NO/cGMP are required to initiate production of cGMP. The PDE5 inhibitor then will augment the effect of these normal mechanisms. Theoretically, then, these drugs should work better in men with partial function than in men with complete lack of ability to initiate an erection. One might also theorize that the drug should work less well in men with a neurogenic source of their problem, such as men with complete cavernous nerve transection during radical prostatectomy, and severe diabetic neuropaths, who have lost the ability to initiate a response. Subgroup analysis of large clinical studies supports these theories.

Sildenafil

Sildenafil was the first PDE5 inhibitor developed for the treatment of ED. It is available in tablets as the drug Viagra (Pfizer), the citrate salt of sildenafil, in 25-, 50-, and 100-mg doses. After oral administration, it is rapidly absorbed, with absolute bioavailability of 40%. Peak serum levels in healthy

volunteers are reached from 30 minutes to 2 hours, with a mean of 1 hour. Fat in the gastrointestinal tract may limit rapidity of absorption speed, delaying the onset of action. The half-life of the drug is 4 hours, and with single daily dosing, there is no accumulation of the drug. It is hepatically metabolized by the cytochrome P450 system, and may have interactions with cimetidine, erythromycin, and protease inhibitors. Lower doses or increased intervals need to be considered with concomitant use of sildenafil with these medications. In addition, in men with hepatic dysfunction or severe renal impairment, the action of the drug may also be prolonged (20).

Sildenafil is highly specific for PDE5. It has been shown to have a mean 50% inhibitory concentration (IC_{50}) of 3.5 nM. It is highly specific for PDE5 when compared to the other PDE inhibitors, and has some slight affinity for PDE6, with an IC_{50} around nine times that of sildenafil (51). This weak affinity for PDE6 is responsible for the low rate of transient disordered color vision.

Although initially developed and tested as an antianginal agent, it was reasoned that there may be beneficial effects on penile tissue chemistry. In the early studies in cardiac patients, it became apparent that this theoretical effect was real, with subjects in those studies reporting the "side effect" of improved potency.

Early studies were performed in the clinic setting to collect objective data supporting the efficacy of sildenafil in augmenting erectile responses. In 1996, Boolell et al. reported that sildenafil caused objective improvement in the ability to maintain an erection as measured by the RigiScan tumescence monitoring device (52). Price et al. reported similar results in a series of diabetic men (53).

These early studies were promising for the use of sildenafil in the clinical treatment of ED, and led to development of phase III multicenter, randomized, placebo-controlled studies, which were performed on a global basis. These rigorous studies were carried out in men with ED defined by the National Institutes of Health consensus conference (53a). The International Index of Erectile Function (IIEF) was used extensively in these studies to determine efficacy. The IIEF has been validated as an accurate and reproducible method of assessing several domains of sexual function (54). IIEF questions 3 (assessing the ability to *obtain* an erection sufficient for penetration) and 4 (assessing the ability to *maintain* an erection following penetration) were primary endpoints in most studies. Scores for each IIEF question range from 1 (indicating nearly absent or absent function) to 5 (indicating nearly always or always present function). A global efficacy question regarding improvement in erections and patient diaries were also recorded. The design of the early sildenafil studies has served as a model for virtually all subsequent studies of this and other PDE5 inhibitors.

Goldstein et al. reported results of two large cooperative U.S. studies for the Sildenafil Study Group (55). The first was a fixed-dose study of 532 men with ED randomized to receive either placebo or 25-, 50-, or 100-mg doses of sildenafil. The mean age of subjects was 57 to 60 years, and approximately 30% had hypertension and 15% had diabetes mellitus. Sildenafil at all doses was markedly better than placebo in improving IIEF scores. For IIEF question 3, the percentage changes from baseline scores for placebo and 25-mg, 50-mg, and 100-mg doses were 5%, 60%, 84% and 100%, respectively. For IIEF question 4, the increases over baseline were 24%, 121%, 133%, and 130%, respectively. Finally, at the end of the 24-week study, improved erections were noted by 25% of men taking placebo versus 56%, 77%, and 84% of men taking 25, 50, and 100 mg of sildenafil, respectively (55).

The dose-escalation portion of the U.S. Sildenafil Study Group included 329 men with ED, and was patterned to predict what would happen in a clinical setting in which physicians may change dosages of medications based on clinical response. Patients were randomized to receive either placebo or 50 mg of sildenafil and increased or decreased dosage based on effectiveness and adverse events. This study also showed significant superiority over placebo for all primary and secondary endpoints (55).

Worldwide, studies have verified the conclusions of these initial large studies (56,57). A recently published comprehensive summary of sildenafil studies details the excellent efficacy seen in all patient populations tested, including those with existing heart disease and those with cardiovascular risk factors (58).

In general, 70% to 78% of men report improvement in erections with sildenafil compared to 20% to 25% of men taking placebo. Most men increase dosage of the drug to 100 mg, with very few decreasing dosage for adverse events. Efficacy appears to be maintained long term, with very stable efficacy over open-label extension studies. Long-term data in open extensions suggest that erections continue to be improved in 99.8% for initial responders, and satisfaction with the treatment is seen in 95.1% of subjects taking the drug for 3 years (58).

Adverse events in sildenafil trials tended to be relatively minor and rarely were a cause for discontinuation of treatment (59). These are listed in Table 11.1.

Vardenafil

At the time of this writing, the PDE5 inhibitor vardenafil (Levitra; Bayer/GlaxoSmithKline) has been launched in Europe and is in final regulatory review by the U.S. Food and Drug Administration. It is being tested at 5-, 10-, and 20-mg doses. Absorption may be slightly more rapid than that of sildenafil, with peak plasma concentrations reached at 0.7 hour, and the half-life may be slightly longer, at 4 to 4.8 hours (60). The half-life may be as long as 6 hours in older patients. Because it is degraded by the cytochrome P450 system, the same drug interactions as sildenafil should be noted.

Vardenafil is a more potent inhibitor of PDE5 than sildenafil, with an IC_{50} for this enzyme of 0.7 nmol per L, as compared with 6.6 nmol per L for sildenafil. There may also be less inhibition of PDE6 when compared to sildenafil (see later discussion). Theoretically, this should translate into less chance of a change in color vision with vardenafil. This has been confirmed in clinical trials.

Porst et al. studied greater than 600 men in a phase 2 investigation (61). Vardenafil 20 mg improved erection in 80% of the participants. Participants were successful in greater than 70% of intercourse attempts. His group also noted effectiveness in all etiologies of ED, and the drug was well tolerated, even in men taking antihypertensive medications (61).

The large North American phase 3 trial of vardenafil was recently published (62). This was a fixed-dose, randomized, placebo-controlled trial of 5, 10, and 20 mg of vardenafil versus placebo. Study design followed the usual pattern, with IIEF questions 3 and 4, Sexual Encounter Profile, and Global Assessment Question as the endpoints. Vardenafil was very significantly superior to placebo in all endpoints measured. At week 24 of the study, 80.7% of those taking 20 mg of vardenafil noted improvement of erection, compared to 22.9% taking placebo. The percentage of intercourse attempts that resulted in successful vaginal penetration was 81.1% for 20 mg of vardenafil and 51.9% for placebo. At the lower dose of vardenafil, the improvement was somewhat less, but still superior to placebo. Table 11.2 lists adverse events reported in this study.

Tadalafil

Tadalafil (Cialis; Lilly ICOS) is a PDE5 inhibitor that is approved for use in Europe, but is still waiting for approval from the U.S. Food and Drug Administration. Doses of 2.5,

TABLE 11.1. *Most commonly reported treatment-related adverse events during placebo-controlled sildenafil studies[a]*

Adverse event	Sildenafil	Placebo
Headache	14.6%	3.3%
Facial flushing	14.1%	1.9%
Dyspepsia	6.2%	0.7%
Dizziness	2.2%	1.1%
Rhinitis	2.6%	0.2%
Abnormal vision	5.2%	0.3%

[a]See ref. 59.

TABLE 11.2. *Adverse events in North American Pivotal Trial of vardenafil at highest dose[a]*

Adverse event	Vardenafil 20 mg	Placebo
Headache	21%	4%
Rhinitis	17%	5%
Cutaneous flushing	13%	0%
Dyspepsia	6%	1%
Sinusitis	5%	1%
Accidental injury	4%	3%
Flu syndrome	2%	1%

[a]See ref. 62.

5, 10, and 20 mg have been investigated. After oral administration of tadalafil, the peak serum concentration is reached in 2 hours. The half-life of the drug is 17.5 hours, leading to a much longer time period of effectiveness. The IC_{50} for PDE5 is higher than that of sildenafil. Tadalafil does not interact with the other PDE enzymes, families 1 through 4 and 6 through 10. However, the IC_{50} for PDE11 is only fivefold higher than that of PDE5, allowing for the potential of cross-reactivity with PDE11 (20).

Tadalafil has undergone clinical testing in men presenting with ED. Porst reported on 179 men randomized to 2, 5, 10, or 25 mg of tadalafil or placebo (63). Again, design of the study was similar to the original sildenafil trials. Total erectile function domain scores on the IIEF (maximum score 30) at study end were 19.3, 22.9, 23.6, and 24.2, respectively, with increasing doses of tadalafil, compared to 14.7 with placebo. The increases were statistically significant for all groups. Erections were improved by the treatment in 51.4%, 59.5%, 80.6%, and 80.6%, respectively, at increasing doses, compared to 17.1% for placebo (63).

Brock et al. performed an integrated analysis of five double-blind, placebo-controlled randomized trials of tadalafil 2.5, 5, 10, and 20 mg (64). There were 1,112 men randomized in the various studies examined, and tadalafil was significantly more effective than placebo in improving erectile function. Increased efficacy of tadalafil was seen with increasing dose of the drug. At the highest dosage range, the mean improvement of the IIEF erectile dysfunction domain (maximum score of 30) was 7.9, compared to 0.6 with placebo. The percentage of intercourse attempts carried to completion was 70% with 20 mg of tadalafil, compared to 31% with placebo. Erections were deemed improved in 81% of men receiving tadalafil 20 mg, compared to 35% on placebo. Table 11.3 lists adverse events related to tadalafil.

Comparison of PDE5 Inhibitors

From the foregoing discussion, it is clear that although the PDE5 inhibitors all have the same goal in therapy, that of inhibition of the PDE5 enzyme in the penile tissue, there are some differences in the agents. The differences have been described in detail in the excellent review article by Corbin and Francis (20). Some of these differences are noted in Tables 11.4 and 11.5.

TABLE 11.3. Adverse events in integrated tadalafil studies at highest two doses[a]

Adverse event	Tadalafil 20 mg	Tadalafil 10 mg	Placebo
Headache	21%	12%	6%
Dyspepsia	17%	9%	2%
Back pain	9%	6%	5%
Rhinitis	5%	6%	4%
Myalgias	7%	5%	2%
Vasodilation	5%	3%	2%

[a]See ref. 64.

TABLE 11.4. Differences in potency and pharmacokinetic properties of phosphodiesterase type 5 inhibitors[a]

Parameter[b]	Sildenafil 100 mg	Vardenafil 20 mg	Tadalafil 20 mg
IC_{50} (nM)	3.5	0.1	6.7
C_{max} (ng/mL)	560	209	378
T_{max} (h)	0.8	0.7	2.0
$T_{1/2}$ (h)	3.7	3.9	17.5

[a]See ref. 20.

[b]IC_{50}, Mean inhibitory concentration for phosphodiesterase type 5; C_{max}, peak plasma concentration; T_{max}, time to C_{max}; $T_{1/2}$, half-life of the agent.

First, there are different potencies in inhibitions of the enzyme among the drugs. Vardenafil is the most potent, as demonstrated by the lowest IC_{50}, the concentration at which the PDE5 enzyme is 50% inhibited. Next most potent is sildenafil, followed by tadalafil. One must keep in mind, however, that potency in inhibiting an enzyme in the laboratory does not necessarily translate into *in vivo* effects, as rate of absorption, bioavailability, rate of elimination, and protein binding are all factors that may affect function in the nonlaboratory setting.

There are pharmacokinetic differences as well. Sildenafil and vardenafil reach peak plasma concentrations in a little less than 1 hour, and perhaps up to 1 hour in several studies. Tadalafil reaches peak plasma concentrations at about 2 hours. The half-lives of sildenafil and vardenafil are similar at around 4 hours, with vardenafil having a somewhat longer half-life in some studies. Tadalafil, on the other hand, has a half-life of 17.5 hours, and even longer in elderly subjects. One can surmise that there may be advantages or disadvantages to this longer presence. It could be argued that the longer half-life simplifies the administration of the drug, with less planning needed for the sexual activity. Conversely, if there are adverse events, the longer duration of the drug may prolong the danger of the side effect. In addition, more

TABLE 11.5. Differences in selectivity of phosphodiesterase type 5 inhibitors (20)[a]

Agent	PDE5	PDE6 (rod)	PDE6 (cone)	PDE11
Sildenafil	3.5	37	34	2730
	(1)	**(11)**	**(10)**	**(780)**
Vardenafil	0.14	3.5	0.6	162
	(1)	**(25)**	**(4)**	**(1,160)**
Tadalafil	6.74	1260	1300	37
	(1)	**(187)**	**(193)**	**(5)**

[a]Results on the top line for each agent are the values of mean inhibitory concentration (IC_{50}) for each of the phosphodiesterase (PDE) enzymes listed. The bold numbers on the bottom are the ratios of the IC_{50} for each enzyme to that for sildenafil. The higher the ratio, the less affinity there is for the enzyme, and the more selective the drug is for PDE5. All agents have virtually no affinity for other families of PDE enzymes not listed here.

continuous levels may theoretically lead to tachyphylaxis or change in regulation of the PDE enzymes themselves. Those espousing this theory would argue that a short-acting agent, such as sildenafil or vardenafil, might be safer because the drug is effectively gone within 12 hours.

There are some selectivity differences noted in Table 11.5. Although all the compounds are highly selective for PDE5 inhibition, there is some affinity for other PDE enzyme families. As noted previously, sildenafil has only tenfold selectivity for PDE5 over PDE6, which is present in the retina, and this is most likely responsible for the disordered color vision seen in some patients. Vardenafil has been stated to have greater selectivity for PDE5 over PDE6, but some studies (see Table 11.5) note a difference between cone and rod enzymes. However, no distorted color vision has been reported in vardenafil studies. Both sildenafil and vardenafil have virtually no affinity for the other PDE families.

Tadalafil shows excellent selectivity for PDE5 when compared to families 1 through 4 and 6 through 10. However, there is only a fivefold selectivity for PDE5 over the newly discovered PDE11 enzyme. The function of PDE11 is not known, but it has been localized in skeletal muscle, cardiac muscle, pituitary gland, and testis, including sperm cells (65). Because the function is not known, we also do not know what will result from inhibition of PDE11.

As far as clinical comparisons go, it is important to realize that at the time of this writing, no direct study to compare efficacies of the different drugs has been performed. Until such direct comparative data are available, we cannot make any comment on which drug may be the preferred agent.

Cardiovascular Safety of PDE5 Inhibitors

The adverse effects of PDE5 inhibitors, save for any cross-reactivity with other PDE families, is due to systemic inhibition of the PDE5 enzyme. This enzyme is present in high levels in the penile smooth muscle, and this allows effect from the oral agent while limiting systemic effects. However, the enzyme is also present in other tissue. For instance, there is PDE5 in the gastroesophageal sphincter, and a PDE5 inhibitor may cause relaxation of the sphincter, reflux, and dyspepsia, which have been seen in the clinical studies (see Tables 11.1 through 11.3).

Type 5 PDE is present in penis, vascular smooth muscle, including pulmonary bed, platelets, and visceral smooth muscle (66). In the vasculature, the effect of these agents is smooth muscle relaxation, causing vasodilation. This gives rise to the most commonly reported adverse events, headache and flushing. These can be bothersome, but certainly not dangerous. However, systemic vasodilation may give rise to changes in cardiovascular physiology that may cause unfavorable changes. We next discuss the evidence for cardiovascular safety of the PDE5 inhibitors. Because most of the clinical data concern sildenafil, most of the data presented here are gleaned from studies of that drug. This does not imply that the other drugs are unsafe, and conversely does not imply that sildenafil results can be generalized to the other drugs. The data are simply not available.

Several studies the of the hemodynamic effects of sildenafil on normal volunteers and men with ischemic heart disease were reported by Jackson et al. (67). Eight healthy volunteers were given intravenous infusions of placebo or 20, 40, or 80 mg of sildenafil. There was a small but statistically significant decrease in blood pressure of between 7 and 9 mm Hg at the two higher doses. There was no difference in orthostatic changes in heart rate or blood pressure between placebo and drug.

The effect of oral sildenafil doses ranging from 50 to 200 mg (twice the highest recommended clinical dose) was tested in eight volunteers. Peak plasma levels were reached in 0.8 to 0.9 hour, and mild blood pressure decreases of 7 to 10 mm Hg were seen, which returned to baseline within 6 hours. No orthostatic changes were seen. In both the oral sildenafil challenge and the intravenous challenge, increasing doses of sildenafil were associated with increasing plasma levels of cGMP, suggesting that inhibition of degradation of cGMP derived from the systemic vascular bed is the cause of the mild hypotension (67). These small changes in blood pressure observed after intravenous or oral administration of the drug appear to be clinically insignificant.

Finally, both invasive and noninvasive cardiac testing in eight men with ischemic heart disease was performed both before and after sildenafil infusion. There was a mild drop in blood pressure and cardiac output, but no change in response to exercise was noted, and heart rate was not affected. There were no clinically relevant changes in electrocardiogram, and no adverse events were noted from the infusion (67).

Because of the potential interaction of sildenafil and organic nitrates due to each drug's relationship to the NO/cGMP pathway in the systemic vascular smooth muscle, data regarding this interaction should be reviewed. In a randomized crossover design, 12 men were administered oral sildenafil 25 mg or placebo three times daily for 4 days to achieve steady-state plasma concentrations (68). On day 4, the subjects received an intravenous infusion of glycerol trinitrate with progressively increasing dose until hypotension was seen. On day 5, a sublingual nitroglycerine tablet was given 1 hour after a sildenafil or placebo dose. Participants were significantly less tolerant of nitrate infusion when taking sildenafil. Decreases in systolic blood pressure after administration of sublingual nitroglycerine were four times greater with sildenafil than placebo. Only single-digit blood pressure drops were seen with concomitant administration of the calcium channel blocker amlodipine (68), which were similar to those seen in the Jackson et al. studies (67).

Other antihypertensive agents seem safer. There are several reports that the incidence of adverse events in sildenafil patients is not different between those taking no antihypertensive medications and those taking different classes of agents or multiple drugs (69–71).

Padma-Nathan et al. reviewed extensive data from pooled studies of sildenafil, both placebo-controlled and open-label design, from premarketing to 4 years postapproval of the drug (59). Pooled data from 35 placebo-controlled studies gave the rates of adverse events listed in Table 11.1. When examining the patient population of 5,918 subjects, it was noted that a large percentage of those individuals had vascular disease or vascular risk factors. There were 1,328 men with diabetes, 1,582 with hypertension, and 582 with documented ischemic heart disease. The rates of treatment-related adverse events were similar to those in the total patient population and those with vascular risk factors. Discontinuation rates due to adverse events were 1.9% in diabetics, 2.3% in hypertensive patients, and 3.6% in those with ischemic heart disease, compared to 2.0% for the general population. Discontinuation rate in the placebo group was 2.3% (59).

In the 4-year summary data, the rate of adverse events in patients taking one, two, or three classes of antihypertensive therapy were compared to that of patients not on antihypertensive therapy; the incidence of treatment-related adverse events was similar among all groups (59).

Zusman et al. reviewed the overall cardiovascular safety of sildenafil in placebo-controlled studies (72). To the time of that publication in 1999, there were 693 patient-years exposure to sildenafil in placebo-controlled studies, 4,220 patient-years in open-label studies, and 349 patient-years of placebo exposure. The incidences of serious cardiovascular events are noted in Table 11.6, which demonstrates that there is no difference in subjects taking sildenafil or placebo. Furthermore, the death rate for all sildenafil subjects was 0.53 per 100 patient-years, compared to 0.57 per 100 patient-years for those taking placebo (72).

Padma-Nathan et al. updated similar information in 2002, and these data are shown in tabular form in Table 11.7. When comparing sildenafil to placebo in controlled studies, there is no difference in the rate of myocardial infarction or all-cause mortality. In open-label studies, the rate of events is even lower (59). Clearly from these data, it appears that sildenafil is safe.

More detailed information regarding effects of sildenafil on patients with documented coronary disease has been recently forthcoming. Herrmann et al. examined the hemodynamic effects of sildenafil in men with severe coronary disease, and found small decreases in peripheral and pulmonary arterial pressures, but no changes in heart rate, cardiac output, and coronary flow reserve (73). Several treadmill studies have

TABLE 11.7. *Incidence of myocardial infarction and all-cause mortality in sildenafil studies*[a]

Outcome examined	N	Events per 100 patient-years
Myocardial infarction		
Placebo	949	0.95
Sildenafil (double-blind)	1644	0.85
Sildenafil (open-label)	10,859	0.53
Sildenafil, total	12,503	0.58
All-cause mortality		
Placebo	949	0.53
Sildenafil (double-blind)	1644	0.55
Sildenafil (open-label)	10,859	0.34
Sildenafil, total	12,503	0.37

[a]See ref. 59.

been performed recently showing no difference between patients administered sildenafil or placebo in rates of angina, time to limiting, and electrocardiogram changes (74,75).

Treatment of Erectile Dysfunction in Cardiac Patients

There is concern in treating patients with ED that this may create an increased risk for cardiac events. This concern arises from two issues. The first is drug toxicity, such as hypotension created by administration of a PDE5 inhibitor. This, as the foregoing data should suggest, is the lesser concern. The other concern is that the exertion related to sexual activity will incite a cardiac event. It has been estimated that relative risk of a myocardial infarction is 2.5 times baseline within 2 hours of sexual activity (76).

Several consensus panels have been convened to examine ED treatment guidelines in patients at risk for cardiovascular events. The most quoted is the Princeton Consensus Panel, which was a multidisciplinary group of cardiologists, internists, urologists, and others (77). The panel suggested that patients be stratified into low-, intermediate-, and high-risk categories. Description of the Princeton Consensus Panel's classification and recommendations for each follows.

Low-risk patients have controlled hypertension, mild and stable angina, successful coronary revascularization, previous uncomplicated infarction, mild cardiac valve disease, or no symptoms but less than three cardiovascular risk factors. The recommendation is that these patients may receive treatments for ED and may resume sexual activity.

High-risk patients include those with unstable angina, uncontrolled hypertension, class III or IV heart failure, recent (less than 2 weeks) infarction, high-risk arrhythmias, obstructive cardiomyopathies, or moderate to severe valvular disease. These patients should not receive treatment for ED and should not attempt sexual activity until treatment changes their cardiac condition to a safer stratification.

Intermediate-risk patients have moderate angina, infarction 2 to 6 weeks old, class II heart failure, low-risk arrhythmias, or three or more cardiovascular risk factors. Prior to initiating sexual activity or treatment for ED, these patients

TABLE 11.6. *Incidence of serious cardiovascular events in phase II and III sildenafil studies*[a,b]

	Placebo	Sildenafil, PC	Sildenafil, open-label
Serious events	4.9	3.9	2.3
Myocardial infarction	1.4	1.7	0.7
Stroke	0.9	0.4	0.3

[a]See ref. 72.
[b]Incidence reported as events per 100 patient-years of exposure; PC, administered during placebo-controlled studies.

should undergo more evaluation with subsequent treatment to improve their situation or to restratify them to low risk.

It is important to reiterate that because of the interaction between organic nitrates and PDE5 inhibitors, any patient taking long-acting nitrates or at risk for requiring sublingual nitroglycerin is not a candidate for this class of drugs. Most of the data regarding nitrate safety have been obtained with sildenafil, but all drugs in this class should be considered contraindicated with nitrates. Studies are ongoing to determine the minimum time between a PDE5 inhibitor administration and nitrate administration that could be safe, but, pending results from such studies, it is best to avoid coadministration.

REFERENCES

1. Laumann EO, Paik A, Rosen RC. Sexual dysfunction in the United States: prevalence and predictors. *JAMA* 1999;281:537–544.
2. Ayta, IA, McKinlay, JB, Krane, RJ. The likely worldwide increase in erectile dysfunction between 1995 and 2025 and some possible policy consequences. *BJU Int* 1999;84:50–56.
3. Guirguis WR. Oral treatment of erectile dysfunction: from herbal remedies to designer drugs. *J Sex Marital Ther* 1998;24:69–73.
4. Ernst E, Pittler MH. Yohimbine for erectile dysfunction: a systematic review and meta-analysis of randomized clinical trials. *J Urol* 1998;159:433–436.
5. Teloken C, Rhoden EL, Sogari P, et al. Therapeutic effects of high dose yohimbine hydrochloride on organic erectile dysfunction. *J Urol* 1998;159:122–124.
6. Montague DK, Barada JH, Belker AM, et al. Clinical Guidelines Panel on Erectile Dysfunction: summary report on the treatment of organic erectile dysfunction. The American Urological Association. *J Urol* 1996;156:2007–2011.
7. Andersson KE, Wagner G. Physiology of penile erection. *Physiol Rev* 1995;75:191–236.
8. Heaton JWP, Morales A, Adams MA, et al. Recovery of erectile function by the oral administration of apomorphine. *Urology* 1995;45:200–206.
9. Lue TF, Zeineh SJ, Schmidt RA, et al. Neuroanatomy of penile erection: its relevance to iatrogenic impotence. *J Urol* 1984;131:273–280.
10. Chuang AT, Steers WD. Neurophysiology of penile erection. In: Carson CC, Kirby RS, Goldstein I, eds. *Texbook of erectile dysfunction.* Oxford: Isis Medical Cedia, 1999:60.
11. Hedlund H, Andersson KE. Comparison of the responses to drugs acting on adrenoreceptors and muscarinic receptors in human isolated corpus cavernosum and cavernous artery. *J Auton Pharmacol* 1985;5:81–88.
12. Cormio L, Edgren J, Lepantalo M, et al. Aortofemoral surgery and sexual function. *Eur J Vasc Endovasc Surg* 1996;11:453–457.
13. Aboseif SR, Lue TF. Hemodynamics of penile erection. *Urol Clin N Am* 1988;15:1–7.
14. Rajfer J, Aronson WJ, Bush PA, et al. Nitric oxide as a mediator of relaxation of the corpus cavernosum in response to nonadrenergic, noncholinergic neurotransmission. *N Engl J Med* 1992;326:90–94.
15. Burnett AL, Lowenstein CJ, Bredt DS, et al. Nitric oxide: a physiologic mediator of penile erection. *Science* 1992;257:401–403.
16. Burnett AL. Nitric oxide in the penis: physiology and pathology. *J Urol* 1997;157:320–324.
17. Palmer RM, Ferrige AG, Moncada S. Nitric oxide release accounts for the biological activity of endothelium-derived relaxing factor. *Nature* 1987;327:524–526.
18. Rajasekaran M, Mondal D, Agrawal K, et al. *Ex vivo* expression of nitric oxide synthase isoforms (eNOS/iNOS) and calmodulin in human penile cavernosal cells. *J Urol* 1998;160:2210–2215.
19. Ignarro LJ, Bush PA, Buga GM, et al. Nitric oxide and cyclic GMP formation upon electrical field stimulation cause relaxation of corpus cavernosum smooth muscle. *Biochem Biophys Res Commun* 1990;170:843–850.
20. Corbin JD, Francis SH. Pharmacology of phosphodiesterase-5 inhibitors. *Int J Clin Pract* 2002;56:453–459.
21. NIH Consensus Development Panel on Impotence. NIH Consensus Conference. Impotence. *JAMA* 1993;270:83–90.
21a. Hatzichristou D, Hatzimouratidis K, Bekas M, et al. Diagnostic steps in the evaluation of patients with erectile dysfunction. *J Urol* 2002;168,615–620.
22. Virag R, Bouilly P, Frydmand D. Is impotence an arterial disorder? A study of arterial risk factors in 440 impotent men. *Lancet* 1985;1:181–184.
23. Feldman HA, Johannes CB, Derby CA, et al. Erectile dysfunction and coronary risk factors: prospective results from the Massachusetts Male Aging Study. *Prevent Med* 2000;30:328–338.
24. Derby CA, Mohr BA, Goldstein I, et al. Modifiable risk factors and erectile dysfunction: Can lifestyle changes modify risk? *Urology* 2000;56:302–306.
25. Burchardt M, Burchardt T, Baer L, et al. (2001). Erectile dysfunction is a marker for cardiovascular complications and psychosocial functioning in men with hypertension. *Int J Impot Res* 2001;13:276–281.
26. Burchardt M, Burchardt T, Baer L, et al. Hypertension is associated with severe erectile dysfunction. *J Urol* 2000;164:1188–1191.
27. Jensen J, Lendorf A, Stimpel H, et al. The prevalence and etiology of impotence in 101 male hypertensive outpatients. *Am J Hypertens* 1999;12:271–275.
28. Brindley GS. Pilot experiments on the actions of drugs injected into the human corpus cavernosum penis. *Br J Pharmacol* 1986;87:495–500.
29. Guay AT, Perez JB, Jacobson J, et al. Efficacy and safety of sildenafil citrate for treatment of erectile dysfunction in a population with associated organic risk factors. *J Androl* 2001;22:793–797.
30. McVary KT, Carrier S, Wessells H. Smoking and erectile dysfunction: Evidence based analysis. *J Urol* 2001;166:1624–1632.
31. Shabsigh R, Fishman IJ, Schum C, et al. Cigarette smoking and other vascular risk factors in vasculogenic impotence. *Urology* 1991;38:227–231.
32. Klein R, Klein BE, Lee KE, et al. Prevalence of self-reported erectile dysfunction in people with long-term IDDM. *Diabetes Care* 1996;19:135–141.
33. Feldman HA, Goldstein I, Hatzichristou DG, et al. Impotence and its medical correlates: results of the Massachusetts Male Aging Study. *J Urol* 1994;151:54–61.
34. Rosen MP, Greenfield AJ, Walker TG, et al. Cigarrette smoking: an independent risk factor for atherosclerosis in the hyogastric-cavernous arterial bed of men with arteriogenic impotence. *J Urol* 1991;145:759–763.
35. Guay AT, Perez JB, Heatley GJ. Cessation of smoking rapidly decreases erectile dysfunction. *Endocrine Pract* 1998;4:23–26.
36. Greenstein A, Chen J, Miller H, et al. Does severity of ischaemic coronary disease correlate with erectile dysfunction? *Int J Impot Res* 1997;9:123–126.
37. Chung WS, Shim BS, Park YY. Hemodynamic insult by vascular risk factors and pharmacologic erection in men with erectile dysfunction: Doppler sonographic study. *World J Urol* 2000;18:427–430.
38. Kirby M, Jackson G, Betteridge J, et al. Is erectile dysfunction a marker for cardiovascular disease? *Int J Clin Pract* 2001;55:614–618.
39. Sullivan ME, Keoghane SR, Miller MAW. Vascular risk factors and erectile dysfunction. *BJU Int* 2001;87:838–845.
40. Hakim LS, Goldstein I. Diabetic sexual dysfunction. *Endocrinol Metab Clin N Am* 1996;25:379–400.
41. Sairam K, Kulinskaya E, Boustead GB, et al. Prevalence of undiagnosed diabetes mellitus in male erectile dysfunction. *BJU Int* 2001;88:68–71.
42. De Angelis L, Marfella MA, Siniscalchi M, et al. Erectile dysfunction and endothelial dysfunction in type II diabetes: a possible link. *Diabetologia* 2001;44:1155–1160.
43. Richardson D, Vinik A. Etiology and treatment of erectile failure in diabetes mellitus. *Curr Diabetes Rep* 2002;2:501–509.
44. Vermeulen A, Kaufman JM, Goemaere S, et al. Estradiol in elderly men. *Aging Male* 2002;5:98–102.
45. Meuleman EJH. Prevalence of erectile dysfunction: need for treatment? *Int J Impot Res* 2002;14[Suppl 1]:S22–S28.
46. Ohl DA, Goldstein I: Vasculogenic impotence. In Ernst CE, Stanley JC, eds. *Current therapy in vascular surgery.* New York: Springer-Verlag, 2000:413–418.

47. Padma-Nathan H, Hellstrom WJG, Kaiser FE, et al. Treatment of men with erectile dysfunction with transurethral alprostadil. Medicated Urethral System for Erection (MUSE) Study Group. *N Engl J Med* 1997;336:1–7.

48. Linet OI, Ogrinc FG. Efficacy and safety of intracavernosal alprostadil in men with erectile dysfunction. The Alprostadil Study Group. *N Engl J Med* 1996;334:873–877.

49. Levine LA, Dimitriou RJ. Vacuum constriction and external erection devices in erectile dysfunction. *Urol Clin N Am* 2001;28:335–341.

50. Anastasiadis AG, Wilson SK, Burchardt M, et al. Long-term outcomes of inflatable penile implants: reliability, patient satisfaction and complication management. *Curr Opin Urol* 2001;11:619–623.

51. Ballard SA, Gingell CJ, Tang K, et al. Effects of sildenafil on the relaxation of human corpus cavernosum tissue *in vitro* and on the activities of cyclic nucleotide phosphodiesterase isozymes. *J Urol* 1998;159:2164–2171.

52. Boolell M, Gepi-Attee S, Gingell JC, et al. Sildenafil, a novel effective oral therapy for male erectile dysfunction. *Br J Urol* 1996;78:257–261.

53. Price DE, Gingell JC, Gepi-Attee S, et al. Sildenafil: study of a novel oral treatment for erectile dysfunction in diabetic men. *Diabet Med* 1998;15:821–825.

53a. National Institutes of Health. NIH Consensus Conference 1993.

54. Rosen RC, Riley A, Wagner G, et al. The international index of erectile function (IIEF): a multidimensional scale for assessment of erectile dysfunction. *Urology* 1997;49:822–830.

55. Goldstein I, Lue TF, Padma-Nathan H, et al. Oral sildenafil in the treatment of erectile dysfunction. Sildenafil Study Group. *N Engl J Med* 1998;338:1397–1404.

56. Hartmann U, Meuleman E, Cuzin B, et al. Sildenafil (Viagra): analysis of preferred doses in a European, 6-month, double-blind, placebo-controlled, flexible dose-escalation study in patients with erectile dysfunction. *Int J Impot Res* 1998;10 [Suppl]:S34.

57. Montorsi F, McDermott TE, Morgan R, et al. Efficacy and safety of fixed-dose oral sildenafil in the treatment of erectile dysfunction of various etiologies. *Urology* 1999;53:1011–1018.

58. Carson CC, Burnett AL, Levine LA, et al. The efficacy of sildenafil citrate (Viagra) in clinical populations: an update. *Urology* 2002;60:12–27.

59. Padma-Nathan H, Eardley I, Kloner RA, et al. A 4-year update on the safety of sildenafil citrate (Viagra). *Urology* 2002;60[suppl]:67–90.

60. Klotz T, Sachse R, Heidrich A, et al. Vardenafil increases penile rigidity and tumescence in erectile dysfunction patients: a RigiScan and pharmacokinetic study. *World J Urol* 2001;19:32–39.

61. Porst H, Rosen R, Padma-Nathan H, et al. The efficacy and tolerability of vardenafil, a new, oral, selective phosphodiesterase type 5 inhibitor, in patients with erectile dysfunction: the first at-home clinical trial. *Int J Impot Res* 2001;13:192–199.

62. Hellstrom WJG, Gittelman M, Karlin G, et al. Vardenafil for treatment of men with erectile dysfunction: efficacy and safety in a randomized, double-blind, placebo-controlled trial. *J Androl* 2002;23:763–771.

63. Porst H. IC351 (tadalafil, Cialis): update on clinical experience. *Int J Impot Res* 2002;14[Suppl]:S57–S64.

64. Brock GB, McMahon CG, Chen KK, et al. Efficacy and safety of tadalafil for the treatment of erectile dysfunction: results of integrated analyses. *J Urol* 2002;168:1332–1336.

65. Fawcett L, Baxendale R, Stacey P, et al. Molecular cloning and characterization of a distinct human phosphodiesterase gene family: PDE11A. *Proc Natl Acad Sci USA* 2000;97:3702–3207.

66. Corbin JD, Francis SH. Cyclic GMP phosphodiesterase-5: target of sildenafil. *J Biol Chem* 1999;274:13729–13732.

67. Jackson G, Benjamin N, Jackson N, et al. Effects of sildenafil citrate on human hemodynamics. *Am J Cardiol* 1999;83:13C–20C.

68. Webb DJ, Freestone S, Allen MJ, et al. Sildenafil citrate and blood-pressure-lowering drugs: results of drug interaction studies with an organic nitrate and a calcium antagonist. *Am J Cardiol* 1999;83:21C–28C.

69. Zusman R, Collins M. Effect of sildenafil on blood pressure in men with erectile dysfunction taking concomitant antihypertensive medications. *J Am Coll Cardiol* 1999;32[Suppl]:238A.

70. Prisant M, Brown M. Sildenafil citrate: well-tolerated by patients with erectile dysfunction taking concomitant antihypertensive therapy. *Am J Hypertens* 1999;12[Suppl]:10A–11A.

71. Kloner R, Brown M. *Safety of sildenafil citrate in men with erectile dysfunction taking multiple antihypertensive agents.* Presented at the 14th annual scientific meeting of the American Society of Hypertension, New York, 1999.

72. Zusman RM, Morales A, Glasser DB, et al. Overall cardiovascular profile of sildenafil citrate. *Am J Cardiol* 1999;83:35C–44C.

73. Herrmann HC, Chang G, Klugherz BD, et al. Hemodynamic effects of sildenafil in men with severe coronary artery disease. *N Engl J Med* 2000;342:1622–1626.

74. Patrizi R, Leonardo F, Pelliccia F, et al. Effect of sildenafil citrate upon myocardial ischemia in patients with chronic stable angina in therapy with beta-blockers. *Ital Heart J* 2001;2:841–844.

75. Arruda-Olson AM, Mahoney DW, Nehra A, et al. Cardiovascular effects of sildenafil during exercise in men with known or probable coronary artery disease: a randomized crossover trial. *JAMA* 2002;287:719–725.

76. Muller JE, Mittleman A, Maclure M, et al. Triggering myocardial infarction by sexual activity. Low absolute risk and prevention by regular physical exertion. Determinants of Myocardial Infarction Onset Study Investigators. *JAMA* 1996;275:1405–1409.

77. DeBusk R, Drory Y, Goldstein I, et al. Management of sexual dysfunction in patients with cardiovascular disease: recommendations of the Princeton Consensus Panel. *Am J Cardiol* 2000;86:175–181.

CHAPTER 12

The Management of Hyperlipidemia and Exercise Therapy in the Treatment of Peripheral Arterial Disease

James J. Maciejko

Key Points

- Atherosclerosis is a diffuse, inflammatory/immune disease affecting primarily large and medium-size muscular arteries.
- Risk factor modification and exercise training are essential components in the management of patients with peripheral arterial disease (PAD).
- Lipid management should be an integral part of the treatment of PAD.
- Lipids are transported via three pathways: exogenous (dietary), endogenous, and reverse cholesterol transport.
- Apolipoproteins direct the metabolic fate of lipoprotiens.
- Elevated lipoprotein(a) is an independent predictor of atherosclerotic cardiovascular disease risk.
- Classes of lipid-lowering agents include statins, niacin, fibrates, resins, and intestinal cholesterol absorption inhibitors.
- The prescription of fluvastatin or rosuvastatin to a patient on warfarin may increase the effect of both drugs.
- Niacin is the only lipid-lowering agent that reduces lipoprotein(a) plasma concentrations.
- Exercise training is superior to medications (i.e., pentoxifylline and cilostazol) for improving maximal walking distance in patients with PAD.

INTRODUCTION

Atherosclerotic peripheral arterial disease (PAD) of the lower extremities is a major clinical problem in most industrialized nations. The presentation varies depending on rate of progression, presence and extent of collateral circulation, activity of the patient, and comorbidities. PAD is commonly associated with coronary artery and cerebral vascular diseases, indicating that the underlying cause, atherosclerosis, is not a focal disease, but rather a diffuse, inflammatory/immune disease involving both large and medium/sized muscular arteries. It is estimated that approximately 8 to 10 million individuals in the United States have PAD (1).

The modifiable risk factors for PAD are the same as those for coronary heart disease (CHD). These risk factors include hyperlipidemia, smoking, hypertension, diabetes mellitus and insulin resistance, hyperhomocysteinemia, obesity, physical inactivity, and personality type. Although several of these risk factors have statistical associations with future atherosclerotic events, many have not yet been established as causally related to the atherosclerotic process. These factors are more appropriately called risk indicators or disease predictors, whereas those factors where causality has been established are better termed risk factors (2). Modification of established risk factors and a walking (exercise) program are the cornerstones of therapy for patients with PAD. The established risk factors are cigarette smoking, diabetes mellitus, hypertension, and abnormalities in lipid metabolism.

Lipid disorders are an important risk factor for CHD and all other types of atherosclerotic cardiovascular disease (ASCVD). Intervention with diet and medications to reduce low-density lipoprotein-cholesterol (LDL-C) concentrations have proven to decrease the risk of future coronary events, stroke, and total mortality in patients with established (CHD) (3–5). Reducing LDL-C concentrations among individuals without clinical evidence of CHD also significantly lowers the risk of developing a coronary heart event (6–7). A large, major clinical trial that demonstrated the relevance of lipid management among patients with PAD (with or without CHD) was the Heart Protection Study (8).

The Heart Protection Study determined that the long-term impact of lipid management among patients with PAD significantly improved all-vascular and nonvascular mortality, and major morbidity outcomes. Of the 20,536 participants in this trial, 2,701 had diagnosed PAD without CHD or other vascular disease. Following 5 years of lipid management with a statin, a highly significant 25% reduction ($p<0.001$) in all vascular events was noted compared to the placebo participants. The Heart Protection Study was the first placebo-controlled, large-scale interventional trial demonstrating the benefit of lipid management for reducing the risk of all clinical ASCVD events in patients with PAD. This study emphasized that lipid management should be an integral part of the treatment program for all individuals with PAD (8).

LIPID AND LIPOPROTEIN METABOLISM

The effective management of patients with lipid abnormalities requires a working knowledge of lipoprotein metabolism. The plasma lipoproteins are macromolecular complexes that constitute the functional units for the transport of hydrophobic lipids in the blood. The major lipoprotein lipids include cholesteryl ester, triglyceride, and phospholipid. Free cholesterol, which makes up only 3% of the total cholesterol concentration in plasma, is located primarily on the surface of lipoproteins. Lipoproteins from normal individuals are classified according to their densities into five major classes: chylomicrons, very low density lipoproteins (VLDL), intermediate-density lipoproteins (IDL), low-density lipoproteins (LDL), and high-density lipoproteins (HDL). The physical and chemical characteristics of the major plasma lipoproteins are presented in Table 12.1

The protein components of lipoproteins are called apolipoproteins. Apolipoproteins, along with free cholesterol and phospholipid, form the outer shell of lipoproteins. Apolipoproteins allow for the structural integrity of lipoproteins, and also play the more important role of directing the metabolic fates of lipoproteins. Several apolipoproteins serve as ligands for lipoprotein receptors, others are cofactors for activating enzymes involved in the metabolism of the lipids within lipoproteins, and still others are important in the cellular internalization of a lipoprotein and the regulation of intracellular lipid synthesis. Normal plasma concentrations, distribution, and major functions for the apolipoproteins are provided in Table 12.2.

Lipoproteins transport lipids to various sites in the body via three pathways: exogenous (dietary) lipid transport, endogenous lipid transport, and reverse cholesterol transport (Figs. 12.1 and 12.2). The exogenous lipid transport pathway is the movement of dietary lipid from the intestine throughout the body and ultimately to the liver. The endogenous lipid transport pathway is the transport of lipids synthesized in the liver to peripheral tissues, and reverse cholesterol transport is the removal of cholesterol from peripheral cells, with subsequent delivery to the liver.

Exogenous Pathway

Dietary fatty acids and monoglycerides, along with dietary and biliary cholesterol, are incorporated into micelles in the intestinal lumen by the action of bile acids. The micelle structure allows intestinal lipid to be absorbed from the lumen into intestinal enterocytes. Fatty acids and monoglycerides are absorbed by passive diffusion, whereas cholesterol is delivered into the enterocyte by a process involving a cholesterol transport protein located in the brush border of the enterocytes lining the lumen of the small intestine. Cholesterol delivered into the enterocyte is subsequently attached to a fatty acid by the enzyme acyl coenzyme A:cholesterol acyltransferase$_2$ (ACAT$_2$), forming cholesteryl ester. This esterification reaction traps cholesterol inside the enterocyte, and prevents it

TABLE 12.1. *Classification and physical–chemical characteristics of plasma lipoproteins[a]*

Lipoprotein[a]	Density (g/mL)	Lipid composition (%)[b]			Protein (%)	Diameter (nm)	Electrophoretic mobility
		C	TG	PL			
Chylomicron	<0.95	5	90	3	2	80–1200	Origin
VLDL	0.95–1.006	20	60	10	10	30–80	Pre-beta
IDL	1.006–1.019	40	35	10	15	23–35	Broad beta
LDL	1.019–1.063	50	5	20	25	18–25	Beta
HDL	1.063–1.21	25	5	25	45	5–12	Alpha

[a]VLDL, very low density lipoprotein; IDL, intermediate-density lipoprotein; LDL, low-density lipoprotein; HDL, high-density lipoprotein.
[b]C, The sum of esterified and free cholesterol; TG, triglyceride; PL, phospholipid.

TABLE 12.2. *The major plasma apolipoproteins*

Apolipoprotein (Apo)	Major lipoprotein affiliation[a]	Function[b]	Normal plasma concentration (mg/dL)
Apo A-I	HDL	Ligand for HDL binding, cofactor for LCAT	140
Apo A-II	HDL	Modulator of LPL and HEL activities	40
Apo A-IV	HDL	Unknown	—
Apo B-48	Chylomicron	Ligand for hepatic remnant receptor (?)	—
Apo B-100	LDL	Ligand for LDL receptor	90
Apo C-I	VLDL	LPL activator	7
Apo C-II	VLDL	LPL activator	5
Apo C-III	VLDL	LPL inhibitor	15
Apo D	HDL	LCAT activator (?), fatty acid facilitator (?)	10
Apo E	Chylomicron, VLDL, IDL, LDL	Ligand for hepatic LDL and LRP receptors	12
Apo(a)	Lp(a)	Structural component for Lp(a)	5

[a]HDL, High-density lipoprotein; LDL, low-density lipoprotein; VLDL, very low density lipoprotein; IDL, intermediate-density lipoprotein; Lp(a), lipoprotein(a).

[b]LCAT, Lecithin:cholesterol acyltransferase; LPL, lipoprotein lipase; HEL, hepatic endothelial cell lipase; LRP, LDL receptor-related protein.

from being pumped back out into the lumen of the intestine. The passively absorbed fatty acids and monoglycerides are reassembled into triglycerides within the enterocyte. The cholesteryl ester, triglyceride, apolipoprotein (apo) B-48, and other apolipoproteins (e.g., A-I, A-II, C-II, C-III, E) are then packaged together in the enterocyte to form triglyceride-rich lipoproteins called chylomicrons. The enterocytes secrete chylomicrons into terminal lymphatics, which transport them into larger and larger lymph vessels, and ultimately into the thoracic duct. From the thoracic duct, the chylomicrons enter the systemic circulation.

As chylomicrons travel through the blood stream, they enter into the capillary beds of tissues and organs, where they undergo catabolism by the enzyme lipoprotein lipase (LPL) (Fig. 12.1). LPL is present on the surface of capillary endothelial cells and requires apo C-II as a cofactor for activation. The principal sites of LPL activity are skeletal muscle, adipose tissue, mammary glands, and the myocardium. LPL hydrolyzes core triglycerides, releasing fatty acids, which either attach to albumin or are taken up by neighboring cells. Several of the surface components (e.g., apolipoproteins, free cholesterol, phospholipid) of chylomicrons are released

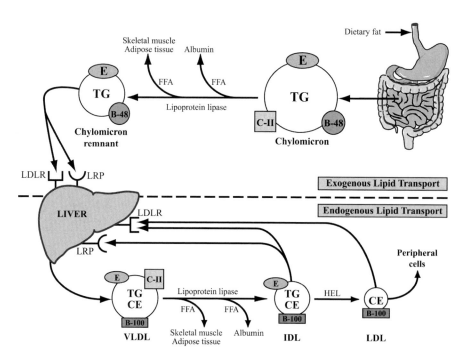

FIG. 12.1. Exogenous and endogenous lipid transport. E, apoE; B-48, apoB-48; C-II, apoC-II, B-100, apoB-100; FFA, free fatty acids; LDLR, low-density lipoprotein (LDL) (apoB/E) receptor; LRP, LDL receptor-related protein; TG, triglyceride; CE, cholesteryl ester; VLDL, very low density lipoprotein; IDL, intermediate-density lipoprotein; HEL, hepatic endothelial cell lipase.

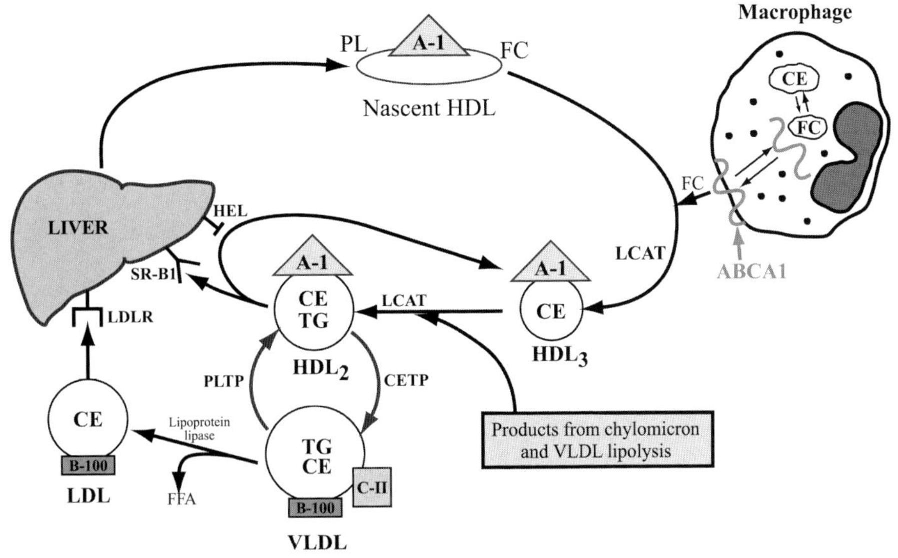

FIG. 12.2. Reverse cholesterol transport. PL, phospholipid; FC, free cholesterol; CE, cholesteryl ester; TG, triglyceride; LCAT, lecithin:cholesterol acyltransferase; ABCA1, adenosine triphosphate (ATP)-binding cassette transporter A1; CETP, cholesteryl ester transfer protein; PLTP, phospholipid transfer protein; FFA, free fatty acids; LDLR, low-density lipoprotein (LDL) receptor; SR-B1, class B, type I scavenger receptor; HEL, hepatic endothelial cell lipase; HDL, high-density lipoprotein; VLDL, very low density lipoprotein; A-I, apoA-1; B-100, apoB-100; C-II; apoC-II.

during hydrolysis of the triglycerides and transferred to HDLs. The triglyceride-depleted chylomicron remnant is released from LPL and rapidly removed from the circulation by the liver. Approximately 70% of chylomicron remnants are removed from the circulation by hepatic receptors designated as LDL receptor-related protein (LRP), and the remaining 30% are removed by the hepatic LDL receptor (LDLR) or what is also called the apo B/E receptor (9). Both receptors appear to recognize apo E on the remnant surface (10).

Chylomicrons are not normally present in the fasting state (i.e., 12-hour fast) because the plasma half-life of a chylomicron is about 30 minutes. Chylomicronemia may occur as a consequence of the genetic absence of LPL or apo C-II, or because of uncontrolled diabetes mellitus, excess alcohol intake, and estrogen or steroid use. Chylomicronemia is not believed to increase the risk for atherosclerosis, although chylomicron remnants may be atherogenic (11).

Endogenous Pathway

VLDL and LDL accomplish the transport of endogenously (i.e., hepatic) synthesized lipid. Hepatic triglycerides are produced from the assembly of free fatty acids and glycerol, and are incorporated into the cores of VLDLs. The size of VLDL is determined by the amount of triglyceride contained in the lipoprotein. Large, triglyceride-rich VLDLs are secreted in situations of excess triglyceride production, including obesity, excessive alcohol consumption, and hyperglycemia resulting from diabetes mellitus. The fatty acids used to manufacture the triglycerides in VLDL are derived from two primary sources. Either they are delivered to the liver via al-

bumin or the liver synthesizes them. Hepatic lipogenesis is the synthesis of fatty acids from glucose, and this pathway is regulated through the interactions of insulin, glucagon, and somatostatin.

Once in the plasma, the metabolic fate of VLDL is similar to that of the chylomicron (12). VLDLs enter the capillary beds of various tissues, and the core triglycerides undergo hydrolysis by LPL, thereby releasing free fatty acids. Surface components (i.e., apolipoproteins, phospholipid, free cholesterol) separate from the hydrolyzing VLDLs and are transferred to HDLs, and the liberated free fatty acids are taken up by surrounding cells or attach to albumin. Following hydrolysis, the remaining remnant lipoprotein particles are called VLDL remnants or intermediate density lipoproteins (IDLs). Normally, 75% of the VLDL remnants are removed from the circulation by hepatic LDL receptors. Approximately 25% bypass this receptor and undergo further hydrolysis and other compositional changes by the hepatic enzyme hepatic endothelial cell lipase (HEL), and become the cholesteryl ester-rich LDLs, whose sole apolipoprotein is apo B-100 (13).

LDLs transport cholesterol to peripheral cells. LDLs travel throughout the bloodstream to the microcirculatory beds of peripheral tissues, where they cross endothelial cells of capillaries and interact with neighboring cells. LDL is internalized into peripheral cells by binding to the LDL receptor located in coated pit regions of cell membranes (14). Once internalized, the LDL is degraded to free cholesterol, free fatty acids, and amino acids. Cholesterol is used by all cells as a structural component of membranes or can be used by some cells for synthetic purposes—steroidogenesis by adrenal and gonadal cells, and bile synthesis by hepatocytes. Cholesterol internalized through this receptor-mediated pathway also regulates both the rate of intracellular cholesterol biosynthesis and the availability of LDL receptors. Increased free cholesterol within a cell downregulates the production of LDL receptors and reduces the activity of the rate-limiting enzyme for cholesterol biosynthesis, 3-hydroxy-3 methylglutaryl-coenzyme A reductase (HMG-CoA reductase). Downregulation of the LDL receptor occurs through the association of free cholesterol with intracellular proteins that reduce the expression of mRNA in the nucleus for LDL-receptor protein synthesis (15). A cholesterol deficiency in the cell will upregulate the production of LDL receptors and stimulate cholesterol biosynthesis. Through this feedback mechanism, it becomes apparent that LDL receptor activity is the prime regulator of plasma LDL-C concentrations. Low or absent LDL receptor activity increases the plasma LDL-C concentration, and because there is virtually no cholesterol from LDL within the cell to downregulate cholesterol biosynthesis, production of cholesterol, even though it is not needed, increases and adds to the hypercholesterolemia.

Among healthy individuals, about 60% of circulating LDL is removed via LDL receptors on the membranes of hepatocytes and about 20% via these receptors located on the cell membranes of peripheral cells. The remaining 20% of LDL is removed from plasma through nonspecific mechanisms (12). The liver can convert LDL-derived cholesterol to bile salts through the action of bile synthase. Peripheral cells that do not use LDL-derived cholesterol for cell membrane development, or, in the case of certain glands, for steroidogenesis, must rely on the presence of HDL to rid themselves of excess cholesterol (i.e., reverse cholesterol transport).

Reverse Cholesterol Transport

HDLs serve in the reverse cholesterol transport pathway (16). HDLs do not contain apo B; instead they contain apo A-I and apo A-II. HDLs are manufactured primarily by the liver, and to some extent by the small intestine, as nascent lipoproteins. These nascent lipoproteins are flat disks containing free cholesterol, phospholipid, and primarily apo A-I. In the periphery, they interact with a membrane-bound transporter protein, adenosine triphosphate (ATP)-binding cassette transporter A1 (ABCA1) (17–20). This interaction allows for the removal of intracellular cholesterol and phospholipid by an active transport pathway. The current concept is that the interaction of nascent HDLs with ABCA1 initiates the shuttling of this transporter protein between the cell membrane and stored intracellular cholesterol pools (18,19). Arriving at the intracellular cholesterol storage pool, ABCA1 accepts cholesterol and shuttles back to the cell membrane, where the cholesterol is transferred to nascent HDLs. As nascent HDLs acquire cholesterol, they disassociate from the ABCA1 transporter proteins, cross capillary endothelial cells, and reenter the circulation, where the enzyme lecithin:cholesterol acyltransferase (LCAT) esterifies free cholesterol to fatty acids (21). The source of fatty acids is albumin. Apo A-I on the surface of nascent HDL acts as a cofactor for LCAT activation, and the transfer of the free fatty acids from albumin for esterification to free cholesterol is thought to involve apo D (22,23). The esterification results in the formation of cholesteryl esters, which change the structure of the nascent HDLs to round lipoproteins. The cholesteryl esters migrate to the center of the lipoprotein, forming a hydrophobic core with a hydrophilic surface made up mainly of phospholipid and apo A-I. These HDLs are now referred to as HDL_3. HDL_3 may acquire additional lipid through accepting surface lipids from hydrolyzing triglyceride-rich lipoproteins (i.e., chylomicrons and VLDL) or by promoting additional efflux of cholesterol from cholesterol-laden peripheral cells. These additional acquisitions result in larger, more lipid-rich HDLs, referred to as HDL_2 (24). It is presumed that the lipidation of nascent HDL by the ABCA1 transport pathway is necessary for the generation of mature HDL particles (i.e., HDL_3 and HDL_2) and the removal of cholesterol from peripheral cells, including macrophages of the arterial wall (18).

The fate of the lipids in HDL_2, which are primarily cholesteryl esters, involves one of three pathways. Cholesteryl esters of HDL_2 can be transferred by means of plasma cholesteryl ester transfer protein (CETP) to VLDL or LDL in exchange for triglyceride and phospholipid (25). Through this pathway, collected cholesterol from peripheral cells is eventually transported to the liver via LDL. CETP activity tends to be high in conditions associated with high triglyceride and low HDL-C concentrations, whereas low CETP activity is associated with lower triglyceride and higher plasma HDL-C concentrations (26). HDL_2 may also be selectively removed by the liver and adrenal glands. A receptor for this process has been identified on hepatocyte and adrenal cell membranes, and is referred to as class B, type I scavenger receptor (SR-BI) (27,28). Binding of HDL_2 to this receptor internalizes the lipoprotein, removing it and the associated cholesteryl ester from the blood. Finally, HDL_2 may interact with the hepatic enzyme HEL, which catabolizes some of the core lipids in HDL_2, resulting in the conversion of the larger HDL_2 to the smaller HDL_3, which are then returned to the circulation (29). The catabolized lipids enter into the hepatocyte and are ultimately excreted in the bile. Most of the variability in the plasma total HDL-C concentration reflects the HDL_2 concentration.

It is of interest to note that mutations in ABCA1 transporter are responsible for Tangier disease, a rare autosomal recessive disorder characterized by a rapid turnover of plasma apo A-I and severe HDL deficiency (30). Despite the marked deficiency of plasma HDL, atherosclerosis is not generally a feature of Tangier disease.

HDL may also have functions unrelated to reverse cholesterol transport that play a role in its antiatherogenic effect. It is believed that HDL may decrease LDL oxidation and may have other antioxidant functions (31). HDLs also appear to decrease the expression of leukocyte adhesion molecules, which are manifested by dysfunctional vascular endothelial cells (32). HDLs may also promote prostacyclin (PGI_2)

synthesis by vascular endothelial cells through supplying these cells with arachidonic acid (33).

Lipoprotein(a)

Another lipoprotein that has clinical relevance, although not considered a major plasma lipoprotein, is lipoprotein(a), or Lp(a) (34). It is recognized as a strong predictor of CHD risk. It was first described in 1963 as lipoprotein antigen or a genetic variant of LDL. This lipoprotein consists of an LDL particle with an apo (a) attached to it by a disulfide bond. Apo (a) is a unique glycoprotein with protein domains, known as kringles, which have structural homology with plasminogen. Apo (a) contains multiple and variable numbers of kringle domains. Variability in the Lp(a) plasma concentration relates to the molecular weight of apo (a), the number of kringle domains, and differences in its hepatic secretion rate (35,36). The physiological function of Lp(a) is not known. The atherogenicity of Lp(a) may be the result of several suggested mechanisms. Increased plasma concentrations may interfere with fibrinolysis or clot lysis (37–39). Like LDL, Lp(a) can be deposited directly in the arterial wall, promoting atherosclerosis, and increased Lp(a) concentrations have been associated with premature CHD in many studies (40–47). A plasma concentration of Lp(a) of greater than 30 mg/dL is considered to be an independent risk factor for atherosclerotic cardiovascular disease. One might consider measuring Lp(a) in the following circumstances:

- Patient or family history of premature ASCVD
- Familial history of marked hyperlipidemia
- Established ASCVD with a normal routine lipid profile
- Hyperlipidemia refractory to statin or resin therapy
- History of recurrent arterial stenosis (48)

MANAGEMENT OF LIPOPROTEIN DISORDERS

The management of lipoprotein disorders is essential for optimal care of patients with PAD disease. The Heart Protection Study clearly demonstrated that LDL-C reduction among individuals with PAD reduces their risk of all vascular events (i.e., CHD, stroke, and PAD events) (8). Therefore, it is essential to evaluate for lipoprotein disorders in all PAD patients.

The third report of the National Cholesterol Education Program (NCEP) provides updated clinical guidelines for lipid testing and management (49). These guidelines have been widely endorsed by other professional organizations including the American Heart Association and the American College of Cardiology (50). The NCEP guidelines maintain that an elevated LDL-C is a major cause of atherosclerosis, and therefore they identify an elevated LDL-C as the primary target of lipid-lowering therapy. The risk classification of LDL-C concentrations is shown in Table 12.3, which also provides the classifications for HDL-C and triglyceride. An LDL-C concentration ≥160 mg per dL is classified as a high-risk value for atherosclerosis, 130 to 159 mg per dL is borderline, 100 to 129 mg per dL is near or above optimal, and an

TABLE 12.3. *National Cholesterol Education Program Adult Treatment Panel III classification of low-density-lipoprotein cholesterol (LDL-C), high-density-lipoprotein cholesterol (HDL-C), and triglyceride*[a]

LDL-C (mg/dL)	
<100	Optimal
100–129	Near or above optimal
130–159	Borderline high
160–189	High
≥190	Very high
HDL-C (mg/dL)	
<40	Low
≥60	High
Triglyceride (mg/dL)	
<150	Normal
150–199	Borderline high
200–499	High
≥500	Very high

[a]See ref. 49.

LDL-C level of less than 100 mg per dL is optimal. A triglyceride concentration of greater than or equal to 150 mg per dL is considered elevated, and an HDL-C concentration less than 40 mg per dL is considered low. A fasting triglyceride concentration in excess of 500 mg per dL is noteworthy because it confers risk of pancreatitis. Other major risk factors for atherosclerosis defined by the NCEP Adult Treatment Panel III (ATP III) include cigarette smoking, hypertension (blood pressure greater than or equal to 140/90 mm Hg or on antihypertensive medication), age (men greater than or equal to 45 years; women greater than or equal to 55 years), and family history of premature CHD (CHD in male first-degree relatives less than 55 years old; CHD in female first-degree relatives less than 65 years old). For each patient, treatment goals and lipid thresholds for initiating drug therapy are based on the presence of CHD or CHD risk equivalents or on the number of major risk factors. Three risk categories are established by the 2001 NCEP guidelines. Risk category 1 includes patients with definite CHD or a CHD risk equivalent. The presence of all clinical forms of atherosclerotic disease (including PAD), diabetes mellitus, or multiple risk factors that confer a 10-year risk for a coronary event of greater than 20% are CHD risk equivalents. It should be emphasized that the presence of a diabetes counts as a CHD risk equivalent because diabetes mellitus confers a risk of a new coronary event within 10 years equal to that of someone with established CHD (51). Individuals with established CHD or a CHD risk equivalent are at high risk for a coronary event and therefore have the lowest LDL-C goal (less than 100 mg per dL).

Risk category 2 consists of individuals without CHD or a CHD risk equivalent but with multiple (greater than or equal to 2) risk factors and in whom the 10-year risk of a coronary event is less than or equal to 20%. The risk is estimated from the Framingham scoring system (49). The major risk factors, exclusive of an elevated LDL-C and diabetes mellitus are used to define risk and the goals and cut points for LDL-C treatment. The LDL-C goal for persons in risk category 2 is less than 130 mg per dL. Risk category 3 consists of persons having no or one risk factor. The majority of individuals in this category have a 10-year risk of a coronary event of less than 10%, and their LDL-C goal is less than 160 mg per dL.

At any plasma LDL-C concentration, the risk for CHD may be increased by the presence of the metabolic syndrome. This syndrome is closely linked to a generalized metabolic disorder called insulin resistance in which the normal actions of insulin are impaired. Whereas some individuals can be genetically predisposed, excess body fat and physical inactivity are the leading promoters for the development of insulin resistance. The NCEP ATPIII guidelines recommend that this syndrome be a secondary therapeutic target for ASCVD risk reduction after LDL-C lowering (49). The metabolic syndrome is clinically characterized by at least three of the following risk factors: abdominal obesity (waist circumference greater than 40 in. in men and greater than 35 in. in women), elevated triglyceride (TG) levels (greater than or equal to 150 mg per dL), low HDL cholesterol (less than 40 mg per dL in men and less than 50 mg per dL in women), hypertension (greater than or equal to 130 mm Hg/greater than or equal to 85 mm Hg), and fasting glucose greater than or equal to 110 mg per dL. The risk of ASCVD due to the metabolic syndrome may also be enhanced by elevated plasma levels of Lp(a) and homocysteine. The presence of an elevated Lp(a) and/or homocysteine concentration suggests a more aggressive treatment strategy is needed in a patient with the metabolic syndrome.

The effective treatment of lipoprotein disorders requires a thorough evaluation of the patient to determine the cause(s) of the dyslipidemia. The accurate identification of the cause(s) for the dyslipidemia allows the physician to select the most appropriate therapeutic options. The evaluation should include a medical history and complete family history of the patient, which are useful for identifying genetic etiology or predisposition to atherosclerosis. Cardiovascular disease risk factors (e.g., obesity, hypertension, diabetes mellitus, smoking) and all medications taken by the patient should be documented.

The physical examination includes assessment for xanthomas, xanthelasmas, corneal arcus, and lipemia retinalis. Tendon xanthomas (present in heterozygous and homozygous familial hypercholesterolemia) are found primarily in Achilles tendons, digital extensor tendons of the hand, and patellar tendons. Tuberous xanthomas (present in dysbetahyperlipoproteinemia) will occur on the knees and elbows, and striate xanthomas may occur in the palmar and digital skin creases. Eruptive xanthomas of the skin can occur with any cause of a marked hypertriglyceridemia (greater than 1,000 mg per dL) and are most commonly found on the back, the shoulders, and the buttocks. Other components of the physical examination should include assessment of blood pressure, body mass index (Kg/m^2), and peripheral pulses (e.g., popliteal, posterior tibial, dorsalis pedis). A cardiovascular examination is also recommended.

The laboratory measurements should include a fasting lipid profile, fasting glucose, creatinine, and thyroid-stimulating hormone (TSH). Creatinine kinase, aspartate, and alanine aminotransferases and alkaline phosphatase should be obtained for patients where lipid-lowering drug therapy will likely be initiated. Assessment of the serum albumin level is advisable for hypertriglyceridemic individuals where the initiation of a fibrate is likely. Additional laboratory tests [e.g., Lp(a), homocysteine, apolipoproteins] should only be ordered in subsets of patients, where in the judgment of the physician, the results may aid in refining the diagnosis or optimizing therapy.

The standard fasting lipid profile assessment includes the measurement of total cholesterol, triglyceride, and HDL-C after an overnight fast of greater than 12 hours using standardized assays. Should triglyceride concentration be less than 400 mg per dL, the LDL-C concentration can be calculated using the Friedewald formula: LDL-C=total cholesterol − HDL-C–triglyceride/5 (52). Direct LDL-C methods involving immunoprecipitation of VLDL and HDL are available, allowing for the measurement of LDL-C in the nonfasting state and in individuals with fasting triglyceride concentrations greater than or equal to 400 mg per dL. In addition, a direct LDL-C can be obtained using ultracentrification. Emerging data suggest that whereas serum apo A-I or apo B-100 concentrations provide little additional information about atherosclerosis risk beyond the fasting lipid profile (53), an elevated Lp(a) is an independent risk factor for CHD, and its measurement may be useful in subsets of patients with PAD, including those with marked hypercholesterolemia and those with essentially normal lipids, or those who are relatively refractory to statin therapy (48).

Following the clinical and laboratory evaluations, the goal is to identify the cause(s) of the dyslipidemia, either primary or secondary, or a combination. This is necessary because the management of a secondary dyslipidemia is, whenever possible, correction of the underlying cause. Several conditions may give rise to secondary dyslipidemia. The most important causes of secondary dyslipidemia are listed in Table 12.4.

Hypothyroidism often causes an elevation of LDL-C and, when accompanied by obesity, elevations of both LDL-C and triglycerides. Generally, correction of the thyroid dysfunction normalizes the lipoprotein abnormality. Because hypothyroidism can be subtle in its clinical presentation, a thyroid-stimulating hormone value should be obtained on all patients with hyperlipidemia.

Renal disorders can cause dyslipidemia. Nephrotic syndrome (protein-losing nephropathy) results in a marked increase in hepatic apo B-100 production with subsequent enhanced secretion of VLDL (54). This manifests as a mixed hyperlipidemia with elevations of the LDL-C and triglyceride levels. Renal insufficiency and especially end-stage renal disease are often associated with hypertriglyceridemia and low HDL-C. Lipoprotein lipase and HEL activities are suppressed in renal insufficiency, which reduces the catabolism of chylomicrons and VLDL and elevates the plasma triglyceride concentration (55).

Diabetes mellitus-induced dyslipidemia occurs in both insulin-dependent (type 1) diabetes and non-insulin-dependent

TABLE 12.4. *Selected causes of secondary dyslipidemia*

Cause	Hypercholesterolemia	Hypertriglyceridemia
Hypothyroidism	•	
Nephrotic syndrome	•	•
Renal insufficiency		•
Diabetes mellitus		•
Obstructive liver disease	• (Lp-X)[a]	
Hepatitis		•
Anorexia nervosa	•	
Hormones		
Estrogen		•
Progesterone	•	
Medications		
Immunosuppressive agents		•
Corticosteroids		•
Thiazides		•
Beta-blockers		•
HIV-protease inhibitors		•
Lifestyle		
Excess alcohol intake		•
Obesity		•
Diet rich in saturated fat	•	
Diet rich in refined carbohydrates		•
Physical inactivity	•	•

[a]Lp-X, An abnormal lipoprotein characterizing obstructive liver disease (59). It is composed of free cholesterol molecules attached to albumin.

(type 2) diabetes (56,57). It may be particularly severe in patients with diabetic ketoacidosis. In poorly controlled type 1 diabetes, the absolute deficiency of insulin causes a reduction in peripheral LPL activity. In addition, the deficiency of insulin leaves the activities of glucagon, cortisol, and growth hormone on peripheral adipocyte hormone-sensitive lipase unopposed, resulting in lipolysis and release of free fatty acids from adipose cells into the circulation. The increased availability of free fatty acids increases hepatic triglyceride synthesis and secretion of triglyceride-enriched VLDL. The combination of decreased peripheral catabolism and increased synthesis leads to the accumulation of VLDL in the circulation, which causes hypertriglyceridemia and a reciprocal decline in HDL-C. The same pathophysiologic mechanisms cause the hypertriglyceridemia in diabetic ketoacidosis. The mechanisms are more pronounced in diabetic ketoacidosis, with massive peripheral lipolysis and hepatic gluconeogenesis. The large amounts of free fatty acids cleared by the liver are both oxidized to ketone bodies and resynthesized into triglycerides. The secretion of hepatic VLDL triglyceride can saturate peripheral LPL, resulting in defective clearance of chylomicrons, which markedly elevates the plasma triglyceride concentration (57).

In type 2 diabetes, hypertriglyceridemia with reciprocal low HDL-C levels is the result of peripheral insensitivity to the action of insulin, accompanied by compensatory hyperinsulinemia (58). The insulin insensitivity inhibits the synthesis and activity of LPL, and consequently impairs the peripheral catabolism of triglyceride-rich lipoproteins (i.e., VLDL and chylomicrons). Hepatocytes remain sensitive to the action of insulin, and therefore the hyperinsulinemia suppresses beta-

oxidation of free fatty acids, shunting them into the synthesis of triglycerides and enhanced production of VLDL. The hypertriglyceridemia with low HDL-C levels in type 2 diabetes is the result of both impaired catabolism and enhanced synthesis of VLDL. Effective glycemic control will usually reduce plasma triglycerides to near-optimal levels.

Obstructive liver disease, especially primary biliary cirrhosis, may lead to the formation of hypercholesterolemia. The hypercholesterolemia is unique and due to the appearance in plasma, for unknown reasons, of an abnormal lipoprotein termed Lp-X (59). This is a large, discoidal lipoprotein particle, enriched in unesterified (or free) cholesterol. Modest hepatoinflammation that can result from excess alcohol intake can lead to hypertriglyceridemia (60). Alcohol also stimulates the production of apo A-1, and therefore ethanol-associated hypertriglyceridemia is usually accompanied by normal or elevated plasma levels of HDL-C. Advanced parenchymal liver disease, such as cirrhosis, diminishes lipoprotein synthesis, leading to hypolipidemia (60).

Anorexia nervosa may cause hypercholesterolemia (61). The mechanism is thought to be due to reduction in the hepatic conversion of cholesterol to bile acids. This results in an increased intrahepatic concentration of cholesterol with a subsequent reduction in the synthesis and expression of LDL receptors. This causes reduced catabolism of plasma LDL and a resulting hypercholesterolemia.

Estrogens may elevate plasma triglycerides through stimulating hepatic triglyceride synthesis, and possibly by antagonizing the action of peripheral LPL (62). Estrogens also stimulate the synthesis and expression of hepatic LDL receptors, leading to lower plasma concentrations. Estrogens increase hepatic production of HDL and inhibit HDL_2 catabolism by HEL, giving rise to increased plasma HDL-C levels. Progesterones antagonize the effect of estrogens on lipoprotein metabolism. Progesterones decrease triglyceride and HDL production by the liver and modestly increase plasma LDL-C concentrations.

Several commonly used medications can adversely affect plasma lipoprotein concentrations. Beta-blockers without intrinsic sympathomimetic activity increase triglyceride and lower HDL-C concentrations. Evidence suggests that beta-blockers inhibit the peripheral action of LPL and therefore retard the catabolism of VLDL triglycerides (61). Thiazide diuretics can increase plasma triglyceride concentrations (63). Corticosteroids increase plasma triglycerides by augmenting the action of insulin on the liver. This causes increased hepatic production of fatty acids and triglycerides. Because the insulin-potentiating action of corticosteroids can also increase the activity of LPL, increased conversion of VLDL to LDL can result in elevated plasma concentration of LDL-C. Antiretroviral therapy such as human immunodeficiency virus-1 protease inhibitors cause secondary hypertriglyceridemia. Treatment with antiretroviral therapy causes increased production of VLDL triglycerides by the liver. This concomitantly results in a decrease in the plasma HDL-C concentrations. The management of the hypertriglyceridemia induced by antiretroviral therapy focuses on the use of fibric acid derivatives. Because they compete with antiretroviral drugs for the same cytochrome P450 metabolic pathway (i.e., 3A4), they must be used with caution, and patients should be carefully monitored for potential adverse reactions (myopathy, hepatoinflammation, cholelithiasis).

Several lifestyle factors can contribute to dyslipidemia. Diets enriched in saturated fats and physical inactivity can lead to elevations in the plasma concentrations of LDL-C and triglycerides. Obesity, diets enriched in refined carbohydrates, and alcohol are common secondary causes of hypertriglyceridemia (64). Alcohol consumption reduces oxidation of free fatty acids by the liver, which stimulates hepatic triglyceride synthesis and VLDL secretion. Regular, modest alcohol intake raises the HDL-C plasma concentration by mechanism(s) not completely understood. Because of the impact of these lifestyle factors on lipoprotein metabolism, lifestyle changes are important in the effective treatment of most lipoprotein disorders.

The NCEP Adult Treatment Panel III recommends, in addition to lipid-lowering medications, a multifaceted lifestyle approach to managing dyslipidemia and reducing the risk for atherosclerosis. This approach has been designated as therapeutic lifestyle changes (TLC) and includes the following:

• Reduced intake of saturated fats (less than 7% of calories) and cholesterol (less than 200 mg per day)
• Therapeutic options for enhancing LDL-C lowering such as the use of plant stanols/sterols (2 g per day) and increased intake of soluble fiber (10 to 20 g per day)
• Weight reduction

TABLE 12.5. *Composition of the therapeutic lifestyle changes diet*

Dietary component	Recommended intake
Total fat	25%–35% of total calories
Saturated and trans fats	<7% of total calories
Polyunsaturated fats	≤10% of total calories
Monounsaturated fats	≤20% of total calories
Carbohydrates	50%–60% of total calories
Protein	15%–20% of total calories
Cholesterol	<200 mg/d
Fiber	20–30 g/d

Adapted from Expert Panel on Detection, Evaluation and Treatment of High Blood Cholesterol in Adults. Executive summary of the third report of the National Cholesterol Education Program (NCEP) Expert Panel on Detection, Evaluation and Treatment of High Blood Pressure in Adults (Adult Treatment Panel III). *JAMA* 2001;285:2486–2497, with permission.

• Increased physical activity (daily energy expenditure from exercise to be at least 200 kcal per day) (49)

At all stages of nutritional counseling, it is recommended that patients be referred to registered dieticians or qualified nutritionists for medical nutrition therapy. The nutrient composition of the TLC diet is summarized in Table 12.5. It is recommended that the prescribed total number of calories ingested per day allow the individual to either attain or maintain an ideal body weight.

Because individuals with PAD are considered to be a CHD risk equivalent, in addition to the therapeutic lifestyle changes, pharmacologic therapy to reach their LDL-C and triglyceride goals is essential. It is important to remind the patient that when lipid-lowering medications are prescribed, attention to therapeutic lifestyle changes should always be maintained. The physician should always reinforce the notion to the patient that the efficacy of the lipid-lowering drug, relies on a prudent diet, an optimal weight, and an active lifestyle.

LIPID-LOWERING PHARMACOLOGY

Five classes of lipid-lowering agents are available in the United States. They include HMG-CoA reductase inhibitors (statins), nicotinic acid (niacin), fibric acid derivatives (fibrates), bile acid sequestrants (resins), and intestinal cholesterol absorption inhibitors. These pharmacologic agents allow drug therapy to be tailored to the specific lipid abnormality of an individual. Lipid-lowering drugs can be given as monotherapy or as combination drug therapy, particularly in individuals with mixed hyperlipidemias or with severe hypercholesterolemia or hypertriglyceridemia. A summary of the lipid-lowering agents for treating dyslipidemia is provided in Table 12.6.

3-Hydroxy-3 Methylglutaryl-Coenzyme A Reductase Inhibitors

HMG CoA reductase inhibitors, or statins, are the most effective of the lipid-lowering medications for reducing plasma

TABLE 12.6. *Drugs affecting lipoprotein metabolism[a]*

Class	Mode of action	Lipid effects	Agents	Side effects
HMG CoA reductase inhibitors (statins)	↓ Cholesterol biosynthesis ↑ LDL receptor activity	↓ LDL (18%–60%) ↑ HDL (5%–15%) ↓ TG (7%–30%)	Lovastatin, pravastatin, simvastatin, fluvastatin, atorvastatin, rosuvastatin	Increase in liver enzymes Myalgia/myositis
Bile acid sequestrants (resins)	Interrupts enterohepatic recirculation of bile acids ↑ Hepatic conversion of cholesterol to bile ↑ Hepatic LDL receptor activity	↓ LDL (15%–30%) ↑ HDL (3%–5%) ↑ TG	Cholestyramine, colestipol, colesevelam HCl	Abdominal discomfort, constipation, nausea Decreases the absorption of other drugs
Fibric acid derivatives (fibrates)	Activates PPARα (increases gene expression for apo A-I, apo A-II, and LPL; downregulates gene expression for apo C-III)	↓ TG (20%–70%) ↑ HDL (10%–20%) ↔,↑ LDL	Gemfibrozil, fenofibrate	↑ Lithogenicity of bile gallstones Dyspepsia Myopathy
Nicotinic acid (niacin)	↓ Mobilization of FFA from peripheral adipose tissue ↓ VLDL synthesis ↓ HDL catabolism	↓ TG (20%–50%) ↑ HDL (15%–35%) ↓ LDL (5%–25%) ↓ Lp(a) (10%–30%)	Extended-release niacin, crystalline niacin, polygel controlled-release niacin	Cutaneous flushing Hepatoinflammation Gastrointestinal distress Hyperuricemia Hyperglycemia
Selective cholesterol absorption inhibitors	Inhibits intestinal cholesterol absorption ↓ Cholesterol content of chylomicrons	↓ LDL (15%–25%) ↓ TG (5%–15%) ↔ HDL	Ezetimibe	Diarrhea, abdominal pain

[a]HMG CoA, 3-Hydroxy-3 methylglutaryl-coenzyme A; LDL, low-density lipoprotein; HDL, high-density lipoprotein; TG, triglycerides; PPARα, peroxisome proliferator-activated receptor α; LPL, lipoprotein lipase; FFA, free fatty acids; VLDL, very low density lipoprotein; Lp(a), lipoprotein(a).

concentrations of LDL-C (65,66). The first of these agents made available by the U.S. Food and Drug Administration (FDA) was lovastatin in 1987. There are six statins (lovastatin, pravastatin, simvastatin, fluvastatin, rosuvastatin and atorvastatin) that have been approved for clinical use (Table 12.7). Statins act primarily in the liver and competitively inhibit HMG CoA reductase, the rate-limiting enzyme in cholesterol biosynthesis. Endogenous cholesterol is synthesized from acetyl CoA through a rate-limiting intermediate step, the conversion of HMG CoA to mevalonic acid, which is catalyzed by HMG CoA reductase. All 27 carbon atoms of

cholesterol are derived from acetyl CoA. Inhibition of HMG CoA reductase by statins dramatically reduces the rate of cholesterol biosynthesis and the concentration of hepatocellular cholesterol. This enhances the expression of the LDL receptor gene and increases the synthesis and manifestation of high-affinity LDL receptors on hepatocyte membranes. The increased hepatic LDL receptor activity enhances the clearance of LDL from the blood. As monotherapy, the reduction in serum LDL-C concentrations induced by treatment with a statin ranges from 18% to about 65%. Although the efficacies of the statins for reducing LDL-C vary substantially, it

TABLE 12.7. *Characteristics of 3-hydroxy-3 methylglutaryl-coenzyme A reductase inhibitors*

Characteristic	Lovastatin	Pravastatin	Simvastatin	Fluvastatin	Atorvastatin	Rosuvastatin
Dose range (mg/d)	10–80	10–40	10–80	20–80	10–80	5–40
Maximum mean low-density-lipoprotein cholesterol reduction (%)	40	32	47	35	60	65
Plasma half-life (h)	2.5	1.0	2.0	0.5	14	19
Effect of food on absorption	Increased absorption	Decreased absorption	None	None	None	None
Penetration across the blood–brain barrier	Yes	No	Yes	No	No	No
Hepatic metabolism of cytochrome P450 isozyme	3A4	None	3A4	2C9	3A4	Minor 2C9
Solubility	Lipophilic	Hydrophilic	Lipophilic	Hydrophilic	Lipophilic	Hydrophilic
Derivation	Fermentation	Fermentation	Fermentation	Synthetic	Synthetic	Synthetic

is important to note that the response to increasing the dose of a statin is not proportional because the dose–response relation for all statins is curvilinear (65). About 85% to 90% of the effectiveness of a statin is in the starting dose. In general, a doubling of the dose above the starting dose decreases plasma LDL-C concentrations by an additional 4% to 6%. Subsequent dose titrations yield smaller and smaller increments of LDL-C lowering.

Lovastatin, pravastatin, and simvastatin are structurally similar and are fungally derived (Table 12.7). Fluvastatin, rosuvastatin and atorvastatin are synthetic statins with distinct structures different from that of the fermentation-derived statins. With the exception of atorvastatin and rosuvastatin which have plasma half-lives of 14 and 19 hours respectively, the half-lives of the other statins range between 0.5 and 2.5 hours when given as once-daily therapy. Statins are more effective when dosed in the evening because of the diurnal rhythm of cholesterol biosynthesis in human beings, which shows enhanced rates of cholesterol biosynthesis at night compared with during the day (66).

With the exception of pravastatin, the statins rely on cytochrome P450 enzyme systems for metabolism (65,66). Fluvastatin is metabolized primarily by the cytochrome P450 2C9 isozyme, whereas lovastatin, simvastatin, and atorvastatin are primarily metabolized by the cytochrome P450 3A4. Pravastatin does not undergo substantial metabolism by the cytochrome P450 system and is excreted as the parent compound by the kidney and, to a lesser extent, the small bowel. Rosuvastatin, a new statin, does not appear to undergo extensive cytochrome P450 metabolism and may therefore have a reduced proclivity for clinically significant interactions with other medications (67,68).

All of the statins modestly lower plasma triglyceride concentrations. The triglyceride-lowering effect is consistent with the known mechanisms of action of these agents to both reduce the hepatic biosynthesis of cholesterol and enhance catabolism of LDL and remnant lipoproteins (e.g., IDL). Statins are not effective for reducing elevated triglycerides due to chylomicronemia. Statins also raise the plasma HDL-C concentration by modest amounts. Although the mechanism(s) for this potentially beneficial effect are unknown, it may involve enhanced production of nascent HDL, because statins raise the plasma concentration of apo A-I by 5% to 10% (69).

The statins as a class have been well tolerated, and significant side effects are quite rare. A review of the five major trials with statins indicates a high degree of safety (70). These trials involved over 30,000 participants, with one-half receiving statin therapy for an average of 5 years. A meta-analysis summarized in the review demonstrated that the incidences of fatal trauma and suicide did not differ between the patients taking a statin and those taking placebo. The incidence of cancer was not different between the two groups. The most common adverse effects associated with statin use included liver transaminase elevation, myalgia [muscle pain or weakness without significant (less than three times the upper limit of normal) serum creatinine kinase elevation], and gastroin-

testinal upset. The rarer side effects include myositis (myalgia with serum creatinine kinase concentrations of greater than 1,000 u per L) and sleep disturbances.

Liver transaminase (alanine aminotransferase and aspartate aminotransferase) elevation (exceeding three times normal) necessitating discontinuation of statin therapy occurs in less than 1% of patients generally taking the higher doses (40 or 80 mg per day). Liver transaminase levels will usually return to normal within 2 weeks following discontinuation of a statin. It is very rare to observe this side effect in individuals treated with starting doses. Minor elevations of liver transaminase concentrations (increases of up to 1.5 times the upper limit of the normal range) can be ignored and are usually transient (66).

Evidence of abnormalities in skeletal muscle function among some patients taking statins manifests in several ways. Some patients may complain of muscle aches and weakness without objective evidence of muscle toxicity (i.e., no increased levels of creatinine kinase). Approximately 10% of patients treated with statins develop this form of myopathy, which suggests that it is related to drug therapy. The etiology of this form of myopathy is unknown, although several case reports (71,72) indicate that it may be due to deleterious effects of statins on the peripheral nervous system. A recent study from Denmark demonstrated an association between idiopathic polyneuropathy and statin use (73). Although the mechanism underlying statin-induced peripheral neuropathy is unknown, two hypotheses have been suggested. Interference with cholesterol biosynthesis through statin-induced inhibition of HMG CoA reductase may alter nerve membrane function because cholesterol is a ubiquitous component of human cell membranes. Statins may also coinhibit the synthesis of the key mitochondrial respiratory chain enzyme ubiquinone, which may disturb neuron energy utilization and thereby induce neuropathy. Structural and functional changes of the neurons exposed long term to statins could be explained by either mechanism. Discontinuation of the statin or reducing the dose will usually resolve this somewhat common, although idiopathic, form of myopathy.

About 1% to 2% of patients treated with statins develop transient high levels of creatinine kinase accompanied by myalgia. This is more objective evidence of true myositis, yet elevations of creatinine kinase can occur periodically from other causes such as increase in activity or exercise level. When statin therapy increases creatinine kinase levels severalfold, reduction in dose is indicated. Rarely (1 in approximately 1,000 patients), statins produce severe myositis. This response can occur without obvious evidence of a precipitating cause. Severe myositis or rhabdomyolysis is manifest by marked discomfort and weakness of skeletal muscle, extreme elevations of creatinine kinase, myoglobinuria, and necrosis of the glomarular membrane. The mechanism for this reaction is not understood. It typically occurs with high plasma concentrations of statins and their metabolites, which presumably act directly on muscle cells. With severe myositis (i.e., rhabdomyolysis), prompt discontinuation of the drug is necessary (66).

Both liver transaminase elevation and myositis occur more commonly among individuals taking higher doses of statins or who are concurrently taking other drugs metabolized by the specific cytochrome P450 isozyme that is responsible for metabolizing the statin. Lovastatin, atorvastatin, and simvastatin are metabolized by the cytochrome P450 3A4 isozyme, and fluvastatin is metabolized by the cytochrome P450 2C9 isozyme. Drugs that are either substrates for or inhibitors of the cytochrome P450 3A4 or 2C9 may retard the metabolism of these statins, thereby increasing their plasma concentrations and potential for side effects. Drugs that either inhibit or are substrates for the cytochrome P450 3A4 isozyme include fibrates, erythromycin, tetracycline, azole antifungals, several calcium channel blockers, HIV-protease inhibitors, and immunosuppressive agents. It is also reported that specific ingredients of grapefruit or grapefruit juice inhibit the cytochrome P450 3A4 isozymes. Therefore, using higher doses of atorvastatin, lovastatin, or simvastatin in an individual concurrently taking one or more of the drugs that require or inhibit the cytochrome P450 3A4 isozyme may lead to increased plasma concentrations of the drugs and increase the risk for hepatotoxicity or myotoxicity. Fluvastatin and warfarin are common substrates for the cytochrome P450 2C9 isozyme. Therefore, prescribing fluvastatin to an individual anticoagulated by warfarin may increase the effects of both drugs. It is advisable to assess the international normalized ratio (INR) and/or partial thromboplastin time (PTT) in a patient who is anticoagulated by warfarin approximately 48 to 72 hours after the initiation of fluvastatin, with appropriate adjustment of the warfarin dose, if necessary.

Sleep disturbances are rare and may occur with the statins that cross the blood–brain barrier, lovastatin and simvastatin. For a patient who experiences a sleep disturbance side effect with lovastatin or simvastatin, the drugs pravastatin, atorvastatin, rosuvastatin, or fluvastatin, which do not cross the blood–brain barrier, may be attempted (74,75).

The statins are useful for treating most primary hypercholesterolemias. The primary hypercholesterolemias include heterozygous familial hypercholesterolemia, familial defective apo B-100, familial combined hyperlipidemia, and polygenic (or common) hypercholesterolemia. It is generally recommended that the starting dose of a statin be initiated. The patient should be followed up in approximately 6 to 8 weeks after statin initiation for assessment of the LDL-C and appropriate safety laboratories including the serum liver transaminases and creatinine kinase concentrations. Should the desired LDL-C concentration be achieved and the safety laboratories be normal, follow-up is recommended biannually. Should the LDL-C concentration not be achieved, the dose of the statin may be increased if the LDL-C level is within 10% of the target. The patient should then be followed up in a subsequent 6 to 8 weeks. However, should the LDL-C concentration not be achieved and the level be greater than 10% from the target, consideration should be given to maintaining the starting dose of the statin and adding a second LDL-lowering agent. Agents for consideration with a statin for additional LDL-C-lowering include the resins, nicotinic acid, and ezetimibe.

Bile Acid Sequestrants

Bile acid sequestrants are anion exchange resins, which are not absorbed from the gastrointestinal tract. The lack of systemic exposure makes these agents useful in special populations such as children, women who are of child-bearing age (or pregnant), and individuals with hepatic or renal dysfunction. These agents act by binding bile in the intestinal lumen, thereby decreasing their normal reabsorption in the terminal ileum and increasing their excretion into the feces (76,77). Normally, 97% of bile acids undergo an enterohepatic recirculation, with only a small percentage being excreted in the feces. By reducing bile acid absorption, resins deplete the hepatic bile acid concentration, resulting in enhanced conversion of cholesterol to bile acids by the action of the enzyme 7-alpha dehydrogenase. The increased conversion of cholesterol to bile (primary glycocholate) reduces the hepatic cholesterol concentration, which stimulates increased synthesis and expression of LDL receptors on hepatic membranes, with subsequent enhanced plasma LDL clearance. In addition, the reduced hepatic cholesterol concentration modestly stimulates hepatic cholesterol and triglyceride biosynthesis, with subsequent VLDL secretion into the blood. However, the increase in LDL receptor expression supersedes the increase in cholesterol biosynthesis, with the net effect being a reduction in plasma total cholesterol and LDL-C levels (77).

The available resins are cholestyramine, colestipol, and colesevelam HCl. A 5-g dose of colestipol is approximately equivalent to a 4-g dose of cholestyramine. When given in doses of 8 to 16 g (cholestyramine) or 10 to 20 g (colestipol) daily, these resins decrease serum LDL-C concentrations by 15% to 20% (78,79). Colesevelam HCl is more potent than either cholestyramine or colestipol. At a dose of 3.8 g per day of colesevelam HCl, plasma LDL-C concentration is reduced by approximately 20% (80).

The major use of a resin is in combination with a statin to provide additional LDL-C reduction (79). This combination is particularly useful for a patient who cannot tolerate a high dose of a statin, or if the statin alone is not sufficient to reduce the LDL-C to the target level. Because resins are nonsystemically acting agents, they do not increase the adverse potential effect of a statin when used in combination. Therefore, it is recommended that a patient be followed up every 6 months when on a statin/resin combination. Resins can be used as monotherapy as previously indicated, and are particularly appropriate for women of childbearing potential, patients who cannot tolerate statins, individuals with hepatic dysfunction, and children with familial hypercholesterolemia. In addition, patients with modest elevations of LDL-C who may not choose to take a systemically acting medication are candidates for monotherapy with resins.

Cholestyramine and colestipol are ion-exchange resins and have the potential to bind other negatively charged drugs including thyroxin, warfarin, statins, calcium channel blockers, beta-blockers, digitalis, thiazides, and valproic acid (66). It is recommended that other drugs be taken 1 hour before or 4 hours after cholestyramine or colestipol. The polymer backbone structure of colesevelam HCl contains quaternary amine pockets. This structure has specific affinity for bile acids at the exclusion of other drugs (80). Therefore, dosing medications at the same time as colesevelam HCl does not appreciably alter their absorption from the intestine. The resins do not interfere with the absorption of fat-soluble vitamins (i.e., A, D, E, and K) in adults unless there is an associated disturbance in bile acid metabolism due to either significant hepatic or small bowel disease (79).

Because resins are nonabsorbable medications, the principal side effects are limited to the gastrointestinal tract. Abdominal discomfort, gas, heartburn, and constipation occur in 50% or more of patients receiving a resin (78). These side effects are less frequent in individuals receiving colesevelam HCl (80). Constipation is the most frequent lower gastrointestinal complaint and can be alleviated by adding soluble fiber (such as one tablespoon of psyllium hydrophilic mucilloid in 8 ounces of water) once or twice daily (81). Soluble fiber also enhances the cholesterol-lowering effects of resins because it possesses independent cholesterol-lowering properties.

Nicotinic Acid (niacin)

Nicotinic acid or niacin is a water-soluble B complex vitamin that, when used in pharmacologic doses, becomes a drug that favorably affects the serum concentrations of lipids and lipoproteins (82). Nicotinic acid is available as immediate-release (crystalline) and sustained-release (slow- or extended-release) preparations.

The lipid-altering effects of nicotinic acid have been recognized for over 45 years. The drug has been widely used to treat hypercholesterolemia, modest hypertriglyceridemia, and mixed hyperlipidemia. The beneficial effects on atherosclerosis have been documented in several clinical endpoint and coronary angiographic trials in which nicotinic acid was used alone or as part of the lipid-lowering drug regimen in patients with hyperlipidemia (83–87).

The mechanism(s) by which nicotinic acid alters the lipid profile have not been well defined. It may involve several actions including partial inhibition of the release of free fatty acids from adipose tissue, which reduces hepatic triglyceride synthesis and secretion of VLDL. It may also increase LPL activity, which would increase the rate of VLDL triglyceride removal from the plasma (88). Nicotinic acid does not appear to affect fecal excretion of fats, sterols, or bile acids. It is the only lipid-lowering agent that reduces Lp(a) plasma concentrations, and it is the most effective agent for raising plasma HDL-C concentrations. These beneficial effects occur through nicotinic acid's ability to reduce hepatic synthesis of Lp(a) (89) and to slow the catabolism of plasma HDL through blocking the activity of the SR-B1 hepatic receptor (90,91).

At doses of 1.5 to 4.5 g per day, crystalline nicotinic acid reduces the LDL-C and triglyceride concentrations by 5% to 21% and by 12% to 30%, respectively. Plasma concentrations of Lp(a) are reduced by 14% to 35% and HDL-C concentrations rise by 16% to 22% (92). Similar changes in plasma lipid and lipoprotein concentrations have also been observed in response to treatment of dyslipidemic individuals with extended-release nicotinic acid (Niaspan). At doses of 1 and 2 g per day, extended-release nicotinic acid reduces LDL-C, Lp(a), and triglycerides by 6% and 15%, by 12% and 28%, and by 20% and 30%, respectively (93). It increases HDL-C plasma concentrations by 24% and 26%, respectively.

Nicotinic acid can be used as monotherapy, in combination with a statin or a resin for treatment of marked hypercholesterolemia and mixed hyperlipidemia, or in combination with a fibrate for treating marked hypertriglyceridemia (66). Because it reduces Lp(a), it can be useful in combination with a statin or resin in hypercholesterolemic patients with elevated concentrations of Lp(a) (79).

Therapy with crystalline nicotinic acid should be started at a low dose given one or two times daily. A common schedule is to begin with 100-mg tablets following meals and to double the dose at intervals of 7 to 10 days. After reaching a dose of 2 g per day, the dose should be maintained for approximately 6 to 8 weeks, at which time the lipid and lipoprotein levels should be reevaluated and the patient examined for adverse reactions including a safety chemistry profile (liver transaminases, glucose, and uric acid). If an adequate reduction of LDL-C or triglyceride has not been achieved and no side effects are evident, the dose may be doubled to approximately 4 g per day. The patient should be monitored every 6 to 8 weeks after each dose increase. Extended-release nicotinic acid (Niaspan, given once daily) at a dose of 1 g per day has a similar effect on the lipid profile as 2 g of crystalline nicotinic acid. This extended-release preparation of nicotinic acid has improved tolerability over crystalline and some sustained-release nicotinic acid preparations. The FDA has issued guidance stating its opposition to the sale of over-the-counter nicotinic acid products for the treatment of hypercholesterolemia. Approved nicotinic acid agents by prescription include Niacor, Niaspan, Nicolar, and Slo-Niacin.

Nicotinic acid is generally not well tolerated. Adverse effects include cutaneous flushing, gastrointestinal distress, liver transaminase elevation, hyperglycemia, and hyperuricemia. These side effects are usually reversible after discontinuation of nicotinic acid. Severe hepatotoxicity has been reported, although rare, and associated with the slow-release preparations (94). Nicotinic acid use should be avoided in individuals with a hypersensitivity to the drug, liver disease, active peptic ulcer disease, hyperuricemia, inflammatory bowel disease, significant glucose intolerance, and diabetes mellitus (relative contraindication). Although nicotinic acid may be used in patients with diabetes mellitus (95), careful monitoring of the diabetic status should be undertaken. Nicotinic acid can raise the blood glucose concentration, and it is not clear whether this is the result of interference with insulin secretion or enhancement of insulin resistance. Mild elevations in the liver transaminases can occur in 2% to 5% of patients taking nicotinic acid, yet these elevations rarely require cessation of treatment. Nicotinic acid can potentiate the effect of warfarin, and therefore the INR should be assessed 2 to 3 days after initiating nicotinic acid in a patient receiving warfarin. Nicotinic acid can also raise the level of uric acid in the blood, and consequently should be avoided in patients with a history of gout.

The most disturbing side effect of nicotinic acid is cutaneous flushing, although the extended-release formulation has modestly reduced this untoward effect (93). Cutaneous flushing is the result of nicotinic acid stimulating prostacyclin production by the endothelial cells of cutaneous blood vessels (96). Premedicating an individual with aspirin (81 to 325 mg) approximately 30 minutes before giving nicotinic acid can mitigate this prostaglandin-mediated symptom. It is also advisable to take nicotinic acid immediately following a meal and to avoid hot liquids, alcohol, and spicy foods to further reduce the potential for cutaneous flushing.

Education, supervision, and monitoring are required for all patients taking nicotinic acid. Because nicotinic acid can be obtained without a prescription, many people take it without physician supervision. Self-medication should be discouraged.

Cholesterol Absorption Inhibitors

Ezetimibe is the first of a new class of selective intestinal cholesterol absorption inhibitors that represent a new option for the pharmacologic treatment of hypercholesterolemia. Ezetimibe selectively inhibits the intestinal uptake and absorption of dietary and biliary cholesterol at the brush border of small intestinal enterocytes, confining cholesterol to the intestinal lumen for subsequent elimination (97–99). Ezetimibe (10 mg per day) reduces cholesterol absorption from the intestine by 25% to 50% (100). Through inhibiting the intestinal absorption of cholesterol, ezetimibe presumably reduces the cholesterol content of chylomicrons and the delivery of cholesterol in the chylomicron remnant to the liver. The reduced delivery of cholesterol reduces intrahepatic cholesterol levels, with upregulation of LDL receptor production and expression, and subsequent increased catabolism of plasma LDL. Although this is its assumed mechanism of action, this issue is being investigated. Ezetimibe does not appear to affect the absorption of fatty acids, monoglycerides, or fat-soluble vitamins (99).

The effectiveness of ezetimibe is predicated on its undergoing glucuronidation in the intestine. The glucuronidated metabolite is more potent than ezetimibe itself in inhibiting intestinal cholesterol absorption (97). Most of the glucuronidated metabolite remains in the intestinal lumen, as opposed to the parent ezetimibe, which repeatedly undergoes enterohepatic recirculation and delivery back to the villi in the intestinal lumen via bile (98). A study of intravenous ad-

ministration of ezetimibe in rats indicated decreased uptake of cholesterol into enterocytes and decreased cholesterol absorption into the plasma and enterohepatic circulation (101).

Ezetimibe given 10 mg once daily reduces the plasma LDL-C and total cholesterol concentrations by 18% and 21%, respectively (102). The drug modestly reduces triglycerides (8%) and has virtually no effect on the HDL-C concentration. Ezetimibe can be administered with or without food, and it has a low potential for drug interactions with cytochrome P450 substrates (99). Choice of morning or evening dosing seems to have no appreciable effect on the lipid-lowering potential of ezetimibe. According to the package insert, no dosage adjustment is necessary in patients with mild hepatic insufficiency or renal insufficiency or in geriatric patients.

Coadministration of ezetimibe with statins (including atorvastatin, simvastatin, lovastatin, and pravastatin) significantly lowered LDL-C 12% to 22% more than statin monotherapy, with no alterations in the pharmacokinetics of either class of agents (103–108). Combination therapy with ezetimibe also significantly increased HDL-C 1% to 3% more and significantly decreased triglycerides 7% to 11% more than statin monotherapy (103,104,106).

Because ezetimibe and its glucuronide conjugate are repeatedly delivered to the intestinal wall by enterohepatic recycling, limited peripheral exposure occurs. Ezetimibe was well tolerated in clinical trials of monotherapy, and had an adverse effect profile similar to that of placebo. The most commonly reported adverse effects in 242 patients taking ezetimibe were headache (9.5%), viral infection (7.9%), arthralgia (3.3%), and upper respiratory tract infection (less than 1%) (102). Analysis of the clinical trials in which ezetimibe (10 mg daily) was added to statins for 8 and 12 weeks showed that the combination was well tolerated, with a safety profile similar to those of the statins alone (103,106).

Fibric Acid Derivates (Fibrates)

The fibric acid derivatives or fibrates are the most effective plasma triglyceride-lowering agents. These agents also effectively raise the HDL-C concentration. Fibrates influence lipoprotein metabolism by activating specific members of the nuclear hormone receptor family called peroxisome proliferator-activated receptors (PPAR). There are three PPAR nuclear receptors, PPARα, PPARβ, and PPARγ. The fibrates activate PPARα, which in turn enhances the gene expression for synthesis of apo A-I, apo A-II, and LPL (109). Additionally, activation of PPARα reduces the gene expression for apo C-III. Apo C-III is an inhibitor of LPL activity (110). Therefore, the primary mechanism for reducing triglycerides by a fibrate is through enhanced hydrolysis of plasma triglyceride-rich lipoproteins in the periphery. Fibrates have also been shown to lower plasma triglycerides through enhancing hepatic oxidative metabolism of fatty acids, resulting in decreased triglyceride synthesis and VLDL secretion (110,111). Enhanced gene expression for the synthesis of apo A-I and apo A-II is responsible, in part, for the increase in the HDL-C plasma concentration. Fibrates have no effect on the plasma Lp(a) concentration.

There are two available fibrates in the United States. Gemfibrozil is given 600 mg twice daily and fenofibrate is given 160 mg once daily. Both are indicated for the management of hypertriglyceridemia. At normal doses, fibrates reduce the serum triglyceride concentration by 20% to 70% and raise the HDL-C concentration approximately 10% to 20% (112–114). Patients with extremely high plasma triglyceride concentrations (greater than or equal to 1,000 mg per dL) generally have low LDL-C, and the LDL-C may increase during treatment with a fibrate in these individuals (114,116). Should the increase be substantial, a low-dose statin or a resin may be added to the regimen.

Fibrates are also useful in patients with combined hyperlipidemia (elevations of LDL and VLDL) and in type III hyperlipidemia (elevation of remnant lipoproteins) (117). In type III hyperlipidemia, fibrates yield marked reductions in plasma remnant lipoproteins and regression of tuberous xanthomas. They are the drugs of choice for treating this dyslipidemia. For combined hyperlipidemia (type II$_b$), they can be added to a statin or bile acid-binding resin. When used in patients with a statin, fenofibrate is preferred to gemfibrozil because it is better tolerated (118). This combination does increase the risk for liver transaminase elevation and myopathy, and therefore patients should be followed up at 3- to 4-month intervals. Because fenofibrate can increase biliary lithogenicity, the safety laboratories should include an alkaline phosphatase in addition to the liver transaminases and creatinine kinase. When combining fenofibrate with a statin, it is recommended that fenofibrate be given once daily in the morning and a short-acting statin (lovastatin, simvastatin, pravastatin, or fluvastatin) be given once daily in the evening (79). This will reduce the risk that plasma levels of fenofibrate and a statin will be concurrently elevated, increasing the potential for side effects. For patients treated with this combination, it is appropriate to start with low doses of the statins and observe the patients clinically for efficacy and safety. It is generally not recommended to prescribe higher doses of a statin with this combination.

Gemfibrozil may be used as monotherapy for treating hypertriglyceridemia or in combination with a resin for the treatment of combined hyperlipidemia. In the primary prevention trail, conducted by the Helsinki Heart Study (119), in dyslipidemic men, gemfibrozil therapy (600 mg twice daily) over 5 years reduced CHD incidence by 34% compared to placebo. Subsequent analyses of the data revealed the greatest benefit was derived by patients with combined hyperlipidemia. The secondary prevention study, the Veterans Administration HDL Intervention Treatment trial (120), observed that gemfibrozil therapy (600 mg twice daily) for 5 years reduced CHD events and stroke by 22% and 28%, respectively, compared to placebo in men with a history of CHD.

The fibrates are generally well tolerated. The adverse effects of fibrates include gastrointestinal upset and discomfort, increased risk of gallstone formation, hepatoinflammation,

and interference with binding of warfarin to albumin. This latter side effect is due to the fact that fibrates and warfarin are largely bound to albumin. These two drugs given concurrently compete for albumin-binding sites, thereby displacing more free drug and increasing the potential for side effects. Therefore, as with fluvastatin and nicotinic acid, when a fibrate is initiated in a patient anticoagulated with warfarin, the INR and/or PTT should be assessed 48 to 72 hours after initiation of the fibrate, with adjustment of the warfarin dose, if necessary. Fibrates have an absolute contraindication in hepatic disease (including primary biliary cirrhosis), chronic renal failure and preexisting gallbladder disease. The drugs should not be used by pregnant women or nursing mothers.

As monotherapy, in addition to monitoring for lipid response, liver transaminases should be assessed 8 weeks after the initiation of fibrate therapy and every 6 months thereafter. When combined with a statin (the fibrate of choice is fenofibrate) or nicotinic acid, follow-up should occur at 8 weeks after adding the fibrate and every 3 to 4 months thereafter. A fibrate/resin combination does not increase the frequency of follow-up beyond what is recommended for a fibrate only.

Combination Lipid-Lowering Therapy

Combination therapy with lipid-lowering agents can include two or, in some cases, three individual lipid-lowering drugs. Combination lipid-lowering therapy may be used for individuals with marked hypercholesterolemia, mixed hyperlipidemia, or more moderate degrees of hyperlipidemia, in which the dose of a single medication needed to achieve the target lipid or lipoprotein level is not tolerated by the patient. For these individuals, a combination of two agents at lower doses will have complementary effects and less potential for side effects. Severe primary hypercholesterolemia is best treated by a combination of a statin with either a resin, nicotinic acid, or ezetimibe (Table 12.8). These combinations can reduce the LDL-C concentration by 65% or more. A resin with nicotinic acid can be considered, and triple therapy using a statin plus a resin and either ezetimibe or nicotinic acid may be necessary for optimal management of some adult patients with heterozygous familial hypercholesterolemia (79). Referral to a lipid specialist is strongly recommended for management of patients requiring such combination therapy.

Mixed hyperlipidemia, where the goal of therapy is to reduce both the LDL-C and triglycerides, may require combined drug therapy. The most effective combination is fenofibrate and a statin. However, this combination is associated with an increased risk of myopathy and hepatoinflammation above what is anticipated with either agent used alone. It is generally recommended that when this combination is used, no more than the starting dose of a statin be given with fenofibrate. Should the LDL-C remain above the target level with this combination, one may consider adding a resin. Other lipid-lowering combinations that can be considered for treating combined hyperlipidemia include a statin and nicotinic acid, or a resin and nicotinic acid. Triglyceride

TABLE 12.8. *Lipid-lowering agents and combinations for treating dyslipidemia*

Dyslipidemia[a]	Monotherapy	Combination therapy options
Hypercholesterolemia (↑LDL-C, normal TG and HDL-C)	Statins, resins, ezetimibe, niacin	Statin + resin Statin + ezetimibe Statin + nicotinic acid Resin + nicotinic acid Statin + resin + nicotinic acid
Hypercholesterolemia with low HDL-C Hypertriglyceridemia	Statins, nicotinic acid Fibrates, nicotinic acid	Statin + nicotinic acid Fibrate + nicotinic acid Fibrate + low-dose statin
Combined hyperlipidemia (↑LDL-C and ↑TG)	Niacin, statins, fibrates	Statin + fenofibrate Statin + nicotinic acid Nicotinic acid + resin Statin + fenofibrate + resin

[a]LDL-C, low-density-lipoprotein cholesterol; TG, triglycerides; HDL-C, high-density-lipoprotein cholesterol.

reduction with either of these two combinations will be less than that of the statin and fenofibrate combination.

Marked primary hypertriglyceridemia including chylomicronemia as observed in type V hyperlipidemia may be treated with a combination of a fibrate and niacin. As with the statin/fibrate combination, it is best to initiate the fibrate once daily in the morning and the niacin once daily in the evening (79). This reduces the risk of plasma levels of the fibrate and niacin being elevated at the same time, and therefore conceptually reduces the risk of side effects.

When combining a systemically acting agent (statin, nicotinic acid, fibrate) with a nonsystemically acting agent (resin, ezetimibe), and after achieving the desired lipid response, follow-up should occur biannually with appropriate safety chemistry assessment. When combining systemically acting agents, more frequent follow-up (e.g., three or four times per year) is advisable.

THE ROLE OF EXERCISE FOR PATIENTS WITH PERIPHERAL ARTERIAL DISEASE

Claudication is a specific symptom of PAD, which results from inadequate delivery of oxygen to muscle cells. It is defined as walking-induced pain in one or both lower extremities that does not abate with continued walking and is relieved only by rest. Claudication is variable, with some patients having only a sense of aching or weakness in the legs with walking, others experiencing a tightening or pressing pain developing in the calves or buttocks, and others feeling a sharp, cramping calf pain that may be excruciating. Symptoms of claudication result in difficulty in carrying out routine daily activities and many patients become deconditioned because of the lack of activity. Exercise therapy along with risk factor modification is an important aspect in the medical management of the patient with PAD and intermittent claudication.

Prospective studies have demonstrated a benefit from exercise therapy in patients experiencing claudication from PAD (121–123). A meta-analysis of both randomized and nonran-

domized trials of exercise training among individuals with claudication indicated that exercise improved symptom-free walking time by an average of 180% (121). The greatest improvements in walking ability occurred when each exercise session lasted more than 30 minutes and sessions were conducted at least three times per week. Another meta-analyses, examining only randomized, controlled trials, concluded that exercise improved maximal walking time by an average of 150% (124). Because pentoxifylline and cilostazol, medications used to treat the symptoms of PAD, increase maximal walking distance by 20% to 60% (average 50%) (125), it is evident that exercise is superior for improving maximal walking ability.

Although the benefit of exercise training in patients with PAD is unequivocal, the precise mechanisms are not completely understood. Several proposed mechanisms include development of collateral blood flow, improvement in vascular endothelial cell function, improved hemorheology, and enhanced oxygen extraction by skeletal muscle (126).

Increase in Collateral Blood Flow

The development of collateral circulation as a result of exercise training results in increased blood flow and oxygen delivery to ischemic extremities. Studies using animal models of occlusive arterial disease demonstrated that exercise training developed collateral circulation and improved blood flow to hind limb muscles of rats (127,128). There are few data, however, demonstrating the development of collateral circulation in response to exercise training in human subjects. Six months of exercise training and conditioning improved functional outcomes and peripheral circulation in patients with intermittent claudication (129). This study showed that exercise increased reactive hyperemic blood flow by 27% and maximal calf blood flow by 30%, and these changes were associated with improved walking ability. Despite this clinical improvement, the ankle–brachial index did not change. Other studies involving human subjects have not been able to document increased lower extremity blood flow following exercise training (130–132). The results of these studies collectively suggest that whereas exercise training may not increase collateral blood flow despite improved walking ability, it may induce redistribution of blood flow from inactive to active muscles. This hypothesis has been supported by animal studies, although not yet confirmed in humans (133).

The evidence for exercise-induced increases in collateral blood flow in patients experiencing claudication from PAD is limited and inconsistent. Therefore, although development of collateral blood flow may be a mechanism for improved walking ability among some individuals experiencing claudication, it is likely that other mechanisms play a role in explaining the large exercise-induced improvements in function and symptoms that occur in patients following exercise training.

Improvement in Endothelial Cell Function

Increased nitric oxide production by vascular endothelial cells is thought to participate in the exercise-induced hyperemia of both the peripheral and coronary artery circulations (134). Nitric oxide, sometimes referred to as endothelial-derived relaxing factor, is a principal mediator of normal vascular tone. It is released continuously by vascular endothelial cells, and in addition to maintaining artery tone, it prevents platelet and leukocyte adhesion to the endothelial surface (135). Atherosclerosis and hypercholesterolemia are associated with dysfunctional endothelial cells and reduced production of nitric oxide. It is possible that reduced nitric oxide production by the vascular endothelial cells lining the arteries of the lower extremities in patients with PAD could impair vasodilation and reduce blood flow.

Using animal models, studies have shown that exercise increases the synthesis and release of nitric oxide and prostacyclin from vascular endothelial cells, which induces vasodilatation and increases blood flow (136). An uncontrolled study of PAD patients experiencing claudication observed that following 6 months of exercise training, endothelial-dependent vasodilation of the lower extremity arteries increased by 61% (137). These data are supported by data from studies conducted in patients with congestive heart failure (138), type 2 diabetes (139), insulin resistance (140), and hypertension (141), which suggest that exercise training improves endothelial-dependent vasodilation.

Exercise training can achieve weight loss with decreases in blood pressure and improvements in the lipid profile and glucose metabolism (142). These salutary metabolic effects may also contribute to enhancing vascular endothelial cell nitric oxide secretion with subsequent vasodilation, increased blood flow, and reduced symptoms of claudication.

Improved Hemorheology

Hemorheology is the study of blood flow in relation to pressure, volume, and resistance, especially in terms of blood vis-

cosity and red blood cell deformation in the microcirculation. It is likely that abnormal hemorheology exists in patients with PAD, because pentoxifylline improves the flow properties of blood in treated PAD patients through decreasing viscosity, improving erythrocyte flexibility, and increasing leukocyte deformability. It has been reported that exercise training may improve abnormal hemorheology (143,144). Two months of exercise training by PAD patients reduced whole blood and plasma viscosity along with a significant increase in pain-free walking (144). This study concluded that hemorheology improved with exercise training to a similar degree that is achieved with medications such as pentoxifylline. In another study, treadmill walking for short periods of moderate intensity by patients with PAD decreased plasma adenosine levels, suggesting decreased ischemia and improved pain-free walking duration (145). Although limited, these data support the notion that exercise training may improve or reverse abnormal hemorheology in patients with PAD.

Metabolic Adaptations and Oxygen Extraction

Exercise training reduces lactate formation, which implies that blood flow and/or oxygen extraction are increased (146,147). Exercise training has also been reported to induce other metabolic adaptations that may account for the improvement in walking ability. Intracellular mitochondrial content and mitochondrial marker enzyme activity is high among healthy individuals who exercise routinely (148). Several reports indicate that either mitochondrial content or mitochondrial marker enzyme activity is increased with exercise training in patients with PAD (149). Such increases could reduce the average path length for oxygen diffusion within the muscle cell and reduce the intracellular adenosine diphosphate concentration, thereby reducing the rate of glycolysis and lactate production (150). Reduced lactate production leads to vasodilation and improved blood flow.

Another metabolic adaptation that could occur with exercise training is reduced plasma acylcarnitine concentrations. Plasma acylcarnitine concentrations, which reflect skeletal muscle metabolic status, are increased at rest and after only 10 minutes of exercise in PAD patients (151). Healthy individuals show no evidence of acylcarnitine accumulation in the blood after 18 minutes of exercise, and only small increases after vigorous exercise. The accumulation of acylcarnitines in the plasma of PAD patients after mild exercise may be a response to hypoxia or reduced skeletal muscle oxygen extraction. These observations suggest that at the point of claudication-induced pain, PAD patients are oxidizing fat in spite of a rising lactate output (152). Sustained exercise training decreases fat oxidation and the resting plasma acylcarnitine concentration in patients with PAD, thereby improving pain-free walking time.

Although the mechanisms for improving symptom-free walking time by exercise training are not completely elucidated, the value of exercise in the treatment of claudication is well documented. Along with smoking cessation and controlling hyperlipidemia, diabetes mellitus, and hypertension, exercise training forms the foundation of medical therapy for PAD patients.

Mode of Exercise Training

Walking is the preferred exercise of choice for patients with PAD (121,126). It is inexpensive, provides improvement in claudication symptoms, and is what patients naturally need to do. Some individuals with PAD may have to climb stairs at home or at work, so it is important to also consider incorporating this type of activity into a training program (153).

Before prescribing an exercise training program, it is prudent to perform treadmill exercise testing with 12-lead electrocardiographic monitoring so that potential cardiac ischemic symptoms and rhythm disturbances may be identified (154,155). Most patients with claudication often have concomitant clinical or occult CHD, hypertension, or adverse cardiovascular and physiological responses during exercise training, and therefore an exercise stress test prior to exercise training is prudent. The exercise stress test will also provide information about thresholds of heart rate and blood pressure responses for use in establishing an exercise prescription. Enrollment of a patient in a medically supervised exercise training program with monitoring of heart rate, blood pressure, and electrocardiogram changes is optimal (154).

At the start of the exercise program, the patient should be instructed to walk at a pace fast enough to bring about claudication-induced pain (moderate to above moderate discomfort) after approximately 100 yards. A walking track or the use of a walking odometer is necessary. The patient should then walk a little farther (i.e., 10 to 20 yards), stop, stand still, and wait until the discomfort ceases. He or she should then continue walking again and repeat this cycle for 30 to 40 minutes. For patients who have access to a treadmill, the exercise program should include establishing a training intensity that produces moderate claudication pain within the first 5 minutes of treadmill walking. The patient should stop and wait until the pain subsides. The patient should then continue walking on the treadmill until the point of claudication-induced pain, and then stop. This cycle should be repeated several times over a 30- to 40-minute period.

Each training session should be approximately 30 to 40 minutes and consist of short periods of treadmill walking interspersed by short rest periods. As the patient's walking ability improves, the exercise workload should be increased by modifying the treadmill incline or speed (or both), or in the case of track walking, the speed, to ensure that the stimulus for producing claudication pain always occurs during the training session. Patients should participate in three to four sessions per week (155). A summary of the key elements of an exercise training program for patients with symptomatic PAD is given in Table 12.9.

Resistance training is generally recommended by the American Heart Association for most patients with other manifestations of cardiovascular disease because of its

TABLE 12.9. *Elements of an exercise training program for patients with symptomatic peripheral arterial disease*

Role of clinician
  Determine that claudication is the major symptom limiting exercise
  Discuss the risks and benefits of therapeutic alternatives, including pharmacologic, percutaneous, and surgical interventions
  Initiate modification of risk factors for systemic atherosclerosis
  Perform treadmill stress testing
  Provide formal referral to a claudication exercise-rehabilitation program
Exercise guidelines for claudication
  Warm-up and cool-down periods of 5–10 min each
  Treadmill and track walking are the most effective exercises for claudication
  Treadmill: The initial workload of the treadmill is to set a speed and grade that elicits claudication symptoms within 5 min
  Track: Patients walk until claudication of moderate severity occurs, then rest either standing or sitting for a brief period to permit symptoms to subside
  The exercise–rest–exercise pattern should be repeated throughout the exercise session
  The initial session should be 30 min of intermittent walking; walking is increased by 5 min each session until 50 min of intermittent walking can be accomplished
  Treadmill or track walking three to five times per week
Frequency: three to five times per week
  Duration: 6 to 8 weeks of supervised training; patients should continue the walking program on their own, with a follow-up at the supervised program at least biannually
Important considerations
  As walking ability improves and a higher heart rate is achieved, the possibility exists that cardiac signs and symptoms may appear; these symptoms should be appropriately diagnosed and treated

Adapted from Robeer GG, Brandsma JW, van den Heuvel SP, et al. Exercise therapy for intermittent claudication: a review of the quality of randomized trials and evaluation of predictive factors. *Eur J Vasc Endovasc Surg* 1998;15:36–43, with permission.

beneficial effects on strength, endurance, flexibility, cardiovascular function, CHD risk factors, and psychosocial well-being. However, for patients with claudication, resistance training does not appear to directly improve walking ability, whereas walking is most effective for improving claudication-limited walking capacity (123). Additionally, many patients with claudication also have reduced muscle mass, strength, and endurance, which could make resistance training extremely difficult.

There are no data to support the efficacy of informal advice about exercise for patients with PAD (156). It is recommended that patients receive supervised, standardized exercise training in a hospital or clinic-based environment (157–159). Following participation in such a program for at least 2 months, some patients may have the ability and desire to continue exercise training either at home or at a health-club facility. However, these individuals should be encouraged to return periodically (e.g., biannually) to the hospital or clinic-based program for evaluation, observation, and, if necessary, refinement of their exercise training program.

About 10% of patients with PAD undergo amputation (160). There is little information about the effectiveness of exercise training for amputees. Arm ergometric stress testing to assess overall cardiovascular status is an alternative for patients who cannot perform the standard treadmill exercise test. Exercise training with the arms in lower extremity amputees may improve cardiovascular endurance and upper-body strength in the poorly conditioned patient (161).

Patients with PAD have a chronic disease characterized by moderate to severe impairment in walking ability. Exercise training produces clinically important improvements in walking efficiency, exercise capacity, and claudication pain severity. These changes in exercise performance can translate into improved activity in the home and work environments. Therefore, a supervised exercise rehabilitation program should be considered an important treatment option for patients experiencing claudication from PAD.

REFERENCES

1. Criqui MH, Fronek A, Barret-Connor E, et al. The prevalence of peripheral arterial disease in a defined population. *Circulation* 1985;71:510–515.
2. Blackburn H. The concept of risk. In: Pearson TA, Criqui MH, Luepker RV, et al., eds. *Primer in preventive cardiology.* Dallas, TX: American Heart Association, 1994:25–41.
3. Scandinavian Simvastatin Survival Study Group. Randomized trial of cholesterol lowering in 4444 patients with coronary heart disease: the Scandinavian Simvastatin Survival Study (4S). *Lancet* 1994;344:1383–1389.
4. Sacks FM, Pfeffer MA, Moye LA, et al. The effect of pravastatin on coronary events after myocardial infarction in patients with average cholesterol levels. *N Engl J Med* 1996;335:1001–1009.
5. The Long-Term Intervention with Pravastatin in Ischaemic Disease (LIPID) Study Group. Prevention of cardiovascular events and death with pravastatin in patients with coronary heart disease and a broad range of initial cholesterol levels. *N Engl J Med* 1998;339:1349–1357.
6. Shepherd J, Cobbe SM, Ford I, et al. Prevention of coronary heart disease with pravastatin in men with hypercholesterolemia. *N Engl J Med* 1995;333:1301–1307.
7. Downs JR, Clearfield M, Weis S, et al. Primary prevention of acute coronary events with lovastatin in men and women with average cholesterol levels. Results of AFCAPS/TexCAPS. *JAMA* 1998;279:1616–1622.
8. Heart Protection Study Collaborative Group. MRC/BHF Heart Protection Study of cholesterol lowering with simvastatin in 20,536 high-risk individuals: a randomized placebo-controlled trial. *Lancet* 2002;360:7–22.
9. Herz J. The LDL-receptor related protein: portrait of a multifunctional receptor. *Curr Opin Lipidol* 1993;4:107–113.
10. Mahley RW. Apolipoprotein E: cholesterol transport protein with expanding role in cell biology. *Science* 1988;240:622–628.
11. Groot PHE, van Stiphout WHJ, Kraus XH, et al. Postprandial lipoprotein metabolism in normolipidemic men with and without coronary artery disease. *Arterioscler Thromb* 1991;11:653–660.
12. Gotto AM, Pownall HJ, Havel RA. Introduction to the plasma lipoproteins. In: Segrest JP, Albers JJ, eds. *Methods of enzymology.* New York: Academic Press, 1986:3–41.
13. Goldberg IJ, Le NA, Paternitti JR, et al. Lipoprotein metabolism during acute inhibition of hepatic triglyceride lipase in the cynomolgus monkey. *J Clin Invest* 1982;70:1184–1190.
14. Brown MS, Goldstein JL. A receptor-mediated pathway for cholesterol homeostasis. *Science* 1986;232:34–47.
15. Brown MS, Goldstein JL. The SREBP pathway: regulation of cholesterol metabolism by proteolysis of a membrane-bound transcription factor (review). *Cell* 1997;89:331–340.
16. Barter PJ, Rye KA. Molecular mechanisms of reverse cholesterol transport. *Curr Opin Lipidol* 1996;7:82–87.
17. Oram JF, Lawn RM, Garvin MR, et al. ABCA1 is the cAMP-inducible apolipoprotein receptor that mediates cholesterol secretion from macrophages. *J Biol Chem* 2000;275:34508–34511.
18. Oram JF, Vaughan AM. ABCA1-mediated transport of cellular cholesterol and phospholipids to HDL apolipoproteins. *Curr Opin Lipidol* 2000;11:253–260.
19. Wang N, Silver DL, Costet P, et al. Specific binding of apoA-I, enhanced cholesterol efflux, and altered plasma membrane morphology in cells expressing ABCA1. *J Biol Chem* 2000;275:33053–33058.
20. Chembenoit O, Hamon Y, Marguet D, et al. Specific docking of apolipoprotein A-I at the cell surface requires a functional ABCA1 transporter. *J Biol Chem* 2002;276:9955–9960.
21. Glomset JA. The plasma lecithin:cholesterol acyltransferase reaction. *J Lipid Res* 1968;9:155–167.
22. Frank PG, Marcel YL. Apolipoprotein A-I: structure–function relationships. *J Lipid Res* 2000;41:853–872.
23. LaRosa JC. Lipid-lowering. In: LaRosa JC, ed. *Medical management of atherosclerosis.* New York: Marcel Dekker, 1998:1–30.
24. Ginsberg HN. Lipoprotein physiology and its relationship to atherogenesis. *Endocrinol Metab Clin North Am* 1990;19:211–224.
25. Fielding CJ, Fielding PE. Intracellular cholesterol transport. *J Lipid Res* 1997;38:1503–1521.
26. Inazu A, Brown ML, Hesler CB, et al. Increased high-density lipoprotein levels caused by a common cholesteryl-ester transfer protein gene mutation. *N Engl J Med* 1990;323:1234–1238.
27. Williams DL, Connelly MA, Temel RE, et al. Scavenger receptor BI and cholesterol trafficking. *Curr Opin Lipidol* 1999;10:329–339.
28. Williams DL, Connelly MA, Temel RE, et al. Scavenger receptor B1 and cholesterol trafficking. *Curr Opin Lipidol* 1999;10:329–339.
29. Ginsberg HN. Lipoprotein metabolism and its relationship to atherosclerosis. *Med Clin North Am* 1994;78:1–20.
30. Funke H. Genetic determinants of high-density lipoprotein levels. *Curr Opin Lipidol* 1997;8:189–196.
31. Parthasarathy S, Barnett J, Fong LG. High-density lipoprotein inhibits the oxidative modification of low-density lipoprotein. *Biochim Biophys Acta* 1990;1044:275–283.
32. Barter PJ, Rye KA. High-density lipoproteins and coronary heart disease. *Atherosclerosis* 1996;121:1–12.
33. Pomerantz KB, Fleisher LN, Tall AR, et al. Enrichment of endothelial cell arachidonate by lipid transfer from high-density lipoproteins: relationship to prostaglandin I_2 synthesis. *Lipid Res* 1985;26:1269–1276.
34. Utermann G. The mysteries of lipoprotein(a). *Science* 1989;246:904–910.
35. Lackner C, Boerwinkle E, Leffert CC, et al. Molecular basis of apolipoprotein(a) isoform heterogenicity as revealed by pulsed-field gel electrophoresis. *J Clin Invest* 1991;87:2153–2161.

36. Boerwinkle E, Leffert CC, Lin J, et al. Apolipoprotein (a) gene accounts for greater than 90% of the variation in plasma lipoprotein(a) concentrations. *J Clin Invest* 1992;90:52–60.
37. Loscalzo J, Weinfeld M, Fless GM, et al. Lipoprotein (a), fibrin binding, and plasminogen activation. *Arteriosclerosis* 1990;10:240–245.
38. Miles LA, Fless GM, Levin EG, et al. A potential basis of the thrombotic risks associated with lipoprotein (a). *Nature* 1989;339:301–303.
39. Hajjar KA, Gavish D, Breslow JL, et al. Lipoprotein (a) modulation of endothelial cell surface fibrinolysis and its potential role in atherosclerosis. *Nature* 1989;339:303–305.
40. Sigurdsson G, Baldursdottir A, Sigvalderson H, et al. Predictive value of apolipoproteins in a prospective survey of coronary artery disease in men. *Am J Cardiol* 1992;69:1251–1254.
41. Jauhiainen M, Koskinen P, Ehnholm C, et al. Lipoprotein (a) and coronary heart disease risk: a nested case–control study of the Helsinki Heart Study participants. *Atherosclerosis* 1991;89:59–67.
42. Ridker PM, Hennekens CH, Stampfer MJ. A prospective study of lipoprotein (a) and the risk of myocardial infarction. *JAMA* 1993;270:2195–2199.
43. Schaefer EJ, Lamon-Fava S, Jenner JL, et al. Lipoprotein (a) levels and risk of coronary heart disease in men. The Lipid Research Clinics Coronary Primary Prevention Trial. *JAMA* 1994;274:999–1003.
44. Cremer P, Nagel D, Labrot B, et al. Lipoprotein Lp(a) as predictor of myocardial infarction in comparison to fibrinogen, LDL cholesterol and other risk factors: results from the prospective Gottingen Risk Incidence and Prevalence Study (GRIPS). *Eur J Clin Invest* 1994;24:444–453.
45. Bostom AG, Gagnon DR, Cupples LA, et al. A prospective investigation of elevated lipoprotein (a) detected by electrophoresis and cardiovascular disease in women. The Framingham Heart Study. *Circulation* 1994;90:1688–1695.
46. Assman G, Schulte H, von Eckardstein A. Hypertriglyceridemia and elevated lipoprotein (a) are risk factors for major coronary events in middle-aged men. *Am J Cardiol* 1996;77:1179–1184.
47. Bostom AG, Cupples LA, Jenner JL, et al. Elevated lipoprotein (a) and coronary heart disease in men aged 55 years and younger. *JAMA* 1996;276:544–548.
48. Futterman LG, Lemberg L. Lp(a)—an independent risk factor for coronary heart disease after menopause. *Am J Crit Care* 2001;10:63–67.
49. Expert Panel on Detection, Evaluation and Treatment of High Blood Cholesterol in Adults. Executive summary of the third report of the National Cholesterol Education Program (NECP) Expert Panel on Detection, Evaluation and Treatment of High Blood Colesterol in Adults (Adult Treatment Panel III). *JAMA* 2001;285:2486–2497.
50. Smith J, Blair SN, Criqui MH, et al. Preventing heart attack and death in patients with coronary disease. *Circulation* 1995;92:2–4.
51. Haffner SM, Lehto S, Ronnemaa T, et al. Mortality from coronary heart disease in subjects with type 2 diabetes and in non-diabetic subjects with and without prior myocardial infarction. *N Engl J Med* 1998;339:229–234.
52. Friedewald WT, Levy RI, Fredrickson DS. Estimation of the concentration of low-density lipoprotein cholesterol without use of the preparative ultracentrifuge. *Clin Chem* 1972;18:499–502.
53. Stampfer MJ, Sacks FM, Salvini S, et al. A prospective study of cholesterol apolipoproteins and the risk of myocardial infarction. *N Engl J Med* 1991;325:373–381.
54. Joven J, Villabona C, Vilella E, et al. Abnormalities of lipoprotein metabolism in patients with the nephrotic syndrome. *N Engl J Med* 1990;323:579–584.
55. Rader DJ, Rosas S. Management of selected lipid abnormalities: hypertriglyceridemia, low HDL cholesterol, lipoprotein (a) in thyroid and renal diseases and post-transplantation. *Med Clin North Am* 2000;84:43–61.
56. Detection and management of lipid disorders in diabetes. *Diabetes Care* 1993;16:828–834.
57. Abbate SL, Brunzell JD. Pathophysiology of hyperlipidemia in diabetes mellitus. *J Cardiovasc Pharmacol Ther* 1990;16:51–57.
58. Taskinen M. Insulin resistance and lipoprotein metabolism. *Curr Opin Lipidol* 1995;6:153–160.
59. Seidel D, Alaupovic P, Furman RH, et al. A lipoprotein characterizing obstructive jaundice. *J Clin Invest* 1970;49:2396–2407.
60. Seidel D. Lipoproteins in liver disease. *J Clin Chem Clin Biochem* 1987;25:541–551.
61. Stone NJ. Secondary causes of hyperlipidemia. *Med Clin North Am* 1994;78:117–141.
62. Knopp RH, Walden CE, Wahl PW, et al. Oral contraceptive and postmenopausal estrogen effects on lipoprotein triglyceride and cholesterol in an adult female population: Relationships to estrogen and progestin potency. *J Clin Endocrinol Metab* 1981;53:1123–1130.
63. Grimm RH, Hunninghake DB. Lipids and hypertension. Implications of guidelines for cholesterol management in the treatment of hypertension. *Am J Med* 1986;80[Suppl 2A]:56–63.
64. Gaziano JM, Manson JE. Diet and heart disease: the role of fat, alcohol and antioxidants. *Cardiol Clin* 1996;14:69–83.
65. Gotto Jr AM. Lipid-regulating drugs and low-density lipoprotein apheresis. In: Gotto Jr AM, Pownall HJ, eds. *Manual of lipid disorders*. Baltimore: Williams & Wilkins, 1992:292–323.
66. Knopp RH. Drug treatment of lipid disorders. *N Engl J Med* 1999;341:493–511.
67. Olsson AG, Pears J, Mizan J, et al. Effect of rosuvastatin on low-density lipoprotein cholesterol in patients with hypercholesterolemia. *Am J Cardiol* 2002;88:504–508.
68. McCormick AD, McKillip D, Butters CJ, et al. *ZD4522—an HMG-CoA reductase inhibitor free of metabolically mediated drug interactions: metabolic studies in human in vitro systems.* Presented at the 29th annual meeting of the American College of Clinical Pharmacology, September 2000, Chicago.
69. Jones P, Kafonek S, Laurora I, et al. Comparative dose efficacy study of atorvastatin versus simvastatin, pravastatin, lovastatin and fluvastatin in patients with primary hypercholesterolemia (the CURVES study). *Am J Cardiol* 1998;81:582–587.
70. Muldoon MF, Manuck SB, Mendelsohn AB, et al. Cholesterol reduction and non-illness mortality: meta-analysis of randomised clinical trials. *Br Med J* 2001;322:11–15.
71. Ahmad S. Lovastatin and peripheral neuropathy. *Am Heart J* 1995;130:1321.
72. Jeppesen U, Gaist D, Smith T, et al. Statins and peripheral neuropathy. *Eur J Clin Pharmacol* 1999;54:835–838.
73. Gaist D, Jeppesen U, Anderson M, et al. Statins and risk of polyneuropathy. A case–control study. *Neurology* 2992;58:1333–1337.
74. Roth T, Richardson GR, Sullivan JP, et al. Comparative effects of pravastatin and lovastatin on nighttime sleep and daytime performance. *Clin Cardiol* 1992;15:426–432.
75. Parinen M, Pihl S, Strandberg T, et al. Comparison of effects on sleep of lovastatin and pravastatin in hypercholesterolemia. *Am J Cardiol* 1994;73:876–880.
76. Grundy SM, Vega GL, Bilheimer DW. Influence of combined therapy with mevinolin and interruption of bile acid reabsorption on low-density lipoproteins in heterozygous familial hypercholesterolemia. *Ann Intern Med* 1985;103:339–343.
77. Gotto AM. Management of dyslipidemia. *Am J Med* 2002;112:105–185.
78. The Lipid Research Clinics Coronary Primary Prevention Trial Result I. Reduction in incidence of coronary heart disease. *JAMA* 1984;251:351–364.
79. Illingworth RD. Management of hypercholesterolemia. *Med Clin North Am* 2000;84:23–42.
80. Davidson MH, Dillon MA, Gordon B, et al. Colesevelam hydrochloride (Cholestagel). A new, potent bile acid sequestrant associated with a low incidence of gastrointestinal side effects. *Arch Intern Med* 1999;159:1893–1900.
81. Maciejko JJ, Brazg R, Shah A, et al. Psyllium for the reduction of cholestyramine associated gastrointestinal symptoms in the treatment of primary hypercholesterolemia. *Arch Fam Med* 1994;3:955–960.
82. Altschul R, Hoffer A, Stephen JD. Influence of nicotinic acid on serum cholesterol in man. *J Arch Biochem Biophys* 1955;54:558–559.
83. Deedwania PC. Clinical perspectives on primary and secondary prevention of coronary atherosclerosis. *Med Clin North Am* 1995;79:973–998.
84. Kwiterovich PO. State of the art update and review: Clinical trials of lipid-lowering agents. *Am J Cardiol* 1998;82:3U–17U.
85. Rossnow JE. The effects of lowering serum cholesterol on coronary heart disease risk. *Med Clin North Am* 1994;78:181–195.
86. Coronary Drug Project Research Group. Clofibrate and niacin in coronary heart disease. *JAMA* 1971;231:360–381.

87. Brown GB, Zhao XQ, Chait A, et al. Simvastatin and niacin, antioxidant vitamins, or the combination for the prevention of coronary disease. *N Engl J Med* 2001;345:1583–1592.

88. Hotz W. Nicotinic acid and its derivatives: a short survey. *Adv Lipid Res* 1983;20:195–217.

89. Carlson LA, Hamsten A, Asplund A. Pronounced lowering of serum levels of lipoprotein Lp(a) in hyperlipidemic subjects treated with nicotinic acid. *J Intern Med* 1989;226:271–276.

90. Shepherd J, Packard CJ, Patsch JR, et al. Effects of nicotinic acid therapy on plasma high-density subfraction and composition and on apolipoprotein A metabolism. *J Clin Invest* 1979;63:858–867.

91. Kamanna V, Kashyap ML. Mechanism of action of niacin on lipoprotein metabolism. *Curr Atheroscler Rep* 2000;2:36–46.

92. Illingworth DR, Stein EA, Metchel YB, et al. Comparative effects of lovastatin and niacin in primary hypercholesterolemia. *Arch Intern Med* 1994;154:1586–1595.

93. Morgan JM, Capuzzi DM, Guyton JR. A new extended-release niacin (Niaspan): efficacy, tolerability and safety in hypercholesterolemic patients. *Am J Cardiol* 1998;82:29U–34U.

94. Mullin GE, Greenson JK, Mitchell MC. Fulminant hepatic failure after ingestion of sustained-release nicotinic acid. *Ann Intern Med* 1989;111:253–255.

95. Grundy SM, Vega GL, McGovern ME, et al. Efficacy, safety and tolerability of once-daily niacin for the treatment of dyslipidemia associated with type 2 diabetes. *Arch Intern Med* 2002;162:1568–1569.

96. Morrow JD, Parsons WG, Roberts LJ. Release of markedly increased quantities of prostagland I_2 *in vivo* in humans following the administration of nicotinic acid. *Prostaglandins* 1989;38:263–274.

97. vanHeek M, France CF, Compton DS, et al. *In vivo* metabolism-based discovery of a potent cholesterol absorption inhibitor, SCH58235, in the rat and rhesus monkey through the identification of the active metabolites of SCH48461. *J Pharmacol Exp Ther* 1997;283:157–163.

98. van Heek M, Farley C, Compton DS, et al. Comparison of the activity and disposition of the novel cholesterol absorption inhibitor, SCH58235, and its glucuronide, SCH60663. *Br J Pharmacol* 2000;129:1748–1754.

99. Knopp RH, Bays H, Manion CV, et al. Effect of ezetimibe on serum concentrations of lipid-soluble vitamins [Abstract]. *Atherosclerosis* 2002;2[Suppl]:90.

100. Sudhop T, Lutjohann D, Kodal A, et al. Inhibition of intestinal cholesterol absorption by ezetimibe in humans. *Circulation* 2002;106:1943–1948.

101. Davis HR, Compton DS, Hoos L, et al. Ezetimibe (SCH58235) localizes to the brush border of small intestinal enterocyte and inhibits enterocyte cholesterol uptake and absorption [Abstract]. *Eur Heart J* 2000;21[Suppl]:636.

102. Bays HE, Moore PB, Drehobl MA, et al. Effectiveness and tolerability of ezetimibe in patients with primary hypercholesterolemia: pooled analysis of two phase II studies. *Clin Ther* 2001;23:1209–1230.

103. Davidson MH, McGarry T, Bettis R, et al. Ezetimibe coadministered with simvastatin in patients with primary hypercholesterolemia. *J Am Coll Cardiol* 2002;40:2125–2134.

104. Ballantyne C, Houri J, Notarbartolo A, et al. Ezetimibe co-administered with atorvastatin in 628 patients with primary hypercholesterolemia [Abstract]. *J Am Coll Cardiol* 2002;39[Suppl A]:227A.

105. Gagne C, Gaudet D, Bruckert E. Efficacy and safety of ezetimibe coadministered with atorvastatin or simvastatin in patients with homozygous familial hypercholesterolemia. *Circulation* 2002;105:2469–2475.

106. Bays H, Weiss S, Gagne C, et al. Ezetimibe added to ongoing statin therapy for treatment of primary hypercholesterolemia [Abstract]. *J Am Coll Cardiol* 2002;39[Suppl A]:245A.

107. Lipka L, Kerzner B, Corbelli J, et al. *Results of ezetimibe coadministered with lovastatin in 548 patients with primary hypercholesterolemia.* Paper presented at the World Congress of Cardiology, May 2002, Sydney, Australia.

108. Melani L, Mills R, Hassman D, et al. *Ezetimibe coadministered with pravastatin in 538 patients with primary hypercholesterolemia.* Paper presented at the World Congress of Cardiology, May 2002, Sydney, Australia.

109. Staels B, Dallongeville J, Auwerx J, et al. Mechanism of action of fibrates on lipid and lipoprotein metabolism. *Circulation* 1998;98:2088–2093.

110. Brown WV, Baginsky ML. Inhibition of lipoprotein lipase by an apoprotein of human very low-density lipoprotein. *Biochem Biophys Res Commun* 1972;46:375–382.

111. Rustaeus S, Lindberg K, Stillemark P, et al. Assembly of very low density lipoprotein: a two-step process of apolipoprotein B core lipidation. *J Nutr* 1999;129[Suppl]:463S–466S.

112. Staels B, Dallongeville J, Auwerx J, et al. Mechanism of action of fibrates on lipid and lipoprotein metabolism. *Circulation* 1998:98:2088–2093.

113. Kremer P, Marowski C, Jones C, et al. Therapeutic effects of bezafibrate and gemfibrozil in hyperlipoproteinemia type IIA and IIB. *Curr Med Res Opin* 1989;11:293–303.

114. Goldberg AC, Schonfeld G, Feldman EB, et al. Fenofibrate for the treatment of type IV and V hyperlipoproteinemias: a double-blind, placebo-controlled, multicenter U.S. study. *Clin Ther* 1989;11:69–83.

115. Hunninghake DB, Peters J. Effects of fibric acid derivatives on blood lipid and lipoprotein levels. *Am J Med* 1987;83[Suppl 5B]:44–49.

116. Wilson DE, Lees RS. Metabolic relationships among the lipoproteins: reciprocal changes in the concentrations of very low- and low-density lipoproteins in man. *J Clin Invest* 1972;51:1052–1062.

117. Kuo PT, Wilson AC, Kostis JB, et al. Treatment of type III hyperlipoproteinemia with gemfibrozil to retard the progression of coronary artery disease. *Am Heart J* 1988;116:85–90.

118. Ellen RLB, McPherson R. Long term efficacy and safety of fenofibrate and a statin in the treatment of combined hyperlipidemia. *Am J Cardiol* 1998;81:60B–65B.

119. Frick MH, Elo O, Haapa K, et al. Helsinki Heart Study: primary prevention trial with gemfibrozil in middle-aged men with dyslipidemia. *N Engl J Med* 1987;317:1237–1245.

120. Rubins HB, Robins SJ, Collins D, et al. Gemfibrozil for the secondary prevention of coronary heart disease in men with low levels of high-density lipoprotein cholesterol. *N Engl J Med* 1999;341:410–418.

121. Gardner AW, Poehlman ET. Exercise rehabilitation programs for the treatment of claudication pain: a meta-analysis. *JAMA* 1995;274:975–980.

122. Regensteiner JG. Exercise in the treatment of claudication: assessment and treatment of functional impairment. *Vasc Med* 1997;2:238–242.

123. Robeer GG, Brandsma JW, van den Heuvel SP, et al. Exercise therapy for intermittent claudication: a review of the quality of randomized clinical trials and evaluation of predictive factors. *Eur J Vasc Endovasc Surg* 1998;15:36–43.

124. Leng GC, Fowler B, Ernst E. Exercise for intermittent claudication. *Cochrane Database Syst Rev* 2000;2:CD000990.

125. Creager MA. Medical management of peripheral arterial disease. *Cardiol Rev* 2001;9:238–245.

126. Stewart KJ, Hiatt WR, Regensteiner JG, et al. Exercise training for claudication. *N Engl J Med* 2002;347:1941–1951.

127. Yang HT, Ogilvie RW, Terjung RL. Training increases collateral-dependent muscle blood flow in aged rats. *Am J Physiol* 1995;268:H1174–H1180.

128. Mathien GM, Terjung RL. Muscle blood flow in trained rats with peripheral arterial insufficiency. *Am J Physiol* 1990;258:H759–H765.

129. Gardner AW, Katzel LI, Sorkin JD, et al. Exercise rehabilitation improves functional outcomes and peripheral circulation in patients with intermittent claudication: a randomized controlled trial. *J Am Geriatr Soc* 2002;49:755–762.

130. Lundgren F, Dahllof AG, Lundholm K, et al. Intermittent claudication — surgical reconstruction or physical training? A prospective randomized trial of treatment efficiency. *Ann Surg* 1989;209:346–355.

131. Johnson EC, Voyles WF, Atterbom HA, et al. Effects of exercise training on common femoral artery blood flow in patients with intermittent claudication. *Circulation* 1989;80[Suppl III]:III-59–III-72.

132. Lundgren F, Dahllof AG, Schersten T, et al. Muscle enzyme adaptation in patients with peripheral arterial insufficiency: spontaneous adaptation, effect of different treatments and consequences on walking performance. *Clin Sci* (Lond) 1989;77:485–493.

133. Terjung RL, Mathien GM, Erney TP, et al. Peripheral adaptations to low blood flow in muscle during exercise. *Am J Cardiol* 1988;62:15E–19E.

134. Kingwell BA. Nitric oxide as a metabolic regulator during exercise: effects of training in health and disease. *Clin Exp Pharmacol Physiol* 2000;27:230–250.

135. Levine CN, Keaney JF, Vita JA. Cholesterol reduction in cardiovascular disease: clinical benefits and possible mechanisms. *N Engl J Med* 1995;332:512–521.

136. McAllister RM, Hirai T, Musch TI. Contributions of endothelium-derived nitric oxide (EDNO) to the skeletal muscle blood flow response to exercise. *Med Sci Sports Exerc* 1995;27:1145–1151.

137. Brendle DC, Joseph LJ, Corretti MC, et al. Effects of exercise rehabilitation on endothelial reactivity in older patients with peripheral arterial disease. *Am J Cardiol* 2001;87:324–329.

138. Hambrecht R, Fiehn E, Weigl C, et al. Regular physical exercise corrects endothelial dysfunction and improves exercise capacity in patients with chronic heart failure. *Circulation* 1998;98:2709–2715.

139. Maiorana A, O'Driscoll G, Cheetham C, et al. The effect of combined aerobic and resistance exercise training on vascular function in type 2 diabetes. *J Am Coll Cardiol* 2002;38:860–866.

140. Lavrencic A, Salobir BG, Keber I. Physical training improves flow-mediated dilation in patients with the polymetabolic syndrome. *Arterioscler Thomb Vasc Biol* 2000;20:551–555.

141. Higashi Y, Sasaki S, Kurisu S, et al. Regular aerobic exercise augments endothelium-dependent vascular relaxation in normotensive as well as hypertensive subjects: role of endothelium-derived nitric oxide. *Circulation* 1999;100:1194–1202.

142. Hiatt WR, Regensteiner JG, Hargarten ME, et al. Benefit of exercise conditioning for patients with peripheral arterial disease. *Circulation* 1990;81:602–609.

143. Neibauer J, Cooke JP. Cardiovascular effects of exercise: role of endothelial shear stress. *J Am Coll Cardiol* 1996;28:1652–1660.

144. Ernst EE, Matrai A. Intermittent claudication, exercise and blood rheology. *Circulation* 1987;76:1110–1114.

145. Capecchi PL, Pasini FL, Cati G, et al. Experimental model of short-time exercise-induced preconditioning in PAD patients. *Angiology* 1997;48:469–480.

146. Sorlie D, Myhre K. Effects of physical training in intermittent claudication. *Scand J Clin Lab Invest* 1978;38:217–222.

147. Ruell PA, Imperial ES, Bonar FJ, et al. Intermittent claudication. The effect of physical training on walking tolerance and venous lactate concentration. *Eur J Appl Physiol Occup Physiol* 1984;52:420–425.

148. Saltin B, Gollnick PD. In: Peachy LD, Adrian RH, Geiger RS, eds., *Handbook of physiology: skeletal muscle.* Baltimore: American Physiological Society, 1983:555–631.

149. Barnard RJ. In: Bouchard C, Shephard RJ, Stephens T, eds., The role of exercise in the treatment of peripheral vascular disease. *Physical Activity, Fitness and Health.* Champaign, IL: Human Kinetics, 1994: 622–632.

150. Yang HT, Dinn RF, Terjung RL. Training increases muscle blood flow in rats with peripheral arterial insufficiency. *J Appl Physiol* 1990;69: 1353–1359.

151. Hiatt WR, Nawaz D, Brass EP. Carnitine metabolism during exercise in patients with peripheral vascular disease. *J Appl Physiol* 1987;62: 2383–2387.

152. Lundgren F, Dahllof AG, Schersten T, et al. Muscle enzyme adaptation in patients with peripheral arterial insufficiency: spontaneous adaptation, effect of different treatments and consequences on walking performance. *Clin Sci* 1989;77:485–493.

153. Jones PP, Skinner JS, Smith LK, et al. Functional improvements following StairMaster vs. treadmill exercise training for patients with intermittent claudication. *J Cardiopulm Rehabil* 1996;16:47–55.

154. American Association of Cardiovascular and Pulmonary Rehabilitation. *Guidelines for cardiac rehabilitation and secondary prevention programs.* Champaign, IL: Human Kinetics, 1999.

155. Kenny WL, ed. *ACSM's guidelines for exercise testing and prescription,* 5th ed. Baltimore: Williams & Wilkins, 1995.

156. Coffman JD. Intermittent claudication—be conservative. *N Engl J Med* 1991;325:577–578.

157. Regensteiner JG, Meyer TJ, Krupski WC, et al. Hospital vs. home-based exercise rehabilitation for patients with peripheral arterial occlusive disease. *Angiology* 1997;48:291–300.

158. Patterson RB, Pinto B, Marcus B, et al. Value of a supervised exercise program for the therapy of arterial claudication. *J Vasc Surg* 1997;25:312–319.

159. Nehler MR, Hiatt WR. Exercise therapy for claudication. *Ann Vasc Surg* 1999;13:109–114.

160. Leng GC, Lee AJ, Fowkes FG, et al. Incidence, natural history and cardiovascular events in symptomatic and asymptomatic peripheral arterial disease in the general population. *Int J Epidemiol* 1996;25:1172–1181.

161. Priebe M, Davidoff G, Lampman RM. Exercise testing and training in patients with peripheral vascular disease and lower extremity amputation. *West J Med* 1991;154:598–601.

CHAPTER 13

Peripheral Arterial Disease

Risk Factor Identification and Modification

Douglas S. Jacoby and Emile R. Mohler, III

Key Points

- Peripheral arterial disease (PAD) results in significant morbidity and mortality, with approximately a threefold risk of death during 10 years, after adjusting for other risk factors.
- PAD has associations with other vascular diseases, and serves as an independent risk factor for coronary artery disease, cerebral vascular disease, and arterial aneurysms.
- Modification of traditional cardiovascular risk factors is critical to improving outcomes, with interventions including promoting smoking cessation, achieving tight glycemic control, correcting dyslipidemia, and optimizing blood pressure.
- Nontraditional risk factors may eventually improve risk stratification and serve as therapeutic targets, but their role requires further investigation.
- Medical management of intermittent claudication relies on exercise training, with the addition of pharmacologic intervention if needed.

INTRODUCTION

Peripheral arterial disease (PAD) results in significant morbidity and mortality throughout industrialized societies. The prevalence of PAD rises sharply with age, with noninvasive testing revealing PAD in 2.5% of the population at ages 40 to 59 years, 8.3% at ages 60 to 69 years, and 18.8% at ages 70 to 79 years (1,2). In addition to age, other major risk factors are smoking and diabetes, with additional risk factors including hypertension and dyslipidemia (3).

Among patients with PAD, approximately 50% are asymptomatic (4). Men with PAD have a 10-year mortality of 61.8%, which is a relative risk (RR) of 3.3 relative to men without PAD. Women have a 10-year mortality of 33.3%, which is a RR of 2.5 relative to women without PAD (1). Despite the prognostic significance of PAD, a recent study of primary care management found that only 49% of physicians knew that their patients had PAD, whereas 83% of the patients knew the diagnosis (5).

Although PAD results in amputations in about 4% to 7% of affected patients, the true burden of morbidity and mortality reflects adverse outcomes throughout the entire cardiovascular system (6). PAD is an independent risk factor for coronary artery disease, cerebrovascular disease, and aneurysmal disease, and in addition has to associations with diabetes and hypertension (4). Despite the prevalence of PAD and associated cardiovascular risk, only approximately 25% of patients are undergoing treatment (4).

The following discussion focuses on risk factors for PAD, and provides evidence that medical management altering these risk factors improves outcomes. When we discuss the data for different risk factors, we will frequently rely on two noninvasive vascular tests to provide a more sensitive measure of PAD than history and physical exam alone. The ankle–brachial index (ABI) is the ratio of the ankle systolic pressure to the brachial artery systolic pressure. An ABI of greater than 0.90 is normal, with 0.7 to 0.89 considered mild and 0.5 to 0.69 moderate. An ABI of less than 0.5 reflects severe PAD, with significant risk of critical limb ischemia (7). In a substudy of the Systolic Hypertension in the Elderly Program (SHEP) trial, an ABI of less than or equal to 0.9 was associated with a mortality relative risk of 3.8 (8). In general, the lower the ABI, the higher is the risk of a cardiovascular event, with the lowest ABIs associated with an annual mortality of 25% (3).

Carotid and femoral intimal–medial thickness (IMT) is a measure of the morphology of the arterial blood vessel wall that appears to detect early atherosclerosis and correlate with risk of future vascular events. In the Arterosclerosis Risk in Communities Study, which included 13,870 participants, mean carotid IMT was significantly greater in patients with clinical cardiovascular disease (9). Studies have specifically examined the relationship between carotid IMT and PAD. The Edinburgh Artery Study, which included 1,106 participants, found an association between carotid IMT and PAD in both asymptomatic patients ($p<0.01$) and symptomatic patients ($p<0.01$) (10). The Rotterdam Study, which included 970 participants, found an association between PAD and a carotid IMT of greater than 0.89 mm (11). The Secondary Manifestations of ARTerial disease (SMART) study demonstrated an association between carotid IMT and abdominal aortic aneurysm (12).

Traditional cardiovascular risk factors (smoking, diabetes, dyslipidemia, hypertension) and nontraditional cardiovascular risk factors [homocysteine, lipoprotein(a), fibrinogen, high-sensitivity C-reactive protein (CRP), and others] affect the development and progression of PAD (Fig. 13.1). The following discussion focuses on risk factor identification and

medical management, followed by therapeutic interventions that decrease mortality and symptoms and increase the quality of life.

RISK FACTOR IDENTIFICATION AND MODIFICATION

Cardiac Disease

The population of adults with PAD overlaps significantly with that with coronary artery disease (CAD). CAD has been found in 29% of patients with PAD, compared to 11% of patients without PAD (2). One study utilizing angiography to diagnose CAD found that 90% of patients with intermittent claudication have CAD (1). In a study of 439 men, an ABI of less than 0.9 was associated with twice the cardiac event rate (13). The increased risk of cardiac events in patients with PAD has been corroborated in many other studies (14).

Because patients with PAD are at high risk for cardiovascular disease and multiple cardiac risk factors, an association with left ventricular dysfunction would not be surprising. Although no study has evaluated PAD alone, a case–control study examined 522 patients presenting to hospital with a stroke, transient ischemic attack, or PAD, and found that left ventricular dysfunction with an ejection fraction of less than 40% was five times more common than in the control subjects (15). Because patients with strokes or PAD often engage in limited physical activity, a majority of these patients were asymptomatic, reflecting hidden left ventricular dysfunction. As modern medicine is refined to identify or target high-risk populations for screening, future research may indicate that patients with PAD are at sufficiently high risk to warrant evaluation with echocardiography even if they are otherwise asymptomatic.

Smoking

Cigarette smoking is the most significant risk factor for PAD, and over 90% of patients referred to vascular clinics in hospitals have a history of smoking (16,17). This association has been known for over 90 years. In 1911, Wilhelm Erb reported that intermittent claudication (IC) was three to six times more likely in patients who smoked relative to nonsmokers. Since that time, many other studies have confirmed the association between smoking and PAD, with RR ranging from 2 to 10 (5,18–30).

There have not been prospective randomized controlled trials to evaluate these associations, but the consistent association in numerous study designs provides support that the association is one of causation. For example, in a study comparing 184 smokers to 56 age-matched nonsmokers, with no additional risk factors in either group, IMT, which reflects peripheral atherosclerosis and is associated with cardiovascular outcomes, showed a significant worsening in smokers for both carotid IMT ($p<0.02$) and femoral IMT ($p<0.0001$), providing further support that this association is dose dependent (31). Thus, progression of PAD is affected by smoking

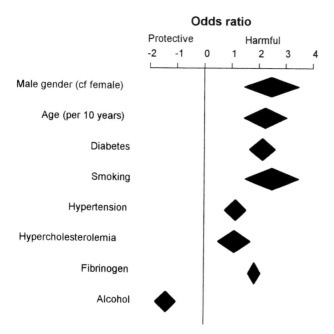

FIG. 13.1. Diagram showing the range of odds ratios for risk factors for progression of peripheral arterial disease. From TransAtlantic Inter-Society Consensus in Supplement to *Journal of Vascular Surgery* 2000;31:517.

quantity and duration, and is correlated with the development of claudication (32). The RR of developing claudication has been estimated at 2.11 for patients smoking more than 20 cigarettes per day, and at 1.75 for those smoking 11 to 20 cigarettes per day (33). Although people exposed to environmental smoke consume a lower amount of toxins than those directly smoking, there is still an increased risk of developing vascular disease, with increased cardiovascular events and PAD.

Beyond the initial development of vascular disease, smoking accelerates the progression of both claudication symptoms and the need for vascular interventions. An exercise study of 138 patients with PAD and stable claudication found that smokers developed symptoms more quickly, and these symptoms persisted for a longer duration (34). In patients with PAD who had undergone surgical revascularization, continuing to smoke more than 15 cigarettes per day increased the probability of requiring an amputation by five times at 2 years and by three times at 5 years (35). Patients with PAD who continue to smoke have a 40% to 50% 10-year mortality, mainly due to myocardial infarction and stroke (20,36).

Smoking cessation appears to lessen the risk of vascular events, slowing the progression to leg ischemia and reducing the risk of myocardial infarction or cardiovascular death (37). Although there are no randomized trials of smoking cessation, many trials have compared patients who quit smoking with those who continued to smoke. Patients who stopped smoking cigarettes improved maximal treadmill walking distance up to 46.7 meters (38), and were less likely to develop rest pain due to ischemia, which occurred in 18% of current smokers versus 9% of those who quit (39).

In order to assist patients with smoking cessation, a complete approach including education, support, and pharmacologic agents provides the highest likelihood of success (Table 13.1). Rather than casually telling patients to stop smoking, medical professionals need to spend several minutes focusing on smoking, just as with other medical problems. Patients must be educated about the extremely high risk of cardiovascular events, particularly patients with PAD. The risk of events falls rapidly with smoking cessation, and symptoms may improve, which may provide important motivation for the patient.

Once the patient understands why smoking cessation is critically important to reduce the risk of a stroke or heart attack, the next step involves employing standard approaches for motivating change. One well-developed model involves moving the patient from precontemplation of change, in this case smoking cessation, to contemplation, to determination, to action, and then finally to maintenance. This model reinforces the need to follow smoking sequentially through multiple office visits. Once the patient reaches the determination stage, the physician should encourage a specific quit date, and contract with the patient to not smoke after that date, not even a single cigarette, without first calling the physician's office to speak with one of the health care providers. Although personal experience indicates that patients rarely actually call the health care provider, this provides an extra safety net and deterrent to help maintain their smoking cessation. Various pharmacologic therapies are available to support patients with smoking cessation. For patients who are driven to smoke predominantly by chemical addiction, nicotine may serve as the best first-line agent. Various different mediums exist, including gum, spray, inhaler, and patch. Nicotine appears to be safe in patients with vascular disease, with no increase in adverse events. Some concern has been raised about long-term nicotine replacement promoting angiogenesis, which accelerates atherosclerosis; however, this should not deter physicians from recommending short-term nicotine replacement to aide smoking cessation (40).

For patients who are more driven to smoke by stress or anxiety, bupropion hydrochloride (Zyban) may be the best first-line agent. One trial compared 12-month abstinence rates using sustained-release buproprion compared to placebo, and found 23% of patients using buproprion were abstinent versus 12% of the placebo group (41). These results are typical for smoking cessation trials, during which nicotine replacement or buproprion consistently increases the smoking cessation rate by approximately 50% to 100%. Nicotine and buproprion can be safely combined to assist patients who need additional pharmacologic help. Many patients may require medication to address anxiety and nicotine addition. By providing a careful well-rounded program to motivate action and maintain cessation through support and pharmacologic assistance, physicians can help patients achieve higher rates of cessation.

TABLE 13.1. *Smoking cessation*

Patient stage	Health provider action
Precontemplation	Educate patient about cardiovascular risk
Contemplation	Reinforce health benefits of smoking cessation
Determination	Explore patient's need for support
	Select pharmacologic agent to assist cessation
	Select date of cessation
	Contract for cessation, with patient to call office before ever smoking again
Action	Arrange health provider phone call to ensure and praise success
Maintenance	Make follow-up appointments and/or phone calls
	Praise patient efforts; quitting is difficult
	Reinforce education on health benefits the patient is receiving

Diabetes

Diabetic patients have two to four times the rate of PAD compared to nondiabetic patients, as well as decreased femoral and pedal pulses and rates of abnormal ankle–brachial indices ranging from 11.9% to 16% (42–45). The Hoorn study found a 7% prevalence of abnormal ankle–brachial indices in nondiabetic patients, whereas diabetic patients on mulitple hypoglycemic medications had a prevalence of 20.9% (46). Diabetic patients are more likely to have infrapopliteal arterial occlusive disease than nondiabetic subjects (47). This PAD correlates with both the duration and severity of diabetes (47). As a result of increased PAD, diabetes results in an increased risk of claudication, with a relative risk of 3.5% in men and 8.6% in women, according the Framingham cohort (21). Diabetes contributes to half of all lower extremity amputations in the United States, with the relative risk of lower extremity amputation ranging from 12 to 40 times higher than in nondiabetic patients (48,49).

No evidence shows that tight glycemic control decreases the incidence of intermittent claudication or critical limb ischemia (50,51). However, because the United Kingdom Prospective Diabetes Study showed that tight control decreases microvascular complications and may reduce myocardial infarction ($p=0.052$), tight control is still strongly recommended (52).

See Chapter 5 for a more detailed discussion of the significance of diabetes and vascular disease.

Dyslipidemia

PAD occurs more frequently in patients with dyslipidemia. In particular, the risk of PAD increases with elevations in total cholesterol (19,22,33), low-density lipoprotein cholesterol (LDL-C), triglycerides (19), and lipoprotein(a) [Lp(a)] (53,54). Every 10-mg per dL increase in total cholesterol raises the likelihood of developing PAD by approximately 10% (44). In a study of 60 subjects aged 32 to 65 years, elevated serum cholesterol was associated with increased carotid and femoral IMT (55,56). In a study of 101 asymptomatic men aged 28 to 60 years with no cardiovascular risk factors other than smoking, hypercholesterolemia was associated with increased carotid and femoral IMT compared to men with normal cholesterol ($p<0.01$) (56,57). Similar to the discussion of total cholesterol, elevations in LDL-C, very low density lipoprotein (VLDL), and triglycerides are also associated with PAD, whereas patients with elevated high-density lipoprotein cholesterol (HDL-C) and apolipoprotein A-1 have a reduced incidence of PAD (54,58).

There is no published prospective, randomized study of lipid-lowering therapy enrolling only patients with PAD. However, published data support lipid modification as an important strategy to reduce cardiovascular events. A meta-analysis of randomized trials of lipid-lowering therapy in patients with PAD reviewed 698 patients who had received therapy lasting from 4 months to 3 years. Therapy included diet, cholestyramine, probucol, and nicotinic acid. Lipid-lowering therapy resulted in a large but nonsignificant reduction in mortality (odds ratio 0.21, 95% confidence interval 0.03 to 1.17). There was little change in nonfatal events (odds ratio 1.21, 95% confidence interval 0.80 to 1.83), though there was a reduction in the severity of claudication. A total of 20,536 patients at high risk for cardiovascular events but without hyperlipidemia, including 2,701 patients with PAD, were randomized to simvastatin in the Heart Protection Study. In this study, there was a statistically significant 18% reduction in cardiovascular death, consistent among all subgroups including those with PAD, and including patients with a LDL-C of less than 116 mg per dL. Two trials showed a significant overall reduction in disease progression on angiogram (odds ratio 0.47, 95% confidence interval 0.29 to 0.77) (59). In the Cholesterol Lowering Atherosclerosis Study, 188 men with both CAD and PVD were randomized to placebo or colestipol plus niacin, in addition to diet therapy. Based on femoral angiography with 1- or 2-year follow-up, the lipid-lowering therapy resulted in a stabilization or regression of atherosclerosis that was statistically significant in proximal segments ($p<0.02$) and moderately severe atherosclerotic segments ($p<0.04$) (60). The Regression Growth Evaluation Statin Study (REGRESS) of 255 men with CAD reported that pravastatin 40 mg per dL reduced the combined carotid and femoral IMT ($p<0.01$) after 2 years (61). In the Scandinavian Simvastatin Survival Study, a post hoc subgroup analysis showed that treatment with simvastatin reduced the likelihood of new or worsening claudication, with RR of 0.6 (confidence interval 0.4 to 0.9) (62).

The effect of Lp(a) reduction on peripheral artery stenosis and claudication symptoms is unclear. In a 2-year study of 42 patients with CAD and elevated total cholesterol and Lp(a) levels who were randomized to simvastatin alone or simvastatin plus biweekly apheresis, Lp(a) levels were unchanged in the simvastatin-alone group, but fell by 20% in the simvastatin-plus-apheresis group. Follow-up ultrasound of femoral and tibial vessels showed a decrease in stenoses in simvastatin plus apheresis from 9 to 7 patients, whereas the simvastatin alone group increased from 6 to 13, $p=0.002$ (63,64). Thus, although no one proposed apheresis as a standard therapeutic intervention, this does suggest a pathogenic role for lipoprotein(a) in PAD.

Overall, dyslipidemia serves as a strong risk factor for the development and progression of PAD, and correcting the dyslipidemia reduces further cardiovascular events. Thus, according the the National Cholesterol Education Program III (NCEP III), patients with PAD have the same goals and management strategies as patients with CAD (65). Specifically, the primary goal is reduce LDL-C levels to below 100 mg per dL. Although therapeutic lifestyle changes including diet and exercise are strongly encouraged, the addition of pharmacologic lipid-modifying agents is usually required. Statin drugs frequently serve as the first-line agent due to their potency in reducing LDL-C levels while having few side effects. Once the statin or other agent is started, it should be titrated in 6-week intervals until the patient has achieved an LDL-C of less than 100 mg per dL. For patients who do not achieve LDL-C goals on a statin, a second agent may be added, such as bile acid-sequestering resins or ezetimibe, which inhibits cholesterol absorption at the brush border of the small intestine. When patients have significantly elevated triglycerides, fibrates may serve as the best primary or secondary agent. For patients with low HDL-C levels, niacin therapy increases HDL-C levels and thereby decreases cardiovascular events.

Once patients have achieved an LDL of less than 100 mg per dL, the NCEP III provides a secondary target for patients with a triglyceride level of greater than 200 mg per dL. This target is a non-HDL-C of less than 130 mg per dL, with non-HDL-C calculated as total cholesterol minus HDL-C. Thus, additional pharmacologic intervention is required for patients with PAD who have triglyceride levels above 200 mg per dL and non-HDL-C that is not less than 130 mg per dL, even if the LDL-C is less than 100 mg per dL. These patients in particular have dyslipidemia profiles that tend to benefit from fibrates or niacin. Finally, for patients with PAD who do not meet any NCEP III criteria for a lipid-modifying agent, there still may be a benefit for starting pharmacologic therapy, particularly a statin. As previously mentioned, the Heart Protection Study found that treating high risk patients with a LDL-C of less than 116 mg per dL reduced cardiovascular death. Thus, although the LDL-C was not strictly at the goal of the current guidelines, statins are likely to benefit patients with PAD even if their lipid profile does not require pharmacologic intervention. See Chapter 12 for more detail about hyperlipidemia.

Hypertension

Hypertension occurs frequently in patients with PAD. Although several studies have concluded that hypertension is not a risk factor for intermittent claudication (20,66), the majority of studies have found that hypertension serves as an independent risk factor, including the Framingham Study and Edinburgh Artery Study. Treating hypertension improves clinical outcomes and leads to reduced carotid IMT. The Celiprolol Intima–Media Enalapril Efficacy Study examined 98 patients with essential hypertension, and found that both celiprolol and enalapril lead to decreased carotid IMT in 9 months (56). In the Verapamil in Hypertension and Atherosclerosis Study, verapamil led to a greater decrease in carotid IMT than chlorthalidone, and this corresponded to a lower cardiovascular event rate ($p<0.05$) (67).

When selecting an antihypertensive agent, there has been some concern that beta-blockers might worsen claudication. In one study, atenolol or nifedipine alone did not affect the maximal treadmill walking distance, but the combination of these drugs reduced maximal treadmill walking by 9% (73). Other studies did not find any adverse impact of beta-blockade, with a meta-analysis indicating they are safe in patients with PAD, except in severe PAD, in which case they should be used cautiously (3,69–70).

Both basic science and clinical investigation indicate that the renin–angiotensin system (RAS) is a major factor in atherothrombosis and may be considered a nontraditional risk factor for PAD. The RAS directly contributes to atherothrombotic events by promoting inflammation, causing endothelial function, reducing fibrinolysis, and facilitating LDL oxidation (7). Angiotensin II, the major effector peptide of RAS, stimulates inflammation by activating the proinflammatory transcription factor nuclear factor-κB. Nitric oxide's ability to protect endothelial function is impaired from the degradation of bradykinin by angiotensin-converting enzyme (ACE) and from oxidative stress generated by angiotensin II. RAS leads to increased plasminogen activator inhibitor-1 and tissue factor activity, which promote thrombosis over fibrinolysis. Finally, angiotensin II enhances the oxidation of LDL and stimulates the uptake of LDL by upregulating its receptor, lactin-like oxidized LDL receptor-1 (LOX-1).

Clinical trials of RAS inhibition in humans have shown decreased cardiovascular events. The Heart Outcomes Prevention Evaluation demonstrated that ACE inhibition with ramipril decreased rates of death and myocardial infarction in high-risk patients without left ventricular dysfunction or heart failure (72). This randomized controlled trial included 9,297 patients with a history of coronary artery disease, peripheral vascular disease, stroke, or two or more cardiovascular risk factors, one of which had to include diabetes. The patients were followed for 5 years for a primary outcome composite of myocardial infarction, stroke, or death from cardiovascular causes. ACE inhibition significantly decreased myocardial infarction, stroke, or death from cardiovascular cause both separately and as the primary outcome composite (RR= 0.78, $p<0.001$). ACE inhibition was beneficial in each of the subgroups of people included in the study, including the 4,051 patients with PAD as evidenced by an ABI of less than 0.9. Of patients receiving placebo, those with PAD reached the primary outcome in 22% of cases, compared with 14.3% of patients without PAD, indicating that even among high-risk patients, PAD is a strong risk factor for cardiovascular events.

See Chapter 8 for more detail about hypertension and PAD.

Nonlipid Serological Risk Factors

The study population from the Physician's Health Study, a prospective randomized trial of aspirin and beta-carotene in 14,916 men without prior cardiovascular disease, was used to evaluate novel risk factors for PAD. One hundred forty men developed intermittent claudication or were hospitalized for peripheral revascularization during the 9 years of follow-up. Using a case–control design, these subjects were matched with 140 controls from the study population who did not develop PAD, with age and smoking status matched (73). Baseline plasma samples from the beginning of the study were used to measure both traditional and novel risk factors. Among the lipid parameters, total cholesterol, HDL, LDL, triglycerides, and apolipoprotein (apo) B-100 were all predictors of risk. The total cholesterol/HDL ratio had the strongest correlation, with little added benefit from adding LDL, apo A-1, or apo B-100 to the analysis. Lp(a) did not add benefit to the standard lipid panel, despite the previously given evidence that lowering Lp(a) reduces the progression of PAD (74). Among the nonlipid parameters, the inflammatory marker CRP was the strongest predictor of risk, with the RR of PAD increasing by each quartile of CRP level from 1.0 at the lowest CRP quartile to 2.1 at the highest. Consistent with other studies showing that fibrinogen is marker of increased cardiovascular events, including increased PAD with fibrinogen polymorphism 455AA, fibrinogen levels also predicted the development of PAD, indicating a possible role for hemostatic factors (22,75–77). Although adding CRP or fibrinogen to the standard lipid panel improved risk prediction, the addition of both agents did not provide significant further risk stratification. Homocysteine did not predict PAD, although several other studies have found an association using carotid and femoral IMT (56).

In contrast to the foregoing study, other case–control and prospective studies showed that high serum homocysteine serves as an independent risk factor for PAD and death due to cardiovascular events (3,78–81). On a pathophysiologic level, homocysteine may serve as a risk factor because it enhances the oxidation of LDL and generation of reactive oxygen species, which causes endothelial dysfunction and inflammation, thereby promoting atherosclerosis (82).

Whereas nonlipid risk factors serve as markers for vascular disease, the clinical question remaining is whether targeting these risk factors will improve the prognosis of patients with PAD. A randomized, double-blind, placebo-controlled trial of pravastatin 40 mg in patients with hypercholesterolemia and PAD found significantly decreased CRP levels (45%) and von Willebrand factor levels (18%) (83). Thus, consistent with our current understanding of the importance of inflammation in atherothrombotic disease, the inflammatory marker CRP levels reflect cardiovascular risk, and fall with risk-reducing treatment. It is still uncertain whether screening with CRP or following CRP levels will help guide cardiovascular risk management more effectively than the routine lipid parameters that are currently the standard of care.

With respect to fibrinogen and other hemostatic factors such as plasminogen activator inhibitor-1 (PAI-1), tissue-type plasminogen activator (TPA), and tissue factor (TF) that are increased in atherosclerosis, there are no clinical trials indicating that altering their levels reflects improved clinical outcomes. However, some evidence comes indirectly from the renin–angiotensin system, which promotes thrombosis by increasing levels of PAI-1, TPA, and TF (71,84,85). Many clinical trials indicate that blockade of the renin–angiotensin system decreases atherothrombotic events. One mechanism by which blocking the renin–angiotensin system may provide vascular protection is by promoting fibrinolysis. Thus, the prognostic role of monitoring hemostatic factor levels requires further investigation.

With respect to homocysteine, because altered B12 metabolism and dietary folate deficiency are two causes of elevated homocysteine levels, supplements of B vitamins and food fortified with folate will lower homocysteine levels (86). However, no clinical trials have demonstrated that lowering homocysteine levels reduces cardiovascular events or surrogate outcomes in patients with PAD (87).

Infection

The role of infection in promoting atherosclerosis and the role of treating infection to prevent cardiovascular events are currently unclear, and therefore current management of PAD does not address infectious disease. However, future research may ultimately indicate a role for antibiotics. *Chlamydia pneumoniae* and cytomegalovirus are associated with atherosclerosis throughout the vascular system, including peripheral arteries (88–90). Although the mechanism by which infection is associated with atherosclerosis is not known, one possibility is stimulation of inflammation. Treating infection with antibiotics showed benefit in two small studies, but not in the larger study Azithromycin in Coronary Artery Disease: Elimination of Myocardial Infection with Chlamydia (91–93).

MEDICAL MANAGEMENT OF CLAUDICATION

Lifestyle Modification: Exercise

In addition to modifying the conventional cardiovascular risk factors mentioned earlier, exercise has been shown to benefit patients with PAD. Exercise recommendations are 35 to 50 minutes, three to five times per week (Table 13.2). Studies of exercise training indicate a 100% to 150% increase in maximal walking distance, improving the quality of life of patients limited by claudication (94). A meta-analysis of patients with claudication that included both randomized and nonrandomized trials showed that exercise training led to a 180% improvement in pain-free walking time and a 120% improvement in maximal walking time (95). These improvements were most significant in patients who exercised three or more times per week for more than 30 minutes at intensities designed to achieve near-maximal pain. Whereas benefits may occur within 4 weeks, improvements were greater in programs lasting six months or longer (96). Another meta-analysis of patients with intermittent claudication limited to

TABLE 13.2. *Exercise program for claudication*

Type of exercise	Treadmill or track walking most effective
Warm-up period	5–10 min
Intensity	Adjust speed and grade to elicit claudication within 3–5 min
Duration	Walk until claudication of moderate severity occurs, then rest and resume walking to achieve 35 min of intermittent walking; over time, increase the duration of intermittent walking to 50 min
Cool-down period	5–10 min
Frequency	Three to five times per week
Supervision	Helps to adjust intensity and manage cardiovascular symptoms

From Stewart KJ, Hiatt WR, Regensteiner JG, et al. Exercise training for claudication. *N Engl J Med* 2002;347:1941–1951, with permission.

randomized controlled trials found a 150% increase in maximal walking time (97). These increases in walking time significantly exceed improvements obtained with pharmacologic agents, which are discussed in the next subsection.

There are many explanations for the benefits of exercise. On a functional level, one can imagine that exercise breaks the cycle of disability that is associated with PAD. Patients with PAD have reduced oxygen delivery and consumption. The peak oxygen consumption of patients with claudication during graded treadmill exercise is 50% of that of age-matched controls (98). This impaired oxygen supply promotes endothelial dysfunction, ischemia, and inflammation, which both accelerates atherosclerosis and diminishes the aerobic capacity of muscles, thereby decreasing walking ability. As patients exercise less, they become more deconditioned and worsen other cardiovascular risk factors such as hyperlipidemia and hypertension, which further promotes worsening PAD, leading to a downward spiral (99).

Exercise programs interfere with this cycle of disability and promote improvement in symptoms. PAD is associated with impaired nitric oxide activity, which results in endothelial dysfunction. Exercise, as well as modification of other cardiovascular risk factors, increases nitric oxide activity, restoring endothelial function (100,101). Muscle metabolism improves, with enhanced oxygen extraction and decreased acylcarnitines, which are associated with further walking ability (102,103). Inflammatory markers such as CRP decrease, in part due to less ischemia at any given workload (104). These changes occurring with exercise lead to decreased oxygen utilization for the same workload, thereby improving walking economy (105). Furthermore, progression of atherosclerosis is also slowed because systemic risk factors are favorably modified, with decreases in weight, blood pressure, glucose, and triglycerides and increases in HDL (106).

Pharmacologic Treatment of Claudication

Pentoxifylline, a methylxanthine derivative, improves the deformability of red blood cells and white blood cells, lowers plasma fibrinogen concentrations, and has antiplatelet effects (107). There are many published studies evaluating pentoxifylline, with a meta-analysis indicating a net benefit of 44 meters in the maximal distance walked on a treadmill (confidence interval 14 to 74) (108). Thus, whereas pentoxifylline appears to offer some benefit to patients with claudication, the benefit is small relative to other interventions, such as exercise, which leads to an improvement of 179 meters (confidence interval 60 to 298) (108).

Cilostazol is a phosphodiesterase type 3 inhibitor that results in increased intracellular cyclic AMP. Cilostazol also inhibits platelet aggregation, the formation of arterial thrombi, and vascular smooth muscle proliferation. Finally, cilostazol causes vasodilation, although, because vasodilator drugs do not improve claudication-limited exercise, this mechanism is unlikely to be responsible for cilostazol's efficacy (3). Four randomized controlled trials have examined cilostazol,

with a total of 1,534 patients with claudication. Cilostazol improved pain-free and maximal walking distance 35% to 50% above placebo, enhanced quality-of-life measures by questionnaires, increased ABI, and raised HDL levels (109–111). Patients with diabetes who were treated with cilostazol showed a significant reduction in the carotid IMT (56). Cilostazol was superior to pentoxifylline (112). Cilostazol is hepatically metabolized by cytochrome P450, and therefore may have drug interactions with similarly metabolized drugs. Side effects are most frequently headache, followed by diarrhea, palpitations, and dizziness. Whereas cilostazol is safe with aspirin, there are no data on combinations with clopidogrel. Finally, due to concern with long-term administration of phosphodiesterase III inhibitors and New York Heart Association class II and IV patients, cilostazol is contraindicated in patients with heart failure, although it has never been studied in this population (113).

Whereas cilostazol is the major drug approved for treatment of claudication in the United States, two other classes of drugs are available in Europe. Naftidrofuryl, which may antagonize 5-hydroxytryptamine, appears to improve pain-free treadmill walking distance, but it does not improve maximal walking distance, according to a critical review of five controlled trials (114). Propionyl levocarnitine may improve the metabolism in ischemic muscles, and has been shown in two trials of 730 patients to increase pain-free and maximal treadmill walking distance, as well as quality of life, more than placebo (115,116).

Prostaglandin drugs, which have antiplatelet and vasodilating properties, showed some promise in improving the walking distance in patients with intermittent claudication when administered intravenously; however, an initial trial using an oral analogue, beraprost, failed to show significant improvement, and was poorly tolerated at high doses due to headache, flushing, and gastrointestinal side effects (117,118). Subsequently, a randomized controlled trial of beraprost in patients with intermittent claudication found a statistically significant improvement in pain-free and maximal walking distance as well as a reduced incidence of cardiovascular events (118). A similar study conducted in the United States did not show any benefit with beraprost compared to placebo in exercise performance (119). Thus, more studies are necessary before prostaglandin therapy can be considered for the treatment of PAD.

Angiogenic growth factors are also being considered as therapy for improving claudication symptoms. Phase I and phase II trials using gene transfer techniques encoding for vascular endothelial growth factor, which is a growth factor that may promote angiogenesis and improve blood flow, indicate safety for clinical use, but efficacy has yet to be proven (120–123).

CARDIOVASCULAR RISK REDUCTION

Patients with PAD have an extremely high risk of future vascular complications and death, and should all be

TABLE 13.3. *Medical management of peripheral vascular disease*

Lifestyle modification
  Smoking cessation
  Exercise
  Diet
  Weight loss
Pharmacotherapy
  Cardiovascular risk reduction
    Lipid modifying agents with low-density lipoprotein goal <100 mg/dL
    Antiplatelet agents
    Angiotensin-converting enzyme inhibitor or angiotensin II receptor blockers
    Agents to control blood pressure, with goal blood pressure <130 mm Hg/85 mm Hg
    Agents to control diabetes, with goal hemoglobin A1c <7%
  Intermittent claudication improvement
  Cilostazol
  Pentoxifylline (second-line agent)
  New and experimental agents

managed with a triad of medicines proven to reduce this risk (Table 13.3). As discussed previously, lipid modification, including modification of HDL and triglycerides as recommended by NCEP III guidelines, is necessary to address in all patients with PAD. Second, unless contraindicated in an individual, all patients with PAD should receive antiplatelet therapy, which reduces cardiovascular events according to multiple studies. See Chapter 14 for more details about different antiplatelet agents. Finally, for the reasons outlined in the section on hypertension, consideration should be given to patients for receiving ACE inhibitors or angiotensin II type 1 receptor blockers, unless a contraindication exists. Inhibition of the renin–angiotensin system has antiatherosclerotic activity, which has been demonstrated in multiple animal models of atherosclerosis and suggested in clinical trials in human. A beta-blocker should be prescribed to all patients with PAD who are scheduled for vascular surgery. Given the associated high risk for cardiovascular events in patients with PAD, those patients who do not receive aggressive risk factor modification will not live long enough to enjoy any intervention afforded them to improve lifestyle.

REFERENCES

1. Criqui MH. Epidemiology and prognostic significance of peripheral arterial disease. *Am J Med Contin Educ Ser* 1998;3–9.
2. Criqui MH, Denenberg JO, Langer RD, et al. The epidemiology of peripheral arterial disease: importance of identifying the population at risk. *Vasc Med* 1997;2(3):221–226.
3. Hiatt WR. Medical treatment of peripheral arterial disease and claudication. *N Engl J Med* 2001;344(21):1608–1621.
4. Becker GJ, McClenny TE, Kovacs ME, et al. The importance of increasing public and physician awareness of peripheral arterial disease. *J Vasc Interv Radiol* 2002;13(1):7–11.
5. Hirsch AT, Criqui MH, Treat-Jacobson D, et al. Peripheral arterial disease detection, awareness, and treatment in primary care. *JAMA* 2001;286(11):1317–1324.
6. Fowkes FG. Epidemiological research on peripheral vascular disease. *J Clin Epidemiol* 2001;54(9):863–868.
7. Schainfeld RM. Management of peripheral arterial disease and intermittent claudication. *J Am Board Fam Pract* 2001;14(6):443–450.
8. Newman AB, Sutton-Tyrrell K, Vogt MT, et al. Morbidity and mortality in hypertensive adults with a low ankle/arm blood pressure index. *JAMA* 1993;270:487–489.
9. Burke GL, Evans GW, Riley WA. Arterial wall thickness is associated with prevalent cardiovascular disease in middle-aged adults. The Atherosclerosis Risk in Communities (ARIC) Study. *Stroke* 1995;26:386–391.
10. Allan PL, Mowbray PI, Lee AJ, et al. Relationship between carotid intima–media thickness and symptomatic and asymptomatic peripheral arterial disease. The Edinburgh Artery Study. *Stroke* 1997;28:348–353.
11. Bots ML, Hoffman A, Grobbee DE. Common carotid intima–media thickness and lower extremity arterial atherosclerosis. The Rotterdam Study. *Arteriosler Thromb* 1994;14:1885–1891.
12. Simmons PC, Algra A, Bots ML, et al. Common carotid intima–media thickness in patients with peripheral arterial disease or abdominal aortic aneurysm: the SMART study. Second Manifestations of ARTerial disease. *Atherosclerosis* 1999;146:243–248.
13. Ogren M, Hedblad B, Isacsson SO, et al. Non-invasively detected carotid stenosis and ischaemic heart disease in men with leg arteriosclerosis. *Lancet* 1993;342(8880):1138–1141.
14. Schainfeld RM. Management of peripheral arterial disease and intermittent claudication. *J Am Board Fam Pract* 2001;14(6):443–450.
15. Kelly R, Staines A, MacWalter R, et al. The prevalence of treatable left ventricular systolic dysfunction in patients who present with noncardiac vascular episodes: a case–control study. *J Am Coll Cardiol* 2002;39(2):219–224.
16. Schainfeld RM. Management of peripheral arterial disease and intermittent claudication. *J Am Board Fam Pract* 2001;14(6):443–450.
17. Fowkes FG. Epidemiological research on peripheral vascular disease. *J Clin Epidemiol* 2001;54(9):863–868.
18. Schroll M, Munck O. Estimation of peripheral arteriosclerotic disease by ankle blood pressure measurements in a population study of 60-year-old men and women. *J Chronic Dis* 1981;34(6):261–269.
19. Hughson WG, Mann JI, Garrod A. Intermittent claudication: prevalence and risk factors. *Br Med J* 1978;1(6124):1379–1381.
20. Reunanen A, Takkunen H, Aromaa A. Prevalence of intermittent claudication and its effect on mortality. *Acta Med Scand* 1982;211(4):249–256.
21. Kannel WB, McGee DL. Update on some epidemiologic features of intermittent claudication: the Framingham Study. *J Am Geriatr Soc* 1985;33(1):13–18.
22. Gofin R, Kark JD, Friedlander Y, et al. Peripheral vascular disease in a middle-aged population sample. The Jerusalem Lipid Research Clinic Prevalence Study. *Isr J Med Sci* 1987;23(3):157–167.
23. Murabito JM, D'Agostino RB, Silbershatz H, et al. Intermittent claudication. A risk profile from the Framingham Heart Study. *Circulation* 1997;96:44–49.
24. Kannel WB. Risk factors for atherosclerotic cardiovascular outcomes in different arterial territories. *J Cardiovasc Risk* 1994;1(4):333–339.
25. Criqui MH, Browner D, Fronek A, et al. Peripheral arterial disease in large vessels is epidemiologically distinct from small vessel disease. An analysis of risk factors. *Am J Epidemiol* 1989;129(6):1110–1119.
26. Gordon T, Kannel WB. Predisposition to atherosclerosis in the head, heart, and legs. The Framingham study. *JAMA* 1972;221(7):661–666.
27. Freund KM, Belanger AJ, D'Agostino RB, et al. The health risks of smoking. The Framingham Study: 34 years of follow-up. *Ann Epidemiol* 1993;3(4):417–424.
28. Ingolfsson IO, Sigurdsson G, Sigvaldason H, et al. A marked decline in the prevalence and incidence of intermittent claudication in Icelandic men 1968–1986: a strong relationship to smoking and serum cholesterol—the Reykjavik Study. *J Clin Epidemiol* 1994;47(11):1237–1243.
29. Weiss NS. Cigarette smoking and arteriosclerosis obliterans: an epidemiologic approach. *Am J Epidemiol* 1972;95(1):17–25.
30. Powell JT, Edwards RJ, Worrell PC, et al. Risk factors associated with the development of peripheral arterial disease in smokers: a case-control study. *Atherosclerosis* 1997;129(1):41–48.

31. van den Berkmortel FW, Smilde TJ, Wollersheim H, et al. Intima–media thickness of peripheral arteries in asymptomatic cigarette smokers. *Atherosclerosis* 2000;150(2):397–401.

32. Cheng KS, Mikhailidis DP, Hamilton G, et al. A review of the carotid and femoral intima–media thickness as an indicator of the presence of peripheral vascular disease and cardiovascular risk factors. *Cardiovasc Res* 2002;54(3):528–538.

33. Bowlin SJ, Medalie JH, Flocke SA, et al. Epidemiology of intermittent claudication in middle-aged men. *Am J Epidemiol* 1994;140(5):418–430.

34. Gardner AW. The effect of cigarette smoking on exercise capacity in patients with intermittent claudication. *Vasc Med* 1996;1(3):181–186.

35. Ameli FM, Stein M, Provan JL, et al. The effect of postoperative smoking on femoropopliteal bypass grafts. *Ann Vasc Surg* 1989;3:20–25.

36. Faulkner KW, House AK, Castleden WM. The effect of cessation of smoking on the accumulative survival rates of patients with symptomatic peripheral vascular disease. *Med J Aust* 1983;1(5):217–219.

37. Hiatt WR. Medical treatment of peripheral arterial disease and claudication. *N Engl J Med* 2001;344(21):1608–1621.

38. Quick CR, Cotton LT. The measured effect of stopping smoking on intermittent claudication. *Br J Surg* 1982;69[Suppl]:S24–S26.

39. Jonason T, Bergstrom R. Cessation of smoking in patients with intermittent claudication. Effects on the risk of peripheral vascular complications, myocardial infarction and mortality. *Acta Med Scand* 1987;221:253–260.

40. Heeschen C, Jang JJ, Weis M, et al. Nicotine stimulates angiogenesis and promotes tumor growth and atherosclerosis. *Nat Med* 2001;7(7):833–839.

41. Hurt RD, Sachs DP, Glover ED, et al. A comparison of sustained-release bupropion and placebo for smoking cessation. *N Engl J Med* 1997;337(17):1195–1202.

42. Abbott RD, Brand FN, Kannel WB. Epidemiology of some peripheral arterial findings in diabetic men and women. *Am J Med* 1990;88:376–381.

43. Meijer WT, Hoes AW, Rutgers D, et al. Peripheral arterial disease in the elderly: the Rotterdam Study. *Arterioscler Thromb Vasc Biol* 1998;18(2):185–192.

44. Hiatt WR, Hoag S, Hamman RF. Effect of diagnostic criteria on the prevalence of peripheral arterial disease. The San Luis Valley Diabetes Study. *Circulation* 1995;91(5):1472–1479.

45. Beckman JA, Creager MA, Libby P. Diabetes and atherosclerosis: epidemiology, pathophysiology, and management. *JAMA* 2002;287(19):2570–2581.

46. Beks PJ, Mackaay AJ, de Neeling JN, et al. Peripheral arterial disease in relation to glycaemic level in an elderly Caucasian population: the Hoorn study. *Diabetologia* 1995;38:86–96.

47. Jude EB, Oyibo SO, Chalmers N, et al. Peripaheral arterial disease in diabetic and nondiabetic patients. *Diabetes Care* 2001;24:1433–1437.

48. Beckman JA, Creager MA, Libby P. Diabetes and atherosclerosis: epidemiology, pathophysiology, and management. *JAMA* 2002;287(19):2570–2581.

49. Nathan DM. Long-term complications of diabetes mellitus. *N Engl J Med* 1993;328(23):1676–1685.

50. Beckman JA, Creager MA, Libby P. Diabetes and atherosclerosis: epidemiology, pathophysiology, and management. *JAMA* 2002;287(19):2570–2581.

51. UK Prospective Diabetes Study Group. UKPDS Blood Pressure Study. *BMJ* 1998;317:703–713.

52. UK Prospective Diabetes Study Group. The UK Prospective Diabetes Study. *Lancet* 1998;352:837–853.

53. Cantin B, Moorjani S, Dagenais GR, et al. Lipoprotein(a). distribution in a French Canadian population and its relation to intermittent claudication (the Quebec Cardiovascular Study). *Am J Cardiol* 1995;75:1224–1228.

54. Johansson J, Egberg N, Johnsson H, et al. Serum lipoproteins and hemostatic function in intermittent claudication. *Arterioscler Thromb* 1993;13(10):1441–1448.

55. Joensuu T. Determinants of femoral and carotid artery atheroscleoris. *J Intern Med* 1994;236:79–84.

56. Cheng KS, Mikhailidis DP, Hamilton G, et al. A review of the carotid and femoral intima–media thickness as an indicator of the presence of peripheral vascular disease and cardiovascular risk factors. *Cardiovasc Res* 2002;54(3):528–538.

57. Gariepy J. Wall thickening of carotid and femoral arteries in male subjects with isolated hyperchlesterolemia. PCVMETRA Group. *Atherosclerosis* 1995;113:141–151.

58. Mowat BF, Skinner ER, Wilson HM, et al. Alterations in plasma lipids, lipoproteins and high density lipoprotein subfractions in peripheral arterial disease. *Atherosclerosis* 1997;131(2):161–166.

59. Leng GC, Price JF, Jepson RG. Lipid-lowering for lower limb atherosclerosis (Cochrane Review). In: *The Cochrane library, issue 4*. Chichester, UK: Wiley.

60. Blankenhorn DH, Azen SP, Crawford DW, et al. Effects of colestipol–niacin therapy on human femoral atherosclerosis. *Circulation* 1991;83:438–447.

61. de Groot E, Jukema JW, Montauban van Swijndregt AD, et al. B-mode ultrasound assessment of pravastatin treatment effect on carotid and femoral artery walls and its correlations with coronary arteriographic findings: a report of the Regression Growth Evaluation Statin Study (REGRESS). *J Am Coll Cardiol* 1998;31:1561–1567.

62. Pedersen TR, Kjekshus J, Pyorala K, et al. Effect of simvastatin on ischemic signs and symptoms in the Scandinavian Simvastatin Survival Study (4S). *Am J Cardiol* 1998;81:333–335.

63. Kroon AA, van Asten WN, Stalenhoef AF. Effect of apheresis of low-density lipoprotein on peripheral vascular disease in hypercholesterolemic patients with coronary artery disease. *Ann Intern Med* 1996;125(12):945–954.

64. Hiatt WR. Medical treatment of peripheral arterial disease and claudication. *N Engl J Med* 2001;344(21):1608–1621.

65. Executive summary of the third report of the National Cholesterol Education Program (NCEP). Expert Panel on Detection, Evaluation, and Treatment of High Blood Cholesterol in Adults (Adult Treatment Panel III). *JAMA* 2001;285(19):2486–2497.

66. Smith GD, Shipley MJ, Rose G. Intermittent claudication, heart disease risk factors, and mortality. The Whitehall Study. *Circulation* 1990;82(6):1925–1931.

67. Zanchetti A, Rosei EA, Dal Palu C, et al. The Verapamil in Hypertension and Atherosclerosis Study (VHAS): results of long-term randomized treatment with either verapamil or chlorthalidone on carotid intima–media thickness. *J Hypertens* 1998;16:1667–1676.

68. Solomon SA, Ramsay LE, Yeo WW, et al. Beta blockade and intermittent claudication: placebo controlled trial of atenolol and nifedipine and their combination. *BMJ* 1991;303:1100–1104.

69. Radack K, Deck C. Beta-adrenergic blocker therapy does not worsen intermittent claudication in subjects with peripheral arterial disease. A meta-analysis of randomized controlled trials. *Arch Intern Med* 1991;151:1769–1776.

70. Dormandy JA, Rutherford RB. Management of peripheral arterial disease (PAD). TASC Working Group. TransAtlantic Inter-Society Concensus (TASC). *J Vasc Surg* 2000;31(1 Pt 2):S1–S296.

71. Schmidt-Ott KM, Kagiyama S, Phillips I. The multiple actions of angiotensin II in atherosclerosis. *Regul Peptides* 2000;93:65–77.

72. The Heart Outcomes Prevention Evaluation Study investigators. Effects of an angiotensin-converting-enzyme inhibitor, ramipril, on cardiovascular events in high-risk patients. *N Engl J Med* 2000;342(3):145–153.

73. Ridker PM, Stampfer MJ, Rifai N. Novel risk factors for systemic atherosclerosis: a comparison of C-reactive protein, fibrinogen, homocysteine, lipoprotein(a), and standard cholesterol screening as predictors of peripheral arterial disease. *JAMA* 2001;285(19):2481–2485.

74. Ridker PM, Stampfer MJ, Rifai N. Novel risk factors for systemic atherosclerosis: a comparison of C-reactive protein, fibrinogen, homocysteine, lipoprotein(a), and standard cholesterol screening as predictors of peripheral arterial disease. *JAMA* 2001;285(19):2481–2485.

75. Kannel WB, Wolf PA, Castelli WP, et al. Fibrinogen and risk of cardiovascular disease. The Framingham Study. *JAMA* 1987;258(9):1183–1186.

76. Smith FB, Lee AJ, Hau CM, et al. Plasma fibrinogen, haemostatic factors and prediction of peripheral arterial disease in the Edinburgh Artery Study. *Blood Coagul Fibrinolysis* 2000;11(1):43–50.

77. Lee AJ, Fowkes FG, Lowe GD, et al. Fibrinogen, factor VII and PAI-1 genotypes and the risk of coronary and peripheral atherosclerosis: Edinburgh Artery Study. *Thromb Haemost* 1999;81(4):553–560.

78. Graham IM, Daly LE, Refsum HM, et al. Plasma homocysteine as a risk

factor for vascular disease. The European Concerted Action Project. *JAMA* 1997;277(22):1775–1781.

79. Malinow MR, Kang SS, Taylor LM, et al. Prevalence of hyperhomocyst(e)inemia in patients with peripheral arterial occlusive disease. *Circulation* 1989;79(6):1180–1188.

80. Kang SS, Wong PW, Malinow MR. Hyperhomocyst(e)inemia as a risk factor for occlusive vascular disease. *Annu Rev Nutr* 1992;12:279–298.

81. Fermo I, Vigano' DS, Paroni R, et al. Prevalence of moderate hyperhomocysteinemia in patients with early-onset venous and arterial occlusive disease. *Ann Intern Med* 1995;123(10):747–753.

82. Welch GN, Loscalzo J. Homocysteine and atherothrombosis. *N Engl J Med* 1998;338(15):1042–1050.

83. Blann AD, Gurney D, Hughes E, et al. Influence of pravastatin on lipoproteins, and on endothelial, platelet, and inflammatory markers in subjects with peripheral artery disease. *Am J Cardiol* 2001;88(1):A7–A92.

84. Soejima H, Ogawa H, Yasue H, et al. Angiotensin-converting enzyme inhibition reduces monocyte chemoattractant protein-1 and tissue factor levels in patients with myocardial infarction. *J Am Coll Cardiol* 1999;34(4):983–988.

85. Vaughan DE. Angiotensin, fibrinolysis, and vascular homeostasis. *Am J Cardiol* 2001;87(8A):18C–24C.

86. Jacques PF, Selhub J, Bostom AG, et al. The effect of folic Acid fortification on plasma folate and total homocysteine concentrations. *N Engl J Med* 1999;340(19):1449–1454.

87. Hiatt WR. Medical treatment of peripheral arterial disease and claudication. *N Engl J Med* 2001;344(21):1608–1621.

88. Elkind MS, Lin IF, Grayston JT, et al. *Chlamydia pneumoniae* and the risk of first ischemic stroke: the Northern Manhattan Stroke Study. *Stroke* 2000;31(7):1521–1525.

89. Siscovick DS, Schwartz SM, Corey L, et al. *Chlamydia pneumoniae*, herpes simplex virus type 1, and cytomegalovirus and incident myocardial infarction and coronary heart disease death in older adults: the Cardiovascular Health Study. *Circulation* 2000;102(19):2335–2340.

90. Muhlestein JB. Chronic infection and coronary artery disease. *Med Clin North Am* 2000;84(1):123–148.

91. Gupta S, Leatham EW, Carrington D, et al. Elevated *Chlamydia pneumoniae* antibodies, cardiovascular events, and azithromycin in male survivors of myocardial infarction. *Circulation* 1997;96(2):404–407.

92. Gurfinkel E, Bozovich G, Daroca A, et al. Randomised trial of roxithromycin in non-Q-wave coronary syndromes: ROXIS Pilot Study. ROXIS Study Group. *Lancet* 1997;350(9075):404–407.

93. Muhlestein JB, Anderson JL, Carlquist JF, et al. Randomized secondary prevention trial of azithromycin in patients with coronary artery disease: primary clinical results of the ACADEMIC study. *Circulation* 2000;102(15):1755–1760.

94. Stewart KJ, Hiatt WR, Regensteiner JG, et al. Exercise training for claudication. *N Engl J Med Online* 2002;347(24):1941–1951.

95. Gardner AW, Poehlman ET. Exercise rehabilitation programs for the treatment of claudication pain. A meta-analysis. *JAMA* 1995;274:975–980.

96. Stewart KJ, Hiatt WR, Regensteiner JG, et al. Exercise training for claudication. *N Engl J Med Online* 2002;347(24):1941–1951.

97. Leng GC, Fowler B, Ernst E. Exercise for intermittent claudication. *Cochrane Database Syst Rev* 2000;CD000990.

98. Hiatt WR, Nawaz D, Brass EP. Carnitine metabolism during exercise in patients with peripheral vascular disease. *J Appl Physiol* 1987;62(6):2383–2387.

99. Stewart KJ, Hiatt WR, Regensteiner JG, et al. Exercise training for claudication. *N Engl J Med Online* 2002;347(24):1941–1951.

100. Harris LM, Faggioli GL, Shaw R. Vascular reactivity in patients with peripheral vascular disease. *Am J Cardiol* 1995;76:207–212.

101. Yataco AR, Corretti MC, Gardner AW, et al. Endothelial reactivity and cardiac risk factors in older patients with peripheral arterial disease. *Am J Cardiol* 1999;83:754–758.

102. Hiatt WR, Regensteiner JG, Wolfel EE, et al. Effect of exercise training on skeletal muscle histology and metabolism in peripheral arterial disease. *J Appl Physiol* 1996;81(2):780–788.

103. Hiatt WR, Regensteiner JG, Hargarten ME, et al. Benefit of exercise conditioning for patients with peripheral arterial disease. *Circulation* 1990;81:602–609.

104. Tisi PV, Shearman CP. Exercise training for intermittent claudication: does it adversely affect biochemical markers of the exercise-induced inflammatory response? *Eur J Vasc Endovasc Surg* 1997;14:344–350.

105. Womack CJ. Improved walking economy in patients with peripheral arterial occlusive disease. *Med Sci Sports Exerc* 1997;29:1286–1290.

106. Stewart KJ, Hiatt WR, Regensteiner JG, et al. Exercise training for claudication. *N Engl J Med Online* 2002;347(24):1941–1951.

107. Hiatt WR. Medical treatment of peripheral arterial disease and claudication. *N Engl J Med* 2001;344(21):1608–1621.

108. Girolami B, Bernardi E, Prins MH, et al. Treatment of intermittent claudication with physical training, smoking cessation, pentoxifylline, or nafronyl: a meta-analysis. *Arch Int Med* 1999;159:337–345.

109. Dawson DL, Cutler BS, Meissner MH, et al. Cilostazol has beneficial effects in treatment of intermittent claudication: results from a multicenter, randomized, prospective, double-blind trial. *Circulation* 1998;98:678–686.

110. Money SR, Herd JA, Isaacsohn JL, et al. Effect of cilostazol on walking distances in patients with intermittent claudication caused by peripheral vascular disease. *J Vasc Surg* 1998;27:267–274.

111. Beebe HG, Dawson DL, Cutler BS, et al. A new pharmacological treatment for intermittent claudication: results of a randomized, multicenter trial. *Arch Intern Med* 1999;159(17):2041–2050.

112. Dawson DL, Cutler BS, Hiatt WR, et al. A comparison of cilostazol and pentoxifylline for treating intermittent claudication. *Am J Med* 2000;109(7):523–530.

113. Hiatt WR, Nehler MR. Peripheral arterial disease. *Advan Intern Med* 2001;47:89–110.

114. Lehert P, Comte S, Gamand S, et al. Naftidrofuryl in intermittent claudication: a retrospective analysis. *J Cardiovasc Pharmacol* 1994;23[Suppl 3]:S48–S52.

115. Brevetti G, Perna S, Sabba C, et al. Effect of propionyl-L-carnitine on quality of life in intermittent claudication. *Am J Cardiol* 1997;79:777–780.

116. Brevetti G, Perna S, Sabba C, et al. Propionyl-L-carnitine in intermittent claudication: double-blind, placebo-controlled, dose titration, multicenter study. *J Am Coll Cardiol* 1995;26:1411–1416.

117. Schainfeld RM. Management of peripheral arterial disease and intermittent claudication. *J Am Board Fam Pract* 2001;14(6):443–450.

118. Lievre M, Morand S, Besse B, et al. Oral beraprost sodium, a prostaglandin I(2) analogue, for intermittent claudication: a double-blind, randomized, multicenter controlled trial. Beraprost et Claudication Intermittente (BERCI). Research Group. *Circulation* 2000;102(4):426–431.

119. Mohler III ER, Hiatt WR, Olin JW, et al. Treatment of intermittent claudication with beraprost sodium, an orally active prostaglandin I2 analogue: a double-blinded, randomized, controlled trial. *J Am Coll Cardiol* 2003;41(10):1679–1686.

120. Schainfeld RM. Management of peripheral arterial disease and intermittent claudication. *J Am Board Fam Pract* 2001;14(6):443–450.

121. Rajagopalan S, Trachtenberg J, Mohler E, et al. Phase I Study of Direct Administration of a Replication Deficient Adenorvirus Vector Containing the VEGF cDNA (CI-1023) to Patients with Claudication. *Am J Cardiol* 2002;90;5:512–516.

122. Mohler ER, Rajagopalan S, Olin JW, et al. Adenoviral-mediated gene transfer of vascular endothelial growth factor in cirtical limb ischemia-safety results from a phase 1 trial. *Vascular Medicine* 2003;8.

123. Rajagopalan S, Mohler ER, Lederman RJ, et al. Regional angiogenesis with vascular endothelial growth factor in peripheral arterial disease: a phase II randomized, double-blind, controlled study of adenoviral delivery of vascular endothelial growth factor 121 in patients with disabling intermittent claudication. *Circulation* 2003;108(16):1933–1938.

CHAPTER 14

Anticoagulant and Antiplatelet Therapy in Peripheral Vascular Disease

James J. Ferguson, III

Key Points

- Circulating platelets adhere to damaged endothelium resulting from vascular injury. These platelets are initially activated and then aggregate.
- Antiplatelet therapy is targeted at platelet activation and aggregation. Medications specific to this action include aspirin, dipyridamole, sulfinpyrazone, cilostazol, thienopyridines and glycoprotein IIb/IIIa antagonists.
- Anticoagulation therapy is aimed at thrombin generation and activity. Medications effective in this action include unfractioned heparin, low-molecular-weight heparin, direct thrombin inhibitors, and warfarin.
- Utilization of anticoagulant and antiplatelet therapy inhibits the ability to form thrombus. This is critical to prevent acute events in patients with atherosclerosis in most vascular beds.
- Heparin-induced thrombocytopenia (HIT) and heparin-induced thrombocytopenia/thrombosis syndrome (HITIS) reduce platelet counts and may induce disseminated thrombosis. Treatment is to discontinue heparin and use a direct thrombin antagonist.

COAGULATION AND PLATELETS

During vascular injury, the endothelial barrier, which separates the tissues of the vessel wall from the circulating blood, is damaged or lost. Subsequently, platelets adhere to exposed collagen, von Willebrand factor, and fibrinogen via specific cell receptors (glycoprotein [GP] Ib and GP Ia/IIa) and are activated via several independent mediators, including thromboxane, serotonin, epinephrine, adenosine diphosphate (ADP), and thrombin. Resultant degranulation releases chemotaxins, clotting factors, and vasoconstrictors, which promote thrombin generation, vasospasm, and subsequent platelet accumulation. The platelet phospholipid membrane both serves as a cofactor potentiating the coagulation process and provides the key surface on which the coagulation cascade enzymes function maximally. Activated platelets are the primary source of the phospholipid surface on which the coagulation cascade proceeds.

Classically, the coagulation system mechanisms have been compartmentalized into an intrinsic pathway (with all of the required factors present in the blood), an extrinsic pathway (with at least some requisite extravascular factors), and a common pathway (into which both former pathways feed). In recent years, however, a new perspective on coagulation has evolved (1), which details three steps: initiation, amplification, and propagation (Fig. 14.1).

Initiation involves injury-related exposure of tissue factor—the major driving force for coagulation—which (via factors VIIa, IX, and X) ultimately generates small amounts of thrombin (Fig. 14.1A). Conceptually, this can be viewed as the "spark" igniting coagulation. In the *amplification* stage (Fig. 14.1B), this small amount of thrombin feeds back via multiple pathways, resulting in the production of large amounts of preassembled coagulation complexes—the "tenase" (and subsequent prothrombinase) complex, which functions as chemically explosive "hand grenades." Specifically,

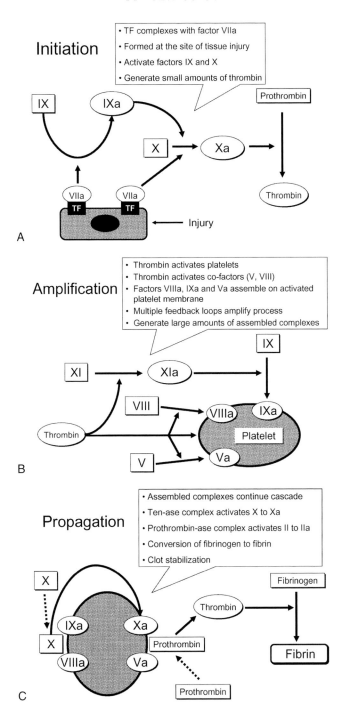

FIG. 14.1. A: In the initiation phase of coagulation, exposure of tissue factor (TF) results in the generation of small amounts of thrombin. **B:** In the amplification phase of coagulation, the previously generated small amounts of thrombin feed back and amplify the formation of large numbers of preassembled complexes on the surface of activated platelets. **C:** In the propagation phase of coagulation, the preassembled complexes are catalyzed to generate large amounts of thrombin, which can either feed back to again amplify the process or proceed through to complete the coagulation process by converting fibrinogen to fibrin, and, ultimately, cross-linked fibrin and a mature thrombus.

thrombin activates platelets and two key cofactors (V and VIII); subsequently, the requisite factors (Va, VIIIa, and IXa) assemble on the activated platelet membrane. Thus, in conjunction with an activated platelet membrane (itself arising from thrombin), the small amount of thrombin generated by the initial injury acts to create large amounts of these prepackaged complexes, which can subsequently "detonate" in the *propagation* phase (Fig. 14.1C). In this final sequence of events, factor X is activated by the "ten-ase" complex (factors VIIIa, IXa, and the activated membrane), with subsequent formation of the prothrombinase complex (factors Xa and Va and the activated membrane). This, in turn, catalyzes the conversion of prothrombin (factor II) to thrombin (factor IIa). This amplified thrombin response then directly catalyzes the conversion of soluble fibrinogen into insoluble fibrin in the final stage of thrombus formation.

Platelets are small, discoid, nonnucleated fragments that circulate in the blood (2). Because of higher shear forces, they tend to be positioned close to the blood vessel wall interface. When circulating platelets encounter a damaged vessel, they adhere to the exposed adhesive glycoproteins, such as GP Ib/and Ia/IIa. Following adhesion, various agonists, including thrombin, collagen, thromboxane A_2, serotonin, epinephrine, and ADP, combine with specific receptors on the platelet's surface to induce platelet activation. These agonist–receptor interactions are coupled through G proteins to generate secondary messengers, which induce structural and morphological changes in the platelets, resulting in the release of platelet granules. During platelet activation, a key receptor on the surface of the platelet, the GP IIb/IIIa receptor, also becomes activated. Although many agonists have the potential to activate platelets, the final common pathway of platelet aggregation proceeds via GP IIb/IIIa (3).

Because they can bind to more than one GP IIb/IIIa receptor, fibrinogen (a dimeric molecule) and von Willebrand factor (a multimeric molecule) act to cross-link platelets, creating an arborizing network of activated platelets at the injury site as platelet aggregation proceeds. Von Willebrand factor, as a multimeric molecule, has more potential binding sites, and hence plays a much more important role, than fibrinogen in mechanical shear-induced platelet aggregation (4). Because an activated platelet membrane is an important cofactor in the generation of thrombosis, the end result of the adhesion/activation/aggregation process is a concentration of activated platelet membrane at the injury site, which allows coagulation to proceed, but confines the coagulation process to the injured surface.

ANTITHROMBOTIC THERAPY

To better conceptualize the actions of the multiple available antithrombotic agents, it is useful to break coagulation into a four-step process: platelet activation, platelet aggregation, thrombin generation, and thrombin activity (Fig. 14.2). All

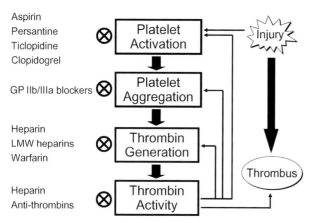

FIG. 14.2. The major groups of antithrombotic therapeutic agents act at one (or more) of four sites in the coagulation process: platelet activation, platelet aggregation, thrombin generation, and thrombin activity. GP, glycoprotein; LMW, low molecular weight.

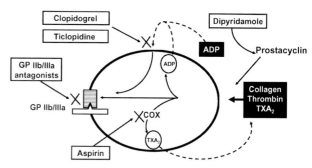

FIG. 14.3. The mechanism of action of the major antiplatelet agents. Aspirin and the thienopyridines interfere with platelet activation, blocking the two primary feedback loops for platelet-induced platelet activation (thromboxane and adenosine diphosphate [ADP], respectively). The glycoprotein (GP) IIb/IIIa antagonists block platelet aggregation, and prevent the assembly of the critical mass of activation platelet membrane necessary to support thrombus formation. TXA$_2$, Thromboxane A$_2$; COX, cyclooxygenase.

available antithrombotic agents act on one (or more) of these four steps.

Antiplatelet Therapy: Targeting Platelet Activation and Aggregation

Aspirin

There are various antiplatelet agents (Table 14.1). Aspirin exerts its antiplatelet effect by acetylating a key serine moiety (serine 530) of cyclooxygenase-1 (COX-1) and preventing the formation of thromboxane A2 from arachidonic acid (Fig. 14.3) (5–9). It has much lesser activity against COX-2. This effect is transient in endothelial cells because the half-life of aspirin is short and the constitutive enzyme rapidly regenerates. In platelets, which have no nuclei and cannot resynthesize mRNA, this effect is irreversible. However, numerous additional thromboxane-independent pathways exist for platelet activation, including ADP (an important additional internal amplification mechanism), serotonin, thombin,

and shear forces (mediated by ADP rather than thromboxane). There also is a significant number of patients who are either completely (approximately 5%) or relatively (approximately 15% to 20%, depending on the test used) resistant to the antiplatelet effects of aspirin (10).

Dipyridamole

Dipyridamole inhibits cyclic adenosine monophosphate phosphodiesterase (11,12). Its mechanism of action is complex, but probably the most important effects relate to the direct release of prostanoids from the endothelium. Dipyridamole may also interfere with platelet function by inhibiting the cellular uptake and metabolism of adenosine, raising the concentration at the platelet vascular interface and increasing the levels of intracellular cyclic adenosine monophosphate in the platelets themselves. Dipyridamole may potentiate the antiplatelet actions of aspirin, although the clinical significance of this remains controversial. It has a terminal half-life of 10 days and is primarily excreted in the bile. Slow uptake

TABLE 14.1. *Antiplatelet agents*

Aspirin	Inhibits platelet cyclooxygenase Blocks thromboxane formation	Inhibits platelet activation, feedback

Thienopyridines
  Ticlopidine
  Clopidogrel
	Interfere with adenosine diphosphate
	  signaling
		Inhibit platelet activation, feedback
		Side effects of neutropenia,
		  thrombocytopenic purpura
		Much lower incidence of side effects
		Faster onset of action

Dipyridamole	Phosphodiesterase inhibitor Stimulates endothelial prostacyclin	Inhibits platelet activation (limited) May synergize with aspirin
Sulfinpyrazone	Inhibits platelet cyclooxygenase Blocks thromboxane formation (limited)	Inhibit platelet activation (limited) [Not currently in general use]
Cilostazol	Phosphodiesterase 3 inhibitor Interferes with internal signaling	Inhibits (somewhat) platelet activation
Glycoprotein IIb/IIIa antagonists	Interfere with fibrinogen, von Willebrand factor binding	Inhibit platelet aggregation

of dipyridamole by the platelets can be due to its binding with plasma proteins. It is also capable of enhancing platelet survival in patients with venous or arterial thrombosis, prosthetic valves, and prosthetic graft. With the advent of other antiplatelet agents such as the thienopyridines (as discussed later), dipyridamole is not used much in patients with coronary artery disease (CAD), but is still utilized (with aspirin) in some patients with cerebrovascular disease. Side effects of dipyridamole include angina pectoris or exacerbation of chest pain, headaches, hypertension, hypotension, ST-T segment changes, and tachycardia. Concurrent use of dipyridamole with aspirin increases the risk of gastrointestinal ulceration and hemorrhage.

Sulfinpyrazone

Sulfinpyrazone is a uricosuric agent, structurally related to phenylbutazone. The mechanism of action is uncertain, but it appears to competitively inhibit platelet cyclooxygenase (13,14). It also reduces thrombus formation on subendothelium, inhibits platelet adhesion to collagen, and may protect endothelium from chemical injury. Sulfinpyrazone is well absorbed orally, and remains strongly bound to plasma proteins; it has a plasma half-life of ≤10 hours. The most beneficial effects of sulfinpyrazone appear to be on prosthetic surfaces rather than on biological surfaces. The clinical benefit has been variable in patients with CAD, with debatable benefit after myocardial infarction (MI), no benefit in preventing stroke, and no benefit in patients with unstable angina pectoris (USA), and is no longer recommended for use an a platelet antagonist.

Thienopyridines (Ticlopidine and Clopidogrel)

The thienopyridines ticlopidine and clopidogrel act to inhibit the platelet 2-methylthio-ADP-binding receptor, although it is unclear whether the exact effect is on receptor expression, function, or occupation (15–22). In response to other stimuli whose actions may, in part, be mediated through ADP released from endogenous platelet granules, thienopyridines also blunt platelet aggregation. Thienopyridines also inhibit platelet aggregation in response to shear stress, and deaggregate platelet thrombus that has already formed. It is generally believed that thienopyridines are biotransformed and activated in the liver; biotransformation of the thienopyridines by the hepatic CP450 system has been well documented, and plasma levels of the parent drug are not detectable 2 hours after oral administration. It has been suggested that both ticlopidine and clopidogrel can interfere with *in vitro* ADP-induced aggregation of washed human platelets, and thus biotransformation may not be a necessary step (18). This effect was not noted when either plasma or albumin was present. Regardless of the exact mechanism, thienopyridines produce a permanent inhibition of the low-affinity ADP receptor, and platelets exposed to thienopyridines are irreversibly inhibited for their lifetime (8 to 10 days).

The onset of action of ticlopidine is about 48 to 72 hours, and it takes about 5 to 6 days to achieve steady-state levels of platelet inhibition. Ticlopidine has also been shown to reduce fibrinogen concentrations and blood viscosity and to increase the filterability of whole blood and red blood cells. Ticlopidine is metabolized in the liver. Adverse effects of ticlopidine include neutropenia, rash, diarrhea, and, rarely, thrombotic thrombocytopenic purpura (TTP) (19).

Clopidogrel bisulfate is a thienopyridine derivative. As compared to ticlopidine, the antiplatelet effects of clopidogrel appear somewhat more rapidly, particularly with oral loading. Clopidogrel is rapidly absorbed after oral administration, reaching peak plasma concentrations approximately 1 hour after an oral dose. Steady-state concentrations are reached after approximately 3 days of consecutive dosing. Food or antacids do not appear to interfere with its absorption or bioavailability. Both clopidogrel and its primary metabolite (a carboxylic acid derivative) are highly protein bound (*in vitro* binding to albumin of 98% and 94%, respectively). There are no significant differences in men and women of the primary metabolite. The drug is well absorbed in the elderly and has comparable pharmacodynamic effects in the elderly as in younger patients. Evaluation of the pharmacodynamic effects of clopidogrel has shown significant inhibition of platelet function within 2 hours of a 400-mg dose, an effect that persists for up to 48 hours. With repeated oral daily doses of 50 to 100 mg, a significant antiplatelet effect is measurable at 48 hours, and reaches steady state 4 to 7 days after initiating therapy. Dose-ranging studies have shown that a clopidogrel dose of 75 mg per day provides a similar degree of platelet inhibition to that achieved with 250 mg twice daily (b.i.d.) of ticlopidine. The side effects of clopidogrel are same as or even milder than those seen with aspirin, and much less frequent than with ticlopidine. The much lower frequency of TTP and bone marrow toxicity, even over an extended period of follow-up, is a major advantage of clopidogrel over ticlopidine (20).

Cliostazol

Cilostazol is a phosphodiesterase type 3 inhibitor, and hence has antiplatelet effects similar to those of dipyridamole (23,24). These effects have not been well characterized when cilostazol is added to aspirin and/or thienopyridines. The therapeutic benefits of cilostazol in patients with peripheral arterial disease (PAD) appear primarily related to symptomatology and walking distance, and may relate more to its vasodilator effects than specific antiplatelet activity.

Glycoprotein IIb/IIIa Antagonists

The platelet GP IIb/IIIa serves as the final common pathway for platelet aggregation and is a principal determinant of arterial thrombus volume and strength (25). Inhibition of GP IIb/IIIa function profoundly alters platelet hemostatic function and prevents thrombus growth. There are three commercially available intravenous agents: abciximab (Reo-Pro) is a chimeric monoclonal Fab fragment, which binds nonspecifically to GP IIb/IIIa; eptifibatide (Integrilin) is a cyclic heptapeptide, which competitively and selectively binds to GP IIb/IIIa; and tirofiban (Aggrastat) is a nonpeptide derivative of tyrosine, which also binds to GP IIb/IIIa in a selective and competitive fashion. Peptide GP IIb/IIIa antagonists contain either the arginine–glycine–aspartic acid (RGD) sequence itself or a similar sequence, such as lysine–glysine-aspartic acid (KGD). Cyclic forms of the peptides are more resistant to degradation than linear peptides, but still have significantly short half-lives because they are broken down in the body. Another factor contributing to their relatively short half-life is renal excretion. The nonpeptide, or peptidomimetic, antagonists are designed to have a spatial and charge conformation that closely resembles that of the RGD-binding sequence. Because peptide and peptidomimetic compounds are competitive antagonists, therapeutic efficacy is dependent on maintaining plasma levels high enough to compete favorably with fibrinogen for GP IIb/IIIa receptor binding. Yet other GP IIb/IIIa antagonists (xemilofiban, orbofiban, sibrafiban, etc.) are prodrugs of peptidomimetic compounds and can be given orally. These oral compounds significantly extend the potential duration of potent antiplatelet inhibition (26–37). These oral agents have been clinically investigated for a number of cardiovascular applications, as will be discussed, but are not commercially available, and are unlikely to be clinically developed.

Anticoagulant Agents: Targeting Thrombin Generation and Thrombin Activity

The addition of anticoagulant therapy to antiplatelet therapy further inhibits the ability to form thrombus in response to injury. Anticoagulant therapy can be utilized to inhibit thrombin generation, thrombin activity, or both (Table 14.2).

Unfractionated Heparin

The most common form of systemic anticoagulation agent is unfractionated heparin (UFH), a heterogeneous mixture of polysaccharides of varying chain lengths, ranging in molecular weight from 5,000 to 30,000 daltons (38–41). UFH exerts its anticoagulant effect by binding via a specific pentasaccharide sequence to antithrombin (an endogenous regulator of coagulation) and, when doing so, results in conformational changes in antithrombin that enhance its affinity for its regulatory targets, thrombin and factor Xa (Fig. 14.4). The binding of thrombin by the heparin–antithrombin complex (by virtue of long heparin saccharide chains) greatly facilitates the interaction between thrombin and antithrombin by placing them in close proximity. In addition to this indirect inhibition of thrombin activity (by ternary complexes of antithrombin–heparin–thrombin), UFH is also an inhibitor of thrombin generation because of the ability of the heparin–antithrombin complex to bind and inhibit activated factor X (Xa), a key component of the prothrombinase complex that converts prothrombin to thrombin.

Unfractionated heparin has a number of significant limitations, which result in unpredictable degrees of anticoagulation and difficulty achieving therapeutic effect. Serum heparin concentration is significantly affected by its high degree of protein binding, and consequently its biological effect can be highly variable. Given its dependence on antithrombin as a cofactor, UFH can also be ineffective when endogenous supplies of antithrombin are depleted. The antithrombotic activity of UFH is further limited by its inability to inactivate clot-bound thrombin (secondary to the fact that the heparin–antithrombin complex is too large to intercalate into the clot). Finally, the heparin–antithrombin complex is inactivated by both platelet factor IV (released from activated platelets and platelet-rich thrombi) and by fibrin II monomers. Thus, a "therapeutic" degree of heparin anticoagulation may be very difficult to achieve and may not be sufficient to prevent propagation of thrombus. As with all anticoagulant therapy, the use of unfractionated heparin carries a risk of bleeding, most frequently at the sites of vascular access. The risk of bleeding is generally proportional to the dose of UFH (as assessed by the activated clotting time) and the use of adjunctive anticoagulant, antiplatelet, and fibrinolytic therapy. Heparin itself is known to activate platelets. A final infrequent, but worrisome, complication of UFH therapy is heparin-induced

TABLE 14.2. Anticoagulant agents[a]

Unfractionated heparin	Indirect thrombin inhibitor (via antithrombin) Blocks thrombin formation	Highly protein bound Activates platelets Risk of HIT
Low-molecular-weight heparins	Indirect thrombin inhibitors (via antithrombin) Block thrombin formation	Shorter saccharide chains Less protein binding Less platelet activation Less risk of HIT
Direct thrombin inhibitors	Not dependent on antithrombin Block thrombin activity Block thrombin-induced platelet activation	No platelet activation No risk of HIT
Warfarin	Interferes with synthesis of vitamin K-dependent factors (II, VII, IX, X, protein C, protein S)	Narrow therapeutic range

[a]HIT, Heparin-induced thrombocytopenia.

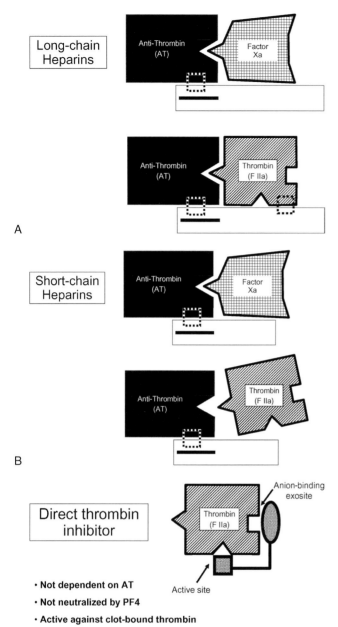

Long-chain
Heparins

Anti-Thrombin
(AT)

Factor
Xa

A

Short-chain
Heparins

Anti-Thrombin
(AT)

Factor
Xa

Anti-Thrombin
(AT)

Thrombin
(F IIa)

B

Direct thrombin
inhibitor

Anion-binding
exosite

Thrombin
(F IIa)

Active site

• **Not dependent on AT**
• **Not neutralized by PF4**
• **Active against clot-bound thrombin**
C • **Less variability of effect**

FIG. 14.4. A: Long-chain heparins bind to antithombin (AT) and markedly increase the inhibition of thrombin (factor IIa [F IIa] and Factor Xa. However, the inhibition of thrombin is chain-length dependent because it also requires the binding of the heparin–antithrombin complex to thrombin, in essence lining it up for inhibition in much the same way that a key is positioned in a lock. **B:** Shorter-chain heparins inhibit factor Xa, which does not need to be precisely lined up with the heparin–antithrombin complex; hence, inhibition of factor Xa is not chain-length dependent. **C:** Direct thrombin inhibitors do not require the intermediary of antithrombin, and act directly to block the actions of thrombin, interfering with the active, catalytic site and, in some cases, the anion-binding exosite as well. They do not act against factor Xa, and thus block thrombin activity rather than thrombin generation. PF4, Platelet factor 4.

thrombocytopenia and the more ominous heparin-induced thrombocytopenia/thrombosis syndrome (42–45).

Low-Molecular-Weight Heparins

As just discussed, the ability of the heparin–antithrombin complex to bind and inhibit thrombin is dependent on the presence of the long heparin saccharide chains (greater than 18 monosaccharide units) (46–48). Conversely, the interaction between the heparin–antithrombin complex and factor Xa is not chain-length dependent. The low-molecular-weight heparins (LMWHs) are derived from chemical cleavage of longer, unfractionated heparin chains, producing shorter saccharide chains (molecular weight ranging from 4,000 to 6,000 daltons). These shorter chain lengths result in a greater degree of factor Xa inhibition (and hence inhibition of thrombin generation) relative to thrombin inhibition (Fig. 14.4B). Shorter chain lengths also convey less protein binding, and therefore more potent, predictable, and sustained anticoagulation. In many circumstances, LMWHs have supplanted UFH as the primary antithrombotic of choice. LMWHs carry the additional advantage of maintaining some downstream antithrombin activity (due to retention of some longer chains) and therefore may still significantly block thrombin activity if large amounts of thrombin are not present. In contrast, pentasaccharide (Arixtra) is a pure Xa inhibitor with no residual downstream thrombin activity (49,50). Heparin and the heparin derivatives are all indirect thrombin and/or factor Xa inhibitors in that they require antithrombin as a cofactor.

Direct Thrombin Inhibitors

The direct-acting thrombin antagonists inhibit the coagulation cascade at multiple points (51–53). In contrast to heparin and heparin derivatives, which act indirectly via antithrombin, the direct thrombin inhibitors directly and specifically inhibit the autocatalytic actions of thrombin and the conversion of fibrinogen to fibrin (Fig. 14.4C). Additionally, thrombin inhibitors block the amplification feedback actions of thrombin and interfere with thrombin-mediated platelet activation. Importantly, unlike heparin, the direct-acting thrombin antagonists do not require antithrombin cofactor for their activity against thrombin, thus allowing for concentration-dependent activity.

The classic example of a thrombin inhibitor is hirudin, an antithrombotic compound derived from the salivary glands of the medicinal leech (*Hirudo medicinalis*). The hirudin molecule consists of two primary parts (both of which have been synthetically altered to form second- and third-generation direct thrombin antagonists): a compact hydrophophic core at the amino-terminal end (which contains the active binding site) and an extremely hydrophilic carboxy-terminal end (which dictates the molecule's solubility and pharmacokinetics). The active binding site of hirudin (forming a highly stable noncovalent complex with thrombin) is irreversible, but has been synthetically altered in subsequently derived products to be either reversible or competitively reversible. Under physiological condition, hirudin exists in multimeric forms; however, hirudin appears to function as a monomer when interacting with thrombin. Hirudin binds both circulating and clot-bound thrombin, and, unlike heparin, neither has significant protein binding nor is inhibited by platelet factor 4. For these reasons, the direct thrombin inhibitors provide a more reliable degree of anticoagulation. Four direct thrombin antagonists are commercially available: desirudin, lepirudin, bivalirudin, and argatroban.

Warfarin

Warfarin and other coumarin anticoagulants inhibit vitamin K-2,3-epoxide reductase in hepatic microsomes, thus interfering with hepatic recycling of vitamin K, which is a necessary cofactor for the synthesis of specific γ-carboxy-glutamic acid residues (54,55). These particular residues are needed for the posttranslational modification of certain proteins synthesized in the hepatocytes, the so-called vitamin K-dependent coagulation factors II, VII, IX, and X and protein C and protein S. Warfarin is water soluble, is completely absorbed from the gastrointestinal tract, and reaches maximal blood concentrations in 90 minutes. It is metabolized by hepatic microsomal enzymes, and is almost totally bound to plasma proteins; consequently, it has a relatively long plasma half-life.

Following a dose of warfarin sufficient to completely block hepatic synthesis of vitamin K dependent proteins, each of the involved clotting factors will disappear from the blood at a speed inversely proportional to its half-life. Thus, the levels of factor VII (with a half-life of 5 hours) will fall very rapidly (with commensurate prolongation of the prothrombin time [PT]), whereas more slowly metabolized coagulation factors, factors IX and X (20 to 60 hours) and prothrombin (100 hours), will fall more slowly. After approximately 5 days, the levels of all involved coagulation factors will have fallen. Because the counterregulatory protein C and protein S also have short half-lives, in the early phases of intiating warfarin therapy, patients may actually be prothrombotic, despite what appears to be a therapeutic PT.

After warfarin therapy is stopped, the individual factors return to normal, also in proportion to their individual rates of synthesis.

Clinical Use of Antithrombotic Agents in Peripheral Vascular Disease Acute Therapy

Anticoagulation for Peripheral Intervention

Percutaneous interventional procedures in peripheral arteries generally employ the same pharmacologic adjuncts as utilized for coronary intervention, where aspirin and unfractionated heparin have been mainstays of procedural anticoagulation (56,57) (Table 14.3). With the advent of stents, many clinicians have generalized from the coronary experience and added adjunctive thienopyridines to aspirin following peripheral stent placement. This remains empiric, and there is ongoing at least one formal randomized, placebo-controlled

TABLE 14.3. *Therapeutic application of antiplatelet and anticoagulant therapy in peripheral arterial disease*

Acute therapy: Procedural anticoagulation (for percutaneous interventions) and other thrombotic exacerbations
  Antiplatelet
    Aspirin
    Aspirin + ticlopidine
    Aspirin + clopidogrel (replacing ticlopidine)
  Anticoagulant
    Unfractionated heparin
    Low-molecular-weight heparins
    Direct thrombin inhibitors
Long-term therapy
  Antiplatelet
    Aspirin
    Ticlopidine
    Clopidogrel (replacing ticlopidine)
    Aspirin + clopidogrel
  Anticoagulant
    Warfarin

trial of adjunctive clopidogrel for 12 months following peripheral stent placement, the Clopidogrel and Aspirin in the Management of Peripheral Endovascular Revascularization study (57a), in 2,000 patients undergoing percutaneous peripheral interventions. In carotid stenting, aspirin and clopidogrel are already fairly routinely used in the short term (with growing long-term experience), and there is emerging experience with combination therapy shortly after carotid endarterectomy (again, with growing long-term use as well). The Clopidogrel and Aspirin in Surgery for Peripheral Arterial Disease trial is a planned test of clopidogrel for 12 months following bypass surgery in 1,600 patients with peripheral arterial disease (57a).

LMW heparins are utilized infrequently for procedural anticoagulation in the periphery, but there is growing experience extending some of the current experience with LMW heparins for coronary intervention (58–64), particularly with more sophisticated anticoagulation monitoring. GP IIb/IIIa antagonists are used relatively infrequently. For coronary applications, they provide substantial reductions in postprocedure creatine kinase MB (CKMB) elevations in higher-risk patients. In the periphery, there is no such enzymatic marker for injury, and they are generally withheld unless there is evidence of visible thrombus or evidence of ongoing thrombus formation. Direct thrombin inhibitors have not been extensively used in the periphery, although there is at least one recent report (63) and an editorial that has advocated further study (64), particularly in light of a recent report documenting the occurrence of procedural complications (primarily bleeding) in a single-center experience with peripheral intervention (65). The Randomized Evaluation in PCI Linking Angiomax to Reduced Clinical Events study was performed in patients undergoing coronary intervention (66), and very little data exist for use in the periphery.

These agents have potential application in patients with impaired renal function and in patients at high risk for bleeding, but more data are needed. Direct thrombin inhibitors are the antithrombotic of choice in patients with heparin-induced thrombocytopenia, as will be discussed.

Long-Term Antiplatelet and Anticoagulant Therapy

Aspirin

Much of the support for the routine use of aspirin in patients with peripheral arterial disease comes from the Antithrombotic Trialists meta-analyses. The first meta-analysis (the Antiplatelet Trialists' Collaboration), published in 1994 and including clinical trials through 1990, demonstrated that oral antiplatelet therapy (primarily aspirin) was effective in preventing recurrent events across a wide range of atherosclerotic vascular disease, primarily coronary and cerebrovascular (67–69). It did deal with poststroke therapy (where aspirin was effective), but did not examine other peripheral arterial disease. A more recent and more comprehensive analysis was undertaken, involving trials through 1997, with additional focus on stroke and peripheral arterial disease, and was published in 2002 (70). The analysis included 287 studies, which involved 135,000 patients in whom antiplatlet therapy was compared with control, and 77,000 patients in whom different antiplatelet regimens were compared (Table 14.4).

Overall, antiplatelet therapy (primarily aspirin) reduced the incidence of any serious vascular event by one-fourth, of nonfatal MI by one-third, of nonfatal stroke by one-fourth, and vascular mortality by one-sixth. The absolute reduction in serious vascular events was 36 per 1,000 treated for 2 years with previous stroke or transient ischemic attack (TIA). In 21 trials of patients with stroke or TIA, antiplatelet therapy reduced vascular events from 21.4% with control to 17.8%. Overall, among 9,214 patients with PAD in 42 trials, there was a relative reduction of 23% in total vascular events (from 7.1% to 5.8%). In 26 trials of patients with intermittent claudication, antiplatelet therapy reduced vascular events from 7.9% with control to 6.4%. Similarly, in 12 trials of patients following surgical grating of peripheral lesions, antiplatelet therapy reduced events from 6.5% to 5.4%, and it reduced events from 3.6% to 2.5% in four trials of patients undergoing peripheral angioplasty. In six trials in patients with carotid disease, antiplatelet therapy reduced events from 12.8% to 10.6%. However, much of the new information about PAD in the recent meta-analysis came from the Atherosclerotic Disease Evolution by Picotamide Trial, which compared the thrombaoxane synthase inhibitor picotamide to placebo (71).

In the meta-analysis, aspirin doses of 75 to 150 mg daily were at least as effective as higher doses. The effects of doses less than 75 mg were less certain. There was no good evidence to support the hypothesis that doses of aspirin ≥1,000 mg daily might be preferable in patients at high risk of stroke. A more recent trial (not included in the meta-analysis) supports this. The Aspirin and Carotid Endarterectomy trial showed that in 2,849 patients undergoing carotid endarterectomy, the composite outcome of MI stroke or death was significantly lower among patients taking 81 or 325 mg of aspirin versus those taking 625 to 1,300 mg (72).

The addition of more oral antiplatelet therapy to aspirin generally appeared to provide some incremental benefit (70). In 25 trials comparing dipyridamole plus aspirin with aspirin alone (involving 10,404 patients), combination therapy was associated with a nonsignificant 6% relative reduction in events (from 12.4% with aspirin to 11.8% with aspirin plus dipyridamole). There was only one trial, the European Stroke Prevention Study 2 (73), that showed benefit in poststroke patients, but that benefit was in recurrent stroke, not MI or vascular death. Stronger data support the addition of ticlopidine or clopidogrel, as will be noted.

Aspirin alone has also been shown to potentially alter the need for revascularization in patients with PAD. The Physicians Health Study (74–76) evaluated the effects of low-dose aspirin (325 mg per day) compared to placebo in 22,071 male physicians who did not have a history of MI or cerebrovascular disease at baseline; the average treatment period was approximately 5 years. The aspirin group had a 46% reduction in the need for surgical limb revascularization, but there was no difference between groups in the incidence of intermittent claudication (74). From the perspective of coronary events, there was a substantial reduction (44%) in the risk of myocardial infarction, but no reduction in the incidence of stroke, all-cause cardiovascular mortality, or the incidence of new angina (76). Thus, long-term aspirin therapy appears to be effective in reducing the incidence of acute thrombotic

TABLE 14.4. *Efficacy of antiplatelet therapy in clinical subgroups in the recent antiplatelet trialists meta-analysis (70)*

Clinical category	Number of trials	Antiplatelet event rate (%)	Control event rate (%)	Percentage odds reduction
Previous myocardial infarction	12	13.5	17.0	25
Previous stroke/transient ischemic attack	21	17.8	21.4	22
Coronary angioplasty	9	2.7	5.5	53
Stable coronary artery disease	7	9.9	14.1	33
Carotid disease	6	10.6	12.8	19
Peripheral arterial disease				
Claudication	26	6.4	7.9	23
Peripheral graft	12	5.4	6.5	22
Peripheral angioplasty	4	2.5	3.6	29
Subtotal	42	5.8	7.1	23

events, but may not affect the progress of the underlying atherosclerotic disease.

In the recently reported African-American Antiplatelet Stroke Prevention Study, aspirin alone (650 mg per day) appeared just as good as ticlopidine (250 mg b.i.d.) in the treatment of 1,809 African-American patients with a recent (7 to 90 days) noncardioembolic ischemic stroke (77). The trial was halted prematurely by the Data Safety and Monitoring Committee on the basis of a futility analysis. The primary outcome of recurrent stroke, MI, or vascular death occurred in 12.3% of the aspirin group and 14.7% of the ticlopidine group (*p*=ns). Adverse events were slightly, but not significantly higher with ticlopidine.

Thienopyridines

Two large studies have examined the utility of ticlopidine in patients with cerebrovascular disease. The Canadian American Ticlopidine Study trial was performed in 1982 to 1986, and compared ticlopidine (250 mg b.i.d.) with placebo in 1,072 patients with a history of recent stroke (1 week to 4 months) (78). Patients were followed for a mean of 2 years following enrollment; the primary endpoint was the composite of ischemic stroke, MI, or vascular death. The placebo group had a primary event rate of 15.3% per year, the ticlopidine group had a primary event rate of 10.8% per year (relative risk reduction [RRR] 23.3%; *p*=0.02). The Ticlopidine Aspirin Stroke Study trial was performed in 1982 to 1987 and compared ticlopidine (250 mg b.i.d.) with aspirin (650 mg b.i.d.) in 3,069 patients with a history of a recent stroke precursor or minor stroke within the last 3 months (79). Patients were followed for a mean of 3.4 years following enrollment; the primary endpoint was the composite of nonfatal stroke and all-cause mortality. The aspirin group had a primary event rate of 19% over 3 years, and the ticlopidine group had a primary event rate of 17% over 3 years (RRR 12%; *p*=0.048).

A single trial has evaluated ticlopidine in unstable angina (80). In an open-label trial, 652 patients with unstable angina were randomized to conventional therapy (excluding aspirin) with or without ticlopidine. At 6 months, there was a 46% RRR for the endpoints of death or nonfatal MI (from 13.6% to 7.3%, *p*=0.009). No study has compared ticlopidine to aspirin in acute coronary syndromes.

The Clopidogrel versus Aspirin in Patients at Risk of Ischemic Events (CAPRIE) trial was a large-scale randomized trial of the safety and efficacy of clopidogrel (75 mg per day) versus aspirin (325 mg per day) in 19,185 patients with atherosclerotic vascular disease followed for up to 3 years (81). The study population included patients with recent ischemic stroke (within 6 months), recent myocardial infarction (within 35 days), or symptomatic peripheral arterial disease. The primary endpoint was the composite incidence of stroke (fatal and nonfatal), myocardial infarction (fatal and nonfatal), and other vascular death. At a mean follow-up of 1.9 years, the clopidogrel group had

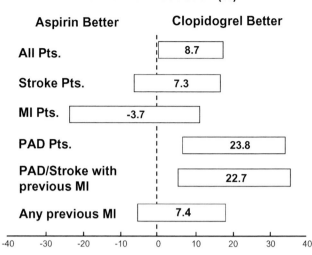

FIG. 14.5. Relative risk reduction in the composite of death, myocardial infarction (MI), and stroke in the major clinical subgroups in the Clopidogrel versus Aspirin in Patients at Risk of Ischemic Events study. Peripheral arterial disease (PAD) patients and patients with multibed vascular disease (and greater atherosclerotic burden) had the greatest relative clinical benefit. (Adapted from CAPRIE Steering Committee. A randomised, blinded trial of clopidogrel versus aspirin in patients at risk of ischemic events (CAPRIE). *Lancet* 1996;348:1329–1339, with permission.)

significantly fewer composite first events (5.32% per year risk vs. 5.83% per year with aspirin; RRR 8.7%; *p*=0.043). The outcome event most dramatically reduced by clopidogrel therapy was myocardial infarction. The greatest relative risk reduction (23.8%) was noted in patients with peripheral arterial disease (Fig. 14.5), in whom the annual event rate was reduced from 4.86% with aspirin to 3.71% with clopidogrel (*p*=0.0028). There were no major differences between the aspirin and clopidogrel groups in terms of safety. The incidence of significant neutropenia was 0.10% in the clopidogrel group and 0.17% in the aspirin group. When patients with coronary disease and either concomitant cerebrovascular disease or peripheral vascular disease were examined, there was striking superiority of clopidogrel in reducing outcome events in this population (relative risk reduction 22.7%). Mechanistically, an important factor may be the key role that ADP plays in shear-induced platelet aggregation. In peripheral vascular disease and coronary artery disease plus disease in other vascular beds, there is a greater atherosclerotic burden, more shear forces, and, probably, a more important role for ADP-induced platelet activation/aggregation. Recent additional analyses of the CAPRIE cohort have documented the significant benefit of clopidogrel over aspirin in patients with a prior history of coronary artery bypass grafting (82) and patients with diabetes (83), and showed the benefits of clopidogrel over aspirin in preventing not only initial events (the primary CAPRIE analysis), but recurrent and total vascular events as well (84).

The Clopidogrel in Unstable angina to Prevent Recurrent ischemic Events (CURE) trial was a multicenter, randomized, double-blind, placebo-controlled study comparing combination therapy with aspirin and clopidogrel versus aspirin alone in patients with acute coronary syndromes (85). A total of 12,562 patients with unstable angina or non-Q wave MI (within 24 hours of their last episode of pain) received aspirin 75 to 325 mg and then were randomized to clopidogrel (300-mg load followed by 75 mg daily) or placebo for 3 months to 1 year. The primary endpoint was a composite of cardiovascular (CV) death, MI, or stroke. The main safety endpoints were major bleeding (disabling or symptomatic intracranial or intraocular bleeding, or transfusion of more than two units of blood) and life-threatening bleeding (hemoglobin decrease of greater than 5 g per dL, hypotension requiring inotropes, bleeding requiring surgery or transfusion of more than four units of blood, or intracranial bleeding).

Seventy-five percent of the patients enrolled in CURE had unstable angina; 25% had an elevated enzyme or troponin level; 94% had an abnormal electrocardiogram; and half had ST-segment deviation. Approximately 30% of the patients underwent revascularization; the mean follow-up was 9 months. Treatment with clopidogrel and aspirin was associated with a 20% relative reduction in the primary endpoint of CV death, MI, or stroke, largely driven by a 23% relative reduction in the incidence of MI. Differences in the other components of the primary endpoint (CV death, stroke, non-CV death) failed to reach statistical significance. There was a 31% reduction in in-hospital refractory ischemia (2.06% to 1.42%, p=0.001) and a 25% reduction in severe ischemia (5.03% to 3.83%, p=0.001). The curves for the primary endpoint began to diverge very early favoring clopidogrel (within the first few hours). At 24 hours, a 20% relative reduction in the composite death, MI, and stroke was also noted. The benefits of clopidogrel were present across all major subgroups: patients with and without major ST-segment deviation, enzyme or troponin elevation, and prior and subsequent revascularization (86). Benefits were also noted in composite events with long-term therapy in addition to in-hospital benefit. Although there was a 34% excess of major bleeding in the clopidogrel arm, there was no significant excess of life-threatening bleeding with combination therapy.

The Clopidogrel for the Reduction of Events During Observation trial demonstrated that long-term therapy following percutaneous coronary intervention with aspirin and clopidogrel was superior to aspirin alone in reducing the 1-year incidence of death, MI, and stroke (87). This reinforces and extends the potential benefits of secondary prevention with more intense oral antiplatelet therapy beyond the acute coronary syndrome population to a larger population of patients with manifest coronary atherosclerotic disease.

The Clopidogrel for High Atherothrombotic Risk and Ischemic Stabilization, Management and Avoidance trial is a currently ongoing prospective, randomized study comparing aspirin alone with aspirin plus clopidogrel (75 mg per day) in patients at risk for vascular events (documented cerebrovas-

cular disease, documented coronary artery disease, symptomatic PAD, or multiple risk factors—two major, one major plus two minor, or three minor). A total of at least 15,200 patients are to be randomized; it is an event-driven trial (1,040 primary events of stroke, MI, or cardiovascular death), and the estimated duration of follow-up is approximately 42 months. Another trial, Management of Atherothrombosis with Clopidogrel in High Risk Patients with Recent TIA or Ischemic Stroke, is examining the utility of clopidogrel in a high-risk stroke/TIA population of approximately 7,600 patients treated and followed for 18 months.

Oral IIb/IIIa Antagonists

There have been five large randomized trials of oral IIb/IIIa antagonists in patients with atherosclerotic disease: the Evaluation of Xemilofiban in Controlling Thrombotic Events trial (7,232 patients undergoing coronary intervention) (33), the Orofiban in Patients with Unstable Coronary Syndromes Thrombolysis in MI trial (10,288 patients following acute coronary syndromes (32), the Sibrafiban Versus Aspirin to Yield Maximum Prevention from Ischemic Heart Events Post Acute Coronary Syndromes (SYMPHONY) trial (9,169 patients following acute coronary syndromes) (34), the SECOND SYMPHONY trial (6,637 patients following acute coronary syndromes) (35), and the Blockade of the GP IIb/IIIa Receptor to Avoid Vascular Occlusion (BRAVO) trial (9,190 high-risk patients following coronary event, cerebrovascular events, or with multibed vascular disease) (36). Despite the fact that these studies all used very powerful antiplatelet agents, all five trials demonstrated a trend toward higher mortality in the IIb/IIIa groups. A recent meta-analysis (37) of four of these studies demonstrated a 37% increase in mortality (p=0.001), and a 40% increase in MI at 30 days (p=0.002) with active therapy. Only one of the five trials, BRAVO, included patients with non-coronary vascular disease as a primary inclusion criterion (36). Of the 9,190 patients enrolled in BRAVO, 3,319 had had a recent cerebrovascular event (within the prior 5 to 30 days), and 1,481 had had other peripheral vascular disease, with either concomitant coronary or cerebrovascular disease. Similar to the overall population, these subgroups showed a trend toward increased mortality with no significant clinical benefit with lotrafiban, although in all patients with cerebrovascular disease there was a nonsignificant trend favoring lotrafiban. A recent trial of the oral GP IIb/IIIa antagonist chromafiban in patients with peripheral vascular disease was also recently halted prematurely because of safety concerns.

Warfarin

The Thrombosis Prevention Trial compared low-intensity warfarin (target international normalized ratio [INR] 1.3 to 1.8), aspirin (75 mg per day), both, or neither in 5,499 men aged 45 to 69 years who were at risk for a first MI, but had not yet had an event (88). The trial was initiated in 1984, initially as a trial of warfarin versus placebo. A total of 1,427 men entered the first nonfactorial portion of the study between 1984 and 1989; the median follow-up was 1.1 years. In 1989, the trial was changed to a factorial comparison of warfarin/placebo and aspirin/placebo; the overall mean follow-up was 6.8 years. The primary endpoint was all ischemic heart disease events, defined as coronary death and fatal and nonfatal MI. In the overall trial, there were a total of 410 primary outcome events. The total primary event rate over the course of the study was 8.4% in the placebo group (1.3% per year). Neither warfarin alone nor aspirin alone significantly reduced outcome events; the primary event rates were similar in both groups: 6.5% overall, or 1.0% per year. Primary outcome events were significantly lower with combination therapy: 5.6% overall, or 0.9% per year, although combination therapy was also associated with a small, but significant increase in the incidence of hemorrhagic stroke (0.1%).

The initial data regarding the role of oral anticoagulants in patients with myocardial infarction came from three randomized trials using moderate-intensity anticoagulation (estimated INR 1.5 to 2.5). Two of these studies, the Medical Research Council Study and the Veterans Administration Cooperative Study (89,90), showed a significant reduction with anticoagulant therapy in the incidence of stroke, but no effect on mortality. The third study, the Bronx Municipal Study (91), showed a significant reduction in mortality with anticoagulant therapy and a nonsignificant trends toward fewer strokes. All three studies showed a reduction in the incidence of pulmonary embolism.

A pooled analysis of data from seven randomized trials published between 1964 and 1980 showed that chronic oral anticoagulant therapy after MI reduced the combined endpoints of mortality and nonfatal reinfarction by approximately 20% over a 1- to 6-year treatment period (92–94). A subsequent comprehensive review of 32 trials also suggested that anticoagulant treatment significantly reduced mortality (95).

Attention then turned to the degree of anticoagulation, with a focus still on patients with coronary artery disease. A review of 19 trials of oral anticoagulants (96) found that in trials with an INR target range of 2.5 to 5, mortality was reduced by approximately 40% and the risk of nonfatal MI was reduced by approximately two-thirds. In contrast, studies with inadequate or poor documentation of the degree of anticoagulation showed no difference in mortality, but did identify a trend in favor of anticoagulant therapy in the prevention of reinfarction.

The beneficial effects of more intense anticoagulant therapy in the postinfarction period have been examined in a number of subsequent studies. The Sixty-Plus Reinfarction Study was limited to patients older than 60 years following an MI who had been treated with oral anticoagulants for at least 6 months prior to enrollment; qualifying patients were then randomized to continue on oral anticoagulant therapy or to have it withdrawn (97). There was a significant reduction in the incidence of reinfarction and stroke in patients ran-

domized to continue warfarin therapy. In the Warfarin Reinfarction Study (WARIS) 1,214 post-MI patients (with no age restriction) were randomized to warfarin (target INR 2.8 to 4.8) or placebo and followed for an average of 37 months (98). There was a highly significant reduction in mortality in the warfarin group (24% relative reduction in the intention-to-treat cohort, and 35% relative reduction in the on-treatment cohort), along with a 50% relative reduction in the incidence of nonfatal reinfarction and a 55% reduction in the incidence of fatal cerebrovascular accident. There was a slightly increased risk of intracranial hemorrhage with warfarin, but this risk was far outweighed by the significant reduction in overall cerebrovascular events. The Anticoagualants in the Secondary Prevention of Events on Coronary Thrombosis (ASPECT) study also had no age restrictions, and randomized patients to higher-intensity warfarin therapy (INR 2.8 to 4.8) or placebo (99). ASPECT demonstrated that warfarin was associated with a 40% relative reduction in the incidence of stroke and a greater than 50% relative reduction in the incidence of reinfarction.

More recently, a number of studies have evaluated a variety of intensities of anticoagulation, either alone or in combination with aspirin, in patients with acute coronary syndromes. The ASPECT II study compared longer-term therapy with warfarin alone (target INR 3.0 to 4.0), aspirin (80 mg per day), and the combination of warfarin (INR 2.0 to 2.5) plus aspirin in 993 patients following an acute coronary syndrome (100). The study was stopped early by the sponsor because of slow recruitment. The composite endpoint of death, MI, and stroke occurred in 9.0% of patients on aspirin alone, 5.0% of those on warfarin alone, and 5.0% of those on warfarin and aspirin. There were slightly higher rates of minor bleeding in the group on combination therapy. The Antithrombotics in the Prevention of Reocclusion in Coronary Thrombolysis II study involved 308 patients with Thrombolysis in Myocardial Infarction grade 3 coronary flow after thrombolysis for ST segment-elevation MI who were randomized to aspirin (160 mg initially followed by 80 mg daily) or to aspirin plus warfarin (INR 2.0 to 3.0) (100). The primary endpoint was the rate of angiographic reocclusion at 3 months. Reocclusion occurred in 30% of the group given aspirin alone, compared with 18% in those given aspirin plus warfarin (a 40% relative reduction). There was an increase in minor but not major bleeding events in the combination therapy group.

The WARIS II trial compared warfarin alone (mean INR 2.8), aspirin alone (160 mg per day), or both (mean INR 2.2; aspirin 75 mg per day) in 3,630 patients less than 75 years of age with acute myocardial infarction (AMI) randomized at the time of hospital discharge and followed up for 2 years (101). The primary endpoint was the first occurrence of the composite of all-cause death, nonfatal reinfarction, or thromboembolic stroke; this occurred in 20% of the patients on aspirin alone, 16.7% of those on warfarin alone, and 15% of those on the combination of both drugs. Combination therapy was significantly superior to aspirin alone ($p=0.0005$), but there was no significant difference between the two warfarin groups. The incidence of major bleeding was 0.15% per year in the aspirin-alone group, 0.58% per year in the warfarin-alone group, and 0.52% per year in the combination group.

Two other recent studies, the Coumadin Aspirin Reinfarction Study (CARS) and the Combined Hemotherapy And Mortality Prevention Study (CHAMP), compared aspirin alone with the combination of aspirin and low-intensity warfarin (lower limit of targeted INR less than 2.0). The CARS study involved 8,803 patients with AMI, and demonstrated that low-fixed-dose warfarin (1 or 3 mg per day) plus aspirin (80 mg) was no more effective than aspirin alone (160 mg) for long-term treatment (102). The incidence of death, recurrent MI, or stroke was 8.6% in the aspirin-alone group and 8.4% in the aspirin-plus-warfarin group after a mean of 14 months of follow-up. The aspirin-plus-warfarin group also was noted to have a significant increase in major bleeding events. The CHAMP study evaluated the relative efficacy and safety of aspirin alone (160 mg per day) and the combination of warfarin (INR 1.5 to 2.5) and aspirin (81 mg per day) in 5,059 patients following MI in an open-label trial (103). There were no differences between the two groups in total mortality (17.3% vs. 17.3%), nonfatal MI (13.1% vs. 13.3%), or nonfatal stroke (4.7% vs. 4.2%). Again, major bleeding was more common in the combination therapy group.

The recent American Heart Association/American College of Cardiology guidelines for warfarin therapy (55) cited a recent meta-analysis of 31 randomized trials of oral anticoagulant therapy published between 1960 and 1999 (104). These studies all involved patients with coronary artery disease treated for ≥3 months. When the results were stratified by the intensity of anticoagulation therapy, high-intensity (INR 2.8 to 4.8) and moderate-intensity (INR 2 to 3) oral anticoagulation regimens reduced the rates of MI and stroke, but increased the risk of bleeding 6.0- to 7.7-fold. In combination with aspirin, low-intensity anticoagulation (INR less than 2.0) was not superior to aspirin alone, whereas moderate- to high-intensity oral anticoagulation and aspirin versus aspirin alone at least showed encouraging trends. There was a modest increase in the bleeding risk associated with the combination.

Three other studies evaluated oral anticoagulant therapy to prevent reinfarction in unstable angina patients over shorter-term time periods. The Organization to Assess Strategies for Ischemic Syndromes (OASIS) pilot study (105), the Antithrombotic Therapy in Acute Coronary Syndromes trial (106), and the OASIS 2 study (107) all suggested that in the short term, oral anticoagulation therapy could reduce the incidence of adverse events in the first 30 days if given in an intermediate INR range (2 to 3), but that the benefits of extended therapy were less well established.

There are relatively few randomized trials of oral anticoagulant therapy in patients with peripheral arterial disease. In a population of patients following surgical revascularization, a relatively high-intensity oral anticoagulant regimen (INR 2.6 to 4.5) was associated with a significant 51% reduction

in mortality (from 6.8% to 3.3% per year), compared with an untreated control group (p < 0.023) (warfarin guidelines) (108). The Arterial Disease Multiple Intervention Trial was a National Institutes of Health-sponsored pilot trial evaluating the use of warfarin, niacin, and an antioxidant "cocktail" in patients with peripheral arterial disease. It was not designed to look at clinical outcomes; instead, it focused on how effective therapy was in affecting laboratory parameters related to treatment; it was designed as a pilot for a later, larger, definitive, efficacy-powered trial. However, the larger-scale subsequent National Institutes of Health-sponsored outcomes-powered trial was never performed.

Heparin-Induced Thrombocytopenia

There are multiple clinical entities that can result in acute reductions in the platelet count, including increased destruction (via both immune and nonimmune mechanisms), decreased production, hypersplenism, hemodilution, post-cardiopulmonary bypass, and artifactual pseudothrombocytopenias. Among the immune causes are drug-induced thrombocytopenias; of these, heparin in a frequent culprit.

Heparin-induced thrombocytopenia (HIT) comes in two forms (109). Type I, which is a mild, nonimmunologic process, is not associated with adverse clinical sequellae, occurs primarily with high-dose intravenous heparin, and relates mainly to mild direct platelet activation by the heparin saccharide chains. Type II HIT, on the other hand, involves more dramatic falls in platelet counts (greater than 50% decrease), can be associated with any dose of heparin and any route of administration, and can be directly associated with severe adverse clinical events. The likelihood of type II HIT varies with the dose of heparin, is substantially greater for UFH than LMWH, and is more prominent with bovine-derived heparin than with porcine-derived heparin. In its most severe form (heparin induced thrombocytopenia thrombosis syndrome [HITTS]) it involves active thrombus formation, which can be severe and even potentially life-threatening.

The first step in the pathogenesis of HIT involves the binding of platelet factor 4 (PF4; secreted from activated platelets) to heparin saccharide chains (110). The heparin–PF4 complexes can elicit an immunoglobulin G (IgG) antibody response, and can result in heparin–PF4–IgG immune complexes. These immune complexes, in turn, can bind to platelets via an Fc receptor, producing activation and degranulation of the affected platelets. This results in the release of even more PF4, and the continuation of a vicious cascade of further platelet activation. Because activation and degranulation are fatal events for a platelet, platelet counts fall as the process accelerates. The thrombotic aspects of this come forth when platelet thrombi (involving aggregated clumps of activated platelets) develop at sites of preexisting pathology and form the nidus for subsequent thrombus formation. The affected areas can include atherosclerotic segments or areas of endothelial injury on otherwise intact blood vessel walls (both arterial and venous).

The clinical syndromes associated with HIT include arterial thrombus, venous thromboembolic events (predominating over arterial events by 4:1, with deep vein thrombosis and pulmonary embolism being the most common complications), skin lesions at heparin injection sites (erythematous plaques or overt skin necrosis), and acute platelet activation syndromes such as acute inflammatory reactions (fever, chills, etc.) or transient global amnesia.

The treatment of HIT and HITTS, until recently, was problematic. On the hand, these patients already had an underlying pathology that necessitated the administration of heparin in the first place. On the other hand, the use of additional heparin was contraindicated in the face of heparin-mediated thrombosis. LMWHs and heparinoids carry less risk of HIT (111), but once thrombocytopenia (and especially thrombosis) is established, these agents are also relatively contraindicated, because they can cross-react with PF4. In patients with a *history* of HIT, very brief short-term heparin infusions could be used for acute circumstances such as percutaneous procedures or cardiopulmonary bypass, but subsequent use of heparin had to be strictly avoided, and a small but finite risk of catastrophic thrombosis remained. Other strategies, such as use of the defibrinogenating agent ancrod, were also employed. The preferred therapy until recently was to promptly initiate oral anticoagulant therapy with warfarin. There were two problems with this approach. First, therapeutic levels of anticoagulation would not be achieved for days, and warfarin was not useful for the acute anticoagulation that was necessary in the face of ongoing thrombus formation. Second, in the early phase of initiating warfarin, patients actually become *more* prothrombotic, in association with falling levels of the vitamin K-dependent counterregulatory protein C and protein S (which have very short half-lives).

The development of the direct-acting thrombin antagonists (desirudin, lepirudin, bivalirudin, and argatroban) has dramatically changed the acute therapeutic approach. Acute, reliable anticoagulation is now possible, without worsening the risk of of thrombotic events (112). Chronic oral anticoagulant therapy may still be warranted, but can be initiated in controlled circumstances, on a background of reliable acute anticoagulation.

SUMMARY

The coagulation process is inherently accelerative. The modern view of coagulation has moved beyond mechanistic sequential pathways to the more important underlying processes of initiation, amplification, and propagation. Platelets and the activated platelet membrane play a key role in thrombus formation, and there is an emerging appreciation of the complex linkages among coagulation, inflammation, and atherosclerosis.

Coagulation can be interrupted in a number of different ways. Aspirin and the thienopyridines block specific pathways of platelet activation (thromboxane and ADP, respectively, two of the key feedback mechanisms), GP IIb/IIIa antagonists block platelet aggregation, Xa inhibitors and warfarin block thrombin generation, and direct thrombin antagonists block thrombin activity. Heparin and LMWHs strike a balance favoring more or less (respectively) anti-IIa/anti-Xa activity ratio.

Much of the clinical application of anticoagulant and antiplatelet agents has focused on coronary and cerebrovascular disease. With our increasing awareness of the importance of other peripheral vascular disease, more and more attention is now focusing on the utility of these agents for this disease as well. In general, anticoagulant and antiplatelet therapy is useful in reducing the manifestations and adverse clinical sequellae of atherosclerotic disease, no matter where it occurs in the body. However, there is no strong evidence supporting their use to prevent the progression of atherosclerotic disease—that is the aim of other therapies discussed in this text. Nevertheless, given the substantial risk that PAD patients have for subsequent coronary or cerebrovascular events, and the frequent overlap of atherosclerotic disease across vascular beds, some form of adjunctive therapy is warranted in most, if not all, of these patients, with more intense therapy applied in higher-risk individuals.

REFERENCES

1. Schafer AI. Coagulation cascade: an overview. In: Loscalzo J, Schafer AI, eds. *Thrombosis and hemorrhage.* Boston: Blackwell Scientific, 1994:3–12.
2. Ferguson JJ, Quinn M, Moake JL. Platelet physiology. In: Ferguson JJ, Chronos NAF, Harrington RA, eds. *Antiplatelet therapy in clinical practice.* London: Martin Dunitz, 2000:15–34.
3. Lefkovits J, Plow EF, Topol EJ. Platelet glycoprotein receptors in cardiovascular medicine. *N Engl J Med* 1995;332:1553–1559.
4. Moake JL, Turner NA, Stathopoulos NA, et al. Shear-induced platelet aggregation can be mediated by vWF released from platelets, as well as by exogenous large or unusually large vWF multimers, requires adenosine diphosphate, and is resistant to aspirin. *Blood* 1988;71:1366–1374.
5. Vane J. Inhibition of prostaglandin biosynthesis as a mechanism of action of aspirin-like drugs. *Nature* 1971;231:232–235.
6. Smith JB, Willis AL. Aspirin selectively inhibits prostaglandin production in human platelets. *Nature* 1971;231:235–237.
7. Pedersen AK, Fitzgerald GA. Dose-related kinetics of aspirin. Presystemic acetylation of platelet cyclo-oxygenase. *N Engl J Med* 1984;311:1206–1211.
8. Patrono C. Aspirin as an antiplatelet drug. *N Engl J Med* 1994;330:1287–1294.
9. Schror K. Aspirin and platelets: the antiplatelet actions of aspirin and its role in thrombosis treatment and prophylaxis. *Semin Thromb Hemost* 1997;23:349–355.
10. Eikelboom JW, Hirsch JH, Weitz JI, et al. Aspirin-resistant thromboxane biosynthesis and the risk of myocardial infarction, stroke, or cardiovascular death in patients at high risk for cardiovascular events. *Circulation* 2002;105:1650–1655.
11. Fitzgerald G. Dipyridamole. *N Engl J Med* 1987;316:1247–1257.
12. Schwartz L, Bourassa MG, Lespérance J, et al. Aspirin and dipyridamole in the prevention of restenosis after percutaneous transluminal coronary angioplasty. *N Engl J Med* 1988;318:1714–1719.
13. Baumgartner HR. Effects of acetyl salicylic acid, sulfinpyrazone and dipyridamole on platelet adhesion and aggregation in flowing native and anticoagulated blood. *Haemostasis* 1979;8:340–352.
14. Cairns JA, Gent M, Singer J, et al. Aspirin, sulfinpyrazone, or both in unstable angina. *N Engl J Med* 1985;313:1369–1375.
15. Schror K. The basic pharmacology of ticlopidine and clopidogrel. *Platelets* 1993;4:252–261.
16. Schror K. Ticlopidine and clopidogrel. In: Ferguson JJ, Chronos NAF,

Harrington RA, eds. *Antiplatelet therapy in clinical practice.* London: Martin Dunitz, 2000:93–113.

17. Ferguson JJ. Clopidogrel. In: Braunwald E, ed. *Harrison's advances in cardiology.* New York: McGraw-Hill, 2002:144–154.

18. Weber AA. Reimann S, Schror K. Specific inhibition of ADP-induced platelet aggregation by clopidogrel *in vitro. Br J Pharmacol* 1999;126:415–420.

19. Kupfer Y, Tessler S. Ticlopidine and thrombotic thrombocytopenic pupura. *N Engl J Med* 1997;337:1245.

20. Bennett CL, Connors JM, et al. Thrombotic thrombocytopenic purpura associated with clopidogrel. *N Engl J Med* 2000;342:1773–1777.

21. Pereillo JM, Maftouh M, Andrieu A, et al. Structure and stereochemistry of the active metabolite of clopidogrel. *Drug Metab Dispos* 2002;30:1288–1295.

22. Savi P, Pereillo JM, Uzbiaga MF, et al. Identification and biological activity of the active metabolite of clopidogrel. *Thromb Hemost* 2002;84:891–896.

23. Kohda N, Tani T, Nakayama S, et al. Effect of cilostazol, a phosphodiesterase III inhibitor, on experimental thrombosis in the porcine carotid artery. *Thromb Res* 1999;159:337–345.

24. Igawa T, Tani T, Chijiwa T, et al. Potentiation of anti-platelet aggregating activity of cilostazol with vascular endothelial cells. *Thromb Res* 1990;57:617–623.

25. Lefkovits J, Plow EF, Topol EJ. Platelet glygoprotein IIb/IIIa receptors in cardiovascular medicine. *N Engl J Med* 1995;332:1553–1559.

26. Simpfendorfer C, Kottke-Marchant K, Lowrie M, et al. First chronic platelet glycoprotein IIb/IIIa integrin blockade: a randomized, placebo-controlled pilot study of xemilofiban in unstable angina with percutaneous coronary interventions. *Circulation* 1997;96:76–81.

27. Kereiakes DJ, Runyon JP, Kleiman NS, et al. Differential dose response to oral xemilofiban after antecedent intravenous abciximab: administration for complex coronary intervention. *Circulation* 1996;94:906–910.

28. Cannon CP, McCabe CH, Borzak S, et al. Randomized trial of an oral platelet glycoprotein IIb/IIIa antagonist, sibrafiban, in patients after an acute coronary syndrome. *Circulation* 1998;97:340–349.

29. ORBIT Investigators. Pharmacodynamic efficacy, clinical safety, and outcomes after prolonged platelet glycoprotein IIb/IIIa receptor blockade with oral xemilofiban. *Circulation* 1998;98:1268–1278.

30. TIMI 12 Investigators. Randomized trial of an oral platelet glycoprotein IIb/IIIa antagonist, sibrafiban, in patients after an acute coronary syndrome. *Circulation* 1998;97:340–349.

31. Muller Thomas H, Weisenberger H, Brickl R, et al. Profound and sustained inhibition of platelet aggregation by fradafiban, a nonpeptide platelet glycoprotein IIb/IIIa antagonist, and its orally active prodrug, lefradafiban, in men. *Circulation* 1997;96:1130–1138.

32. Cannon CP, McCabe CH, Wilcox RG, et al. Oral glycoprotein IIb/IIIa inhibition with orbofiban in patients with unstable coronary syndromes (OPUS-TIMI 16) trial. *Circulation* 2000;102:149–156.

33. O'Neill WW, Serruys P, Knudtson M, et al. Long term treatment with a platelet glycoprotein-receptor antagonist after percutaneous coronary revascularization: evaluation of oral xemilofiban in controlling thrombotic events. EXCITE Trial Investigators. *N Engl J Med* 2000;342:1316–1324.

34. SYMPHONY Investigators. Comparison of sibrafiban with aspirin for prevention of cardiovascular events after acute coronary syndromes: a randomized trial: sibrafiban versus aspirin to yield maximum protection from ischemic heart events post acute coronary syndromes. *Lancet* 2000;335:337–345.

35. Second SYMPHONY Investigators. Randomized trial of aspirin, sibrafiban or both for secondary prevention after acute coronary syndromes. *Circulation* 2001;103:1727–1733.

36. Topol EJ, Easton DE, Harrington R, et al. Randomized, double-blind, placebo-controlled international trial of the oral IIb/IIIa antagonist lotrafiban in coronary and cerebrovascular disease. *Circulation* 2003;108:399–406.

37. Chew DP, Bhatt DL, Sapp S, et al. Increased mortality with oral platelet glycoprotein IIb/IIIa antagonists: a meta-analysis of phase III multicenter randomized trials. *Circulation* 2001;103:201–206.

38. Hirsh J. Heparin. *N Engl J Med* 1991;324:1565–1574.

39. Hirsh J, Warkentin TE, Raschke R, et al. Heparin and low molecular weight heparin: mechanisms of action, pharmacokinetics, dosing considerations, monitoring, efficacy, and safety. *Chest* 1998;114:489S–510S.

40. Hirsch J, Fuster V. Guide to anticoagulant therapy. Part I: heparin. *Circulation* 1994;89:1449–1468.

41. Hirsh J, Anand SS, Halperin JL, et al. Guide to anticoagulant therapy: heparin. *Circulation* 2001;103:2994–3018.

42. Becker PS, Miller VT. Heparin-induced thrombocytopenia. *Stroke* 1989;20:1449–1459.

43. Aster RH. Heparin-induced thrombocytopenia and thrombosis. *N Engl J Med* 1995;332:1374–1376.

44. Warkentin TE, Levine MN, Hirsh J, et al. Heparin-induced thrombocytopenia in patients treated with low-molecular-weight heparin or unfractionated heparin. *N Engl J Med* 1995;332:1330–1335.

45. Brieger DB, Mak KH, Kottke-Marchant K, et al. Heparin-induced thrombocytopenia. *J Am Coll Cardiol* 1998;31:1449–1459.

46. Fareed J, Hoppensteadt DA, Walenger JM. Current perspectives on low molecular weight heparins. *Semin Thromb Heamost* 1993;19 (Suppl 1):1–11.

47. Weitz J. Low-molecular-weight heparins. *N Engl J Med* 1997;337:688–698.

48. Young E, Wells P, Holloway S, et al. *Ex-vivo* and *in-vitro* evidence that low molecular weight heparins exhibit less binding to plasma proteins than unfractionated heparin. *Thromb Hemost* 1994;71:300–304.

49. Turpie AG. Pentasaccharides. *Semin Hematol* 2002;39:158–171.

50. Chew JW. Fondaparinux: a new antithrombotic agent. *Clin Ther* 2002;24:1757–1769.

51. Lefkovits J, Topol E. Direct thrombin inhibitors in cardiovascular medicine. *Circulation* 1994;90:1522–1536.

52. Becker RC, Cannon CP. Hirudin: its biology and clinical use. *J Thromb Thrombolysis* 1994;1:7–16.

53. The Direct Thrombin Inhibitor Trialists' Collaborative Group. Direct thrombin inhibitors in acute coronary syndromes: principal results of a meta-analysis based on individual patients' data. *Lancet* 2002;359:294–302.

54. Whitlon DS, Sadowski JA, Suttie JW. Mechanisms of coumarin action: significance of vitamin K epoxide reductase inhibition. *Biochemistry.* 1978;17:1371–1377.

55. Hirsh J, Fuster V, Ansell J, et al. AHA/ACC Foundation guide to warfarin therapy. *Circulation* 2003;107:1692–1711.

56. Popma JJ, Weitz J, Bittl JA, et al. Antithrombotic therapy in patients undergoing coronary intervention. *Am Heart J* 1999;137:250–257.

57. Kleiman NS. Putting heparin into perspective: its history and the evolution of its use during percutaneous coronary intervention. *J Invasive Cardiol* 2000;12[Suppl F]:20F–26F.

57a. Bhatt DL, Topal ES. Scientific and therapeutic advances in antiplatelet therapy. *Nat Rev Drug Discov* 2003;2:15–28.

58. Chen WH, Lau CP, Lau YK, et al. Stable and optimal anticoagulation is achieved with a single dose of intravenous enoxaparin in patients undergoing percutaneous coronary intervention. *J Invasive Cardiol* 2002;18:439–442.

59. Wong GC, Giugliano RP, Antman EM. Use of low molecular weight heparins in the management of acute coronary syndromes and percutaneous coronary intervention. *JAMA* 2003;289:331–342.

60. Kereiakes DJ, Grines C, Fry E, et al. Enoxaparin and abciximab adjunctive pharmacotherapy during percutaneous coronary intervention. *J Invasive Cardiol* 2001;13:272–278.

61. Kereiakes DJ, Montalescot G, Antman EM, et al. Low-molecular-weight heparin therapy for non-ST-elevation acute coronary syndromes and during percutaneous coronary intervention: an expert consensus. *Am Heart J* 2002;144:615–624.

62. Kadakia RA, Ferguson JJ. Use of enoxaparin in patients undergoing percutaneous coronary intervention. *Crit Pathways Cardiol* 2003;2:1–6.

63. Allie DE, Lirtzman MD, Wyatt CH, et al. Bivalirudin as a foundation anticoagulant in peripheral vascular disease: a safe and feasible alternative for renal and iliac interventions. *J Invasive Cardiol* 2003;15:334–342.

64. Bhatt DL. Heparin in peripheral vascular intervention—time for a change? *J Invasive Cardiol* 2003;15:249–250.

65. Shammas NW, Lemke JH, Dippel EJ, et al. In-hospital complications of peripheral vascular interventions using unfractionated heparin as the primaryanticoagulant. *J Invasive Cardiol* 2003;15:242–246.

66. Lincoff AM for the REPLACE-2 Investigators. The REPLACE-2 trial: bivalirudin and provisional GPIIb/IIIa blockade compared with heparin and planned GPIIb/IIIa blockade during percutaneous coronary intervention [Online Abstract]. *Circulation* 2002;106:2986-a.

67. Antiplatelet Trialists' Collaboration. Collaborative overview of randomized trials of antiplatelet therapy. I. Prevention of death, myocardial infarction, and stroke by prolonged antiplatelet therapy in various categories of patients. *BMJ* 1994;308:81–106.

68. Antiplatelet Trialists' Collaboration. Collaborative overview of randomized trials of antiplatelet therapy. II. Maintenance of vascular graft or arterial patency by antiplatelet therapy. *BMJ* 1994;308:159–68.

69. Antiplatelet Trialists' Collaboration. Collaborative overview of randomized trials of antiplatelet therapy. III. Reduction in venous thrombosis and pulmonary embolism by antiplatelet prophylaxis among surgical and medical patients. *BMJ* 1994;308:235–246.

70. Antithrombotic Trialists' Collaboration. Collaborative meta-analysis of randomized trials of antiplatelet therapy for prevention of death, myocardial infarction, and stroke in high risk patients. *BMJ* 2002;324:71–86.

71. Balsano F, Violi F, ADEP Group. Effects of picotamide on the clinical progression of peripheral vascular disease. A double-blind placebo-controlled study. *Circulation* 1993;87:1563–1569.

72. Taylor DW, Barnett HJM, Ferguson GG, et al. Low dose and high dose acetylsalicylic acid for patients undergoing carotid endarterectomy: a randomized controlled trial. *Lancet* 1999;353:2179–2184.

73. Diener HC, Cunha L, Forbes C, et al. European Stroke Prevention Study 2. Dipyridamole and acetylsalicylic acid in the secondary prevention of stroke. *J Neurol Sci* 1996;143:1–13.

74. Goldhaber SZ, Manson JE, Stampfer MJ, et al. Low-dose aspirin and subsequent peripheral artrial surgery in the Physicians' Health Study. *Lancet* 1992;340:143–145.

75. Physicians' Health Study Research Group. Final report on the aspirin component of the ongoing Physicians' Health Study. *N Engl J Med* 1989;321:129–135.

76. Ridker PM, Manson JE, Buring JE, et al. The effect of chronic platelet inhibition with low-dose aspirin on atherosclerotic progression and acute thrombosis: Clinical evidence from the Physicians' Health Study. *Am Heart J* 1991;122:1588–1592.

77. Gorelick PB, Richardson D, Kelly M, et al. Aspirin and ticlopidine for prevention of recurrent stroke in black patients: a randomized trial. *JAMA* 2003;289:2947–2957.

78. Gent M, Blakely JA, Easton JD, et al. The Canadian American Ticlopidine Study (CATS) in thromboembolic stroke. *Lancet* 1989;1:1215–1220.

79. Ticlopidine Aspirin Stroke Study Group. A randomized trial comparing ticlopidine hydrochloride with aspirin for the prevention of stroke in high-risk patients. *N Engl J Med* 1989;321:501–507.

80. Balsano F, Rizzon P, Violi F, et al. Antiplatelet treatment with ticlopidine in unstable angina: a controlled multicenter clinical trial. The Studio della Ticlopidina nell'Angina Instabile Group. *Circulation* 1990;82:17–26.

81. CAPRIE Steering Committee. A randomised, blinded trial of clopidogrel versus aspirin in patients at risk of ischemic events (CAPRIE). *Lancet* 1996;348:1329–1339.

82. Bhatt DL, Chew DP, Hirsch AT, et al. Superiority of clopidogrel versus aspirin in patients with prior cardiac surgery. *Circulation* 2001;103:363–368.

83. Bhatt DL, Marso SP, Hirsch AT, et al. Amplified benefit of clopidogrel versus apririn in patients with diabetes mellitus. *Am J Cardiol* 2002;90:625–628.

84. Ferguson JJ, Villareal RP, Massin EK. The effect of clopidogrel vs aspirin on recurrent clinical events and total vascular mortality: results from the CAPRIE study. *J Am Clin Cardiol* 2001;37[Suppl A]:336A.

85. CURE Study Investigators. Effects of clopidogrel in addition to aspirin in patients with non-ST segment elevation acute coronary syndromes. *N Engl J Med* 2001;345:494–502.

86. Mehta SR, Yusuf S, Peters RJG, et al. Efects of pretreatment with clopidogrel and aspirin followed by long-term therapy in patients undergoing percutaneous coronary interventions: the PCI-CURE study. *Lancet* 2001;358:527–533.

87. Steinhubl SR, Berger PB, Mann JT, et al. Early and sustained dual oral antiplatelet therapy following percutaneous coronary intervention: A randomized controlled trial. *JAMA* 2002;288:2411–2420.

88. The Medical Research Council's General Practice Research Framework. Thrombosis prevention trial: Randomised trial of low intensity oral anticoagulation with warfarin and low-dose aspirin in the primary prevention of ischaemic heart disease in men at increased risk. *Lancet* 1998;351:233–241.

89. Veterans Administration Cooperative Study. Anticoagulants in acute myocardial infarction: results of a cooperative clinical trial. *JAMA* 1973;225:724–729.

90. Medical Research Council Group. Assessment of short-term anticoagulant administration after cardiac infarction: Report of the Working Party on Anticoagulant Therapy in Coronary Thrombosis. *Br Med J* 1969;1:335–342.

91. Drapkin A. Merskey C. Anticoagulant therapy after acute myocardial infarction. *JAMA* 1972;222:541–548.

92. Cairns JA, Hirsh J, Lewis Jr. HD, et al. Antithrombotic agents in coronary artery disease. *Chest* 1992;102:456S–481S.

93. Goldberg RJ, Gore JM, Dalen JE, et al. Long term anticoagulant therapy after acute myocardial infarction. *Am Heart J* 1985;109:616–622.

94. Leizorovicz A, Boissel JP. Oral anticoagulant in patients surviving myocardial infarction. *Eur J Clin Pharmacol* 1983;24:333–336.

95. Chalmers TC, Matta RJ, Smith Jr. H, et al. Evidence favoring the use of anticoagulants in the hospital phase of acute myocardial infarction. *N Engl J Med* 1977;297:1091–1096.

96. Loeliger EA. Oral anticoagulation in patients surviving myocardial infarction: a new approach to old data. *Eur J Clin Pharmacol* 1984;26:137–141.

97. The Sixty Plus Reinfarction Study Research Group. A double-blind trial to assess long-term oral anticoagulant therapy in elderly patients after myocardial infarction. *Lancet* 1980;2:989–994.

98. Smith P, Arnesen H, Holme I. The effect of warfarin in mortality and reinfarction after myocardial infarction. *N Engl J Med* 1990;323:147–152.

99. ASPECT Research Group. Effect of long-term oral anticoagulant treatment on mortality and cardiovascular morbidity after myocardial infarction. *Lancet* 1994;343:499–503.

100. Ferguson JJ. Meeting highlights: highlights of the 22nd congress of the European Society of Cardiology. *Circulation* 2001;104:e41–e45.

101. Ferguson JJ. Meeting highlights: highlights of the XXIII congress of the European Society of Cardiology. *Circulation* 2001;104:e111–e116.

102. Coumadin Aspirin Reinfarction Study (CARS) Investigators. Randomised double-blind trial of fixed low-dose warfarin with aspirin after myocardial infarction. *Lancet* 1997;350:389–396.

103. Fiore LD, Ezekowitz MD, Brophy MT, et al. Departmentof Veterans Affairs Cooperative Program clinical trial comparing combined warfarin and aspirin with aspirin alone in survivors of acute myocardial infarction: primary results of the CHAMP study. *Circulation* 2002;105:557–563.

104. Anand S, Yusuf S. Oral anticoagulation in patients with coronary artery disease. *J Am Coll Cardiol* 2003;41:62S–69S.

105. Anand SS, Yusuf S, Pogue J, et al. Long-term oral anticoagulant therapy in patients with unstable angina or suspected non–Q-wave myocardial infarction: Organization to Assess Strategies for Ischemic Syndromes (OASIS) pilot study results. *Circulation* 1998;98:1064–1070.

106. Cohen M, Adams PC, Parry G, et al. Combination antithrombotic therapy in unstable rest angina and non–Q-wave infarction in nonprior aspirin users: primary end point analysis from the ATACS trial. *Circulation* 1994;89:81–88.

107. The Organization to Assess Strategies for Ischemic Syndromes (OASIS) Investigators. Effects of long-term, moderate-intensity oral anticoagulation in addition to aspirin in unstable angina. *J Am Coll Cardiol* 2001;37:475–484.

108. Chesney CM, Elam MB, Herd JA, et al. Effect of niacin, warfarin, and antioxidant therapy on coagulation parameters in patients with peripheral arterial disease in the Arterial Disease Multiple Intervention Trial (ADMIT). *Am Heart J* 2000;140:631–636.

109. Brieger DB, Mak KH, Kottke-Marchant K, et al. Heparin-induced thrombocytopenia. *J Am Coll Cardiol* 1998;31:1449–1459.

110. Amiral J, Bridey F, Wolf M, et al. Antibodies to macromolecular platelet factor 4–heparin complexes in heparin-induced thrombocytopenia: a study of 44 cases. *Thromb Haemost* 1995;73:21–28.

111. Warkentin TE, Levine MN, Hirsh J, et al. Heparin-induced thrombocytopenia in patients treated with low-molecular-weight heparin or unfractionated heparin. *N Engl J Med* 1995;332:1330–1335.

112. Lewis BE, Wallis DE, Berkowitz SD, et al. Argatroban anticoagulant therapy in patients with heparin-induced thrombocytopenia. *Circulation* 2001;103:1838–1843.

CHAPTER 15

Noninvasive Diagnosis of Peripheral Vascular Disease

Keith A. Mauney

Key Points

- Noninvasive peripheral vascular testing combines nearly equal measures of art and science. A detailed understanding of the nuances of available technologies and their limitations will ensure diagnostic accuracy and efficiency.
- Physiological peripheral vascular tests measure physical processes, but their output is framed in anatomic equivalents; anatomic imaging studies are often thought of in physiological terms. Data from either approach alone can be misleading.
- Peripheral arterial testing can be conducted at three levels of interrogation, but each level may require different combinations of tests. Limited testing may overlook processes that carry strategic impact; excessive and unnecessary testing will trigger resistance of another kind: political and regulatory. Cardiovascular noninvasive testing, with its enormous annual price tag, is now the most closely monitored and dynamically regulated field in health care, apart from ionizing-related technology.

OVERVIEW

Noninvasive peripheral vascular tests are among the most helpful tools available to the practitioner and are among the easiest to use. For the patient presenting with overt or suspected claudication, the initial workup can be accomplished in a single visit. Similarly, for the patient with nonspecific limb swelling and pain, consideration of large-vessel deep vein thrombosis can be dealt with as efficiently. Although originally developed and introduced by vascular surgeons, the technology can and has been mastered by physicians of nearly every specialty, and today its decreased cost has placed it within reach of anyone willing to commit to its proper use. Once considered the exclusive providence of the specialist, this technology has become the twenty-first century equivalent of the stethoscope, further extending the reach of the front-line clinician.

MISSION

Although it is referred to as a laboratory, the vascular testing center is anything but. It is both practical and efficient to think of the service as a unique paramedical consultation; it requires interplay between the participants to achieve maximum benefit. Any discussion of technical procedures would be misplaced without first defining the proper mission of this noninvasive vascular laboratory service. Much has been accomplished regarding the credentialing of professionals and facilities performing these tests, but the proper channeling of appropriate candidates for testing will remain the strategic focus of Medicare and everyone who follows its lead. The goal is a simple one, and it has defined the course that federal regulations governing it have taken over the decades:

1. Define the nature of the suspected vascular disorder.
2. Localize and classify any vascular diseases that might be found.
3. Conduct a physiological, functional analysis of the condition.
4. Define a program of treatment.

Consequent to this elementary algorithm, the ordering clinician must specify precisely in writing the disorder to be defined and the specific tests to be performed. In more obscure or complex cases, informal discussion of the case directly with the technical staff can significantly streamline decision making, originating at both ends. The vascular technologist brings to the bedside not only the usual specialized knowledge, but also vast clinical experience in the contextual aspects of vascular diagnosis. Both novice and experienced physicians have found this resource one to be carefully cultivated.

LOWER EXTREMITY ARTERIAL OCCLUSIVE DISEASE

Capillary perfusion requires a satisfactory pressure gradient between arteriolar inflow and venule outflow, a relationship affected by both arterial *and* venous pressure. In the event that this gradient falls too low, microcirculatory flow continues, but is rerouted through metarioles, with nonnutritive consequences. The differential diagnosis of ischemia therefore includes consideration of both arterial inflow pressure and venous outflow resistance.

LEG CLAUDICATION

The goal for the complete workup of the patient with suspected arterial insufficiency has three parts: prevent (or prescribe the most conservative approach to) limb loss, relieve activity-limiting symptoms, and strategically improve overall circulatory capacity. True claudication is a syndrome and is distinguished by four features: (a) the absence of symptoms at rest; (b) the onset of limb pain, tension, or other discomfort with a definable level of activity; (c) progression of severity to the point of intolerance, forcing the subject to stop; and (d) relief of symptoms after a period of rest. Inarticulate patients often paint a vague or misleading picture of their condition and physical findings may lead in several directions.

Differential diagnosis of arterial insufficiency can be established at three different levels of involvedness (arbitrarily defined here by level):

Level I: Ankle–brachial index
Level II: Complete segmental limb assessment
Level III: Physiological response provocation

An understanding of the precision technique and its acceptable variations is absolutely essential to interpreting and applying the test data.

Level I. The Ankle–Brachial Index

The ankle–brachial index (ABI) concept is simple: Systolic blood pressure at the ankle should be nearly equal to or higher than that of the arms. The increased resistance imposed by the greater length of passage to the legs creates a relatively higher systolic pressure even though cardiac output remains constant. In the normal, resting state, the ankle–brachial index should be greater than 0.90–0.95 (1–5); however, accu-

rate measurement depends on several factors, among them specialized equipment. For this reason, even a limited diagnostic inquiry must meet the same stringent standards as a full-blown workup. Pneumatic cuff artifact can induce significant error by two means: Cuff width is inappropriate or the length of the bladder is insufficient to encircle the ankle. In typical cases where a standard exam-room blood pressure cuff is used, ankle pressures may be underestimated. In addition, the physician may have experience with the portable Doppler stethoscope, often used on a vascular service. In spite of its versatility, this instrument may not meet federal standards of practice when submitting a claim for reimbursement; specialized direction-sensing instruments with hardcopy output must be used for formal documentation of disease. Fortunately, all the equipment discussed in this section is inexpensive, virtually indestructible, and simple to use.

The ABI is conducted with the patient at physical and psychological rest in an environment conducive to both. Ideally, the subject is positioned supine, but relevant measurement can be obtained in a semi-Fowler's or even sitting position provided that the final interpretation states the nonstandard condition. The objective is to measure the higher of two ankle pressures in the limb and compare it to the higher of the two arm pressures.* Ten- or 12-cm-wide cuffs are applied to the arms and ankles, for the latter at least 1 cm proximal to the malleolar prominence. The direction-sensing Doppler probe is hand held at an oblique angle over the interrogating artery distal to the cuff. This may be any suitable site for each brachial pressure, and specifically over the dorsalis pedis and posterior tibial artery for each ankle pressure. A lateral branch of the plantar arch (between the elevator ligaments for the fourth and fifth digits) may be substituted for an undetected dorsalis pedis, and the peroneal artery may be used in the event one of the tibial branches cannot be found. Once a reasonably strong signal is acquired, the cuff is inflated to suprasystolic pressure (obliterating the signal); cuff pressure is slowly bled and the signal reacquired at the level of systolic cuff pressure. Complicating what appears to be an easy task is the fact that diseased-vessel Doppler signals may be faint and can be masked in such cases by venous or collateral plantar arch flow. The determination of systolic pressure is rightfully made by the audible analysis of a skilled, experienced listener, but validated by an astute clinician.

Diabetic vessels may or may not undergo partial or complete segmental calcification, creating a potential for false elevation of pneumatically derived pressures. This elevation may be so extreme as to disappear beyond the upper end of the pressure scale (clearly indicating an invalid measurement), or it may be subtler, creating only a slight false elevation of

---

*Both the anterior and posterior tibial arteries normally supply the plantar arch; the peroneal branch does not normally contribute significant blood pressure to the foot. Because forefoot and digital arteries derive their pressures from the arch, the higher inflow pressure of either inflow vessel at the ankle is appropriate for use. Separately, with regard to the arms, the two brachial pressures may be unequal, but should never reflect a higher cardiac pressure gradient than did actually exist.

TABLE 15.1. *Criteria for ankle–brachial index (ABI) analysis*

ABI	Technical analysis[a]
>0.90–0.95	No resting evidence of peripheral arterial occlusive disease
(0.95–0.90)–0.50	Probable single-level lower extremity arterial occlusive disease
<0.50	Probable multilevel lower extremity arterial occlusive disease

[a]The terms no resting evidence and single- or multilevel arterial occlusive disease historically imply the presence of a pressure-reducing effect somewhere proximal to the site of detection (6–9). In the forging of this terminology, ABI results were compared to long-leg arteriography: Films showing predominantly a single site of high-grade obstruction correlated strongly with moderately reduced ankle–brachial ratios. The concept of high-grade obstruction has commonly been referred to as *hemodynamically significant,* and it is still considered by many to apply to any vascular diameter reduction of >70%–80%. Such a lesion would produce a perfusion-threatening pressure drop downstream, thus triggering some interventive response. However, the term indirectly creates the expectation of the finding of a single-site, high-grade obstruction when in fact no single lesion exists. Likewise, a significant pressure drop in the principal vessel does not necessarily draw a short, straight line from the patient to invasive intervention: Collateral flow may satisfactorily reconstitute pressure to maintain perfusion in many sedentary individuals for the rest of their life. Distal vascular pressure can also drop secondary to the cumulative effects of lesser degrees of stenosis in series, and changes in cardiac output can alter the microvascular consequence of either type of pattern, including lesser degrees of obstruction. Differentiation of focal versus tandem lesion effects becomes important when deciding among treatments: angioplasty, bypass, and/or exercise rehabilitation. For these reasons, it is preferred that use of the term hemodynamically singnificant be clarified whenever used. Noninvasive test results should report objective findings as detected and avoid the general use of the clinically ambiguous term.

pressure. Any leg pressures obtained from diabetic patients, regardless of numeric value, should be considered illegitimate. In such cases, other, less inconsistent tests such as Doppler waveform analysis, toe pressures, and volume plethysmography should be used; each will be discussed separately within this section.

Once the resting ABI data have been evaluated for credibility, technical results can be classified as shown in Table 15.1.

Before declaration of a final report, the ABI ratio must be correlated with analysis of the Doppler arterial waveforms used to obtain pressures. Normal peripheral arterial Doppler waveforms demonstrate a tri- or biphasic pattern (Fig. 15.1). In such cases, there is abundant pressure, creating a rapid systolic acceleration curve, which is quickly detained by the usually high level of distal vascular resistance. The secondary diastolic reversal is derived from the considerable reserve of blood pressure, which propels the arrested blood slightly backward, toward the low-resistance renal and visceral circulation. In the case of a distensible artery, early

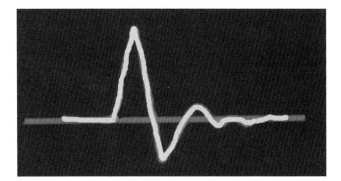

FIG. 15.1. Normal triphasic Doppler waveform.

diastolic recoil of the distended perimeter provides a gentle pressure boost, which may generate enough force to mount late forward movement and thus a third distinct component. Either tri- or biphasic arterial waveforms are considered unremarkable at rest (although the suggestion of decreased vascular compliance may be noted in the case of the latter; its clinical significance is anecdotal). A monophasic waveform (Fig. 15.2) predicts a pressure-reducing phenomenon at or proximal to the site of detection. The overtly changed features (prolonged acceleration/deceleration slopes and absence of diastolic components) are accounted for by the deprivation of pressure energy, depleted at one or more proximal sites of stenosis. It is important to remember that degradation of pressure energy occurs to some degree at every site of vessel narrowing, and a single large-scale event or multiple smaller ones can produce that significant poverty. The Doppler waveform degrades to its monophasic state at or distal to the site of the most proximal significant pressure depletion. Further broadening of the waveform with or without persistent elevation above the zero baseline suggests an increasingly severe degree of stenosis, or occlusion. There are, however, no objective, reproducible data to permit its distinct stratification.

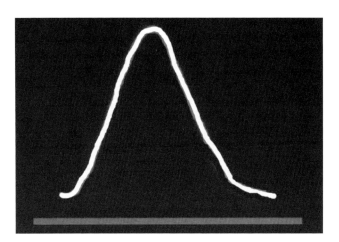

FIG. 15.2. Dampened, or monophasic, Doppler waveform, compatible with a pressure-reducing phenomenon at or anywhere proximal to its site of detection.

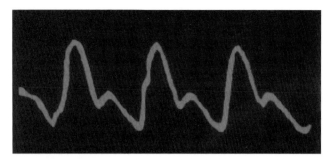

FIG. 15.3. Normal pulse volume recording waveform; note the evident dicrotic notch.

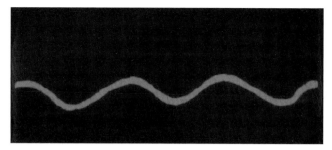

FIG. 15.5. Occlusive pulse volume recording waveform.

The two elements of the ABI test battery reinforce each other with objective pressure and physiological flow data at the ankle, either excluding or paving the way for further non-invasive studies to localize problems to better plan care. However, there are two remaining problems. First is the credibility issue attached to blood pressures from the diabetic patient. Second is the fact that the ABI provides reference only to blood flow to the ankle; its value in predicting nutritive flow through the foot to the toes is random. The vascular laboratory's respective answers to these problems are ankle volume plethysmography and the measurement of systolic toe blood pressure.

Volume plethysmography (also referred to as pulse volume recording [PVR] or pressure cuff recording [PCR]) is a tool as simple to describe as it is difficult to pronounce. The test is based on the fact that blood is essentially incompressible. Therefore, when a given stroke volume of blood enters the systemic arterial tree, the pressure shock wave creates a nearly identical time–volume displacement curve throughout the entire vessel. This curve closely approximates the intraarterial pressure trace derived by invasive means (Fig. 15.3). Studies comparing pulse volume waveforms to long-leg arteriography have shown a favorable correlation of the dicrotic (double beat) notch to vessels absent more than 70%- to 80%-diameter stenosis (10,11). Likewise, the

dicrotic notch appears to disappear at the location along the leg where systolic pressure begins to significantly drop (Fig. 15.4). Like the Doppler waveform, once the notch is lost it is not recovered at any distal site. Much conflicting data have been produced over the decades regarding the value of other features of the additionally degraded volume pulse waveform (Figs. 15.5 and 15.6). Detailed discussion of the suggested stratification of disease by these means is beyond the scope of this work. In essence, a volume pulse waveform with a notch (however indiscernible) implies the absence of pressure-reducing stenosis; absence of the notch in a nonobese limb, however, strongly supports it.

In the actual test procedure, a pneumatic cuff is placed to encircle the entire limb at a designated segment and is then inflated to supravenous pressure (approximately 55 mm Hg). The force of blood within *all* arterial vessels beneath the cuff creates a transient spike in cuff air pressure over time. The momentary changes are measured by an air pressure transducer, which outputs a signal to a display device and strip chart recorder for analysis. This test differs significantly from the ankle pressure measurement method in two very important ways. With volume plethysmography, the character of *both* the primary vessel *and* collateral flow channels can be studied; Doppler-assisted pressure measurement reports only the vessel studied. Likewise, the influence of diabetic vessel calcification is wasted on volume plethysmography; blood flow that might be slightly restricted by stiff vessel walls

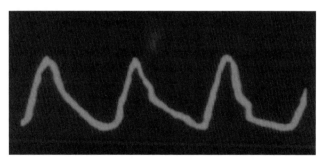

FIG. 15.4. Stenotic pulse volume recording waveform. A clear notch is absent, but the waveform contour is still narrow. This finding may be explained by a low signal-to-noise ratio, a special problem with large limbs. Substantiation of this finding with Doppler and pressure data is strongly recommended.

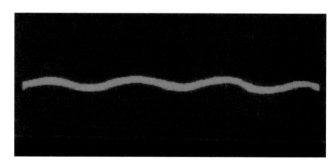

FIG. 15.6. Absent pulse volume recording waveform; further degradation of the waveform likely parallels the physiological basis seen in the Doppler waveform, but the specific categorization of severity remains anecdotal.

is theoretically rerouted through collateral vessels with no effect on the overall volume flow profile over time. However, as impressive as its credentials sound, the practical limitation of arterial plethysmography is its complete subjectivity and limited sensitivity in obese limbs.

Toe blood pressure is the last and most often overlooked element of the leg arterial study. Many clinicians consider the data important only in the context of wound healing and therefore do not include them as part of the arterial test battery. Neither the national consensus of vascular surgeons nor Medicare agrees with this posture. The former recommends that toe pressure data be included as a part of every arterial exam (limited or complete), and the latter requires documentation of it as part of the basis for reimbursement. Ankle pressure measurements stop at the ankle and may be artificially elevated in the diabetic subject. The digital arteries appear to be among the last to calcify in these individuals and may thus be the only credible witnesses to document the fact and severity of peripheral atherosclerosis (2,3,7,8, 12–32).

The arteries of the toes are the most remote from the heart and thus suffer the cumulative consequences of virtually every sort and site of vascular resistance. A drop in precapillary perfusion pressure to less than 30 to 40 mm Hg will lead to metarteriolar shunting and nonnutritive flow. Trophic cutaneous change, especially thinning of the epidermis, often precedes frank necrosis by years, increasing susceptibility to otherwise innocent injury and/or leading to direct ulceration. Although it is true most foot ulcers are largely venous in origin, arterial inflow must be evaluated carefully as part of the initial workup for wound care.

Various testing centers have proposed different methods for distal limb perfusion assessment, including forefoot pressure measurement, toe–ankle indices, and even toe–brachial indices. Measurement of cutaneous blood flow using xenon-133 clearance times, transcutaneous oxygen partial pressure measurement, and even laser Doppler velocimetry have been described, but none share the endorsement accorded to direct toe pressure measurement by the American and European vascular community.

The process requires a special pneumatic cuff (ranging from 1.5 to 5 cm wide) whose bladder is long enough to encircle the entire digit. An infrared-emitting/sensing diode is attached lightly to the skin and is used solely as a pulse detector, similar to the role of the Doppler probe in limb pressures. Infrared light penetrates the subcutaneous bed and is unaffected by skin color, thickness, or maceration. Its sensitivity to low-flow states is remarkable, allowing credible measurements even in extremely low flow states. The only special technical consideration meriting caution is undetectable cutaneous flow secondary to vasoconstriction in an excessively cool environment. This may be of more than casual concern if the procedure is being performed in the usually frosty radiology department.

Only a single digit need be measured to yield a credible estimate of plantar arch inflow pressure unless there is evidence of digital artery occlusion. Studies worldwide have shown that local wound healing is likely to fail when digital artery systolic pressure falls below 40 to 50 mm Hg in nondiabetic individuals. Diabetic patients appear to require a digital systolic pressure of 50–60 mm Hg or greater to support local tissue healing.

These data offer unique, powerful, and convincing information to help predict the healing potential of the patient with dry digital gangrene or the candidate for forefoot versus below-knee amputation (2,12,13,15,17,18,24,28,30, 33–35) (Table 15.2).

Level II. Complete Segmental Limb Assessment

The individual test elements already described can be used in combination to isolate significant limb pressure gradients to specific functional compartments. The physiological picture created in *this* process foretells the likely anatomic image

TABLE 15.2. *Criteria for toe blood pressure analysis*

	Digital systolic pressure (mm Hg)	Technical analysis
Nondiabetic patient	>40–50	Digital pressure probably adequate to support local tissue healing (in this nondiabetic patient)[a]
	<40–50	Digital pressure probably inadequate to support local tissue healing (in this nondiabetic patient)
Diabetic patient	>50–60	Digital pressure probably adequate to support local tissue healing (in this diabetic patient)
	<50–60	Digital pressure probably inadequate to support local tissue healing (in this diabetic patient)

[a]It is recommended that this parenthetical language be included in any final report to indicate the current assumption regarding the patient's diabetic state.

TABLE 15.3. *Analysis of segmental limb pressures*

Cuff site	Significance of gradient		Cuff site
Ankle (1 cm above the malleolar head) Below knee (1 cm below the patella)	>30-mm Hg gradient: distal limb obstruction	>30-mm Hg gradient: popliteal level obstruction	Ankle (1 cm above the malleolar head) Below knee (1 cm below the patella)
Above knee (1 cm above the patella)	>30-mm Hg gradient: superficial femoral artery obstruction		Above knee (1 cm above the patella)
High thigh (at the upper margin of the leg) Higher arm pressure		<30-mm Hg *above* the higher recorded pressure of both arm pressures: ileofemoral arterial obstruction[a]	High thigh (at the upper margin of the leg) Higher arm pressure

[a]These criteria apply to use of 10-cm-wide cuffs below the knee, 12-cm-wide cuffs above it. Obese patients may require a 30- to 40-cm-wide cuff for thigh pressure measurement; in this case, the thigh–arm gradient is significant if the thigh pressure is >30 mm Hg *below* the higher arm pressure. Regardless of cuff widths used, bilateral thigh–arm pressure gradients cannot differentiate bilateral ileofemoral from aortoiliac arterial occlusive disease.

that may later appear on the arteriogram, thus permitting accurate and conservative management of the patient early in the course of disease. It also assists in translating the terms *good, fair,* and *poor, or one-, two-,* and *three-vessel runoff below the knee,* into a more objective physiological term, a fact of great benefit when contemplating whether and where to amputate.

The ankle–brachial examination is now extended: Blood pressure cuffs are positioned at four limb sites (Table 15.3). Cuff-to-cuff gradients in excess of 30 mm Hg predict significant pressure loss at the site of detection; only adjacent cuffs on the same leg are examined cross-limb comparisons at the same cuff level are not considered. Special consideration is given to the relationship between the thigh and the higher arm pressure. Additionally, bilateral brachial pressures are compared: A gradient in excess of 30 mm Hg is compatible with a subclavian or brachiocephalic pressure-reducing stenosis (Table 15.3).

As with the ABI, Doppler waveforms are obtained to substantiate pressure measurement data. Optimal signals are documented at both tibial sites and popliteal, superficial femoral, and common femoral sites. Monophasic transition at any level is compatible with detection of a pressure-reducing process at that site. Doppler and segmental pressure data occasionally conflict, due most often to cuff artifact with the latter, particularly in obese patients. In these cases, the Doppler waveform is accorded the greater credibility. Diabetic subjects may also require substitution of segmental pressure data with volume plethysmography waveforms. In every case, toe systolic pressure should be obtained.

Level III. Physiological Response Provocation

The resting study can be augmented when necessary through active or reactive hyperemia testing. In either case, arterio-

lar dilation is achieved to lower vascular resistance; during this state there is a natural lowering of limb blood pressure. The fundamental objective purpose of the test is to monitor the postprocedure time to recovery. Ankle–brachial indices are recorded at rest and immediately posthyperemia, then at 5-minute intervals thereafter. A normal individual will recover to 95% of the resting ABI within 1 minute; patients with pressure-reducing processes require longer, the recovery time loosely related to the magnitude of flow deprivation. Measurements are repeated until the ABI has recovered to at least 80% of its baseline value.

Active hyperemia requires physical exercise of the legs to create a local oxygen deficit. The subject usually walks on a treadmill at a comfortable (and individually prescribed) workload, usually against an increasing incline. A treadmill is unnecessary, of course, provided the subject is exercised to the point of maximum limb tolerance. Regardless of how it is achieved, active participation of the entire cardiovascular/pulmonary system is preferred, as a complete functional picture can be gleaned. It permits validation of cause and effect in spurious symptomatic individuals, and can also document maximum limb tolerance (for serial comparison in exercise rehabilitation patients). One potentially significant drawback is the induction of myocardial ischemia or rhythm disturbances in subjects with covert coronary artery disease. Although no formal consensus has been established regarding cardiac monitoring and staff qualifications for low-impact exercise testing, the medical/legal risk remains.

Reactive hyperemia offers a suitable alternative to exercise, provoking an identical pressure drop by differing means. The physiologic mechanism of response differs from the cumulative vasoactive metabolic process: In the presence of decreased wall tension, the smooth muscle of the arteriolar walls relaxes immediately, in proportion to the drop in pressure. In this case, baseline ABI data are properly recorded

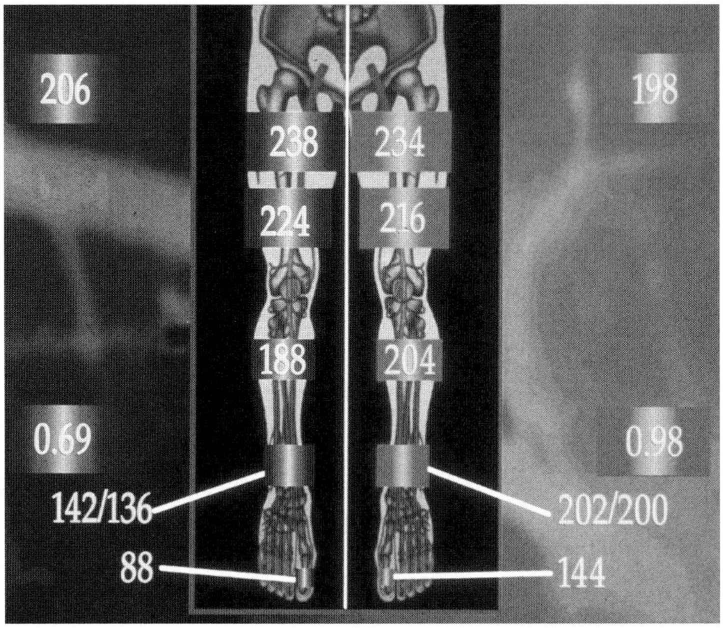

FIG. 15.7. Case data: resting segmental pressures.

and limb pressure is then dropped to zero by an occlusive cuff placed on the high thigh for a period of 3 to 5 minutes. The cuff is released, and then staged postocclusive ABI ratios are acquired. Results are interpreted in the same manner as with exercise testing.

Today most centers performing hyperemia studies use active hyperemia for functional classification pre- or postintervention or to differentiate neurogenic from ischemic vascular symptoms.

Case Example

A 71-year-old white women presents with bilateral right greater than left leg cramping at night and when walking through her house. She is nondiabetic with history of uncontrolled hypertension for 10 years; she quit smoking 10 years ago (Fig. 15.7). Pressure data in this nondiabetic subject should be credible. Resting systolic arterial pressures are shown as acquired from each level (arms at upper corners, dorsalis pedis/posterior tibial measurements at each ankle). ABI values appear in inset boxes at each ankle. No significant brachial gradient is noted. The right ABI suggests single-level arterial obstruction; the left ABI is normal in this resting state. A significant pressure gradient is detected between the right above-knee and below-knee cuffs, compatible with popliteal arterial occlusive disease. Digit pressures appear probably adequate to support local healing bilaterally (Fig. 15.8). Doppler waveform analysis is credible in diabetic and nondiabetic individuals but reveals only information from the vessel studied; indirect assessment of collateral potential cannot be objectively inferred with this technique in the resting state. Triphasic or biphasic waveforms indicate normal resting limb hemodynamics. Monophasic transition is noted

at the right popliteal level, again compatible with popliteal arterial obstruction.

Least accurate of all as a stand-alone procedure, volume pulse waveforms may play a contributory role in the clarification of conflicting pressure data, particularly in diabetics (Fig. 15.9). Their predictive value in excluding pressure-reducing lesions far exceeds their accuracy in detecting them. Absence of a dicrotic notch implies the presence of obstructive disease, but credibility is dubious in the presence of obesity. The notch is absent at the right ankle and both sites below the left knee. The conflict these findings present is superceded by the Doppler and pressure findings, both considered more reproducibly credible in nondiabetic cases. In any event, the findings of toe systolic pressures in excess of levels required for local tissue healing indicate no immediate threat to resting tissue perfusion.

Conclusions. 1. Probable right popliteal arterial occlusive disease. 2. Digit pressures probably adequate to support local tissue healing, bilaterally. 3. Further clarification of functional capacity and elucidation of collateral potential could be gathered by active or reactive hyperemia testing.

Summary

The clinical workup of lower limb ischemia involves a series of analytical processes, each with different degrees of objectivity. The noninvasive differential diagnosis differs depending on the specific questions to be answered; therefore, informal consultation with the vascular laboratory staff on complex or bewildering cases will often bring more productive results than blind ordering of tests. The vascular technologist inevitably spends more time with the patient in a more relaxed environment, conducive to communication, and may uncover symptoms or factors unexplored by the busy

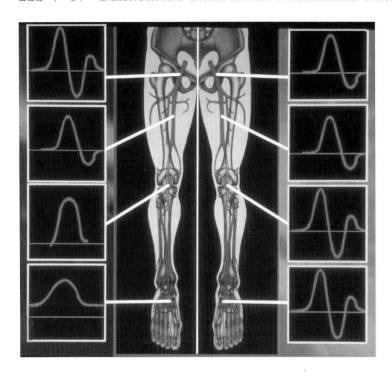

FIG. 15.8. Case Data: resting Doppler waveforms.

physician. Though the protocols described in Table 15.4 represent minimum documentation standards for the complete exam, it is wise to develop a close working relationship with the technical laboratory staff to allow expansion of the process when indicated. Especially important in this regard is the potential use and role of duplex ultrasound imaging.

DUPLEX ARTERIAL IMAGING

High-resolution ultrasound imaging of carotid vessels first appeared in 1978; Doppler technology was integrated into the instrument a year later, thus creating the term used today. Though the concept of direct noninvasive vascular imaging is enticing and the pictures produced from color Doppler display are engaging, duplex ultrasound is limited in its contribution. Its role is complementary to physiological testing and in many cases it may provide an additional unique perspective.

Imaging alone produces a limited and static picture. Atherosclerosis in the legs is a diffuse process: For every atherosclerotic plaque that can be seen and measured, there are many others whose physiological effects can be neither

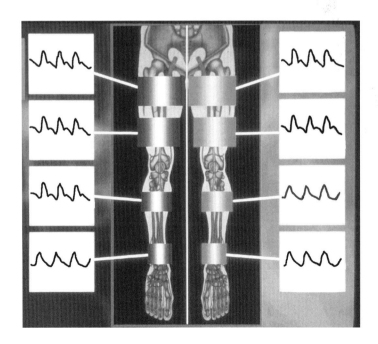

FIG. 15.9. Case data: resting pulse volume waveforms.

TABLE 15.4. *Noninvasive physiological test battery protocol*

Vascular history/physical exam? *Nondiabetic*
?
Segmental limb pressures and/or
volume plethysmography
?
Doppler waveforms
?
Toe pressures
?
(*Elective*)
Active hyperemia or reactive hyperemia

Vascular history/physical exam? *Diabetic*
?
Volume plethysmography
?
Doppler waveforms
?
Toe pressure
?
(*Elective*)
Active hyperemia or reactive hyperemia

quantified nor ignored. Imaging resolution is spectacular in optimal circumstances, but practically limited or noncontributory in most others. Achromatic (gray-scale) Doppler waveform analysis is conducted in the same manner as previously described. Color Doppler adds only subjective information, which may serve to narrow the anatomic survey for focal high-grade stenosis (Fig. 15.10). None of these elements is genuinely unique in the diagnostic process, but special use of

them may elucidate findings derived by physiological means. The one piece of flow data that duplex imaging alone can provide, however, is the ability to estimate actual blood velocity at nearly any location in the leg (Fig. 15.11). This can be quite powerful in the serial follow-up of bypass and stent procedures. Apart from this, the multimedia display can be helpful in the diagnosis and management of false aneurysm, arteriovenous fistula, popliteal or other aneurysm, Baker's cyst, and even abscess. A summary of potential uses is listed in Table 15.5.

A summary of technical findings and specific report language for all of the procedures described is presented in Table 15.6.

EVALUATION OF PELVIC ARTERIAL INSUFFICIENCY: ERECTILE DYSFUNCTION

The process of erection involves a host of interactive factors, only one of which is arterial supply. However, for many patients presenting with proximal limb arterial occlusive disease (and for many more without it), the finding of erectile impotence is common. A combination of physiological and duplex technology may offer some diagnostic clues in these cases.

The penile–brachial index (PBI) is simple, reasonably objective, and can be performed quickly and unobtrusively with no special preparation. It may often be conducted as an extension of the Level II or Level III arterial examination where aortoiliac or ileofemoral involvement is suspected.

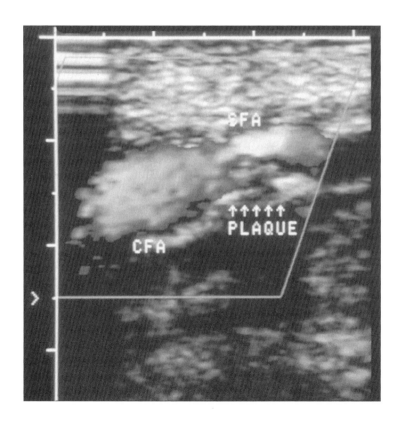

FIG. 15.10. Color Doppler at a nonstenotic site. In this case, physical narrowing of the vessel is easily seen; no turbulence is noted in the color display. This finding alone may be misleading: It requires correlation with flow velocity data to confirm waveform and velocity identity.

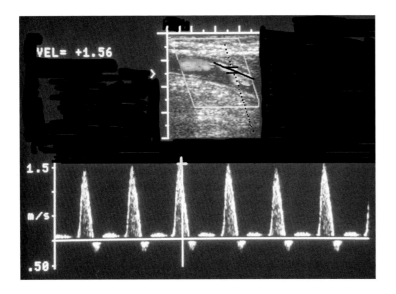

FIG. 15.11. Doppler duplex at stenosis. The unique contribution afforded is the ability to detect *focal* high-grade stenosis (greater than 70% to 80%-diameter loss). The effect of tandem lesions proximal to the site of sampling, each of which is insufficient by it-self to produce detectable flow acceleration, may reveal damping of the Doppler waveform at the point of pressure reduction.

Interrogation of the internal iliac distribution is relevant because these vessels can be stented, achieving a more natural solution than might be prescribed otherwise. A special blood pressure cuff is used, long enough to encircle the entire shaft and thus compress all four penile arteries simultaneously. An infrared cutaneous flow sensor is attached to the skin distally and resting systolic pressure is recorded. Ankle–brachial index data are also obtained for corroboration. Normal values for the PBI were originally derived from men less than 40 years of age and are shown in Table 15.7 (7,11,14,31,35–48). These criteria dif-

fer from the ABI in that the penis lies closer to the heart than the ankles: the less the distance traveled by blood, the less is the resistance and thus the lower is the systolic pressure.

The positive threshold criterion for older patients (presumably greater than or equal to 70 years) may be lower than stated here. Although published data are largely contradictory, informal consensus of the vascular community suggests that a PBI of as low as 0.5 to 0.55 may still be regarded as normal. There is additional information available on these select cases, particularly if the erection is incomplete or unsustained

TABLE 15.5. *Uses of duplex ultrasound imaging in arterial occlusive disease*

Identify focal high-grade stenosis in native, bypassed, or stented vessels	Color Doppler mapping of the entire vessel segment may reveal turbulence in the otherwise laminar-flow vessel; focal doubling of peak systolic velocity is evident
Survey for intermediate-level obstruction (>50%–70%-diameter stenosis)	Color Doppler reveals turbulence, but focal systolic velocity does not double
False aneurysm and abscess	An ectopic collection of clotted/liquid blood is seen adjacent to an artery; color Doppler reveals a systolic jet, agitating the extravascular contents; differential diagnosis is abscess; clinical correlation required
Arteriovenous fistula	Direct color Doppler mapping of the vessel shows arteriovenous communication at the involved site; achromatic Doppler demonstrates low arterial resistance proximal to the fistula, normal high resistance distal to it; Doppler patterns in the vein are normal distal to the fistula and become dramatically high velocity and pulsatile proximal to it
Popliteal or other aneurysm	Focal dilation of the affected vessel is confirmed by imaging; the intact vessel wall perimeter can be identified
Baker's cyst	Extravasated synovial fluid can be imaged in the region of the bursal head (which may even displace the location of the popliteal vessels); achromatic Doppler waveform analysis may reveal a monophasic waveform with extreme leg extension
Popliteal entrapment	The achromatic Doppler waveform may undergo positional monophasic transition with protracted leg extension; color Doppler may reveal turbulence in the same state

TABLE 15.6. Protocol for reporting non-duplex peripheral arterial testing

Report text	Doppler waveform analysis	Volume plethysmography (pulse volume recording, pressure cuff recording)	Segmental limb pressures	Toe pressures	Duplex arterial assessment
Normal: No resting evidence of (pressure-reducing) arterial occlusive disease, bilaterally	Doppler arterial waveforms may be either bi- or triphasic	Waveforms will demonstrate the presence (however scant) of a discernible dicrotic notch	The ABI will be normal; there is no evidence of a >30-mm Hg pressure gradient between ipsilateral adjacent cuffs; the high thigh pressure is ≥30 mm Hg greater than the higher arm pressure	In nondiabetics, the toe pressure will be at least 50 mm Hg; in diabetics, it will be >60 mm Hg	Normal: (Study is described as complete or incomplete, specifying any segments not clearly evident.) No evidence of flow-accelerating arterial stenosis compatible with >70% diameter stenosis; Doppler waveform analysis at each principal site is unremarkable; conclusion: no resting evidence of pressure-reducing arterial stenosis in accessible sites
Abnormal: (Right leg/left leg): Probable (left/right)/ileofemoral/ common femoral, femoropopliteal, popliteal, tibial/distal limb) arterial occlusive disease. If there are findings compatible with bilateral ileofemoral arterial involvement, they may also be described as possible aortoiliac arterial occlusive disease, though the findings cannot distinguish the two	The Doppler waveform will be monophasic at the most proximal site of pressure-reducing arterial occlusive disease; it will not recover; further degradation of the waveform may occur at additional sites of stenosis, but objective evidence does not exist	The volume pulse waveform will lose its notch at the most proximal site of pressure-reducing arterial occlusive disease; however, the notch may be missing in the absence of stenosis; the most likely cause is large limb girth; it is also possible that stenosis of as little as 60% diameter loss can produce a positive finding, particularly in the presence of low cardiac output	The ankle–brachial index will be abnormal, indicating either single- or multilevel arterial occlusive disease; There will be a >30-mm Hg pressure gradient between one or more pairs of ipsilateral adjacent cuffs; the high thigh pressure (if measured with the standard-width cuff) may be <30 mm Hg higher than the higher of the two arm cuffs (indicating likely ileofemoral vs. common femoral arterial occlusive disease	In nondiabetics, the toe pressure will be <50 mm Hg; in diabetics, it will be <60 mm Hg	Abnormal: Flow acceleration is detected at (specify location) compatible with >70% focal diameter stenosis Doppler waveforms may be abnormal in the absence of detected focal disease. If so, monophasic transition of the Doppler waveform at the (specify level) is compatible with pressure-reducing stenosis at this site; additional, more distal processes cannot be excluded by this test

TABLE 15.7. *The penile–brachial index*

>0.6–0.65	No resting evidence of pelvic arterial insufficiency to account for erectile dysfunction
<0.6–0.65	Probable pelvic arterial inflow insufficiency

during the physical activity of intercourse. In such cases, the patient may have a penile venous leak, permitting loss of corpus cavernosal blood volume. This volume loss may or may not be adequately resupplied from the internal iliac system at rest. In the case where turgidity is maintained satisfactorily in the quiescent state, but lost under strenuous activity, a pelvic arterial steal circumstance may be the cause. Active or reactive hyperemia provocation of the limbs creates a similar physiological circumstance and may uncover a likely, albeit indirect source of the problem. The ABI and PBI are both acquired with the legs in resting and posthyperemic states. Normal potent individuals should demonstrate a hyperemic response, increasing penile pressures by approximately 20%. Impotent individuals demonstrate no increase, or even a decrease in penile pressure by at least 15% (35,49,50).

LOWER EXTREMITY VENOUS ASSESSMENT

Duplex ultrasound imaging is ideally suited for deep vein imaging of the legs. It is portable, fast, and usually credible in the deep vessels from thigh to knee. In the evaluation of deep vein thrombosis (DVT), the diagnostic premise is straightforward: the deep vein is imaged in a transverse plane and is normally seen to collapse as transient surface pressure is applied to it with the ultrasound probe. Diagnostic criteria can be reduced to this single statement: Patent vessels collapse completely; veins with clot do not. In theory, visualization of clot should be the ideal standard; in practice, ultrasound is blessed to be able to produce any image from the deep vessel in the swollen or obese leg. For decades, studies have equated the accuracy of duplex ultrasound to venography in the veins between the inguinal ligament and the knee. Both tests appear to be equally inaccurate (± 50% sensitivity and specificity) in the calf. Regardless of the accepted accuracy of ultrasound, the standard vascular laboratory examination typically stops at the thigh. In cases where the study is extended into the pelvis and even the inferior vena cava, images are often uninterpretable or inconclusive. If possible, however, the examination should include all of the IVC, even above the diaphragm.

There are more challenges: previously established DVT cannot be absolutely differentiated from acute DVT, particularly when the latter involves a recanaluted vein. In spite of these shortcomings, duplex imaging remains a valuable tool for elucidating marginal symptoms or signs of DVT and is absolutely essential in the documentation of deep vein valve incompetence, especially in the complete workup of wound-healing potential.

VENOUS IMAGING

Venous imaging comprises two parts. First, the deep veins of the leg are imaged (and compressed) at approximately 2- to 3-cm intervals, beginning at the inguinal ligament and usually terminating at the thigh. The technologist records images in the resting and compressed states at no less than three sites in the thigh and separately at the popliteal vein. The three paired deep veins of the calf may or may not be interrogated depending on the institutional protocol; many laboratories elect to document only the posterior tibial veins (often the only credible images seen), if attempted at all. There may be renewed interest in calf vein assessment because recent multicenter data have shown that long-term, low-dose coumadin therapy significantly reduces the risk of pulmonary embolus in patients with prior DVT (51). Unfortunately, no technological breakthroughs in ultrasound imaging appear on the horizon to make diagnosis in the calf any simpler.

Deep vein valve incompetence is another matter. Doppler ultrasound does not depend on the high levels of signal-to-noise ratio that imaging requires to produce credible data. This procedure is performed as a second part of the duplex venous examination (and is required by Medicare to be documented for reimbursement). Four sites are tested: posterior tibial vein, popliteal, superficial femoral, and common femoral. An image of the vessel confirms the identity of the vessel studied. The character and direction of venous flow are documented during separate compression maneuvers, distal and proximal to the site interrogated. Normally (in the absence of outflow obstruction), compression *distal* to a site causes venous velocity to increase. The magnitude of change is variable from person to person, but its response should be approximately symmetric with the same site on the opposite (and theoretically unaffected) limb. Proximal site compression is clinically more instructive: the back pressure produced in this maneuver should close the unidirectional bicuspid valves of the vein, arresting completely all venous flow. Incompetent veins permit augmented velocity in the reverse direction, a fact easily detected by either achromatic or color Doppler. In the event that flow signals are inconclusive due to extremely deep vessels, direction-sensing continuous-wave Doppler can be substituted. Its higher transmitted power and superior sensitivity atone for the fact that no image can be simultaneously acquired.

Venous Doppler findings are reported as a technical summary. Augmentation findings are regarded as subjective because complex flow patterns with collateral venous flow typically obfuscate any rational conclusion. Deep vein valve incompetence is reported as present or absent at each of the sites tested.

Although national standards are proposed and encouraged through the Intersocietal Commission for Vascular

TABLE 15.8. *Venous imaging and data analysis/report protocol*[a]

Protocol	Technical comments
Step 1: Longitudinal survey	
Survey the vessel longitudinally from inguinal ligament to knee to rule out any evidence of partial or complete DVT in the large veins	Surface compression could dislodge the clot one is trying to document; if image detail is poor, use color or power/angio Doppler to inspect for any apparent filling defect
Step 2: Systematic examination	
Begin in transverse at the inguinal ligament: press slowly and steadily inward until the vein completely collapses; start at the level of the common femoral vein and move down the limb at 2- to 3-cm increments; press inward until the vein collapses completely, and release	Though one is compressing every few centimeters, formal documentation is necessary only in the proximal, mid, and distal thigh and the popliteal vein; calf veins are optional (if performed, document proximal, mid, and distal calf compression)
Step 3: Popliteal vein	
Continue to as close to the knee as possible, then move to the popliteal space; press inward as before	Hint: Mature collateral veins surrounding the popliteal suggest either established or acute calf or popliteal obstruction
Step 4: Calf veins	
At this point in the study, the calf veins are optional, depending on the physician's preference; they will likely be best imaged with the limb in a dependent position, or supine with a venous tourniquet applied above the knee	The risk of complication from anticoagulant therapy is the same as or greater than the risk of life-threatening pulmonary embolus; conservative management may be used, but with the caution that calf DVT can propagate to the popliteal with more serious risk
Step 5: Saphenous vein	
Alternate, indirect method to determine calf vein DVT: image the greater saphenous vein near the ankle in a longitudinal view and inspect the resting color Doppler flow pattern (the limb may be either supine or dependent); normally the vein flow is somewhat quiet and symmetric with the opposite limb; in the event the flow pattern is high velocity and continuous, and is asymmetric with the opposite leg, it represents increased shunting of blood from the deep system as a result of its reduced total cross-section area	This method is highly subjective; the greater the experience of the technologist, the more credible is the likely diagnosis; three things can shunt blood from deep veins to the superficial: (a) partial or complete calf vein DVT, (b) previous DVT, which may or may not have resolved to some degree, and (c) compression on the deep calf veins from muscular edema (from any cause)
Step 6: Compression/augmentation	
Medicare requires documentation of flow patterns; this includes the vein's response to distal and proximal limb compression maneuvers	The purpose of this aspect of the exam is to establish or rule out the finding of deep venous valve incompetence; though there is no simple intervention for deep vein valve incompetence, its documentation paves the way for insurance reimbursement for medical therapies that are often related to complications from extreme or chronic cases
Place the probe either longitudinal or transverse on the vein at each of the following veins: common femoral, superficial femoral, popliteal, and posterior tibial; at each site, squeeze gently but steadily on the muscular part of the limb distal, and then proximal; document the effect of each of the two maneuvers at each separate vein site	

Interpretive criteria	Comments
Data are *adequate* or *inadequate* for diagnosis; *credible* evidence of *complete* vessel wall collapse establishes a patent vein	Crystal-clear evidence will be rare; depend on the visual evidence from live inspection or from videotape of the wall's dynamic response to compression
DVT is *present* or *absent, partial,* or *complete* at the specified limb level	The interpretation should summarize technical findings, even if normal; end the report with a final conclusion for quick reference

Deep vein valve incompetence is reported as such at each limb

Sample report language

Normal example

Findings: Manual compression of the deep venous system is achieved at each of the seven levels imaged in both legs. No evidence of either partial or complete deep vein obstruction, bilaterally. No evidence of deep vein valve incompetence, bilaterally
Conclusion: No evidence of DVT or deep vein valve incompetence, bilaterally

Abnormal example

Findings: Incomplete surface compression of the right popliteal vein is compatible with partial vein thrombosis. All other sites tested above and below this point respond normally. Deep vein valve incompetence is noted only at the posterior tibial vein level. The left leg findings are unremarkable
Conclusion: Evidence of partial right popliteal vein DVT; right tibial vein valve incompetence

Abnormal example

Manual compression of the deep venous system is achieved from the common femoral to the popliteal vein levels, bilaterally. Direct imaging of the calf veins is precluded by obesity and swelling. Greater saphenous vein flow patterns are enhanced in the right calf, compatible with deep vein shunting, secondary to partial or complete venous system obstruction. No evidence of deep vein valve incompetence, bilaterally
Conclusion: No evidence of large vessel DVT in either leg; indirect evidence compatible with right calf vein DVT. No evidence of deep vein valve incompetence, bilaterally

[a]DVT, Deep vein thrombosis.

Laboratories, protocols for data acquisition and methods of reporting vary dramatically among institutions. A recommended strategy for both protocol and reporting is summarized in Table 15.8 (see Chapter 39).

REFERENCES

1. Aboyans V, Lacroix P, Preux PM, et al. Variability of ankle-arm index in general population according to its mode of calculation. *Int Angiol* 2002;21:237–243.
2. Andersen HJ, Nielsen PH, Bille S, et al. The ischaemic leg: a long-term follow-up with special reference to the predictive value of the systolic digital blood pressure. Part I: No arterial reconstruction. *Thorac Cardiovasc Surg* 1989;37:348–350.
3. Broderick GA. Evidence based assessment of erectile dysfunction. *Int J Impot Res* 1998;10[Suppl 2]:S64–S73; discussion, S77–S79.
4. Brooks B, Dean R, Patel S, et al. TBI or not TBI: that is the question. Is it better to measure toe pressure than ankle pressure in diabetic patients? *Diabet Med* 2001;18:528–532.
5. Goldstein I, Siroky MB, Nath RL, et al. Vasculogenic impotence: role of the pelvic steal test. *J Urol* 1982;128:300–306.
6. Engel G, Burnham SJ, Carter MF. Penile blood pressure in the evaluation of erectile impotence. *Fertil Steril* 1978;30:687–690.
7. Nielsen PH, Andersen HJ, Bille S, et al. The ischaemic leg: a long-term follow-up with special reference to the predictive value of the systolic digital blood pressure. Part II: After arterial reconstruction. *Thorac Cardiovasc Surg* 1989;37:351–354.
8. Takasaki N, Kotani T, Miyazaki S, et al. Measurement of penile brachial index (PBI) in patients with impotence. *Hinyokika Kiyo* 1989;35:1365–1368.
9. Wabrek AJ, Shelley MM, Horowitz LM, et al. Noninvasive penile arterial evaluation in 120 males with erectile dysfunction. *Urology* 1983;22:230–234.
10. Kawai M, Moriguchi S, Ikezawa T, et al. A study of ankle and toe pressure prediction following aortofemoral bypass. *Vasa* 1988;17:162–167.
11. Puppo P, de Rose AF, Pittaluga P, et al. Penile–brachial pressure index as a guide for the dosage of intracavernous injection of papaverine. *Eur Urol* 1988;14:210–213.
12. Adera HM, James K, Castronuovo Jr JJ, et al. Prediction of amputation wound healing with skin perfusion pressure. *J Vasc Surg* 1995;21:823–828; discussion, 828–829.
13. Apelqvist J, Castenfors J, Larsson J, et al. Wound classification is more important than site of ulceration in the outcome of diabetic foot ulcers. *Diabet Med* 1989;6:526–530.
14. Austoni E, Colombo F. Impotence from the 70's through the 90's: 20 years of evolution of diagnosis and therapy. *Arch Ital Urol Nefrol Androl* 1992;64:231–237.
15. Belch JJ, Diehm C, Sohngen M, et al. Critical limb ischaemia: a case against Consensus II. *Int Angiol* 1995;14:353–356.
16. Bird CE, Criqui MH, Fronek A, et al. Quantitative and qualitative progression of peripheral arterial disease by non-invasive testing. *Vasc Med* 1999;4:15–21.
17. Boeckstyns ME, Jensen CM. Amputation of the forefoot. Predictive value of signs and clinical physiological tests. *Acta Orthop Scand* 1984;55:224–226.
18. Carser DG. Do we need to reappraise our method of interpreting the ankle brachial pressure index? *J Wound Care* 2001;10:59–62.
19. Chiu RC, Lidstone D, Blundell PE. Predictive power of penile/brachial index in diagnosing male sexual impotence. *J Vasc Surg* 1986;4:251–256.
20. Dow JA, Gluck RW, Golimbu M, et al. Multiphasic diagnostic evaluation of arteriogenic, venogenic, and sinusoidogenic impotency. Value of noninvasive tests compared with penile duplex ultrasonography. *Urology* 1991;38:402–407.
21. Feinglass J, McCarthy WJ, Slavensky R, et al. Effect of lower extremity blood pressure on physical functioning in patients who have intermittent claudication. The Chicago Claudication Outcomes Research Group. *J Vasc Surg* 1996;24:503–511; discussion, 511–512.
22. Goss DE, de Trafford J, Roberts VC, et al. Raised ankle/brachial pressure index in insulin-treated diabetic patients. *Diabet Med* 1989;6:576–578.
23. Holstein P. The distal blood pressure predicts healing of amputations on the feet. *Acta Orthop Scand* 1984;55:227–233.
24. Johansson KE, Marklund BR, Fowelin JH. Evaluation of a new screening method for detecting peripheral arterial disease in a primary health care population of patients with diabetes mellitus. *Diabet Med* 2002;19:307–310.
25. Kawai M. Pelvic hemodynamics before and after aortoiliac vascular reconstruction: the significance of penile blood pressure. *Jpn J Surg* 1988;18:514–520.
26. Kempczinski RF Segmental volume plethysmography in the diagnosis of lower extremity arterial occlusive disease. *J Cardiovasc Surg* (Turin) 1982;23:125–129.
27. Kirby KA, Arkin DB, Laine W. Digital systolic pressure determination in the foot. *J Am Podiatr Med Assoc* 1987;77:340–342.
28. Kroger K, Stewen C, Santosa F, et al. Toe pressure measurements compared to ankle artery pressure measurements. *Angiology* 2003;54:39–43.
29. Larsson J, Apelqvist J, Castenfors J, et al. Distal blood pressure as a predictor for the level of amputation in diabetic patients with foot ulcer. *Foot Ankle* 1993;14:247–253.
30. Michaels J. Second European consensus document on chronic critical limb ischaemia. *Eur J Vasc Surg* 1993 Mar;7(2):223.
31. Pozin AA, Korshunov NI. Non-invasive diagnosis of lesions of peripheral blood vessels in patients with diabetes mellitus. *Klin Med* (Moscow) 1991;69:53–555.
32. Williams LR, Flanigan DP, et al. Prediction of improvement in ankle blood pressure following arterial bypass. *J Surg Res* 1984;37:175–179.
33. Apelqvist J, Castenfors J, Larsson J, et al. Prognostic value of systolic ankle and toe blood pressure levels in outcome of diabetic foot ulcer. *Diabetes Care* 1989;12:373–378.
34. Nicoloff AD, Taylor Jr LM, Sexton GJ, et al. Relationship between site of initial symptoms and subsequent progression of disease in a prospective study of atherosclerosis progression in patients receiving long-term treatment for symptomatic peripheral arterial disease. *J Vasc Surg* 2002;35:38–46; discussion, 46–47.
35. Setacci C, Giubbolini G, Romei R, et al. Penile–brachial pressure index as an expression of the degree of hypogastric circulatory insufficiency. *Angiologia* 1984;36:293–296.
36. Bone GE, Pomajzl MJ. Toe blood pressure by photoplethysmography: an index of healing in forefoot amputation. *Surgery* 1981;89:569–574.
37. Carter SA. Ankle and toe systolic pressures comparison of value and limitations in arterial occlusive disease. *Int Angiol* 1992;11:289–297.
38. Chiu AW, Chen KK, Chen MT, et al. Penile brachial index in impotent patients with coronary artery disease. *Eur Urol* 1991;19:213–216.
39. Di Nardo E, Spigonardo F, Kester G, et al. Arterial pressure in the toes of patients with obliterative arteriopathy of the legs. *Ann Ital Chir* 1984;56:81–86.
40. Duprez D, Missault L, Van Wassenhove A, et al. Comparison between ankle and toe index in patients with peripheral arterial disease. *Int Angiol* 1987;6:295–297.
41. Elliott BM, Collins Jr GJ, Youkey JR, et al. The noninvasive diagnosis of vasculogenic impotence. *J Vasc Surg* 1986;3:493–497.
42. Kalani M, Brismar K, Fagrell B, et al. Transcutaneous oxygen tension and toe blood pressure as predictors for outcome of diabetic foot ulcers. *Diabetes Care* 1999;22:147–151.
43. Lepantalo M, Kangas T, Pietila J, et al. Non-invasive characterisation of angiopathy in the diabetic foot. *Eur J Vasc Surg* 1988;2:41–45.
44. Robinson LQ, Woodcock JP, Stephenson TP. Duplex scanning in suspected vasculogenic impotence: a worthwhile exercise? *Br J Urol* 1989;63:432–436.
45. Schwartz AN, Lowe MA, Ireton R, et al. A comparison of penile brachial index and angiography: evaluation of corpora cavernosa arterial inflow. *J Urol* 1990;143:510–513.
46. Setacci C, Giubbolini G, Campoccia G, et al. Sexual impotence of vascular etiology in arterial obstructive disease of the legs. *Boll Soc Ital Biol Sper* 1983;59:1603–1608.

47. Strandness Jr DE, Sumner DS. Noninvasive methods of studying peripheral arterial function. *J Surg Res* 1972;12:419–430.
48. Ubbink DT, Tulevski II, den Hartog D, et al. The value of non-invasive techniques for the assessment of critical limb ischaemia. *Eur J Vasc Endovasc Surg* 1997;13:296–300.
49. Bell D, Lewis R, Kerstein MD. Hyperemic stress test in diagnosis of vasculogenic impotence. *Urology* 1983;22:611–613.
50. Gelin J, Jivegard L, Taft C, et al. Treatment efficacy of intermittent claudication by surgical intervention, supervised physical exercise training compared to no treatment in unselected randomised patients: I. One year results of functional and physiological improvements. *Eur J Vasc Endovasc Surg* 2001;22:107–113.
51. Ridker PM, Goldhaber SZ, Danielson E, et al. PREVENT Investigators. Long-term, low-intensity warfarin therapy for the prevention of recurrent venous thromboembolism. *N Engl J Med* 2003 Apr10; 348(15):1425–1434. Epub 2003 Feb 24.

CHAPTER 16

Optimal Endovascular Therapy for Lower Extremity Revascularization

Christopher J. White

Key Points

- Aortoiliac balloon angioplasty procedural success rate is greater than 90% and compares favorably with aortofemoral bypass.
- The long term patency of femoral–popliteal balloon angioplasty depends on clinical (i.e., diabetes) as well as anatomic variables (distal runoff).
- In femoral–popliteal lesions, self-expanding stents are preferred due to the risk of sent compression resulting in stent fracture or collapse. In addition, stents have longer patency than balloons in longer lesions.
- The procedural success rate for tibioperoneal angioplasty is about 85%, and 1- to 2-year patency rates range between 45% and 85%. Appropriate patient selection is critical for these lesions.
- Percutaneous revascularization therapy is rapidly replacing surgical therapies as the initial treatment of choice for lower extremity vascular disease.

INTRODUCTION

Peripheral vascular transluminal angioplasty is a safe and effective means of restoring blood flow in selected patients with symptomatic lower extremity ischemia (1). The benefits of balloon angioplasty in patients with iliac and femoral artery lesions have been documented in randomized trials (2–4). The long-term results of angioplasty for selected stenoses and occlusions of the lower extremity compare favorably with the surgical results, and the morbidity, costs, and hospital stay associated with angioplasty are less than those of surgical treatment (5–8). The selection of patients for lower extremity angioplasty should be guided by, but not limited to, accepted indications established for the surgical treatment of patients with peripheral vascular disease. Accepted indications for performing angioplasty include lifestyle-limiting or progressive claudication, ischemic pain at rest, nonhealing ischemic ulcerations, and gangrene. Before attempting angioplasty, it is important that the angiographic anatomy of the inflow vessels and outflow vessels be demonstrated.

A favorable procedural result is more likely for stenoses than total occlusions, for aortoiliac than femoral–popliteal disease, and in patients with claudication rather than limb salvage situations (6,9). In general terms, the long-term patency of peripheral vessels treated with balloon angioplasty is also influenced by both clinical and anatomic variables (6). Long-term patency rates tend to be higher in nondiabetic male claudicators with aortoiliac disease and discrete stenoses with good distal runoff. Conversely, restenosis is more likely to occur in diabetic female patients with critical limb ischemia, femoral–popliteal or tibioperoneal disease, diffuse and lengthy occlusive lesions, and poor distal runoff.

AORTOILIAC INTERVENTION

Aortoiliac Balloon Angioplasty

Ideal lesion subsets for iliac percutaneous transluminal angioplasty (PTA) have been proposed (Table 16.1). The

TABLE 16.1. *Iliac balloon angioplasty lesion criteria*

Favorable iliac percutaneous transluminal angioplasty	Unfavorable iliac percutaneous transluminal angioplasty
Stenoses	Occlusion
Noncalcified	Long lesions (≥5 cm)
Discrete (≤3 cm)	Aortoiliac aneurysm
Two or three runoff vessels	Atheroembolic disease
Nondiabetic patients	Extensive bilateral aortoiliac disease

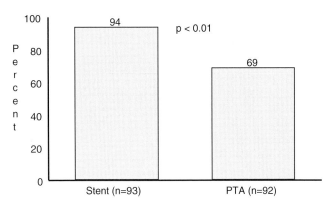

FIG. 16.2. Randomized trial of iliac stents versus percutaneous transluminal angioplasty (PTA). (Adapted from Richter GM, Noeldge G, Roeren T, et al. First long-term results of a randomized multicenter trial: iliac balloon-expandable stent placement versus regular percutaneous transluminal angioplasty. In: *Stents: state of the art and future developments.* Morin Heights, Canada: Polyscience, 1995:30–35, with permission.)

procedural success rate of balloon angioplasty for these "optimal" aortoiliac stenoses is expected to be greater than 90%, with a 5-year patency rate of successfully dilated lesions between 80% and 85%. The procedural success rate and long-term patency rates are lower for occlusions, which have a 33% to 85% procedural success rate and a 75% to 100% patency rate at 2 to 4 years (7,10).

These results compare favorably to the surgical results in patients undergoing aortoiliac and aortofemoral bypass operations, which have a 74% to 95% 5-year patency (6). In a series of 105 consecutive patients undergoing aortofemoral bypass (58% for symptomatic claudication), the operative mortality was 5.7%, the early graft failure rate was 5.7%, and the 2-year patency was 92.8% (11). In a randomized comparison of PTA versus surgery for 157 iliac lesions, there was no difference in the 3-year cumulative rate for study-related deaths, amputations, and revascularization failure between surgery (81.8%) and PTA (73.1%) (*p*=0.41) (Fig. 16.1) (3). The recommendation, based on clinical trials, is to perform the percutaneous therapy before surgical therapy if a patient is a candidate for either procedure (3,4).

Aortoiliac Stents

The use of either balloon-expandable or self-expanding metal stents has improved the results of balloon angioplasty of these vessels (Fig. 16.2) (12–14). Because iliac vessels are large in diameter (greater than 7 mm), the risk of thrombosis or restenosis after iliac placement of metallic stents is low. Balloon-expandable stents have greater radial force and allow for greater precision during placement, which is useful for ostial lesions. Self-expanding stents are more flexible and can be more easily delivered from the contralateral femoral access site. The self-expanding stents easily adapt to normal vessel tapering and are suited to longer lesions, in which the proximal vessel may be several millimeters larger than the distal vessel. There has been debate about whether stent architecture or stent materials (i.e., nitinol vs. stainles steel) had any affect on restenosis rates. Recently, the results of the Cordis Randomized Iliac Stent Project (CRISP) trial were presented, and failed to show any difference in outcomes between nitinol (Smart; Cordis, Miami Lakes, FL) and stainless steel (Wallstent; Boston Scientific Corp., Watertown, MA) stents at 1 year (Fig. 16.3) (15).

Primary placement (without regard to the predilation balloon-result) of balloon-expandable stents has been evaluated in a multicenter trial for iliac placement in 486 patients followed for up to 4 years (mean 13.3 ± 11 months) (16). Using a life-table analysis, it was found that clinical benefit was present in 91% of the patients at 1 year, 84% at 2 years, and 69% at 43 months of follow-up. The angiographic patency rate of the iliac stents was 92%. Complications occurred in 10% of patients and were predominantly related to the arterial access site. Five patients suffered thrombosis of the stent, four of whom were recanalized with thrombolysis and balloon angioplasty.

Stent placement for suboptimal angioplasty results (provisional stent placement) has been reported with the Palmaz

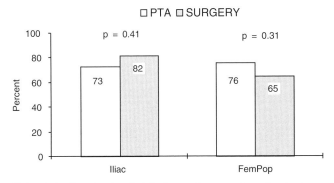

FIG. 16.1. Randomized trial of percutaneous transluminal angioplasty (PTA) versus surgery. Three-year-event-free survival. FemPop, femoropopliteal. (Adapted from Wilson SE, Wolf GL, Cross AP. Percutaneous transluminal angioplasty versus operation for peripheral arteriosclerosis. Report of a prospective randomized trial in a selected group of patients. *J Vasc Surg* 1989;9–19, with permission.)

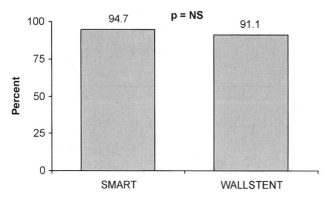

FIG. 16.3. Bar graph showing the 1-year results of the Cordis Randomized Iliac Stent Project trial (15). Restenosis, death, and target vessel revascularization.

stent in 184 iliac lesions after failed or suboptimal balloon angioplasty outcomes (17). The clinical results demonstrated a 91% procedural success rate and a 6-month patency rate of 99% for iliac lesions. Long-term follow-up demonstrated a 4-year primary patency rate of 86% and a secondary patency rate of 95% for iliac lesions.

Excellent results for provisional stent placement with self-expanding Wallstents have been reported in patients following failed or suboptimal angioplasty in iliac lesions (18). Vorwerk and colleagues demonstrated excellent outcomes for provisional iliac stent placement with the self-expanding Wallstent in aortoiliac lesions (19). They reported patency at 1 year of 95%, at 2 years of 88%, and at 4 years of 82% in 118 treated lesions (19).

Debate continues regarding the benefit of primary versus provisional stent placement. In a meta-analysis of more than 2,000 patients from eight reported angioplasty (PTA) series and six stent series, a statistically significant advantage for immediate procedural success and a 43% reduction in long-term (4-year) failures for aortoiliac stent placement were found compared to balloon angioplasty alone. A report from a European randomized trial of primary iliac (Palmaz) stent placement versus balloon angioplasty demonstrated a 4-year patency of 94% for the stent group versus a 69% patency for the balloon angioplasty group (Fig. 16.2) (20).

In a randomized trial of iliac PTA with provisional stenting versus primary stenting in iliac arteries, pressure gradients across the lesions after primary stent placement (5.8 ± 4.7 mm Hg) were significantly lower than after balloon angioplasty alone (8.9 ± 6.8 mm Hg), but not after provisional stenting (5.9 ± 3.6 mm Hg) in the PTA group (21). The procedural success rate, defined as a postprocedural gradient less than 10 mm Hg, revealed no difference between the two treatment strategies (primary stenting=81% vs. PTA plus provisional stenting=89%). By employing a provisional stenting strategy, stent placement was avoided in 63% of the lesions, and still achieved an equivalent hemodynamic result compared to primary stenting. Long-term follow-up will be necessary to evaluate the efficacy of this approach.

Iliac stent placement is useful to gain vascular access via iliac obstructive lesions for intraaortic balloon counterpulsation. Iliac stent placement can be a valuable adjunctive procedure to lower extremity surgical bypass. In selected patients, a combined approach using angioplasty and surgery can be a safe and effective method of revascularization (22) (see Chapter 34).

FEMORAL–POPLITEAL INTERVENTION

Femoral–Popliteal Balloon Angioplasty

Indications for femoral–popliteal revascularization include lifestyle-limiting claudication that has failed medical therapy and critical limb ischemia. Percutaneous angioplasty has a primary success rate between 70% and 97% for femoropopliteal atherosclerotic lesions, with the success rate being higher for stenoses than for total occlusions (23,24). Reported patency rates for successfully dilated femoral–popliteal lesions range between 50% and 70% at 3 to 5 years (7). These results compare favorably with the results of infrainguinal surgical bypass.

A randomized trial comparing balloon angioplasty to surgery for patients with femoropopliteal lesions showed equivalent hemodynamic improvement compared to surgery, and angioplasty was equally as durable as a surgical bypass procedure (3,4). There was no significant difference between the two groups after 3 years of follow-up for study-related deaths, amputations, and late interventions (Figs. 16.4 and 16.5) (3,4). In the case of a failed angioplasty, the patient still had the option of surgical therapy without placing at the patient at higher risk of limb loss or surgical failure. The authors concluded that in lesions that are amenable to either angioplasty or surgery, angioplasty should be selected for its lower morbidity and cost and equivalent long-term results and durability (3,4).

The long-term patency of femoropopliteal angioplasty depends on clinical as well as anatomic variables (25–27). Clinical factors that negatively affect long-term patency of PTA

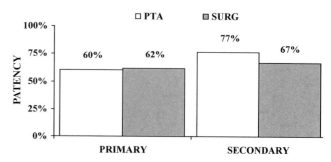

FIG. 16.4. Randomized trial of percutaneous transluminal angioplasty (PTA) versus surgery (SURG). (Adapted from Holm J, Arfidsson B, Jivegard L, et al. Chronic lower limb ischaemia. A prospective randomized controlled study comparing the 1-year results of vascular surgery and percutaneous transluminal angioplasty (PTA). *Eur J Vasc Surg* 1991;5:517–522, with permission.)

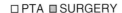
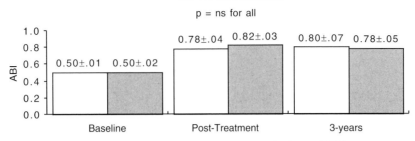

FIG. 16.5. Randomized trial of percutaneous transluminal angioplasty (PTA) versus surgery. Ankle–brachial index (ABI) results. (Adapted from Wilson SE, Wolf GL, Cross AP. Percutaneous transluminal angioplasty versus operation for peripheral arteriosclerosis. Report of a prospective randomized trial in a selected group of patients. *J Vasc Surg* 1989;9:1–9, with permission.)

include female sex, diabetes, and the presence of rest pain or threatened limb loss. Technical factors that correlate with long-term failure of angioplasty include longer lesion length, multiple versus single lesions, lesion eccentricity, and a poor angiographic appearance postangioplasty.

The status of the distal runoff vessels in the tibial vessels also affects the long-term success of PTA in the femoropopliteal vessels. In one study of 370 patients undergoing angioplasty for lower limb ischemia, patients with no or one-vessel runoff had a 3-year patency of only 25%, compared with 78% in patients with two- or three-vessel runoff (26). Minar and colleagues analyzed restenosis at 2 years in 207 patients following successful femoropopliteal angioplasty, and used a multivariate analysis to assess variables affecting restenosis (Table 16.2) (28) (see Chapter 23).

Femoral–Popliteal Stents

Self-expanding stents are preferred in this location because of the risk of stent compression or damage from external

TABLE 16.2. *Variables affecting restenosis following femoropopliteal angioplasty*

	Two-year patency (%)	p
Claudication	64	0.06
Limb threat	50	
Two- or three-runoff	68	0.02
No or one-vessel runoff	49	
Stenosis (single)	74	0.06
Stenosis (multiple)	63	
Occlusion (<10 cm)	59	0.06
Occlusion (≥10 cm)	47	
Diabetes (+)	68	0.05
Diabetes (−)	54	
Male patient	68	0.06
Female patient	56	

Adapted from Minar E, Ahmadi A, Koppenstemer R, et al. Comparison of effects of high-dose and low-dose aspirin on restenosis after femoropopliteal percutaneous transluminal angioplasty. *Circulation* 1995;91:2167–2173, with permission.

trauma for balloon-expandable stents. Early nonrandomized clinical series suggested that superficial femoral artery (SFA) stent placement could be accomplished with a very high primary success rate, and that the restenosis rates were lowest in the larger-diameter arteries and shorter lesions, and with fewer stents placed (17,18). In contrast to the results of SFA balloon angioplasty, primary patency with stent placement was minimally affected by clinical indication and lesion morphology (29). The 3-year patency rates for SFA stents in the patients with a stenosis and claudication was 66%, compared to 63% in patients with an occlusion and limb-threatening ischemia. Compared to SFA balloon angioplasty, stent placement yielded statistically better results in patients with occlusions and critical limb ischemia (29).

The U.S. Food and Drug Administration approved the IntraCoil stent (Sulzer, Minneapolis, MN) in 2001 for the primary treatment of symptomatic atherosclerotic disease in the femoral–popliteal arteries. This was based on data from 266 patients entered into a pivotal U.S. randomized trial. Patients were included in the trial if they had (a) symptomatic leg ischemia and they were candidates for balloon angioplasty, (b) stenoses 15 cm long or occlusions 12 cm long, and (c) a target lesion proximal to the tibial artery bifurcation. At 9 months there was no difference in target lesion revascularization between the stent group (14.3%) and the balloon group (16.1%, *p*=ns); however for the longer lesion lengths, there was an apparent advantage for the stent (Figs. 16.6 and 16.7).

The current evidence-based recommendation regarding femoral–popliteal artery stents is to use them in a "provisional" strategy. That is, stents should be used, in general, to salvage a failed balloon angioplasty result in femoral–popliteal arteries. An exception to this may be in patients with longer lesions, those with occlusions, and those with limb-threatening ischemia, where there is some evidence of superior stent performance compared to balloon angioplasty (29).

Drug-Eluting Stents

Most recently, data on a small number (*n*=36) of patients randomized to either a bare metal self-expanding stent or a

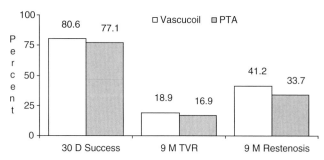

FIG. 16.6. VascuCoil pivotal Food and Drug Administration approval data. PTA, percutaneous transluminal angioplasty; 30 D Success, 30-day success; 9 M TVR, 9-month target vessel revascularization; 9 M Restenosis, 9-month restenosis. p=ns for all.

drug-eluting (sirolimus) self-expanding stent (Smart) have been reported (30). At 6 months, the restenosis rate was 0% in the sirolimus group and 23.5% in the uncoated stent group (p=0.10). There were no occlusions in the sirolimus group, whereas one patient in the uncoated stent group had an occlusion (30).

Brachytherapy Trials

A randomized trial comparing brachytherapy (BT; ^{192}Ir, 12 Gy) and balloon angioplasty (PTA+BT) to balloon angioplasty (PTA) in 113 patients demonstrated a benefit for the brachytherapy group (31). The overall recurrence rate at 6 months was 28.3% in the PTA+BT group versus 53.7% in the PTA group (p<0.05). Trials are underway to investigate the utility of brachytherapy for in-stent restenosis (31,32).

Laser-Assisted Angioplasty

There has been the expectation that by "debulking" atherosclerotic plaque, the primary patency of the SFA could be

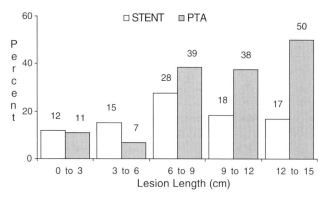

FIG. 16.7. VascuCoil pivotal Food and Drug Administration approval data for restenosis stratified by lesion length. PTA, percutaneous transluminal angioplasty.

improved. The Peripheral Excimer Laser Angioplasty trial randomized 251 patients to either PTA or laser-assisted PTA in patients with claudication and a total SFA occlusion (33). There was no difference in clinical events or patency rates at 1 year of follow-up. There is no convincing evidence that laser-assisted angioplasty adds any benefit to conventional therapy (33,34). The one area in which the laser may be of help is in crossing total occlusions that are not crossable with a guidewire (see Chapter 33).

Cutting Balloon Angioplasty

The cutting balloon is approved in the coronary circulation for "undilatable" lesions (35,36). There is no good evidence base to extend the indications for this device beyond that. Certainly, there is no evidence to suggest benefit for placing undersized coronary cutting balloons in large peripheral arteries or in large peripheral stents with in-stent restenosis.

TIBIOPERONEAL INTERVENTION

Tibioperoneal Angioplasty

Below-knee angioplasty has been generally reserved for cases of threatened limb loss because of the technical difficulty of using conventional peripheral angioplasty equipment in these vessels and the fear of potential limb loss should a complication occur. Although published experience is limited, the procedural success rate for tibioperoneal angioplasty is about 85%, and the 1- to 2-year patency rate ranges between 40% and 85% (37,38).

The use of coronary angioplasty equipment has improved the results of below-knee intervention. In 111 patients with tibioperoneal angioplasty for claudication (47%), tissue loss (27%), or rest pain (26%), Dorros and coworkers (39) had a primary success rate of 90% for all lesions, including 99% for stenoses and 65% for occlusions. At the time of hospital discharge, 95% of the patients were symptomatically improved. This evidence supports the contention that angioplasty of the tibioperoneal vessels should not necessarily be reserved for limb salvage situations; however, caution is advised in patient selection because the surgical options are limited if angioplasty fails.

Optimal treatment of infrapopliteal disease requires appropriate patient and lesion selection for treatment. Focal stenoses have the best outcomes, with fewer than five separate lesions associated with a higher success rate. Success is measured by relief of rest pain, healing of ulcers, and avoiding amputation, not by long-term vessel patency. When trying to heal ulcers, the basic principle is that it takes more oxygenated blood flow to heal a wound than to maintain tissue integrity (40). Current trials suggest that percutaneous therapy can result in long-term limb salvage in more than 80% of patients and should be considered the current standard of treatment in patients with limb-threatening ischemia who are candidates for endovascular intervention (40,41).

CONCLUSION

Percutaneous revascularization therapy is rapidly replacing surgical therapies as the initial treatment of choice for lower extremity vascular diseases. Of the new devices, stents appear to have improved the outcomes for iliac lesions, but their role in infrainguinal revascularization should be limited to bailout use, after failed or failing angioplasty. Adjunctive devices and procedures such as atherectomy, lasers, brachytherapy, and cutting balloons have a very limited role in the treatment of lower extremity ischemic lesions and should only be used after failure of balloon angioplasty. The emergence of drug-eluting stents, with their antirestenotic properties, is eagerly awaited. If drug-eluting stents prove to be as effective in preserving late patency as they have in coronary arteries, this would establish the primacy of percutaneous therapy for lower extremity revascularization.

REFERENCES

1. Isner JM, Rosenfield K. Redefining the treatment of peripheral artery disease. Role of percutaneous revascularization. *Circulation* 1993;88:1534–1557.
2. Whyman MR, Kerracher EMG, Gillespie IN, et al. Randomised controlled trial of percutaneous transluminal angioplasty for intermittent claudication. *Eur J Vasc Surg* 1996;12:167–172.
3. Wilson SE, Wolf GL, Cross AP. Percutaneous transluminal angioplasty versus operation for peripheral arteriosclerosis. Report of a prospective randomized trial in a selected group of patients. *J Vasc Surg* 1989;9:1–9.
4. Holm J, Arfvidsson B, Jivegard L, et al. Chronic lower limb ischaemia. A prospective randomized controlled study comparing the 1-year results of vascular surgery and percutaneous transluminal angioplasty (PTA). *Eur J Vasc Surg* 1991;5:517–522.
5. Johnston KW, Rae M, Hogg-Johnston SA, et al. 5-year results of a prospective study of percutaneous transluminal angioplasty. *Ann Surg* 1987;206:403–413.
6. Johnston KW. Balloon angioplasty: predictive factors for long-term success. *Semin Vasc Surg* 1989;3:117–122.
7. Cassarella W. Noncoronary angioplasty. *Curr Prob Cardiol* 1986;11:141–174.
8. Tegtmeyer CG, Hartwell GD, Selby GB, et al. Results and complications of angioplasty in aortoiliac diseases. *Circulation* 1991;83:153–160.
9. Wilson SE, Sheppard B. Results of percutaneous transluminal angioplasty for peripheral vascular occlusive disease. *Ann Vasc Surg* 1990;4:94–97.
10. Gallino A, Mahler F, Probst P, et al. Percutaneous transluminal angioplasty of the arteries of the lower limbs: a 5 year follow-up. *Circulation* 1984;70:619–623.
11. Ameli FM, Stein M, Provan JL, et al. Predictors of surgical outcome in patients undergoing aortobifemoral bypass reconstruction. *J Cardiovasc Surg* 1990;31:333–339.
12. Sullivan TM, Childs MB, Bacharach JM, et al. Percutaneous transluminal angioplasty and primary stenting of the iliac arteries in 288 patients. *J Vasc Surg* 1997;25:829–839.
13. Laborde JC, Palmaz JC, Rivera FJ, et al. Influence of anatomic distribution of atherosclerosis on the outcome of revascularization with iliac stent placement. *J Vasc Interv Radiol* 1995;6:513–521.
14. Palmaz JC, Garcia OJ, Schatz RA, et al. Placement of balloon-expandable intraluminal stents in iliac arteries: first 171 procedures. *Radiology* 1990;174:969–975.
15. Cordis Randomized Iliac Stent Project. (CRISP). Presentation at the annual meeting of the Society of Interventional Radiology, 2003. Available at http://www.jnj.com/news/jnj—news/20030331—124524.htm
16. Palmaz JC, Laborde JC, Rivera FJ, et al. Stenting of the iliac arteries with the Palmaz stent: experience from a multicenter trial. *Cardiovasc Intervent Radiol* 1992;15:291–297.
17. Henry M, Amor M, Ethevenot G, et al. Palmaz stent placement in iliac and femoropopliteal arteries: primary and secondary patency in 310 patients with 2–4 year follow up. *Radiology* 1995;197:167–174.
18. Zollikofer C, Antonucci F, Pfyffer M, et al. Arterial stent placement with use of the Wallstent: midterm results of clinical experience. *Radiology* 1991;179:449–456.
19. Vorwerk D, Gunther RW, Schurmann K, et al. Aortic and iliac stenosis: follow-up results of stent placement after insufficient balloon angioplasty in 118 cases. *Radiology* 1996;198:45–48.
20. Richter GM, Noeldge G, Roeren T, et al. First long-term results of a randomized multicenter trial: iliac balloon-expandable stent placement versus regular percutaneous transluminal angioplasty. In: . . . ed., *Stents: state of the art and future developments.* Morin Heights, Canada: Polyscience, 1995:30–35.
21. Tetteroo E, Haaring C, van der Graaf Y, et al. Intraarterial pressure gradients after randomized angioplasty or stenting of iliac artery lesions. Dutch Iliac Stent Trial Study Group. *Cardiovasc Intervent Radiol* 1996;19:411–417.
22. Perler BA, Williams GM. Does donor iliac artery percutaneous transluminal angioplasty or stent placement influence the results of femorofemoral bypass? Analysis of 70 consecutive cases with long-term follow up. *J Vasc Surg* 1996;24:363–370.
23. Capek P, McLean GK, Berkowitz HD. Femoropopliteal angioplasty: factors influencing long-term success. *Circulation* 1991;83[Suppl I]:70–80.
24. Morgenstern B, Getrajdman GI, Laffey KJ, et al. Total occlusions of the femoropopliteal artery: high technical success rate of conventional balloon angioplasty. *Radiology* 1989;172:937–940.
25. Stokes KR, Strunk HM, Campbell DR, et al. Five-year results of iliac and femoropopliteal angioplasty in diabetic patients. *Radiology* 1990;174:977–982.
26. Jens WD, Armstrong S, Cole SEA, et al. Fate of patients undergoing transluminal angioplasty for lower-limb ischemia. *Radiology* 1990;177:559–564.
27. Hewes RC, White Jr RI, Murray RR, et al. Long-term results of superficial femoral artery angioplasty. *Am J Radiol* 1986;146:1025–1029.
28. Minar E, Ahmadi A, Koppensteiner R, et al. Comparison of effects of high-dose and low-dose aspirin on restenosis after femoropopliteal percutaneous transluminal angioplasty. *Circulation* 1995;91:2167–2173.
29. Muradin GSR, Bosch JL, Stijnen T, et al. Balloon dilation and stent implantation for treatment of femoropopliteal arterial disease: meta-analysis. *Radiology* 2001;221:137–145.
30. Duda SH, Pusich B, Richter G, et al. Sirolimus-eluting stents for the treatment of obstructive superficial femoral artery disease. *Circulation* 2002;106:1505–1509.
31. Minar E, Pokrajac B, Maca T, et al. Endovascular brachytherapy for prophylaxis of restenosis after femoropopliteal angioplasty: results of a prospective randomized study. *Circulation* 2000;102:2694–2699.
32. Waksman R, Laird JR, Jurkovitz CT, et al. Peripheral Artery Radiation Investigational Study (PARIS) investigators. Intravascular radiation therapy after balloon angioplasty of narrowed femoropopliteal arteries to prevent restenosis: results of the PARIS feasibility clinical trial. *J Vasc Interv Radiol* 2001;8:915–921.
33. Scheinert D, Laird Jr JR, Schroder M, et al. Excimer laser-assisted recanalization of long, chronic superficial femoral artery occlusions. *J Endovasc Ther* 2001;8:156–166.
34. Steinkamp HJ, Rademaker J, Wissgott C, et al. Percutaneous transluminal laser angioplasty versus balloon dilation for treatment of popliteal artery occlusions. *J Endovasc Ther* 2002;9:882–888.
35. Vorwerk D, Gunther RW, Schurmann K, et al. Use of a cutting balloon for dilatation of a resistant venous stenosis of a hemodialysis fistula. *Cardiovasc Intervent Radiol* 1995;18:62–64.
36. Engelke SC, Morgan RA, Belli AM. Using 6-mm cutting balloon

angioplasty in patients with resistant peripheral artery stenosis: preliminary results. *AJR Am J Roentgenol* 2002;179:619–623.

37. Schwarten DE, Cutcliff WB. Arterial occlusive disease below the knee: treatment with percutaneous transluminal angioplasty performed with low-profile catheters and steerable guide wires. *Radiology* 1988;169:71–74.

38. Matsi PJ, Manninen HI, Suhonen MT, et al. Chronic critical lower-limb ischemia: prospective trial of angioplasty with 1–36 months of follow-up. *Radiology* 1993;188:381–387.

39. Dorros G, Lewin RF, Jamnadas P, et al. Below-the-knee angioplasty: tibioperoneal vessels, the acute outcome. *Catheter Cardiovasc Diagn* 1990;19:170–178.

40. Dorros G, Jaff MR, Dorros AM, et al. Tibioperoneal (outflow lesion) angioplasty can be used as primary treatment in 235 patients with critical limb ischemia. Five-year follow-up. *Circulation* 2001;104:2057–2062.

41. Soder HK, Manninen HI, Jaakkola P, et al. Prospective trial of infrapopliteal artery balloon angioplasty for critical limb ischemia: angiographic and clinical results. *J Vasc Interv Radiol* 2000;11:1021–1031.

CHAPTER 17

Imaging of Peripheral Arterial Disease

George Gordon Hartnell and Julia Gates

Key Points

- In the diagnosis of renal artery stenosis, false-positive computed tomography (CT) angiography (CTA) and contrast-enhanced magnetic resonance angiography (MRA) results are commonly due to poor technique or lack of patient cooperation.
- Less invasive imaging modalities for the diagnosis of peripheral arterial disease include CTA and MRA.
- Carotid artery disease may often be diagnosed by using Doppler ultrasound alone.
- Use of multidetector CT units allows for accurate three-dimensional reconstruction of vessels from any perspective.
- CTA is excellent for imaging larger vessels and intraabdominal vessels and for making assessments after stent placement.
- Two-dimensional time-of-flight MRA is susceptible to signal loss, which may result in overestimation of severity of the stenosis or may suggest complete occlusion.
- Imaging of the renal arteries is more difficult due to their small size, resulting in reduced precision in assessing stenosis.
- Contrast agents include iodinated agents, carbon dioxide, and gadolinium-based agents.

INTRODUCTION

The assessment of peripheral arterial disease (PAD) by imaging has undergone substantial changes over the last decade. There have been major changes in both imaging techniques and therapeutic options. Whereas at one time, imaging required film screen angiography with large volumes of contrast media, it is now possible to acquire images less invasively with computed tomography (CT) angiography (CTA) or magnetic resonance angiography (MRA). The introduction of digital subtraction arteriography (DSA) has allowed the use of smaller catheters and reduced contrast volumes. With the development of safer contrast agents, this has allowed more accurate definition of many aspects of PAD (1). Besides being safer, the newer contrast agents are much better tolerated (2,3). The number of therapeutic options for treating PAD has increased both as a consequence of new endovascular techniques, such as stenting and stent grafting (4,5), and developments in surgical techniques (e.g., bypass

grafts can be anastomosed to distal vessels less than 1 mm diameter) (6).

When choosing a technique for imaging PAD, several issues must be addressed, and these are outlined in the following subsections.

Information

What information is required?

What is the most appropriate imaging technique (Table 17.1)?

Is the clinical problem due to large-vessel disease, an inflow problem? Would the diagnosis be as well or better made with MRA or CTA, rather than conventional catheter arteriography? Both MRA and CTA can provide important three-dimensional (3D) information for stent grafting, for example (7,8).

Is small vessel disease the concern, an out-flow problem? In a patient with resting ischemia, distal small vessel

TABLE 17.1. *Choice of techniques for imaging different types of peripheral arterial disease[a]*

Clinically problem	First-line technique	Supplementary
Acute aneurysm/dissection (thoracic aorta)	CTA, TEE	DSA, MRI/MRA
Chronic aneurysm/dissection (thoracic aorta)	MRI/MRA, CTA	TEE, TTE, DSA
AAA	MRI/MRA, CTA	US[b], DSA
AAA pre-stent graft	CTA	DSA, MRI/MRA
AAA post-stent graft	CTA	DSA, MRI/MRA
Carotid artery stenosis	DUS, CE-MRA	MRI/MRA, DSA, CTA
RAS	CE-MRA, CTA	DSA, MRI/MRA
RAS post-stent	CTA	DSA
Intermittent claudication	CE-MRA, MRA	ToF MRA, DSA, CTA
Resting leg ischemia	CE-MRA, DSA	ToG MRA

[a]AAA, abdominal aortic aneurysm; CE-MRA, contrast-enhanced magnetic resonance angiography ($\pm$ time-of-flight magnetic resonance angiography); CTA, computed tomography angiography; DSA, digital subtraction arteriography; DUS, Doppler ultrasound; MRI/MRA, combination of magnetic resonance imaging, cine magnetic resonance angiography, and CE-MRA; TEE, transesophageal echocardiography; ToF, time-of-flight; TTE, transthoracic echocardiography; US, ultrasound.
[b]Best for screening for AAA.

disease would be best evaluated with either DSA or MRA (9,10).

Therapy

What are the available therapeutic options? There is no value, for instance, to imaging a submillimeter-size target vessel in a patient with resting ischemia and tissue loss if there is no surgeon available who can perform a distal anastomosis to a vessel of this size.

Special Clinical Considerations

Are there major comorbidities or problems with vascular access that might affect procedural safety?

The presence of certain conditions (e.g., renal insufficiency, major allergies, congestive heart failure) may favor the use of MRA or carbon dioxide DSA to avoid the risks of using conventional contrast agents.

If there is no safe arterial access, noninvasive imaging with CTA or MRA may be preferable. Patients with a wide range of metallic implants may be unsuitable for MRA, as are patients with claustrophobia.

Resources

What expertise and imaging equipment are available? The best possible performance of each technique is not necessarily available at every institution.

INFORMATION REQUIRED FROM IMAGING OF PERIPHERAL ARTERIAL DISEASE

The information required from diagnostic imaging varies with the type of PAD being investigated and will determine

the imaging approach used. For the purposes of this discussion, it is assumed that patients have either symptomatic disease or are being investigated following positive findings on other screening procedures, such as segmental pressure or duplex Doppler imaging. In this situation it is important to not only make a diagnosis of PAD, which can usually be made clinically, but to accurately stage the disease to allow planning of the best approach to treatment.

Intermittent Claudication

In patients who have intermittent claudication, significant obstructive disease is often limited to only one level, mainly either the iliac arteries or the femoral arteries. There is usually good runoff to the tibial arteries. Therefore, the obstructed vessels being imaged are typically between 4 and 10 mm in diameter. The distal vessels are unobstructed, 2 to 4 mm in diameter, and the 3D anatomy is relatively uncomplicated. Treatment options by angioplasty, stenting, or bypass grafting require definition of the type of lesion (stenosis or occlusion), configuration (concentric, eccentric, calcified, ulcerated), length of the lesion, and adequacy of the distal runoff. This type of clinical problem is easily addressed by CTA, MRA, and DSA, although both MRA and CTA have limited capability to define stenosis morphology in smaller vessels. Both CTA and MRA deal well with aortoiliac occlusive disease and have very similar accuracies (7,11,12). MRA and DSA are preferable in assessing the entire aortodistal circulation (9,10).

Although CTA can be used, the spatial resolution in the longitudinal axis is limited by the heat capacity of the x-ray tube. Current CT scanners do not match the longitudinal resolution of DSA and MRA over long distances (typically better than 2.5 line pairs per mm for DSA, 1 to 1.5 mm in slice thickness for MRA, and 3 mm for CTA), and are not recommended for patients with suspected infrapopliteal obstruction (13). Most patients with claudication do not have significant infrapopliteal obstruction, and their more proximal disease can be adequately imaged by CTA (13).

Critical Peripheral Ischemia

The situation is different in patients with rest pain or tissue loss; there is usually obstructive PAD at multiple levels. This impairs flow of contrast agents distally, reducing image contrast. In addition, smaller vessels are typically involved, especially in patients with diabetes. Therefore, higher spatial and contrast resolution imaging is required. Because these patients are often in pain and have difficulty keeping still, good temporal resolution is also required, which may not be possible with CTA or MRA. In these patients it is necessary to provide good information concerning the following factors:

- In-flow (aortoiliac) obstruction and suitability for endovascular treatment.
- Distal bypass targets, including the *dorsalis pedis* artery and plantar arteries.
- Length of diseased segments.
- Adequacy of runoff vessels beyond the site of any lesions to be treated by endovascular techniques or bypass grafting.

These patients tend to be sicker, with more comorbidities, than patients with intermittent claudication. This may make the use of large volumes of iodinated contrast for CTA inappropriate, and some MRA techniques may be inadequate to show distal bypass target vessels accurately. Although claims have been made for the accuracy of MRA for assessing the infrapopliteal arteries (9,14), the correlative conventional arteriography or DSA used to validate these studies is often inadequate to serve as a true gold standard (10,15,16).

Aneurysmal Disease

In patients with aneurysmal disease, CTA and MRA have largely replaced catheter arteriography (11,17–19). Good definition of complex 3D anatomy is easier with CTA (Fig. 17.1) or MRA (8), although rotational angiography may provide similar information when available. For stent graft patients, it is also important to identify the relationship of calcification to landing sites, which is not so easy with catheter angiography or MRA, and to define the relationship of the stent graft to the aneurysm after deployment (Fig. 17.2). It should be remembered that for some surgeons, ultrasound remains the only imaging study required prior to repair of an abdominal aortic aneurysm in otherwise uncomplicated patients.

The relationship of major branch vessels (e.g. renal arteries, internal iliac arteries) to the aneurysm is best achieved by 3D CTA (Fig. 17.1) or MRA (usually CTA for stent grafting), whereas the single-projection image provided by catheter angiography may be misleading (17). Both CTA and mag-

netic resonance imaging (MRI)/MRA have been shown to be more accurate in the diagnosis and assessment of abdominal and thoracic aortic aneurysms than has catheter aortography (17–21).

Renal Artery Disease

The problems of reliable renal artery imaging are related to the size of the renal arteries (typically the diameter of the proximal renal arteries is 4 to 6 mm), respiratory motion, variant anatomy (e.g., multiple renal arteries), position deep in the abdomen, and complex 3D anatomy. With good technique, both CTA (Fig. 17.2) and MRA (Fig. 17.3) should be nearly as accurate as DSA. The same considerations apply to assessing mesenteric artery anatomy. Certain conditions can limit the diagnostic yield for some modalities; for example, the reliable diagnosis of fibromuscular dysplasia by CTA and MRA remains a challenge.

Although there are many patients with hypertension or renal insufficiency who would benefit from screening, catheter arteriography usually is not justified by the low probability of finding treatable renovascular disease. Both CTA and contrast-enhanced (CE)-MRA are appropriate screening tests in this situation; CE-MRA is preferable in patients with renal insufficiency (22). In routine use, these techniques should have significantly greater accuracy than radionuclide or Doppler methods and provide useful anatomic information to guide intervention (23).

With good technique, especially when using a submillimeter-resolution matrix, a normal CTA or CE-MRA should effectively rule out treatable atherosclerotic renal artery stenosis (22,24). False-positive results remain common due to poor patient cooperation (especially breath holding), variant anatomy, poor-contrast bolus, and inappropriate technique. In borderline cases, invasive measurement of pressure gradients may be required to determine the significance of a lesion. The use of renal vein renin sampling is somewhat controversial.

After renal artery stenting, CE-MRA images are compromised by signal loss around the stent. In this situation, CTA is the noninvasive imaging method of choice to detect restenosis (25).

Carotid Artery Disease

Carotid bifurcation disease differs from other types of PAD in that it is readily accessible to accurate high-resolution assessment by Doppler ultrasound (DUS). Frequently, arteriographic imaging is not required. In expert hands, DUS is accurate and, unless there are atypical features, usually arteriographic imaging provides little additional information. Further imaging is indicated if the quality of DUS is thought to be inadequate or if DUS is discordant with other findings. Another imaging technique may also be used if there is a degree of stenosis close to the level where an intervention is thought appropriate (e.g., 70%). Some feel that although

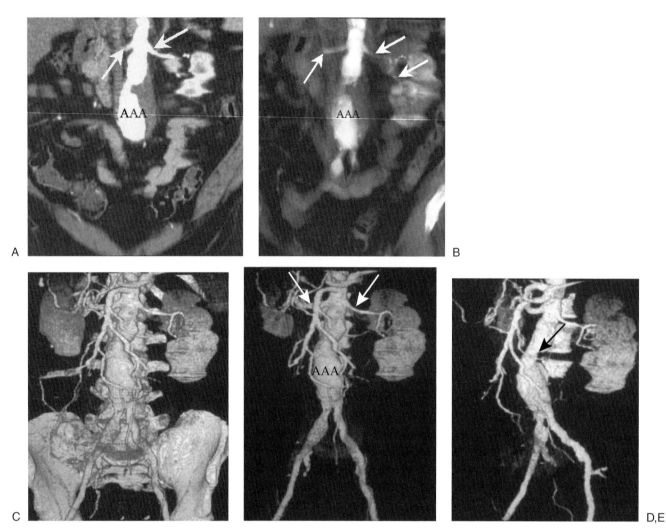

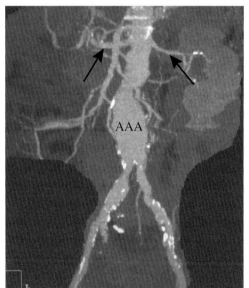

FIG. 17.1. A: Stages in three-dimensional (3D) computed tomography angiography–multiplanar reconstruction (MPR): When voxel dimensions are nearly equal, the 3D data can be viewed from any required perspective without loss of image quality. Here a 3-mm-thick coronal MPR shows the relationship of the renal artery origins (*arrows*) to the neck of an abdominal aortic aneurysm (AAA). **B:** Stages in 3D CTA–thick MPR: The thickness of MPR can be changed depending on the information to be displayed. Here a 25-mm-thick coronal MPR shows the relationship of the renal artery origins (*arrows*) to the neck of the AAA (compared with 5-mm MPR thickness in panel A). More of the renal arteries (*arrows*) and AAA is shown, but superimposition of structures obscures some detail. **C:** Stages in 3D CTA–volume rendering techniques (VRT): The 3D data set can be represented such that all voxels over a certain attenuation are visualized in a 3D model. Different attenuation ranges can be color coded to identify different structures. With CTA not only are vessels shown, but so are other high-attenuation structures, such as bone. These may obscure detail, as shown here. **D:** Stages in 3D CTA: editing VRT images. The 3D data set can be edited to remove overlying bones, as shown here. In this image, the bones of the spine and pelvis seen in panel C have been removed to show the vascular anatomy more clearly. This shows the relationship of the renal arteries (*arrows*) to an infrarenal AAA and a dilated right common iliac artery. **E:** Stages in 3D CTA: rotation. The 3D data set represented by this VRT image can be rotated to view the anatomy from any desired perspective. Here a left anterior oblique gives a better view of the aneurysm neck (*arrow*). **F:** Stages in 3D CTA: maximum intensity projection (MIP). The 3D data can also be presented as a MIP in which it is possible to "see through" lower-attenuation tissues to the higher attenuation of contrast in the arteries. This also allows demonstration of calcification superimposed on the arterial anatomy. As with VRT, image quality is improved by editing to remove overlying high-attenuation structure, such as bones. Here the bulk of the spine and the pelvic bones has been edited out of the data set, allowing clear assessment of the aorta between the renal arteries (*arrows*) and the neck of the AAA.

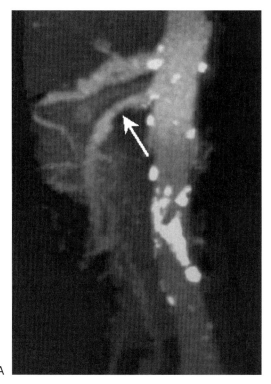
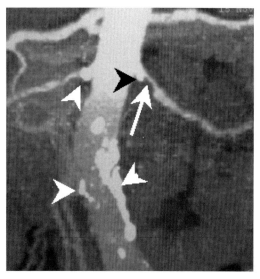

A

B

FIG. 17.2. A: Visceral artery computed tomography angiography. The three-dimensional image data in a CTA can be viewed from any perspective. Unlike conventional angiography, a single CTA can be used to evaluate multiple vessels, which may have perpendicular origins, as with the renal and mesenteric arteries. This sagittal maximum intensity projection (MIP) image from a CTA evaluation for mesenteric ischemia shows a 50% proximal, eccentric superior mesenteric artery stenosis (*arrow*). The adjacent celiac artery is not obstructed, making significant ischemia due to proximal stenosis unlikely. **B:** Renal artery CTA. The same data from the CTA shown in panel A can be viewed from an orthogonal perspective to assess the renal arteries. The coronal MIP shows an unexpected severe eccentric, proximal stenosis of the left renal artery (*arrow*) and less severe narrowing on the right. There is heavy calcification in the wall of the aorta and the renal artery origins (*arrowheads*). The reduction in contrast density between the upper and the lower part of the image is due to clearance of the contrast column from the aorta, reflecting too long a delay between contrast injection and starting the CTA acquisition.

multilevel disease is uncommon, it occurs with sufficient frequency to justify further imaging with CTA, MRA, or catheter arteriography.

In many centers, CTA or MRA has largely replaced catheter carotid arteriography. When properly performed, both techniques can assess the severity of bifurcation disease as well as demonstrate tandem lesions above or below the carotid bifurcation (26). The small but significant risk of stroke associated with catheter carotid arteriography (27) is also a good reason for using CTA or MRA. In most institutions, MRA has been established as the usual correlative imaging technique; equivocal results (i.e., possibility of a "string sign") can be further evaluated in selected patients with DSA.

Follow-up of Interventions

Similar considerations apply following an arterial intervention. Peripheral revascularization by endovascular or open

surgical methods can usually be monitored by noninvasive ultrasound techniques. If there is evidence of restenosis or occlusion, then the same imaging methods used to make the original diagnosis are usually most appropriate and allow for easier comparison of imaging.

Subsequent to a carotid artery intervention, DUS is usually adequate for follow-up. It is only when evaluating an intraabdominal procedure that more expensive imaging by CTA, MRA, or angiography is usually required. In this context, the presence of metal either in stents or surgical material may cause significant artifacts that can limit the utility of MRA, although this is less of a problem with CE-MRA. CTA is usually the most appropriate method for evaluating patients with renal or aortoiliac stents or stent-grafts. Not only is CTA relatively accurate for evaluating in-stent restenosis, it is also accurate for detecting endoleaks, graft thrombosis (Fig. 17.4), changes in vessel size, and changes in stent or stent-graft configuration (Fig. 17.5).

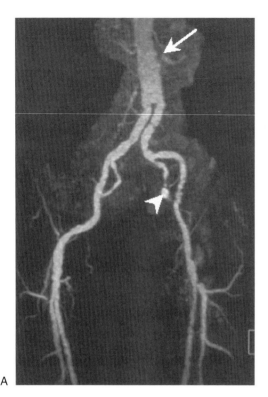

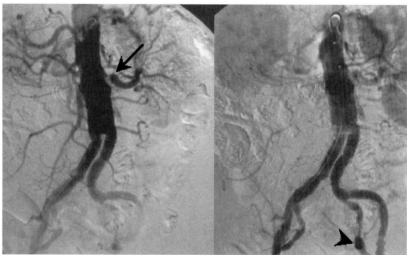

A   B

FIG. 17.3. A: View of the of the abdomen and pelvis obtained using three-dimensional contrast-enhanced magnetic resonance angiography (CE-MRA) in a patient with bilateral claudication. This developed years after an aortobifemoral bypass graft for iliac artery stenosis. The effective field of view (45 × 45 cm) is larger than that provided by the 16-in. image intensifier used for digital subtraction arteriography (DSA) (as shown in panel B). An asymmetric field of view with a 512 matrix was used. Image quality is sufficient to show a left renal artery stenosis (*arrow*), a left internal iliac artery aneurysm (*arrowhead*), a patent aortobifemoral bypass graft with no evidence of stenosis, and mild left external iliac artery ulceration. **B:** Two images from a DSA aortogram showing the same information as the CE-MRA shown in panel A. However, two images are required to show the left renal artery stenosis (*arrow*), the left internal iliac artery aneurysm (*arrowhead*), the patent bypass graft with no evidence of stenosis, and the mild left external iliac artery ulceration.

COMPUTED TOMOGRAPHY ANGIOGRAPHY

The development of CTA was made possible by technical developments in CT scanners that allow both large volumes to be imaged using thin sections (as small as 1 mm or less for some applications) and the presentation of information in near isometric volumes of information (voxels). Generally, this type of CT scanning uses spiral (also referred to as helical) scanning, which continuously acquires information while the x-ray source rotates around the patient. Initially, a single row of x-ray detectors was used, limiting the area of coverage and/or spatial resolution. Now multidetector units with up to 64 rows of detectors are available. When combined with larger x-ray tubes with very high heat capacities, this allows extensive anatomic coverage or high–spatial-resolution CTA, depending on the problem to be evaluated.

The data provided can be represented as single axial images, as with conventional CT. With older CT scanners, each voxel (volume of data) had significant thickness along the longitudinal or z-axis (typically 5 to 10 mm, compared with 1 to 2 mm height and width), making 3D reconstruction unsat-

isfactory for imaging all but the largest vascular structures. With current multidetector CT units, voxel dimensions are similar or equal (isometric) along all three axes (x, y, z). This allows accurate imaging when reconstructed and viewed from any perspective (Fig. 17.1). For small-diameter vessels, such as renal arteries, submillimeter voxel dimensions should be used. Several techniques are widely used to present these data (28).

Multiplanar Reconstruction

Multiplanar reconstruction (MPR) is a two-dimensional (2D) technique used to view any desired 2D slice or section from a 3D data set. When near-isometric voxels are acquired, the spatial resolution and image quality are the same for any orientation of the image. The use of MPR facilitates a view of relevant anatomy from an appropriate perspective; for example, the relationship between renal artery origins and the neck of an aortic aneurysm can be assessed (Fig. 17.1A). Generally, thin sections are used; the use of thicker sections may superimpose too much information and obscure detail

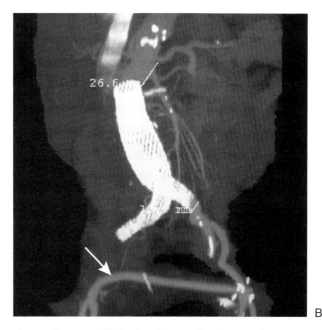

FIG. 17.4. A: Volume-rendered computed tomography angiogram (CTA) showing aortic stent graft (Aneuryx). The upper end of the graft has migrated caudally and there has been thrombosis of the right limb of the graft, necessitating a femorofemoral crossover bypass graft (*arrow*). The limbs of the stent graft were crossed deliberately at the time of insertion. **B:** Maximum intensity projection CTA showing an aortic stent graft. This image more clearly shows the relationship of the upper end of the stent graft to the renal arteries, allowing easy measurement of the graft migration. The spatial resolution of this study is sufficient to show the corrugations in the femorofemoral crossover bypass graft (*arrow*).

(Fig. 17.1B). Curved MPR sections can be generated manually or automatically to follow tortuous anatomy (Figs. 17.5D, 17.5E).

Maximum Intensity Projection

In maximum intensity projection (MIP), the highest attenuation voxels along any ray (line) through the image are identified and projected into a 3D image; the image can be rotated and viewed from any appropriate direction (Figs. 17.1F and 17.2). This method is also widely used in MRA (Fig. 17.3), where the highest signal voxels form the image (29).

Surface-Shaded Display

In the surface-shaded display (SSD) technique, all voxels with an average attenuation above a certain level are represented as a 3D image that can be rotated in any direction, and an imaginary source of illumination is used to provide a perspective of the surface of the 3D object (Fig. 17.6). This technique has been largely replaced by volume-rendering techniques.

Volume-Rendering Techniques

Volume-rendering techniques (VRTs) are developments of the SSD approach. Volumes with a certain range of attenu-

ations are assigned a color and are presented as a 3D image that can be rotated (Fig. 17.1). Colors and threshold attenuations can be varied depending on the application (24,28). This technique can be used for CTA; for imaging the airways, bowel, and bone; and for many other applications.

All 3D reconstruction techniques benefit from editing of the 3D data set to remove areas of high attenuation (e.g., bone for CTA) or signal (e.g., fat for MRA) from the image, which might obscure the area of interest (Fig. 17.1).

The use of 3D reconstruction facilitates understanding of spatial relationships and allows evaluation of very large quantities of imaging data. Typically, CTA covering 50 cm of the abdomen and pelvis and using a slice thickness of 2 mm can generate more than 250 images. A complete aortofemoral runoff covering greater than 1 m with 3.2-mm sections, reconstructed at 1.6 mm, would generate nearly 700 images (13). Although these images may need to be reviewed to identify other abnormalities, the vascular anatomy is usually best understood by reviewing the MPR and 3D images. The choice of technique depends on the problem to be addressed; usually, multiple methods are used.

The position of CTA relative to MRA and conventional arteriography for the diagnosis of PAD is not constant. Developments in each technique alter this relationship constantly (Tables 17.1 through 17.4). In general, CTA is excellent for imaging larger vessels and intraabdominal vessels, and for assessing the results of stent or stent-graft placement (Table 17.2). At the time of writing, CTA is recommended as a

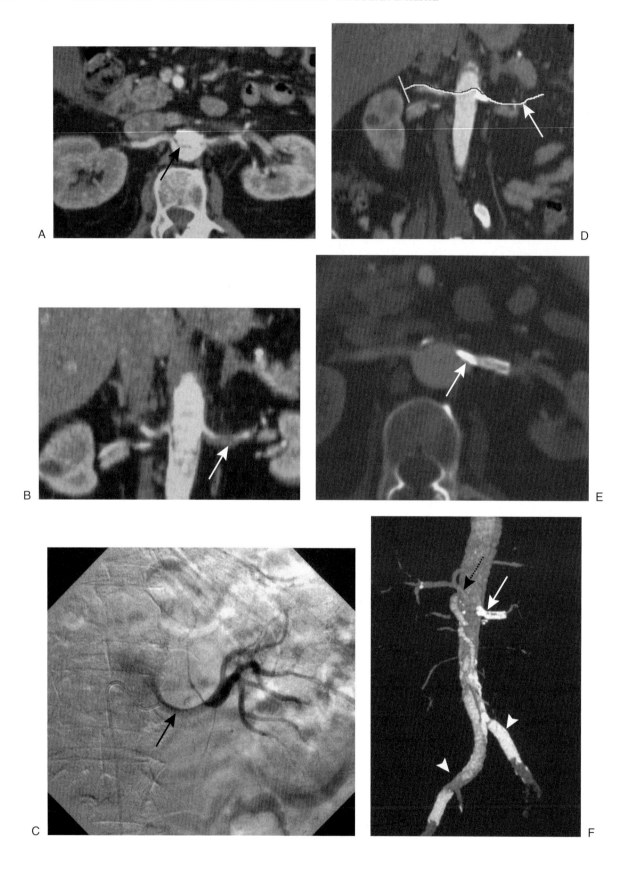

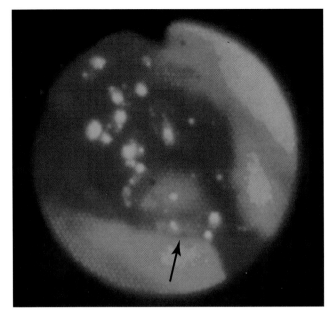

COLOR FIG. 2.3. Angioscopic view of thrombus totally occluding the superficial femoral artery in a patient presenting with acute limb ischemia. The thrombus is reddish brown superimposed on a yellow plaque with protruding lipid core (*arrow*) into the lumen. (From Seeger JM, Abela GS. Angioscopy as an adjunct to arterial reconstructive surgery. *J Vasc Surg* 1986;4:315–320, with permission.)

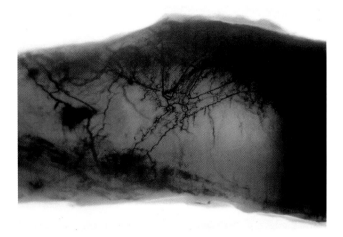

COLOR FIG. 2.7. Vasa vasorum in plaque removed from the superficial femoral artery of a patient at postmortem. The vasa vasorum is stained with India ink, demonstrating a profuse network of small vessels with areas of vessel disruption evidenced by leaking of the ink into the plaque. (Courtesy of Drs. Erico Barbieri and George Abela.)

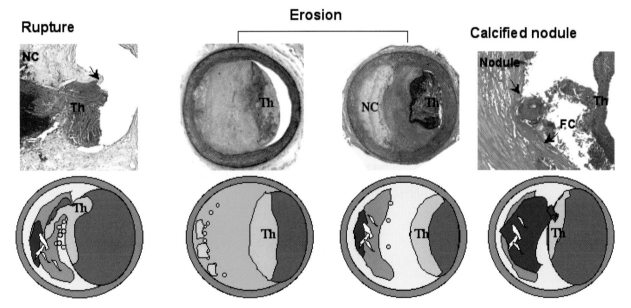

COLOR FIG. 2.9. Atherosclerotic lesions with luminal thrombi. Ruptured plaques (*arrow*) have thin, fibrous caps (*FC*) with luminal thrombi (*Th*) (**left**). These lesions often have a necrotic core (*NC*) containing large numbers of cholesterol crystals and thin, fibrous caps (less than 65 mm). The fibrous cap is thinnest at the site of rupture and consists of a few collagen bundles and rare smooth muscle cells. Plaque with thrombus at a site of surface erosion can also be detected (**middle**). Occasionally, plaques with calcified nodules protruding into the lumen can be seen at sites of plaque disruption (**right**). (From Virmani R, Kolodgie FD, Burke AP, et al. Lessons from sudden coronary death. A comprehensive morphological classification scheme for atherosclerotic lesions. *Arterioscler Thromb Vasc Biol* 2000;20:1262–1275, with permission.)

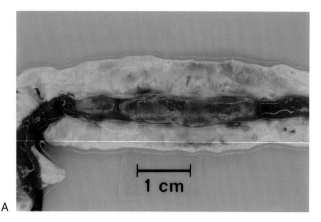

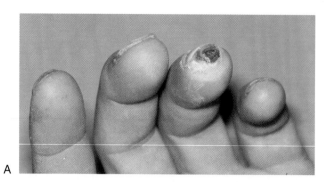

A

COLOR FIG. 7.4. A: Ischemic digital ulceration in a left-hand-dominant automotive mechanic from repetitive blunt trauma to the hand.

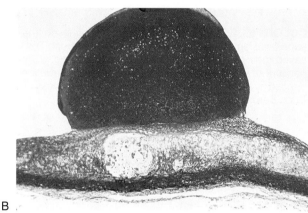

B

COLOR FIG. 2.12. Gross and histologic images of platelet-rich thrombi from an atherosclerotic model of plaque disruption and thrombosis. **A:** Large, white, platelet-rich thrombus with red thrombus attached on either side in the midthoracic aorta of an atherosclerotic rabbit triggered with Russell viper venom and histamine. **B:** Light micrograph of a thrombus attached to the thoracic aorta (Masson's trichrome, magnification 16 X). A cavity is noted below the thrombus, and the intimal surface is markedly thinned. (From Abela GS, Picon PD, Friedl SE, et al. Triggering of plaque disruption and arterial thrombosis in an atherosclerotic rabbit model. *Circulation* 1995;91:776–784, with permission.)

A

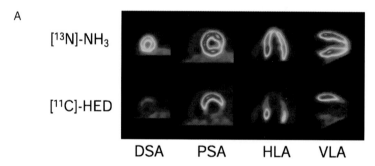

$[^{13}N]$-NH$_3$

$[^{11}C]$-HED

DSA   PSA   HLA   VLA

COLOR FIG. 10.3. *High-risk cardiac sympathetic dysinnervation complicating diabetes.* **A:** Position emission tomography with (^{11}C)hydroxyephedrine [(^{11}C)HED] was used to quantitate regions of cardiac sympathetic denervation in a 24-year-old patient with type 1 diabetes and symptomatic autonomic and peripheral neuropathy. All cardiovascular reflex tests were abnormal, and the patient suffered from orthostatic hypotension and painful diabetic neuropathy. Blood flow images of the left ventricle appear normal (infact resting perfusion is increased in subjects with cardiovascular autonomic neuropathy, secondary to tachycardia), but abnormalities of tracer retention are extensive, with only the proximal myocardial segments being visualized. DSA, Distal short axis; PSA, proximal short axis; HLA, horizontal long axis; VLA, vertical long axis.

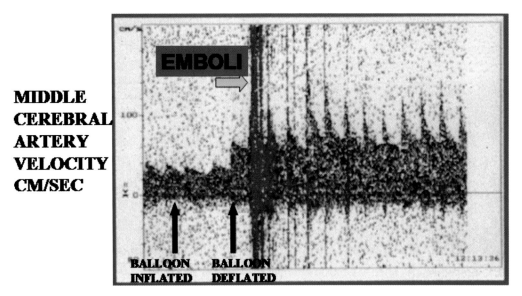

MIDDLE CEREBRAL ARTERY VELOCITY CM/SEC

COLOR FIG. 21.2. Transcranial Doppler demonstrating embolization with balloon deflation.

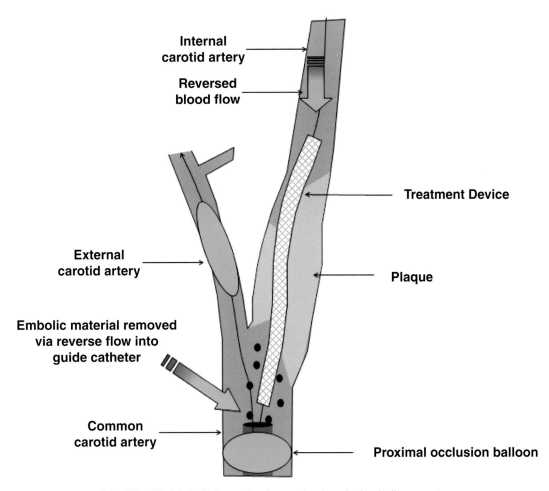

COLOR FIG. 21.4. Schematic of a proximal occlusion balloon system.

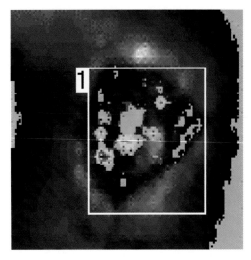

COLOR FIG. 31.1. A laser Doppler image perfusion scan of a diabetic foot ulcer wound bed on the first day of biological collagen dressing.

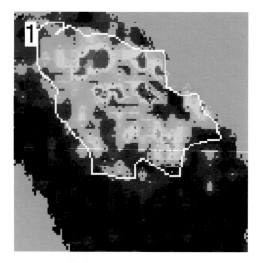

COLOR FIG. 31.2. Increase in angiogenesis in the wound bed after 21 days of biological collagen dressing therapy.

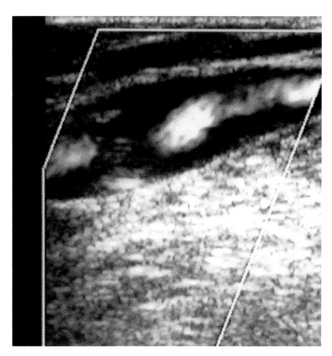

COLOR FIG. 39.1. Duplex image of reflux at the saphenofemoral valve. This is the cause of the prominent medial thigh varicosity.

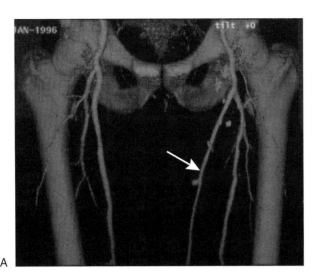 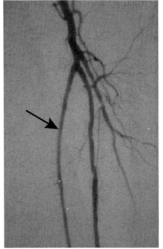

A   B

FIG. 17.6. A: Surface-shaded display (coronal SSD with anterior illumination). This image from a patient with a femoropopliteal bypass graft shows a patent graft (*arrow*) with no anastomotic narrowing. This image was acquired with an older spiral computed tomography scanner, and consequently to achieve adequate resolution, only a limited area could be imaged during a single acquisition. **B:** Selective DSA image confirms that the bypass graft (*arrow*) is patent with no proximal obstruction.

first-line technique for assessment of aortic aneurysms or dissection, aortoiliac disease, aortic arch disease, and renal artery stenosis (Fig. 17.2), as well as the detection of pulmonary arterial emboli and the assessment of live renal donors (11,21,24). It is the preferred method for monitoring changes after aortic stent-graft placement and after other interventions where metal devices are deployed (Figs. 17.4 and 17.5). This is provided there are no contraindications to giving a relatively large bolus of an iodinated contrast agent (typically 100 to 150 mL) and assumes that the patient can keep still with respiration suspended for the duration of the scan (typically 20 to 30 seconds for abdominal CTA).

In addition to these applications, CTA, albeit usually as a second-line imaging procedure, can be used to evaluate PAD affecting the infrainguinal arteries and carotid arteries as well as bypass grafts (Fig. 17.6). MRA is very good for both of these applications, especially when using contrast-enhanced

sequences. MRA does not have the limitations of contrast toxicity, radiation, and spatial resolution when imaging smaller vessels (Tables 17.2 through 17.4). This is important when evaluating stenosis of the carotid and tibial arteries. As already discussed, the need to cover a very long area, with reduced *z*-axis resolution due to the need for increased slice thickness, limits the utility of lower limb CTA.

MAGNETIC RESONANCE ANGIOGRAPHY

There are three basic types of MRA: time-of-flight (ToF), phase-contrast (PC), and contrast-enhanced (CE) MRA. Although all have their place in the assessment of PAD, we will concentrate on ToF MRA and CE-MRA techniques (Tables 17.3 and 17.4). Phase-contrast MRA methods are more difficult to implement and are mainly used for targeting a particular area of abnormality or for measuring flow.

←

FIG. 17.5. A: Axial source image from computed tomography angiogram (CTA) showing aortic dissection extending into both renal arteries. There is near occlusion of the left renal artery, and the right renal artery arises from the false lumen (*arrow*). **B:** Coronal multiplanar reconstruction (MPR) image (created from the same three-dimensional data set as in panel A) confirms that the right renal artery is patent but the left renal artery is nearly occluded (*arrow*). **C:** Selective digital subtraction arteriography confirms the CTA findings of eccentric narrowing and near occlusion of the left renal artery (*arrow*). This was treated by stent placement. **D:** Following extensive reconstruction with multiple stents and aortic fenestration, the patient returned for a routine follow-up CTA. This image shows the position (*arrow*) of a curved MPR (shown in panel E) to assess the left renal artery stent. **E:** Curved MPR (in the position shown in panel D) shows that the left renal artery stent has been compressed (*arrow*) by the dissection flap. **F:** Volume-rendered image from the follow-up CTA illustrated in panels D and E, showing the position of the compressed left renal stent along with bilateral iliac artery stents (*arrowheads*). The edges of the dissection flap are shown; the full extent of the dissection was best shown by MPR. Note the common origin of the superior mesenteric and celiac arteries (*dashed arrow*).

TABLE 17.2. *Attributes of computed tomography angiography for imaging peripheral arterial disease (13)*

Positive
  Quick imaging, image acquisition <60 sec, <30 min room time
  Multiple reconstruction methods
  Good visualization of calcified lesions
  Assessment of adjacent nonvascular anatomy
  Good spatial resolution for smaller areas of coverage
  Can be used on most patients
Negative
  Radiation
  Potential for contrast toxicity
  Time-consuming three-dimensional reconstruction
  Limited longitudinal (*z*-axis) spatial resolution for larger areas of coverage

Time-of-flight MRA uses signal related to the passage of spin in blood flow into the imaging slice. Data can be acquired for sequential thin slices (typically 3 to 5 mm slice thickness) for 2D ToF or for a large slab for 3D ToF (typically 0.5 to 1.5 mm slice or partition thickness). The 2D techniques are used for larger fields of view, such as thoracic, abdominal, and peripheral imaging (Fig. 17.7). Variations of this technique can be used to provide cine images to assess flow patterns (which can also be done with PC-MRA). The limitation of 2D ToF is susceptibility to signal loss due to complex flow patterns, such as those occurring at a stenosis. This leads to varying degrees of overestimation of the severity of the stenosis, and may suggest complete occlusion in the presence of a stenosis (Fig. 17.7). The thicker slices required to achieve adequate signal-to-noise ratios limit spatial resolution in the longitudinal or *z* axis.

Three-dimensional ToF MRA is more useful for examining smaller areas, such as the carotid bifurcation. Imaging time reduces the usefulness of 3D ToF MRA for evaluating larger

TABLE 17.3. *Attributes of time-of-flight magnetic resonance angiography for imaging peripheral arterial disease*

Positive
  Unlimited anatomic coverage, provided adequate time is available
  Quick maximum intensity projection image processing
  Good axial spatial resolution, especially when surface coils are used
  No contrast agents
  Flow direction information
Negative
  Very time-consuming (one leg runoff may take up to 1 h)
  Sensitive to patient movement
  Signal loss from metal implants (stents, etc.) may affect image quality
  Flow-related artifacts (turbulent flow, reverse flow direction from collaterals) reduce longitudinal (*z*-axis) spatial resolution
  Overestimates the degree of stenosis (two dimensional more so than three dimensional)

TABLE 17.4. *Attributes of contrast-enhanced magnetic resonance angiography (CE-MRA) for imaging peripheral arterial disease[a]*

Positive
  Wide coverage; coverage is increased if stepping is available for runoff imaging
  Quick maximum intensity projection image processing
  Good axial and longitudinal (*z*-axis) spatial resolution, especially with surface coils
  More robust than ToF MRA
  Better stenosis/occlusion definition than ToF MRA, as CE-MRA is relatively insensitive to flow-related signal loss
  Less toxic contrast agents than for computed tomography angiography
  Quick imaging, image acquisition <60 sec, <30 mins room time
Negative
  Implants may contraindicate magnetic resonance imaging
  Claustrophobia may cut short the examination
  Signal loss from metal implants (stents, etc.) may affect image quality (less of a problem than with ToF MRA)
  Sensitive to patient movement, especially when using subtraction techniques
  Expensive contrast agents

[a]ToF MRA, Time-of-flight magnetic resonance angiography.

areas, as does susceptibility to motion; patient immobilization in a dedicated coil is beneficial. The smaller voxels used for 3D ToF MRA reduce susceptibility to flow-related artifacts, allowing more precise assessment of a stenosis. Overall, spatial resolution is superior to 2D ToF MRA.

Contrast-Enhanced MRA

Good quality CE-MRA requires MR imagers with higher performance than is needed for conventional MRA. Very fast and powerful amplifiers are required to allow fast imaging using short echo (TE) and repetition times (TR). With this approach, a bilateral femoral runoff study that might take more than 1 hour with 2D ToF MRA can be completed in less than 1 minute of imaging time using 3D CE-MRA and a stepping table (30). Aortic imaging can be even faster, with subsecond CE-MRA removing the need for breath holding (31). The intravascular contrast medium contains gadolinium. Although gadolinium-based agents are more expensive than conventional iodinated contrast agents, they are less toxic and are given in smaller volumes (typically 40 mL for CE-MRA compared with 130 mL for CTA).

The best 3D CE-MRA imaging generally uses a subtraction technique. This is achieved by first taking a mask image without contrast; contrast is injected via a peripheral vein; arrival of contrast in the area of interest is monitored using real-time imaging; when contrast fills the area of interest, the 3D gradient echo imaging sequence is initiated to collect the image data. The contrast image is subtracted from the mask image, leaving a high-contrast image of the vessels (Figs. 17.3 and 17.8). Using varying delays allows imaging of either the

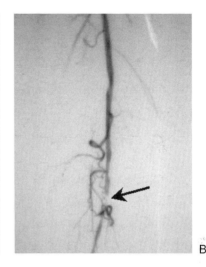

FIG. 17.7. A: Two-dimensional magnetic resonance angiography (MRA) shows a short stenosis or occlusion (*arrow*) in the right superficial femoral artery (SFA) and a longer occlusion in the left SFA (*between arrowheads*). Short, severe stenoses cannot be differentiated from occlusion using this type of MRA. **B:** Selective DSA of the right SFA illustrated in panel A, confirming the presence of a short, complete occlusion (*arrow*). Although the MRA shows the occlusion and one collateral vessel, the full extent of the collateral circulation bridging the lesion is not shown.

arteries or veins, as appropriate. Multiple acquisitions after a single injection allow multiphase imaging of arteries and veins.

In addition to MRA, other MRI techniques may be useful for vascular imaging in PAD. This is especially so with aortic imaging, where T1-weighted MRI (spin–echo or turbo spin–echo sequences) is used show the true size of aneurysms (which may be underestimated by MRA, as this only shows the patent lumen of a vessel). Using this approach, studies have shown MRI and MRA to be as accurate as any other technique for identifying and staging both abdominal and thoracic aortic disease (17,18). In patients with suspected inflammatory or mycotic aneurysms, the use of T2-weighted imaging (such as short inversion time inversion recovery [STIR] or turbo STIR) or delayed contrast enhancement shows areas of high signal (32).

The imaging of peripheral arteries by ToF MRA was widely used until the advent of CE-MRA (9,33). Even when CE-MRA is available, it may not be possible to adequately evaluate the complete peripheral circulation from the aorta to the feet. In this situation, targeted ToF MRA prior to CE-MRA can allow a complete examination.

For carotid artery imaging, the ability to use high-resolution 3D ToF MRA, with dedicated neck coils, allows accurate detection and quantification of a stenosis at the level of the carotid bifurcation (26). Examination with CE-MRA provides more robust imaging from the aortic arch to the circle of Willis.

MRA is a good method for screening for renal artery stenosis affecting the more proximal parts of the renal arteries (Fig. 17.3). Although this can be done with ToF MRA, more of the renal arteries can be seen by CE-MRA. Demonstration of a normal proximal renal artery effectively excludes significant atherosclerotic renal artery stenosis. The ability to exclude stenosis due to fibromuscular dysplasia is less well defined. The problem with screening for renal artery stenosis is one of specificity. Imaging the renal arteries is made difficult by their small size (4 to 6 mm, and as small as 1 mm for multiple renal arteries, an anatomic variant), perpendicular origin from the aorta (causing flow disturbances), and depth within the abdomen (requiring a larger field of view, which reduces spatial resolution). As a result of these factors, areas of reduced signal mimicking stenosis are relatively common, especially in patients who cannot keep still or cannot suspend respiration. In addition, too often, inappropriate imaging protocols are used, which have inadequate spatial resolution or use inadequate contrast doses for the MR imager and sequences used.

DIGITAL SUBTRACTION ARTERIOGRAPHY

Digital subtraction artheriography (DSA) uses computer subtraction of a noncontrast (mask) image from a contrast image to create an image of vessels. Although this increases contrast resolution compared with conventional film screen angiography (the previous, widely used technique), the spatial resolution of DSA is inferior to that of conventional angiography. In most circumstances related to investigating PAD, the benefits of increased contrast resolution outweigh the cost of reduced spatial resolution (Fig. 17.9). The benefits include need for less concentrated contrast medium (reduced risk and discomfort), faster imaging (being a digital technique), and better definition of areas with limited flow (e.g., tibial

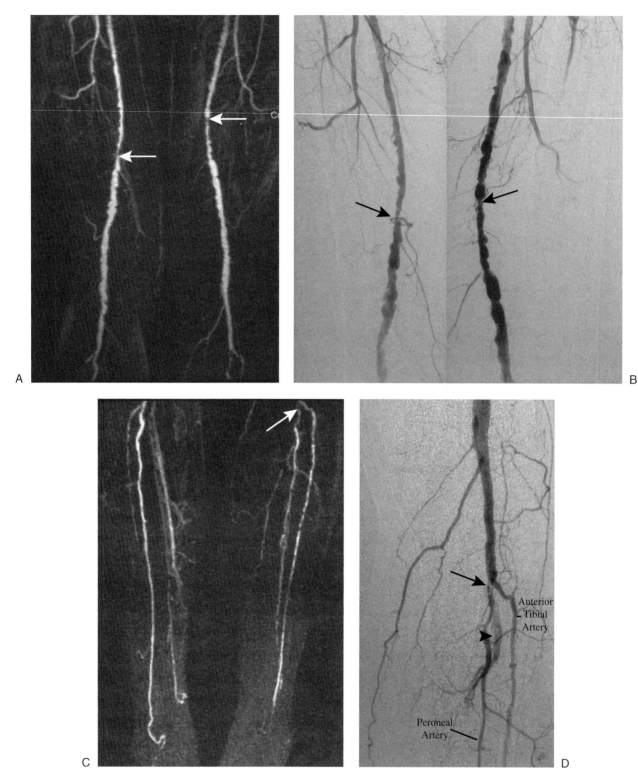

FIG. 17.8. A: Three-dimensional contrast-enhanced magnetic resonance angiography (3D CE-MRA) of the femoral arteries in a patient with severe bilateral claudication. There are bilateral short stenoses (*arrows*) and extensive ulceration. With this type of acquisition, short lesions, including areas of ulceration, are better shown than with time-of-flight MRA. By using an asymmetric field of view with a 512 matrix and coronal acquisition, the voxels are nearly isometric with dimensions of about 1 mm, allowing accurate representation of ulceration as shown here. **B:** Two images from bilateral selective digital subtraction arteriography (DSA) of the superficial femoral arteries show very similar appearances to the CE-MRA image (panel A). In particular, the degree of ulceration, stenosis (*arrows*), and position of branch vessels are confirmed by the DSA images. This allows assessment for and accurate planning of any intervention.

(Continued)

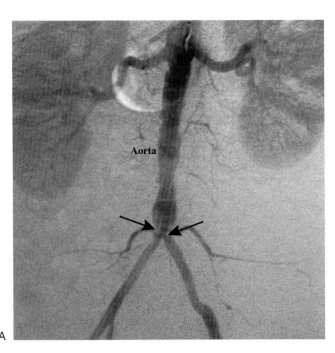

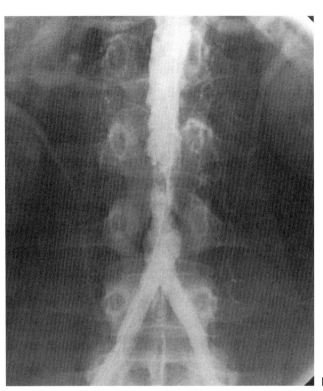

A

B

FIG. 17.9. A: Conventional digital subtraction arteriography (DSA) aortogram (30 mL of half-strength contrast at 15 mL/sec) shows bilateral stenosis of the origins of the common iliac arteries (*arrows*). Not only is the aorta easy to see, but the major branches are also well shown. **B:** Film screen aortogram following bilateral iliac stenting (40 mL of full-strength contrast at 20 mL/sec). Due to a generator fault, DSA could not be used for this final image. Although the aorta and iliac arteries can be seen adequately, the image is not as clear as the image in panel A, despite using much more contrast.

arteries beyond occlusions). The use of the subtraction technique renders DSA susceptible to movement artifacts, which can mimic or mask abnormalities (Figs. 17.10 and 17.11).

There are several reasons for the continued use of DSA as a diagnostic tool even with the availability of good quality CTA or MRA (Table 17.5). DSA is often cited as the reference standard for arterial imaging. Spatial resolution is several times better than with CTA or MRA. This status is probably justified, provided the arteriography is performed correctly. Certainly, digital arteriography should be available for peripheral imaging and interventions. It is too often assumed that arteriography is a standardized technique; this is not the case (15,16). Many variables affect arteriographic quality (10).

The standards for imaging equipment quality for imaging PAD have been well described (34) and can be summarized as follows:

- A moving-top table or a stepping gantry is required
- A spatial resolution is required of at least (a) 2.5 line pairs per mm for a 14-in. (36-cm) field of view (FOV), (b) 3.3 line pairs per mm for a 9-in. (23-cm) FOV, and (c) 4.6 line pairs per mm for a 6-in. (15-cm) FOV.
- Digital imaging capabilities with at least a 14-in. image intensifier should be included in all peripheral vascular and interventional suites.
- Digital imaging requires a 1,024 × 1,024 image matrix with a monitor capable of displaying this matrix.

FIG. 17.8. (*continued*) **C:** 3D CE-MRA of the tibial arteries acquired during the same contrast injection as in panels A, B, using a moving-table technique. At this level, the spatial resolution is often inadequate to show the necessary detail to plan distal bypass grafting. The foot vessels are not well shown, due to slow flow delivering the contrast. On the left, there appears to be stenosis of the tibioperoneal trunk (*arrow*) and occlusion of the posterior tibial artery. **D:** Image from a selective DSA (12 mL of contrast injected into the left external iliac artery) of the left tibial arteries, showing a similar appearance to the CE-MRA image. The tibioperoneal trunk stenosis is confirmed (*arrow*), as is the occlusion of the posterior tibial artery. The DSA also reveals a small arteriovenous fistula (*arrowhead*), not shown by CE-MRA.

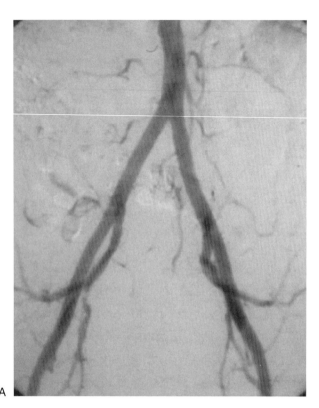
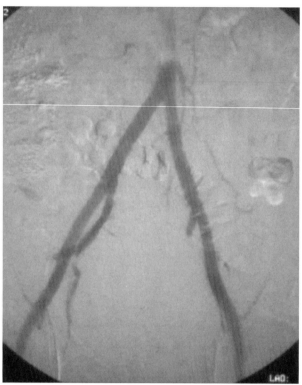

A
B

FIG. 17.10. A: Conventional contrast digital subtraction arteriography (DSA) showing pelvic arteries (anteroposterior projection; 20 mL at 10 mL/sec; half-strength Optiray 350). Good breath holding is required to minimize movement artifact, especially due to overlying bowel gas. If there is excessive peristalsis, glucagon (0.25 mg intravenously) can be used to minimize this. **B:** Carbon dioxide DSA (anteroposterior projection; 60 mL of CO_2 injected into the distal aorta) showing the pelvic arteries, compared to the conventional contrast DSA shown in panel A). Although the internal iliac artery branches are not fully shown, the common and external iliac arteries, the areas of interest, are shown well enough to exclude significant obstruction.

- The equipment should be operable in fluoroscopic and pulsed radiographic modes.
- The equipment should acquire and display at least 5 frames per second in 1,024 × 1,024 mode.

Numerous factors affect the quality of digital arteriography, including the following:

- Spatial resolution (usually limited by the digital matrix).
- Very short exposure time to minimize blurring due to movement.
- Density and volume of contrast administered.

- Level of the contrast injection; the closer the injection to the site of imaging, the better.
- Obstructions between the site of the injection and the image acquisition.
- Electronic postprocessing to enhance edges (this also enhances the effect of image noise).
- Imaging matrix (1,024 × 1,024 is recommended).
- Number of gray-scale levels (256 minimum, eight-bit imaging).

Digital subtraction arteriography is the preferred arteriographic method for the following reasons:

FIG. 17.11. A: Carbon dioxide digital subtraction arteriography (DSA) (40 mL of CO_2 injected into the right external iliac artery), showing the proximal superficial femoral artery (SFA) with minor proximal narrowing (***). Orientation is right anterior oblique (RAO) 10 deg, to profile the origin of the *profunda femoris* artery (*arrow*). **B:** Carbon dioxide DSA (40 mL of CO_2 injected into the right external iliac artery), showing mid-distal SFA with more minor narrowings. Orientation is RAO 10 deg to maintain alignment with panel A and to project the SFA (*arrow*) away from the density of the shaft of the femur. **C:** Carbon dioxide DSA (40 mL of CO_2 injected into the right external iliac artery), showing the popliteal artery (*arrow*). Orientation is anteroposterior with respect to the axis of the knee joint, but requires 20° RAO angulation of the image intensifier to achieve this. (***Continued***)

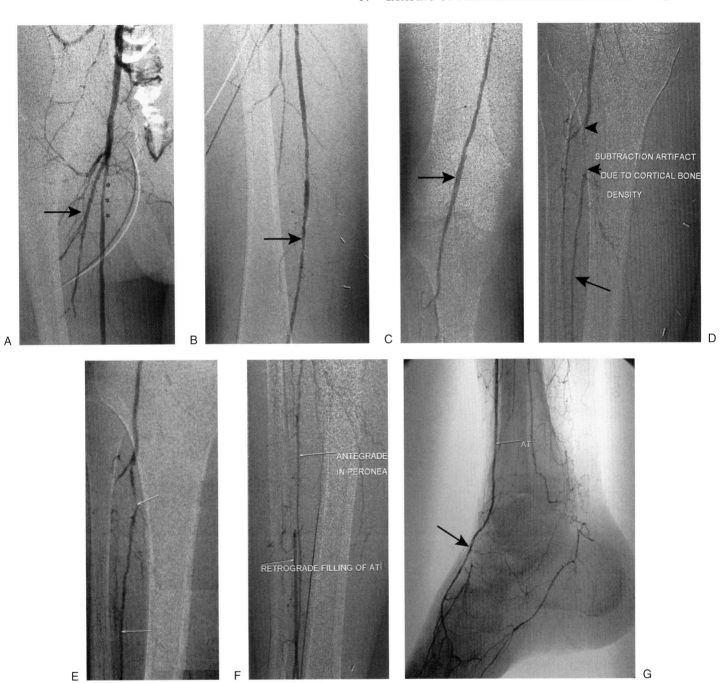

FIG. 17.11. (*continued*) **D:** Carbon dioxide DSA (40 mL of CO_2 injected into the right external iliac artery), showing the distal popliteal artery and the origins of the tibial arteries. The lower image contrast of CO_2 contributes to a subtraction artifact (*between arrowheads*), which obscures the tibioperoneal trunk, which is superimposed on the slight movement of the cortical bone of the proximal tibia. The peroneal artery (*arrow*) is patent. **E:** Carbon dioxide DSA (40 mL of CO_2 injected into the right external iliac artery) at the same level as in panel D. The degree of obliquity has been increased to project the tibioperoneal trunk away from the cortical bone causing the artifact in panel D. The tibioperoneal trunk is now shown to be patent with a distal stenosis (*arrow*). **F:** Carbon dioxide DSA (40 mL of CO_2 injected into the right external iliac artery) of the distal calf, showing antegrade flow in the peroneal artery and retrograde filling of a significant caliber anterior tibial artery. This vessel would be shown by contrast-enhanced magnetic resonance angiography (MRA), but, because of the reversal of flow direction, would not be shown by time-of-flight MRA. The image intensifier has been angled to separate the tibia and fibula, which also reduces overlap of the tibial arteries. **G:** Conventional DSA with the foot imaged in a lateral orientation. At this level, distal to a significant obstruction, the image quality of CO_2 DSA is often inadequate. A small volume (16 mL) of isoosmolar iodinated contrast (Iodixanol) provides much better image quality and more reliable assessment of distal targets for bypass grafting (in this case the *dorsalis pedis* artery; *arrow*).

TABLE 17.5. *Attributes of intraarterial digital subtraction arteriography for imaging peripheral arterial disease*

Positive
  Wide coverage; coverage is increased if stepping is available for runoff imaging
  Images immediately available
  Minimal postprocessing
  Best spatial resolution
  Robust; can be used for sick or unstable patients
  Smaller contrast volume than for computed tomography angiography
  Less-toxic contrast agent available (CO_2) than for computed tomography angiography
  Quick imaging, image acquisition milliseconds, <30–50 min room time
  Allows intervention at same time as diagnostic procedure
Negative
  Risks of arterial puncture and catheter manipulation ($<1\%$ major complication rate)
  Long procedure if difficult access
  Extra cost, mainly related to recovery time following arterial puncture
  Contrast toxicity (minimized by good preparation)
  Radiation

- Better contrast resolution (which compensates for poorer spatial resolution than conventional film screen arteriography).
- Rapid speed of image acquisition and review.
- Lower contrast volumes or concentrations, reduced patient risk and discomfort.
- Better contrast resolution allows use of nonstandard contrast agents such as gadolinium and carbon dioxide (Figs. 17.10 and 17.11).
- Digital image analysis allows objective measurements of lesion severity.
- Pulsed fluoroscopy allows reduction in radiation dose.
- Digital imaging allows road mapping and similar aids to endovascular intervention.
- Easier image storage (digital).

To take full advantage of the benefits of DSA, special attention should be paid to details of technique. To minimize vessel trauma, the smallest catheters compatible with contrast flow rates required should be used (typically 4 French). Nonselective injections should only be used for imaging the extremities when obstructive disease is relatively symmetrical and proximal (e.g., femoropopliteal disease, patients with claudication). Injections should be as selective as compatible with safety and anatomy in patients with resting ischemia due to multilevel disease, especially in those with distal (tibial) disease. The closer the injection to the site of interest, the less contrast volume is required. The more proximal the injection, the poorer is the image quality (Fig. 12).

Low-osmolality contrast agents should be used to minimize patient discomfort and movement (and to reduce the risk of allergy or renal failure). Appropriate angulation of the imaging equipment should be used to demonstrate the

anatomy clearly (e.g., separate the tibial arteries, profile tortuous iliac arteries). Patient positioning and immobilization should be optimized to define lesions (Figs. 17.9 and 17.10). This is more difficult with nonselective injections. Both lesions and normal anatomy need to be shown; often the most important information concerns patency of target vessels beyond a lesion (e.g., tibial runoff vessels to level of the midfoot, plantar arch, or *dorsalis pedis*). Variant anatomy, which is common and may not be obvious with noninvasive techniques, should be clearly defined (35).

Full evaluation of the femoral circulation requires imaging from the aorta to the feet. The DSA examination can be modified if some information has already been provided by CE-MRA, with areas of concern imaged by DSA. This may especially be an issue in characterizing lesion length and morphology when deciding on the most appropriate intervention. Other aspects of peripheral DSA technique that require careful attention, especially with some angiographic equipment, include the following (10):

- Biplane imaging for complex lesions or anatomy (e.g., eccentric lesions, obstructive aortoiliac disease, foot target vessels).
- Pressure measurements (e.g., obstructive aortoiliac disease pre- and postintervention).
- Adequate injection rates, volumes, and concentration; volumes should be increased for distal imaging and for imaging beyond obstructive disease (Fig. 17.12).
- Image collimation (to avoid "burn-out" or artifactual vessel attenuation; Fig. 17.12).
- Filters and other devices may need to be employed to improve image quality (Fig. 17.12).
- Pharmacologic flow augmentation may be required (e.g., intraarterial papaverine).
- Dorsiflexion to ensure adequate opacification of the *dorsalis pedis* artery (Fig. 17.13).

ALTERNATIVE CONTRAST AGENTS FOR ARTERIOGRAPHY

The development of DSA has allowed the use of other agents as contrast media for arteriography. Although these agents provide less image contrast than iodinated agents, in selected cases they may provide adequate information at lower risk.

Carbon Dioxide

The use of CO_2 is increasing in patients with renal insufficiency or allergy to iodinated contrast agents. Even when the quality of CO_2 DSA becomes degraded for very distal imaging, it can allow a substantial reduction in the dose of conventional contrast used (Fig. 17.11). A special medical grade of CO_2 should be used, which has fewer impurities than conventional CO_2 supplies. Medical-grade CO_2 is appropriate for arterial imaging below the diaphragm. Although dedicated injection systems are available, provided care is taken

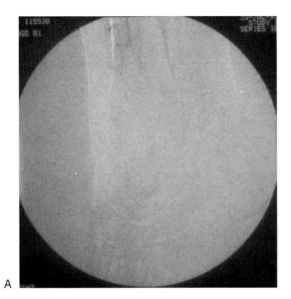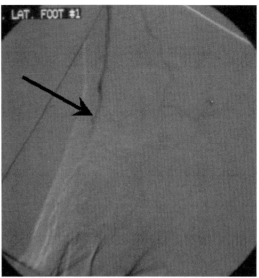

A   B

FIG. 17.12. A: Image from digital subtraction arteriography (DSA) of the right foot obtained at another hospital. There is plantar flexion, inadequate contrast density, and poor collimation. There is no visible target artery for bypass. On the basis of this study, the patient was advised to have an amputation. **B:** Image from DSA of the right foot shown in panel A obtained with appropriate dorsiflexion, adequate contrast density, and correct collimation. The *dorsalis pedis* (*arrow*) is now visible as a target artery for bypass. This patient went on to have a successful femorodistal bypass graft and avoided amputation.

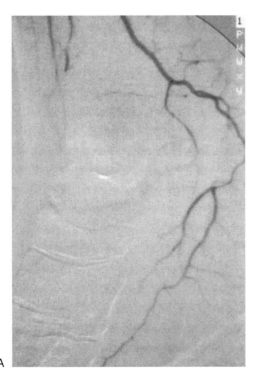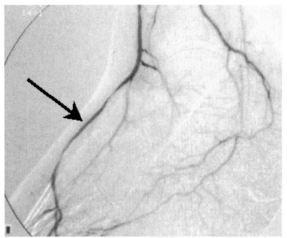

A   B

FIG. 17.13. A: Image quality affects patient management and outcomes. Image from digital subtraction arteriography (DSA) of the plantar-flexed right foot in a patient with critical ischemia and nonhealing ulcer. There is no target artery visible in the foot. Consequently, this patient had a femoroperoneal bypass graft (the peroneal artery is a less durable and successful target vessel in these patients). **B:** The following year, the patient shown in panel A returned for evaluation following occlusion of the femoroperoneal bypass. Angiography was performed using the same DSA technique, but with correct dorsiflexion of the foot, a *dorsalis pedis* artery is now visible (*arrow*). This vessel was used as a target for successful distal bypass grafting.

to avoid contamination with air, these are not necessary. Because CO_2 has no significant viscosity, very small catheters (3 French or smaller) can be used. Image contrast can be improved by changing the radiographic technique [reducing peak voltage (expressed as kilovoltage, kVp) and increasing current (expressed in milliamperes-seconds, mAs)].

The use of CO_2 requires careful attention to patient positioning and the highest quality radiography. For example, placing the patient in the Trendelenberg position facilitates distal femoral arteriography. Selective injection, with tailoring of the volume injected to the area under review, improves image quality and reduces discomfort. Minimum opacification and stacking software may also improve image quality. It is important to allow the CO_2 to disperse between injections. Injections in rapid succession may lead to a gas lock, which can cause ischemia; blood flow is required to clear the gas. Multiple bubbles, especially beyond an obstruction, take longer to disperse. Abdominal injections should be used carefully, as excess CO_2 in the mesenteric arteries may clear slowly.

Gadolinium-Based Agents

Gadolinium is a rare earth element, which is also radiodense. The concentrations of agents used for CE-MRA can also be used for selective DSA in patients with a contraindication to iodinated contrast agents. Image contrast can be improved by changing the radiographic technique (i.e., the peak voltage is increased by about 10 kVp). Unlike CO_2, gadolinium-based agents can be used for selective carotid and other DSA above the diaphragm.

The absolute reduction in risk for renal failure is unclear, and there may be no benefit when compared with equally attenuating amounts of iodinated nonionic contrast media, especially if an isoosmolar agent is used (36). There seems to be a significant benefit in patients with allergy to iodinated contrast. The safe dose range is unknown, but it is generally recommended that the total dose not exceed 60 mL. No gadolinium-based agent is approved by the Food and Drug Administration for this application.

APPENDIX. RISK REDUCTION FOR PATIENTS AT HIGH RISK FOR ADMINISTRATION OF IODINATED CONTRAST MEDIA (COMPUTED TOMOGRAPHY ANGIOGRAPHY OR DIGITAL SUBTRACTION ARTERIOGRAPHY)

Patients with a History of Allergy or Related Conditions Prior to Administration of Iodinated Contrast Media

The following information is based on the considerations in ref. 37.

Allergies are phenomena such as asthma, urticaria (hives), eczema, rhinitis, allergic conjunctivitis, hypotension, and so on, resulting from exposure to an agent (such as drugs, seafood, and other chemicals). Previous exposure to contrast media without adverse effect does not reduce the risk associated with these conditions and does not remove the need for steroid prophylaxis.

Situations requiring steroid prophylaxis include the following:

- Allergies to contrast media and any other drugs.
- Allergies to foods (especially shellfish) or any other identifiable environmental agent.
- Significant asthma/atopy.

In all of these situations one should use nonionic contrast media (38) and the following premedication (37):

- Prednisone* 30 to 40 mg × 3, orally, over 36 hours, or 50 mg × 2, orally, over 24 hours.
- Diphenhydramine (Benadryl) 25 to 50 mg, intravenously, on-call. Divided dose in borderline hypotensive, elderly, or fragile patients, as the blood pressure can drop precipitously. Other, similar antihistamines may be used.
- +/− Hydrocortisone, 200 mg, intravenously, on-call in emergencies (although steroids given less than 6 hours before exposure probably have little or no effect).

Renal Insufficiency

The presence of renal insufficiency increases the risk of iodinated contrast media causing renal failure, especially in patients with diabetes mellitus. Vigorous hydration with intravenous saline (39) is recommended, although the risk to nondiabetics with normal renal function is small. In patients with an elevated baseline creatinine (greater than 1.5 mg per dL), N-acetyl-cysteine (600 mg × 3, orally, over 24 hours) significantly reduces the risk of renal failure (40,41).

Use of nonionic contrast agents should be routine in these patients, and many researchers recommend the use of isoosmolar contrast agents (3).

Metformin

The risk of metformin causing lactic acidosis is small, except in patients with renal failure. Because of the risk of contrast agents precipitating renal insufficiency in diabetics, it is recommended that agents containing metformin be discontinued or not taken on the day of any procedure requiring the administration of radiographic contrast. Metformin should be withheld for at least 48 hours after the procedure and only restarted once it has been determined that renal function, as measured by serum creatinine, is unchanged and normal.

---

*Equivalent doses of methyl-prednisolone (Solumedrol; Medrol) or dexamethasone (Decadron) are acceptable. The approximate conversion relation is 20 mg of hydrocortisone (Solucortef; Cortef) = 5 mg of prednisone (Deltasone) = 4 mg of methyl-prednisolone (Medrol) = 0.75 mg of dexamethasone (Decadron).

REFERENCES

1. Alson MD, Lang EV, Kaufman JA. State of the art: pedal arterial imaging. *J Vasc Interv Radiol* 1997;8:9–18.
2. Rudnick MR, Goldfarb S, Wexler L, et al. Nephrotoxicity of ionic and nonionic contrast media in 1196 patients: a randomized trial. *Kidney Int* 1995;47:254–261.
3. Aspelin P, Aubry P, Fransson SG, et al. Nephrotoxic effects in high-risk patients undergoing angiography. *N Engl J Med* 2003;348:491–499.
4. Uher P, Nyman U, Forssell C, et al. Percutaneous placement of stents in chronic iliac and aortic occlusive disease. *Eur J Vasc Endovasc Surg* 1999;18:114–121.
5. Parodi JC. Endovascular stent graft repair of aortic aneurysms. *Curr Opin Cardiol* 1997;12:396–405.
6. Berceli SA, Chan AK, Pomposelli FB, et al. Efficacy of dorsal pedal artery bypass in limb salvage for ischemic heel ulcers. *J Vasc Surg* 1999;30:499–508.
7. Willman JK, Wildermuth, Pfammatter T, et al. Aortoiliac and renal arteries: prospective intraindividual comparison of contrast-enhanced three-dimensional MR angiography and multi-detector row CT angiography. *Radiology* 2003;226:798–811.
8. Thurnher SA, Dorffner R, Thurnher MM, et al. Evaluation of abdominal aortic aneurysm for stent-graft placement: comparison of gadolinium-enhanced MR angiography versus helical CT angiography and digital subtraction angiography. *Radiology* 1997;205:341–352.
9. Baum RA, Rutter CM, Sunshine JH, et al. Multicenter trial to evaluate vascular magnetic resonance angiography of the lower extremity. American College of Radiology Rapid Technology Assessment Group. *JAMA* 1995;274:875–880.
10. Gates G, Hartnell GG. Optimized diagnostic arteriography in high risk patients with severe peripheral vascular disease. *Radiographics* 2000;20:121–133.
11. Rubin GD, Shiau MC, Leung AN, et al. Aorta and iliac arteries: single versus multiple detector-row helical CT angiography. *Radiology* 2000;215:670–676.
12. Torreggiani WC, Varghese J, Haslam P, et al. Prospective comparison of MRA with catheter angiography in the assessment of patients with aorto-iliac occlusion before surgery or endovascular therapy. *Clin Radiol* 2002;57:625–631.
13. Ofer A, Nitecki SS, Linn S, et al. Multi-detector CT angiography of peripheral vascular disease: a prospective comparison with intraarterial digital subtraction angiography. *Am J Roentgenol* 2003;180:719–724.
14. Kreitner KF, Kalden P, Neufang A, et al. Diabetes and peripheral arterial occlusive disease: prospective comparison of contrast-enhanced three-dimensional MR angiography with conventional digital subtraction angiography. *Am J Roentgenol* 2000;174:171–179.
15. Hartnell GG. Contrast angiography and MR angiography: still not optimum. *J Vasc Interv Radiol* 1999;10:99–100.
16. Hartnell GG. MR angiography compared with digital subtraction angiography. *Am J Roentgenol* 2000;175:1188–1189.
17. Ecklund KE, Hartnell GG, Hughes LA, et al. MR angiography as the sole method for evaluating abdominal aortic aneurysms: correlation with conventional techniques and surgery. *Radiology* 1994;192:345–350.
18. Hartnell GG, Finn JP, Zenni M, et al. Magnetic resonance imaging of the thoracic aorta: a comparison of spin echo, angiographic and breathhold techniques. *Radiology* 1994;191:697–704.
19. Prince MR. Gadolinium-enhanced MR aortography. *Radiology* 1994; 191:155–164.
20. Nienaber CA, von Kodolitsch Y, Nicolas V, et al. The diagnosis of thoracic aortic dissection by noninvasive imaging procedures. *N Engl J Med* 1993;328:1–9.
21. Costello P, Ecker C, Tello R, et al. Assessment of the thoracic aorta by spiral CT. *Am J Roentgenol* 1992;158:1127–1130.
22. Tan KT, van Beek EJR, Brown PWG, et al. Magnetic resonance angiography for the diagnosis of renal artery stenosis: a meta-analysis. *Clin Radiol* 2002;57:617–624.
23. Sharafuddin MJ, Stolpen AH, Dixon BS, et al. Value of MR angiography before percutaneous renal artery angioplasty and stent placement. *J Vasc Interv Radiol* 2002;13:901–908.
24. Kuszyk BS, Heath DG, Johnson PT, et al. CT angiography with volume rendering for quantifying vascular stenoses: *in vitro* validation of accuracy. *Am J Roentgenol* 1999;173:449–455.
25. Mallouhi A, Rieger M, Czermak B, et al. Volume rendered multidetector CT angiography: noninvasive follow-up of patients treated with renal artery stents. *Am J Roentgenol* 2003;180:223–239.
26. Saouaf R, Grassi CJ, Hartnell GG, et al. Complete MR angiography and Doppler ultrasound as the sole imaging modalities prior to carotid endarterectomy. *Clin Radiol* 1998;53:579–586.
27. North American Symptomatic Carotid Endarterectomy Trial Collaborators. Beneficial effects of carotid endarterectomy in symptomatic patients with high-grade carotid stenosis. *N Engl J Med* 1991;125:445–453.
28. Cody DD. Image processing in CT. *Radiographics* 2002;22:1255–1268.
29. Lewin JS, Laub G, Hausman R. Three dimensional time-of-flight MR angiography: applications in the abdomen and thorax. *Radiology* 1991;179:261–264.
30. Loewe C, Schoder M, Rand T, et al. Peripheral vascular occlusive disease: evaluation with contrast enhanced moving-bed MR angiography versus digital subtraction angiography in 106 patients. *Am J Roentgenol* 2002;179:1013–1021.
31. Finn JP. Baskaran, V, Carr JC, et al. Thorax: low dose contrast-enhanced three-dimensional MR angiography with subsecond temporal resolution—initial results. *Radiology* 2002;224:896–904.
32. Tennant WG, Hartnell GG, Baird RN, Horrocks M. Radiologic investigation of abdominal aortic aneurysm disease: Comparison of three modalities in staging and the detection of inflammatory change. *J Vasc Surg* 1993;17:703–709.
33. Owen RS, Carpenter JP, Baum RA, et al. Magnetic resonance imaging of angiographically occult runoff vessels in peripheral arterial occlusive disease. *N Engl J Med* 1992;326:1577–1581.
34. AHA Inter-Council Report on Peripheral and Visceral Angiographic and Interventional Laboratories. Optimal resources for the examination and endovascular treatment of the peripheral and visceral vascular systems. *Circulation* 1994;89:1481–1493.
35. Kadir S. *Atlas of normal and variant angiographic anatomy.* Philadelphia: WB Saunders, 1991:148–156.
36. Nyman U, Elmstahl B, Leander P, et al. Gdolinium contrast media for DSA in azotemia. Are they really safer than iodinated agents? *Acad Radiol* 2002;9[Suppl]:S528–S530.
37. Thomsen HS, Morcos SK, for Contrast Media Safety Committee, European Society of Urogenital Radiology. Prevention of generalized reactions to CM. *Acad Radiol* 2002;9[Suppl]:S443–S435.
38. Steinberg EP, Moore RD, Powe NR, et al. Safety and effectiveness of high-osmolality as compared with low-osmolality contrast material in patients undergoing cardiac angiography. *N Engl J Med* 1992;326:425–430.
39. Solomon R, Werner C, Mann D, et al. Effects of saline, mannitol, and furosemide on acute decreases in renal function induced by radiocontrast agents. *N Eng J Med* 1994;331:1416–1420.
40. Tepel M, van der Giet M, Schwarzfeld C, et al. Prevention of radiographic-contrast-agent-induced reductions in renal function by acetylcysteine. *N Engl J Med* 2000;343:180–184.
41. Shyu KG, Cheng JJ, Kuan P. Acetylcysteine protects against acute renal damage in patients with abnormal renal function undergoing a coronary procedure. *J Am Coll Cardiol* 2002;40:1383–1388.

CHAPTER 18

Physiology of Renal Artery Disease

Michael G. Dickinson, Cheryl L. Laffer, and Fernando Elijovich

Key Points

- Renovascular hypertension is the most common correctable secondary cause of hypertension.
- The incidence of renovascular hypertension is probably around 4% of the general population, but could approach 15% to 30% in patients with coronary artery disease.
- Research into renovascular hypertension has provided most of our current knowledge of the physiology of hypertension and the renin–angiotensin–aldosterone system.
- The presentation and response to therapy of patients with renal artery stenosis can vary depending on which of the recognized stages of renal artery stenosis is being observed.
- There is a key interplay between renin/angiotensin and sodium intake in the mechanism and maintenance of hypertension.
- An understanding of the glomerular hemodynamic effects of various commonly used medications is essential when caring for patients with vascular disease.
- Recent research suggests that oxidative metabolism and specifically nitric oxide may play an important role in the pathophysiology and response to therapy of renal artery stenosis.

INTRODUCTION

The kidneys are highly vascular organs, which receive 20% of the cardiac output. It is thus obvious that the study of vascular diseases cannot be deemed complete without thorough assessment of (a) the impact of vascular diseases on the renal vasculature and (b) the effect of changes in renal physiology on the structure and function of the blood vessels. Much of the groundwork for our current understanding of the relationship between blood pressure regulation and renal disease was laid by studies on the pathophysiology of renal artery stenosis. Thus, this chapter, which is devoted to a review of renal physiology in the setting of vascular disease, focuses on the pathophysiological mechanisms involved in the stenosis of the main renal arteries. We also review a variety of other diseases of the renal vasculature not covered elsewhere in this text (see Chapter 19). Issues of diagnosis and management of renal artery stenosis are covered in a subsequent chapter and thus not addressed here.

STENOSIS OF THE MAIN RENAL ARTERIES

Prevalence and Incidence

Renovascular hypertension is considered the most common correctable secondary cause of hypertension. However, the actual incidence and prevalence of renal artery stenosis and renovascular hypertension are difficult to determine. The reasons for this are multiple. First, patients with essential hypertension often have atherosclerosis, and thus atherosclerotic involvement of the renal arteries, which is not necessarily the cause of their hypertension. For example, in 1,651 patients with a single plane screening renal arteriogram performed during cardiac catheterization, 30% had at least some degree of stenosis, 15% had a stenosis of greater than 50%, and among the latter, 47% did not have hypertension (1), an observation consistent with experimental studies indicating that a stenosis needs to be about 70% to cause blood pressure elevation (2). Second, prevalence studies in the general population are not feasible because the detection of renal artery stenosis requires expensive and invasive testing. Third, percentages derived from renal angiograms (the gold-standard diagnostic test) overestimate prevalence because they introduce sampling bias (only patients with vascular disease will undergo these tests). Although it would be expected that autopsy studies avoid such bias, one study of 221 patients older than 50 years detected stenoses greater than 50% of luminal diameter in 27% of the entire cohort, and in 53% of subjects with a diastolic blood pressure greater than 100 mm Hg (3). These high prevalences probably reflect the fact that the patients had died while hospitalized, hence were likely to have a high incidence of vascular disease. A larger autopsy study (n = 5,000) suggested an overall prevalence of 4%, more likely to represent the actual figure in the general population (4).

Historical Basis of Research into Renovascular Disease and Renovascular Hypertension

Study of experimentally induced stenosis of the main renal arteries has provided much of our understanding of the mechanisms of hypertension. Dr. Harry Goldblatt, while a medical resident, followed the course of uremia in a patient who had become anephric due to a surgical accident. He was impressed by the fact that the patient did not develop hypertension, as opposed to his experience with most uremic deaths. He concluded that the kidneys must be present for hypertension to develop, and therefore that a diseased kidney had to be linked to the cause of hypertension (5). Goldblatt developed a method to induce varying degrees of renal artery stenosis in dogs and so created several classical models of experimental hypertension. In the one-stenosed, one-nonstenosed kidney model (two kidney one clip, or 2K1C), the main characteristic is that the nonischemic kidney retains the ability to excrete salt. In contrast, in the bilaterally stenosed kidneys model (two kidney two clip) and in its analogous one kidney one clip model (1K1C), in which dogs first undergo unilateral nephrectomy, all renal functional tissue is subject to the hemodynamic consequences of the clipping, and renal excretory function is impaired (6). This work not only established that hypertension could be induced by stenoses of the renal arteries, but also suggested that the kidney was producing a substance responsible for the hypertension because constriction of the renal vein along with that of the renal artery did not result in hypertension. Eventually, two independent groups (Braun-Menendez in Argentina and Page and Helmer in the United States) identified an alcohol-soluble peptide that was responsible for the blood pressure elevation and named it after the original terms *angiotonin* and *hypertensin,* using the consensus word *angiotensin.*

Gavras et al., working with the Goldblatt models in rats, unraveled their mechanisms even further (7). They provided a definitive explanation for the differences in renin dependence of blood pressure observed between the 2K1C and 1K1C models. In 2K1C, renin secretion from the stenotic

kidney raises blood pressure, which in turn produces pressure natriuresis by the unclipped kidney (i.e., a net fluid and sodium loss). Because this pressure natriuresis results in contracted plasma volume, renin secretion from the clipped kidney is persistently stimulated. Thus, renin dependence of blood pressure in 2K1C is maintained for a long period, until the unclipped kidney loses excretory capacity (7). In contrast, in the 1K1C model, all renal tissue (i.e., the solitary kidney) is hypoperfused, that is, downstream to the clip, and therefore pressure natriuresis cannot take place because the ischemic kidney is not exposed to the increased systemic arterial pressure. This leads to sodium retention and volume expansion, which shut off renin secretion. Therefore, renin dependence of blood pressure is short lived in this model, and hypertension becomes sodium and volume dependent in the face of renin levels that are no longer measurably increased (8).

Stages of Renal Vascular Hypertension

In light of the understanding provided by Gavras's group on the differences between the 2K1C and 1K1C Goldblatt models in rats, the physiology of renal vascular hypertension is best understood by grouping the clinical presentation into three stages (9):

Phase I
  • Increased renin and angiotensin II levels
  • Blood pressure tends to be angiotensin-converting enzyme inhibitor (ACE-I) responsive
  • Closest animal model is 2K1C Goldblatt
Phase II
  • Renin and angiotensin II levels return toward normal
  • Increased extracellular fluid volume is present
  • Blood pressure tends to be not as responsive to ACE-I
  • Closest animal model is 1K1C Goldblatt
Phase III
  • Hypertension is not reversible by correction of the stenosis

Phase I

The pathophysiology of this phase is analogous to that of the 2K1C model in the rat and is applicable to unilateral renal artery stenosis in humans (whether dysplastic or atherosclerotic), at least in its early stages before the unaffected kidney loses excretory function due to hypertensive nephrosclerosis or other hormonal mechanisms to be described.

Figure 18.1 depicts the renin–angiotensin–aldosterone system in the setting of a significant (greater than 70% narrowing) unilateral renal artery stenosis. The stenosis leads to reduction in renal perfusion pressure, which in turn diminishes glomerular filtration rate and the filtered solute load. Reduced distal delivery of sodium and consequently of its tubular cell transport are the signals sensed by macula densa cells, which in turn trigger renin release from the granular

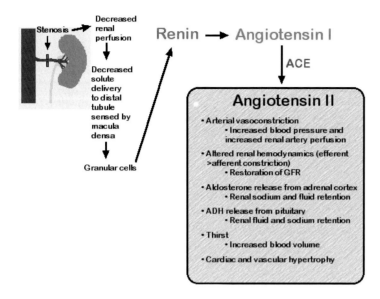

FIG. 18.1. Hormonal effects of clipping of the renal artery. The clip on the artery causes a reduction in blood flow to the kidney. This results in a net reduced glomerular filtration rate (GFR), causing decreased solute delivery to the distal renal tubule. This is sensed by the specialized tubular cells (macula densa). This stimulus from the macula densa causes the granular cells to release renin. Renin causes angiotensinogen to be converted to angiotensin I, which results in increased angiotensin II, the effects of which are summarized. ACE, angiotensin-converting enzyme.

cells of the juxtaglomerular apparatus. Increased circulating renin converts its substrate (angiotensinogen) into the inactive decapeptide angiotensin I, which is further cleaved by ACE into the powerful vasoconstrictor octapeptide angiotensin II. The classical actions of this peptide (systemic vasoconstriction and fluid preservation via aldosterone stimulation and tubular effects) result in increased blood pressure, which restores renal perfusion pressure of the affected kidney at the expense of systemic hypertension.

Intrarenally (Fig. 18.2), angiotensin II also exerts significant glomerular hemodynamic effects, but they have different consequences in the stenosed and nonstenosed kidney. Angiotensin II is a vasoconstrictor of both glomerular arterioles, but its effect is greater in the efferent than in the afferent vessel. In the stenosed kidney, the consequent decrease in glomerular pressure runoff results in relative preservation of glomerular filtration rate (GFR) despite reduced renal plasma flow. In contrast, in the nonstenosed kidney, both the increased systemic pressure and the efferent vasoconstriction mediated by angiotensin II lead to glomerular hypertension, supranormal GFR, and a net diuretic effect (so-called pressure natriuresis). Pressure natriuresis prevents the volume expansion that would occur in response to impaired renal blood flow and maintains or even reduces plasma volume. This allows for continued renin secretion by the stenosed kidney, accounts for blood pressure dependence on renin during phase I renovascular hypertension, and explains the antihypertensive effect of ACE inhibitors in this situation.

Figure 18.3, adapted from an experiment with conscious dogs that underwent ligature of one renal artery, depicts the systemic hemodynamics of phase I (i.e., 2K1C model). The increase in blood pressure is paralleled by an increase in total peripheral resistance, without significant change in cardiac output. Anderson and coworkers further showed that the increased total systemic vascular resistance of 2K1C correlated with circulating angiotensin II levels, and calculated that 25% was attributable to the stenotic kidney, 15% to the nonstenotic kidney, and 60% to the nonrenal vasculature (10).

Not shown in Fig. 18.3 is the fact that volume expansion is not a major component in the initial phases of 2K1C hypertension. However, the initial increase of plasma renin activity gradually starts drifting back toward normal after a few weeks, foretelling the end of phase I, and the shift of blood pressure dependence from renin to volume. Accordingly, in the experiment by Anderson et al., angiotensin II levels decreased over time, whereas systemic vascular resistance remained increased, indicating the development of a nonangiotensin component to the hypertension. Consistent with these observations, captopril decreased blood pressure in the initial stages of the experiment, but its antihypertensive effect diminished over time. The non-angiotensin II component that maintains hypertension when renin and angiotensin levels are falling is thought to be volume expansion. Even before loss of excretory capacity of the unclipped kidney by hypertensive damage, its pressure natriuresis may be counteracted by two powerful sodium-reabsorptive influences of angiotensin II: direct tubular actions and stimulation of aldosterone secretion. Ensuing volume expansion leads to the end of phase I and to volume dependence of blood pressure.

FIG. 18.2. Glomerular hemodynamics in renal artery stenosis (RAS) under a variety of states. Case 1. Normal state: Glomerular filtration is driven by the pressure balance achieved by renal perfusion pressure plus the balance between arteriolar tone before (afferent arteriole) and after (efferent arteriole) the glomerulus. Case 2. Renal artery stenosis: Stenosis reduces the flow of blood to the glomerulus. Neurohormonal influences (especially angiotensin II) result in greater efferent vasoconstriction than afferent vasoconstriction. The net balance is a relative preservation of intraglomerular pressure (**Continued**)

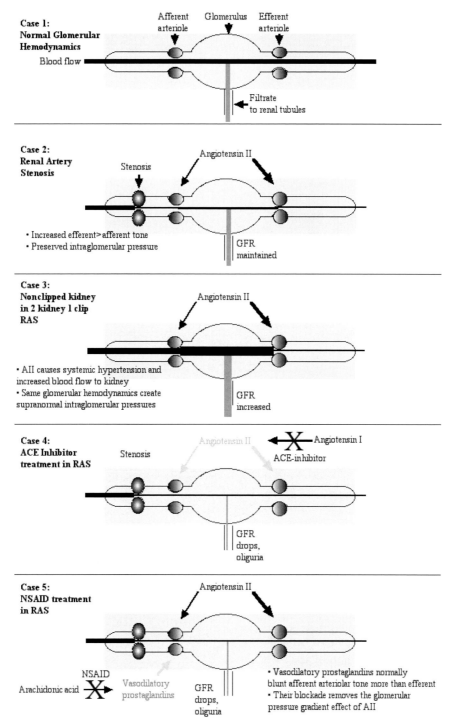

FIG. 18.2. (*continued*) (filtration pressure) and therefore preserved glomerular filtration rate (GFR). Case 3. Normal kidney in a patient with renal artery stenosis on contralateral side: Contralateral kidney causes the same neurohormonal influences as in case 2 as well as systemic hypertension. The result is increased renal perfusion pressure plus even greater intraglomerular pressure because of the efferent/afferent arteriolar balance. The glomerular hypertension likely results in renal injury as well as supranormal glomerular filtration rate, termed pressure natriuresis. AII, Angiotensin II. Case 4. Angiotensin-converting enzyme (ACE) inhibition in renal artery stenosis removes the efferent/afferent gradient, and therefore intraglomerular pressure drops and GFR drops, resulting in oliguria. Case 5. Nonsteroidal antiinflammatory drug (NSAID) treatment in renal artery stenosis: Vasodilatory prostaglandins normally blunt the effects of angiotensin (AII). These prostaglandins affect afferent tone more than efferent tone, and therefore the blockade of their production will result in a disproportionate afferent arteriolar vasoconstriction. There is no longer a difference between efferent and afferent vasoconstriction, and therefore the intraglomerular pressure drops and GFR drops, and oliguria results.

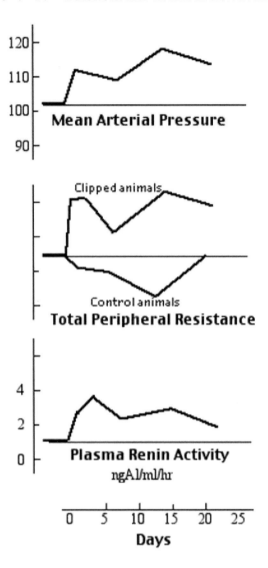

• Cardiac output remained unchanged in both groups

• Plasma renin activity remained at baseline in control animals

FIG. 18.3. Effect of clipping the left renal artery in the conscious dog (with other kidney intact): the two kidney one clip Goldblatt hypertension model. In this model, the blood pressure rises and is maintained at an elevated state. This is done mostly by an increase in total peripheral resistance, as cardiac output remained stable in both the clipped dogs and the control dogs. Plasma renin activity is elevated, but gradually starts to drift back toward normal. (Adapted from Anderson, WP, Ramsey DE, Takata M. Development of hypertension from unilateral renal artery stenosis in conscious dogs. *Hypertension* 1990;16:441-451, with permission.)

Additional mechanisms contribute to blood pressure dependence on the renin–angiotensin system in early 2K1C hypertension. In a 2K1C model produced by clipping the rat aorta below the right but above the left renal artery, Martinez and coworkers showed that the hypertensive animals exhibited increased vascular responsiveness to angiotensin II infusion compared to controls (11). This increased vascular responsiveness to angiotensin II was associated with reduced nitric oxide synthase mRNA levels and activity. Both vascular hyperresponsiveness and nitric oxide synthase changes were prevented by pretreatment of the animals with the angiotensin II AT1 receptor blocker losartan. On the other hand, N^G-nitro-L-arginine methyl ester (L-NAME), a nitric oxide synthase inhibitor, was capable of inducing angiotensin II vascular hyperreactivity in control but not hypertensive rats, indicating that nitric oxide synthase activity was already impaired in the hypertensive animals (11). In summary, these data indicate that angiotensin-mediated suppression of nitric oxide vasodilation contributes to exaggerated vascular reactivity to angiotensin II, thus enhancing the role of the latter in the early phase of renovascular hypertension.

Studies in humans also support abnormalities of the nitric oxide vasorelaxant system in renovascular hypertension. Higashi et al. (12) demonstrated reduced forearm blood flow responses to acetylcholine but not to isosorbide. These data indicate that endothelium-dependent (i.e., nitric oxide-dependent) vasodilation is impaired in patients with renovascular hypertension. In contrast, endothelium-independent vasodilatory capacity is preserved, as demonstrated by the experiments with the nitric oxide donor isosorbide. Renal angioplasty restored acetylcholine responsiveness to normal levels in these patients, suggesting that their endothelial dysfunction is linked to the abnormalities of the renin–angiotensin system induced by the renal artery stenosis (12). It is likely that deficiency of the nitric oxide system in an angiotensin II-dependent model of hypertension is due to increased reactive oxygen species. In the study by Higashi et al., several indicators of oxidative stress (such as 8-HO-2-deoxyguanosine) were found to be elevated in patients with renovascular hypertension and they correlated with the magnitude of the abnormal response to acetylcholine. There is ample experimental evidence indicating that angiotensin II is a powerful activator of NADH/NADPH oxidase activity, leading to the generation of superoxide, reduction of nitric oxide levels, and increased markers of oxidative stress (13).

At least part of the increase in oxidative stress produced by angiotensin may be due to its stimulation of the synthesis of aldosterone. Virdis et al. gave angiotensin II infusions to rats, and showed that the increases in biochemical markers of oxidative stress and activity of NADPH oxidase could be blocked by spironolactone (14). In contrast, a similar reduction of blood pressure by hydralazine did not diminish angiotensin II-induced oxidative stress, indicating that the effect was specific for the aldosterone receptor blocker. Moreover, infusion of aldosterone produced the same results as that of angiotensin II, indicating that this mineralocorticoid may also be responsible for increased oxidative stress and vascular hyperreactivity to angiotensin II in renovascular hypertension (14).

Finally, a role for the sympathetic nervous system in the maintenance of hypertension in the 2K1C model is highly controversial. Neither renal denervation in Goldblatt's experiments (6) nor the combination of propranolol and phentolamine in 2K1C rats (15) affected the development or maintenance of hypertension, suggesting that the sympathetic nervous system was not an important contributor. However, human studies of catecholamine kinetics with radiotracers demonstrated that there is increased cardiac norepinephrine spillover in renovascular hypertension, suggesting that at least cardiac (if not systemic) sympathetic overactivity is present in these patients (16). The reasons for variable results on the role of the sympathetic nervous system in renovascular hypertension have been reviewed by Grassi et al., and include the facts that sympathetic activity (a) closely relates to and varies with that of the renin–angiotensin system, (b) is a late phenomenon in the progression of renovascular hypertension, and (c) may be increased regionally (e.g., in the heart), but not systemically (17).

Phase II

The pathophysiology of this phase is analogous to that of the 1K1C model in the rat and is applicable to bilateral renal artery stenosis in humans, but only when the narrowing of the main artery of both kidneys is hemodynamically significant. This is not always true in human renovascular hypertension. In elderly patients with bilateral atherosclerotic disease of the renal arteries, it is more common that the stenosis is hemodynamically significant on only one side. When such is the case, the patients behave, from the functional point of view, as if the lesion were unilateral and the pathophysiology is that of phase I. Phase II of renovascular hypertension may also be reached from phase I, as a consequence of the development of hypertensive nephrosclerosis in the nonstenosed kidney, a phenomenon that is a function of time and of the severity of blood pressure elevation. Once established and significant, widespread arteriolar nephrosclerosis of the nonstenosed kidney is functionally equivalent to having stenosed its main renal artery.

Figure 18.4 depicts data in uninephrectomized dogs with stenosis of the remaining kidney (1K1C model). This is analogous to human bilaterally significant renal artery stenosis because all functional renal tissue is downstream to the stenosis, that is, hypoperfused with diminished glomerular pressure. The figure shows that renin and aldosterone stimulation are transient and short lived. Levels return to normal as a consequence of expansion of plasma volume due to diminished salt and water excretion by the hypoperfused kidney. That is, the 1K1C model lacks the phenomenon of pressure natriuresis because this requires an unclipped kidney subject to the increased systemic pressure (as discussed in the 2K1C model). However, when the 1K1C animal is sub-

jected to salt restriction to prevent sodium retention despite renal dysfunction, renin secretion is sustained, and the pathophysiology mimics that of the 2K1C animal. Consistent with these observations, Gavras et al. demonstrated that an ACE inhibitor reduced blood pressure of 1K1C rats only if they had been salt depleted for 4 weeks prior to clipping, but not if the clipped animals had been previously maintained on a normal salt diet (8). The antihypertensive effect of ACE inhibitors in salt-depleted, 1K1C rats was completely abolished by restoration of sodium balance by a high-salt diet (8).

An equivalent interplay between salt and the renin–angiotensin system was demonstrated by Gavras et al. in the late stages of 2K1C hypertensive rats, once angiotensin II tubular actions or aldosterone counteracted pressure natriuresis or after hypertensive nephrosclerosis of the unclipped kidney reduced its excretory function (7). As discussed previously, renin levels fell at this stage and blockade of the renin–angiotensin system lost effectiveness, mimicking the situation in 1K1C rats. However, if these animals were subjected to dietary salt depletion or diuretic treatment, their plasma renin activity and angiotensin II levels rose and the effectiveness of blockade of the renin–angiotensin system was restored (7).

Figure 18.5 depicts a pressure natriuresis curve, which demonstrates the experimental relationship between sodium intake and the impact of angiotensin II and ACE inhibition. Angiotensin II increases blood pressure at all levels of sodium intake, but this effect is significantly enhanced with higher sodium intake. Angiotensin-converting enzyme inhibitors lower blood pressure, and this effect is most enhanced in the setting of lower sodium intake.

Finally, a role for endothelin has been described in the development and maintenance of hypertension and as a growth-promoter determining organ hypertrophy in 1K1C but not 2K1C rats (18). This is consistent with observations in many other experimental hypertensive models, indicating that overexpression of endothelial endothelin and its participation in hypertension and vascular remodeling are much more important in salt-dependent (e.g., deoxycorticosterone-salt, aldosterone-induced, Dahl salt-sensitive, insulin-resistant, and 1K1C models) than in salt-independent or renin-dependent forms of hypertension (e.g., spontaneously hypertensive rat, 2K1C, and L-NAME-induced) (19).

The relevance of these observations to human renovascular hypertension is unclear, perhaps because most studies have been conducted in patients with unilateral renal artery stenosis. Plasma levels of endothelin in these patients have been found to be either normal (20–22) or elevated (23,24), renal levels vary, and urinary excretion is high, but normalizes 1 month after angioplasty (20,23,24). Renal vein concentrations of endothelin do not differ between the stenosed and the nonstenosed kidney. In contrast, endothelin synthesis of patients with renovascular hypertension seems to reflect systemic influences unrelated to the underlying pathophysiology of blood pressure elevation. For example, plasma endothelin

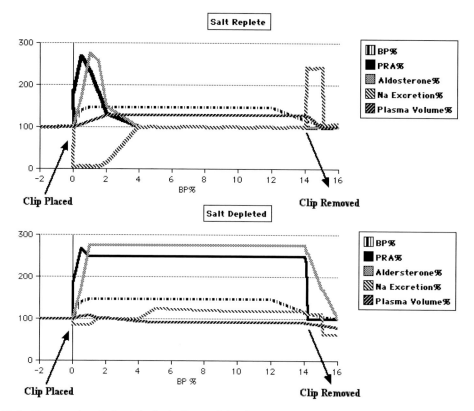

FIG. 18.4. Hormonal and physiological effects of the Goldblatt one kidney one clip hypertension model. Normal state: When the clip is placed, plasma renin activity (PRA) and aldosterone levels peak, resulting in marked reduction in sodium excretion and expansion of plasma volume. Once plasma volume is increased, the PRA and aldosterone return near baseline at a new volume-expanded and hypertensive steady state. Salt depleted: When a clip is placed, PRA and aldosterone levels peak, but volume expansion cannot occur and elevated blood pressure (BP) is maintained by continued elevations of PRA, aldosterone, and angiotensin II. Clip removal: BP immediately returns toward normal, and volume expansion and hormonal elevations resolve, but BP drop occurs more quickly than resolution of these initial driving forces. (Adapted from Berger AC. The Goldblatt Memorial Lecture, part I: experimental renovascular hypertension, *Hypertension* 1979:1:447–445, with permission.)

relates to the magnitude of insulin resistance (22) and with the magnitude or number of sites involved by the atherosclerotic process (25). Moreover, endothelin levels do not predict the response to therapy (21) after renal revascularization. Finally, plasma endothelin correlates with the degree of stenosis of the renal artery in patients with unilateral, but not bilateral renal artery stenosis (23), which is opposite to what would be expected from the observations in experimental 1K1C and 2K1C models.

Phase III

Irreversible renal damage occurs in the late stages of the natural history of renovascular hypertension. At this point, correction of the renal artery stenosis does not cure or ameliorate the hypertension. This indicates that blood pressure elevation is now maintained by mechanisms other than those triggered by the initial etiology of the disease and analogous to those of hypertension in chronic renal failure of any cause. Lack of

responsiveness to the anatomic correction of the narrowing of the renal artery is what defines Phase III of renovascular hypertension.

Progressive renal damage of the nonstenosed kidney is attributable to the effect of chronic sustained hypertension. Transmission of elevated systemic blood pressure plus the efferent arteriolar vasoconstrictor effect of angiotensin II leads to increased glomerular pressure. The magnitude of this increase is the major correlate of anatomic renal damage. Pathology of the nonclipped kidney of 2K1C rats at 11 weeks discloses multiple abnormalities, including glomerular injury, tubulointerstitial injury, tubulointerstitial cell proliferation, dense focal interstitial monocyte and macrophage influx, increased deposition of types I and IV collagen, and increased cellular expression of desmin and actin (26). Because these abnormalities are absent in the clipped kidney, whereas both kidneys are exposed to the same circulating levels of renin, angiotensin II, and aldosterone, it is most likely that the histological changes of the nonclipped kidney are

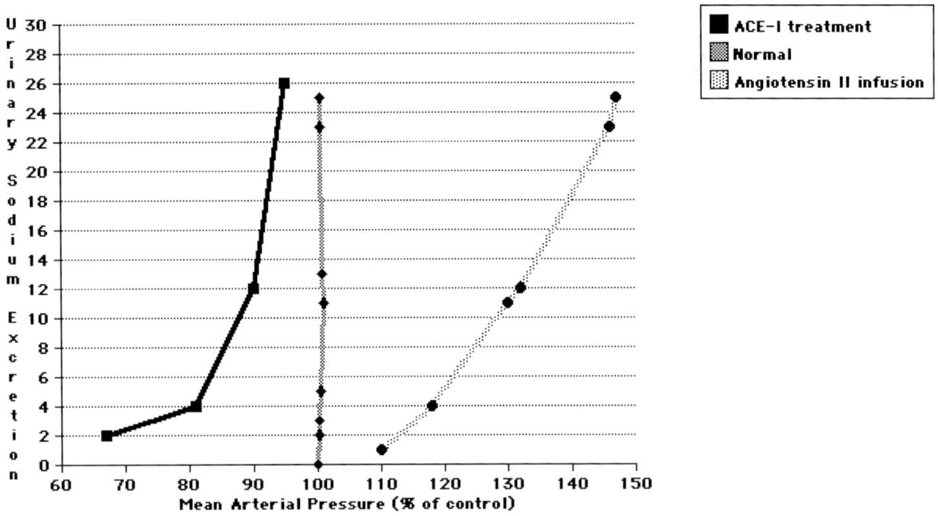

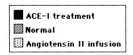

FIG. 18.5. Salt loading pressure natriuresis curves. Data points represent conditions with increasing intake of sodium. (a) Normal state: Sodium intake is tightly linked to sodium excretion. Blood pressure is tightly maintained regardless of sodium intake. (b) Angiotensin causes salt-sensitive hypertension. Increasing sodium intake causes increased blood pressure. Increased sodium excretion occurs only at the state of higher blood pressure. (c) Angiotensin-converting enzyme inhibitor (ACE-I) lowers blood pressure at all levels, but especially at low sodium intake. Increasing sodium intake minimizes the hypotensive effect of ACE inhibition. (Adapted from Guyton AC, Hall JE, Coleman TG, et al. The dominant role of the kidneys in long term arterial pressure regulation in normal hypertesnive states. In: Laragh JH, Brenner BM, eds., *Hypertension: pathophysiology, diagnosis, and management,* 2nd ed. New York: Raven Press, 1995:1311–1326, with permission.)

entirely attributable to the elevation of arterial and glomerular pressures.

The role of glomerular hypertension in determining progressive renal damage in the nonclipped kidney of renovascular hypertension (and in other diseases of the kidney) is illustrated by the depiction of the actions of pharmacologic agents in Fig. 18.2. ACE inhibitors, by diminishing angiotensin II, reverse efferent arteriolar vasoconstriction and decrease intraglomerular pressure. In the nonclipped kidney, these agents will reduce supranormal GFR; therefore, their effect on glomerular hemodynamics will protect against long-term glomerular damage. In contrast, in the clipped kidney, maintenance of GFR in the face of reduced renal blood flow is dependent on efferent arteriolar angiotensin II vasoconstriction; therefore, ACE inhibitors will reduce glomerular function in this kidney. This is of clinical relevance in bilateral, hemodynamically significant renal artery stenosis. In these patients, all GFR is dependent on intrarenal angiotensin II; therefore, use of ACE inhibitors may precipitate acute renal insufficiency with azotemia and oliguria.

Similar hemodynamic consequences as those produced by efferent arteriolar vasodilation may be induced by afferent arteriolar vasoconstriction. This is the main effect produced by nonsteroidal antiinflammatory agents (NSAIDs) on glomerular hemodynamics. These drugs reduce the intrarenal synthesis of prostaglandin E2 (PGE2) and PGI2, vasodilatory prostaglandins that normally counteract the vasoconstrictor

effect of angiotensin II on the afferent arteriole. Removal of this vasodilatory tone by NSAIDs leads to afferent arteriolar vasoconstriction and a fall in GFR. This is the mechanism by which NSAIDs can also lead to azotemia and acute renal failure.

Dihydropyridine calcium channel blockers preferentially dilate the afferent arteriole. Therefore, in the setting of angiotensin II-dependent maintenance of GFR, their administration has the potential to increase glomerular pressure, and, thus, injury. Nitrendipine given to rats with renovascular hypertension increased diuresis, GFR, and protein excretion, and led to increased glomerular volume and injury, despite no appreciable change in systemic arterial pressure. Pretreatment of the animals with enalapril not only reduced blood pressure, but also prevented all adverse renal events due to ensuing treatment with nitrendipine (27).

These observations make it apparent why an understanding of the relationships among glomerular hemodynamics, glomerular pressure, glomerular filtration rate, and the diverse effects of pharmacologic agents on glomerular arterioles is indispensable for the judicious use of these therapeutic agents in renovascular hypertension and renal disease in general.

Progressive renal damage of the stenosed kidney is attributable to ischemia. Chade et al. demonstrated that the clipped kidney of renovascular hypertensive pigs releases profibrotic factors and develops parenchymal fibrosis (28), concomitant with increases in PGF2α–isoprostane, a marker of oxidative stress. Isoprostane plasma levels continue to increase in the later phase of the hypertension, when renin levels have returned to normal, and they correlate with the continued increase in systemic arterial pressure (29), indicating that oxidative stress is involved in the chronic phase of renovascular hypertension. Renal fibrosis is much enhanced when these experiments are conducted in hypercholesterolemic pigs (30). This observation has improved our understanding of the mechanisms by which atherosclerotic renal artery disease, the most prevalent form of renovascular hypertension, leads to ischemic nephropathy and end-stage renal disease in patients with multiple cardiovascular risk factors.

Physiological Responses to Removal of the Stenosis

Involvement of additional counterregulatory mechanisms, unrelated to the renin–angiotensin–aldosterone system, but also participating in the pathophysiology of renal artery stenosis, was inferred from experiments in which early removal of the clip led to normalization of the hypertension. Brice et al. noticed that after removing the clip in 2K1C rats, blood pressure sustained a rapid fall in the first hour and then a more gradual one to full normalization in 24 hours (31). Surprisingly, plasma renin concentration took 3 hours to return to normal levels, and vascular tissue (aortic) levels did not normalize until 24 hours after unclipping. Because the decline in blood pressure preceded that of plasma renin, they suggested that the kidney had released a plasma vasodepressor substance on removal of the clip. Russell et al. showed that unclipping resulted in reduction of blood pressure beyond that produced by angiotensin receptor blockers (32), supporting the view that mechanisms other than normalization of the renin–angiotensin–aldosterone system participated in the decline in blood pressure produced by unclipping. Muirhead et al. attributed this effect of unclipping to a substance released from renal medullary interstitial cells that they named the antihypertensive neutral renomedullary lipid (ANRL) (33). However, this putative lipid vasodilator was never fully characterized. In contrast, others have shown that inhibitors of nitric oxide synthase significantly blunt the magnitude of the blood pressure decline following unclipping (34), indicating that nitric oxide may participate in the blood pressure response to this intervention. In summary, the current understanding of the antihypertensive effect of unclipping in 2K1C is that there is a combined effect of the reduction in the tone of the renin–angiotensin system and an increased vasodilatory effect of increased nitric oxide production and perhaps other, as-yet-unidentified vasodilators.

Causes of Renal Artery Stenosis

Atherosclerotic Renal Artery Stenosis

Atherosclerosis is the most common cause of a stenosis of the main renal arteries. The risk factors and the epidemiology are the same as those for atherosclerosis elsewhere in the body. The clinical presentation of unilateral renal artery stenosis may be that of (a) onset of new hypertension in a patient older than 55 to 60 years, when onset of essential hypertension is not that common, (b) abrupt worsening of blood pressure in a previously known hypertensive patient, and (c) progressive renal insufficiency not accounted for by the severity of hypertension or intercurrent diseases. Sudden onset or worsening of hypertension is thought to be due to plaque rupture with sudden worsening of the degree of stenosis. Bilateral disease can share all of the clinical features, but also presents as "flash" pulmonary edema because of the combination of increased afterload (hypertension) and preload (volume expansion). The diagnosis and management of atherosclerotic disease of the renal arteries are discussed in detail in Chapter 19.

Fibromuscular Dysplasia

Fibromuscular dysplasia is a noninflammatory, nonatherosclerotic vascular disease affecting medium to small vessels. It results in fibromuscular alterations in the intimal and/or medial layers of the renal artery, which produce obstruction to arterial blood flow (35–37). Figure 18.6 depicts angiograms illustrating its most common forms. Medial fibroplasia is the most common type (70% to 85% of the cases), and is almost exclusively seen in young women (diagnosis generally made between the ages of 25 and 50 years). The "string-of-beads" appearance in the angiogram is due to actual aneurysmatic dilation of multiple sections of the artery at points where the integrity of the medial layer is disrupted. Because these are real aneurysms, the "beads" are wider (i.e., of larger diameter) than the unaffected renal artery. Medial fibroplasia seldom causes progressive renal insufficiency. Angioplasty or surgical repair is indicated primarily for the relief of hypertension when it is not controlled by medical therapy.

Perimedial fibroplasia is the second-most-common type (10% to 25% of cases), is seen in younger women (ages 15 to 30 years), and is usually bilateral, with highly stenotic lesions. The "string-of-beads" appearance in this entity is due to "denting" of the lumen by hypertrophic medial fibrous tissue. That is, the "beads" are not aneurysms, but pseudoaneurysms instead. Therefore, as opposed to the angiographic aspect of medial fibroplasias, the beads of perimedial fibroplasias are smaller than (or of equal size as) the unaffected portions of the renal artery. Perimedial fibroplasia has a high rate of progression to renal failure, and angioplasty or surgical intervention is indicated for its prevention.

The previous two forms of fibromuscular dysplasia involve the main renal arteries and/or their branches in a fairly widespread manner. In contrast, two additional forms of fibromuscular dysplasia (called intimal fibroplasia and medial

Type	Frequency	Risk of progression	Threat to renal function	Description	Image
Medial fibroplasia	70%–85%	++	−	Beaded stenoses with aneurysmal dilatations larger than normal artery	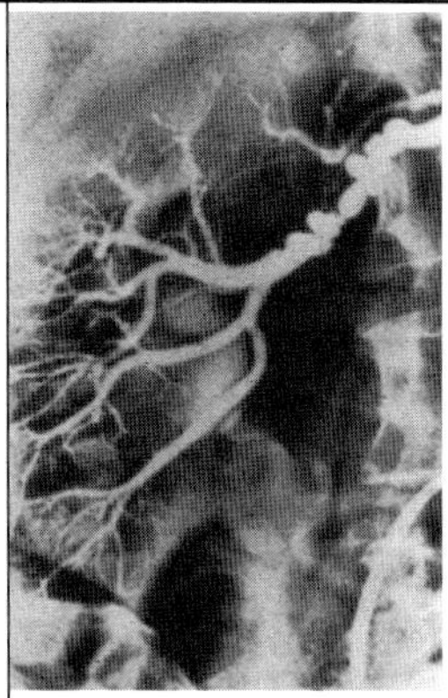
Perimedial fibroplasia	10%–25%	++++	++++	Beaded stenoses with aneurysmal dilatations smaller than normal artery	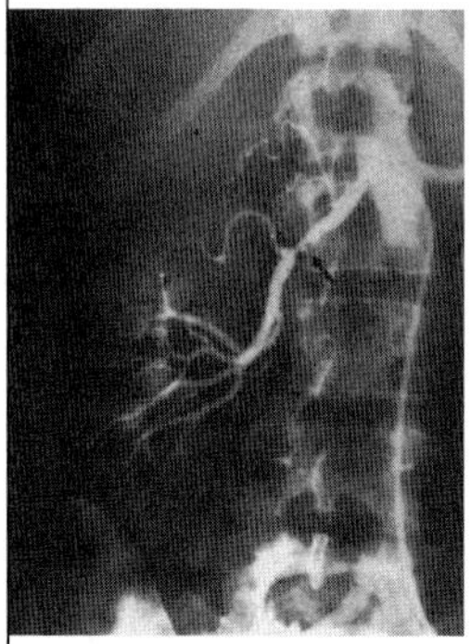
Intimal fibroplasia and medial hyperplasia	10%	++++	++++	Very tight stenoses	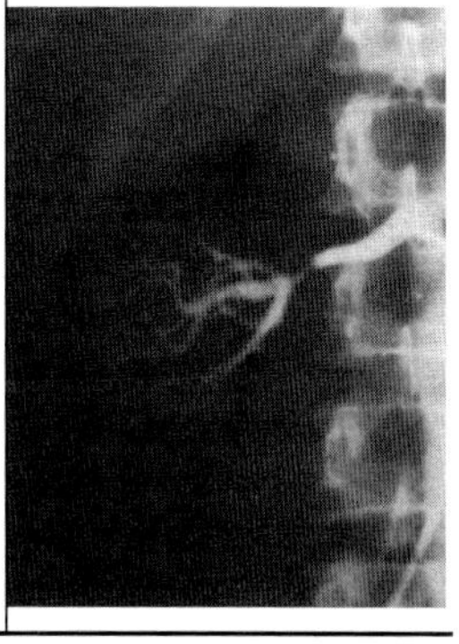

FIG. 18.6. Examples of various types of renal artery fibromuscular dysplasia, including medial fibroplasia, perimedial fibroplasia, intimal fibroplasia, and medial hyperplasia. (Images reprinted from Pohl MA. Renal artery stenosis, renal vascular hypertension and ischemic nephropathy. In: Schrier RW, Gottschalk CW, eds., *Diseases of the kidney,* 6th ed. Boston:Little Brown, 1997:1367–1427, with permission.)

hyperplasia) are characterized by a localized high-grade stenosis on angiogram. They are usually seen by pediatricians in children and adolescents, and they have a high rate of progression with total occlusion of the vessel and renal failure. Therefore, angioplasty or surgical repair is always indicated (38).

It is apparent from the clinicopathological description of the multiple forms of fibromuscular dysplasia that this disease should be suspected when the onset of hypertension occurs before the fourth decade, that is, before the usual age of onset

for essential hypertension, particularly in women, and especially in otherwise healthy individuals without atherosclerotic vascular disease. In this sense, fibromuscular dysplasia is the mirror image of atherosclerotic renal artery stenosis. The latter may produce hypertension in the middle aged or in the elderly, but must be definitely suspected when blood pressure elevation first occurs after age 60 years, particularly in an individual without family history of hypertension, or with any other manifestation or physical finding suggestive of atherosclerotic vascular disease (e.g., coronary, carotid, or femoral bruits), or with hypertension refractory to treatment.

Thromboembolic Renal Injury

Thromboembolic disease is another vascular cause of renal injury. The heart is the most common source of renal thromboemboli (39). Cardiac entities known to be complicated by renal embolism include atrial fibrillation, left ventricular intracavitary thrombi secondary to myocardial infarction or dilated cardiomyopathy, septic vegetations of bacterial endocarditis (particularly fungal), aseptic vegetations (Libman-Sacks in systemic lupus erythematosus endocarditis, and marasmic endocarditis in patients with terminal malignant disease), and the rare paradoxical emboli from deep vein thrombosis in subjects with a patent foramen ovale. In severe atherosclerotic disease of the abdominal aorta, abdominal aortic aneurysms and renal artery aneurysms can embolize into the kidney. The guide wire or the actual catheter may produce dislodgment of a plaque during diagnostic angiography or cardiac catheterization. In all these situations, embolic material may consist of a clot, dislodged fragments of an atherosclerotic plaque, or both (40–42). A microvascular form of atheroembolism, cholesterol embolism, is discussed later in this chapter.

The presenting symptoms of renal embolization depend on the size of the embolus and the extent and severity of the parenchymal involvement. Large emboli may mimic the presentation of a renal colic, with flank and abdominal pain, nausea, vomiting, and hematuria (hemorrhagic infarct) with or without associated fever. Anuric acute renal failure has been reported in bilateral massive embolism and in embolism of a solitary kidney. Oliguria can result from unilateral embolism, however, presumably secondary to spasm of the contralateral kidney. Smaller emboli (clot or plaque) may present as relatively rapid loss of renal function and refractory hypertension.

The gold standard for diagnosis of renal embolism is the renal angiogram (43), but other radiological techniques may provide enough indirect evidence when the diagnosis is suspected on clinical grounds. For example, renal ultrasound may show a triangular echogenic mass, representing a hemorrhagic infarct. Nuclear renograms and computed tomography (CT) scans with contrast will show decreased perfusion of the affected area of the kidney, with characteristic rim enhancement in the latter. These alternative tests often permit avoiding the risk of use of intravenous contrast in a condition with already compromised renal function. Angiography should therefore be reserved for the few cases in which the diagnosis is unclear despite the use of noninvasive imaging techniques, particularly when an accurate diagnosis will determine therapeutic choices.

The treatment of renal thromboembolism is long-term anticoagulation, with the duration of therapy being determined by the underlying cause and the potential for recurrent events. From a comprehensive review of the literature, Nicholas and DeMuth recommended that large unilateral emboli be also treated with intravenous, and large bilateral emboli with intraarterial, thrombolytic therapy (44). In both cases, percutaneous endovascular intervention may have to be pursued for the preservation of renal function (44).

Renal Artery Thrombosis

Renal artery thrombosis is a complication that occurs in 1% to 3% of cases of severe blunt abdominal trauma (45). It can also be the consequence of inflammatory vascular diseases and hypercoagulable states (42). Unilateral renal artery thrombosis is more common on the right renal artery, for reasons not well understood, but bilateral disease has also been reported. Clinical presentation is characterized by flank and abdominal pain associated with nausea, vomiting, and fever. Diagnosis is usually made by a CT scan that is characterized by lack of renal parenchymal enhancement with contrast and lack of visualization of the collecting system. Treatment modalities include surgical repair, thrombolytic therapy, and angioplasty.

Vasculitis

A variety of vasculitic processes involving medium-size or conduit arteries can also cause obstruction of the renal arteries (46). The characteristic involvement of the renal circulation in polyarteritis nodosa is the presence of multiple renal artery aneurysms, usually intrarenal, and in large branches of first or second order. This involvement of the renal circulation is so classic that renal angiogram is used as a diagnostic test to confirm the presence of polyarteritis nodosa, even when the disease is suspected on the basis of nonrenal, systemic manifestations. Complications of these renal aneurysms include narrowing or occlusion of the involved arterial branches.

Takayasu's arteritis is often thought of as a disease of the aortic arch and upper extremity arteries. However, it is not uncommon that the abdominal aorta and its branches are the primary locations of the disease or are involved jointly with the arch vessels. Renal artery stenosis and occlusion are often a component of Takayasu's arteritis of the abdominal aorta (47). Interpretation of the impact of the vasculitides on renal function and blood pressure is complicated by the fact that these conditions may also cause glomerulonephritis. A thorough clinical evaluation is usually needed to sort out the relative contribution of the vascular and glomerular components of the disease to the renal insufficiency and hypertension observed during the course of these disorders.

OTHER IMPORTANT CONDITIONS OF THE RENAL VASCULATURE

Renal Vein Thrombosis

Renal vein thrombosis is usually a complication of the nephrotic syndrome, especially the one produced by membranous glomerulopathy (42). Acute renal vein occlusion generally presents as acute flank pain (which may mimic a renal colic), costovertebral angle tenderness, and gross hematuria. Subacute or slowly developing occlusions may be asymptomatic and sometimes only suspected by a marked increase in the degree of proteinuria. Factors that may contribute to thrombosis of the renal veins in the setting of nephrotic syndrome include urinary loss of low–molecular-weight antithrombotic factors, increased hepatic production of prothrombotic factors, thrombocytosis, increased platelet aggregation, hemoconcentration due to edema, and thrombogenic effects of direct immunologic injury or steroid treatment.

Renal vein thrombosis has also been reported in association with trauma, oral contraceptive use, corticosteroid treatment, direct tumor extension from renal cell carcinoma, and dehydration in infants. CT scan is the diagnostic test of choice, and may show enlarged and distended renal veins or may allow for direct visualization of the thrombi. Hydronephrosis secondary to renal vein thrombosis may be detected by renal ultrasound, whereas the intravenous pyelogram will show decreased or absent visualization of the collecting system of the affected kidney. The treatment for renal vein thrombosis is long-term anticoagulation.

Atheroembolic Renal Injury

Cholesterol embolism of the kidneys, although an embolic disorder, is described separately from renal thromboembolism because it is a peculiar entity that affects the renal microcirculation and has unique clinical features. It is a complication of procedures or therapies that have the potential to dislodge or destabilize atherosclerotic plaques (e.g., arteriography, vascular surgery, anticoagulation, and thrombolytic treatment) (48), leading to embolization of cholesterol crystals. These crystals lodge in the arteriolar bed and act as foreign bodies, triggering a fibrotic inflammatory reaction, which leads to vascular injury. The clinical presentation is characterized by a triad of (a) livedo reticularis representing crystal embolization to the extremities, (b) acute renal failure representing embolization to the kidneys, and (c) eosinophilia, eosinophiluria, or both, which are manifestations of the inflammatory process. This complication must be suspected when a patient develops progressive renal dysfunction after angiography, vascular surgery, or treatment with anticoagulants or thrombolytics, and is often missed by attributing renal injury to contrast nephropathy. Clues to its diagnosis include peripheral eosinophilia (70% to 80% of cases), eosinophiluria, evidence for extrarenal embolic injury (e.g., livedo reticularis, gastrointestinal bleeding, retinal emboli), later onset than contrast nephropathy (e.g., 1 to 4 weeks after the inciting event), and continued progressive renal decline. It is more common in men than in women and in whites than in blacks. Diabetes, hypertension, aortic aneurysm, and advanced age (it is rare before age 50 years) are considered risk factors for its development. The diagnosis can be confirmed by a cutaneous or renal biopsy in which either the cholesterol crystals or the clefts left by them are

visualized. Taking the skin biopsy from a site of suspected embolic injury has a better likelihood of demonstrating the diagnosis than kidney biopsies because renal cholesterol embolism has a random spotty distribution. Although there has been the suggestion that corticosteroids and plasmapheresis may be effective treatments, results are controversial and options are limited (49). Pretreatment with statins may stabilize atherosclerotic plaques in patients at risk, but this suggestion has not been proved in prospective studies. Because anticoagulation is known to precipitate atheroembolic events, its avoidance, if at all possible, is recommended before vascular procedures.

SUMMARY

This review of the pathophysiology of renal artery stenosis and other diseases of the renal vessels is intended to provide the basic tenets on which the diagnosis and management of these patients is predicated, as is discussed in subsequent chapters of this book. In brief, we have tried to convey the following:

1. The history of the unraveling of the pathophysiology of renal artery stenosis provides much more than a mere understanding of renovascular hypertension. It was the study of this pathology that led to the current understanding of the renin–angiotensin–aldosterone system and of important mechanisms involved in hypertension and cardiovascular disease in general. Ongoing research in this field continues to uncover the participation of novel mechanisms in renal pathophysiology and its relationship with blood pressure regulation. Taking this historical background into consideration, it is clear that the physician interested in renal disease, cardiovascular disease, or hypertension must always pay attention to ongoing research in the pathophysiology of renal artery stenosis because it has the potential to continue providing novel insights into the mechanisms of these multiple disorders.

2. Specific study of the differential pathophysiology of the 2K1C and 1K1C models and the interplay between sodium and renin for blood pressure maintenance provides the clinician with an understanding of the variation in presentation, clinical features, and response to treatment observed in the diverse forms of human renovascular hypertension in its different stages. Furthermore, the same interplay between sodium and the renin–angiotensin system provides a conceptual framework for understanding essential hypertension.

3. Review of the effect of widely used agents (e.g., angiotensin converting-enzyme inhibitors, dihydropyridine calcium channel blockers, aldosterone antagonists, and nonsteroidal antiinflammatory drugs) on glomerular hemodynamics was intended to provide the clinician with the necessary ammunition for judicious use of these agents in hypertension and renal disease.

4. We also reviewed how some unresolved puzzles in the renin–angiotensin-based physiology of renal artery stenosis

(e.g., unexplained effects of unclipping) led to the discovery of counterregulatory influences mediated by systems that are now in the forefront of the understanding of multiple cardiovascular and renal function phenomena, namely the counterregulatory endothelial vasodilator system mediated by nitric oxide, and its regulation by angiotensin II-induced production of oxygen radicals and superoxide anion. Oxidative stress and endothelial dysfunction may account for many previously not fully understood phenomena, such as the establishment of an irreversible phase of renovascular hypertension and the relationship between cardiovascular risk factors and ischemic nephropathy.

5. In reviewing the most common causes of renal artery occlusive disease (atherosclerosis and fibromuscular dysplasia), we provided a brief discussion of their usual forms of presentation, clinical characteristics, differential demographics, and diagnostic features as an introduction to Chapter 19 in which these issues will be discussed in depth. Finally, we reviewed other, less common entities in which circulatory or systemic disorders compromise the renal vasculature to provide clinicians with a differential diagnostic framework that goes beyond the usual causes of renovascular disease.

REFERENCES

1. Harding MB, Smith LR, Himmelstein SI, et al. Renal artery stenosis: prevalence and associated risk factors in patients undergoing routine cardiac catheterization. *J Am Soc Nephrol* 1992;2:1608–1616.
2. Imanishi M, Akabane S, Takamiya M, et al. Critical degree of renal artery stenosis that causes hypertension in dogs. *Angiology* 1992;43:833–842.
3. Holley KE, Hunt JC, Brown Jr AL, et al. Renal artery stenosis, a clinical–pathologic study in normotensive and hypertensive patients. *Am J Med* 1964;37:14–22.
4. Sawicki PT, Kaiser S, Heinemann L, et al. Prevalence of renal artery stenosis in diabetes mellitus—an autopsy study. *J Intern Med* 1991;229:489–492.
5. Barger AC. The Goldblatt Memorial Lecture, part I: experimental renovascular hypertension. *Hypertension* 1979;1:447–455.
6. Goldblatt H, Lynch J, Hanzal RF, et al. Studies on experimental hypertension. *J Exp Med* 1933;59:347–379.
7. Gavras H, Brunner HR, Thurston H, et al. Reciprocation of renin dependency and sodium volume dependency in renal hypertension. *Science* 1975;188:1316–1317.
8. Gavras H, Brunner HR, Vaughan D, et al. Angiotensin–sodium interaction in blood pressure maintenance of renal hypertensive and normotensive rats. *Science* 1973;180:1369–1372.
9. Brown JJ, Davies DL, Morton JJ, et al. Mechanism of renal hypertension. *Lancet* 1976;1:1219–1221.
10. Anderson WP, Ramsey DE, Takata M. Development of hypertension from unilateral renal artery stenosis in conscious dogs. *Hypertension* 1990;16:441–451.
11. Martinez Y, Martinez S, Meaney Y, et al. Angiotensin II type 1 receptor blockade restores nitric oxide-dependent renal vascular responses in renovascular hypertension. *J Cardiovasc Pharmacol* 2002;40:381–387.
12. Higashi Y, Sasaki S, Nakagawa K, et al. Endothelial function and oxidative stress in renovascular hypertension. *N Engl J Med* 2002;346:1954–1962.
13. Cifuentes ME, Rey FE, Carretero OA, et al. Upregulation of p67(phox) and gp91(phox) in aortas from angiotensin II-infused mice. *Am J Physiol* 2000;279:H2234–H2240.
14. Virdis A, Nevers MF, Amiri F, et al. Spironolactone improves angiotensin-induced vascular changes and oxidative stress. *Hypertension* 2002;40:504–510.
15. Nystrom HC, Jia J, Johansson M, et al. Neurohormonal influences on maintenance and reversal of two-kidney one-clip hypertension. *Acta Physiol Scand* 2002;175:245–251.
16. Petersson MJ, Rundqvist B, Johansson M, et al. Increased cardiac sympathetic drive in renovascular hypertension. *J Hypertens* 2002;20:1181–1187.
17. Grassi G, Esler M. The sympathetic nervous system in renovascular hypertension: lead actor or "bit" player? *J Hypertens* 2002;20:1071–1073.
18. Li JS, Knafo L, Turgeon A, et al. Effects of endothelin antagonism on blood pressure and vascular structure in renovascular hypertensive rats. *Am J Physiol* 1996;271:H88–H93.
19. Elijovich F, Laffer CL. Participation of renal and circulating endothelin in salt-sensitive essential hypertension. *J Hum Hypertens* 2002;16:459–467.
20. Cecioni I, Modesti PA, Poggesi L, et al. Endothelin-1 urinary excretion, but not endothelin-1 plasma concentration, is increased in renovascular hypertension. *J Lab Clin Med* 1999;134:386–391.
21. Teunissen KE, Postma CT, van Jaarsveld BC, et al. Endothelin and active renin levels in essential hypertension and hypertension with renal artery stenosis before and after percutaneous transluminal renal angioplasty. *J Hypertens* 1997;15:1791–1796.
22. Zaporowska-Stachowiak I, Głuszek J, Chodera A. Comparison of the serum insulin and endothelin level in patients with essential and renovascular hypertension. *J Hum Hypertens* 1997;11:795–800.
23. Takeda M, Saito K, Tsutsui T, et al. Plasma endothelin-1 level in patients with renovascular hypertension—does the kidney with stenosis of the renal artery upregulate production of endothelin-1? *Eur J Med Res* 1997;2:315–320.
24. Poch E, Jimenez W, Feu F, et al. Increased plasma endothelin concentration in atherosclerotic renovascular hypertension. *Nephron* 1995;71:291–296.
25. Lerman A, Edwards BS, Hallett JW, et al. Circulating and tissue endothelin immunoreactivity in advanced atherosclerosis. *N Engl J Med* 1991;325:997–1001.
26. Eng E, Veniant M, Floege J, et al. Renal proliferative and phenotypic changes in rats with two kidney, one clip Golblatt hypertension. *Am J Hypertens* 1994;7:177–185.
27. Wenzel UO, Helmchen U, Schoeppe W, et al. Combination treatment of enalapril with nitrendipine in rats with renovascular hypertension. *Hypertension* 1994;23:114–122.
28. Chade AR, Rodriguez-Porcel M, Grande JP, et al. Distinct renal injury in early atherosclerosis and renovascular disease. *Circulation* 2002;106:1165–1171.
29. Lerman LO, Nath KA, Rodriguez-Porcel M, et al. Increased oxidative stress in experimental renovascular hypertension. *Hypertension* 2001;37:541–546.
30. Chade AR, Rodriguez-Porcel M, Grande JP, et al. Mechanisms of renal structural alterations in combined hypercholesterolemia and renal artery stenosis. *Arterioscler Thromb Vasc Biol* 2003;23:1295–1301.
31. Brice JM, Russell GI, Bing RF, et al. Surgical reversal of renovascular hypertension in rats: changes in blood pressure, plasma and aortic renin. *Clin Sci* 1983;65:33–36.
32. Russell GI, Bing RF, Thurston H, et al. Surgical reversal of two-kidney one clip hypertension during inhibition of the renin–angiotensin system. *Hypertension* 1982;4:69–76.
33. Muirhead EE, Byers LW, Pitcock JA, et al. Derivation of neutral antihypertensive lipid from renal venous effluent in rats. *Clin Sci* 1981;61:331s–333s.
34. Huang WC, Tsai RY, Fang TC. Nitric oxide modulates the development and surgical reversal of renovascular hypertension in rats. *J Hypertens* 2000;18:601–613.
35. Begelman, SM, Olin, JW. Fibromuscular dysplasia. *Curr Opin Rheumatol* 2000;12:41–47.
36. Luscher TF, Lie JT, Stanson AW, et al. Arterial fibromuscular dysplasia. *Mayo Clin Proc* 1987;62:931–952.
37. Morris CS, Rimner JM. Diagnostic and therapeutic angiography of the renal circulation. In: Schrier RW, Gottschalk CW, eds., *Diseases of the kidney*, 6th ed. Boston: Little Brown, 1997:411–434.
38. Pohl MA. Renovascular hypertension and ischemic nephropathy. In:

Wilcox C, ed., *Atlas of diseases of the kidney,* vol 3. Philadelphia: Current Medicine, 1999:3.1–3.22.

39. Hoxie HJ, Coggin CB. Renal infarction: statistical study of two hundred and five cases and detailed report of an unusual case. *Arch Intern Med* 1940;65:587–593.

40. Argiris A. Splenic and renal infarctions complicating atrial fibrillation. *Mt Sinai J Med* 1992;64:342–349.

41. Lllach F, Nikakhtar B. Renal thromboembolism, atheroembolism, and renal vein thrombosis. In: Schrier RW, Gottschalk CW, eds., *Diseases of the kidney,* 6th ed. Boston: Little Brown, 1997:411–434.

42. Yudd M, Lllach F. Vascular complications involving the renal vessels. In: Brenner BM, ed., *Brenner & Rector's the kidney,* 6th ed. Philadelphia: WB Saunders, 2000:1537–1562.

43. Peterson NE, McDonald DF. Renal embolization. *J Urol* 1968;100:140–145.

44. Nicholas GG, DeMuth WE. Treatment of renal artery embolism. *Arch Surg* 1994;119:278–285.

45. Stables DP, Porches RF, DeVillera Van Nierkerk J. Traumatic renal artery occlusion: 21 cases. *J Urol* 1974;115:229–235.

46. Balow JE, Fauci AS. Vasculitic diseases of the kidney. In: Schrier RW, Gottschalk CW, eds., *Diseases of the kidney,* 6th ed. Boston: Little Brown, 1997:1851–1878.

47. Hall S, Barr W, Lie JT, et al. Takayasu arteritis. A study of 32 North American patients. *Medicine* (Baltimore) 1985;64:89–99.

48. Dupont PJ, Lightstone L, Chitterbuck EJ, et al. Cholesterol emboli syndrome. *Br Med J* 2000;321:1065–1067.

49. Hasegawa M, Kawashima S, Shikano M, et al. The evaluation of corticosteroid therapy in conjunction with plasma exchange in the treatment of renal cholesterol embolic disease. A report of 5 cases. *Am J Nephrol* 2000;20:263–267.

CHAPTER 19

Renal Artery Stenosis

Diagnosis and Management

Michael G. Dickinson, Uma Krishnan, Greg Houlihan, and Craig M. Walker

---

Key Points

- Renal artery stenosis is a common problem in patients with vascular disease.
- Atherosclerotic renal artery stenosis is a progressive disorder, and is reflected by changes in renal function and size.
- Clinical prediction models are available that help to select which patients should be tested for renal artery stenosis.
- Noninvasive diagnostic testing for renal artery stenosis is institution dependent, but is generally either magnetic resonance angiography or duplex renal ultrasound.
- Revascularization of stenosed renal arteries can be done with angioplasty with an initial success rate of 80% to 90%.
- Angioplasty plus stenting can obtain initial technical success rates of close to 100%.
- In-stent restenosis after stenting may occur in 10% to 20% of cases, and therefore continued surveillance for recurrence is recommended.
- Revascularization is associated with reductions in blood pressure, number of medications needed for blood pressure control, and preservation of renal function in those with declining renal function.
- Initial complications of revascularization including worsening renal function can be observed, and careful technique should be followed to minimize these complications.
- Few prospective randomized clinical trials comparing medical management and revascularization have been performed, and it is hoped that ongoing trials will better define which patients are best helped by revascularization.

INTRODUCTION

Renal artery stenosis is the most common correctable cause of secondary hypertension. It results in volume expansion and can worsen congestive heart failure and can result in flash pulmonary edema. It likely plays a significant role in the development of chronic renal insufficiency and end-stage renal failure in certain patients. The hypertension from renal artery stenosis worsens the prognosis of other vascular diseases. The elevated neurohormones in renal artery stenosis have been shown to cause endothelial dysfunction and may be associated with accelerated vascular disease systemically. Renal artery stenosis is therefore an important issue for consideration in the management of any patient with vascular disease.

The causes of renal artery stenosis are listed in Table 19.1. In Chapter 18, the epidemiology and pathophysiology of renal artery stenosis and the presentation and diagnosis of the nonatherosclerotic causes of renal artery stenosis were reviewed. More than 90% of all renovascular lesions are caused by atherosclerosis (1). This chapter reviews practical aspects in the management of patients with atherosclerotic

TABLE 19.1. *Causes of renal artery stenosis*

Atherosclerosis
Fibromuscular dysplasia
Aortic or renal artery dissection
Vasculitis (Takayasu's arteritis)
Thrombotic or cholesterol embolization
Collagen vascular disease
Neurofibromatosis
Trauma
Posttransplantation stenosis
Postradiation

Adapted from Vashist A, Heller EN, Brown EJ, et al. Renal artery stenosis: a cardiovascular perspective. *Am Heart J* 2002;143:559–564.

renal artery stenosis. We review the natural history of the disease, detection and screening for the disease, and options for management of the disease. We consider the risks and benefits of revascularization and some of the debate that has centered around it.

GENERAL CHARACTERISTICS OF ATHEROSCLEROTIC RENAL ARTERY STENOSIS

Atherosclerotic renal artery stenosis is generally ostial in nature. The site of the stenosis is not specific to the renal artery, and commonly involves the adjacent portion of the abdominal aorta as well. The stenosis most commonly affects the proximal 2 cm of the renal artery. Bifurcation sites also are common locations for stenosis. Distal renal artery or branch involvement is uncommon. In patients over 50 years of age, bilateral disease is common (2). As discussed in Chapter 18, the incidence and prevalence in the general population are difficult to ascertain, but may be about 4% (3). The prevalence in patients with other evidence of vascular disease is likely higher (25% to 50%), as given in Table 19.2.

NATURAL HISTORY

Atherosclerotic renal artery stenosis (RAS) is a chronic and progressive disease. Most studies (over a variable follow-up period) estimate the risk of radiological progression of

TABLE 19.2. *Prevalence of renal artery stenosis in select populations*

Patient population studied	Prevalence (%)
Patients who died while hospitalized	27
Routine cardiac catheterization patients	25
Patients having peripheral angiography	50
Patients starting renal dialysis	16–20
Patients older than age 60 years on dialysis	25–30

Adapted from McLaughlin K, Jardine AG, Moss JG. ABC of arterial and venous disease—renal artery stenosis. *BMJ* 2000;320:1124–1128.

atheromatous renal artery stenosis to be about 50%. The risk is dependent on the initial severity of the lesion. The rate of total occlusion of a renal artery with greater than 60% stenosis is about 5% a year (2). Progression of renal artery stenosis may not be clinically evident, as adequacy of blood pressure control does not necessarily reflect progression of disease. Declining renal function (increasing serum creatinine) or decreasing renal size may, however, be a better marker for progression. In a retrospective series of 85 patients with RAS followed for 52 months, 44% demonstrated progression of RAS, and 16% demonstrated progression to total occlusion (4). Reduction in kidney size and increase in serum creatinine were good clinical markers for progressive atherosclerotic renal artery disease, but adequacy of blood pressure (BP) control was not. The likelihood of progression was higher for those with a baseline stenosis greater than 75% than for those with lesser degrees of stenosis. A prospective study used duplex ultrasound follow-up on 84 patients (139 arteries) who did not have revascularization, and showed 42% progression at 2 years. The total occlusion rate at 2 years was 11% (5). Patients with bilateral renal artery stenosis are more likely to develop renal insufficiency, and those who have an occluded renal artery are at high risk for progression to end-stage renal failure. Patients with bilateral disease who have one of the arteries completely occluded have a rate of end-stage renal failure of 50% at 2 years. The rate of loss of functional renal tissue (implied by loss of renal size of greater than 1 cm at 1 year after diagnosis) is about three times higher for patients with bilateral disease than for those with unilateral disease (43% vs. 13%) (2).

DIAGNOSIS OF RENAL ARTERY STENOSIS

Clinical Presentation

The first step in the diagnosis of renal artery stenosis is to consider the diagnosis. Patients with renal artery stenosis may present with hypertension, renal insufficiency, or acute pulmonary edema. Clinical examination often shows bruits over major vessels, including the abdominal aorta (a feature of widespread atherosclerosis), although the classic finding of lateralizing bruits over the renal arteries is uncommon. Renal artery stenosis can be predicted just as accurately by key clinical parameters such as advanced age, recent onset of hypertension, female sex, presence of atherosclerosis, smoking, abdominal bruits, elevated creatinine, and hypercholesterolemia. Figure 19.1 compares the characteristics of patients with renal artery stenosis with patients with essential hypertension. Renal artery stenosis should be a consideration in any patient with vascular disease who has significant hypertension.

Importance of Patient Selection for Testing

For a screening test it is important to consider the sensitivity, specificity, and predictive values of the investigation as well as prevalence of the target disease in the population to

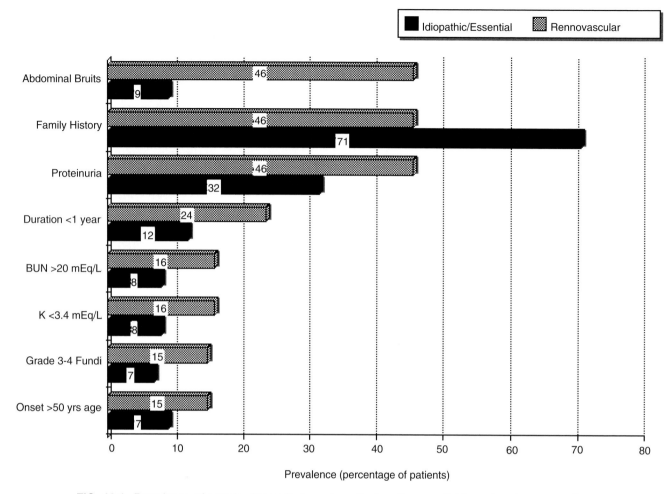

FIG. 19.1. Prevalence of certain clinical features in patients with essential hypertension versus those with renovascular hypertension. Presence of abdominal bruits, proteinuria, recent onset of hypertension, and comcomitant renal insufficiency is suggestive of renal artery stenosis. Family history of hypertension is more suggestive of essential hypertension. BUN, blood urea nitrogen; K, serum potassium. (Adapted from Simon N, Franklin SS, Bleifer KH, et al. Clinical characteristics of renovascular hypertension. *JAMA* 1972;220:1209–1218.)

be screened. In a nonselected hypertensive population, the prevalence of renovascular hypertension (RVH) is low (1% to 5%). For an investigation with a sensitivity and specificity of 90%, such a low prevalence results in the investigation having only a 20% positive predictive value. This is diagrammed in Fig. 19.2. As the disease prevalence increases, the predictive value of the test improves. For this reason guidelines have been published to suggest which patients have a high enough pretest probability of disease to warrant testing. Table 19.3 lists the Joint National Committee (JNC) VI guidelines for screening (6). One portion of the Dutch Renal Artery Stenosis Intervention Cooperative (DRASTIC) trial was designed to find an optimal strategy for diagnosing renal artery stenosis in their population of 1,133 hypertensive patients. These patients with preserved renal function were referred for analysis because of difficult-to-treat hypertension or creatinine elevations with attempted treatment with angiotensin-converting enzyme (ACE) inhibitors (7). Using factors including smoking

TABLE 19.3. *Joint National Committee VI guidlines for clinical clues to renal artery stenosis*

Onset of hypertension before age 30 years, especially without a family history, or recent onset of significant hypertension after age 55 years
An abdominal bruit, particularly if it continues into diastole and is lateralized
Accelerated or resistant hypertension
Recurrent (flash) pulmonary edema
Renal failure of uncertain cause, especially with a normal urinary sediment
Coexisting diffuse atherosclerotic vascular disease, especially in heavy smokers
Acute renal failure precipitated by antihypertensive therapy, with angiotensin-converting enzyme inhibitors or angiotensin receptor blockers

Adapted from The sixth report of the Joint National Committee on Prevention, Detection, Evaluation, and Treatment of High Blood Pressure. *Arch Intern Med* 1997;152:2413–2446.

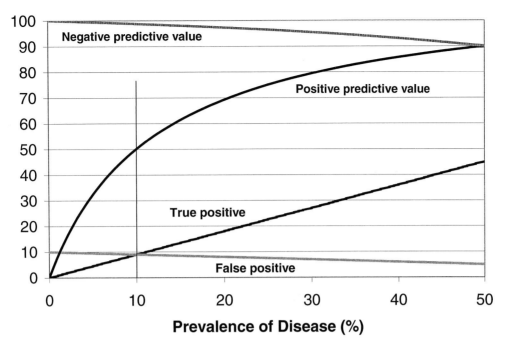

FIG. 19.2. Impact of disease prevalence on the rate of false positives and true positives with a test with 90% sensitivity and 90% specificity. At low prevalence of disease, false positives become much more significant. Even with 90% sensitivity, in populations with a prevalence of 10% or less, those who test positive are as likely not to have disease as they are to have disease. As the pretest probability improves, so does the predictive value of the test. Screening tests for renal artery stenosis should be reserved for those patient populations with >30% prevalence of disease.

status, age, body mass index, and serum creatinine, they devised an algorithm to screen for renal artery stenosis. They developed a clinical prediction rule that had a 72% sensitivity and a 90% specificity (about those of renal scintigraphy).

The number of coronary arteries with significant stenosis is also an independent predictor of RAS, with a relative risk of 2.1 (each diseased coronary artery doubles the likelihood that renal artery stenosis is present) (8). Other vascular diseases are a strong predictor of the presence of disease. In a study of 395 vascular disease patients, the prevalence of RAS was 38% in patients with abdominal aortic aneurysm, 33% in those with aortoiliac occlusive disease, 39% in those with lower extremity occlusive disease, and 50% if the diagnosis was suspected prior to the angiogram (9). Therefore, difficult-to-control hypertension or progressive renal insufficiency in these patient populations should raise a high clinical suspicion for renal artery stenosis.

Diagnostic Tests

Investigative tests include color duplex ultrasonography, captopril renography, magnetic resonance arteriography (MRA), and spiral computed tomography (CT). The standard against which all tests are compared is selective renal arteriography.

Regardless of which test is used, the degree of stenosis that is regarded as significant remains controversial. The value of greater than 75% stenosis is operationally used by most clinicians to indicate a significant stenosis. It is important to appreciate that relying on the degree of stenosis to make a management decision should be treated with caution because other factors contribute to pressure reduction, such as length of stenosis, contour, and distal vascular resistance. Limitations in the use of degree of stenosis are highlighted by the fact that not every patient with RAS has renovascular hypertension. The sensitivity and specificity of some of these tests are summarized in Table 19.4. Each of these tests is reviewed in turn.

TABLE 19.4. Screening tests for renal artery disease

Test	Sensitivity (%)	Specificity (%)
Captopril-stimulated plasma renin activity	73–100	72–95
Renal vein renin	64	87
Captopril renography	90–93	93–98
Intravenous urography	59	89
Duplex and Doppler sonography	84–95	81–98

From The sixth report of the Joint National Committee on Prevention, Detection, Evaluation and Treatment of High Blood Pressure. *Arch Intern Med* 1997;152:2413–2446.

Captopril Renography

Renal scanning with [99m]technetium-diethylenetriamine-pentacetic acid (^{99m}Tc-DTPA) (10) and [99m]technetium-mercaptoacetyl triglycerine ^{99m}Tc-MAG$_3$ (11) is both noninvasive and safe even in patients with renal insufficiency. ^{99m}Tc-DTPA is filtered by the kidney and not reabsorbed, and therefore may serve as a marker for glomerular filtration rate, whereas ^{99m}Tc-MAG$_3$ is both filtered and secreted into the tubules, and may serve as a marker for renal plasma flow. The rationale of performing scans after ACE inhibition derives from the fact that reduction of angiotensin II in the stenotic kidney reduces the glomerular filtration rate (GFR) by reducing efferent arteriolar vasoconstriction, resulting in delayed isotope excretion. The accuracy of this test decreases in patients with increasing serum creatinine values, particularly in excess of 180 μmol/L (12). Captopril renograms have been criticized in that patients (who often have difficult-to-control hypertension) need to be off of angiotensin II inhibition or blockade for a period of time prior to the testing. Furthermore, recent reports have suggested that captopril renography may not be as sensitive or specific in actual practice as previously reported (13). One such review, of 89 patients who underwent both captopril renography and renal angiography, demonstrated a sensitivity of 74% and a specificity of only 59%. The patient population studied had a high prevalence of renal artery stenosis (43%). In spite of this, the positive predictive value was only 58% and the negative predictive value only 75% (14). Based on this study as well as the availability of better, easier-to-perform tests, the captopril renogram is no longer one of the diagnostic tests of choice for renal artery stenosis.

Duplex Ultrasonography

Color and power Doppler (ultrasonic duplex scanning with pulsed-wave Doppler) is a very popular and commonly used screening tool. It has the advantage of providing information on renal arterial blood flow as well as structural data on the kidneys (size, anomalies, etc.) in a painless, noninvasive method without contrast exposure. Further, it can be done for follow-up in patients who have had metal stents implanted. Two types of Doppler ultrasound criteria are used for the detection of RAS (15). Proximal criteria rely on the Doppler-determined peak systolic velocity (after angle correction) and the renal–aortic ratio (RAR) of peak systolic velocities (ratio of peak renal systolic velocity to peak aortic systolic velocity). The usual standards for this measure are noted in Table 19.5 (16). If the peak systolic velocity in the abdominal aorta

TABLE 19.5. *Doppler criteria for diagnosis of renal artery stenosis*[a]

Renal artery stenosis	Renal artery PSV	Renal to aortic ratio of PSV
Proximal criteria[b]		
Normal (0%)	<180 cm/s	<3.5
<60%	≥180 cm/s	<3.5
≥60%	< or ≥180 cm/s	≥3.5
Occlusion (100%)	No signal	No signal
Distal criteria		
Renal artery Doppler pressure rise time		
Normal (no signficant stenosis)	<0.07s	
Abnormal (stenosis likely present)	>0.07s	
Renal resistive index[c]		
Normal (resistance due to distal microvasculature) >0.45		
Abnormal (stenosis likely present; resistance due to proximal macrovasculature)	<0.45	

[a]The proximal criteria have demonstrated validity in the prediction of renal artery stenosis. The distal criteria are less well developed, but may be helpful in predicting which patients might respond to revascularization. A high renal resistive index suggests that the resistance to blood flow is present in both systole and diastole, and implicates resistance in the microvasculature (sum of the glomeruli, etc.) Such microvasculature resistance is what would be expected in chronic renal diseases such as diabetic nephropathy and hypertensive nephrosclerosis and thus patients with such a high index likely have other renal disorders, which will prevent improvement of hypertension or reduction of renal failure with macrovascular revascularization procedures.

[b]PSV, Peak systolic velocity.

[c]Determine Doppler end diastolic velocity (EDV) and maximal systolic velocity (MSV), and calculate renal resistive index (RRI) by RRI = 1 − (EDV/MSV). A difference of 0.15 in the RRI between kidneys is suggestive of a unilateral renal artery stenosis (stenosis in the kidney with the lower RRI).

Adapted from Rundback JH, Sacks D, Kent KC, et al. Guidelines for the reporting of renal artery revascularization in clinical trials. *J Vasc Interv Radiol* 2002;13:959–974.

is low (less than 40 cm per second), the RAR cannot be used, and identification of an at-least 60% renal artery stenosis is based on the finding of a localized high-velocity jet and post-stenotic turbulence. The sensitivity and specificity of duplex ultrasonography are quite variable and are technician dependent, but in an experienced hand both are somewhere between 80% and 95%. A recent study by Olin et al. demonstrated a sensitivity of 98%, a specificity of 98%, positive predictive value of 99%, and a negative predicative value of 97% for duplex ultrasound when compared to renal angiography (17).

The distal (or intraparenchymal) criteria are related to a slow rise of the peak velocity on pulsed-wave Doppler analysis distal to the stenosis. This is similar to the phenomena of pulsus tardus et parvus noted with aortic stenosis. It is measured as a prolonged time to peak systolic velocity (a rise time of greater than 0.07 seconds is abnormal) (16). The time to peak systolic velocity has not, however, been proven to be as reliable an indicator as the proximal criterion (the RAR) (18). What has been thought to be of value is the use of the renal resistive index. The calculation of the renal resistive index is reviewed in Table 19.5. This index is meant to reflect the vascular tone (resistance) in the microvasculature of the kidney beyond the level of the renal artery stenosis. If the resistive index is high, this would suggest that there is significant renovascular disease unrelated to the renal artery stenosis, such as would be seen with hypertensive nephrosclerosis. A renal resistive index of greater than 0.8 has been shown to predict those patients who will not have improved blood pressure or renal function from correction of a renal artery stenosis (19). A renal resistive index of less than 0.45 is suggestive of the diagnosis of renal artery stenosis, and a difference in the resistive index of greater than 0.15 between kidneys is suggestive of a unilateral renal artery stenosis (stenosis in the kidney with the lower resistive index) (16).

Magnetic Resonance Angiography

Magnetic resonance angiography (MRA) is a noninvasive technique that requires neither ionizing radiation nor nephrotoxic contrast. MRA has been advocated as a screening test in high-risk individuals with impaired renal function (20). It has the advantage of being able to provide direct visualization of proximal renal artery lesions as well as an assessment of renal size. It also has the capability of providing information on blood flow rate and GFR (21). Results are best for proximal lesions, however, and more-distal lesions (beyond the first half) and accessory renal arteries were traditionally missed, although sensitivity has continued to improve. It is thought to have a sensitivity of 90% to 100% (15). In practice MRA tends to err on the side of sensitivity with a potential for false positives, but this is also becoming less prevalent as better technology and software continue to be developed. As another benefit of MRA, one study using MRA demonstrated that patients who had MRA prior to renal artery angioplasty had reduced contrast exposure and shorter procedure durations. This suggests that MRA can provide important information in procedural planning that may reduce contrast exposure and improve procedural success (22). The primary limitations of MRA tend to be availability and cost.

Spiral Computed Tomography Angiography

Spiral computed tomography (CT) provides good visualization of the renal blood supply and is minimally invasive (23,24). The main drawback is that the contrast injection has to be maintained over a 20- to 30-second period, resulting in large contrast volumes of 130 to 150 mL. The risk of nephrotoxicity in high-risk patients is substantial. It should probably not be considered in patients with a creatinine greater than 3.0 mg per dL. It is, however, considered to be one of the best tests for sensitivity and specificity.

Blood Tests

Various tests have been used to assess for RAS serologically. The simplest test is to observe for an increase in serum creatinine with ACE-inhibitor treatment. Plasma renin levels have also been measured (especially by looking at captopril-augmented plasma renin activity). Renal vein renin sampling for lateralization has been used. Unfortunately, none of these tests has proved to have a sufficient sensitivity or specificity to advocate their routine use.

Which Test is the Best Noninvasive Test?

Figure 19.3 demonstrates the reciever-operator characteristic curves from a meta-analysis of 66 different trials for the commonly used tests (25). The highest diagnostic accuracies were obtained from CT angiography and gadolinium-enhanced MRA. Ultrasonography was not as good as MRA or CT angiography, but was better than captopril renography. There was, however, considerable variability in the reported sensitivity and specificity for ultrasonography, reflecting the fact that these techniques may be center and operator dependent. In deciding on the best test for an individual patient, it is important to consider then the local availability and reliability of each of these tests, as well as the patients ability to tolerate the intravenous contrast of CT angiography and the confinement and costs of magnetic resonance imaging/MRA. In most centers, MRA and renal duplex ultrasonography have become the standards for screening, depending on test availability and technician expertise.

MANAGEMENT OF RENAL ARTERY STENOSIS

Medical Management

Good medical management is an important part of the care of a RAS patient. This includes tight blood pressure control with the use of ACE inhibitors or angiotension blockers as long as these medications do not cause significant azotemia. Minor increases in creatinine or small declines in GFR are not considered a contraindication to the use of these agents, but

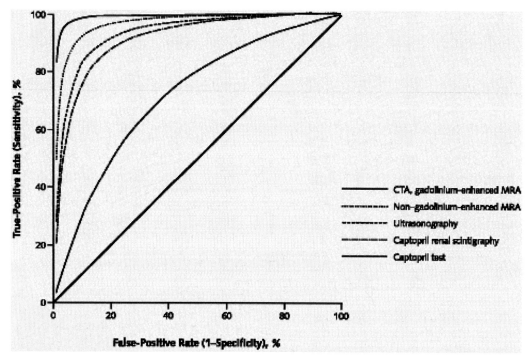

FIG. 19.3. Reciever-operator curves for noninvasive tests for renal artery stenosis. Computed tomography angiography (CAT) and gadolinium-enhanced magnetic resonance angiography (MRA) both have the highest diagnostic reliability, followed closely by non-gadolinium-enhanced MRA and then ultrasonography. (From Boudewijn G, Vasbinder C, Nelemans J, et al. Diagnostic tests for renal artery stenosis in patients suspected of having renovascular hypertension: a meta-analysis. *Ann Intern Med* 2001;135:401–411, with permission.)

an increase of creatinine of greater than 0.5 mg per dL with start of the medication is generally thought severe enough to not use the medication (26). Salt restriction and diuretic use may improve the effectiveness of angiotensin blockade in controlling blood pressure because these patients are generally volume expanded, and reduction of sodium and volume status may restore the effectiveness of angiotensin blockade. Bilateral renal artery stenosis and RAS in an individual with a single kidney will be more likely to present with azotemia with ACE inhibition, and these conditions represent a relative contraindication to angiotensin II blockade/inhibition. Aggressive risk factor modifications such as tight control of lipids and smoking cessation are important. It is also important to understand that these patients are at high risk for other vascular events, including coronary artery disease and myocardial infarction (27), and therefore cardiovascular risk factor modification, antiplatelet treatment, and vigilance for concomitant coronary or peripheral vascular disease are indicated.

Revascularization

The Debate: To Revascularize Or Not?

Revascularization is controversial. Everyone agrees that an open renal artery is better than a closed renal artery, but the debate centers around whether opening the artery will be associated with any change in clinical outcome (or perhaps

might be associated with clinical worsening.) The current Medicare-approved indications for revascularization are as follows:

1. Diastolic blood pressure greater than 100 mm Hg on three or more medications
2. Episodes of flash pulmonary edema
3. Progressive renal dysfunction
4. Unstable angina with resistant hypertension

Options available for renal artery revascularization include surgery (endarterectomy, aortorenal bypass) and percutaneous transluminal angioplasty with or without stent deployment. Balloon angioplasty of the renal arteries was first performed by Gruntzig (28) in 1978 and remains the treatment of choice for fibromuscular dysplasia. With the advent of stenting, angioplasty and stenting has gradually superseded surgery as a treatment of choice for atherosclerotic renal artery stenosis (29). The judgment of success or failure of revascularization is based on two issues: (a) technical success in reopening and maintaining an open vessel, and (b) improvement in clinical status (hypertension or renal insufficiency).

Technical Success

The technical success of balloon angioplasty without stenting is between 80% and 90% with limitations because of the high incidence of ostial disease. Angioplasty plus stenting

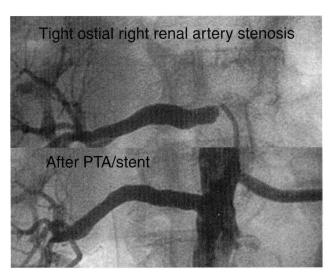

FIG. 19.4. Angiogram of severe right renal artery stenosis and the results obtained from renal percutaneous transluminal artery (PTA) angioplasty and stent placement. (Images used by permission of J. K. Ford, MD, The Heart Group, Padukah, Kentucky.)

achieves much higher technical success (Figs. 19.4 and 19.5). A meta-analysis in the early 1990s found the overall rate of residual stenosis (greater than 50%) from balloon angioplasty without stenting was 12% (30). The largest review of balloon angioplasty and stenting looked at 1,417 angioplasties carried out in 20 centers with significant experience in renal interventional procedures. That study showed a higher over-

all rate of technical failure of angioplasty of 30%. The failure rate in ostial stenoses was even higher at 45%. In that series, 563 cases of RAS treated with angioplasty plus stenting had much better technical success, with an initial success rate approaching 100% (31). In-stent restenosis (neointimal proliferation), however, was a problem occurring in 23% of the cases. Two other studies noted restenosis rates of 11% (32) (on ultrasound at 6 months) and 19% (33) (on angiogram at 8 months). In summary, because of recoil and the ostial nature of renal artery stenosis, the initial technical success of balloon angioplasty is about 80% to 90%. With modern stenting techniques, an excellent technical result (approaching 100%) can be obtained, but with around 10% to 20% incidence of in-stent restenosis. Renal stent restenosis can usually be treated with repeat angioplasty or expansion of a second stent inside the original stent, but this suggests that vigilance is warranted for the occurrence of such restenosis. Follow-up is generally done by duplex ultrasonography at 6 months after revascularization and then annually thereafter. Drug-eluting stents, now in use for coronary disease, may become a therapeutic intervention for RAS in the future.

Complications

The reported complications of renal artery angioplasty and stenting include reduction in renal function (azotemia), cholesterol embolization, renal infarction, renal artery dissection, and renal hematoma. The complication rate has been reported at 23%, with a 4% rate of serious complications (embolization, renal infarcts, and serious renal artery dissection) (31). The primary complication making up most of the 23% is observed reduction in renal function following renal artery revascularization. This azotemia is thought to result from a combination of contrast nephropathy and microembolization of atheromatous material with engagement of the guide catheter. The complication rate is one of the key factors now influencing the balance of overall benefit from revascularization. If there was a 0% incidence of postrevascularization azotemia or decline of renal function, there would be a lot more enthusiasm for revascularizing patients. It is therefore essential to consider the causes of the complications and what can be done to minimize them.

Prevention of Embolization of Atheromatous Material

Keeley and Grines demonstrated in coronary angiography that scraping of visible aortic debris is common (greater than 50% of the time) (34). This incidence could be higher with renal angiography and intervention because of the highly atherosclerotic nature of the abdominal aorta. Furthermore, atheromatous microemboli may be clinically silent in the coronary circulation, but could trigger significant glomerular injury in the kidneys. We suggest that this complication might be avoided (or minimized) by following the approach outlined in Fig. 19.6. This approach tends to avoid catheter manipulation in the abdominal aorta, which generally has a higher burden of atheromatous plaque. Meticulous

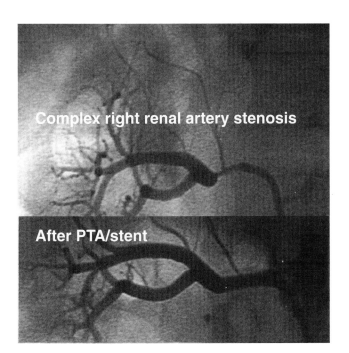

FIG. 19.5. Angiogram of complex renal artery stenosis and the results obtained from renal percutaneous transluminal artery (PTA) angioplasty and stent placement. (Images used by permission of J. K. Ford, MD, The Heart Group, Padukah, Kentucky.)

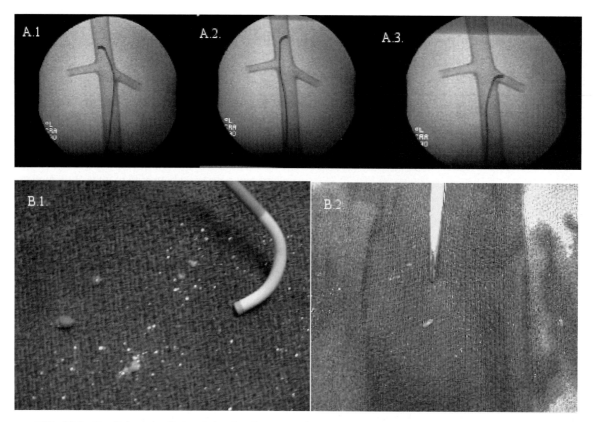

FIG. 19.6. Cardiology Institute of the South approach to renal artery revascularization in to minimize atheroemboli. **A.1–A.3:** All manipulations of the guide catheter should be done in the thoracic aorta, which is generally less atherosclerotic and therefore less likely to dislodge atheromatous material. These images show rotation of the guide catheter being done in the thoracic aorta and then being slowly withdrawn to engage the renal artery. **B.1, B.2:** All catheters should be fully aspirated with the aspirate being pushed down the waste port prior to injecting into the renal artery. These images demonstrate debris collected from the aspiration of guide catheters during renal artery intervention. (Images are courtesy of Dr. Craig Walker.)

attention to catheter aspiration and flushing the aspirate into the waste port will reduce the amount of atheromatous material injected down the renal artery. In the future, distal protection devices such as a filter wire or balloon obstruction devices may become commonplace in renal artery interventions and reduce this complication further, which likely will improve outcomes.

Prevention of Contrast Nephropathy

In some of the classic clinical trials, the amounts of contrast that were used were quite high (on the order of 150 to 200 cc). In common practice, efforts should be made to minimize contrast exposure. It is not uncommon to be able to perform a renal artery intervention with as little as 15 to 20 cc of contrast. To achieve this, however, bony landmarks must be used for catheter and stent positioning instead of multiple contrast injections. Exploiting the data provided by previously obtained noninvasive imaging studies is helpful and reduces the number of diagnostic angiograms and the amount of contrast used (22). Hydration before and after the procedure and possibly the use of *n*-acetylcysteine may fur-

ther help to reduce this complication (especially if higher contrast use is expected).

Therapeutic Results

Several series have published promising results from renal artery angioplasty and stenting in terms of improved hypertension control and prevention of loss of renal function. Ziakka and colleagues followed 107 consecutive hypertensive patients with atheromatous RAS treated with renal percutaneous transluminal angioplasty (PTA) for 12 months (35). Following treatment, blood pressure fell to normal levels in 10 (8.8%) patients and improved in 76 (67.3%), and renal function improved or remained stable in 74% of patients. Renal PTA proved most beneficial in atheromatous RAS patients with stenosis in a single functioning kidney as well as in those who presented with signs of sodium and water retention, such as that seen in patients with signs of heart failure.

Lederman et al. reported a series of 363 procedures using angioplasty and stenting (36). In this series there was excellent technical success, with a good result in 100% of the procedures. Postprocedure azotemia occurred in 12%, but persisted in only 2%. Overall renal function in those with baseline renal insufficiency, improved in 19%, remained stable in 54%, and deteriorated in 27%. There was a significant reduction in systolic and diastolic blood pressure from an average of 164 mm Hg to 142 mm Hg ($p<0.001$) over the approximately 16 months of follow-up (36).

One of the largest series on the effectiveness of renal artery stenting comes from Dorros et al. and the Multicenter Registry (37). This registry was a voluntary multicenter registry of Palmaz–Schatz stent revascularization of 1,058 patients followed over 4 years of follow-up (37). The participants in this registry had significant reductions in systolic blood pressure (from 168 ± 27 to 147 ± 21 mm Hg), diastolic blood pressure (84 ± 15 to 78 ± 12 mm Hg), and the number of blood pressure medications (2.4 ± 1.2 to 2.0 ± 1.0, $p<0.05$) used. Serum creatinine decreased from 1.7 ± 1.2 to 1.3 ± 0.8 mg per dL. Those patients with poor renal function and bilateral disease had a poor survival, and revascularization did not seem to improve their survival. The rest of the patients seemed to benefit from the procedure.

The results of ten descriptive studies of renal artery stenting (416 arteries, 379 patients) were reviewed by Isles et al. (38) Initial technical success was high, at 96% to 100%. Restenosis rates at 6 to 12 months were about 16%. Hypertension was cured in 9%. Renal function improved in 26%, stabilized in 48%, and deteriorated in 26%. They also noted that if renal function had been declining prior to the stenting, the rate of decline seemed to be slowed by stenting. This trend of slowing of decline of renal function in those patients who have declining renal function has been supported by two other trials. Watson et al. observed an improvement in renal function after stenting in 18 of 33 patients, and the decline in function was slowed or stopped in the rest (39). Beutler et al. followed 63 patients who were stented, and noted this same benefit in those with declining renal function (40). In those, however, who had stable renal dysfunction prior to the procedure, stenting did not seem to provide any benefit (40).

Unfortunately, there have not been many randomized controlled trials on the benefits or risks of renal artery revascularization. Those that have been done have shown improvements in the ability to manage hypertension, but have not demonstrated improvements in the harder endpoints of mortality or morbidity (41). The DRASTIC study group (42) performed a prospective randomized trial of renal angioplasty versus medical management in 106 patients with renal artery stenosis and difficult-to-manage hypertension or documented creatinine increase with ACE-inhibitor treatment. The angioplasty-treated patients ended up needing fewer medications for treatment of their hypertension (2.1 vs. 3.2, $p<0.001$). There was no difference, however, in the blood pressure control obtained or in renal function between the two groups. The investigators concluded that, "In the treatment of patients with hypertension and renal-artery stenosis, angioplasty has little advantage over antihypertensive-drug therapy." There were, however, several problems with this study, including the fact that it was held at 26 centers, averaging only two patients at each center,

over a 6-year period. Furthermore, many of the patients had less than critical stenosis (10% had less than 50% stenosis), and nearly half of the medical therapy cohort ended up having angioplasty after the first 3 months because of failure to control blood pressure or decreased renal function.

The Scottish and Newcastle Renal Artery Stenosis Collaborative Group randomized 55 patients with diastolic blood pressure greater than 95 mm Hg on two or more medications and 50% stenosis of a renal artery to stenting versus continued medical management. The stented group had a statistically greater drop in blood pressure ($p<0.05$, with blood pressure drop corrected for the medical group response of 26/10 mm Hg). There was, however, no difference in major outcome events (death, myocardial infarction, heart failure, stroke, or dialysis) in the stent group (43).

Renal artery angioplasty and stenting for improvement of hypertension may not always be successful. The reasons for this failure of benefit are likely threefold:

1. Many patients may be in a later stage of the disease and will have already developed hypertensive nephrosclerotic changes (especially in the contralateral kidney), and thus even with restored renal flow, the physiology (of hypertensive renal insufficiency) to perpetuate the hypertension is still in place. It is possible that earlier intervention may have proved beneficial. Furthermore, in the future, use of certain noninvasive indicators such as the ultrasound-derived renal resistive index may help to predict those more likely to respond to revascularization.

2. Some patients may not have hypertension as a result of renal artery stenosis. As reviewed in Chapter 18, patients with essential hypertension often have atherosclerotic vascular disease and may have renal artery stenosis that was not the cause of their hypertension. In some of the studies, revascularization was performed for stenosis of greater than 50%, even though many experts suggest that hypertension does not result until a stenosis is greater than 70%. Perhaps better results would be obtained if revascularization is reserved for those with a higher degree of stenosis.

3. Medical management of hypertension has improved to the point where the various medications available are good enough to get blood pressure control in spite of the renal artery stenosis. Such medical management may prevent the end-organ damage of uncontrolled hypertension, but does not appear to be as beneficial in preserving renal function in patients who are experiencing a decline in renal function.

In summary, percutaneous angioplasty without stenting obtains a technically good result approximately 80% to 90% of the time. Addition of stenting increases this success rate to close to 100%, but in-stent restenosis can be expected to occur in about 10% to 20% of cases. Blood pressure control generally improves postrevascularization with a reduced need for blood pressure medications. "Cure" of hypertension is observed in less than 10% of those revascularized. Renal function can be improved or the rate of decline of renal

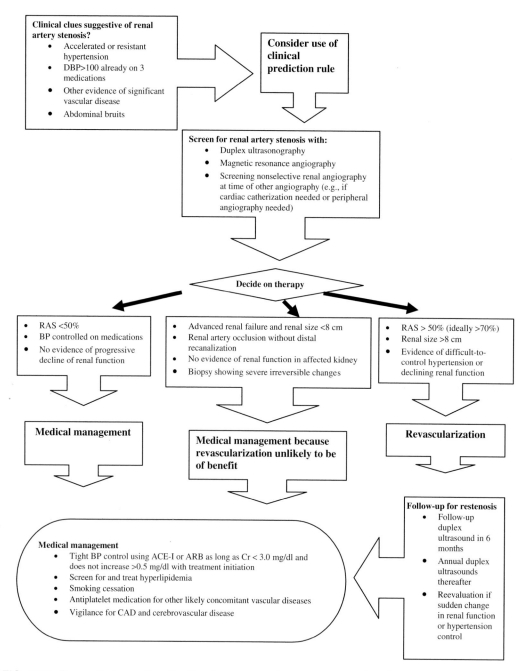

FIG. 19.7. Suggested algorithm for the diagnosis and management of patients with suspected renal artery stenosis. DBP, Diastolic blood pressure; RAS, renal artery stenosis; BP, blood pressure; ACE-I, angiotensin-converting enzyme inhibitor; ARB, angiotensin receptor blocker; Cr, creatinine; CAD, coronary artery disease. (Adapted from Jaff MR. Hypertension and renal artery stenosis: a complex clinical scenario. *J Am Osteopath Assoc* 2002;100[10]S5–S9; and McLaughlin K, Jardine AG, Moss JG. ABC of arterial and venous disease—renal artery stenosis. *BMJ* 2000;320:1124–1128; with permission.)

function slowed, and this appears to be especially beneficial in those with declining renal function. Approximately one-fourth of patients will experience a decline in renal function after revascularization, and this may reflect complications from the procedure (atheroemboli, contrast nephropathy), or may just reflect the continued course of their renal disease. Improvements in technique as described here may, however, reduce this complication rate significantly. Figure 19.7 is a

summary of the recommended diagnostic and therapeutic measures that should be considered for a patient with suspected renal artery stenosis.

Surgical versus Percutaneous Revascularization

Weibull et al. studied 58 patients with unilateral RAS (lesion less than 1 cm from aorta), positive renal vein renins, and severe hypertension, and randomized them to PTA (no stents) or surgery (44). This was followed by routine angiography after 2 years. The initial technical success was higher with surgery than PTA (97% vs. 83%, *p*=0.19), as was the 2-year primary patency (96% vs. 75%, *p*=0.05). The secondary patency (allowing one additional surgery or PTA) was comparable (97% vs. 90%, *p*=0.61) between surgery and PTA. The overall clinical outcome was not different between the groups, however. The rate of hypertension being improved or cured was 90% for PTA and 86% for surgery. These results suggest that a technically better result can be obtained from surgery, but that the overall clinical outcome is not necessarily improved with surgical revascularization. Furthermore, with the addition of stenting, the initial technical success rates of the percutaneous approach are now much higher, and therefore stenting has replaced surgery in the vast majority of cases.

THE FUTURE

Various unpublished initiatives are under way to provide an evidence base. The Action on Secondary Prevention through Intervention to Reduce Events (ASPIRE) trials enrolled patients who underwent stenting after suboptimal balloon angioplasty; this was a nonrandomized safety and efficacy study. Preliminary data on 208 patients presented at the 2002 American Heart Association Scientific Sessions revealed a 16.8% 9-month restenosis rate (45). A trial in the planning stage, Cardiovascular Outcome in Renal Atherosclerotic Lesions (CORAL), is designed to compare medical therapy versus medical therapy plus stenting. Randomized Comparison of Safety and Efficacy of Renal Stenting (RESIST) is an ongoing trial comparing renal stenting with or without distal protection and with or without glycoprotein IIb/IIIa inhibition to assess renal function. The design problems facing these studies are substantial, including the need for a sensitive endpoint to assess the affect of intervention on the kidney. In an attempt to provide a level playing field with well-designed enrollment criteria, study populations, and outcomes reporting, a consortium of American Heart Association councils and the Society of Interventional Radiology FDA Device Forum Committee have published guidelines for future trials (46). Until there is clarity provided by these trials, the clinician will be forced to continue practice based on existing standards, waiting for evidence to support the therapeutic alternatives.

SUMMARY

Renal artery stenosis is a common problem in the population of patients with vascular disease. Its detection requires a high index of suspicion along with appropriate selection of patients for testing. Figure 19.7 summarizes the management of a patient with suspected renal artery stenosis. The initial noninvasive diagnostic test of choice is institution dependent, but is generally either magnetic resonance angiography or renal duplex ultrasonography. Decisions on revascularization are based on the patient's clinical scenario. Patients with difficult-to-control hypertension or those with progressively declining renal function might be helped by renal artery revascularization. Renal artery stenting appears to be an effective strategy, and gives high levels of initial technical success. Careful technique during renal artery stenting may help to prevent complications. Renal artery stenting does have a problem with restenosis, thus requiring careful patient follow-up. It is also hoped that future technologies (such as drug-eluting stents) will reduce these restenosis rates and make the technology even more appealing. Ongoing studies should help to further define which patients benefit from revascularization.

REFERENCES

1. Haller C. Arteriosclerotic renal artery stenosis: conservative versus interventional management. *Heart* 2002;88:193–197.
2. McLaughlin K, Jardine AG, Moss JG. ABC of arterial and venous disease: renal artery stenosis. *BMJ* 2000;320:1124–1127.
3. Sawicki PT, Kaiser S, Heinemann L, et al. Prevalence of renal artery stenosis in diabetes mellitus—an autopsy study. *J Intern Med* 1991;229:489–492.
4. Schreiber MJ, Pohl MA, Novick AC. The natural history of atherosclerotic and fibrous renal artery disease. *Urol Clin North Am* 1984;11:383–392.
5. Zierler RE, Bergelin RO, Isaacson JA, et al. Natural history of atherosclerotic renal artery stenosis: a prospective study with duplex ultrasonography. *J Vasc Surg* 1994;19:250–258.
6. The sixth report of the Joint National Committee on Prevention, Detection, Evaluation and Treatment of High Blood Pressure. *Arch Intern Med* 1997;152:2413–2446.
7. Krijnen P, Van Jaarsveld BC, Steyerberg EW, et al. A clinical prediction rule for renal artery stenosis. *Ann Intern Med* 1998;129:705–711.
8. Uzu T, Inoue T, Fujii T, et al. Prevalence and predictors of renal artery stenosis in patients with myocardial infarction. *Am J Kidney Dis* 1997;29:733–738.
9. Olin JW, Melia M, Young JR, et al. Prevalence of atherosclerotic renal artery stenosis in patients with atherosclerosis elsewhere. *Am J Med* 1990;88[1N]:46N–51N.
10. Blaufox MD, Dubovsky EV, Hilson AJW, et al. Report of working party on radionuclide of choice: captopril renogram consensus conference. *Am J Hypertens* 1991;4:S747–S748.
11. Dondi M. Captopril renal scintigraphy with ^{99m}Tc-mercaptoacetyltriglycerine (^{99m}Tc-MAG3) for detecting renal artery stenosis. *Am J Hypertens* 1991;4:S737–S740.
12. Mann SJ, Pickering TG, Sos TA, et al. Captopril renography in the diagnosis of renal artery stenosis: accuracy and limitations. *Am J Med* 1991;90:30–40.
13. Setaro JF, Saddler MC, Chen CC, et al. Simplifed captopril renography in diagnosis and treatment of renal artery disease. *Hypertension* 1991;18:289–298.
14. Huot SJ, Hannson JH, Dey H, et al. Utility of captopril renal scans for detecting renal artery stenosis. *Arch Intern Med* 2002;162:1981–1984.
15. Zucchelli P. Hypertension and atherosclerotic renal artery stenosis: diagnostic approach. *J Am Soc Nephrol* 2002;13:S184–S186.
16. Rundback JH, Sacks D, Kent KC, et al. Guidelines for the reporting of renal artery revascularization in clinical trials. *J Vasc Interv Radiol* 2002;13:959–974.
17. Olin JW, Piedmonte MR, Young JR, et al. The utility of duplex ultrasound scanning of the renal arteries for diagnosing significant renal artery stenosis. *Ann Intern Med* 1995;122:833–838.
18. Kliewer MA, Tupler RH, Carroll BA, et al. Renal artery stenosis: analysis of Doppler waveform parameters and tardus–parvus pattern. *Radiology* 1993;189:779–787.
19. Radermacher J, Chavan A, Bleck J, et al. Use of Doppler ultrasonography to predict the outcome of therapy for renal-artery stenosis. *N Engl J Med* 2001;344:410–417.
20. Debain JF, Spritzer CE, Grist TM, et al. Imaging of the renal arteries: value of MR angiography. *AJR Am J Roentgenol* 1991;157:981–990.

21. Gedroyc WM, Neerhut P, Negus R. Magnetic resonance angiography of renal artery stenosis. *Clin Radiol* 1995;50:436–439.
22. Sharafuddin MJ, Stolpen AH, Dixon BS, et al. Value of MR angiography before percutaneous transluminal renal artery angioplasty and stent placement. *J Vasc Interv Radiol* 2002;13:901–908.
23. Farres MT, Lammer J, Schima W, et al. Spiral computed tomographic angiography of the renal arteries: a prospective comparison with intravenous and intra-arterial digital subtraction angiography. *Cardiovasc Intervent Radiol* 1996;19:101–106.
24. Beregi JP, Ekohen M, Deklunder G, et al. Helical CT angiography compared with arteriography in the detection of renal artery stenosis. *AJR Am J Roentgenol* 1996;163:867–872.
25. Boudewijn G, Vasbinder C, Nelemans J, et al. Diagnostic tests for renal artery stenosis in patients suspected of having renovascular hypertension: a meta–analysis. *Ann Intern Med* 2001;135:401–411.
26. Vashist A, Heller EN, Brown EJ, et al. Renal artery stenosis: a cardiovascular perspective. *Am Heart J* 2002;143:559–564.
27. Gross CM, Kramer J, Waigand J, et al. Relation between arteriosclerosis in the coronary and renal arteries. *Am J Cardiol* 1997;80:1478–1481.
28. Gruntzig A, Kuhlmann U, Rutolf U, et al. Treatment of renvascular hypertension with percutaneous transluminal dilation of a renal artery stenosis. *Lancet* 1978;1:801–802.
29. Baim DS, Grossman W. *Grossman's cardiac catheterization, angiography, and intervention,* 6th ed. Philadelphia: Lippincott Williams & Wilkins, 2000.
30. Ramsey LE, Waller PC. Blood pressure response to percutaneous transluminal angioplasty for renovascular hypertension: an overview of published series. *BMJ* 1990;300:569–672.
31. Rees CR. Stent for atherosclerotic renovascular disase. *J Vasc Interv Rad* 1999;10:689–705.
32. Morganti A. Renal angioplasty: better for treating hypertension or for rescuing renal function? *J Hypertens* 1999;17:1659–1665.
33. Klow NE, Paulsen D, Vatne K, et al. Percutaneous transluminal renal artery angioplasty using the coaxial technique. *Acta Radiol* 1998;39:594–600.
34. Keeley EC, Grines CL. Scraping of aortic debris by coronary guiding catheters. A prospective evaluation of 1000 cases. *J Am Coll Cardiol* 1998;32:1861–1865.
35. Ziakka S, Belli AM, Kong TK, et al. Percutaneous transluminal renal artery angioplasty: who benefits most? *Int J Clin Pract* 2002;56:649–654.
36. Lederman RJ, Mendelsohn FO, Santos R, et al. Primary renal artery stenting: characteristics and outcomes after 363 procedures. *Am Heart J* 2001;142:314–323.
37. Dorros G, Jaff M, Mathiak L, He T, et al. Multicenter Palmaz stent renal artery stenosis revascularization registry report: four year follow up of 1,058 successful patients. *Cathet Cardivasc Intervent* 2002;55:182–188.
38. Isles CG, Roberston S, Hill D. Management of renovascular disease: a review of renal artery stenting in ten studies. *Q J Med* 1999;92:159–167.
39. Watson PS, Hadjipetrou P, Cox SV, et. al. Effect of renal artery stenting on renal function and size in patients with atherosclerotic renovascular disease. *Circulation* 2000;102:1671–1677.
40. Beutler JJ, van Ampting JMA, Van de Ven PJG, et al. Long-term effects of arterial stenting on kidney function for patients wtih ostial atherosclerotic renal artery stenosis and renal insufficiency. *J Am Soc Nephrol* 2001;12:1475–1481.
41. Haller, C. Arteriosclerotic renal artery stenosis: conservative versus interventional management. *Heart* 2002;88:193–197.
42. van Jaarsveld BC, Krijnen P, Pieterman H, et al. The effect of balloon angioplasty on hypertension in atherosclerotic renal-artery stenosis. Dutch Renal Artery Stenosis Intervention Cooperative Study Group. *N Engl J Med* 2000;342:1007–1014.
43. Webster J, Marshall F, Abdalla M, et al. Randomized comparison of percutaneous angioplasty vs continued medical therapy for hypertensive patients with atheromatous renal artery stenosis. Scottish and Newcastle Renal Artery Stenosis Collaborative Group. *J Hum Hypertens* 1998;12:329–335.
44. Weibull H, Bergqvist D, Bergentz SE, et al. Percutaneous transluminal renal angioplasty versus surgical reconstruction of atherosclerotic renal artery stenosis: a prospective randomized study. *J Vasc Surg* 1993;18:841–850.
45. Giri S, Rosenfield K, Eisenhauer AC, et al. A study to evaluate the safety and effectiveness of renal artery stenting after failed angioplasty: acute and follow-up results of quantitative renal angiography in the ASPIRE2 trial. *Circulation* 2002;106:II714.
46. Rundback JH, Sacks D, Kent KC, et al. Guidelines for the reporting of renal artery revascularization in clinical trials. American Heart Association. *Circulation* 2002;106:1572–1585.

CHAPTER 20

Atherosclerotic Subclavian Artery Disease and Revascularization

Andrew C. Eisenhauer and James A. Shaw

Key Points

- Subclavian stenosis is important in patients with atherosclerotic cardiovascular disease not only because of the symptoms it may cause, but also because of compromise of the internal mammary artery that is frequently used as a conduit for myocardial revascularization.
- However, because symptoms of subclavian obstruction may be subtle or may mimic those of other syndromes, the condition is underdiagnosed.
- The diagnosis of subclavian obstruction first requires a high level of suspicion that prompts appropriate questioning and physical examination. Noninvasive ultrasound and radiographic imaging, although sometimes useful, play a lesser role.
- Although surgical revascularization has been the traditional mode of therapy, interventional techniques are becoming the mainstay of current therapy and have been show to be safe, effective, and durable.

INTRODUCTION

Subclavian artery stenosis, although relatively uncommon, is increasing in clinical importance, particularly due to the very common use of the left internal mammary artery for coronary artery bypass grafting. This condition thus warrants screening and early detection, as current treatment options are relatively noninvasive, safe, and effective. This chapter describes the different clinical symptoms with which patients with subclavian and brachiocephalic disease can present and the treatment options, including percutaneous and open surgical procedures and the relative advantages and disadvantages of both. There is some discussion about emerging technologies and how they may benefit future therapy. A detailed description of how to perform percutaneous subclavian revascularization is given and includes case examples.

INCIDENCE AND CLINICAL DIAGNOSIS

Significant atherosclerotic obstructive disease of the brachiocephalic or subclavian artery is reportedly uncommon, ac-

counting for about 17% of symptomatic extracranial cerebrovascular disease (1,2), with the majority of subclavian stenoses occurring on the left side. However, with the use of internal mammary conduits for coronary artery bypass (3) and the return of many of these patients to coronary angiography because of recurrent symptoms from attrition of associated saphenous vein grafts, the recognition of this problem is increasing. Thus, disease of the subclavian or brachiocephalic vessels can present with a variety of symptoms related to reduced blood flow to areas either directly or indirectly supplied by these vessels.

The "subclavian steal syndrome" arises because of reversal of flow in the vertebral artery as blood is shunted into the brachial circulation (1,4,5) so as to provide adequate arm perfusion. These patients can present with dizziness, syncope, and vertigo related to inadequate perfusion of the posterior cerebral circulation in what is termed vertebrobasilar insufficieny (2,6). Arm claudication can also occur on the side of the subclavian/brachiocephalic lesion with the patient complaining of cramping arm pain with upper limb exercise relieved with rest. Upper extremity ischemic symptoms may occur as a result of ipsilateral claudication related to arm exercise. Ischemia may also result from distal embolization to the digits (7). In the current era of coronary artery bypass surgery, the concept of total arterial revascularzation (3) is now the goal for many surgeons, with the belief that this will provide better long-term patency rates than is possible using saphenous veins as conduits. Thus, the left internal mammary graft is used in the majority of patients, and results in significant improvements in cumulative survival and a reduction in the risk of late myocardial infarction compared to using saphenous vein as a conduit (8,9). The right internal mammary is also now more commonly used (10). However, the prevalence of subclavian artery stenosis in patients undergoing myocardial revascularization is approximately 0.5% to 1.1% (11–13), and if these lesions are not treated prior to coronary surgery, the patients may develop coronary-subclavian steal, where the proximal subclavian stenosis will cause reversal of flow in the internal mammary artery and ischemia of the myocardium supplied by the bypass graft (11,14,15), resulting in the patient presenting with recurrent angina. Similarly, patients who undergo axillofemoral bypass surgery may have unrelieved claudication or graft compromise due to an unrecognized proximal subclavian stenosis.

CLINICAL EXAMINATION

There are only a few clinical signs to help in diagnosing this condition. The most sensitive one is a reduced blood pressure measurement in the limb on the side of the lesion. It is thus important to check patients' blood pressures in both arms, especially those with coronary disease who may require coronary artery bypass grafting in the future or have had it in the past. Should there be disease in both arms, blood pressure may have to be measured in the lower limbs so as to get an accurate recording. Any blood pressure difference between the upper limbs greater than 20 mm Hg suggests subclavian/brachiocephalic disease, and, if clinically indicated, a diagnosis should be sought. The presence of a bruit over the involved vessel is another indicator of the presence of a stenosis. The "labile" blood pressure in these individuals has been dependent on the arm in which it has been taken and not on true variability in true blood pressure. A subclavian lesion is unlikely to be the only atherosclerotic lesion, and thus a full examination of the vasculature is required looking for evidence of carotid, renal, and femoral bruits as well as the presence or absence of pulses in the lower limbs. Occasionally, patients with diffuse atherosclerosis will have "four-limb" obstruction, in which no extremity reflects an accurate central blood pressure.

INDICATIONS FOR REVASCULARIZATION

Once a patient has presented with symptoms believed to be due to the subclavian/brachiocephalic obstruction, it is most likely he or she will require revascularization, whether by percutaneous means or open surgical technique, to alleviate the symptoms. Rarely, patients will improve with conserva-

tive therapy, which largely involves aggressive risk factor modification (16,17).

Prior to performing any revascularization procedure, it is important to assess carefully the patient's true subjective level of disability, as symptoms may range from none to recurrent transient ischemic attacks, stroke, life-threatening syncope, or limb-threatening ischemia. In many instances, the mere presence of a chronic asymptomatic stenosis or occlusion does not justify attempted revascularization. In contrast, revascularization of some asymptomatic patients may be warranted to enable the use of the internal mammary artery for coronary bypass, or, in the case of multilimb occlusive disease, permit accurate blood pressure measurement. It is particularly important to consider the risk–benefit tradeoff in the asymptomatic patient.

There are patients with clear symptoms of arm claudication who are neither bothered nor disabled by them. In these situations, once patients have been informed of the cause of the pain and are confident that there is no underlying illness such as a neurological problem, and it is not restricting their lifestyle, many will elect a conservative approach, and thus avoid the small but real risk of morbidity involved with a revascularization procedure. Similarly, patients with isolated subclavian obstruction and mild symptoms of vertebrobasilar insufficiency may opt for conservative therapy, especially in light of the lack of clear evidence that atherosclerotic subclavian obstruction associated with stable symptoms will commonly progress to limb or central nervous system-threatening ischemia. Thus, revascularization should only be recommended for symptom relief, as there is no evidence it can prevent death or disability.

NONINVASIVE EVALUATION

Although the diagnosis of aortic arch vessel obstruction is primarily clinical and is based on history and careful physical examination, noninvasive evaluation adds important anatomic and functional information that should be obtained before performing elective revascularization. Symptoms of vertigo in these individuals are often ascribed to labyrinthitis or benign positional vertigo, and arm claudication is frequently misinterpreted as radicular pain or referred discomfort from cervical degenerative disk or joint disease. The appropriate suspicion of obstructive arterial disease, coupled with a careful physical examination, may lead to an appropriate diagnosis.

Despite the fact that the history and physical examination are the keys to making the diagnosis, the noninvasive vascular laboratory plays a complementary role. However, symptoms of dizziness and/or vertigo are common in the elderly, and thus many of these individuals may have a coexistent subclavian lesion that can be unrelated to the symptoms. In these cases, the provocation of symptoms and demonstration of reversal of vertebral flow with arm exercise may confirm the relationship between the obstructive lesion and the symptom. The question of concomitant carotid disease may be addressed by a vascular laboratory examination.

Furthermore, although the true "subclavian" portion of the subclavian artery is difficult to image, the presence of an abnormal waveform or flow acceleration can allow confirmation of a suspected stenosis, rule out contralateral disease, and provide an objective baseline from which to measure the results of therapy. Noninvasive techniques can also interrogate the axillary, brachial, and more distal arteries to exclude the presence of more distal disease, which could be confusing at the time of revascularization.

Magnetic resonance angiography (MRA) is another noninvasive imaging modality that can diagnose disease of the extracranial cerebrovascular vessels (18,19). MRA is becoming more widely available and more sensitive and specific at diagnosing subclavian, brachiocephalic, and carotid disease. Its use is restricted by cost, and for certain patients it is contraindicated, such as those with permanent pacemakers and defibrillators in place and those with claustrophobia. However, its use in diagnosing these lesions will continue to expand as it becomes more widely available and affordable. It is advantageous in that it is able to produce good anatomic information in a noninvasive way without using any iodinated contrast.

After revascularization, an ultrasound should be performed early to be used as a baseline. Studies performed after this should be compared with the initial postprocedure study and can be used as a guide to the development of restenosis. As will be discussed, should a stent restenose, it is preferable to treat the lesion prior to the stent occluding totally.

CONTEMPORARY SURGICAL THERAPY

A variety of surgical techniques have been developed in the setting of obstructive atherosclerotic disease, including transthoracic procedures and the recently more favored carotid–subclavian bypass and axilloaxillary bypass. However, even with less invasive extraanatomic, extrathoracic reconstructions, the morbidity and mortality are not insignificant.

Our group has reviewed the surgical literature on the results of nearly 2,000 patients accumulated over 25 years looking at acute success and immediate and late complications (20). The majority of these studies were retrospective series from various institutions with no prospective randomized trials comparing surgery to any other form of therapy or comparing different surgical procedures. Preprocedural symptoms, diagnostic evaluation, and concomitant medical illnesses were inconsistently described. The methods by which one procedure was chosen over another were variable, and the rationale for performing (or not performing) associated carotid endarterectomy in patients with combined carotid disease was not uniformly stated.

The combined initial technical success rate in the surgical groups was high (mean 96%). The major complication of stroke was reported in 3% and death in 2% of cases (20). Of the series in which overall complications were tabulated and in which adverse events of any kind were reported, there was an overall complication rate of 16%. Some reported surgical complications included stroke, myocardial infarction, hemorrhage, phrenic nerve palsy, Horner's syndrome, delayed wound healing, infection, graft thrombosis, and others pertaining to general anesthesia. Risk factors associated with complications suggested that open-chest procedures are associated with a higher mortality and morbidity than are extrathoracic bypasses.

Follow-up was largely clinical, which is adequate to follow recurrence of symptoms, but did not absolutely confirm patency of the treated segment. The development of collaterals may mask the brachiobrachial pressure differential of a stenosed or occluded bypass. Of the documented technically successful procedures, 12% developed recurrence at a mean follow-up of 50 months (20).

Reports of surgical experience continue to become available, and the results have been similar. Berguer and colleagues presented their series of patients undergoing transthoracic (21) and cervical (22) reconstruction of occlusive disease of the supraaortic trunks. Perioperative morbidity and mortality was 16% in the first series and 4.3% in the second. Similarly, Taha and colleagues, in a series of 42 patients with both transthoracic and extraanatomic bypass approaches, reported a combined stroke and death rate of 4.3% with an 80% 3-year patency (23). Azakie published the results of 94 patients in whom endarterectomy using a transthoracic approach was the most common procedure performed (24). The perioperative death rate was 3% and the stroke rate was 4% (24). In a small series of 18 patients, one death and two strokes were reported (25).

These recent results show that surgical approaches to revascularization of the proximal aortic arch vessels still carry a risk of stroke approaching 5% and a mortality greater than 2%. Often, these series involve a transthoracic approach, and it is likely that this invasive technique coupled with the patients' associated coronary and panvascular disease confers this risk. By contrast, in a series of patients with subclavian disease treated with axilloaxillary bypass (and thus not needing a transthoracic approach), there was only a 1.6% perioperative mortality and no strokes (26). However, this extraanatomic reconstruction may be less durable, and is certainly problematic should coronary bypass surgery ever be required.

Recent retrospective series looked at patients who underwent subclavian to carotid bypass using polytetrafluoroethylene (PTFE) grafts only (27,28). Paty et al. looked at all ten patients over a 10-year period who had undergone subclavian arterial reconstruction specifically for coronary subclavian steal syndrome (27). Interestingly, in nine of the patients percutaneous revascularization had been attempted. In seven of the cases, the lesions could not be successfully crossed with a wire, and in two cases, a stent was placed in the setting of a recent total occlusion, but the stent occluded within 24 hours. PTFE grafts were placed successfully in all ten patients, and in one patient, a concomitant carotid endarterectomy was performed for high-grade stenosis. In this small cohort, there were no cardiac or neurological complications postoperatively, and at a mean follow-up of 43 months all bypasses had remained patent (27). In study of 51 patients with symptomatic subclavian disease who were all treated with carotid subclavian bypass (PTFE), there was no perioperative stroke or death. Ten-year primary and secondary patency rates were 92% and 95%, respectively (28).

PERCUTANEOUS INTERVENTIONS IN THE SUBCLAVIAN ARTERY

Balloon angioplasty for subclavian artery stenosis was described in the early 1980s, with subsequent reports showing that acute success and patency rates at follow-up were comparable to those with surgery. Furthermore, there was a low rate of complications and infrequent mortality (29,30). There was initial concern about the potential for distal embolization and stroke, uncertain long-term patency, and difficulty in treating total occlusions. This, in conjunction with given improvements in anesthetic and operative technique, short hospital stays, and early discharge, led many practitioners to continue to regard surgery as the standard therapy against which endovascular methods must be compared.

However, in many other similar-size arteries, vascular stenting has nearly eliminated acute closure, diminished distal embolization, improved medium-term patency, and provided the ability to recanalize chronic total occlusions, enabling percutaneous revascularization to rival surgical techniques in certain situations. The use of vascular stents has become the leading primary endovascular treatment for atherosclerotic obstructive disease of branches of the aorta including the subclavian and carotid arteries. Numerous large series show that carotid stenting is a successful procedure with a low stroke rate and good long-term patency (31,32), and a randomized "high-risk" trial reported favorable results with stenting compared to carotid endarterectomy (Stenting and Angioplasty with Protection in Patients at High Risk for Endartarectomy [SAPPHIRE]. Additional trials are in progress comparing carotid stenting with endarterectomy (33).

Data for percutaneous treatment of the subclavian/brachiocephalic vessels is limited largely due to both the rarity of the disease and limited indications for treating it when it occurs. In our comparison of the reports of surgery versus angioplasty/stenting of this condition, we chose to evaluate simpler but more uniformly reported endpoints of technical success (the ability to perform the planned procedure yielding target lesion revascularization and survival to discharge), patient death, stroke, and patency of the treated segment (20).

In the studies in which stenting was performed, there were no uniformly evaluated/reported procedural complications, but adverse events were reported in 6% (20). Similarly, the overall incidence of postprocedure complications such as vascular access difficulty, hemorrhage, pseudoaneurysm, transfusion, or contrast-mediated transient renal insufficiency is not known. Of the nearly 100 patients represented in the reports, technical success was achieved in 97%. No strokes or deaths occurred. Follow-up data were available in about two-thirds of technically successful cases at a mean duration of 16.8 months. Occlusion or restenosis was reported in 6%. Following publication of this report, there were editorials from interventionalists to broaden the horizons of interventional therapy (34) and from surgeons to proceed with caution (35).

The reports of vascular stenting continue to suggest that perioperative strokes are quite uncommon. Al-Mubarak et al. reported no strokes in their series of 38 patients (29), and strokes occurred in only 0.9% of subclavian procedures described by Henry et al. (30). In addition, treatment failures, when they occurred, were limited to totally occluded arteries. Primary patency ranged from 94% at 20 months to 75% at 8 years; overall patency ranged from 100% at 20 months to 90% at 8 years (29).

There have been some conflicting reports regarding the efficacy of stent implantation. There are concerns about not only long-term patency, but also durability of the stent due to wire fracture at the site of flexion and compression (36). Motarjeme reported disappointing patency rates for balloon angioplasty alone in a group of patients with total occlusions of the subclavian (37), whereas Henry et al. reported good short and intermediate results in both those who underwent angioplasty alone and those who had angioplasty and stenting (30). A European series retrospectively reviewed 115 patients with subclavian disease treated percutaneously (38). The procedures were performed between 1984 and 1998, and all patients after January 1, 1996, routinely received Palmaz stents; none were implanted before this date. Successful revascularization was achieved in 98 patients. There were no periprocedural deaths, 1 patient had a transient ischemic attack from the left vertebral artery and 2 patients had emboli, 1 to the renal and 1 to the mesenteric arteries. All 3 patients recovered completely from these events. Although patency rates were significantly higher at 1 year in the stented group compared to those only treated with angioplasty (95% vs. 76%), by 4 years of follow-up, there was more restenosis in the stented patients (38). Furthermore, a multivariate model of predictors of restenosis in this study included lesion length, residual stenosis after angioplasty, and stent implantation (38). However, this analysis is limited by the large difference in patient numbers in the two groups (26 in the stented group vs. 72 in the angioplasty group) and the fact that stents were only placed after 1996 and in all patients. By this time, technological advances had made it easier to open totally occluded vessels, which were previously rarely successfully treated percutaneously. Thus, many of these lesions in the stented arm had other factors increasing their risk of restenosis and would not have been successfully treated percutaneously prior to the introduction of stents.

CONCLUSION: SURGERY OR STENTING?

Although the surgical series report impressive results, there is no randomized trial comparing surgery versus percutaneous therapy, and thus there is no good evidence that one therapy, is definitively better than the other. The data suggest that when surgery is performed, carotid–subclavian bypass using a PTFE graft carries the lowest perioperative risk and best long-term patency (27,28).

Interestingly, examination of the recently published series of percutaneous subclavian treatment continues to suggest that the rate of periprocedure stroke may be lower with catheter-based revascularization (30). In sofar as comparison is possible, overall (primary and secondary) patencies remain roughly equivalent between surgical and interventional treatment. Surgery offers greater technical success in the treatment of total occlusions, and it may be required to achieve symptomatic relief should catheter revascularization prove unsuccessful (30). Reports of successful treatment of aneurysmal disease suggests that ectatic segments and traumatic disruption may be treated routinely by percutaneous techniques (39).

We believe the choice should be made once patient preference and the relative expertise of the various specialists—vascular surgeons, interventional radiologists, and cardiologists—in treating subclavian/brachiocephalic disease are taken into consideration. When it is feasible from a technical point of view and clinically indicated, we recommend stenting as the first choice of therapy. Furthermore, should the angioplasty be unsuccessful acutely, the surgical option is still available at no increased risk. In cases where there is restenosis of the stent months following the procedure, treatment options include repeat angioplasty and stenting as has been described (40) or surgery.

POTENTIAL NEW DEVELOPMENTS

With the increasing frequency of percutaneous therapies and evolution of the equipment, in particular the widespread use of endovascular stents, these procedures have become safer, easier, and more successful. However, the major limitation with the use of stents is the problem of restenosis (41,42). Angiographic restenosis varies depending on both the diameter of the vessel and the length of stent used, being significantly higher when small-diameter, longer stents are used. From retrospective studies, in-stent restenosis in the subclavian artery appears to be on the order of 10% to 20% (29,38). Recent studies in the coronary circulation have shown significant reduction in in-stent restenosis in patients treated with stents coated with the immunosuppressant agent sirolimus (43). This agent, which is a macrolide antibiotic, inhibits cytokine-stimulated proliferation of T lymphocytes by blocking the cell cycle, and has widespread antiproliferative and antiinflammatory effects (44). Although data in the noncoronary circulation are limited, one study in patients with superficial femoral artery dis ease showed a higher in-stent mean lumen diameter in the drug-eluting stent arm than in the bare stent arm (45). Thus, in the subclavian vessels, where angiographic restenosis is relatively low, trials need to be performed to examine how much, if any, benefit will be achieved with drug-eluting stents and whether there will be sufficient benefit to justify the additional costs of these newer devices.

INTERVENTIONAL TECHNIQUE

Initially, balloon angioplasty of the subclavian or brachiocephalic arteries was largely limited by the available equipment. Large-shaft (greater than 5 French) balloon dilatation catheters accepted 0.035-in guidewires, and guiding catheters were large, difficult to deliver, and hard to image through. Access was either from the femoral approach or the ipsilateral arm (brachial or axillary artery). The balloon catheters were difficult from the brachial approach unless a cutdown was used, and the lack of good guiding catheters made it necessary either to have an additional arterial access for imaging or to exchange catheters frequently. Nevertheless, it was often possible to access, cross, and dilate these lesions successfully. With the advent of stenting, more precise angiographic placement was required, and guiding catheters through which contrast angiography could be performed became necessary. Operators began to adapt techniques developed in coronary angioplasty to the problem, and to develop guiding catheters and modified thin-walled vascular sheaths to deliver balloons and stents to the target. At the same time, there was slow but continual reduction of balloon shaft diameter and overall deflated balloon profile.

Prior to commencing the intervention, most operators recommend performing an aortogram with digital subtraction angiography in the left anterior oblique or right posterior oblique projection. This allows visualization of the arch, proximal, and mid great vessels. Such a study is important to define the extent of atherosclerotic involvement of the aorta in addition to the target artery. It allows one to avoid areas that appear particularly diseased or friable while selectively cannulating the target vessel. In addition, in the case of total occlusions, "late" filming defines the length of the occlusion, the type and degree of collateralization, and possible branch vessel involvement. The ability to perform digital subtraction studies is critical. This technique permits the use of dilute contrast and reduced contrast loads. It allows the more sensitive visualization of poorly opacified distal collaterals and can permit reduced overall radiation exposure to the patient and operator.

Aortography also gives the operator valuable information on the potential difficulty of stable cannulation of the arch vessels. Congenital abnormalities of the origin of the great vessels are identified. However, more commonly, variation in configuration of the normal anatomic arrangement presents the greatest challenge.

Figure 20.1A shows the arch from a patient who presented with unstable angina 8 years post-coronary artery bypass grafting. The other vein grafts were patent, but a significant lesion was seen in the left subclavian, causing coronary-subclavian steal. The aortogram in this patient is an example of a relatively "normal" arch. The aorta is not uncoiled, and the origin of the brachiocephalic trunk is high lying above the

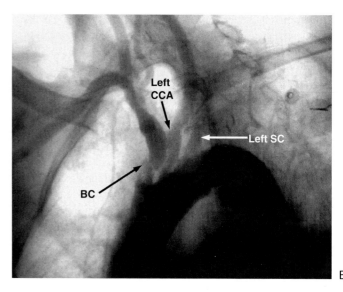

A

B

FIG. 20.1. A: An arch aortogram in the left anterior oblique (LAO) view. This arch shows the origin of the brachiocephalic (BC), left common carotid (CCA), and left subclavian (SC). A severe stenosis can be seen in the ostium of the left subclavian. This shows a relatively "normal" arch. The aorta is not uncoiled, and the origin of the brachiocephalic trunk is high lying above the apex of the arch. **B:** An arch aortogram in the LAO projection. The brachiocephalic (BC), left common carotid (CCA), and left subclavian (SC) (which is occluded proximally) are labeled. This arch illustrates the "difficult" arch configuration, particularly for access to the innominate/right subclavian, the origin of which lies inferior to the apex of the arch, and the origins of all the great vessels are displaced rightward.

apex of the arch. The catheter pathways to the great vessels are all relatively straight, facilitating instrumentation, guidewire manipulation, and crossing power.

Figure 20.1B shows an arch aortogram taken from a patient who presented with acute pulmonary edema and had difficult-to-record blood pressure. Noninvasive imaging had shown significant left subclavian and brachiocephalic disease, and thus it was impossible to get accurate blood pressure measurements from either arm. Brachiocephalic revascularization was performed so that accurate blood pressures could be recorded from the right arm and treatment monitored accurately. As is seen from this image, this arch illustrates the "difficult" arch configuration, particularly for access to the innominate/right subclavian. The innominate origin lies inferior to the apex of the arch, and the origins of all the great vessels are displaced rightward. This configuration makes cannulation of the vessels with stiff guiding catheters or sheaths, especially from the groin, more difficult, and in cases like these, using access from the brachial or radial artery should be considered.

After aortography, the target vessel is cannulated selectively. There are various techniques for performing this, and the choice will depend on exactly where the lesion is, the severity of the stenosis, and how difficult crossing this may be and tortuosity of the aorta.

Our preferred method is to cannulate the vessel with an angiographic catheter (5 or 6 French) and through this either pass an exchange length 0.018-in. guidewire or, if one is concerned about delivery of a long, large-diameter sheath (Shuttle, Cook, Inc., Bloomington, IN), use a 0.035-in. Amplatz wire for extra support. The angiographic catheter is

then exchanged out over the wire for either a guide or a Shuttle sheath. Other operators cannulate the origin of the target vessel directly with a guiding catheter (8 to 10 French) in a similar fashion to the way in which one would cannulate a coronary artery. Some prefer to insert the sheath they will use for stent delivery (6 to 8 French) and, through this, cannulate the target with a smaller (4 to 6 French) angiographic catheter. From the femoral approach, there is a wide variety of catheters that may be used depending on operator preference, target vessel location, arch configuration, and experience. Neuroangiographic catheters (e.g., the DAV and VTK catheters (Cook Inc., Bloomington, IN) as well as the commonly used JR4 catheter) can be used to engage the origin of the subclavian brachiocephalic vessels usually without too much difficulty.

An angiographic disadvantage of the isolated arm (axillary, brachial, or radial) approach is that visualization of the lesion must be via retrograde injection of contrast. When using this interventional approach, it is often desirable to perform an arch aortogram first, without crossing or instrumenting the lesion. This may be possible using small-caliber catheters from the contralateral arm or from the groin. Occasionally, however, there is complete occlusion of all other potential access vessels. In this event, options include foregoing aortography or crossing the lesion and then performing it.

Another important consideration for catheter choice is the configuration of the aortic arch. The left subclavian is usually relatively easy to approach and can be cannulated with a variety of visceral, coronary, or neuroangiographic catheter shapes. As one moves more proximally in the arch, uncoiling, dilatation, or a low-lying origin can make access to the brachiocephalic and right subclavian vessels more difficult. Although it is almost always possible to cannulate with a small-caliber angiographic catheter, subsequent guide catheter or sheath placement may be more difficult especially in the situation of a very low lying brachiocephalic origin, as noted previously. Experience, newly designed sheaths and guides, and the brachial approach can simplify these difficulties.

Chronic total occlusions, which constitute a significant percentage of symptomatic subclavian lesions, merit special consideration. These lesions are firm and often require considerable force to cross even with a stiff, hydrophilic guidewire. Classically, a catheter or long sheath is passed from the groin and engages the "nubbin," or stump, of the total occlusion. A local angiogram is performed and the lesion is probed with a hydrophilic guidewire (Glidewire, Terumo/Boston Scientific, Natick, MA). If the wire can be passed into the distal vessel, a 4 or 5 French catheter (usually a hydrophilic Glidecath, Terumo/Boston Scientific, Natick, MA) is advanced across the total occlusion and its intraluminal position confirmed by the measurement of a distal perfusion pressure waveform, the withdrawal of arterial blood, and contrast injection. Guidewire and balloon catheter exchange is then possible, and one can proceed with the intervention. However, should it not be possible to get through the occlusion from the femoral approach, a combined antegrade and retrograde approach is necessary. To do this, the placement of a radial, brachial, or axillary sheath and Glidecath can provide the back-up needed to cross the occlusion retrogradely. Once passed, the intraluminal position of the catheter must also be confirmed by the measurement of aortic pressure, the withdrawal of arterial blood, and the injection of contrast material. The stenosis will then usually yield to the passage of the Glidecath. On rare occasions, the end of the guidewire that has crossed the lesion may have to be snared and then exteriorized. With control of both ends of a long guidewire, a balloon catheter should be worked across the lesion. There have also been occasions when a chronic total occlusion has developed a tiny recanalized channel that is visible only on selective digital subtraction angiography of the "stump" with high magnification. In this situation, the use of a hydrophilic 0.014-in. coronary wire (such as a Graphix Intermediate SciMed/Boston Scientific Natick, MA or a CrossWire [Terumo/Boston Scientific, Natick, MA]) to cross the lesion, followed by predilatation with a small (2 to 3 mm) coronary balloon, can create an initial channel to allow for passage of 4 French Glidecath and wire exchange. After a channel has been created and stable guidewire position achieved, the lesion is "predilated" as one would after the initial crossing of a non-totally occluded stenosis.

In the case of stenoses, the lesion is usually crossed with an atraumatic steerable guidewire, predilated with a slightly undersized balloon, and then stented with a stent sized on a balloon with a 1:1 balloon artery ratio. In the past, most operators used 0.035-in. guidewires and 5 French Shaft balloon catheters both to predilate and deploy stents. Increasingly, operators are using smaller (0.018-in.) guidewires and smaller

shaft diameter balloons. Rugged, high-pressure, 0.018-in. balloons are available from a variety of manufacturers, and a 0.014-in. monorail stent system with inflated balloon diameters of up to 7 mm are available. In addition, several self-expanding stent systems can be used. Most operators favor balloon-expandable stents at aortoostial locations because they tend to be easier to more accurately position, whereas self-expanding stents are reserved for long-segment disease or situations where more flexibility and rebound are needed. Despite the improvement in equipment, complications can still occur, and great care needs to be taken to prevent them from happening and to be able to deal with them should they be encountered.

Subclavian and brachiocephalic trunk interventions should be considered "cerebrovascular" in all patients. Even in those with documented ipsilateral retrograde vertebral flow, it is possible that this flow will reverse immediately after initial dilatation of the subclavian, and thus the potential for embolization always exists. Care must be taken when manipulating the guide to prevent excessive plaque disruption because embolization of the plaque carries potentially severe cerebrovascular consequences, which are usually irreversible. Although total occlusions can usually be pierced, dilated, and stented, the risk of embolization, guidewire exit, distal dissection, and/or mediastinal hemorrhage must be considered. The operator must be prepared to tamponade vessel perforation with balloon occlusion pending surgical closure or to place a covered stent to treat this complication.

Precise stent placement is crucial. In aortoostial lesions, the chosen stent should protrude 1 to 3 mm into the aorta to ensure good coverage of the vessel ostium. Furthermore, it is important to ensure that stents are positioned fastidiously so that they do not compromise the origins of branch vessels that may be vital to cerebral or cardiac blood supply. Thus, when treating the brachiocephalic artery, extreme care must be taken to avoid compromising the origin of the common carotid artery. Operators must also take care to identify and angiographically isolate the origin of the vertebral and internal mammary arteries to avoid inadvertent occlusion of the origins of these vessels. In cases where there is long-segment disease or chronic total occlusion, the assessment of collateral flow to the arm and the posterior fossa is important. For example, consider a proximal total occlusion of the left subclavian artery in a situation where the major collateral to the arm is the left vertebral. Recanalization and stenting of the left subclavian and inadvertent occlusion of the vertebral will likely augment flow into the arm and relieve arm symptoms. However, the anatomy of the contralateral vertebral system and/or anterior–posterior (carotid–vertebrobasilar) collateral flow may determine the adequacy of perfusion to the posterior circulation and thus the fate of the patient's vertebrobasilar symptoms.

CASE EXAMPLES

Case 1 is that of a patient with unstable angina 7 years post-coronary artery bypass grafting. Although all the saphenous vein grafts were patent, there was a severe subclavian stenosis

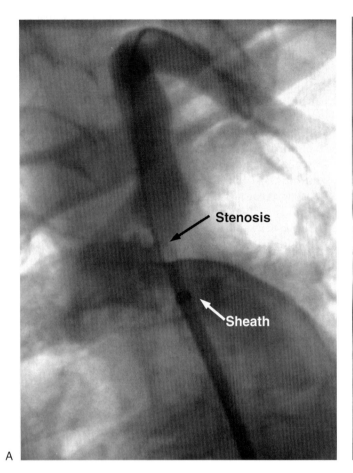

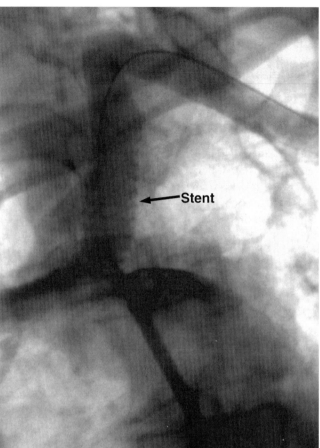

FIG. 20.2. A: A tight ostial stenosis can be seen at the origin of the left subclavian. A delivery sheath proximal to the lesion is labeled and there is an 0.035-in. wire across the lesion. **B:** The lesion has been successfully stented with a 10 × 28 mm Omnilink stent (Guidant Corp., Indianapolis, IN). The ostium of the lesion is covered with the proximal stent protruding into the aorta by 2–3 mm.

proximal to the left internal mammary which was supplying the left anterior descending artery (Fig. 20.2A). This was successfully treated with balloon angioplasty and stenting. As can be seen, poststenting there was an excellent angiographic result (Fig. 20.2B), and symptoms resolved.

Case 2 is the patient whose is shown Fig. 20.1B. The patient presented with recurrent pulmonary edema, and echocardiogram showed normal left ventricular function with moderate to severe left ventricular hypertrophy and mild aortic stenosis. Cardiac catheterization revealed only minor irregularities of the coronary arteries, but extremely elevated central aortic pressures. It was later appreciated that the patient's arm blood pressure recordings were significantly lower than was seen at catheterization. An MRA was performed, which showed occluded left subclavian and tight proximal brachiocephalic disease. It was believed that the uncontrolled blood pressure, which could not be easily monitored, was the cause of the pulmonary edema, and percutaneous revascularization was planned. From the arch aortogram, the occlusion of the left subclavian and the significant lesion in the right brachiocephalic were evident. There was also evidence of an ostial right vertebral lesion and disease in the left internal carotid

artery (see Fig. 20.3). Due to the "difficult" arch anatomy, the radial approach was chose to perform the intervention. Figure 20.3B shows the long delivery sheath coming from the arm with the stent across the lesion. The brachiocephalic artery was stented with a 9 × 28 mm Omnilink stent (Guidant Corp., Indianapolis, IN), and, as can be seen on the arch aortogram done post-stenting, there is no residual stenosis in the brachiocephalic, but a tight vertebral artery lesion remains (Fig. 20.3C). Given the patient's significantly reduced cerebral perfusion, it was decided to treat the vertebral lesion; a JR4 guide was advanced from the arm and engaged the origin of the vertebral artery (Fig. 20.3D). This was then stented with a 6 × 12 mm Herculink stent (Guidant Corp., Indianapolis, IN) (Fig. 20.3E). One year post-stenting, with more accurate monitoring and control of the blood pressure, the patient has had no recurrent presentations with pulmonary edema and no central nervous system symptoms.

Case 3 is an example of patient who presented with recurrent angina 6 months following placement of a subclavian stent that had been originally placed because of coronary subclavian steal syndrome. Figure 20.4A shows evidence of severe in-stent restenosis. This was treated with repeat

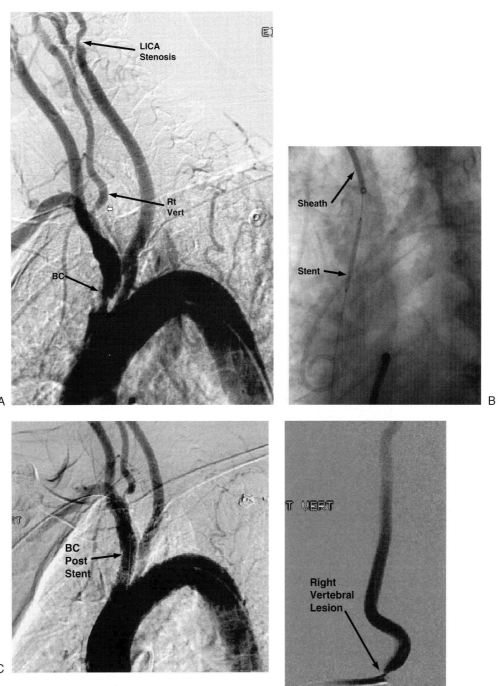

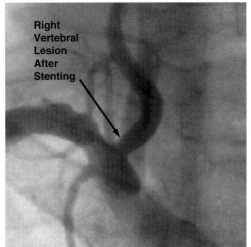

FIG. 20.3. A: An arch with a patient with significant arch vessel disease. A tight lesion in the brachiocephalic (BC) trunk is shown; there is also a lesion at the ostium of the right vertebral and the left internal carotid artery (LICA). **B:** The brachiocephalic lesion treated from a radial approach. The delivery sheath is seen in the right subclavian, and a stent is across the lesion ready to be deployed. **C:** In the aortogram following stenting of the brachiocephalic (BC), a successful angiographic result is seen. **D:** A JR4 guide, also from the radial approach, has selected the right vertebral in the patient following the brachiocephalic stent. A severe ostial stenosis is seen. **E:** A nonselective angiogram of the right subclavian following stenting of the vertebral artery, showing a successful angiographic result.

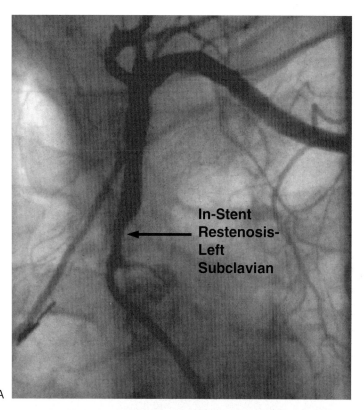

In-Stent
Restenosis-
Left
Subclavian

A

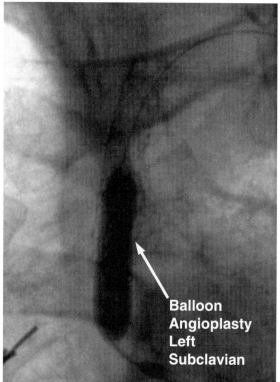

Balloon
Angioplasty
Left
Subclavian

B

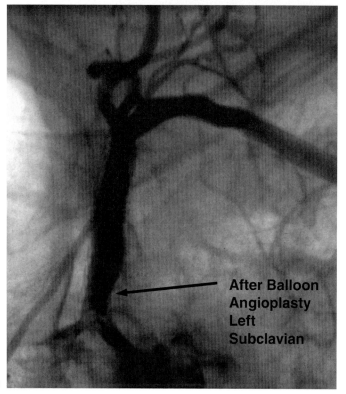

After Balloon
Angioplasty
Left
Subclavian

C

FIG. 20.4. A: An angiogram of the left subclavian showing severe in-stent restenosis in the proximal part of a previously deployed stent. **B:** A balloon inflated inside the stent at the site of the restenotic lesion. **C:** The lesion following successful balloon angioplasty. Minimal residual stenosis is now seen.

angioplasty (Fig. 20.4B), with a good angiographic result (Fig. 20.4C) and resolution of symptoms.

SUMMARY AND CONCLUSIONS

Proximal obstruction of aortic arch branch vessels supplying the upper limb extremities may present with a variety of symptoms. Diagnosis is normally made with a thorough history and physical examination, with a blood pressure difference between the two arms being a strong clue to the presence of unilateral disease. Noninvasive imaging and angiography can be performed to confirm the diagnosis. When considering the treatment options, clinicians should attempt to achieve the greatest patient benefit while minimizing risk.

Before the advent of percutaneous techniques, surgical treatment for these patients was advocated, and extrathoracic procedures emerged as the favorite because of relatively low morbidity and mortality. However, surgical procedures are still associated with a risk of periprocedural complications and do not guarantee a durable result. There are no published prospective, comparative studies on the surgical treatment of subclavian or brachiocephalic artery obstruction.

Percutaneous revascularization with stenting has become an alternative because of its simplicity and equivalent rate of complications compared to surgery. Several studies have reported initial success and mid-term patency rates similar to those of surgery. In addition, compared to balloon dilatation alone, stenting may reduce the long-term risk of particulate material embolization and achieve anatomically and physiologically superior results.

Overall, the results of percutaneous stenting compare favorably with the surgical experience. However, these conclusions are made largely from retrospective data, and there are no prospective, randomized clinical trials of the two forms of therapy. Precise comparison is confounded by the lack of similar patient selection criteria, inclusion bias, and recorded endpoints.

There is no proof that one form of therapy is superior to another. Furthermore, it is unlikely that this question will be addressed by prospective, randomized trials, and catheter-based techniques are increasingly advocated as first-line therapy [46]. Clinicians must weigh personal, institutional, and collective experience and individual patient wishes in determining the best treatment for a given individual.

REFERENCES

1. Tyras DH, Barner HB. Coronary-subclavian steal. *Arch Surg* 1977;112:1125–1127.
2. Fields WS, Lemak NA. Joint study of extracranial arterial occlusion. VII. Subclavian steal—a review of 168 cases. *JAMA* 1972;222:1139–1143.
3. Tatoulis J, Buxton BF, Fuller JA, et al. Total arterial coronary revascularization: techniques and results in 3,220 patients. *Ann Thorac Surg* 1999;68:2093–2099.
4. Editorial. A new vascular syndrome: "The subclavian steal." *N Engl J Med* 1961;265:912.
5. Reivich M. Reversal of blood flow through vertebral artery and its effects on cerebral circulation. *N Engl J Med* 1961;265:878–885.
6. Smith JM, Koury HI, Hafner CD, et al. Subclavian steal syndrome. A review of 59 consecutive cases. *J Cardiovasc Surg (Turino)* 1994;35:11–14.
7. Bryan AJ, Hicks E, Lewis MH. Unilateral digital ischaemia secondary to embolisation from subclavian atheroma. *Ann R Coll Surg Engl* 1989;71:140–142.
8. Cameron A, Kemp Jr HG, Green GE. Bypass surgery with the internal mammary artery graft: 15 year follow-up. *Circulation* 1986;74:III30–III36.
9. Loop FD, Lytle BW, Cosgrove DM, et al. Influence of the internal-mammary-artery graft on 10-year survival and other cardiac events. *N Engl J Med* 1986;314:1–6.
10. Buxton BF, Ruengsakulrach P, Fuller J, et al. The right internal thoracic artery graft—benefits of grafting the left coronary system and native vessels with a high grade stenosis. *Eur J Cardiothorac Surg* 2000;18:255–261.
11. Olsen CO, Dunton RF, Maggs PR, et al. Review of coronary-subclavian steal following internal mammary artery–coronary artery bypass surgery. *Ann Thorac Surg* 1988;46:675–678.
12. Singh RN. Atherosclerosis and the internal mammary arteries. *Cardiovasc Intervent Radiol* 1983;6:72–77.
13. Kay HR, Korns ME, Flemma RJ, et al. Atherosclerosis of the internal mammary artery. *Ann Thorac Surg* 1976;21:504–507.
14. Breall JA, Kim D, Baim DS, et al. Coronary-subclavian steal: an unusual cause of angina pectoris after successful internal mammary-coronary artery bypass grafting. *Cathet Cardiovasc Diagn* 1991;24:274–276.
15. Granke K, Van Meter Jr CH, White CJ, et al. Myocardial ischemia caused by postoperative malfunction of a patent internal mammary coronary arterial graft. *J Vasc Surg* 1990;11:659–664.
16. Ackermann H, Diener HC, Seboldt H, et al. Ultrasonographic follow-up of subclavian stenosis and occlusion: natural history and surgical treatment. *Stroke* 1988;19:431–435.
17. Moran KT, Zide RS, Persson AV, et al. Natural history of subclavian steal syndrome. *Am Surg* 1988;54:643–644.
18. Cosottini M, Zampa V, Petruzzi P, et al. Contrast-enhanced three-dimensional MR angiography in the assessment of subclavian artery diseases. *Eur Radiol* 2000;10:1737–1744.
19. Cosottini M, Pingitore A, Puglioli M, et al. Contrast-enhanced three-dimensional magnetic resonance angiography of atherosclerotic internal carotid stenosis as the noninvasive imaging modality in revascularization decision making. *Stroke* 2003;34:660–664.
20. Hadjipetrou P, Cox S, Piemonte T, et al. Percutaneous revascularization of atherosclerotic obstruction of aortic arch vessels. *J Am Coll Cardiol* 1999;33:1238–1245.
21. Berguer R, Morasch MD, Kline RA. Transthoracic repair of innominate and common carotid artery disease: immediate and long-term outcome for 100 consecutive surgical reconstructions. *J Vasc Surg* 1998;27:34–41; discussion, 42.
22. Berguer R, Morasch MD, Kline RA, et al. Cervical reconstruction of the supra-aortic trunks: a 16-year experience. *J Vasc Surg* 1999;29:239–246; discussion, 246–248.
23. Taha AA, Vahl AC, de Jong SC, et al. Reconstruction of the supra-aortic trunks. *Eur J Surg* 1999;165:314–318.
24. Azakie A, McElhinney DB, Higashima R, et al. Innominate artery reconstruction: over 3 decades of experience. *Ann Surg* 1998;228:402–410.
25. Linguish J, Criado E, Keagy BA. Innominate artery occlusive disease: management with central reconstructive techniques. *Surgery* 1997;121:556–562.
26. Mingoli A, Sapienza P, Feldhaus RJ, et al. Long-term results and outcomes of crossover axilloaxillary bypass grafting: A 24-year experience. *J Vasc Surg* 1999;29:894–901.
27. Paty PS, Mehta M, Darling RC, et al. Surgical treatment of coronary subclavian steal syndrome with carotid subclavian bypass. *Ann Vasc Surg* 2003;17:22–26.
28. AbuRahma AF, Robinson PA, Jennings TG. Carotid-subclavian bypass grafting with polytetrafluoroethylene grafts for symptomatic subclavian artery stenosis or occlusion: a 20-year experience. *J Vasc Surg* 2000;32:411–418; discussion, 418–419.
29. Al-Mubarak N, Liu MW, Dean LS, et al. Immediate and late outcomes of subclavian artery stenting. *Catheter Cardiovasc Interv* 1999;46:169–172.
30. Henry M, Amor M, Henry I, et al. Percutaneous transluminal

angioplasty of the subclavian arteries. *J Endovasc Surg* 1999;6:33–41.

31. Roubin GS, New G, Iyer SS, et al. Immediate and late clinical outcomes of carotid artery stenting in patients with symptomatic and asymptomatic carotid artery stenosis: a 5-year prospective analysis. *Circulation* 2001;103:532–537.

32. Yadav JS, Roubin GS, Iyer S, et al. Elective stenting of the extracranial carotid arteries. *Circulation* 1997;95:376–381.

33. Roubin GS, Hobson 2nd RW, White R, et al. CREST and CARESS to evaluate carotid stenting: time to get to work! *J Endovasc Ther* 2001; 8:107–110.

34. White CJ. The times they are a-changin'. *J Am Coll Cardiol* 1999;33: 1246–1247.

35. Hollier LH. Combining endovascular and surgical techniques: the best of both worlds. *J Endovasc Surg* 1998;5:333–334.

36. Phipp LH, Scott DJ, Kessel D, et al. Subclavian stents and stent-grafts: cause for concern? *J Endovasc Surg* 1999;6:223–226.

37. Motarjeme A. Percutaneous transluminal angioplasty of supra-aortic vessels. *J Endovasc Surg* 1996;3:171–181.

38. Schillinger M, Haumer M, Schillinger S, et al. Risk stratification for subclavian artery angioplasty: is there an increased rate of restenosis after stent implantation? *J Endovasc Ther* 2001;8:550–557.

39. Szeimies U, Kueffer G, Stoeckelhuber B, et al. Successful exclusion of subclavian aneurysms with covered nitinol stents. *Cardiovasc Intervent Radiol* 1998;21:246–249.

40. Bates MC, AbuRahma AF, Stone PA. Restenting for subclavian in-stent restenosis with symptomatic recurrent coronary-subclavian steal. *J Endovasc Ther* 2002;9:676–679.

41. Fischman DL, Leon MB, Baim DS, et al. A randomized comparison of coronary-stent placement and balloon angioplasty in the treatment of coronary artery disease. Stent Restenosis Study Investigators. *N Engl J Med* 1994;331:496–501.

42. Serruys PW, de Jaegere P, Kiemeneij F, et al. A comparison of balloon-expandable-stent implantation with balloon angioplasty in patients with coronary artery disease. Benestent Study Group. *N Engl J Med* 1994;331:489–495.

43. Morice MC, Serruys PW, Sousa JE, et al. A randomized comparison of a sirolimus-eluting stent with a standard stent for coronary revascularization. *N Engl J Med* 2002;346:1773–1780.

44. Curfman GD. Sirolimus-eluting coronary stents. *N Engl J Med* 2002; 346:1770–1771.

45. Duda SH, Pusich B, Richter G, et al. Sirolimus-eluting stents for the treatment of obstructive superficial femoral artery disease: six-month results. *Circulation* 2002;106:1505–1509.

46. Gray WA, DuBroff RJ, White HJ. Clinical problem-solving. A common clinical conundrum. *N Engl J Med* 1997;336:1008–1011.

CHAPTER 21

Cerebral Vascular Disease

Patricia A. Gum, Alex Abou-Chebl, and Jay S. Yadav

Key Points

- Cerebrovascular disease is the second-leading cause of death worldwide.
- Risk factors of cerebral vascular disease include hypertension, atherosclerosis, diabetes, hyperlipidemia, stroke, inflammation, and smoking.
- Rapid and early recanalization is critically important for the effective therapy of acute ischemic stroke.
- Distal embolization is a problem with any treatment for atherosclerotic disease, and embolization into the cerebral vascular system can be of particular consequence.
- The percutaneous treatment of carotid atherosclerotic disease is safe, is the preferred approach to high-surgical-risk patients, and may prove to have much wider application.

INTRODUCTION

Cerebrovascular disease is a major cause of morbidity and mortality; it is second only to cardiovascular disease as a cause of death worldwide (1). In the United States, stroke is the third-leading cause of death, and was responsible for 167,661 deaths in the year 2000. More than 750,000 people experience either an initial or recurrent stoke each year, and more than $51 billion dollars was spent on the diagnosis and treatment of stroke in the year 2000. Additionally, the effects of stroke are not limited to the acute clinical and financial consequences. There are significant long-term effects related to stroke. Nearly one-fourth of all stroke patients die within 1 year following the event, and the prognosis is worse for those who are older than 65 years (2). For those who survive, the long-term clinical ramifications of stroke are not insignificant. Stroke is the number one cause of long-term disability, with 20% of victims still requiring institutional care 3 months after the event.

Although strokes may be caused by either hemorrhage or ischemia, an overwhelming majority (80%) of strokes are ischemic in origin. Of these, 25% to 30% are due to a vascular stenosis or occlusion. Much work has been done to elucidate the underlying causes of these stenoses, and several therapies have been developed for treatment.

RISK FACTORS

The common and internal carotid arteries consist of an intima, a media, and an adventitia, similar to the makeup of the coronary arteries. Atherosclerotic disease in the carotid arteries is therefore, not surprisingly, very similar to that in the coronary arteries. Atheromatous plaque accumulates most commonly in areas of turbulent flow, such as the bifurcations. The material collected after carotid stenting with distal emboli prevention devices (EPD) contains lipid vacuoles, fibrin, platelets, and foam cells (3). Approximately 50% to 60% of patients with carotid disease also have severe coronary stenosis. However, the presence of coronary artery disease is not as clear a marker for carotid disease. Only 5% to 10% of patients with coronary artery disease also have severe carotid atherosclerosis (4).

Of the associated cardiovascular risk factors that can be modified, hypertension has the highest population-attributable risk. Compared with normotensive individuals, people with hypertension are at four times greater risk of stroke (5). The associated risk is consistent across geographic areas and populations (6). Systolic hypertension, in particular, appears to have a stronger negative association than diastolic hypertension (7). However, treatment of hypertension, both systolic and diastolic, imparts a significant and timely

295

reduction in the risk of stroke (8,9). The Systolic Hypertension in the Elderly Program proved an associated reduction for the risk of both hemorrhagic and ischemic stroke with the treatment of systolic hypertension to treatment goals (10,11).

The risk imparted by tobacco use is closely correlated with the amount of abuse. Heavy smokers are at twice the relative risk of stroke as light smokers. The risk of stroke, however, is significantly reduced within 2 years of smoking cessation, and returns to baseline at 5 years after cessation (12).

Diabetes has been shown to not only increase the risk of stroke, but also to increase the mortality secondary to stroke (13). It independently increased the relative risk of stroke from one and one-half times to three times above control in cohort studies (14,15). More recent work has also linked insulin resistance with both an increased risk of carotid atherosclerosis and stroke. There is also evidence that the treatment of insulin resistance decreases this risk (16). Similarly, the UK Prospective Diabetes Study demonstrated a reduction in strokes associated with the treatment of diabetes (17).

Although there has been some debate concerning the associated risk of hyperlipidemia and stroke, several studies have demonstrated this risk and a reduction in this risk with treatment (18–20). More specifically, the use of 3-hydroxy-3-methylglutaryl coenzyme A reductase inhibitors (statins) has been shown to be of benefit in reducing stroke and treating carotid atherosclerosis. Three separate meta-analyses have demonstrated a reduction in stoke with the use of statins (21–23). Statins have also been shown to positively affect vessel wall thickness, luminal area, and progression of intimal–medial thickness (24–26).

Similar to recent work in the coronary realm, inflammation has been shown to be associated with an increased risk of carotid atherosclerosis (27). Elevated serum markers of inflammation such as C-reactive protein and fibrinogen are associated with an increased morbidity and mortality risk after an ischemic stroke during long-term follow-up (28) (see Chapter 2).

There are also several nonmodifiable factors that impart an increased risk of cerebral vascular disease. Race has a significant impact on stroke risk. Blacks below age 85 years are at higher risk of stroke than to non-Hispanic whites, and blacks are more likely to die secondary to complications from a stroke than are whites (2). Stroke risk increases in a stepwise fashion in both women and men in relation to age. The age-adjusted incidence (per 100,000) of stroke is highest in black men (323), followed by black women (260), white men (167), and white women (138) (2).

Beyond the traditional risk factors for atherosclerotic disease, the presence of either physical signs or symptoms bears an increased risk of stroke. A carotid bruit is the physical examination hallmark of carotid atherosclerosis. Although carotid bruits are not predictive of the severity of atherosclerosis, they are associated with a greater risk of stroke, myocardial infarction, and death (12,29). Moreover, once carotid atheromatous lesions have formed, the degree of stenosis and its associated symptoms are predictive of the risk of stroke

(29). For an asymptomatic carotid stenosis of at least 60%, the yearly risk of stroke is 2.1% (30). The risk of death increases in concordance with increasing stenosis severity as well. The adjusted relative risk of death for stenoses less than 45% is 1.32, for stenoses of 45% to 74% it is 2.22, and for stenoses of 75% to 99% it is 3.24 (31). The addition of symptoms dramatically increases the risk associated with carotid stenosis. The risk of stroke following a transient ischemic attack was 40% in the Framingham study, and two-thirds of these strokes occurred within the first 6 months (32). In the North American Symptomatic Carotid Endarterectomy Trial (NASCET) a symptomatic carotid stenosis of greater than 70% was associated with a 26% risk of ipsilateral stroke over 2 years in medically treated patients, and a 50% to 69% symptomatic stenosis carried a 22.2% risk of ipsilateral stroke (33).

TREATMENT STRATEGIES

Acute Stroke Treatment

Intravenous Thrombolysis for Acute Ischemic Stroke

Rapid and early recanalization is critically important for the effective therapy of acute ischemic stroke. Advances in thrombolytic therapy for acute ischemic stroke have been tempered by the risk of intracranial hemorrhage (ICH), which is fatal in the majority of cases. In 1995, the results of the National Institutes of Neurologic Disorders and Stroke (NINDS) trial of intravenous (IV) thrombolysis with recombinant tissue plasminogen activator (tPA) in acute stroke were published (34). This landmark study proved the efficacy of IV tPA (0.9 mg per kg, maximum 90 mg, given 10% as a bolus and the remainder infused over 1 hour) within 3 hours of stroke onset in a mixed stroke population. Despite a tenfold increased risk of symptomatic brain hemorrhage (6% vs. 0.6%), treated patients had a 10% to 13% absolute increase in complete neurological recovery compared to control patients (13). This was the first positive study evaluating acute stroke therapy. Nonetheless, almost 7 years after Food and Drug Administration (FDA) approval, less than 2% of all acute stroke patients in the United States were being treated with IV tPA (35). There are multiple reasons for this underutilization, but the major limitation is the narrow treatment window of 3 hours from symptom onset to treatment initiation. The restrictions imposed by this narrow treatment window have led to further investigation evaluating the use of thrombolytic therapy beyond 3 hours. Although a meta-analysis of IV thrombolysis in acute stroke showed that there may be a slight overall benefit for IV thrombolysis in patients treated between 3 and 6 hours (36), six multicenter trials have been unable to show an overall benefit for IV thrombolysis initiated after 3 hours from stroke onset (37–42). Most recently, the primary endpoints of the European Cooperative Acute Stroke Study II (ECASS II) and the North American Altepase Thrombolysis for Acute Noninterventional Therapy in Ischemic Stroke (ATLANTIS) trial were also negative beyond 3 hours (40) (see Chapter 22 for more details on thrombolysis).

Intraarterial Thrombolysis for Acute Ischemic Stroke

Only two studies have evaluated the safety and efficacy of intraarterial (IA) thrombolysis in a randomized fashion: the Prolyse in Acute Cerebral Thromboembolism (PROACT) I and II trials. In PROACT I, the safety and recanalization efficacy of recombinant pro-urokinase (r-pro-UK) was examined in 40 patients with acute ischemic stroke due to middle cerebral artery (MCA) occlusion of less than 6 hours duration (43). Mechanical disruption of the clot was not permitted, and all patients also received IV heparin, in various dose tiers. The findings of this first study were the foundation for the follow-up clinical efficacy trial, PROACT II, which was launched in February 1996 (44). PROACT II was also a randomized, controlled trial with a similar patient selection as PROACT I, with the exception of excluding patients with early signs of an infarct in greater than one-third of the MCA territory (the ECASS criteria) (39) on the initial computed tomography (CT) scan. The treatment group received a dose of 9 mg of r-pro-UK infused over 2 hours directly into the MCA. "Low-heparin" doses (2,000 U IV bolus followed by 500 U per hour for 4 hours) were used in the treatment and control groups because of the significantly higher ICH rates seen with higher doses in the safety study. A total of 180 patients were randomized. For the r-pro-UK-treated patients, there was a 15% absolute benefit (58% relative benefit) in the functional outcome measure at 3 months ($p=0.04$). On average, 7 patients with MCA occlusion would require IA thrombolysis for 1 to benefit. Recanalization rates were 66% at 2 hours for the treatment group and 18% for the placebo group ($p<0.001$), but the Thrombolysis in Myocardial Infarction (TIMI) 3 (complete recanalization) (45) rate was only 19% with r-pro-UK. Symptomatic brain hemorrhage occurred in 10% of the r-pro-UK group and 2% of the control group. Considering the later time to treatment and greater baseline stroke severity in PROACT II, the symptomatic brain hemorrhage rate, compares favorably with the rates in the IV tPA trials, 6% in the NINDS trial, 9% in ECASS II, and 7% in ATLANTIS (34,37,40). As in the NINDS trial, there was an overall benefit from IA therapy despite the higher brain hemorrhage rate, and there was no excess mortality (24% with treatment vs. 27% in control patients). Despite the positive results of the PROACT II trial, r-pro-UK does not have FDA approval, so IA thrombolysis remains an investigational treatment. In many academic centers, however, IA thrombolysis with a variety of thrombolytic agents remains the de facto standard of care for patients with severe ischemic stroke of less than 6 hours duration.

Stroke Prevention

Percutaneous Treatment for Carotid Stenosis

Percutaneous transluminal angioplasty (PTA) of the carotid artery was first reported in human patients by Mullan et al. (46) and Kerber et al. (47) in 1980. Widespread controversy followed the early forays into the investigation of this procedure. However, event rates comparable to carotid endarterec-

tomy were reported in Kachel's 1996 review of more than 500 carotid angioplasties (48). Since that time, advances in the field have led to carotid artery angioplasty being supplanted by the strategy of carotid stenting (CAS) with distal emboli prevention for the elective treatment of carotid stenosis.

Many of the associated problems of carotid angioplasty including vessel recoil and dissection have been successfully addressed with the use of stents (Fig. 21.1). However, some unique lessons came to light with the initial use of stents in the carotid artery. Both the external compression and torsion forces that affect the carotid artery make balloon-expandable stents a poor choice for carotid artery stenting. Although these stents can be positioned with relative ease and precision, external compression forces can deform the stent and lead to lumen impingement (49). Self-expanding elgiloy stents (Wallstent : Boston Scientific, Natick, MA) or nitinol stents (Precise : Cordis Endovascular, Miami Lakes, FL, Memotherm, Acculink Guidant, St. Paul, MN, Endostent : Endotex, Cupertino, CA, etc.) are therefore better suited for carotid arteries because they continue to exert outward forces resisting external compression.

The first reports of the use of stents for the treatment of carotid artery disease were published by Mathias (50) and Marks et al. (51). There have been several large-scale observational series reported subsequently documenting a low periprocedural event rate and restenosis rate. The majority of the patients included in these series were at high surgical risk for carotid endarterectomy (CEA). The results of these series as well as the major CEA trials are summarized in Table 21.1.

In 1996, Diethrich et al. published the first large-scale series of patients treated with carotid artery stenting (52). The investigators treated 117 carotid artery lesions in 31 symptomatic and 79 asymptomatic patients with percutaneous stenting (52). Treatment was considered successful in 109 (99%) of those treated. There were 7 resultant strokes and 1 death within the first 30 days of follow-up. During a mean follow-up of 7.6 months, no additional neurological events or deaths occurred, and the stent patency rate was 96.6%.

In 1997, Yadav et al. published the first protocol-driven study with independent neurological assessment prior to and following the procedure (53). This was a landmark study, and set the standard for a multidisciplinary, investigationally sound approach in evaluating percutaneous carotid intervention. The authors reported the results from 107 consecutive patients (126 stenoses), the majority of whom met NASCET exclusion criteria for CEA, who were treated with percutaneous carotid angioplasty and elective stenting. The procedure was successful in all instances, and the 30-day risk of major stroke or death was 2.4%. Of the 61 patients who underwent follow-up angiography at 6 months, 3 demonstrated angiographic restenosis. Wholey et al. twice published global reviews of carotid stenting performed worldwide. Their most recent work, published in 2000, reported the results of 5,210 carotid stents placed in 4,757 patients (54). Technical success was achieved in 98.4%. The 30-day risk of stroke was 4.2% (2.7% minor and 1.5% major),

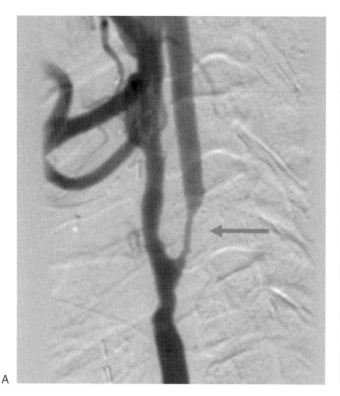
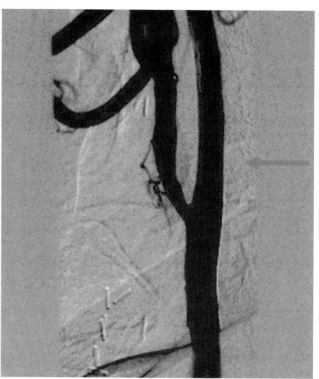

FIG. 21.1. A: Internal carotid artery stenosis prior to treatment. **B:** Internal carotid artery after treatment with carotid artery stenting.

and the mortality rate was 0.86%. Restenosis occurred in 2.0% and 3.5% of patients at 6- and 12-month follow-ups, respectively.

The most recent registry results reported are from the single-arm Acculink for Revascularization of Carotids in High-Risk Patients study. The preliminary 30-day results of 437 patients were reported at the American College of Cardiology 2003 Annual Scientific Sessions. Patients enrolled in the study had a symptomatic carotid stenosis of at least 50%

or an asymptomatic carotid stenosis of at least 80%, and at least one clinical feature that would classify them as high risk. Procedural success was achieved in 92.7% and the combined stroke or death rate was 6.6%. Stroke, death, or myocardial infarction occurred in 7.8%. In subgroup analysis, those patients requiring dialysis were at highest risk, with a combined stroke or death rate of 28.6%, whereas those with a history of restenosis after previous CEA had only a 0.7% risk of stroke or death.

TABLE 21.1. *Carotid artery stenting registries and surgical carotid endarterectomy trial outcomes*

Study[a]	Procedure[b]	Lesions	Lesion severity	Symptoms	Success (%)	Stroke (%)	Myocardial infarction (%)	Death (%)	Restenosis (%)	Follow-up
ECST[c] (62)	CEA	1,807	All	Yes	*	6.6	—	1.0	—	6 yr
NASCET[c] (33)	CEA	328	70%–99%	Yes	99.6	5.5	0.9	0.3	?	8 yr
		430	50%–69%	Yes	99.6	5.6	—	1.2	?	8 yr
ACAS[c] (30)	CEA	757[d]	60%–99%	No	—	2.3	—	0.2	?	2.7 yr
Diethrich[e] (52)	CAS	117			99.1	8.3	0	0.9	1.7	7.6 mo
Yadav[e] (53)	CAS	126			100	6.3	—	0.8	4.9	6 mo
Wholey[e] (63)	CAS	114			95	3.5	0.9	1.9	1.0	6 mo
Wholey, global experience[e] (54)	CAS	5,210			98.4	4.21	—	0.86	3.5	1 yr
Shawl[e] (64)	CAS	192			99	2.9	0	0	2	19 mo
Gupta[e] (65)	CAS	100			100	1	—	0	1	12.1 mo
Reimers[e] (66)	CAS	88			97.7	1.2	2.3	0	0	30 d

[a]ECST, European Carotid Surgery Trialists; NASCET, North American Symptomatic Carotid Endarterectomy Trial; ACAS, Asymptomatic Carotid Atherosclerosis Study.
[b]CEA, Carotid endarterectomy; CAS, carotid stenting.
[c]All were "low risk" as defined in the text.
[d]Most patients were considered to be "high risk" as defined in the text.
[e]Of 825 randomized to surgery, only 757 were treated with CEA.

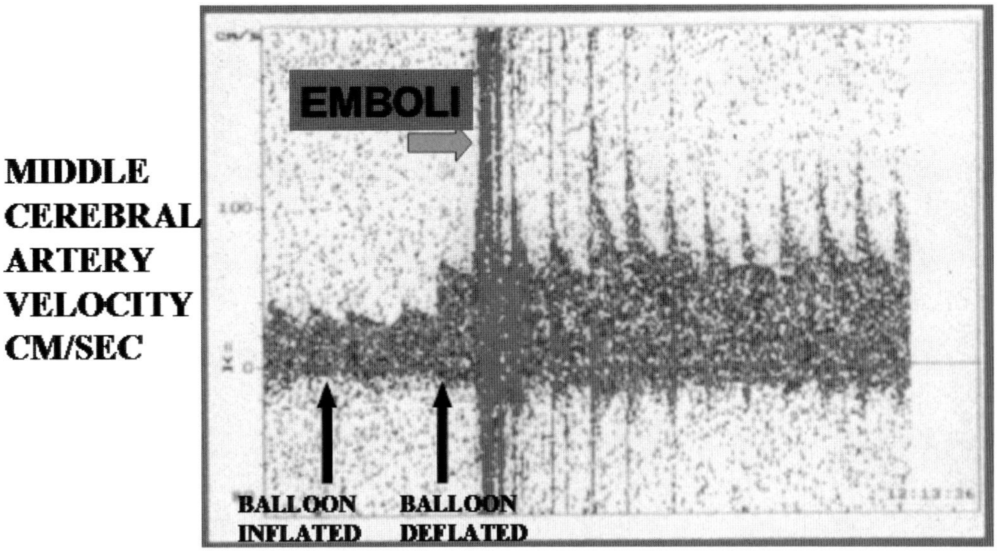

MIDDLE
CEREBRAL
ARTERY
VELOCITY
CM/SEC

EMBOLI

BALLOON
INFLATED

BALLOON
DEFLATED

FIG. 21.2. (See Color Fig. 21.2.) Transcranial Doppler demonstrating embolization with balloon deflation.

Emboli Prevention Devices

Distal embolization is a problem with any treatment for atherosclerotic disease. Embolization into the cerebral vascular system, however, can be of particular consequence. Cerebral ischemia in the setting of CAS occurs almost exclusively with stent delivery and postdilatation. Transcranial Doppler easily detects the occurrence of microemboli during carotid artery stenting and CEA (Fig. 21.2) (55,56). The amount of embolization detected during CEA by transcranial Doppler has been correlated with neurological morbidity (57–59). With this in mind, several devices designed to prevent embolization of procedure-related debris during angioplasty and stenting have been developed. There are three major types of EPD devices, the distal occlusive balloon, the proximal occlusive balloon, and the filter wire.

The PercuSurge GuardWire (Medtronic, Santa Rosa, CA) (Fig. 21.3) is the archetypical distal occlusive balloon EPD. A low-pressure balloon is located at the distal tip of a hollow wire. The stenosis is crossed with this wire, positioning the occlusion balloon distal to the lesion. The occlusion balloon is then inflated, preventing antegrade flow through the internal carotid artery. The occlusion balloon traps debris released during the percutaneous procedure in the internal carotid artery, which is then aspirated prior to deflation of the balloon. This system benefits from a low crossing profile and superior wire flexibility. However, the occlusive nature of this device may not be well tolerated in patients without good collateral flow. Furthermore, there is potential for debris to lodge in the "suction shadow" of the balloon, making it inaccessible for aspiration. This debris can then propagate distally after the occlusion balloon is deflated. Although the distal occlusion balloon is compliant, if care is not taken to secure the wire and prevent movement of this balloon during equipment exchanges, the distal internal carotid artery can be damaged at the site of balloon occlusion by the device.

Additionally, precise localization of the lesion for treatment with angioplasty or stenting can be difficult after inflation of the distal occlusion balloon because antegrade flow of both blood and contrast is halted.

Proximal occlusion balloon systems work by creating retrograde flow in the internal carotid artery, which prevents emboli from traveling to the cerebral circulation (Fig. 21.4). This device requires a 10 French arterial access sheath and femoral venous access. Like the GuardWire, this device depends on occlusive balloons to prevent distal embolization of debris. One is located in the distal common carotid artery and a second in the external carotid artery. This creates a reversal of the pressure gradient in the internal carotid artery and subsequent flow reversal. However, either the common or the

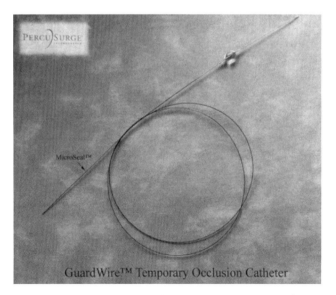

FIG. 21.3. The PercuSurge GuardWire distal emboli prevention system. (Courtesy of Medtronic, Santa Rosa, CA.)

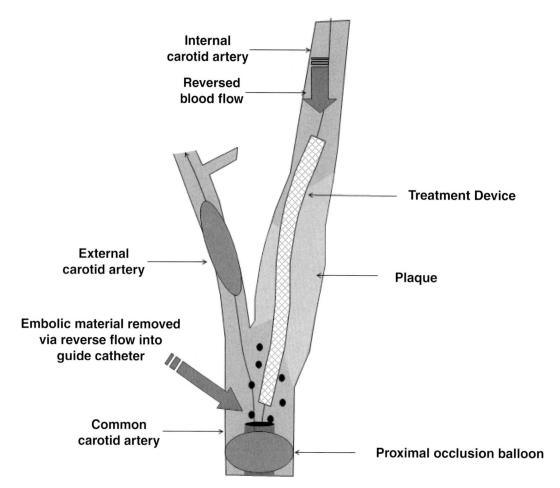

Internal carotid artery

Reversed blood flow

Treatment Device

External carotid artery

Plaque

Embolic material removed via reverse flow into guide catheter

Common carotid artery

Proximal occlusion balloon

FIG. 21.4. (See Color Fig. 21.4.) Schematic of a proximal occlusion balloon system.

external carotid artery can be damaged by the occlusion balloon. Good collateral circulation is also critical because there is no antegrade flow in the treated carotid artery during the length of the procedure. Examples of these devices include the Parodi (Arteria Medical Science Inc, San Francisco, CA) and MOMA (Luvatec, Ron Cadelle, Italy) devices.

There are several examples of the distal filter wire system. The first system designed to conform to the artery and allow both trapping of microemboli and maintenance of antegrade blood flow through the filter was the AngioGuard Emboli Capture Guidewire (Cordis, Miami, FL) (Fig. 21.5). Distal filter devices allow blood flow to be preserved during the intervention, and therefore do not impede visualization of the lesion with contrast material or lead to ischemia. Disadvantages of filters include a larger crossing profile, which may necessitate predilatation prior to placement of the filter distal to the lesion. Additionally, some lesions may release a large embolic load during treatment. If this occurs, the filter may fill with embolic debris, resulting in decreased blood flow through the filter. This can be associated with the patient becoming symptomatic, and always necessitates aspiration of the stagnant column of blood in the internal carotid artery prior to capture of the filter (unpublished data). Many other filter devices, such as Accunet (Guidant), FilterWire EX

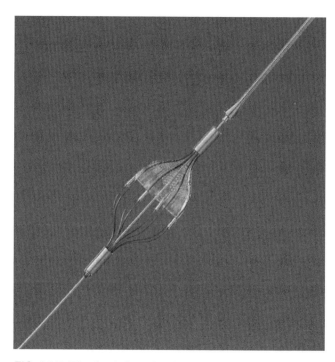

FIG. 21.5. The AngioGuard emboli guidewire system. (Courtesy of Cordis, Miami, FL).

TABLE 21.2. *Emboli prevention device experience*

Study	Number of procedures	Device[a]	Thirty-day events (includes procedural) (%)			
			Major stroke	Minor stroke	Death	All
Henry (67)	184	GuardWire	0.5	0	0.5	1
Al-Mubarak (68)	164	NeuroShield	0	1.2	1.2	2.4
Whitlow (69)	75	GuardWire	0	0	0	0
Reimers (66)	88	Filters (three types)	0	1	0	1
MacDonald (70)	50	NeuroShield	0	2	4	6
Cremonesi (71)	30	TRAP VFS	NA	NA	NA	0
All	591		0.2	0.7	0.2	1.6

[a]GuardWire: Medtronic, Santa Rosa, CA; NeuroShield: MedNova, Galway, Ireland; TRAP VFS, TRAP vascular filtration system: ev3 Inc., Plymouth, MN.

(Boston Scientific Natick, MA), Sulzer-IntraGuard (IntraTherapeutics), MDT-Filte (Medtronic, Minneapolis, MN), Microvena-Trap (Microvena, White Bear Lake, MN), and Mednova (Abbott/Mednova Chicago, IL/Galway, Ireland), have been under investigation.

There are several case series documenting experience with these devices as adjunctive therapy during carotid stenting. The results of these series as well as the outcomes of the major CEA trials are outlined in Table 21.2. Results from these studies demonstrate the efficacy of EPD in reducing procedural stroke compared to retrospective cohorts who did not have a EPD used. Additionally, the outcomes in these series are comparable to those in the CEA trials. The use of EPDs has thus become the clinical standard of care, and all randomized trials comparing carotid stenting with CEA use EPDs. There are no studies comparing different EPDs for safety and efficacy.

Comparison of Carotid Artery Stenting and Carotid Endarterectomy

Percutaneous-based therapy is widely accepted as an alternative to surgical revascularization in coronary artery disease. However, the safety and feasibility of CEA made the early forays into the investigation of carotid angioplasty and stenting controversial. Despite this furor, the less invasive nature of a percutaneous strategy and positive early results made it evident that this procedure was worthy of investigation. Although registries provided early documentation of the feasibility and safety of percutaneous carotid intervention, carotid stenting needed direct prospective, randomized comparison with the historic gold standard surgery. Two major studies directly comparing CEA and percutaneous treatment in a prospective, randomized manner have been completed. The results of these two trials are summarized in Table 21.3.

The Carotid and Vertebral Artery Transluminal Angioplasty Study was a randomized, prospective, multicenter trial designed to compare surgical CEA with the endovascular strategy of angioplasty and provisional stenting (60). There was no difference between the two treatment groups with regard to stroke or mortality. Although the percutaneous treatment group was more likely to experience angiographic restenosis, this did not parlay into an increased ipsilateral stroke rate over 3 years of follow-up. Bleeding and cranial nerve palsies were more common in those treated with CEA. Critics of this trial have questioned the higher than expected complication rate associated with CEA. The event rates may more accurately reflect the real-world risk associated with CEA. Conversely, there were several limitations with the percutaneous method employed. Stents were placed in only

TABLE 21.3. *Thirty-day events from the CAVATAS and SAPPHIRE trials[a]*

		Death	Stroke	Myocardial infarction	Death/any stroke	Death/myocardial infarction/stroke	Cranial nerve palsy	Significant hematoma[b]	Severe restenosis[c]
CAVATAS (60)	Endovascular (251 pts)	3%	4%	—	10%	—	0	1%	14%
	CEA (253 pts)	2%	4%	—	10%	—	9%	7%	4%
p		NS	NS	—	NS	—	<0.001	<0.0015	<0.001
SAPPHIRE (randomized pts) (61)	Endovascular (156 pts)	0.6%	3.8%	2.6%	3.8%	5.8%	5.3%	10.6%	—
	CEA (151 pts)	2.1%	5.3%	7.3%	6.6%	12.6%	0	8.3%	—
p		0.36	0.59	0.07	0.46	0.047	<0.01	0.56	—

[a]CAVATAS, Carotid and Vertebral Artery Transluminal Angioplasty Study; SAPPHIRE, Stenting and Angioplasty with Protection in Patients at High Risk for Endartectomy trial; pts, patients; CEA, carotid endarterectomy.
[b]Major bleeding as measured in SAPPHIRE.
[c]Restenosis measured at 1 year in CAVATAS.

25% of those undergoing percutaneous revascularization, and EPDs were not utilized during any of the percutaneous treatments.

The Stenting and Angioplasty with Protection in Patients at High Risk for Endarterectomy trial recently cemented the role of carotid stenting for carotid stenosis in high-risk patients. The 30-day perioperative outcomes were reported at the American Heart Association Scientific Sessions, Chicago, November 2002 (61). Entry criteria included the presence of either an asymptomatic stenosis of at least 80% by ultrasound or a symptomatic stenosis of at least 50%. All patients enrolled were at increased risk for CEA secondary to a comorbid condition. These conditions included restenosis after previous CEA, congestive heart failure, severe coronary artery disease, previous radical neck surgery or radiation therapy, chronic obstructive pulmonary disease, contralateral carotid artery occlusion, and age greater than 80 years. There were three arms to this trial. In total, 307 patients were randomly assigned to either carotid angioplasty and stenting with emboli protection or CEA. Those patients who, in the opinion of a vascular surgeon, were not surgical candidates and therefore not eligible for randomization could be enrolled in a percutaneous registry (409 patients). Likewise, patients not considered appropriate for percutaneous therapy were enrolled in a surgical registry (17 patients). The primary endpoint was 30-day major adverse cardiovascular events (MACE), including death, stroke, or myocardial infarction. Those patients undergoing percutaneous treatment had a markedly reduced 30-day MACE rate compared to the CEA group (5.8% vs. 12.6%, $p=0.047$). Major bleeding events and transient ischemic attack rates were not significantly different between the two groups (major bleeding 8.3% vs. 10.6%, $p=0.56$; transient ischemic attack 3.8% vs. 2.0%, $p=0.5$). Carotid stenting was also superior to CEA in associated rates of cranial nerve injury (0% vs. 5.3%, $p<0.01$). Restenosis rates have not yet been released. This trial clearly demonstrated a reduction in risk of MACE for high-risk patients treated with carotid stenting compared to conventional CEA.

Several trials to evaluate the percutaneous treatment of carotid artery atherosclerosis are ongoing. One of the most important trials ongoing is the Carotid Revascularization Endarterectomy vs. Stent Trial. This is a multicenter, randomized trial to compare CEA with carotid artery stenting using EPDs in low-risk (i.e. NASCET-eligible) patients. Although this trial has been plagued by funding and enrollment difficulties, it has the potential to provide information on a much wider patient population than has previously been evaluated in a randomized manner.

SUMMARY

From an invasive standpoint, the percutaneous treatment of carotid atherosclerotic disease has had significant advances since its advent in 1980. It has proven to be a safe and pre-

ferred approach to high-surgical-risk patients and may prove to have much wider application. Further investigation is ongoing concerning different patient populations and various devices that may expand the potential uses of this technique. Because this procedure has the potential for significant complications, adequate training and certification will be necessary to ensure optimal patient outcomes.

REFERENCES

1. Murray CJ, Lopez AD. Mortality by cause for eight regions of the world: Global Burden of Disease Study. *Lancet* 1997;349:1269–1276.
2. American Heart Association. *Heart disease and stroke statistics—2003 update*. Dallas, TX: Author.
3. Angelini A, Reimers B, Della Barbera M, et al. Cerebral protection during carotid artery stenting: collection and histopathologic analysis of embolized debris. *Stroke* 2002;33:456–461.
4. Hertzer NR, Beven EG, Young JR, et al. Coronary artery disease in peripheral vascular patients. A classification of 1000 coronary angiograms and results of surgical management. *Ann Surg* 1984;199:223–233.
5. Gorelick PB. Stroke prevention. *Arch Neurol* 1995;52:347–355.
6. Sacco RL, Boden-Albala B, Abel G, et al. Race–ethnic disparities in the impact of stroke risk factors: the northern Manhattan stroke study. *Stroke* 2001;32:1725–1731.
7. Staessen JA, Gasowski J, Wang JG, et al. Risks of untreated and treated isolated systolic hypertension in the elderly: meta-analysis of outcome trials. *Lancet* 2000;355:865–872.
8. Collins R, Peto R, MacMahon S, et al. Blood pressure, stroke, and coronary heart disease. Part 2. Short-term reductions in blood pressure: overview of randomised drug trials in their epidemiological context. *Lancet* 1990;335:827–838.
9. MacMahon S, Peto R, Cutler J, et al. Blood pressure, stroke, and coronary heart disease. Part 1. Prolonged differences in blood pressure: prospective observational studies corrected for the regression dilution bias. *Lancet* 1990;335:765–774.
10. SHEP Cooperative Research Group. Prevention of stroke by antihypertensive drug treatment in older persons with isolated systolic hypertension. Final results of the Systolic Hypertension in the Elderly Program (SHEP). *JAMA* 1991;265:3255–3264.
11. Perry Jr HM, Davis BR, Price TR, et al. Effect of treating isolated systolic hypertension on the risk of developing various types and subtypes of stroke: the Systolic Hypertension in the Elderly Program (SHEP). *JAMA* 2000;284:465–471.
12. Wolf PA, D'Agostino RB, Kannel WB, et al. Cigarette smoking as a risk factor for stroke. The Framingham Study. *JAMA* 1988;259:1025–1029.
13. Bell DS. Stroke in the diabetic patient. *Diabetes Care* 1994;17:213–219.
14. Barrett-Connor E, Khaw KT. Diabetes mellitus: an independent risk factor for stroke? *Am J Epidemiol* 1988;128:116–123.
15. Elkind MS, Sacco RL. Stroke risk factors and stroke prevention. *Semin Neurol* 1998;18:429–440.
16. Kernan WN, Inzucchi SE, Viscoli CM, et al. Insulin resistance and risk for stroke. *Neurology* 2002;59:809–815.
17. UK Prospective Diabetes Study Group. Tight blood pressure control and risk of macrovascular and microvascular complications in type 2 diabetes: UKPDS 38. UK Prospective Diabetes Study Group. *BMJ* 1998;317:703–713.
18. 4S Study Group. Randomised trial of cholesterol lowering in 4444 patients with coronary heart disease: the Scandinavian Simvastatin Survival Study (4S). *Lancet* 1994;344:1383–1389.
19. Lipid Study Group. Prevention of cardiovascular events and death with pravastatin in patients with coronary heart disease and a broad range of initial cholesterol levels. The Long-Term Intervention with Pravastatin in Ischaemic Disease (LIPID) Study Group. *N Engl J Med* 1998;339:1349–1357.
20. Sacks FM, Pfeffer MA, Moye LA, et al. The effect of pravastatin on

coronary events after myocardial infarction in patients with average cholesterol levels. Cholesterol and Recurrent Events Trial investigators. *N Engl J Med* 1996;335:1001–1009.

21. Blauw GJ, Lagaay AM, Smelt AH, et al. Stroke, statins, and cholesterol. A meta-analysis of randomized, placebo-controlled, double-blind trials with HMG-CoA reductase inhibitors. *Stroke* 1997;28:946–950.

22. Bucher HC, Griffith LE, Guyatt GH. Effect of HMGCoA reductase inhibitors on stroke. A meta-analysis of randomized, controlled trials. *Ann Intern Med* 1998;128:89–95.

23. Hebert PR, Gaziano JM, Chan KS, et al. Cholesterol lowering with statin drugs, risk of stroke, and total mortality. An overview of randomized trials. *JAMA* 1997;278:313–321.

24. Corti R, Fayad ZA, Fuster V, et al. Effects of lipid-lowering by simvastatin on human atherosclerotic lesions: a longitudinal study by high-resolution, noninvasive magnetic resonance imaging. *Circulation* 2001;104:249–252.

25. Corti R, Fuster V, Fayad ZA, et al. Lipid lowering by simvastatin induces regression of human atherosclerotic lesions: two years' follow-up by high-resolution noninvasive magnetic resonance imaging. *Circulation* 2002;106:2884–2887.

26. Mercuri M, Bond MG, Sirtori CR, et al. Pravastatin reduces carotid intima–media thickness progression in an asymptomatic hypercholesterolemic Mediterranean population: the Carotid Atherosclerosis Italian Ultrasound Study. *Am J Med* 1996;101:627–634.

27. Magyar MT, Szikszai Z, Balla J, et al. Early-onset carotid atherosclerosis is associated with increased intima–media thickness and elevated serum levels of inflammatory markers. *Stroke* 2003;34:58–63.

28. Di Napoli M, Papa F, Bocola V. Prognostic influence of increased C-reactive protein and fibrinogen levels in ischemic stroke. *Stroke* 2001;32:133–138.

29. Norris JW, Zhu CZ, Bornstein NM, et al. Vascular risks of asymptomatic carotid stenosis. *Stroke* 1991;22:1485–1490.

30. Executive Committee for the Asymptomatic Carotid Atherosclerosis Study Group. Endarterectomy for asymptomatic carotid artery stenosis. *JAMA* 1995;273:1421–1428.

31. Joakimsen O, Bonaa KH, Mathiesen EB, et al. Prediction of mortality by ultrasound screening of a general population for carotid stenosis: the Tromso Study. *Stroke* 2000;31:1871–1876.

32. Whisnant JP, Homer D, Ingall TJ, et al. Duration of cigarette smoking is the strongest predictor of severe extracranial carotid artery atherosclerosis. *Stroke* 1990;21:707–714.

33. North American Symptomatic Carotid Endarterectomy Trial Collaborators. Beneficial effect of carotid endarterectomy in symptomatic patients with high-grade carotid stenosis. *N Engl J Med* 1991;325:445–453.

34. National Institute of Neurological Disorders and Stroke rt-PA Stroke Study Group. Tissue plasminogen activator for acute ischemic stroke. *N Engl J Med* 1995;333:1581–1587.

35. Alberts MJ. tPA in acute ischemic stroke: United States experience and issues for the future. *Neurology* 1998;51:S53–S55.

36. Wardlaw JM, del Zoppo G, Yamaguchi T. Thrombolysis for acute ischaemic stroke. *Cochrane Database Syst Rev* 2000:CD000213.

37. Clark WM, Wissman S, Albers GW, et al. Recombinant tissue-type plasminogen activator (alteplase) for ischemic stroke 3 to 5 hours after symptom onset. The ATLANTIS Study: a randomized controlled trial. Alteplase Thrombolysis for Acute Noninterventional Therapy in Ischemic Stroke. *JAMA* 1999;282:2019–2026.

38. Donnan GA, Davis SM, Chambers BR, et al. Streptokinase for acute ischemic stroke with relationship to time of administration: Australian Streptokinase (ASK) Trial Study Group. *JAMA* 1996;276:961–966.

39. Hacke W, Kaste M, Fieschi C, et al. Intravenous thrombolysis with recombinant tissue plasminogen activator for acute hemispheric stroke. The European Cooperative Acute Stroke Study (ECASS). *JAMA* 1995;274:1017–1025.

40. Hacke W, Kaste M, Fieschi C, et al. Randomised double-blind placebo-controlled trial of thrombolytic therapy with intravenous alteplase in acute ischaemic stroke (ECASS II). Second European–Australasian Acute Stroke Study Investigators. *Lancet* 1998;352:1245–1251.

41. Multicenter Acute Stroke Trial—Europe Study Group. Thrombolytic therapy with streptokinase in acute ischemic stroke. *N Engl J Med* 1996;335:145–150.

42. Multicenter Acute Stroke Trial—Italy (MAST-I) Group. Randomised controlled trial of streptokinase, aspirin, and combination of both in treatment of acute ischaemic stroke. *Lancet* 1995;346:1509–1514.

43. del Zoppo GJ, Higashida RT, Furlan AJ, et al. PROACT: a phase II randomized trial of recombinant pro-urokinase by direct arterial delivery in acute middle cerebral artery stroke. PROACT Investigators. Prolyse in Acute Cerebral Thromboembolism. *Stroke* 1998;29:4–11.

44. Furlan A, Higashida R, Wechsler L, et al. Intra-arterial prourokinase for acute ischemic stroke. The PROACT II study: a randomized controlled trial. Prolyse in Acute Cerebral Thromboembolism. *JAMA* 1999;282:2003–2011.

45. TIMI Study Group. The Thrombolysis in Myocardial Infarction (TIMI) trial. Phase I findings. *N Engl J Med* 1985;312:932–936.

46. Mullan S, Duda EE, Patronas NJ. Some examples of balloon technology in neurosurgery. *J Neurosurg* 1980;52:321–329.

47. Kerber CW, Cromwell LD, Loehden OL. Catheter dilatation of proximal carotid stenosis during distal bifurcation endarterectomy. *AJNR Am J Neuroradiol* 1980;1:348–349.

48. Kachel R. Results of balloon angioplasty in the carotid arteries. *J Endovasc Surg* 1996;3:22–30.

49. Mathur A, Dorros G, Iyer SS, et al. Palmaz stent compression in patients following carotid artery stenting. *Cathet Cardiovasc Diagn* 1997;41:137–140.

50. Mathius K. Percutaneous angioplasty in supra-aortic artery disease. In: Roubin GS, Califf R, O'Neill W, et al., eds., *Interventional cardiovascular medicine: principles and practice.* New York: Churchill Livingstone, 1994:745–775.

51. Marks MP, Dake MD, Steinberg GK, et al. Stent placement for arterial and venous cerebrovascular disease: preliminary experience. *Radiology.* 1994;191:441–446.

52. Diethrich EB, Ndiaye M, Reid DB. Stenting in the carotid artery: initial experience in 110 patients. *J Endovasc Surg* 1996;3:42–62.

53. Yadav JS, Roubin GS, Iyer S, et al. Elective stenting of the extracranial carotid arteries. *Circulation* 1997;95:376–381.

54. Wholey MH, Wholey M, Mathias K, et al. Global experience in cervical carotid artery stent placement. *Catheter Cardiovasc Interv* 2000;50:160–167.

55. McCleary AJ, Nelson M, Dearden NM, et al. Cerebral haemodynamics and embolization during carotid angioplasty in high-risk patients. *Br J Surg* 1998;85:771–774.

56. Markus HS, Clifton A, Buckenham T, et al. Carotid angioplasty. Detection of embolic signals during and after the procedure. *Stroke* 1994;25:2403–2406.

57. Jansen C, Ramos LM, van Heesewijk JP, et al. Impact of microembolism and hemodynamic changes in the brain during carotid endarterectomy. *Stroke* 1994;25:992–997.

58. Gaunt ME, Martin PJ, Smith JL, et al. Clinical relevance of intraoperative embolization detected by transcranial Doppler ultrasonography during carotid endarterectomy: a prospective study of 100 patients. *Br J Surg* 1994;81:1435–1439.

59. Ackerstaff RG, Jansen C, Moll FL, et al. The significance of microemboli detection by means of transcranial Doppler ultrasonography monitoring in carotid endarterectomy. *J Vasc Surg* 1995;21:963–969.

60. CAVATAS Investigators. Endovascular versus surgical treatment in patients with carotid stenosis in the Carotid and Vertebral Artery Transluminal Angioplasty Study (CAVATAS): a randomised trial. *Lancet* 2001;357:1729–1737.

61. Yadav JS. *Stenting and angioplasty with protection in patients at high risk for endarterectomy.* Presented at the American Heart Association scientific sessions, Chicago, November 2002.

62. European Carotid Surgery Trialists' Collaborative Group. MRC European Carotid Surgery Trial: interim results for symptomatic patients with severe (70–99%) or with mild (0–29%) carotid stenosis. *Lancet* 1991;337:1235–1243.

63. Wholey MH, Jarmolowski CR, Eles G, et al. Endovascular stents for carotid artery occlusive disease. *J Endovasc Surg* 1997;4:326–338.

64. Shawl F, Kadro W, Domanski MJ, et al. Safety and efficacy of elective carotid artery stenting in high-risk patients. *J Am Coll Cardiol* 2000;35:1721–1728.

65. Gupta A, Bhatia A, Ahuja A, et al. Carotid stenting in patients older than 65 years with inoperable carotid artery disease: a single-center experience. *Catheter Cardiovasc Interv* 2000;50:1–8; discussion, 9.

66. Reimers B, Corvaja N, Moshiri S, et al. Cerebral protection with filter devices during carotid artery stenting. *Circulation* 2001;104:12–15.

67. Henry M, Henry I, Klonaris C, et al. Benefits of cerebral protection during carotid stenting with the PercuSurge GuardWire system: midterm results. *J Endovasc Ther* 2002;9:1–13.

68. Al-Mubarak N, Colombo A, Gaines PA, et al. Multicenter evaluation of carotid artery stenting with a filter protection system. *J Am Coll Cardiol* 2002;39:841–846.

69. Whitlow PL, Lylyk P, Londero H, et al. Carotid artery stenting protected with an emboli containment system. *Stroke* 2002;33:1308–1314.

70. Macdonald S, Venables GS, Cleveland TJ, et al. Protected carotid stenting: safety and efficacy of the MedNova NeuroShield filter. *J Vasc Surg* 2002;35:966–972.

71. Cremonesi A, Castriota F. Efficacy of a nitinol filter device in the prevention of embolic events during carotid interventions. *J Endovasc Ther* 2002;9:155–159.

CHAPTER 22

Intracranial Interventions

Thomas C. Piemonte, Timothy Alikakos, and Ayman Iskander

Key Points

- Technical advances (including flexible stents, hydrophilic wires, distal protection devices, etc.) have provided the cardiologist with the tools needed for interventional procedures in the peripheral circulation.
- Atherosclerotic lesions at the base of the skull and intracranial vasculature are still underdiagnosed.
- The formation of thrombus in relation to a significant stenosis leading to subsequent embolism is the most common stroke mechanism.
- Lesions are classified into three types: type A (less than 5 mm in length), type B (5 to 10 mm), and type C (greater than 10 mm).
- Collaboration with neurologists and careful attention to blood pressure are essential in intracranial procedures.
- Twenty billion dollars is spent annually on cerebrovascular ischemic disease.
- Medical therapy may decrease the risk of thromboembolism, but does not prevent low-flow ischemia.

INTRODUCTION

The emerging field of interventional neuroradiology has been complex, demanding, and technically challenging. Although pioneered by procedurally based radiologists, a multidisciplinary approach involving the neurologist, the neurosurgeon, the interventional neuroradiologist, and the interventional cardiologist has promised to provide the best results in our hospital.

Because of her or his procedural skills and training as a vascular specialist, the interventional cardiologist plays an increasingly important role in the care of the stroke patient. Collaboration among subspecialists is especially important in interventional neuroradiology procedures because the patient is often very ill with multiple medical problems, presenting clinical challenges to the cardiologist, the neurologist, and the radiologist alike.

The technical advances introduced in the cardiac catheterization laboratory over the last several years—flexible stents, hydrophilic wires, and distal protection devices, to name a few—have provided the cardiologist with the tools needed

for interventional procedures in the peripheral circulation. Intracranial vascular intervention is no exception.

The cardiologist has much to learn from her or his neurological and radiological colleagues, especially in the clinical presentation of the stroke patient and the complex variations in neuroanatomy. Similarly, the cardiologist has much to offer her or his colleagues because of her or his skill in managing the medically related vascular issues involved in all these patients.

This chapter discusses the role of the interventional cardiologist in the care of the stroke patient with intracranial disease. Its scope is limited to intracranial lesions and it does not address internal carotid interventions (see Chapter 21 for carotid interventions).

INTRACRANIAL DISEASE AND THE STROKE PATIENT

Atherosclerotic lesions of the skull base and the intracranial vasculature are not commonly observed because, in part, they are still underdiagnosed in the United States. In North America, 500,000 new strokes and 150,000 stroke-related deaths occur each year. Of these new strokes, intracranial stenosis causes approximately 50,000 ischemic presentations or 10% of all strokes.

This presentation is more prevalent in blacks, Hispanics, and Asian populations. Failure of medical therapy in these patients portends a poor natural history, with the likelihood of a transient ischemic attack or stroke of at least 50%. More worrisome, the median time to any adverse event is only 1 month.

Overall, $20 billion is spent annually on cerebrovascular ischemic disease in the United States. Treatment for the stable patient with intracranial disease, however, remains largely empirical. The patient is first given a trial of medical therapy. Such a regimen may include antiplatelet medications such as aspirin, or a thienopyridine. Anticoagulants such as warfarin, which have been shown to have a slightly greater effectiveness for large artery disease in retrospective trials, are untested in intracranial disease. If medical therapy fails, an interventional approach may be indicated if the patient remains symptomatic.

Several studies have demonstrated the natural history of intracranial lesions when treated medically. The Warfarin–Aspirin Symptomatic Intracranial Disease study (1), funded by the National Institutes of Health, showed a yearly stroke rate of 7.8% in vertebral and 10.7% in basilar circulations. In a separate study of 66 patients with an intracranial stenosis of greater than 50%, Marzewski et al. reported that 12.1% of patients had transient ischemic attacks (TIAs) and 15.2% had a stroke during follow-up of nearly 4 years (2). Although the presence of cerebrovascular disease is associated with an increased risk of morbidity and mortality from stroke, non obstructive cerebrovascular disease (<50% stenosis) carries a relatively low risk of a cerebrovascular event.

Similarly, surgical approaches have been disappointing. The International Cooperative Study of Extracranial/Intracranial Arterial Anastomosis (3) showed that surgical bypass therapy was not very effective; it documented an 8% to 10% stroke rate per year. In light of these discouraging data, catheter-based therapy has been tried in an attempt to improve patient outcome.

CLINICAL EFFECTIVENESS OF INTRACRANIAL ANGIOPLASTY

Early work in cerebrovascular angioplasty established the feasibility of endovascular treatment of cerebral ischemia related to atherosclerotic stenotic lesions of cervical carotid, subclavian, and vertebral origin. The formation of thrombus in relation to a significant stenosis leading to subsequent embolism is the most common stroke mechanism, although in some instances, hemodynamically significant stenosis can also lead to low-flow ischemia, especially if collateral blood flow is not present. This phenomenon of diminished blood flow has been documented in several case reports. The New England Medical Center Posterior Circulation Stroke Registry, in a review of posterior circulation stroke, noted the importance of low-flow hemodynamics in the posterior circulation (3a).

Medical therapy may decrease the risk of thromboembolism, but may not prevent low-flow ischemia. Although preliminary retrospective evidence favors anticoagulation over antiplatelet as best medical therapy, this is the subject of ongoing trials. Angioplasty provides direct treatment of the lesion and can prevent either mechanism of ischemia.

Angioplasty of the extracranial vessels is associated with lower risk than that in intracranial segments, perhaps because the presence of the muscularis and advential layers in the walls of the extracranial vessels—unlike intracranial vessels—making vessel rupture less likely. Shortcomings of percutaneous transluminal angioplasty are elastic recoil, severe dissection, arterial rupture, acute closure, distal embolization, and high late restenosis leading to stroke. Complication rates are thought to vary from 9% to 38%.

If complications are avoided, endovascular treatment of cerebrovascular lesions is quite effective. It improves the clinical status and symptoms of the patient as well as the angiographic appearance of the lesion. It provides increased distal perfusion. As a result, the incidence of TIA and stroke is reduced.

In the series by Marks et al. 23 patients treated by intracranial angioplasty followed for a mean of 3 years had a cerebrovascular accident rate of 3.2% per year in the target vessel territory, much lower then historical controls (4). Connors and Wojack (5) published their series of 50 symptomatic patients undergoing intracranial angioplasty, concluding with an 8% restenosis rate at 3 to 12 months and no major neurological events after treatment. Similar results were seen in the vertebral basilar system. Nahser et al. presented their series of 20 patients with lesions in the vertibrobasilar vasculature (6). They showed a procedural success rate of 86% with complete relief of presenting symptoms (6).

LESION CLASSIFICATION

It appears that intracranial angioplasty decreases significantly with operator experience and advances in endovascular equipment.

Mori et al. documented the outcome of 42 patients with 42 lesions greater than 70% stenosis. They segregated the lesions into three classes according to length, eccentricity, and degree of obstruction, as follows (7):

Type A: Length 5 mm or less, concentric or moderately eccentric, and less than totally occlusive.

Type B: Length 5 to 10 mm, extremely eccentric, or totally occlusive but less than 3 months in duration.

Type C: More than 10 mm in length, greater than 90% angulation, excessively tortuous, or totally occlusive for more than 3 months.

TABLE 22.1. *Intracranial angioplasty outcome according to lesion class[a]*

	Class A	Class B	Class C
Success rate (%)	92	86	33
Risk of fatal or nonfatal stroke or bypass surgery (%)	8	26	87
Restenosis rate at 1 year (%)	0	33	100

[a] Type A: ≤5 mm in length, concentric or moderately eccentric, and less than totally occlusive. Type B: 5–10 mm in length, extremely eccentric, or totally occlusive, but <3 months in duration. Type C: >10 mm in length, >90% angulation, excessively tortuous, or totally occlusive for >3 months.
Adapted from Mori T, Fukuoka M, Kazita K, et al. Follow-up study after intracranial percutaneous transluminal cerebral balloon angioplasty. *Am J Neuroradiol* 1998;19:1525–1533.

Success rate, risk of fatal or nonfatal stroke or bypass surgery, and restenosis rate at 1 year according to lesion type are shown in Table 22.1. Based on these results, Mori et al. recommended intracranial angioplasty on type A lesions only (7).

PERIPROCEDURAL MANAGEMENT

Collaboration with neurological colleagues is essential for the optimal care of these patients. Neurological evaluation by experienced clinicians and special attention to vasculature access by the interventionalist will minimize complication rates in this high-risk subset of patients.

Pretreatment with aspirin and cloplidogrel is recommended, although no randomized trials exist to guide treatment in this group of patients. The data used to support pretreatment are derivative from coronary trials (Clopidogrel in Unstable angina to Prevent Recurrent Events [CURE], Clopidogrel for Reduction of Events During Extended Observation [CREDO]) supporting the pretreatment with antiplatelet agents. Posttreatment, clopidogrel should be continued for at least 1 month (to allow for endothelialization) and aspirin indefinitely.

After intervention is completed, these patients are frequently treated with 24 hours of heparin, or longer (72 hours) if clot is associated with the lesion or visualized during the procedure. Partial thromboplastin time is maintained at 60 to 80 seconds. Early sheath removal is preferred, and can be achieved with minimal disruption of the anticoagulation therapy, when femoral closure devices are used.

The adjunctive use of glycoprotein IIb/IIIa inhibitors is unstudied, but empiric use of intravenous or intrarterial abciximab appears useful in those patients who have demonstrated thrombus angiographically. These patients present challenging management issues as the interventionalist struggles to balance vessel patency with the avoidance of vascular complications.

Careful attention to blood pressure control is essential. Ideally, these patients should have systolic pressures in the upper range of normal in the attempt to promote blood flow through the treated lesion and avoid a low-flow, static state, which would favor thrombosis.

INTERVENTIONAL TECHNIQUES

The cerebral and intracranial vasculature is unforgiving territory for the proceduralist. Careful wire and catheter manipulation is mandatory. Microcatheters, soft-tipped wires, low-profile balloons, and flexible stents promise to make this procedure safer, but the need for special attention to procedural details cannot be overemphasized. Avoidance of unnecessary wire movement during exchanges requires skill, and positioning of the wire in the lumen of the target vessel rather than a branch or perforator artery is more important than the need to do so in the coronary tree. The smaller intracerebral branches are prone to rupture, spasm, and dissection.

Any of these complications may be catastrophic and irreversible.

Coaxially placed soft-tipped guiding catheters minimize ostial dissections. Standard 0.014-in. angioplasty wires and balloons are used to dilate atherosclerotic lesions. Care should be taken to avoid oversizing the lesion, as this will markedly increase the complications encountered. "Perfection is the enemy of the Good" is especially true in the interventional neuroradiology suite; it may be necessary to accept a suboptimal result that appears underdilated rather than risk a more aggressive balloon dilatation. In general, multiple low-pressure inflations are used to dilate lesions secondary to vasospasm, whereas high-pressure inflations (8 to 10 atm) are needed to dilate more calcified atherosclerotic lesions.

Self-expanding stents are used in carotid interventions to avoid compression. Compared with self-expanding stents, balloon-expandable stents are preferred in the intracranial vasculature because of their smaller size, flexibility, and ease of placement. There has been no experience with heparin-coated or drug-eluting stents.

ANTICOAGULATION IN THE INTERVENTIONAL NEURORADIOLOGY SUITE

Endovascular neurointerventional procedures are associated with a risk for ischemic complications, some of which are hemodynamic in origin, but the majority of which are due to thromboembolic complications. Ischemic events complicate 8.2% of coil embolizations (8). Balloon and coil occlusion of aneurysms and parent arteries are associated with 11% and 19% risk of thromboembolic complication, respectively (8). Several factors contribute to thromboembolic risk, including disruption of the lesion by guide wires or catheters resulting in distal embolization; intimal injury caused by balloon inflation; and exposure of highly thrombogenic subendothelial elements like collagen, von Willebrand factor, and tissue factor, which invite platelet aggregation. Contrast dye, catheters, guidewires, and stents can be potentially thrombogenic (9). Arterial thrombus occurring in the setting of endovascular interventions is usually white thrombus comprising densely packed platelets and fibrin. Improved procedural techniques, using better equipment (guides, wires) and distal protection devices, and the incorporation of aggressive antithrombotic therapy, have lowered the rate of ischemic complications.

Randomized trials addressing antithrombotic and antiplatelet therapy in intracranial endovascular interventions are lacking. Therefore, most of the recommendations are empiric, mainly derived from coronary and extracranial experience.

Aspirin irreversibly inhibits cyclooxygenase-1 enzyme (10,11), which is necessary for the production of thromboxane A_2 (see Chapter 14). This vasoconstrictor promotes platelet activation. Aspirin also inhibits collagen-induced platelet activation (11). It should be noted that aspirin does not inhibit thromboxane A_2-independent platelet aggregation; therefore, it is considered a weak antiplatelet drug (11). The antiplatelet effect of aspirin lasts for 7 to 10 days; major side effects are well known including bleeding and peptic ulcer disease. All patients should receive 160 to 325 mg of aspirin prior to the procedure unless contraindicated.

Thienopyridine derivatives (ticlopidine and clopidogrel) exert their effect by blocking the binding of adenosine diphosphate (ADP) to platelet receptors, hindering platelet activation (12,13). They also inhibits ADP-induced platelet–fibrinogen binding, thus preventing platelet aggregation. Platelet inhibition is irreversible and lasts for the 7- to 10-day life span of platelets. Clopidogrel (250 mg twice daily) has been largely replaced ticlopidine because of the side effects of neutropenia and thrombotic thrombocytopenic purpura (TTP). Clopidogrel is administered as 75 mg daily; a 300-mg loading dose can be used if the procedure is planed in less than 6 days. Unlike the situation for ticlopidine, neutropenia and TTP are extremely rare, but rash is occasionally seen (14,15). Laboratory (16) and clinical evidence (17–19) suggests a synergism between aspirin and thienopyridines, and therefore combination antiplatelet therapy is generally advocated.

Unfractionated heparin (UFH) binds to antithrombin III (heparin cofactor II) and inhibits the conversion of prothrombin to thrombin, thus preventing fibrin formation. It also inhibits clotting factors XII, XI, IX, and X (20). In addition to its anticoagulation effects, heparin possesses antiplatelet effect via the inhibition of thrombin-mediated platelet activation.

During neurointervention procedures, heparin is given as 30 to 100 units per kg to maintain an activated clotting time (ACT) between 300 and 350 seconds (or 250 seconds if glycoprotein IIb/IIIa inhibitors are used), and then hourly ACT checks are performed, with additional heparin (typically 1,000 to 2,000 units) given to maintain the therapeutic ACT. It is not necessary to continue heparin postprocedure unless long-term anticoagulation is desired or suboptimal results are obtained requiring anticoagulation. Major side effects include bleeding and heparin-induced thrombocytopenia (HIT). Os-teoporosis can complicate prolonged therapy. Because of its binding to plasma proteins and other cells, UFH demonstrates variable pharmacokinetics.

Low-molecular weight heparin (LMWH) predominantly inhibits factor Xa with no effect on thrombin. It has the advantage of being more predictable; monitoring is not essential. The incidence of side effects with LMWH, mainly HIT, is somewhat less than with UFH. Enoxaparin and dalteparin are both available, but more data exist with the use of enoxaparin (21,25). It is usually given in a dose of 1 mg subcutaneous twice daily, although intravenous enoxaparin has been used in coronary interventions (26). Recently, anti-factor Xa assays became available for monitoring response (usually greater than 0.5 IU per mL) if clinically indicated.

Because UFH and LMWH are ineffective against clot-bound thrombin, direct thrombin inhibitors (DTIs) may have an adjunctive role in endovascular interventions. Hirudin, lepirudin, and most recently bivalirudin have been studied in coronary interventions. Unlike heparin, direct thrombin inhibitors have the advantage of inhibiting clot-bound thrombin, independent of antithrombin III, and without being subjected to deactivation by platelet factor 4. They are indicated in patients with HIT or patients with increased bleeding risk. Oral DTI (ximelagatran) has been shown to be noninferior to coumadin in stroke prevention (27,28). Its use in intracranial interventions has not been tested.

Warfarin exhibits an inhibitory effect on the vitamin K-dependent clotting factors II, VII, IX, and X. Its role in stoke prevention is well documented, but has no place acutely in endovascular procedures.

The final common pathway in platelet aggregation is the cross-linkage of platelets via fibrinogen through glycoprotein (GP) IIb/IIIa receptors located on the surface of platelets. This step is inhibited by GP IIb/IIIA receptor antagonists. Abciximab is a Fab fragment of monoclonal antibody that irreversibly inhibits platelet aggregation and also inhibits vitronectin. It is given as a 0.25-μg per kg loading dose followed by infusion of 0.125 μg per kg per minute for 12 hours. Eptifibatide, a peptide, and tirofiban, a synthetic derivative, reversibly inhibit GP IIb/IIIa receptors. With both agents possessing a half-life of 2 to 2.5 hours, platelets regain their function in 4 to 6 hours. Despite their extensive evaluation in coronary intervention (29–39), GP IIb/IIIa receptor blockers have not been a subject of intense investigation in neurovascular interventions. Initial but limited experience with abciximab has been reported (40). Use of abciximab in neurovascular interventions has been associated with a nonsignificant lower frequency of ischemic stroke in higher risk patients given abciximab (3%) compared to lower risk patients not given abciximab (12%), at the expense of increased intracranial hemorrhage (ICH) (5%) (41). Qureshi et al. reported seven cases of fatal ICH during neurointerventional procedures associated with use of abciximab (42). Of the seven procedures, three were intracranial. Intraarterial abciximab, however, has been used to treat thrombotic burden during neurovascular interventions with some success.

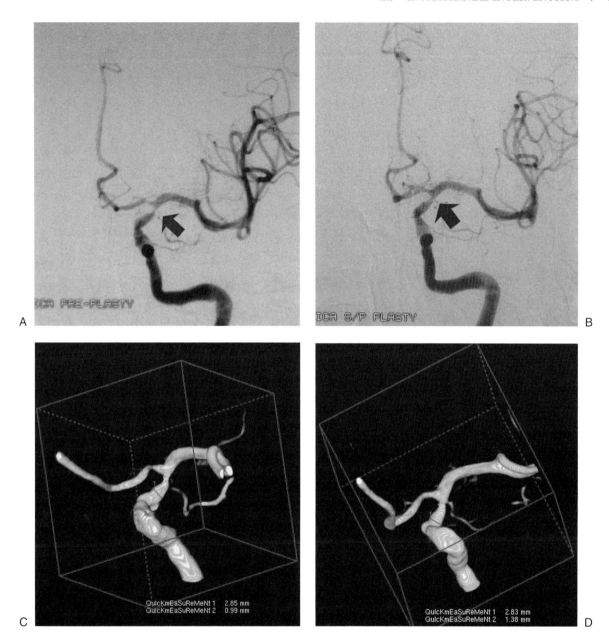

FIG. 22.1. A: Severe stenosis of the supraclinoid portion of the left internal carotid artery. **B:** Postangioplasty image showing modest increase in minimal luminal diameter (MLD). **C:** Three-dimensional reconstruction image preangioplasty. **D:** Three-dimensional reconstruction image postangioplasty demonstrating the improvement in MLD.

Intravenous eptifibatide was shown to be safe in a small pilot study of ten patients (43).

THROMBOLYSIS IN ACUTE STROKE

Fibrinolytic agents work by enhancing the conversion of the proenzyme plasminogen into the active form plasmin, which in turn lyses the fibrin clot into degradation products. Urokinase in no longer available, and prourokinase (pro-UK) is not commercially available. Native recombinant tissue plasminogen activator (rt-PA), alteplase (Activase) and the newer generation reteplase (Retavase) and tenecteplase (TNKase)

are available. Alteplase has a short half-life of 2 to 5 minutes, whereas the newer generation drugs have a longer half-life of 16 to 18 minutes (44).

Three large trials showed promising results with the use of intravenous (IV) rt-PA in acute ischemic stroke (45–47), which led to its approval by the Food and Drug Administration. A significant limitation in the use of IV fibrinolytics is the short 3-hour therapeutic window, which restricted its use to less than 2% of ischemic stroke patients in U.S. community hospitals (48,49) and 6% in university hospitals (50).

A meta-analysis of 14 published trials of thrombolytics raised concern about an increase in mortality and an

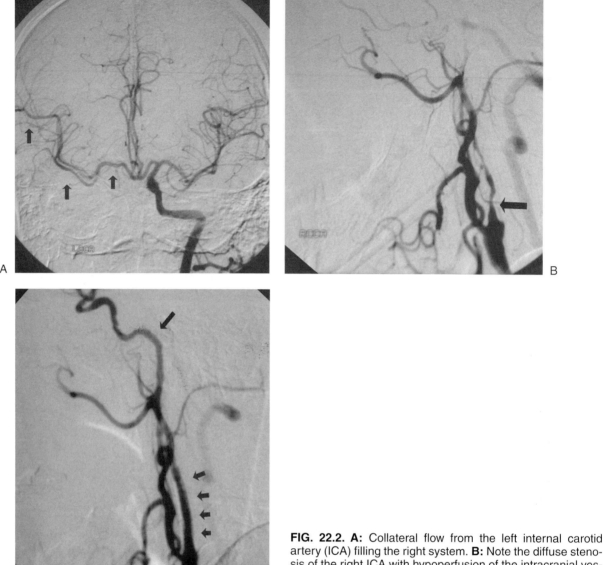

FIG. 22.2. **A:** Collateral flow from the left internal carotid artery (ICA) filling the right system. **B:** Note the diffuse stenosis of the right ICA with hypoperfusion of the intracranial vessels. **C:** Successful stenting of the extracranial (*short arrows*) and intracranial (*long arrow*) ICA with improved perfusion.

increase in symptomatic ICH occurring in 10% of patients allocated to thrombolytics versus 3% of patients allocated to control (51). Although this did not reach statistical significance, investigators are seeking other options, such as catheter-based approaches (primary stroke intervention). Early experience with intraarterial thrombolytics was promising, with recanalization rates of 72% (range 40% to 100%) and a 20% (0% to 67%) incidence of ICH (52).

The Prolyse in Acute Cerebral Thromboembolism (PROACT) trail was the first randomized trial of pro-UK verses placebo, and involved 40 patients treated within 6 hours of a middle cerebral artery (MCA) stroke (53). Recanalization was achieved in 58% of the pro-UK group versus 14.3% of the placebo group ($p=0.17$) (53). A nonsignificant trend for increased ICH was observed in 42.3% of the

treated group versus 7.1% of the placebo group, and symptomatic ICH occurred in 15.4% and 7.1%, respectively (53). This study was followed by a larger multicenter randomized study, PROACT II (54), which enrolled 180 patients within 6 hours of an MCA stroke. Recanalization was higher in the pro-UK group than in the heparin group (54). More patients experienced slight or no neurological disability at 90 days in the pro-UK group (40%) than in the heparin group (25%, $p=0.04$) (54). Despite there being no difference in mortality, there was a non-statistically significant trend toward more symptomatic ICH in the pro-UK group (10%) versus the heparin group (2%, $p=0.06$) (54). In the Emergency Management of stroke study, combination IV and intraarterial (IA) t-PA was used in 17 patients, whereas 18 patients received only IA t-PA and placebo (55). The recanalization rate was higher in the combination arm (54%) versus patients

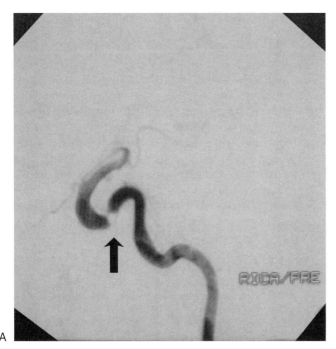

A

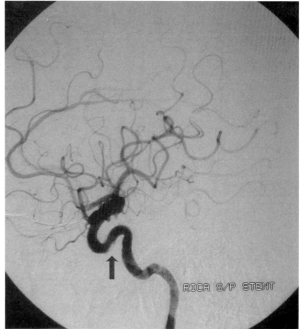

B

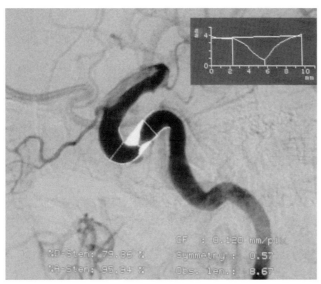

C

FIG. 22.3. **A:** Tight stenosis of the cavernous portion of the right internal carotid artery. **B:** Note the poststent result with widely patent middle cerebral artery. **C:** In-stent restenosis observed on routine follow-up.

in the placebo–IA arm (10%, p=0.03) (55). Despite a lack of difference between the two groups in the rate of symptomatic ICH at the prespecified 24 and 72 hours, mortality tended to be higher in the combination arm (p=0.06) (55).

A hybrid technique involving mechanical clot disruption with the use of IA fibrinolytic was attempted (56,57). In one study, 19 patients received a maximum of 4 U of IA reteplase, with a complete or near-complete recanalization rate of 84% and neurological improvement occurring in 63% at 7 to 10 days (58). Asymptomatic ICH occurred in 3 patients (16%) with an overall mortality of 53% and a functional independency of 37% (58).

The utilization of IA fibrinolytic therapy appears to offer an attractive alternative to systemic therapy in patients presenting 3 hours or more after the onset of the event or who

recently underwent surgery. Caution with patient selection should be exerted to minimize bleeding risk.

CASE DEMONSTRATIONS

The following case presentations demonstrate the clinical decision-making process necessary to ensure safety, and highlight salient points specific to intracranial interventions.

Case 1

A 76-year-old patient admitted because of progressive hemiparesis despite full anticoagulation therapy. Angiography showed a severe stenosis of the supraclinoid portion of the left internal carotid artery with poor filling of the anterior cerebral artery (Fig. 22.1A). There was poor collateral flow from the right internal carotid artery. The right vertebral artery, however, provided collaterals to the left posterior and left anterior circulation via leptomeningeal collaterals. With a 0.014-in. agility wire, a 2.5-mm compliant balloon, and an Envoy guiding catheter (Cordis, Miami, FL), the lesion was dilated using a conservative approach with an intent to "underdilate" the lesion in hope of avoiding intimal dissection (Fig. 22.1B). The patient did well during the procedure and was free of symptoms when seen at 1 year follow-up.

Computer-generated three-dimensional reconstruction prior to and after intervention helps to correctly size vessels and delineate tortuosity not clearly appreciated by angiography (Fig. 22.1C,D).

Case 2

A 73-year-old man with a known right carotid artery stenosis presented with temporary loss of right-sided vision. His visual deficit had progressed over the last 6 months.

Angiography showed a marked narrowing of the right internal carotid artery extending to the cavernous segment of the vessel (Fig. 22.2A). The ophthalmic artery could be partially visualized from collaterals from the external carotid artery. In addition, there was good collateral flow from the left internal carotid artery (Fig. 22.2B).

With a 0.014-in. wire and low-pressure balloon inflations, the lesions were predilated prior to placement of three stents: 2.5 mm × 12 mm, 4.0 mm × 12 mm (both balloon expandable), and 6 mm × 30 mm self-expanding distal to proximal (Fig. 22.2C). Antegrade flow to the middle cerebral artery was visualized post-stent placement indicating improvement in ophthalmic flow. The patient's visual symptoms improved postprocedure.

Case 3

A 65-year-old man presented with retroorbital pain and obscured vision on the right side. Magnetic resonance imaging was negative for evidence of stroke; magnetic resonance arteriography showed a severe narrowing in the cavernous portion of the internal carotid artery. Angiography revealed a patent vertebral system with collateral flow to the middle cerebral artery branches from a large posterior communicating artery. There was also contralateral filling to the right side from the anterior communicating artery.

The right internal carotid artery was imaged. Flow was markedly diminished, with stagnation of dye indicating a severe stenosis at the level of the cavernous segment (Fig. 22.3A). The supraclinoid segment of the internal carotid artery and the ophthalmic artery were barely opacified. An agility 0.014-in. guide wire and a 2.5-mm balloon were used to predilate the lesion. A 4.0 mm × 9.00 mm Penta stent (Guidant Corp., St. Paul, MN) was placed without difficulty (Fig. 22.3B). The patient returned for routine follow-up angiography 11 months later. An in-stent restenosis was ob-

served. The patient was asymptomatic, and therefore no intervention was performed (Fig. 22.3C).

SUMMARY

The interventional cardiologist needs to be a vascular specialist who understands the clinical and technical aspects of caring for the stroke patient. Collaboration with neurologists and interventional neuroradiologists is essential if we hope to make progress in this evolving field. The cardiologist's familiarity with the limits of technology and the neuroradiologist's appreciation of complex anatomy combine different skills in a creative and effective way. All of this makes for a safer procedure for the patient.

REFERENCES

1. The Warfarin–Aspirin Symptomatic Intracranial Disease (WASID) Study Group. Prognosis of patients with symptomatic vertebral or basilar artery stenosis. *Stroke* 1998;29:1389–1392.
2. Marzewski DJ, Furlan AJ, St Louis P, et al. Intracranial internal carotid artery stenosis: longterm prognosis. *Stroke* 1982;13:821–824.
3. EC/IC Bypass Study Group. Failure of extra-intracranial arteries bypass to reduce the risk of ischemic stroke—result of an international randomized trial. *N Eng J Med* 1985;31:1191–1200.
3a. Chaves CJ, Caplan LR, Chung CS, et al. Cerebellar infarcts in the New England Medical Center Posterior Circulation Stroke Registry. *Neurology* 1994;44(8):1385–1390.
4. Marks MP, Marcellus M, Norbash AM, et al. Outcome of angioplasty for atherosclerotic intracranial stenosis. *Stroke* 1999;30:1065–1069.
5. Connors III JJ, Wojak JC. Percutaneous transluminal angioplasty for intracranial atherosclerotic lesions: evolution of technique and short-term results. *J Neurosurg* 1999;91:415–423.
6. Nahser HC, Henkes H, Weber W, et al. Intracranial vertebrobasilar stenosis: angioplasty and follow-up. *Neuroradiology* 2002;21:1293–1301.
7. Mori T, Fukuoka M, Kazita K, et al. Follow-up study after intracranial percutaneous transluminal cerebral balloon angioplasty. *Am J Neuroradiol* 1998;19:1525–1533.
8. Qureshi AI, Luft AR, Sharma MBS, et al. Prevention and treatment of thromboembolic and ischemic complications associated with endovascular procedures: Part II. Clinical aspects and recommendations. *Neurosurgery* 2000;46:1369–1376.
9. Qureshi AI, Luft AR, Sharma MBS, et al. Prevention and treatment of thromboembolic and ischemic complications associated with endovascular procedures: Part I. Pathophysiological and pharmacological features. *Neurosurgery* 2000;46:1344–1359.
10. Roth GJ, Stanford N, Majerus PW. Acetylation of prostaglandin synthase by aspirin. *Proc Natl Acad Sci USA* 1975;72:3073–3076.
11. Theroux P. Antiplatelet therapy: do the new platelet inhibitors add significantly to the clinical benefit of aspirin? *Am Heart J* 1997;134[Suppl]:S62–S70.
12. Harker LA, Bruno JJ. Ticlopidine's mechanism of action on platelets. In: Hass WK, Easton JD, eds., *Ticlopidine, platelets and vascular diseases.* New York, Springer-Verlag, 1993:41–59.
13. Sharis PJ, Cannon CP, Loscalzo J. The antiplatelet effects of ticlopidine and clopidogrel. *Ann Intern Med* 1998;129:394–405.
14. Bennett CL, Connors JM, Carwile JM, et al. Thrombotic thrombocytopenic purpura associated with clopidogrel. *N Engl J Med* 2000;342:1773–1777.
15. CAPRIE Steering Committee. A randomized, blinded, trial of clopidogrel versus aspirin in patients at risk of ischemic events (CAPRIE). *Lancet* 1996;348:1329–1339.
16. Harker LA, Marzec UM, Kelly AB, et al. Clopidogrel inhibition of stent, graft, and vascular thrombogenesis with antithrombotic enhancement by aspirin in nonhuman primates. *Circulation* 1998;98:2461–2469.
17. Karrillon GJ, Morice MC, Benveniste E, et al. Intracoronary stent implantation without ultrasound guidance and with replacement of conventional anticoagulation by antiplatelet therapy: 30-day clinical outcome of the French Multicenter Registry. *Circulation* 1996;94:1519–1527.

18. Goods CM, al-Shaibi KF, Liu MW, et al. Comparison of aspirin alone versus aspirin plus ticlopidine after coronary artery stenting. *Am J Cardiol* 1996;78:1042–1044.

19. Hall P, Nakamura S, Maiello L, et al. A randomized comparison of combined ticlopidine and aspirin therapy versus aspirin therapy alone after successful intravascular ultrasound-guided stent implantation. *Circulation* 1996;93:215–222.

20. Hirsh J. Heparin. *N Engl J Med* 1991;324:1565–1574.

21. Zed PJ, Tisdate JE, Borzak S. Low-molecular weight heparins in the management of acute coronary syndromes. *Arch Int Med* 1999;159: 1849–1857.

22. Antman EM, Handin R. Low-molecular weight heparins. *N Engl J Med* 1997:337:688–698.

23. Bucklye MM, Sorkin EM. Enoxaparin: a review of its pharmacological and clinical application in prevention and treatment of thromboembolic disorders. *Drugs* 1992;44:465–497.

24. The Thrombolysis in Myocardial Infarction (TIMI) 11A Trial Investigators. Dose-ranging trial of enoxaparin for unstable angina. *J Am Coll Cardiol* 1997;29:1574–1582.

25. Antman EM, McCabe CH, Gurfinkel EP, et al. A comparison of low-molecular weight heparin with unfractionated heparin for unstable angina/non-Q-wave myocardial infarction: results of the TIMI 11B. *Circulation* 1999;100:1593–1601.

26. Rabah MM, Premmereur J, Graham M, et al. Usefulness of intravenous enoxaparin for percutaneous coronary intervention in stable angina pectoris. *Am J Cardiol* 1999;84:1391–1395. ,

27. Gustafsson D. The pharmacodynamics and pharmacokinetics of the oral direct thrombin inhibitor ximelagatran and its active metabolite melagatran: a mini-review. *Thromb Res* 2003;109[Suppl 1]:S9–S15.

28. Petersen P, Grind M, Adler J. SPORTIF II Investigators. Ximelagatran versus warfarin for stroke prevention in patients with nonvalvular atrial fibrillation. SPORTIF II: a dose-guiding, tolerability, and safety study. *J Am Coll Cardiol* 2003;41:1445–1451.

29. EPIC Investigators. Use of a monoclonal antibody directed against the platelet glycoprotein IIb/IIIa receptor in high-risk coronary angioplasty. *N Engl J Med* 1994;330:956–961.

30. EPILOG Investigators. Platelet glycoprotein IIb/IIIa receptor blockade and low-dose heparin during percutaneous coronary revascularization. *N Engl J Med* 1997;336:1689–1696.

31. EPISTENT Investigators. Enhancement of the safety of coronary stenting with the use of abciximab, a platelet glycoprotein IIb/IIIa inhibitor. *Lancet* 1998;352:87–92.

32. The CAPTURE Investigators. Randomised placebo-controlled trial of abciximab before and during coronary intervention in refractory unstable angina: the CAPTURE study. *Lancet* 1997,349:1429–1435.

33. Gibson CM, Goel M, Cohen DJ, et al. Six-month angiographic and clinical follow-up of patients prospectively randomized to receive either tirofiban or placebo during angioplasty in the RESTORE trial. Randomized Efficacy Study of Tirofiban for Outcomes and Restenosis. *J Am Coll Cardiol* 1998;32:28–34.

34. The RESTORE Investigators. Effects of platelet glycoprotein IIb/IIIa blockade with tirofiban on adverse cardiac events in patients with unstable angina or acute myocardial infarction undergoing coronary angioplasty. Randomized Efficacy Study of Tirofiban for Outcomes and REstenosis. *Circulation* 1997;96:1445–1453.

35. The PURSUIT Trial Investigators. Inhibition of platelet glycoprotein IIb/IIIa with eptifibatide in patients with acute coronary syndromes. Platelet glycoprotein IIb/IIIa in unstable angina: receptor suppression using integrelin therapy. *N Engl J Med* 1998;339:436–443.

36. The PRISM Study Investigators. A comparison of aspirin plus tirofiban with aspirin plus heparin for unstable angina. *N Engl J Med* 1998;338:1498–1505.

37. The PRISM-PLUS Study Investigators. Inhibition of the platelet glycoprotein IIb/IIIa receptor with tirofiban in unstable angina and non-Q-wave myocardial infarction. *N Engl J Med* 1998;338:1488–1497.

38. Cannon CP, Weintraub WS, Demopoulas LA, et al. Comparison of early invasive and conservative strategies in patients with unstable angina and non-ST segment elevation myocardial infarction treated with the glycoprotein IIb/IIIa inhibitor tirofiban. *N Engl J Med* 2001;344:1879–1887.

39. The PARAGON Investigators. International, randomized, controlled trial of lamifiban (platelet glycoprotein IIb/IIIa inhibitor), heparin, or both in unstable angina. *Circulation* 1998;97:2386–2395.

40. Qureshi AI, Suri FK, Khan J, et al. Abciximab as an adjunct to high risk carotid or vertibrobasilar angioplasty: preliminary experience. *Neurosurgery* 2000;46:1316–1325.

41. Qureshi AI, Suri FK, Ali Z, et al. Carotid angioplasty and stent placement: a prospective analysis of perioperative complications and impact of intravenously administered abciximab. *Neurosurgery* 2002;50:466–475.

42. Qureshi AI, Saad M, Zaidat OO, et al. Intracerebral hemorrhage associated with neurointerventional procedures using combination of antithrombotic agents including abciximab. *Stroke* 2002;33:1916–1919.

43. Qureshi AI, Ali Z, Suri FK, et al. Open-label phase I clinical study to assess the safety of intravenous eptifibatide in patients undergoing internal carotid artery angioplasty and stent placement. *Neurosurgery* 2001;48:998–1005.

44. The Global Use of Strategies to Open Occluded Coronary Arteries (GUSTO III) Investigators: A comparison of reteplase with alteplase for acute myocardial infarction: *N Engl J Med* 1997;337:1118–1123.

45. The National Institute of Neurological Disorders and Stroke rt-PA Stroke Study Group: Tissue plasminogen activator for acute ischemic stroke. *N Engl J Med* 1995;333:1581–1587.

46. Hacke W, Kaste M, Fieschi C, et al. Randomised double-blind placebo-controlled trial of thrombolytic therapy with intravenous Alteplase in acute ischaemic stroke (ECASS II). Second European–Australasian Acute Stroke Study Investigators. *Lancet* 1998;352:1245–1251.

47. Albers GW, Bates VE, Clark WM, et al. Intravenous tissue-type plasminogen activator for treatment of acute stroke: the Standard Treatment with Alteplase to Reverse Stroke (STARS) study. *JAMA* 2000;283:1145–1150.

48. Katzan IL, Furlan AJ, Lloyd LE, et al. Use of tissue-type plasminogen activator for acute ischemic stroke: the Cleveland area experience. *JAMA* 2000;283:1151–1158.

49. Chiu D, Krieger D, Villar-Cordova C, et al. Intravenous tissue plasminogen activator for acute ischemic stroke: feasibility, safety, and efficacy in the first year of clinical practice. *Stroke* 1998;29:18–22.

50. Hoffman JR. Tissue plasminogen activator for acute ischemic stroke: is the CAEP position statement too negative? *Can J Emerg Med* 2001;3:183–185.

51. Wardlaw JM, Sandercock PA, Berge E. Thrombolytic therapy with recombinant tissue plasminogen activator for acute ischemic stroke: where do we go from here? A cumulative meta-analysis. *Stroke* 2003;34:1437–1442.

52. Wilkins RH, Rengachary SS, eds. *Neurosurgery*, 2nd ed., Vol II, Part VII, *Vascular disease of the nervous system.* New York: McGraw-Hill, 1995.

53. del Zoppo GJ, Higashida RT, Furlan AJ, et al. PROACT: a phase II randomized trial of recombinant pro-urokinase by direct arterial delivery in acute middle cerebral artery stroke—PROACT Investigators: Prolyse in Acute Cerebral Thromboembolism. *Stroke* 1998;29:4–11.

54. Furlan A, Higashida R, Wechsler L, et al. Intra-arterial prourokinase for acute ischemic stroke: the PROACT II study—a randomized controlled trial: Prolyse in Acute Cerebral Thromboembolism. *JAMA* 1999;282:2003–2011.

55. Lewandowski CA, Frankel M, Tomsick TA, et al. Combined intravenous and intra-arterial r-TPA versus intraarterial therapy of acute ischemic stroke: Emergency Management of Stroke (EMS) Bridging Trial. *Stroke* 1999;30:2598–2605.

56. Barnwell SL, Clark WM, Nguyen TT, et al. Safety and efficacy of delayed intraarterial urokinase therapy with mechanical clot disruption for thromboembolic stroke. *AJNR Am J Neuroradiol* 1994;15:1817–1822.

57. Ringer AJ, Qureshi AI, Fessler RD, et al. Angioplasty of intracranial occlusion resistant to thrombolysis in acute ischemic stroke. *Neurosurgery* 2001;48:1282–1290.

58. Qureshi AI, Siddiqui AM, Suri MF, et al. Aggressive mechanical clot disruption and low-dose intra-arterial third-generation thrombolytic agent for ischemic stroke: a prospective study. *Neurosurgery* 2002;51:1319–1327.

CHAPTER 23

Iliofemoral Disease

James D. Joye and Mehran Moussavian

> **Key Points**
>
> - The ankle–brachial index (ABI) is an excellent initial screening test for high-risk asymptomatic patients and for patients with symptoms of intermittent claudication.
> - Exercise ABI is a more useful diagnostic tool for evaluation of peripheral arterial disease (PAD).
> - Segmental pressures can determine the level and the extent of the arterial occlusive disease.
> - Ultrasonography is an invaluable diagnostic tool for vascular imaging, lesion location, hemodynamic measurements, and, occasionally, lesion morphology.
> - Angiography is considered the gold standard for imaging and diagnosis of PAD.
> - Computed tomography and magnetic resonance arteriography have revolutionized the diagnostic imaging capabilities in diagnosis and evaluation of iliofemoral disease.
> - Bifurcation lesions of the aortoiliac junction are typically approached via bilateral retrograde common femoral artery access.

It is well established that atherosclerosis is a common systemic disease involving the coronary and the peripheral circulation. Manifestations of coronary artery disease (CAD) and peripheral arterial disease (PAD) frequently coexist because the risk factors, including age, diabetes, tobacco abuse, hypertension, and hyperlipidemia, are similar in both. Iliofemoral vascular disease occurs as result of chronic, progressive arterial stenosis, which may be clinically silent in some patients, whereas others may experience symptoms ranging from life-altering intermittent claudication to limb-threatening ischemia.

Essentially all patients with symptoms of PAD should be screened. Because most patients are asymptomatic and the disease progression is slow, many patients are undiagnosed and untreated. Diagnosis in this patient subset can only be made by screening high-risk patients with noninvasive testing. These patients include the elderly, those with a history of CAD or cerebrovascular disease (CVD), and patients with risk factors for PAD. The prevalence of PVD increases with age, and is greater than 20% in patients older than 70 years, compared to 3% in patients younger than 59 years (1). Noninvasive studies combined with sophisticated imaging capa-

bilities improve diagnostic assessment, but can also be used to follow patients for disease progression or recurrence (restenosis) after an interventional or a surgical procedure. A thorough history and physical examination, in conjunction with ankle–brachial index (ABI), exercise test, segmental pressures, segmental volume plethysmography, and/or duplex ultrasonography will identify the location and severity of disease in a majority of patients with iliofemoral disease (1,2). In patients where the results of these tests are insufficient, or additional information is required prior to surgical or percutaneous intervention, fruitful information can be obtained from computed tomography (CT) scan or contrast-enhanced magnetic resonance arteriography (MRA). It is hypothesized that with the aging population, the incidence and the complexity PVD will continue to increase. It is imperative for the interventional cardiologist to become familiar with various diagnostic tests for risk stratification and management strategies. The diagnosis of PAD, including iliofemoral arterial disease, has profound implications because it is associated with a 50% incidence of cardiovascular morbidity and mortality (3,4).

The iliofemoral arterial segment is a common site for development of atherosclerosis. Endothelial injury and

314

dysfunction as result of lipid accumulation, chronic inflammation, and oxidative stress represent the early stage of atherosclerosis. In contrast to coronary circulation, acute events are rare and are not associated with plaque rupture. In the peripheral circulation, the proximal segments, particularly at bifurcation points, are highly susceptible to development of atherosclerotic plaques. In advanced cases, there is marked reduction of luminal vessel diameter, resulting in decreased perfusion pressure to the distal circulation. In some patients, especially diabetics, the disease process may be more pronounced and extend to the femoropopliteal and tibioperoneal segments. Symptoms include claudication of the buttocks, thighs, and calves classically occurring with exertion and subsiding with rest. Men may present with impotence. Symptoms may be absent, however, due to development of collateral circulation despite presence of hemodynamically significant lesions. In severe cases where collateral circulation is inadequate, symptoms can occur at rest and be associated with musculoskeletal and metabolic abnormalities of the lower extremity (5).

Although patient history is an important tool for diagnostic purposes, leg symptoms are variable and may not be classic for intermittent claudication (6). Both patient and physician awareness of PAD are low, often resulting in missed opportunities to diagnosis PAD. Consequently, the Rose Questionnaire, the Edinburgh Questionnaire, and the San Diego Questionnaire have been developed and tested to improve the diagnosis of claudication. Compared to a history obtained by a physician, the questionnaires are more sensitive and specific for the diagnosis of intermittent claudication. Prior to embarking on additional diagnostic tests, the physician should differentiate between symptoms of true claudication versus pseudoclaudication due to lumbar spinal canal compression (1).

The physical examination of iliofemoral vascular segment includes palpation of femoral and distal pulses and auscultation of the femoral arteries. Diminished or absent pulses can usually locate the site of arterial stenosis. Absence of femoral artery pulse, for example, strongly suggests iliofemoral arterial stenosis. Bruits detected during auscultation are a result of accelerated blood velocity and turbulence at the location of the stenosis. A femoral artery bruit may be appreciated in iliofemoral artery stenosis, and can be an early diagnostic clue in asymptomatic patients. The combination of claudication and an abnormal femoral artery examination markedly increases the specificity and positive predictive value of iliofemoral arterial disease. Other pertinent physical findings include muscle atrophy in severe aortic or iliofemoral disease, skin changes from loss of hair and pallor, ischemic ulcers, and even gangrene (1,6,7) (see Chapters 3 and 4).

ANKLE–BRACHIAL INDEX

The ABI is an excellent initial screening test for high-risk asymptomatic patients, and for patients with symptoms of intermittent claudication. It is a simple diagnostic test and can

TABLE 23.1. *Correlation of ankle–brachial index (ABI) with symptoms and arterial lesion severity*

ABI	Symptoms	Disease severity
>1.3	Indeterminate	Medial wall calcification; nondiagnostic
0.9–1.25	Asymptomatic	No hemodynamically significant lesions
0.6–0.9	Claudication	Single-segment stenosis or collaterals present
0.30–0.60	Claudication	Multiple-segment disease
0.15–0.30	Resting pain	Multiple-segment total occlusions, good distal runoff
<0.15	Impending tissue loss	Multiple-segment total occlusions, poor distal runoff

be done readily in the office setting. The premise is a decline in systolic blood pressure at sites beyond an arterial narrowing. As the severity of stenosis increases, there is a marked reduction in systolic pressure distal to the stenosis (Table 23.1). A low systolic pressure ratio between the brachial and the ankle arteries can establish the presence of PAD. The test is performed by placing a pneumatic cuff around the ankle, which is inflated and subsequently deflated. The ankle pressure is checked with an ultrasound probe over the dorsalis pedis or posterior tibial artery. Brachial pressure can be obtained in the usual manner with a stethoscope. An ABI of 1 is considered normal and an ABI of less than 0.9 is indicative of PAD. An ABI of less than 0.4 indicates severe occlusive disease. Studies comparing the sensitivity of the Edinburgh Questionnaire to the ABI have shown the ABI to be a more accurate diagnostic test because many asymptomatic patients have an ABI of less than 0.9 despite a normal questionnaire. The ABI can be used to follow patients and monitor disease progression, and is a powerful marker of prognosis. Epidemiologic studies have confirmed elevated risk in cardiovascular patients and overall mortality in patients with low ABI. In a study by McKenna et al. patients with an ABI less than 0.4 had 5-year survival of 44% and a relative risk of mortality of 3.4 compared to patients with an ABI greater than 0.85 (8). The ABI is easy to perform and is inexpensive, but it does have its limitations. A resting ABI can be falsely normal despite significant iliac artery disease. It can be abnormally high (greater than 1.3) in diabetic patients due to calcification of the media in the tibial and peroneal arteries, which may not compress normally. As an alternative, measurement of toe pressure can be used in this setting because digital arteries are not affected by calcification (1,8) (see Chapter 15).

EXERCISE TREADMILL TESTING

Exercise ABI is a more useful diagnostic tool for evaluation of PAD. In some circumstances, arterial narrowing of less than 70% may not impede blood flow or cause symptoms at resting conditions. Exercise will alter the blood flow dynamics across a fixed stenotic lesion causing a dramatic fall in the ankle systolic pressure. During the rest period, the systolic pressure recovery time may become prolonged and not return immediately after exercise. Exercise testing elicits symptoms and can provide objective evidence of functional limitation and exercise capacity. In absence of PAD, the ankle systolic pressure is normal with exercise. The test is performed with a patient walking on a treadmill at 2 mph with a 12-deg grade for 5 minutes, or until development of claudication. The ankle pressure is recorded in a supine position after completion of exercise (1).

SEGMENTAL PRESSURES AND SEGMENTAL VOLUME PLETHYSMOGRAPHY

Once the diagnosis of PAD has been established by ABI, segmental limb pressures can determine the level and the extent of the arterial occlusive disease. The test is performed with four cuffs placed around the thigh, the calf, the ankle, and the digit. Typically, a pressure of 20 mm Hg or greater between segments in the same leg or at the same level in the opposite leg is suggestive of arterial narrowing. For example, segmental pressure gradients at the thigh reflect aortoiliac or iliofemoral disease. It is important to recognize that arterial occlusive disease can affect pressure as well as blood flow velocity across a fixed stenosis. Whereas segmental pressures detect pressure changes in limb segments, segmental volume plethysmography identifies patterns of blood flow velocities that can aid in lesion location. Normal arterial velocity is a triphasic pattern consisting of an early systolic forward flow, a reverse flow in diastole, and a late systolic forward flow. The presence of a flow-limiting lesion will blunt the amplitude of the velocity waveform. In a complete occlusion, the waveform is undetectable (1,9,10).

ULTRASOUND

Ultrasonography is an invaluable diagnostic tool for vascular imaging, lesion location, hemodynamic measurement, and, occasionally, lesion morphology. To accomplish this, B-mode imaging, pulse-wave Doppler, continuous-wave Doppler, and color mode display are used to image the vascular anatomy from the aorta to the popliteal artery. In evaluation of iliofemoral arterial disease, the transducer is placed on the femoral artery, and the technician typically images from the femoral artery to the aorta. Doppler waveform and peak systolic velocities (PSV) are obtained. As noted previously, arterial blood flow is triphasic, and attenuation of the waveform or an increasing PSV, due to increase in blood flow across a stenosis, is characteristic of a vascular occlusive lesion. The degree of stenosis can be estimated by comparing the PSV at the lesion to the PSV of a normal vessel segment proximal to the stenosis. The severity of the stenosis is graded as normal, 20% to 50%, 50 to 99%, or occluded depending on the PSV measurement. Normal PSV is less than 100 cm per second. Doubling of PSV is suggestive of a stenosis of 50%

to 99%. In an occluded arterial segment, a Doppler flow is not observed. Duplex scanning is highly accurate in peripheral arterial imaging. A comparative study of duplex scanning with angiography for detection of greater than 50% stenosis showed a sensitivity of 67% to 90% and a specificity of 90% to 98% for the iliofemoral arterial segments (9,11,12).

Ultrasonography is also used to follow patients longitudinally, particularly those who had a surgical or percutaneous intervention. Duplex scanning is commonly used for graft surveillance after surgical revascularization. The long-term patency of venous grafts can be extended if intervention is initiated prior to thrombosis of the graft. Similarly, restenosis or disease progression can be identified in patients with previous percutaneous intervention (13) (see Chapter 15).

ANGIOGRAPHY

Arterial angiography is considered the gold standard for imaging and diagnosis of PAD. It allows definition of the peripheral anatomy including the location, the severity, the morphology, and the extent of PAD. Angiography also delineates arterial inflow and outflow of a stenotic lesion, as well as the presence or absence of collateral circulation to the ischemic zone, which can assist in formulation of treatment strategies. Unrecognized and untreated lesions at the inflow and outflow can affect the short- and long-term success of revascularization. Estimation regarding long-term patency after percutaneous revascularization can be derived by angiographic lesion characteristics such lesion length and chronicity, inferred by presence or absence of collaterals. Angiography is an invasive, expensive diagnostic test associated with low morbidity and mortality. It is usually performed prior to embarking on percutaneous or surgical treatment. It may be indicated in situations where noninvasive test results are inadequate or conflicting. In obese patients, for example, duplex scanning of the iliac artery can be difficult and inaccurate. Angiography is performed with a pigtail catheter placed in the abdominal aorta, followed by selective engagement and angiography of the iliofemoral vessels with an end-hole catheter. Thirty-degree right anterior oblique and left anterior oblique views are sufficient for iliofemoral imaging. Contralateral oblique separates the external–internal bifurcation, and ipsilateral oblique separates the superficial femoral and the profunda artery bifurcation. Most complications are related to vascular access sites and include hematomas, thromboses, and pseudoaneurysms.

COMPUTED TOMOGRAPHY ANGIOGRAPHY AND MAGNETIC RESONANCE ANGIOGRAPHY

Recent technological advances in CT and MRA have revolutionized the diagnostic imaging capabilities in diagnosis and evaluation of iliofemoral arterial disease. Both studies can reconstruct high-definition, three-dimensional arterial imaging of the vascular tree from the abdominal aorta and its major branches, to the lower extremity digits. MRA has unique advantages including the use of nonnephrotoxic contrast agents, lack of invasive techniques, and no exposure to ionizing radiation. Both imaging modalities have been validated to be highly accurate with high sensitivity and specificity in comparative studies with conventional angiography. A recent prospective study of 18 patients comparing multidetector CT angiography to digital subtraction angiography (DSA) showed a sensitivity of 90.9% and a specificity of 92.4% for CT angiography (14). In study of 50 patients, CT angiography had a sensitivity of 100% for diagnosis for femoral artery disease when compared to DSA (15). CT studies are completed more rapidly and are less costly than DSA. Links and colleagues reported a sensitivity of 100% and a specificity of 83% in detection of iliofemoral arterial stenosis greater than 50% using contrast-enhanced gadolinium MRA (16). Patency of various stents was correctly identified using contrast-enhanced MRA. Limitations of MRA include long examination time, cost, availability of software for image acquisition, and single intensity dropouts caused by preexisting stents; artifacts are more severe in bare-metal stents and are minimal in nitinol stents (14–17). Although astonishing advance in CT and contrast-enhanced MRA imaging are emerging, it is unlikely these tests will substitute for the initial screening and diagnostic tests such as ABI and Doppler scan examination (see Chapter 17).

ARTERIAL ACCESS

Most endovascular procedures utilize conventional retrograde common femoral arterial access. This procedure is performed under the typical Seldinger technique and provides a basis for initial lesion assessment. A complete set of lower extremity angiograms is generally attainable with this technique. Not all interventional procedures, however, are ideally performed with such an approach, and the ability comfortably to access arteries with more advanced techniques is critical.

The antegrade common femoral approach is often the access technique of choice in patients with extensive femoropopliteal stenosis or occlusive disease. The skin entry site for the antegrade approach is often several finger breadths above the femoral crease, but the arterial entry site remains safely within the confines of the common femoral artery. Needle passage is anterior to the inguinal ligament and is best performed with a short sheath until accurate access is achieved. This approach is contraindicated in obese patients, and care must be taken to avoid vascular access trauma.

For some patients, a retrograde popliteal approach is necessary. This is especially true with occlusive disease that involves the origin of the superficial femoral artery (SFA), and in cases that cannot be performed from above without subintimal entrapment. The patient must be placed in a prone position, and a micro puncture set is typically utilized. Having a contralateral sheath from above is often useful to fluoroscopically guide popliteal access. Again, short sheaths are generally recommended until safe entry has been achieved.

Iliac interventions may also require brachial artery access to successfully approach bifurcation lesions and occlusions. This can be performed with a percutaneous puncture, but given the diffuse nature of disease in PVD patients, we recommend a cut-down and subsequent primary vessel repair. Support of procedures from the brachial approach often benefits from placement of long sheaths to the terminal aorta. With the brachial approach, axillary puncture and its complications can generally be avoided.

LESION-SPECIFIC APPROACHES

Bifurcation lesions of the aortoiliac junction are typically approached via bilateral retrograde common femoral artery access. This enables simultaneous dilation and stenting with a "kissing technique." Occasionally the brachial approach from above is needed; however, the sheath diameter required for simultaneous catheter placement in both iliac arteries generally exceeds the tolerance of the brachial artery. The brachial access site in bifurcation lesions is thus most useful for angiographic guidance of the procedure from below. If the common iliac lesion involves the origin of the vessel and the contralateral limb is uninvolved, we still recommend bilateral access and reconstruction of both arteries to avoid meaningful plaque shift.

Common iliac lesions that do not involve the vessel origin can be approached retrograde, from the brachial site, or via the contralateral femoral approach. With the advent of more flexible angioplasty and stent platforms, the retrograde site is no longer the sole entry site needed. In the case of occlusive common iliac disease, a retrograde common femoral artery (CFA) access site and either a contralateral or a brachial site is desirable. The latter serves as an angiographic guide, and is occasionally needed to cross lesions that cannot be traversed from below.

Internal iliac artery stenoses involving the origin of the vessel are not uncommon, and are a viable target for endovascular procedures that seek to resolve hip and buttocks claudication. Due to the degree of angulation seen in such vessels, the ideal access approach is via the contralateral CFA or the brachial site. In either case, placement of a sheath in the mid common iliac artery or selective engagement in the internal iliac artery will provide the needed support and visualization needed to successfully recanalize the vessel.

External iliac lesions are not uncommon, and can also be approached via numerous entry sites. Stenoses that involve the origin of the vessel are best approached contralaterally or from a retrograde site. Lesions that are more distal and encroach on the common femoral artery are ideally tackled from a contralateral or brachial point of entry. Occlusions, as in common iliac disease, often benefit from dual access from below and above, in any combination.

Disease of the common femoral artery must, by virtue of the lesion location, be approached from a remote access site. Either the contralateral CFA or the brachial site is ideal. Care must be taken to protect the profunda femoris, and dual wiring of the profunda and the SFA is recommended. Interventions involving the profunda should also be performed from a remote access site.

Peripheral vascular disease involving the SFA is preferably approached from a contralateral approach. The two main

TABLE 23.2. *Morphological stratification of iliac lesions: TransAtlantic Inter-Society Concensus type[a]*

A	Single stenosis <3 cm of CIA or EIA (unilateral/bilateral)			
B	Single stenosis 3–10 cm in length, not extending into CFA	Total of two stenosis <5 cm long in the CIA and/or EIA and not extending into the CFA	Unilateral CIA occlusion	
C	Bilateral, 5- to 10-cm-long stenosis of the CIA and/or EIA, not extending into the CFA	Unilateral EIA occlusion not extending into the CFA	Unilateral EIA stenosis extending into the CFA	Bilateral CIA occlusion
D	Diffuse, multiple unilateral stenoses involving the CIA, EIA, and CFA (>10 cm)	Unilateral occlusion involving both the CIA and EIA or bilateral EIA occlusions	Diffuse disease involving the aorta and both iliac arteries	Iliac stenoses in a patient with an abdominal aortic aneurysm or other lesion requiring aortic iliac surgery

[a]CIA, common iliac artery; EIA, external iliac artery; CFA, common femoral artery.

reasons behind this strategy are complication driven. First, the antegrade approach is known to carry a much higher rate of access site bleeding and serious hemorrhage. Second, on completion of a successful SFA procedure, one would prefer to not have to apply direct upstream pressure with sheath removal or in relation to a groin hematoma. Heavily calcified, diffusely stenosed, and chronically occluded vessels, however, may require an antegrade puncture. In cases with occlusion, a retrograde popliteal puncture may be needed to complete the planned intervention. This is especially the case with ostial SFA occlusion, and guide wire entrapment in the subintimal plane when lesion crossing is attempted from above.

ILIOFEMORAL INTERVENTION: THE TRANSATLANTIC INTER-SOCIETY CONCENSUS STUDY

The TransAtlantic Inter-Society Concensus (TASC) group has developed a set of guidelines to direct appropriate intervention in lesions of the iliofemoral vasculature based on lesion type (18–20). These guidelines serve as a reference point to highlight current data and outcomes in lesion subsets and outline the preferred approach between endovascular and surgical options. In general, type A lesions are best treated with endovascular techniques, and type D lesions are ideally suited for conventional surgery. Type b and c lesions represent those in which a clear preference is not apparent. The morphological stratification of lesions in the iliac and femoropopliteal segments is summarized in Tables 23.2 and 23.3, respectively.

It is worth noting that the TASC guidelines are recommendations, and individual decisions must weigh a variety of factors. In addition, newer technologies have been developed since the writing of these guidelines that may alter their interpretation. Endovascular approaches to iliofemoral lesions can thus be entertained in the vast majority of lesions in all lesion types if the risks of surgical intervention are deemed too ominous to be realistically carried out. TASC type D iliac lesions can virtually all be approached via percutaneous intervention. TASC type D femoropopliteal lesions similarly can undergo endovascular repair, with the exception of occlusions

TABLE 23.3. *Morphological stratification of femoropopliteal lesions: TransAtlantic Inter-Society Concensus type[a]*

A	Single stenosis ≤3 cm in length, not at the origin of the SFA or distal popliteal artery			
B	Single stenosis or occlusions 3–5 cm long, not involving the distal popliteal artery	Heavily calcified stenosis ≤3 cm in length	Multiple lesions, each <3 cm (stenoses or occlusions)	Single or multiple lesions in the absence of continuous tibial runoff to improve inflow for distal surgical bypass
C	Single stenosis or occlusion >5 cm	Multiple stenoses or occlusions, each 3–5 cm, with or without heavy calcification		
D	Complete CFA or SFA occlusions or complete popliteal and proximal trifurcation occlusions			

[a]SFA, superficial femoral artery; CFA, common femoral artery.

that cannot be successfully crossed or those that suffer recurrent restenosis. Given the significant morbidity and mortality associated with true surgical bypass, and imperfect long-term patency of native and especially prosthetic grafts, we feel the best indication for surgical bypass is a failed endovascular procedure (see Chapter 16).

ILIAC ANGIOPLASTY AND STENTING

The acute and long-term results of iliac intervention are generally excellent and support an endovascular approach. The Dutch Iliac Trial demonstrated similar outcomes in patients randomized to percutaneous transluminal angioplasty (PTA) with bailout stenting versus those treated with primary stenting (21). The acute procedural success in most iliac lesions can be expected in the range of 90%, and restenosis in these larger-diameter vessels is typically less than 10% (22,23). Due to the propensity of iliac arteries to dissect, we generally recommend stenting in most cases to preserve acute outcomes and to protect distal flow and vital side branches. The type of stent utilized varies with lesion location.

In iliac lesions that involve the origin of the common iliac arteries, we generally recommend reconstructing the bifurcation with balloon-expandable stents using the kissing stent technique (24). This requires simultaneous inflation and deflation of the stents to ensure optimal luminal gain (Fig. 23.1). The stents are typically placed 5 to 10 mm into the distal aorta to ensure that the origin of the lesions is adequately dilated. Balloon-expandable stents offer the advantage of better visualization, more accurate placement, and superior radial strength. Lesions that involve the body of the common iliac arteries can be treated with a variety of stents; however, our preference is to use balloon expandable stents for the aforementioned reasons.

In treating internal iliac lesions, we again prefer balloon-expandable stents. At this location, proper positioning of the stent and radial strength are mandatory. Generally, only the ostia of the hypogastric arteries are deemed viable targets. Lesions that involve the bifurcation of the internal and the external iliac artery are treated much like the common iliac bifurcation with kissing techniques. The external iliac artery, distal to the proximal-most segment, represents a shift in technology. Although balloon-expandable technology performs well, we prefer self-expanding stents. These vessels have a notoriously high rate of dissection and not infrequent perforation with aggressive techniques. We therefore prefer to predilate with undersized balloons, deploy self-expanding stents across the entirety of the lesion safely into normal reference segments, and postdilate only after the stent is in place (Fig. 23.2). Care is taken to avoid dilating outside the margins of the stent to avoid edge effects.

COMMON FEMORAL INTERVENTION

The common femoral artery represents a unique endovascular challenge. Because this is often the site of repeated access

and is a flexion point, care is taken to avoid stenting at all cost. We therefore strive to achieve reasonable acute results with balloon angioplasty only, and often will accept less than ideal angiographic results. When stenting is mandated due to significant residual plaque burden or high-grade dissection, we prefer the use of self-expanding stents with a coil configuration. These stents have a very open design, which allows for flexibility and, if necessary, subsequent access at a later date.

PROFUNDA FEMORIS

The profunda is a target that must be approached with great care. Profundaplasty is a time-tested procedure whose main utility is in the treatment of limb salvage (25). In patients with high-grade lesions of the profunda and coexistent occlusion of the SFA, a simple angioplasty can restore normal collateral flow distally and alleviate rest pain. The acute results seen with profundaplasty are often angiographically unsatisfactory. Nonetheless, the goal of therapy should be directed at a functional result, and stenting should never be performed. Assessment of postinterventional pressure gradients are often quite useful in guiding the final outcome of the procedure. In cases that fail to achieve the desired endpoint, referral for bypass or endarterectomy should be considered.

FEMOROPOPLITEAL ANGIOPLASTY AND STENTING

The results of infrainguinal intervention vary greatly depending on lesion morphology, location, degree of disease, length of disease, and status of runoff vessels. The general approach to lesions in this territory consists of angioplasty only, with stenting reserved as a bailout procedure for suboptimal acute results (Fig. 23.3). Acute success with PTA alone ranges from 20% to 90% depending on lesion and vessel characteristics. Meaningful dissection is common and occurs in greater than 40% of cases (26). Numerous studies have evaluated angioplasty in a variety of lesion subsets. It is well understood that those that are less durable include lesions at the adductor hiatus, heavily calcified stenoses, and occlusions, and those that have poor runoff. Johnston showed that angioplasty in stenoses with good runoff was successful at 1 year in 74% of patients, whereas occlusions with poor runoff succeeded in only 43% (27). At 5 years, these figures were more dramatically divergent, with success rates of 53% and 16% in the same respective categories. Muradin et al. similarly demonstrated modest 3-year primary patency rates with angioplasty in a meta-analysis of 19 contemporary studies, with results ranging from 30% to 61% (28).

When stenting is employed, the hard rule is to use self-expanding stents due to the compressible nature of these vessels. There has been much debate on stainless steel designs versus nitinol-based platforms, but no head-to-head comparison has been carried out. Unlike in coronary arteries, where stents have made a significant impact on restenosis

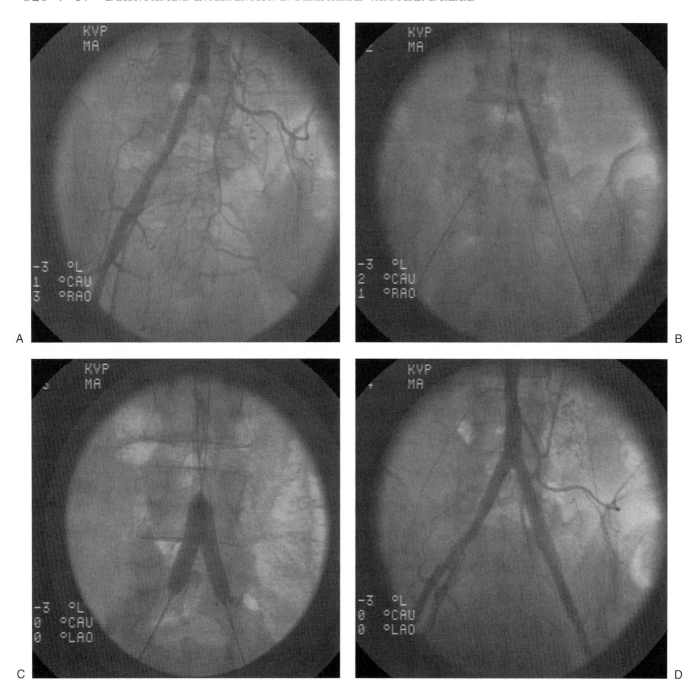

FIG. 23.1. A: Angiogram depicting a chronic, total occlusion of the left common iliac artery in a middle-aged smoker with left lower extremity claudication; note that the right iliac origin is largely devoid of disease. **B:** Bilateral femoral access is used and angioplasty is performed to recanalize the diseased segment. **C:** Kissing stent technique with balloon-expandable stents is performed. Even though the right system is not diseased, both vessels are treated to avoid plaque shift. Care must be taken to extend the stents into the terminal aorta, and stent delivery balloons are simultaneously inflated and deflated. **D:** Final angiogram.

rates, stents in the infrainguinal space have not made a great impact. Whereas restenosis rates with PTA alone average approximately 50% at 1 year, the combination of angioplasty and stenting yields a restenosis rate of approximately 40%. Stents in femoropopliteal vessels generate a greater neointimal response, which largely detracts from the superior acute

luminal gain they initially produce. A meta-analysis of stenting in infrainguinal lesions showed a primary patency rate at 3 years of approximately 60% (28). In longer occlusions, the results are more ominous. Gray and Olin reported primary patency of only 22% in 55 patients with occlusions with a mean lesion length of 16.5 cm (29). Mewissen reported more

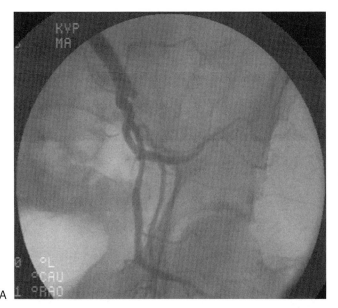

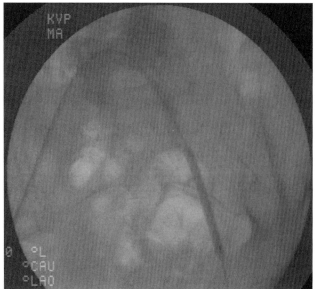

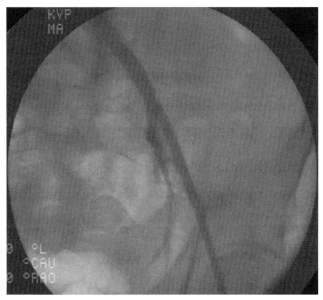

FIG. 23.2. **A:** Angiogram showing total occlusion of the left external iliac artery extending into the common femoral artery in an elderly woman with left lower extremity claudication. **B:** After safe wire passage to the true lumen distally, angioplasty is performed. **C:** Placement of self-expanding nitinol stents is limited to the external iliac artery, and the common femoral artery is left unstented with an excellent angiographic outcome.

favorable short-term results with newer nitinol-based stent platforms; however, primary patency at 2 years is still slightly better than 60% (29a). The only trial in support of Food and Drug Administration-approved stent for femoropopliteal disease showed a target lesion revascularization rate of 18.2% at 9 months in lesions that averaged only 3.8 cm (30). Clearly there is a need for newer strategies to improve late outcomes with endovascular interventions in the infrainguinal arteries (see Chapters 16 and 34).

SPECIAL CONSIDERATIONS: ILIOFEMORAL OCCLUSIONS

Endovascular approaches to occluded iliofemoral arteries represent a distinct set of challenges. The general approach to occluded arteries of the lower extremities utilizes the subin-timal approach, first popularized by Bolia et al. in 1990 (31). It is virtually impossible to traverse a chronic total occlusion in this space and simultaneously remain within the borders of the lumen throughout the length of the lesion. Therefore, the subintimal technique involves passing a hydrophilic wire and catheter through the length of the occlusion in the subintimal compartment (Fig. 23.4). The wire is advanced until it buckles at the origin of the occlusion and a small loop at the end of the wire is formed. The loop is then advanced until it creates a cleavage plane between the plaque and the subintimal layer. The wire and catheter are then passed with minimal steering across the length of the occlusion until the loop reenters the true lumen distally. This technique succeeds in approximately 80% of cases and is followed by angioplasty and stenting of the occluded segment. When this technique is utilized in iliac occlusions, one must be prepared for

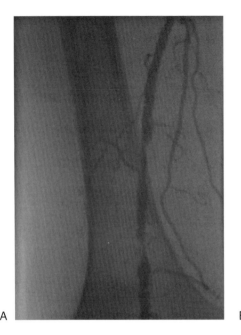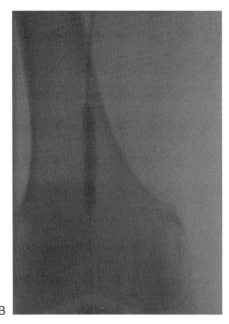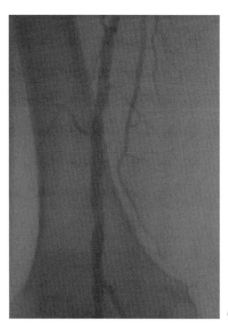

A   B   C

FIG. 23.3. A: Baseline angiogram of an elderly man with limb-threatening, ischemia, revealing tandem lesions of the left popliteal artery. **B:** Angioplasty is performed with an appropriate-size balloon; note that the intention at this location is to achieve a stent-free result. **C:** Final angiogram after angioplasty alone.

unexpected vascular perforation, and access to covered stents are mandatory. Perforation of femoropopliteal lesions is less common and rarely requires acute intervention. PTA results in long occlusions are quite dismal, with an 80% restenosis rate at 1 year. Stenting improves this outcome somewhat, but requires vigilant surveillance with ultrasonography, aggressive antiplatelet regimens, and attention to stent strut fracture. Newer techniques are being developed to maintain luminal position while crossing occlusions. The experience with optical coherence reflectometry and blunt dissection techniques is too premature to comment on.

One new technology that enables successful crossing of occlusions is the CrossPoint TransAccess catheter (Transvascular Inc., Menlo Park, CA). This device comprises a catheter with a hollow-tube reentry needle and integral intravascular ultrasound (IVUS) probe for guidance. In the minority of cases using the subintimal approach that dead end in a subintimal pouch, this catheter routinely allows for reentry into the true lumen. The catheter is advanced to the entrapped segment and IVUS imaging allows for visualization of the adjacent true lumen. This allows for precise delivery of the hollow-tube needle through the intima and back into the lumen (Fig. 23.5). A guide wire can then be advanced through the needle and the procedure can be completed. This enabling technology has significantly improved the acute success of endovascular interventions in occluded vessels.

THE PROMISE OF NEW TECHNOLOGY

The last few years has been marked by an increased awareness of the problem of claudication and alternative endovas-

cular methods for its treatment. Historically, there has been a general reluctance to treat infrainguinal lesions due to suboptimal acute and long-term results with existing methods. Recent technologic advances, however, are changing the way we strategize and approach such lesions.

One of the more significant advances in peripheral vascular intervention has been the development of cryoplasty. Cryoplasty is a new form of angioplasty, which simultaneously dilates the target vessel and freezes the arterial segment to $-10°C$ using nitrous oxide. Cryoplasty has reduced arterial dissection rates to less than 10% (from greater than 40% with PTA), and thereby limits the need for stenting (32). Because the cold reaction alters the morphology of elastin fibers in femoropopliteal vessels, the acute result is stentlike in appearance without the implantation of a foreign body (Fig. 23.6). The late impact of cryoplasty is to induce surrounding smooth muscle cells into an apoptotic life cycle (programmed cell death), which appears to favorably affect restenosis rates. Target lesion revascularization rates with cryoplasty at 9 months are less than 15%, and late angiographic restenosis rates at 18 months are less than 20% (32,33). This represents a major departure from expected outcomes with conventional therapies in femoropopliteal lesions.

A resurgence of atherectomy techniques is also affecting the manner in which we approach femoropopliteal disease. Excimer laser atherectomy has been evaluated in infrainguinal and infrapopliteal targets with interesting results. Although the results of the Peripheral Excimer Laser Atherectomy Trial failed to show a restenosis benefit in SFA lesions, it clearly facilitated improved acute results. In addition to limiting stent use, this form of atherectomy converts

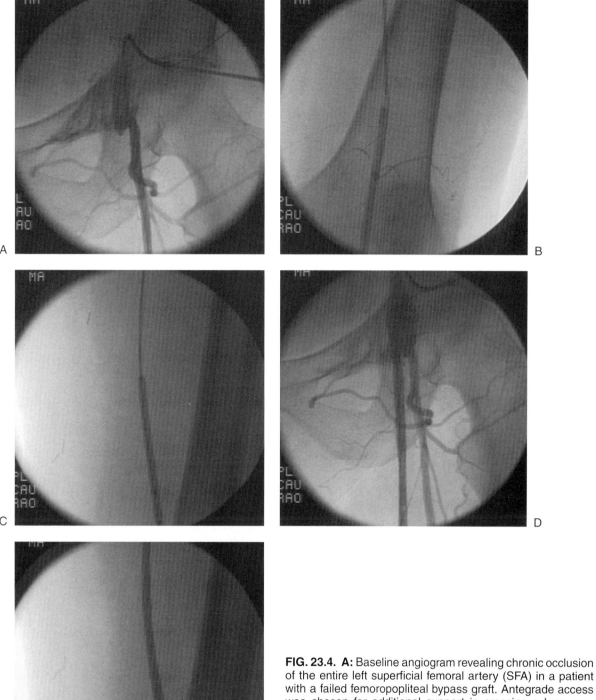

FIG. 23.4. **A:** Baseline angiogram revealing chronic occlusion of the entire left superficial femoral artery (SFA) in a patient with a failed femoropopliteal bypass graft. Antegrade access was chosen for additional support in crossing a long segment of occlusion. **B:** After subintimal passage of a hydrophilic wire, a glide catheter contrast injection confirms return to the true lumen of the left popliteal artery. **C:** Angioplasty of the length of the occlusion is performed. **D:** After placement of self-expanding stents throughout the diseased segment, the final angiogram shows a widely patent proximal SFA. **E:** Final angiogram of the distal SFA.

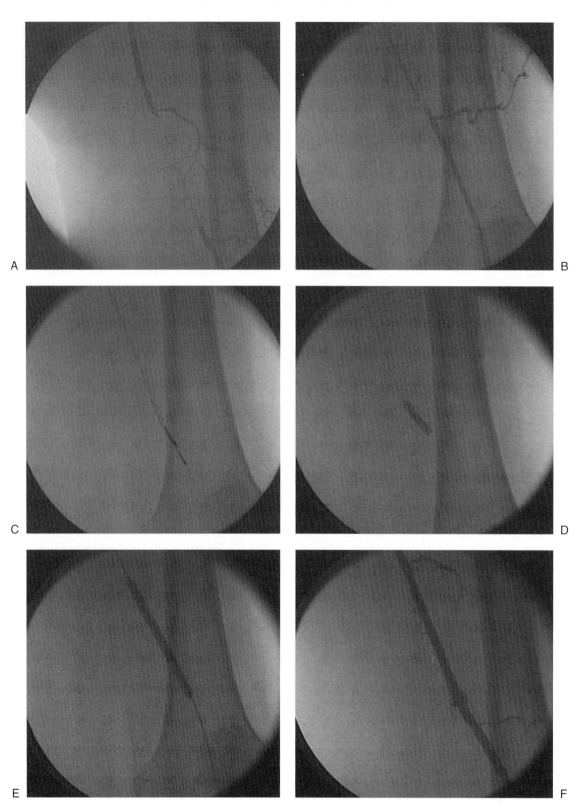

FIG. 23.5. A: Baseline angiogram revealing a segmental occlusion of the distal left superficial femoral artery (SFA) at the level of the adductor canal. **B:** Attempts to cross the occlusion using the subintimal approach fail, leaving the catheter entrapped in the subintimal space adjacent to the left popliteal artery at the site of reconstitution. **C:** Angiographic appearance of the CrossPoint TransAccess catheter (Transvascular Inc., Menlo Park, CA) with deployment of the nitinol hypotube needle laterally. **D:** After safely reentering the true lumen with intravascular ultrasound guidance, dilation of the reentry site is performed with a coronary balloon to facilitate stenting. **E:** Angioplasty of the occluded segment is performed. **F:** After stenting with a self-expanding platform, the final angiogram depicts a widely patent distal left SFA.

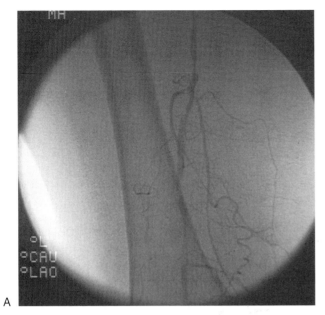

A

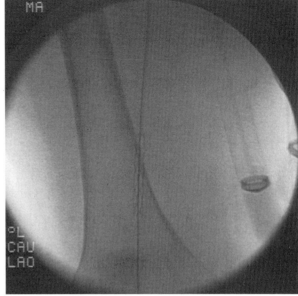

B

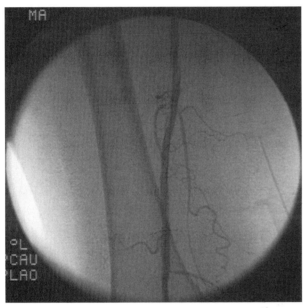

C

FIG. 23.6. **A:** Baseline angiogram showing diffuse femoro-popliteal disease in an elderly woman with advanced right lower extremity claudication. **B:** Cryoplasty is performed across the length of the diseased segment with simultaneous dilation to 8 atm with delivery of −10°C using nitrous oxide. **C:** Final angiogram after stand-alone cryoplasty reveals a widely patent arterial segment without dissection and with a stentlike angiographic appearance.

occlusions to stenoses, and has the added benefit of fulgurating fibrin-laden clots, which typically are harbored within long occlusions. Results in limb salvage applications have been even more impressive, with observed salvage rates in excess of 90%. The SilverHawk atherectomy catheter (Fox-Hollow Technologies, Redwood City, CA) is a newer entrant in the atherectomy field. This device has the ability to significantly debulk lesions and improve luminal dimensions. The late impact of this approach is yet to be realized; however, it, too, has limited the need for stenting. Histological and genomic evaluation of harvested tissues can now be performed, and may yield a broader understanding of the restenosis process and its modulation.

Newer iterations of stents are also being examined in femoropopliteal lesions. The emergence of stent grafts has

raised the possibility of performing *in situ* bypass procedures via endovascular techniques. Late patency in limited studies is encouraging (34). Novel self-expanding nitinol stent platforms are also showing promise in improving long-term patency compared to prior outcomes associated with stents in this area. The impact of drug-eluting stents in the peripheral field also holds great potential. Early results from the SIROCCO (Sirolimus-Coated Cordis SMART Nitinol Self-expandable stent for the treatment of obstructive femoral artery disease) trial suggest that we may soon possess a stent-based approach to femoropopliteal disease that is durable (35). If these results approach those seen in coronary artery applications, a much broader group of patients with infrainguinal disease may be successfully treated with endovascular techniques.

CONCLUSION

The approach to iliofemoral arterial occlusive disease is a challenge that is best managed by a collaborative approach from many disciplines. Endovascular procedures must be supported with reliable and expert surgical back-up. Similarly, proper technique and judgment are fostered by the combined teaching of vascular surgeons, interventional radiologists, interventional cardiologists, and vascular medicine specialists. As the face of the endovascular interventionalist changes, we must all find a way to cooperate for the best interest and outcome of our patients.

REFERENCES

1. Weitz J, Byrne J, Clagett P, et al. Diagnosis and treatment of chronic arterial insufficiency of the lower extremities: a critical review. *Circulation* 1996;94:3026–3049.
2. Hirsch A, Criqui MH, Treat-Jacobson D, et al. Peripheral arterial disease detection, awareness, and treatment in primary care. *JAMA* 2001;286:1317–1324.
3. Vogt MT, Cauley JA, Newman AB, et al. Decreased ankle/arm blood pressure index and mortality in elderly women. *JAMA* 1993;270:465–469.
4. Criqui MH, Langer RD, Fronek A, et al. Mortality over a period of 10 years in patients with peripheral arterial disease. *N Engl J Med* 1992;326:381–386.
5. Regensteiner JG, Wolfel EE, Brass EP, et al. Chronic changes in skeletal muscle histology and function in peripheral arterial disease. *Circulation* 1993;87:413–421.
6. McDermott MM, Greenland P, Liu K, et al. Leg symptoms in peripheral arterial diseases: associated clinical characteristics and functional impairment. *JAMA* 2001;286:1599–1606.
7. Criqui MH, Fronek A, Klauber M, et al. The sensitivity, specificity, and predictive value of traditional clinical evaluation of peripheral arterial disease: results from noninvasive testing in a defined population. *Circulation* 1985;71:516–522.
8. McKenna M, Wolfson S, Kuller L. The ratio of ankle and arm arterial pressure as an independent predictor of mortality. *Atherosclerosis* 1991;87:119–128.
9. Strandness D. Noninvasive vascular laboratory and vascular imaging. In: Young R, Olin J, Bartholomew J, eds. *Peripheral vascular disease*, 2nd. ed. St. Louis, MO: Mosby, 1996:33–64.
10. MacDonald N. Pulse volume plethysmography. *J Vasc Technol* 1994; 18:241–248.
11. Whelan J, Barry M, Moir J. Color flow Doppler ultrasonography: comparison with peripheral arteriography for the investigation of peripheral vascular disease. *J Clin Ultrasound* 1992;20:369–374.
12. Kohler T, Nance D, Cramer M, et al. Duplex scanning for diagnosis of aortoiliac and femoropopliteal disase: a prospective study. *Circulation* 1987;76:1074–1080.
13. Bandyk DF. Ultrasonic duplex scanning in the evaluation of arterial grafts and dilatations. *Echocardiography* 1987;4:251–264.
14. Amos O, Nitecki S, Linn S, et al. Multidetector CT angiography of peripheral vascular disease: a prospective comparison with intraarterial digital subtraction angiography. *AJR Am J Roentgenol* 2003;180:719–724.
15. Rieker O, Schmiedt W, von Zitzewitz H, et al. Prospective comparison of CT angiography of the legs with intraarterial digital subtraction angiography. *Am J Roentgenol AJR* 1996;166:269–276.

16. Links J, Steffens J, Brossmann J, et al. Iliofemoral arterial occlusive disease: contrast-enhanced MR angiography for preinterventional evaluation and follow-up after stent placement. *Radiology* 1999;212:371–377.
17. Rofsky N, Adelman M. MR angiography in the evaluation of atherosclerotic peripheral vascular disease. *Radiology* 2000;214:325–338.
18. Dormandy JA, Rutherford RB. Management of peripheral arterial disease (PAD). TransAtlantic Inter-Society Concensus (TASC). Section B: intermittent claudication *Eur J Vac Endovasc Surg* 2000;19[Suppl A]:S47–S114.
19. Dormandy JA, Rutherford RB. Management of peripheral arterial disease (PAD). TransAtlantic Inter-Society Concensus (TASC). *Eur J Vasc Endovasc Surg* 2000;19 [Suppl A]:S1–S250.
20. Dormandy JA, Rutherford RB. Management of peripheral arterial disease (PAD). TASC Working Group. TransAtlantic Inter-Society Consensus (TASC). *J Vasc Surg* 2000;31[1 Pt 2]:S1–S296.
21. Tetteroo E, van der Graaf Y, Bosch JL, et al. Randomised comparison of primary stent placement versus angioplasty followed by selective stent placement in patients with iliac artery occlusive disease. *Lancet* 1998;351:1153–1159.
22. Henry M, Amor M, Ethevenot G, et al. Percutaneous endoluminal treatment of iliac occlusions: long term follow-up in 105 patients. *J Endovasc Surg* 1998;5:228–235.
23. Sullivan TM, Childs MB, Bacharach JM, et al. Percutaneous transluminal angioplasty and primary stenting of the iliac arteries in 288 patients. *J Vasc Surg* 1997;25:829–838.
24. St Goar FG, Joye JD, Laird JR. Percutaneous arterial aortoiliac intervention. *J Interv Cardiol* 2001;14:533–537.
25. Dacie JE, Daniell SJ. The value of percutaneous transluminal angioplasty of the profunda femoris artery in threatened limb loss and intermittent claudication. *Clin Radiol* 1991;44:311–316.
26. Zorger N, Manke C, Lenhart M, et al. Peripheral balloon angioplasty: effect of short versus long balloon inflation times on the morphologic results. *J Vasc Radiol* 2002;13:355–359.
27. Johnston KW. Factors that influence the outcome of aortoiliac and femoropopliteal percutaneous transluminal angioplasty. *Surg Clin North Am* 1992;72:843–850.
28. Muradin GS, Bosch JL, Stijnen T, et al. Balloon dilation and stent implantation for treatment of femoropopliteal artery disease: meta–analysis. *Radiology* 2001;221:137–145.
29. Gray BH, Olin JW. Limitations of percutaneous transluminal angioplasty with stenting for femoropopliteal arterial occlusive disease. *Semin Vasc Surg* 1997;10:8–16.
29a. Mewissen, MW. Self-Expanding Stents in the Femoropopliteal Segment: Technique and Midterm Results. Advanced Endovascular Therapies and All That Jazz 2002. New Orleans, LA.
30. Ansel GM, Botti Jr CF, George BS, et al. Clinical results for the training-phase roll-in patients in the intracoil femoropopliteal stent trial. *Catheter Cardiovasc Interv* 2002;56:443–449.
31. Bolia A, Miles KA, Brennan J, et al. Percutaneous transluminal angioplasty of occlusions of the femoral and popliteal arteries by subintimal dissection. *Cardiovasc Intervent Radiol* 1990;13:357–363.
32. Laird JR, Biamino G. Interim results of the CryoVascular peripheral balloon catheter system safety registry. Transcatheter Cardiovascular Therapeutics, Washington DC.
33. Fava M, Loyola S, Joye JD, et al. Femoropopliteal cryoplasty: long-term results of first in man experience. Society for Interventional Radiology 2003. Saltlake City VT.
34. Jahnke T, Andresen R, Muller-Hulsbeck S, et al. Hemobahn stent-grafts for treatment of femoropopliteal arterial obstructions: midterm results of a prospective trial. *J Vasc Interv Radiol* 2003:14:41–51.
35. Duda SH, Pusich B, Richter G, et al. Sirolimus-eluting stents for the treatment of obstructive superficial femoral artery disease: six month results. *Circulation* 2002;106:1505–1509.

CHAPTER 24

Transradial Approach for Catheterization

Technique and Limitations by Unusual Anatomy

Gérald R. Barbeau

Key Points

- For our group, the transradial approach is the preferred site of entry in 97% of patients for coronary angiography and intervention.
- A limitation of this approach includes a definite learning curve mainly because of difficult anatomy.
- Special attention to the vascular anatomic variations is critical to avoid complications with the transradial approach.
- Overall, the complication rate is 3% to 5% of all transradial procedures, the majority of these being uneventful.

INTRODUCTION

Percutaneous coronary angiography using the radial artery was first reported by L. Campeau from the Montreal Heart Institute in 1989 (1). He reported in his paper that despite the use of small catheters, spasms were more frequent than when the procedure was done from the femoral access. Loss of radial pulse was also seen in 6%, without clinical sequelae, in patients selected with patent arterial arch assessed with Allen's test. With the availability of smaller guiding catheters (6 French) for angioplasty and stenting, the percutaneous transradial approach (PTRA) was tested for coronary angioplasty and stenting by Kiemeneij and Laarman in 1994 (2). The main advantage of PTRA appeared to be the easy compressibility of the radial artery, and thus the low bleeding rate in this era of stenting under aggressive anticoagulation.

Disadvantages of PTRA included a steep learning curve and technical failure in the range of 1% to 5%. Technical failures were associated mainly with anatomic variations such as radial loops and spastic radial artery. In a previous series from our center, vascular anomalies were seen in 2.4% of patients, corresponding well with the incidence of technical

failure reported in the literature (3). Nevertheless, several groups adopted and refined the PTRA technique to the point that it became in our center the entry site of choice for 97% of patients. This chapter summarizes the transradial approach technique with special attention to vascular anomalies.

METHODS

Screening for Transradial Approach

To avoid ischemic complications of the hand, PTRA should only be performed in patients with patent palmar arterial arches. The modified Allen's test, which measures the amount of time to achieve maximal palmar blush after release of the compression of ulnar artery with continuing occlusive pressure of the radial artery, is usually performed to assess patency of the palmar arterial arches (see Chapter 3). To maximize blushing, the hand is forcefully closed in a fist before arterial compression and opened before release of the ulnar artery compression. Patients with hand blushing in 9 seconds or less are candidates for PTRA. This modified Allen's test is subjective at best, and reported accepted limits vary from 5 to more than 15 seconds.

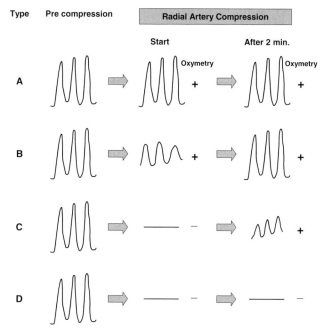

FIG. 24.1. The four types of palmar arch patency findings with plethysmography and oxymetry as recorded with the finger clamp applied on the thumb. (Reprinted from Transradial Approach by Gerald Barbeau. In: Nguyen TN, Saito S, Hu D, et al., eds., *Practical handbook of advanced interventional cardiology*. Amonk, NY: Futura, 2001:23.

Another method is to evaluate the palmar arch patency with plethysmography and oxymetry tests. Plethysmography readings with the clamp applied on the thumb during radial artery compression are divided in four types: type A, no dampening of pulse tracing; type B, dampening of pulse tracing; type C, loss followed with recovery of pulse tracing within 2 minutes; type D, loss of pulse tracing without recovery within 2 minutes. Oxymetry is either positive or negative during radial artery compression. Based on this technique, in a series of 1,010 consecutive patients referred to our catheterization lab, patients were considered suitable for PTRA with plethysmography type A, B, or C and positive oxymetry readings (Fig. 24.1). With these criteria, only 1.5% of patients were excluded for either right or left PTRA (4). The clear advantage of this objective test is that lab personnel with very brief training can perform it.

Standard Technique, Right Percutaneous Transradial Approach

The right arm is placed in a semiabducted position with slight wrist overextension, without constraint (5). In our institution, right radial and bilateral femoral entry sites are disinfected with proviodine and prepared for possible access in case of PTRA failure or need for intraaortic balloon counterpulsation. Local skin anesthesia is obtained with 2% lidocaine injected subdermal with a 25-gauge needle, and a small (1 mm) incision is made with #11 surgical blade. The radial artery is punctured with a 19-gauge open needle or an 18-gauge Insyte catheter (BD, Franklin Lakes, NJ) to obtain a pulsatile blood flow. The artery is cannulated with a 45-cm, 0.019- to 25-in. straight, non-Teflonized guidewire advanced without force. A short (15 cm) 4 to 5 French sheath is then inserted. The arm is then positioned alongside the patient. Verapamil (2.5 mg) is injected through the side arm of sheath. Heparin sulfate (70 units per kg) is given intravenously in all cases. Right PTRA is usually more convenient to the physician, especially if the physician is right handed or if the patient is very obese. Most radial coronary catheters are designed for right PTRA. Also, the left radial artery remains intact to serve as a conduit in case of coronary artery bypass grafting.

Left Percutaneous Transradial Approach

The radial puncture is done on the left side of the patient. The rest of the procedure is the same as for the right procedure except that the left arm is flexed over the abdomen after sheath and guidewire insertion. For patient comfort, a small cushion is placed under the flexed left arm and elbow. For the rest of the procedure, the operator is positioned on the right side of the patient as usual. Left PTRA is the approach of choice for left internal mammary artery angiography. Other indications for left access include highly positioned left coronary venous or radial bypass, patients with pneumonectomy, very old or hypertensive patients with extreme aortic tortuosity, and, sometimes, patient preference.

Catheter Advancement

In all cases, the initial 4 or 5 French diagnostic catheter, loaded with a 150-cm, 0.035-in. Teflonized J-guidewire, is

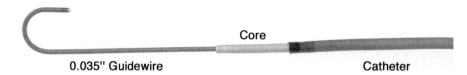

FIG. 24.2. Hydrophilic coated guiding catheter with inner core and standard 0.035-in. guidewire. (Reprinted from Barbeau GR. Radial loops and extreme vessels tortuosity in transradial approach: advantage of hydrophilic-coated guidewires and catheters. *Catheter Cardiovasc Interv* 2003;59:442–450, with permission.)

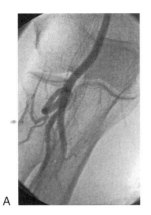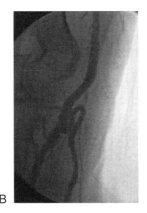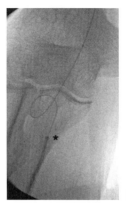

A B C

FIG. 24.3. Anterior (**A**) and (**B**) lateral angiograms of radial artery showing a radial artery loop in a 65-year-old man. A hydrophilic coronary guidewire was used with success, followed with unsuccessful progression of a 5-Fr diagnostic catheter (**C**) (*asterisk*). The procedure was completed via the femoral artery.

introduced into the introducer sheath and the guidewire advanced without fluoroscopy and without undue force. The patient is then asked to take a deep breath while the guidewire is advanced into the ascending aorta under fluoroscopy. This, as well as selective coronary canulation, are best accomplished in the left anterior oblique projection. If there is difficult or no progression of the guidewire, a radial or innominate/subclavian artery angiography is carefully performed with a multipurpose catheter to evaluate the anatomic abnormality and to avoid traumatic manipulation of guidewire. In case of difficult wire advancement, a hydrophilic guidewire (Glidewire, Terumo Inc., Tokyo, Japan) or a hydrophilic coronary guidewire is used (Choice PT, Boston Scientific Corporation-Scimed, Natick, MA). If coronary anatomy reveals lesions suitable for immediate intervention, the diagnostic catheter is exchanged for the appropriate 5 to 8 French sheath and guiding catheter. All catheter exchanges are performed over the standard 150-cm, 0.035-in. Teflonized J-guidewire to avoid renegotiating the critical radiohumeral junction.

Hydrophilic-Coated Catheters

As will be shown in many cases, use of hydrophilic-coated, 6 French guiding catheters (Envy, Cook Inc., Bloomington, IN) makes the procedure easier and without patient discomfort despite the presence of vascular loops, stenosis, or marked tortuosity. Hydrophilic-coated catheters greatly facilitate catheter advancement and manipulation. This catheter also has an inner coaxial catheter accommodating the standard guidewire, straightening distal curves and giving more body to the catheter. The end-hole of the inner catheter is tapered to match the 0.035-in. standard guidewire, making sheathless insertion possible (Fig. 24.2). This is useful to avoid the extra diameter induced by the introducer sheath in smaller radial arteries. In addition, the presence of this

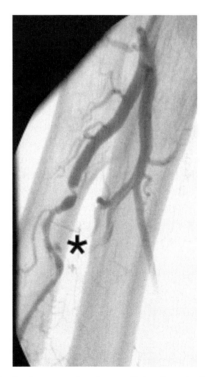

FIG. 24.4. Angiogram showing radial artery tortuosity and spasm/stenosis in a 76-year-old male patient. A small perforation (*asterisk*) was noted after unsuccessful attempts done with a hydrophilic guidewire. A hydrophilic coronary guidewire was used with success followed with passage of a 5-Fr diagnostic catheter. No clinical entry site complications occurred. (Reprinted from Barbeau GR. Radial loops and extreme vessels tortuosity in transradial approach: advantage of hydrophilic-coated guidewires and catheters. *Catheter Cardiovasc Interv* 2003;59:442–450, with permission.)

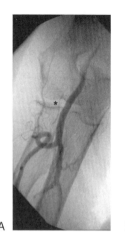 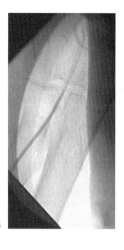 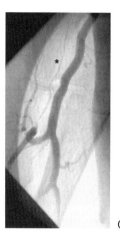

A   B   C

FIG. 24.5. **A:** Angiogram of the radial artery with a short diameter loop in a 74-year-old woman **B:** A hydrophilic coronary guidewire was used with passage of a 4-Fr diagnostic catheter resulting in straightening of the radial loop. A hydrophilic-coated 6-Fr guiding catheter was advanced without any friction or pain. **C:** Following coronary angioplasty, radial artery angiogram was repeated after catheter pull-back to ensure the integrity of the loop. Note the remnant artery in panels A and C (*asterisk*). (Reprinted from Barbeau GR. Radial loops and extreme vessels tortuosity in transradial approach: advantage of hydrophilic-coated guidewires and catheters. *Catheter Cardiovasc Interv* 2003;59:442–450, with permission.)

inner core in the hydrophilic-coated catheter makes a seamless transition between the 0.035-in. standard guidewire and the distal catheter opening, potentially reducing scraping of vessels' inner surface with production of debris (6).

Postprocedure Care

Once the procedure is completed, the arterial sheath is immediately removed and a localized pressure dressing is applied over the puncture site with a compression band (HemoBand, HemoBand Corp., Portland, OR). Pressure dressing is checked every 30 minutes until hemostasis. Following hemostasis, a small dressing is applied over the puncture site. A slightly elastic dressing bandage can be applied for prevention of bleeding or in case of discrete hematoma and for patient comfort. To encourage ambulation immediately after the procedure, we remove all the intravenous lines in the catheterization lab and encourage liberal fluid intake. To avoid bleeding complications, it is of utmost importance to have well-trained personnel who is familiar with the transradial approach and able to recognize early signs of complications. If severe forearm bleeding should occur, especially

if distant from the puncture site, local pressure is applied at suspected bleeding sites with monitoring of finger oxymetry. Supplemental measures are to lower blood pressure, reverse heparin with protamine, and massage the site to diffuse the hematoma under tension. If a compartment syndrome develops with associated hand ischemia, urgent fasciotomy for pressure release may become necessary.

RESULTS OF PREVIOUS STUDIES

The percutaneous transradial approach is successful in approximately 93% to 99% of cases. Predictors of failure are female gender, older age, low body mass index, and lack of operator experience in performing PTRA (7). Causes of failure include inability to puncture, anatomic variation and vascular tortuosity, spasm, and pain. Radial artery thrombosis has been observed in 3% to 6% of procedures. Predictors of radial thrombosis are larger sheath size and lower doses of heparin (8). Omission of heparin results in a very high rate of thrombosis (70%) (9). Radial artery thrombosis is asymptomatic in patients with a patent palmar arterial arch (10). In a large series of 7,049 procedures, vascular complications, such as

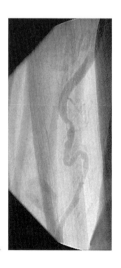 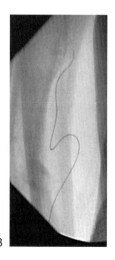 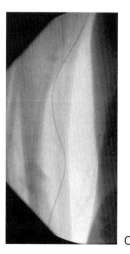

A   B   C

FIG. 24.6. **A:** After unsuccessful progression of the standard guidewire and glidewire, the right radial artery angiogram showed a tortuous and stenotic/spastic mid radial artery in a 79-year-old male patient. After negotiating the tortuosity under fluoroscopy using a coronary hydrophilic guidewire (**B**), the 4-Fr diagnostic catheter was advanced and the coronary angiogram completed (**C**).

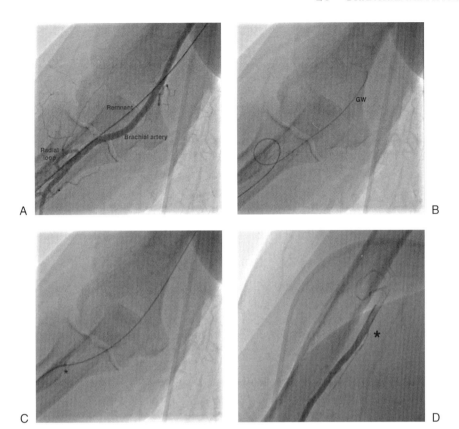

A

B

C

D

FIG. 24.7. A: Radial loop with patent remnant artery noted after unsuccessful catheter advancement over a hydrophilic coronary guidewire in an 82-year-old woman. B: Successful advancement of a hydrophilic coronary guidewire (GW) through the radial loop (C) with straightening with the hydrophilic-coated catheter. D: Origin (*asterisk*) of the small remnant artery at the mid brachial artery level.

hematoma under tension and volar compartment syndrome, were extremely rare (less than 1 per 3,000) despite immediate sheath withdrawal under full heparinization, thrombolytics, and/or potent platelet glycoprotein (Gp) IIb/IIIa receptor blockers (11). PTRA was not associated with increased radiation when compared with transfemoral and transbrachial approaches (12). The success rate was also similar in another comparison study with transbrachial and transfemoral approaches (13). This approach was also perceived as ideal for out-patient PTCA and stenting (14). In a randomized study of radial and femoral approaches, Cooper et al. demonstrated a strong patient preference for the transradial approach as-

sociated with a significant reduction in total hospital cost (15). The radial artery is prone to spasm triggered by fear, anxiety, failed puncture, pain, or rough manipulation of the guidewire or introducer sheath. Pain during sheath removal is seen in a significant number of patients, especially female patients with smaller body size; however, the availability of the hydrophilic-coated sheath has considerably reduced the discomfort associated with sheath removal (16). Finally, the possibility of radial artery atherosclerosis progression after transradial catheterization remains an unresolved question, especially in diabetics in whom coronary bypass with a radial artery conduit is considered (17).

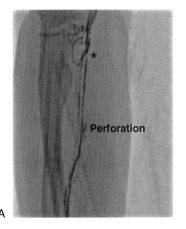

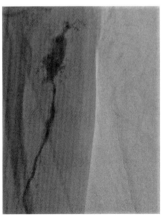

A

B

FIG. 24.8. A: Radial artery angiogram showing a hypoplastic radial artery with associated spasm (*asterisk*) and perforation in a 65-year-old woman. B: Attempts to advance a hydrophilic guidewire resulted in radial artery perforation successfully treated by short-duration local pressure. No clinical sequelae occurred.

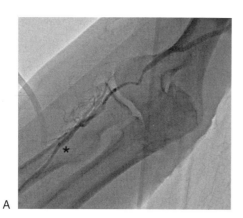 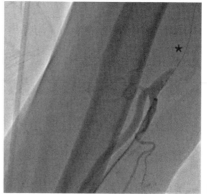

FIG. 24.9. A: Radial artery angiogram with diagnostic catheter (*asterisk*) in a 75-year-old male patient demonstrating spasms and tortuosity in a small radial artery. **B:** Following advancement of a coronary guidewire (*asterisk*), a proximal takeoff of the radial artery is seen at the mid portion of the brachial artery.

ANATOMIC ANOMALIES

Radiobrachial Loops

Of the vascular anomalies, radial loops are the most frequently encountered vascular abnormality and one of the main causes of PTRA failure (Fig. 24.3). In a recent paper by Yokoyama et al., evaluation with two-dimensional echo prior to PTRA is suggested to identify and exclude approximately 5% of patients with forearm vascular anomalies such as radial loops and hypoplastic radial artery (18). However, such preevaluation makes the PTRA procedure less appealing. In the majority of cases, a radial loop anomaly can be managed successfully (3,19). To avoid traumatic manipulation of the guidewire, avoidance of any resistance and early use of angiography to identify any problem cannot be overly emphasized. Use of a hydrophilic guidewire to facilitate the procedure has been suggested, but, as shown in Fig. 24.4, manipulation of hydrophilic wires can induce subintimal dissection and vessel perforation, especially in small muscular radial sidebranches. Use of a hydrophilic 0.014-in. coronary guidewire makes the wire more steerable and allows dye injection through a Y-connector for road mapping (3). Radioulnar loops are usually straightened easily with successive passage of the guidewire and catheter without any consequences,

as exemplified in Fig. 24.5. However, even if successful in negotiating and straightening the radioulnar loop, these procedures are often associated with spasms, pain, and longer duration, especially in catheter rotation, making catheter advancement difficult, if not impossible. If excessive pain is encountered despite use of hydrophilic-coated catheters, the author usually proceeds to the contralateral side or to the femoral approach.

Radial Artery Stenosis–Tortuosity

These anomalies are frequent and make guidewire advancement sometimes more difficult and painful (Figs. 24.4 and 24.6). Once again, angiography can help to understand the anatomy and to choose appropriate catheters. Additional use of vasodilators (isosorbide dinitrate, verapamil) is suggested as well as use of hydrophilic-coated catheters to avoid spasm and pain.

Remnant Artery

It is important to note that a remnant artery is often present at the mid portion of the radial loop with possible advancement of coronary guidewire, but usually not of the catheter. The

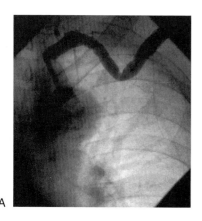 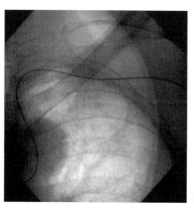

FIG. 24.10. A: Angiogram demonstrating a severe tortuosity and bend in the mid left subclavian artery in a 65-year-old male patient. **B:** Because of pain and difficulty manipulating the diagnostic catheter, the procedure was completed easily with a hydrophilic-coated guiding catheter. (Reprinted from Barbeau GR. Radial loops and extreme vessels tortuosity in transradial approach: advantage of hydrophilic-coated guidewires and catheters. *Catheter Cardiovasc Interv* 2003;59:442–450, with permission.)

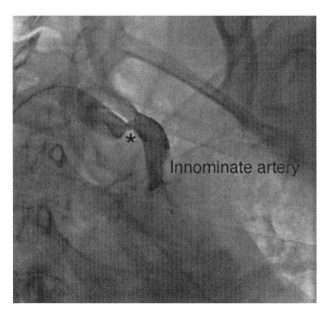

FIG. 24.11. Right subclavian artery angiogram in right anterior oblique projection illustrating a severe stenosis (*asterisk*) with a 120-mm Hg pressure gradient in a 53-year-old woman. The stenosis was suspected after difficult advancement of the guidewire into the ascending aorta.

Radial Artery Perforation

These perforations are usually well tolerated and must be prevented with gentle wire manipulation and early use of angiography. In case of minor perforation, careful observation in the cath lab and on the ward is necessary to identify ongoing bleeding (Fig. 24.8). The procedure can usually be completed with evaluation of the bleeding by angiography at the end of the procedure. In case of ongoing bleeding, local pressure with a blood pressure cuff or elastic bandage is done. Treatment with protamine to reverse heparin effect and blood pressure control are used in most severe cases of forearm bleeding, as in patients treated with GP IIb-IIIa receptor blockers or thombolysis.

Radiobrachial Anomaly

Sometimes, the origin of the radial artery is more proximal than usual, originating up to the lower portion of the axillary artery or the proximal brachial artery. In these circumstances, the radial artery tends to be smaller in diameter and more prone to spasm (Fig. 24.9). Use of smaller catheters (4 to 5 French) or hydrophilic-coated catheters facilitates successful completion of the PTRA procedure.

remnant artery usually has a mid-humeral junction with the brachial artery (Fig. 24.7). Sometimes a catheter can be advanced in the remnant artery to reach the aorta with resultant pain and spasm during the procedure and on the pullback. The spasm on pullback can result in avulsion of the artery with severe bleeding in the arm.

Subclavian/Innominate Tortuosity–Stenosis

Intrathoracic vessel tortuosity is also associated with pain and frequent failure to advance catheter and obtain proper coronary alignment during the transradial approach. These

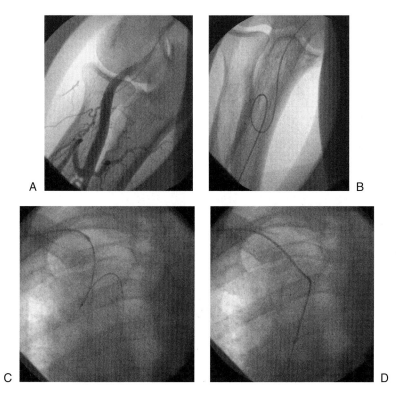

FIG. 24.12. A: Radial artery angiogram in a 66-year-old male patient showing a definite radiobrachial loop, (**B**) successfully crossed after several attempts with a hydrophilic-coated guidewire. **C:** Important tortuosity was also seen in the innominate artery making catheter movement difficult **D:** A 6-Fr hydrophilic-coated guiding catheter was advanced easily without introducer sheath through the radial loop as well as the severe tortuosity of the innominate artery. (Reprinted from Barbeau GR. Radial loops and extreme vessels tortuosity in transradial approach: advantage of hydrophilic-coated guidewires and catheters. *Catheter Cardiovasc Interv* 2003;59:442–450, with permission.)

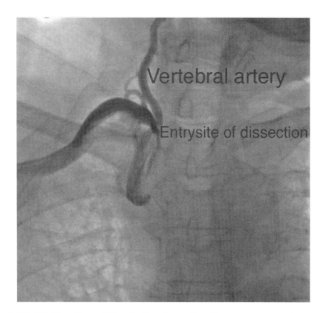

FIG. 24.13. After difficulty in advancing the coronary catheter into the ascending aorta, right subclavian artery angiogram resulted in a proximal dissection at the level of the vertebral artery. The procedure was successfully completed via the femoral approach with no further clinical sequelae in this 76-year-old woman.

anomalies are more frequent in older patients and in patients with a long history of hypertension (Figs. 24.10 and 24.11). Sometimes, more than one site of tortuosity is seen, making the use of hydrophilic-coated catheter mandatory (Fig. 24.12).

Subclavian/Innominate Dissection

Difficult wire and catheter advancement in tortuous vessels can sometimes induce dissection. In such cases, extreme care should be taken in evaluation with angiography to avoid ag-

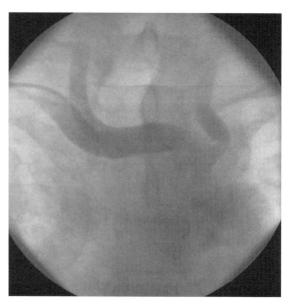

FIG. 24.14. Right innominate arteriogram showing a shared origin with the left carotid artery.

gravating unnoticed dissection (Fig. 24.13). However, the clinical course is usually benign due to the retrograde nature of the dissection.

Aberrant Right Subclavian Artery

An aberrant right subclavian artery is occasionally encountered from right PTRA (20). This anomaly can be suspected by the sinuous course of the catheter in the ascending aorta in anteroposterior or left anterior oblique projections (Fig. 24.14). Selective angiography of the right subclavian artery will reveal its course and relation with left carotid and left subclavian arteries. In the case of a retroesophagal right subclavian artery (arteria lusoria), selective angiography of the

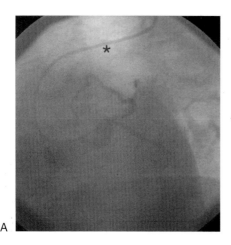
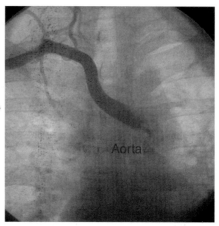

FIG. 24.15. A: Coronary angiogram in left anterior oblique caudal projection showing the typical inverted "S" appearance of the catheter (*asterisk*) in aberrant (arteria lusoria) right subclavian artery. **B:** Right subclavian arteriogram showing its aberrant origin distal to the left subclavian artery.

coronary arteries is more challenging (Fig. 24.15). In this case, catheter exchanges are performed over guidewires left in the ascending aorta.

CONCLUSIONS

This chapter described several cases of anatomic variations and complications occurring in PTRA. Limitations of this approach include a definite learning curve mainly because of difficult anatomy. Although not exhaustive, the list of vascular anomalies given here represents the most frequent causes of pain and failure associated with PTRA. Nevertheless, this represents overall only 3% to 5% of all PTRA procedures, the majority of these being uneventful. Use of early upper arm angiography as well as hydrophilic equipment has allowed greater success rate in a subset of patients previously considered difficult if not impossible.

The PTRA procedure is considered one of the safest entry sites for angiography and coronary angioplasty. In addition, because of an extremely low bleeding rate, it is the only access site compatible with immediate postprocedure ambulation and it is ideal for outpatient interventions. The greater part of vascular complications such as dissection or perforation can be managed conservatively.

REFERENCES

1. Campeau L. Percutaneous radial artery approach for coronary angiography. *Catheter Cardiovasc Diagn* 1989;16:3–7.
2. Kiemeneij F, Laarman GJ. Percutaneous transradial artery approach for coronary Palmaz–Schatz stent implantation. *Am Heart J* 1994;128:167–174.
3. Barbeau G. Radial loops and extreme vessel tortuosity in the transradial approach: advantage of hydrophilic-coated guidewires and catheters. *Catheter Cardiovasc Interv* 2003;59:442–450.
4. Barbeau G, Arsenault F, Larivière M, et al. A new and objective method for transradial approach screening: comparison with the Allen's test in 1010 patients. *J Am Coll Cardiol* 2001;37:34A.
5. Barbeau GR, Carrier G, Ferland S, et al. Right transradial approach for coronary procedures: preliminary results. *J Invasive Cardiol* 1996;8 [Suppl D]:19D–21D.
6. Keeley EC, Grines CL. Scraping of aortic debris by coronary guiding catheters: a prospective evaluation of 1,000 cases. *J Am Coll Cardiol* 1998;32:1861–1865.
7. Barbeau G, Gleeton O, Roy L, et al. Predictors of failure of transradial approach: a multivariate analysis of a large series. *Circulation* 1999;100:I-306.
8. Barbeau G, Bilodeau S, Carrier G, et al. Predictors of radial artery thrombosis after transradial approach: a multivariate analysis of a large series. *J Am Coll Cardiol* 2000;35:A-32.
9. Spaulding C, Lefevre T, Funck F, et al. Left radial approach for coronary angiography: results of a prospective study. *Catheter Cardiovasc Diagn* 1996;39:365–370.
10. Stella PR, Kiemeneij F, Laarman GJ, et al. Incidence and outcome of radial artery occlusion following transradial artery coronary angioplasty. *Catheter Cardiovasc Diagn* 1997;40:156–158.
11. Barbeau G, Gleeton O, Roy L, et al. Transradial approach for coronary interventions: procedural results and vascular complications of a series of 7049 procedures. *Circulation* 1999;100:I-306.
12. Mann 3rd JT, Cubeddu G, Arrowood M. Operator radiation exposure in PTCA: comparison of radial and femoral approaches. *J Invasive Cardiol* 1996;8 [Suppl D]:22D–25D.
13. Kiemeneij F, Laarman GJ, Odekerken D, et al. A randomized comparison of percutaneous transluminal coronary angioplasty by the radial, brachial and femoral approaches: the access study. *J Am Coll Cardiol* 1997;29:1269–1275.
14. Kiemeneij F, Laarman GJ, Slagboom T, et al. Outpatient coronary stent implantation. *J Am Coll Cardiol* 1997;29:323–327.
15. Cooper CJ, El-Shiekh RA, Cohen DJ, et al. Effect of transradial access on quality of life and cost of cardiac catheterization: a randomized comparison. *Am Heart J* 1999;138:430–436.
16. Dery JP, Simard S, Barbeau GR. Reduction of discomfort at sheath removal during transradial coronary procedures with the use of a hydrophilic-coated sheath. *Catheter Cardiovasc Interv* 2001;54:289–294.
17. Gobeil J, Plante S, Barbeau GR, et al. Ultrasonic assessment of radial atherosclerosis changes following transradial angiography, angioplasty in diabetic patients. *Circulation* 1999;100:I-144.
18. Yokoyama N, Takeshita S, Ochiai M, et al. Anatomic variations of the radial artery in patients undergoing transradial coronary intervention. *Catheter Cardiovasc Interv* 2000;49:357–362.
19. Louvard Y, Lefevre T. Loops and transradial approach in coronary diagnosis and intervention. *Catheter Cardiovasc Interv* 2000;51:250–252.
20. Abhaichand RK, Louvard Y, Gobeil JF, et al. The problem of arteria lusoria in right transradial coronary angiography and angioplasty. *Catheter Cardiovasc Interv* 2001;54:196–201.

CHAPTER 25

Complications of Interventional Treatment of Peripheral Vascular Disease

James D. Joye and Mahmoud Eslami-Farsani

Key Points

- This chapter presents an overview of the complications of vascular interventional procedures and their prevention and management.
- Dissection is usually caused by plaque fracture, intimal splitting, and localized medial dissection.
- Distal embolization during intervention of certain arteries may result in major clinical events.
- Arterial perforation is a complication seen in percutaneous treatment of peripheral arterial disease. This is often due to poor vascular compliance, extensive calcification, and complex lesions.
- Complications of vascular access—carotid, brachiocephalic, mesenteric, aortic, renal, iliac, infrainguinal, and infrapopliteal—important in vascular interventional procedures are described.
- A broad armamentarium of stents, catheters, and wires can be used to avoid and treat complications in peripheral procedures.

INTRODUCTION

As the number of vascular interventional procedures in the United States has increased, the number of complications encountered by physicians has also increased. Many of the complications that occur are common to most vascular interventional procedures (1–4). This chapter presents an overview of complications and techniques to prevent them, reduce their occurrence, and manage them.

The incidence of complications related to vascular interventional procedures is dependent on many different factors. Patient population is probably the most important one. Patients referred for vascular intervention represent a subgroup that tends to be older and usually carries serious morbid disease. Older patients at high risk for conventional surgery because of cardiopulmonary illness are now increasingly referred for percutaneous procedures. They usually have extensive occlusive arterial disease requiring multilevel treatment involving thrombolytic therapy, angioplasty, and stent placement. Diffuse atherosclerosis accompanied by dense and heavy plaque burden with end-stage arteries is commonly seen in these patients. Other comorbidities such as diabetes mellitus, chronic renal insufficiency, and hypertension are also frequently seen in these patients. In addition, such patients are two to four times more likely to have a history of myocardial infarction, angina, congestive heart failure, and stroke. Higher rates of silent ischemia have also been observed in these patients. Therefore, some complications may be expected as patients tend be older, have diffuse arterial disease, and carry multiple comorbidities.

The past decade witnessed a dramatic increase in technology and development of medical devices used in treatment of coronary atherosclerosis disease. The development of technology in treatment of peripheral vascular disease, however, has lagged behind, which has resulted in a higher rate of complications. Only recently have medical devices for the sole purpose of peripheral intervention been developed, and as new technology develops, the safety and efficacy of such devices increase. The use of a new device, however, is associated with a higher rate of complication due to lack of operator experience. The skills required for use of a new device will develop over time depending on an operator's frequency of use as well as the operator's dexterity and skills.

DISSECTION

Dissection during peripheral intervention can and will occur in every vascular bed. Dissection is usually caused by plaque fracture, intimal splitting, and localized medial dissection. The factors that can contribute to an increased risk of dissection are multiple. Calcific, eccentric, long lesions tend to be at higher risk for dissection. Diffuse and complex lesions with heavy plaque burden are also prone to dissection. Lesions that are on vessel curvature and bifurcation lesions may easily dissect with balloon injury. Balloon oversizing is an independent predictor of dissection, and larger-diameter balloons tend to have a higher rate of dissection. High-pressure inflations, particularly when noncompliant balloons and the kissing balloon technique are used, can also result in dissection.

Dissection of peripheral arteries can lead to extension of the dissection and flow impairment in a critical side branch and adjacent vascular territory. Dissection in certain arteries is of special concern. For example, dissection of the subclavian artery can involve the internal mammary or vertebral artery,

and dissection of the renal artery may result in distal, spiral dissection and sudden loss of blood flow to a kidney. Common iliac dissection (Fig. 25.1) can lead to involvement of the internal iliac and the common femoral artery. Dissection of the carotid artery may result in cerebrovascular accident requiring emergent surgery. The decision for the treatment of dissection at the site of a lesion depends on its extent and likelihood of flow impairment. Limited retrograde dissection in a vessel usually has a benign course and will likely heal by itself. On the other hand, an antegrade dissection may extend and cause limitation of flow as high-velocity flow enters the false channel, threatening its patency.

A number of different steps can be taken to reduce the incidence of dissections. Attempt should be made to match the balloon diameter to the disease-free distal reference segment (balloon to artery ratio=1). Use of long balloons to cover both the proximal and distal edges of lesions, cutting balloon for calcified lesions, and low-pressure inflations can reduce the rate of dissection in peripheral interventions. Predilation with smaller-diameter balloons not only prevents overstretching of arteries, but helps to determine the lesion's compliance. Prolonged inflations may acutely produce an improved angiographic response, but do not result in improved outcomes or derail inherent recoil. Once peripheral interventions are complicated by dissection, different strategies may be applied for their management. Small retrograde dissections may be left alone because they pose little or no risk. Complex, long lesions may be managed by prolonged balloon

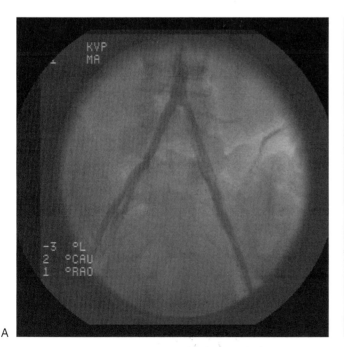

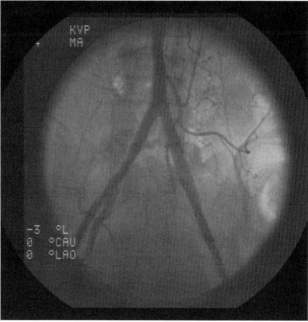

A

B

FIG. 25.1. A: Angiogram revealing dissection of the left common iliac artery with extension into the external iliac and obliteration of the internal iliac in a 57-year-old male smoker following angioplasty of segmental occlusion of the left common iliac. **B:** Angiogram showing the final result following balloon-expandable kissing-stent reconstruction of the common iliac bifurcation and self-expanding nitinol stenting of the dissected arterial segment.

inflations. Dissection planes usually close and tamponade by use of prolonged inflations. Stents play an important role in the management of dissections. Antegrade dissections, and dissections with flow impairment or vessel closure, should all be considered for stent placement.

PERFORATION

Arterial perforation is another complication seen in percutaneous treatment of peripheral arterial disease. Poor vascular compliance, extensive calcification, and complex lesions commonly seen in peripheral arterial disease all contribute to an increased likelihood of perforations. Lesion morphology including eccentricity, length, and anatomic location (bifurcation disease, lesion located on an angulated segment) can also contribute to an increased risk of perforation. In addition, balloon rupture, use of devices that alter the integrity of vascular wall, and use of hydrophilic or stiff wires have been associated with higher rate of perforation.

In our experience, peripheral arteries such as external iliac, common femoral, and popliteal arteries are particularly at higher risk of perforation (Fig. 25.2). Higher rates of perforation have been reported in iliac arteries particularly in patients taking steroids. Perforation of renal arteries is very rare, but can be fatal due to retroperitoneal bleeding. Carotid perforation is also rarely seen, and lower-pressure inflation during postdilatation is recommended.

Unlike some dissections, which can be left alone and treated conservatively, all perforations need to be managed aggressively. Initially, balloon tamponading at the perforation site should be applied. This reduces the active bleeding, but rarely seals the perforation; thus additional intervention is mandatory. If prolonged balloon inflation fails to seal the perforation, a covered stent should be placed across the perforation. In our experience, almost all perforations can be sealed using a covered stent. Rarely, covered stents fail and an immediate surgical treatment becomes necessary.

DISTAL EMBOLIZATION

Almost all percutaneous interventions are known to be associated with thromboembolic or atheroembolic events. Many of these embolic events are unlikely to have any adverse clinical sequelae and may go unnoticed due to small size of the particles. However, larger emboli may result in ischemic events requiring intervention. The incidence of embolization during peripheral intervention is not well known, but is thought to be between 2% and 5%.

Distal embolization during intervention of certain arteries may result in major clinical events. Cerebrovascular accidents and transient ischemic attacks can occur during carotid intervention. This is a major source of morbidity and mortality, and all efforts must be made to prevent it. Intervention of the subclavian artery can result in a posterior cerebrovascular accident due to embolization to the posterior circulation. Embolization during renal artery intervention may not manifest any immediate clinical adverse effects, but it may limit the end results. Manipulation of catheters in the aorta or aortic

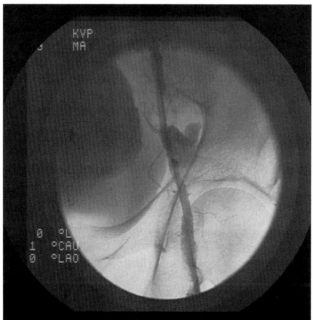
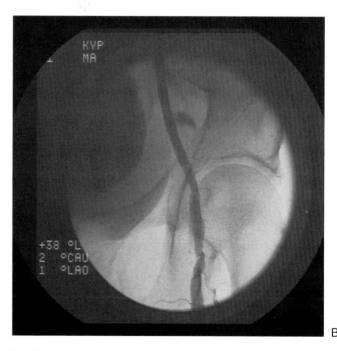

A   B

FIG. 25.2. A: Contralateral angiogram of the left groin after a complex femoropopliteal procedure performed with an antegrade puncture, revealing perforation of the distal left external iliac artery with extravasation of contrast and evolving retroperitoneal hemorrhage. **B:** Angiogram demonstrating complete sealing of the perforation site following prompt deployment of a covered stent.

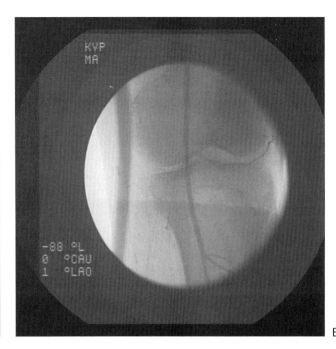

FIG. 25.3. A: Angiogram depicting acute thromboembolic occlusion of the terminal popliteal artery and tibioperoneal vessels after angioplasty and stenting of a long-segment chronic total occlusion of the superficial femoral artery. **B:** Following catheter-directed thrombolysis in the angiographic suite with continued overnight infusion, the angiogram the following morning reveals complete resolution of thrombus with restored distal flow.

intervention can also be associated with distal embolization. Abrupt downstream occlusion of the infrapopliteal arteries is not uncommon with recanalization of chronic total occlusions of the iliofemoral vessels due to inherent fibrin-laden thrombus within the occluded segment (Fig. 25.3). Small emboli may travel to any vascular bed causing abrupt closure of vessels. Trash toe syndrome can result if digital arteries are involved. The most extreme but rarely seen consequences of distal embolization are gangrene and ischemic ulceration.

Several steps can be taken to reduce the risk of distal embolization. All lesions, particularly lesions at high risk of embolization (i.e., fresh, friable thrombus), should be approached carefully. Catheter, wire, and balloon manipulation should be kept to a minimum to reduce the likelihood of lesion disruption. Advancement and removal of catheters should be done over a wire, particularly in patients with tortuous and aneurysmal aorta. Moreover, backbleeding of the guiding catheter should be done after wire pullback to allow removal of particles and air bubbles. Use of protection devices has been recently shown to decrease the incidence of embolization. Protection devices should be considered in peripheral interventions where there is a likelihood of embolization.

Management of distal embolization varies depending on the size of the emboli and the vessel occluded. Small emboli affecting terminal arterial branches causing necrosis are usually managed conservatively. Embolectomy catheters may be necessary to remove large emboli affecting medium to large arteries. Catheter-guided thrombolytic therapy with continuous infusion for 8 to 24 hours can restore perfusion in an acute occlusive event.

VASCULAR ACCESS COMPLICATION

Complications of vascular access are the most common complications encountered in patients undergoing peripheral intervention. The incidence of access complication varies between 2% and 13%. Hematoma, ecchymosis, and pseudoaneurysms are among the frequently seen complications. Most of these are self-limiting, but they can be a source of considerable discomfort. Retroperitoneal bleeding, on the other hand, is a formidable and sometimes fatal complication of vascular access, which can go undetected long after procedure.

Patient body habitus and other characteristics play a significant role in the development of vascular complications. Obese or hypertensive patients are at higher risk of complications, as are patients who are confused or restless. Patients with peripheral vascular disease have calcified, friable arteries, which can be easily damaged. Puncture site is another important factor in development of access complication. For example, retrograde puncture of the femoral artery can result in retroperitoneal bleeding if the vessel is inadvertently punctured above the inguinal ligament. Antegrade common femoral artery puncture is also known to be more likely to result in complication due to a variety of factors (Fig. 25.4). Brachial artery access, on the other hand, has a very low risk of complication. Other factors such as level of

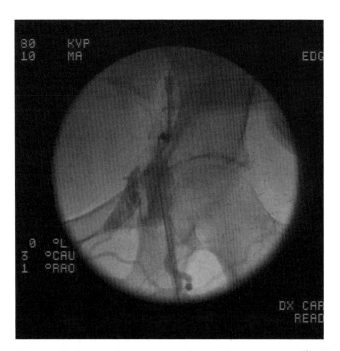

FIG. 25.4. Antegrade puncture of the left common femoral artery in a patient with a failed femoropopliteal bypass graft resulted in perivascular extravasation of contrast and hematoma formation during attempts to advance the sheath into the residual stump of the left superficial femoral artery.

anticoagulation, operator experience, and size of the introducer sheath all play a role in incidence of access complication.

Management of the access site at the end of a peripheral intervention should be considered as important as the intervention itself. If the access site is not managed properly, it can turn a successful intervention into an emergent surgery. A number of different arterial closure devices are available to assist with hemostasis.

Endovascular complications vary with each vascular bed, and a broad knowledge of potential problems is critical. This requires a firm understanding of the anatomy and physiology of each target vessel, as well as an appreciation for the optimal technical approach. The best way to avoid complications is to anticipate potential problem areas. A heavy emphasis is placed on vascular access. Percutaneous entrance and exit are critical, as is intravascular catheter access to vascular structures once the procedure is underway. Knowing the tolerance limits of various vessels and appreciating the impact of calcification, tortuosity, and diffuse disease can help to avert disaster.

CAROTID COMPLICATIONS

The carotid artery is a controversial endovascular target. Data continue to emerge, however, in strong support of carotid artery stenting. Patients referred for carotid artery stenting are typically of the highest risk as mandated by most protocols. In such a cohort of patients, virtually any complication

must be expected (5). Of course the risk of stroke and death is paramount. Embolic protection devices have favorably affected the former (6–8). Nonetheless, lesions that are echolucent, bulky, and high grade should be approached with extra caution. Death in carotid stenting can arise from major cardiovascular accident (CVA), hyperperfusion syndrome with intracranial hemorrhage (9), and myocardial infarction. Embolic protection is designed to prevent major CVA and has proven to be efficacious (10–12). Hyperperfusion syndrome should be anticipated in any patient with a high-grade stenosis and hypertension. This is especially true in patients with contralateral occlusion. In such patients, aggressive modulation of hemodynamics is crucial (13). Patients with recurrent disease after endarterectomy and those with lesions that spare the carotid bulb can safely have their blood pressure lowered preprocedure because they are unlikely to develop the major hemodynamic changes seen with *de novo* bifurcation lesions. Myocardial infarction in carotid stent patients is not surprising given the fact that 50% of these patients have concomitant coronary artery disease. Proper screening and preoperative assessment of ischemia are therefore critical. The wide hemodynamic swings provoked by carotid stenting can serve to trigger an infarct in a patient with high-grade coronary lesions. Dilation of the carotid bulb will routinely provoke a marked drop in blood pressure and a short period of asystole or profound arteriovenous block. Anticipating these problems and dealing with them promptly can make the difference between a successful procedure and a poor outcome. Early in one's experience, preadministration of 1.0 mg of atropine and/or temporary pacemaker placement is a reasonable approach. The bradycardic impact of dilation is typically short lived, however, and we typically reserve such measures for only the most fragile patients. More important is rapid administration of pressor agents. Short-acting agents such as neosynephrine often suffice, but a significant minority require a dopamine infusion, occasionally for 24 to 36 hours. There are several vessel-specific complications to be aware of as well (14). Overdilation of a stenosis, as in any vascular bed, can and will provoke perforation. Accepting a mild residual stenosis in a densely calcified lesion is a far better outcome. Typically, we do not exceed 6-mm-diameter balloons during postdilation, and we take care to size the balloon for the cervical portion of the distal artery rather than fall into the trap of sizing to the bulb or immediately distal vessel where poststenotic dilation is prevalent. Embolic protection systems and stents introduce another set of potential problems. Occlusion balloon protection can evoke transient ischemic attacks and seizures in a small minority of patients. Prompt aspiration and deflation are sometimes needed, as is the occasional administration of benzodiazepines. Filters can overfill and at times need to be aspirated prior to recapture. Circulatory control devices may also create cerebrovascular changes. Any protection device can cause dissection or spasm of the distal artery, and care must be taken to place them in the proper location and to deploy them according to the vessel size. Contrast itself can become problematic if overutilized. Contrast encephalopathy is a rare consequence, but its clinical expression is acutely impossible to separate from true embolic events.

BRACHIOCEPHALIC COMPLICATIONS

Interventions involving the great vessels must be undertaken with care so as to avoid significant sequelae (15–17). Embolization can occur to the carotids, vertebrals, mammaries, and upper extremities. Selective use of protection devices in such cases is advisable. Fortunately, with true steal phenomena, retrograde flow in the vertebral artery is often protective of the posterior fossa, at least until the microvasculature resets its tone. Aggressive intervention in high-grade lesions and occlusions can also provoke perforation and hemothorax. Access to covered stents is mandatory in such cases. Dissection is not uncommon, especially in the subclavian artery (Fig. 25.5). Such tears will occasionally extend into the vertebral artery and internal mammary and provoke ischemia or acute occlusion. To limit these events, we generally predilate with a small-diameter balloon to facilitate stent placement prior to optimal postdilation. As in other vessels, postdilation is best kept within the margins of the stent to avoid edge dissections. Stenting of the origin of the great vessels must take into account the possibility of plaque shift and impingement of neighboring vessels. This is especially true of ostial left subclavian lesions because the left common carotid artery is often immediately adjacent.

MESENTERIC COMPLICATIONS

Patients with true mesenteric ischemia are critically dependent on the flow achieved through the target vessel. Because of the inferior takeoff of these vessels, a brachial approach is generally advised. Failure to achieve necessary support from a femoral approach can increase the likelihood of damaging the ostium, embolizing debris, and migrating the stent to an undesirable location. Although distal embolization and mesenteric ischemia are rare events, meticulous technique is needed to avoid life-threatening complications (18,19). Stenting of mesenteric vessels, especially in the superior mesenteric artery, should be limited to the ostial position to avoid side branch occlusion and to preserve surgical options. Careful wire manipulation is critical, especially in the celiac branches, due to the fragile nature of the vascular beds of the liver and the spleen.

AORTIC COMPLICATIONS

Endovascular treatment of disease of the aorta has gained great attention as an alternative to open surgical repair. Dilation of stenoses and grafting of aneurysms must be undertaken with special care (20–23). Interventions in the stenotic aorta carry the risk of embolization to the mesentery and lower extremities. In friable, ulcerated lesions, the use of covered stents may limit these occurrences. Because of the large profile of devices needed for such interventions, vascular access complications are heightened. Vascular surgical assistance or standby is suggested. Perforation is rare but catastrophic. Again, access to covered stent platforms and vascular surgical expertise are critical to patient safety. Care must be taken when stenting the aorta that clinically significant side branches are not covered. This can provoke mesenteric and/or lower extremity ischemia. Stent embolization is also not unheard of because the larger-diameter stents must

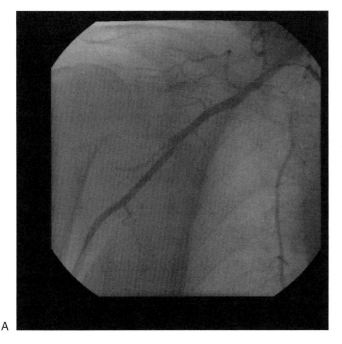
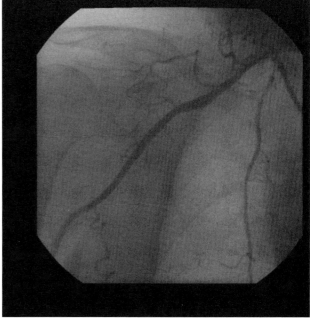

A   B

FIG. 25.5. A: Angioplasty of a distal right subclavian artery stenosis resulted in profound dissection of the lesion. **B:** Angiographic result after placement of a self-expanding stainless steel stent.

be hand-crimped onto the balloon. When possible, safe passage to the target through an appropriate-size sheath may minimize this problem.

RENAL COMPLICATIONS

Renal artery stent procedures are often described as entry level or simple. This is not meant to imply that they are devoid of complications. Renal arteries have a propensity to dissect, especially in the mid-section of the primary artery, where the vessel is tortuous and thin walled (Fig. 25.6). For these reasons, it is recommended that balloons not extend any more distally than necessary, and predilation should be geared to permit safe entry of stents rather than to optimally dilate. Prompt recognition of distal dissection and tacking up the distal extent promptly are critical. Dissection can also involve the surrounding perirenal aorta. This is usually provoked by overdilation and fortunately is not often associated with clinical sequelae. We rarely dilate renal arteries beyond 6 mm and never exceed 7 mm for this reason. Embolization probably occurs to some degree in all renal procedures. Perhaps 15% to 20% of the time, this results in suboptimal long-term results such as declining renal function, protein spilling, and persistent hypertension (24,25). In the future, embolic protection systems will be specifically tailored to renal arteries and will likely have a significant clinical impact. Like other aortoostial interventions, emboli to the distal aorta and its tributaries can occur (26–28). This can result in mesenteric ischemia, sloughing of the perineum, and blue toe syndrome. Perforation of renal arteries is also known

to occur on rare occasions. Caution with densely calcified lesions and access to covered balloon-expandable stents is advised. Flank pain during balloon inflation is a reliable indicator that the adventitia is being stretched, and additional dilation force does little to improve the angiographic results, but significantly increases the risk of trauma. Avoidance of hydrophilic wires is also wise because distal migration of such wires can perforate smaller distal vessels and provoke a capsular hematoma. Care in engaging the renal artery itself is important because plaque shift can occur. In arteries that are difficult to selectively enter, we advise wiring the artery through the diagnostic catheter and then exchanging over the wire for a guide catheter. Failure to do so can result in sufficient plaque shift with the larger-diameter catheter to the extent that the ostium of the vessel can acutely occlude and prompt the need for emergent surgical bypass.

ILIAC COMPLICATIONS

Iliac interventions are routinely performed for the relief of lower extremity claudication. Results tend to be quite durable; however, complications are not uncommon (29–32). Dissection is an almost expected consequence of balloon dilation in the iliac tree. Preventing extension of the dissection into the hypogastric arteries, aorta, and common femoral arteries is critical. Because of the propensity to dissect, we again prefer to underdilate as a prelude to stenting, and postdilate within the margins of the stent. The external iliac artery must be handled with extra care. These vessels are often tortuous and are extremely fragile, especially in their diseased

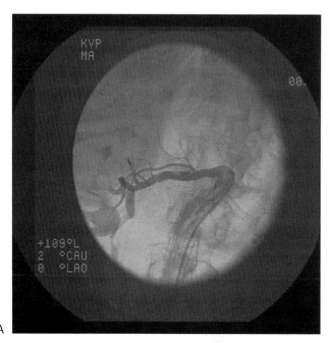

A

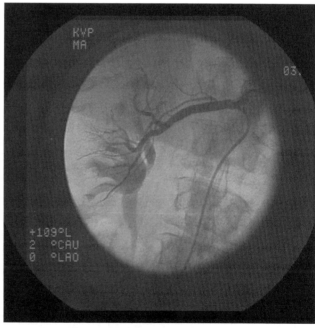

B

FIG. 25.6. A: Complex dissection of the mid-right renal artery secondary to catheter tip trauma induced during selective placement of a Simmons 1 catheter. **B:** Final angiogram following successful stenting of the right renal artery.

state. Perforation of the external iliac artery can occur without warning and occasionally from a seemingly innocent dilation. Access to covered stents for this application is critical to rapidly curtail extravasation of blood into the retroperitoneal space. Special care should also be afforded the internal iliac arteries. Acute obstruction of the sole remaining patent internal iliac can result in nagging hip and buttocks claudication, impotence, and, more importantly, mesenteric ischemia. Bifurcation lesions of the origin of the common iliac arteries require special attention. When reconstructing the carina with balloon-expandable stents, one should not oversize the dilation balloons lest one create trauma to the aorta. A general rule of thumb is that the combined diameter of the two iliac balloons in a kissing balloon approach should not exceed 1.2 times the diameter of the distal aorta. In dealing with chronic occlusions of the iliac arteries, perforation is more prevalent, and consideration of covered stents should be made. Care must also be taken to not miss flaps on the proximal and distal margins related to wire passage. Failure to stent these margins often results in acute closure. Chronic occlusions may also harbor fibrin-laden clot, and thrombotic occlusion of a seemingly perfect angiographic result is not unheard of.

INFRAINGUINAL COMPLICATIONS

Infrainguinal interventions are among the more difficult endovascular procedures. Femoropopliteal lesions have a dense plaque burden and are prone to calcification. The most feared complication of a lower extremity procedure is limb loss. This is quite rare and is nearly completely avoidable with strict attention to anticoagulation and critical respect for the profunda femoris. Interventions in the common femoral artery and ostial superficial femoral artery should be performed with great care to avoid plaque shift and dissection, which can jeopardize the profunda. Stenting across the profunda is generally forbidden. Dissection throughout the femoropopliteal arteries occurs in nearly 50% of cases. Most can be readily dealt with by stent deployment. Stents themselves have introduced a new set of problems including the recent discovery of strut fractures (33). Complications in this femoropopliteal arteries are much more common when dealing with chronic occlusions. In such cases, aggressive wire and catheter techniques are often employed, and the subintimal approach is common. Vessel perforation can occur and result in thigh hematoma, arteriovenous fistulae, and compartment syndrome. Prompt recognition of these problems and definitive resolution is necessary (34,35). Thrombosis is also a major problem in femoropopliteal interventions. The two main sources of clot are from within the course of an occlusion and related to stagnant flow from either poor runoff or upstream compromise. To avoid inflow problems, we recommend the routine use of the crossover technique. Antegrade punctures are notoriously difficult to manage postprocedure, and the compression required to achieve hemostasis will occasionally provoke thrombosis of an otherwise satisfactory outcome. More aggressive anticoagulation is reasonable for patients with poor runoff. One other sequela to be aware of in patients that undergo recanalization of chronic occlusions is the development of ankle edema. This is an expected outcome and represents hyperemia. In some patients, however, restoring normal arterial flow will unmask venous insufficiency, and the edema can be permanent and quite bothersome.

INFRAPOPLITEAL COMPLICATIONS

Below-the-knee interventions are typically reserved for cases of limb salvage and nonhealing ulcers (36,37). Such patients are generally quite ill, frequently diabetic, and have very extensive disease. The procedures are often longer due to the need to establish continuous in-line flow to the distal foot. Complications in such an environment are not surprising. Dissection planes and intimal flaps can acutely interrupt flow and accelerate limb loss if not dealt with properly. Stenting below the knee is generally taboo. However, in cases where flow is impaired and failure to restore flow may have dire consequences, stents must be deployed. Perforation is not uncommon in the tibial vessel related to their small diameter, dense disease, and rampant calcification (Fig. 25.7). Thrombus formation is always a concern, as is distal embolization of clot and atheroma. The tibial vessels also tend to be very reactive and are distally prone to intense spasm. The use of small-wire systems, aggressive anticoagulation, vasodilators, and properly sized balloons are just a few of the maneuvers that will reduce the frequency of unfavorable outcomes.

TEN MUST-HAVE TOOLS TO STAY OR GET OUT OF TROUBLE

When starting a peripheral intervention program, one needs to have access to a broad array of technology to succeed. Some of these devices are intended to prevent trouble and facilitate safe endovascular work, and others are necessary to resolve crisis and assure patient safety. The best way to avoid complications in peripheral procedures is to anticipate them and strategize accordingly.

1. The advent of covered stents has made a major impact on the resolution of acute arterial perforation and dissection. Access to self-expanding and balloon-expandable covered stents allows for minimization of retroperitoneal bleeding in iliac procedures, organ salvage in renal procedures, and prevention of extravasation and the need for emergent surgical repair. These devices may also be useful in limiting embolization from aortic procedures and are an essential tool in dealing with aneurysmal disease.
2. Access to an array of self-expanding bare metal stents is also useful in preventing problems. These devices can be applied when needed in potentially compressible locations for better maintenance of patency. We frequently utilize these devices in distal subclavian lesions and external iliac lesions with minimal predilation to ward off

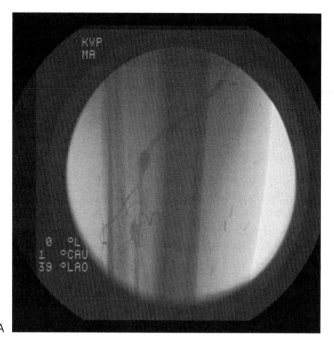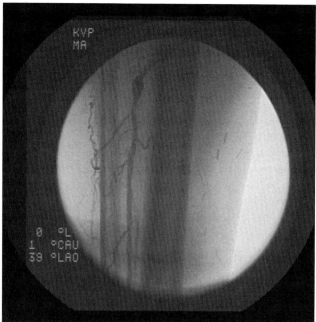

A   B

FIG. 25.7. A: Angiogram showing perforation of the left posterior tibial artery following cutting balloon dilation of a high-grade stenosis distal to a femorotibial bypass in a patient with limb-threatening ischemia. **B:** Final angiogram after prolonged balloon inflation and reversal of anticoagulation.

problematic dissection. Access to self-expanding, nitinol coil stents is also critical for common femoral and popliteal procedures that are threatened by flow-limiting dissection.

3. Hydrophilic wires and exchange catheters are a mainstay in endovascular procedures. Although they must be treated with respect, they allow for easier access to targets beyond tortuous arterial segments. They are also the tools of choice for subintimal crossing of total occlusions.

4. A variety of guide wires is also necessary to safely perform interventions in the peripheral vasculature. This includes extra support wires to allow placement of catheters in difficult anatomy, as well as small-wire systems for safely dealing with more delicate targets such as renal arteries and tibial vessels.

5. A broad selection of sheaths will facilitate successful and safe interventions. In particular, one should have access to reliable crossover sheaths, and sheaths of a variety of lengths and French sizes. Longer sheaths are useful in navigating the aortic arch in the brachial approach and in supporting infrapopliteal and carotid procedures from the femoral approach. As in any intervention, optimal sheath or guide support can mitigate complications.

6. Embolic protection devices are mandatory for carotid interventions. They have had a significant impact on the safety of carotid stent procedures, and are likely to have similar benefits in other vascular targets such as renal arteries.

7. Reentry catheters are a new set of devices that add further safety and predictability to endovascular treatment of to-

tal occlusions. With these devices, one can reenter the true lumen from an entrapped subintimal position without the risk of perforation or compromise of meaningful collateral branches.

8. There are vascular targets that are clearly better off with a nonstent solution. Newer atherectomy devices that can debulk lesions may limit the need for stents, and newer forms of angioplasty such as cryoplasty and cutting balloons may significantly reduce dissection rates. The use of these devices in common femoral, popliteal, and tibioperoneal lesions in particular may provide for a safer, more effective outcome.

9. Access to technology that effectively deals with thrombus is critical to the safe completion of many interventions. The combined use of declotting catheters and pharmacologic agents such as thrombolytics, and antiplatelet agents can restore flow in an acutely occluded vessel.

10. Closure devices may allow for safer completion of procedures. Properly applying the many devices available may reduce the incidence of hematoma formation and pseudoaneurysms. These devices are particularly useful in large-diameter punctures and antegrade sticks.

CONCLUSION

Complications in endovascular approaches to peripheral vascular disease are not uncommon. Critical to improved outcomes and safety is a thorough understanding of the anatomy and physiology of the peripheral vasculature. Proper training and case selection are also mandatory. A broad knowledge of treatment options and available technologies will combine to make procedures safer and more beneficial for all patients.

REFERENCES

1. Belli AM, Cumberland DC, Knox AM, et al. The complication rate of percutaneous peripheral balloon angioplasty. *Clin Radiol* 1990;41:380–383.
2. Kaufman J, Moglia R, Lacy C, et al. Peripheral vascular complications from percutaneous transluminal coronary angioplasty: a comparison with transfemoral cardiac catheterization. *Am J Med Sci* 1989;297:22–25.
3. Katzen BT. Percutaneous transluminal angioplasty for arterial disease of the lower extremities. *Am J Roentgenol* 1984;142:23–25.
4. Kitchens C, Jordan Jr W, Wirthlin D, et al. Vascular complications arising from maldeployed stents. *Vasc Endovascular Surg* 200;36:145–154.
5. Tan KT, Cleveland TJ, Berczi V, et al. Timing and frequency of complications after carotid artery stenting: what is the optimal period of observation? *J Vasc Surg* 2003;38:236–243.
6. Kastrup A, Groschel K, Krapf H, et al. Early outcome of carotid angioplasty and stenting with and without cerebral protection devices: a systematic review of the literature. *Stroke* 2003;34:813–819.
7. Cho L, Yadav JS. Embolization in atherosclerosis. *Neuroimaging Clin North Am* 2002;12:365–372.
8. Ohki T, Veith FJ, Grenell S, et al. Initial experience with cerebral protection devices to prevent embolization during carotid artery stenting. *J Vasc Surg* 2002;36:1175–1185.
9. Nikolsky E, Patil CV, Beyar R. Ipsilateral intracerebral hemorrhage following carotid stent-assisted angioplasty: a manifestation of hyperperfusion syndrome—a case report. *Angiology* 2002;53:217–223.
10. Qureshi AI, Suri MF, Ali Z, et al. Carotid angioplasty and stent placement: a prospective analysis of perioperative complications and impact of intravenously administered abciximab. *Neurosurgery* 2002;50:466–473.
11. Qureshi AI, Luft AR, Sharma M, et al. Prevention and treatment of thromboembolic and ischemic complications associated with endovascular procedures: Part II. Clinical aspects and recommendations. *Neurosurgery* 2000;46:1360–1375.
12. McCabe DJ, Brown MM, Clifton A. Fatal cerebral reperfusion hemorrhage after carotid stenting. *Stroke* 1999;30:2483–2486.
13. Qureshi AI, Luft AR, Sharma M, et al. Frequency and determinants of postprocedural hemodynamic instability after carotid angioplasty and stenting. *Stroke* 1999;30:2086–2093.
14. Dorros G. Complications associated with extracranial carotid artery interventions. *J Endovasc Surg* 1996;3:166–170.
15. Sullivan TM, Gray BH, Bacharach JM, et al. Angioplasty and primary stenting of the subclavian, innominate, and common carotid arteries in 83 patients. *J Vasc Surg* 1998;28:1059–1065.
16. Al-Mubarak N, Liu MW, Dean LS, et al. Immediate and late outcomes of subclavian artery stenting. *Catheter Cardiovasc Interv* 1999;46:169–172.
17. Gonzales A, Gil-Peralta A, Gonzales-Marcos JR, et al. Angioplasty and stenting for total symptomatic atherosclerotic occlusion of the subclavian or innominate arteries. *Cerebrovasc Dis* 2002;13:107–113.
18. Cognet F, Ben Salem D, Dranssart M, et al. Chronic mesenteric ischemia: imaging and percutaneous treatment. *Radiographics* 2002;22:863–879.
19. Matsumoto AH, Angle JF, Spinosa DJ, et al. Percutaneous transluminal angioplasty and stenting in the treatment of chronic mesenteric ischemia: results and long-term follow-up. *J Am Coll Surg* 2002;194[1 Suppl]:S22–S31.
20. Hamdan MA, Maheshwari S, Fahey JT, et al. Endovascular stents for coarctation of the aorta: initial results and intermediate-term follow-up. *J Am Coll Cardiol* 2001;38:1518–1523.
21. Nyman U, Uher P, Lindh M, et al. Primary stenting in infrarenal aortic occlusive disease. *Cardiovasc Intervent Radiol* 2000;23:97–108.
22. Nawaz S, Cleveland T, Gaines P, et al. Aortoiliac stenting, determinants of clinical outcome. *Eur J Vasc Endovasc Surg* 1999;17:351–359.
23. Naslund TC, Edwards Jr WH, Neuzil DF, et al. Technical complications of endovascular abdominal aortic aneurysm repair. *J Vasc Surg* 1997;26:502–509.
24. Sabeti S, Schillinger M, Mlekusch W, et al. Reduction in renal function after renal arteriography and after renal artery angioplasty. *Eur J Vasc Endovasc Surg* 2002;24:156–160.
25. Bush RL, Najibi S, MacDonald MJ, et al. Endovascular revascularization of renal artery stenosis: technical and clinical results. *J Vasc Surg* 2001;33:1041–1049.
26. Lim ST, Rosenfield K. Renal artery stent placement: indications and results. *Curr Interv Cardiol Rep* 2000;2:130–139.
27. Burket MW, Cooper CJ, Kennedy DJ, et al. Renal artery angioplasty and stent placement: predictors of favorable outcome. *Am Heart J* 2000;139[1 Pt 1]:64–71.
28. Novick AC. Complications during renal artery stent placement for atherosclerotic ostial stenosis. *J Urol* 1998;159:2245–2246.
29. Timaran CH, Stevens SL, Freeman MB, et al. Predictors of adverse outcome after iliac angioplasty and stenting for limb-threatening ischemia. *J Vasc Surg* 2002;36:507–513.
30. Scheinert D, Schroder M, Ludwig J, et al. Stent-supported recanalization of chronic iliac artery occlusions. *Am J Med* 2001;110:708–715.
31. Burns BJ, Phillips AJ, Fox A, et al. The timing and frequency of complications after peripheral percutaneous transluminal angioplasty and iliac stenting: is a change from inpatient to outpatient therapy feasible? *Cardiovasc Intervent Radiol* 2000;23:452–456.
32. Formichi M, Raybaud G, Benichou H, et al. Rupture of the external iliac artery during balloon angioplasty: endovascular treatment using a covered stent. *J Endovasc Surg* 1998;5:37–41.
33. Babalik E, Gulbaran M, Gurmen T, Ozturk S. Fracture of popliteal artery stents. *Circ J* 2003;67:643–645.
34. Werner GS, Ferrari M, Figulla HR. Superficial femoral artery rupture after balloon angioplasty: treatment with implantation of a balloon-expandable endovascular graft. *J Vasc Interv Radiol* 1999;10:1115–1117.
35. Hayes PD, Chokkalingam A, Jones R, et al. Arterial perforation during infrainguinal lower limb angioplasty does not worsen outcome: results from 1409 patients. *J Endovasc Ther* 2002;9:422–427.
36. Dorros G, Jaff MR, Dorros AM, et al. Tibioperoneal (outflow lesion) angioplasty can be used as primary treatment in 235 patients with critical limb ischemia: a five-year follow-up. *Circulation* 2001;104:2057–2062.
37. Dorros G, Lewin RF, Jamnadas P, et al. Below-the-knee angioplasty: tibioperoneal vessels, the acute outcome. *Catheter Cardiovasc Diagn* 1990;19:170–178.

CHAPTER 26

Renal Injury Following Contrast Agents

Peter A. McCullough

> **Key Points**
>
> - Renal dysfunction is accurately recognized by calculating the estimated glomerular filtration rate (eGFR) from the age, serum creatinine, gender, race, and weight of the patient, and not from the serum creatinine alone
> - Radiocontrast nephropathy and other major adverse cardiac events after angioplasty begin to occur at eGFR rates of less than 60 mL per minute per 1.73 m^2.
> - Beyond serum creatinine, chronic kidney disease is a unique vascular pathobiological state, which confers the highest cardiac event rates of any patient population and has, as a central feature, pathological intrarenal vasoconstriction in response to iodinated contrast
> - Radiocontrast nephropathy prevention can be achieved with (a) hydration to a target urine output of greater than 150 mL per hour for the first 6 hours after the procedure, (b) use of iodixanol as the preferred contrast agent, (c) limiting contrast volume to less than 100 mL, (d) spacing out second contrast procedures more than 10 days from each other, and (e) administering N-acetylcysteine 600 mg orally twice a day (two doses prior and two doses after contrast exposure).

THE CARDIORENAL INTERSECTION

The modern-day first-world epidemics of obesity and hypertension are central drivers of a secondary epidemic of combined chronic kidney disease (CKD) and cardiovascular disease (CVD) (1). Among those with diabetes for 25 years or more, the prevalence of diabetic nephropathy in type 1 and type 2 diabetes is 57% and 48%, respectively (2). Approximately half of all cases of end-stage renal disease (ESRD) are due to diabetic nephropathy, with most of these cases driven by obesity-related type 2 diabetes and hypertension. With the graying of America and cardiovascular care shifting toward the elderly, there is an imperative to understand why decreasing levels of renal dysfunction act as a major adverse prognostic factor after contrast exposure with or without peripheral or percutaneous coronary intervention (PCI). Acute renal failure, as the most proximal renal event, is predictable, and highlights an opportunity for preventive measures, which are outlined in this chapter.

CHRONIC KIDNEY DISEASE AND CARDIOVASCULAR RISK

Chronic kidney disease is defined through a range of estimated glomerular filtration rate (eGFR) values by the National Kidney Foundation Kidney Disease Outcomes Quality Initiative as depicted in Fig. 26.1 (3). Most studies of cardiovascular outcomes have found that a breakpoint for the development of radiocontrast nephropathy (RCN), later restenosis, recurrent myocardial infarction (MI), diastolic/systolic congestive heart failure (CHF), and cardiovascular death occurs below an eGFR of 60 mL per minute per 1.73 m^2, which roughly corresponds to a serum creatinine (Cr) of greater than 1.5 mg per dL in the general population (4–7). Because Cr is a crude indicator of renal function, and often underestimates renal dysfunction in women and the elderly, calculated measures of eGFR or creatinine clearance (CrCl) by the Cockroft–Gault equation or by the Modification of Diet in Renal Disease (MDRD) equations, now available on

Stages of Chronic Kidney Disease (CKD)

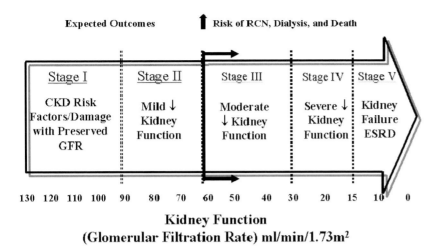

FIG. 26.1. The classification of chronic kidney disease (CKD) according to the National Kidney Foundation Kidney Disease Outcomes Quality Initiative. Increased rates of adverse events are generally seen below an estimated glomerular filtration rate of 60 mL/min/1.73 m². RCN, Radiocontrast nephropathy; GFR, glomerular filtration rate; ESRD, end-stage renal disease. (Adapted from National Kidney Foundation. Clinical practice guidelines for chronic kidney disease: evaluation, classification, and stratification. *Am J Kidney Dis* 2002;2[Suppl 1]: S46–S75, with permission.)

personal digital assistants, are the preferred methods of estimating renal function (3a). The following MDRD equation for CrCl is the preferred method because it does not rely on body weight (3):

$$CrCl = 186.3 * [serum\ creatinine^{-1.154}] * [age^{-0.203}]$$

Calculated values are multiplied by 0.742 for women and by 1.21 for African Americans.

In addition, microalbuminuria at any level of eGFR is considered to represent CKD, and has been thought to occur as the result of hyperfiltration in the kidneys due to diabetes and hypertension-related changes in the glomeruli (8). There have been several definitions developed for microalbuminuria (8). A simple definition for microalbuminuria is a random urine albumin/creatinine ratio (ACR) of 30 to 300 mg per g. An

ACR of greater than 300 mg per g is usually considered a marker of gross proteinuria. It is critical to understand that the risk of RCN is related in a curvilinear fashion to the eGFR, as shown in Fig. 26.2 (9). There are several leading explanations for why CKD is such a potent risk factor for adverse outcomes after cardiovascular events including RCN: (a) excess comorbidities in CKD patients including older age and diabetes, (b) underutilized end-organ protective strategies in CKD patients, or therapeutic nihilism, (c) excess toxicities from conventional therapies used including radiocontrast material and antithrombotics, and (d) the unique pathobiology of the CKD state, which includes intrarenal vasoconstriction when exposed to iodinated contrast agents (10).

SMALL RISES IN CREATININE ARE LINKED TO POOR LONG-TERM OUTCOMES

We and others have demonstrated that the overall risk of RCN, defined as a transient rise in Cr greater than 25% above the baseline occurs in approximately 13% of nondiabetics and 20% of diabetics undergoing PCI (Fig. 26.2) (11). Fortunately, RCN leading to dialysis is rare (0.5% to 2.0%); when it occurs, however, it is related to catastrophic outcomes, including a 36% in-hospital mortality rate, and a 2-year survival of only 19% (11). Transient increases in Cr are directly related to longer intensive care unit and hospital ward stays (3 and 4 more days, respectively) after bypass surgery (12). Recently, it has been shown that even transient rises in Cr translate into differences in adjusted long-term outcomes after PCI (Fig. 26.3) (13,14). What is going on in this population? The leading theory is that when renal function declines, the associated abnormal vascular pathobiology accelerates, and hence the progression of CVD events occurs at a higher rate. This raises the intriguing issue of end-organ protection (10).

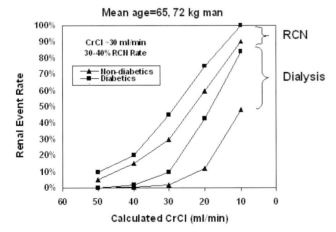

FIG. 26.2. Validated risk of acute renal failure requiring dialysis after diagnostic angiography and ad hoc angioplasty. This assumes a mean contrast dose of 250 mL and a mean age of 65 years. RCN, Radiocontrast nephropathy; CrCl, creatinine clearance. Data adapted from refs. 11 and 13.

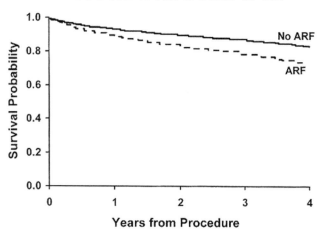

FIG. 26.3. Adjusted, long-term outcomes in 7,586 patients with and without acute renal failure after angioplasty ($p < 0.0001$). Acute renal failure is defined as a 0.5-mg/dL rise in serum creatinine after percutaneous coronary intervention. MI, Myocardial infarction; ARF, acute renal failure. (Adapted from Rihal CS, Textor SC, Grill DE, et al. Incidence and prognostic importance of acute renal failure after percutaneous coronary intervention. *Circulation* 2002;105:2259–2264, with permission.)

RATIONALE FOR RENAL END-ORGAN PROTECTION FOR INTERVENTION PATIENTS

End-organ protection for CKD patients at risk (eGFR less than 60 mL per minute per 1.73 m^2) can be thought of in three separate spheres: (a) long-term cardiorenal protection, (b) removal of renal toxins, and (c) prevention measures carried out before PCI. Long-term cardiorenal protection involves two important concepts: blood pressure control in CKD to a target of approximately 125/75 mm Hg (14), and use of an agent that blocks the renin–angiotensin system (RAS), such as an angiotensin-converting enzyme inhibitor (ACEI) or an angiotensin receptor blocker (ARB) as the base of therapy (15). Importantly, both agents cause a chronic rise in Cr greater than 25% above the baseline in cardiovascular patients (16). It has been shown that, despite the rise in Cr, there are large benefits to ACEI/ARB agents with respect to a reduction in new cases of ESRD, CHF, and cardiovascular death (17–23). It has been sufficiently demonstrated that these benefits extend to nondiabetics and to African Americans with CKD (22,23). Removal of toxins largely refers to the discontinuation of nonsteroidal antiinflammatory agents, aminoglycosides, and cyclosporin. These agents all complicate cardiovascular procedures and increase the risk of RCN. Prevention measures done prior to PCI include hydration, measures to reduce the direct cellular toxicity of the contrast, and, importantly, measures to reduce the intrarenal vasoconstriction that occurs uniquely in CKD patients when exposed to iodinated contrast (9). Based on the totality of evidence, if a patient can be carried through a cardiovascular procedure

(PCI or bypass surgery) without a rise in Cr, one can expect a shorter length of stay and improved long-term survival.

UNIQUE VASCULAR PATHOBIOLOGY IN CHRONIC KIDNEY DISEASE

Going beyond serum creatinine, as renal function declines, there are a host of abnormalities that develop including changes in coagulation, fibrinolysis, lipids, endothelial dysfunction, homocysteine, anemia, calcium/phosphorus balance, and many other factors that have been related to CVD (10). The leading hypotheses include chronic hyperactivation of the RAS leading to adverse cardiac remodeling, accelerated atherosclerosis, and symptomatic events (10). There is a growing body of evidence that erythropoietin deficiency and anemia are related to adverse ventricular remodeling and cardiac failure (24). Hyperhomocystinemia is an obvious therapeutic target for future trials in vascular disease given its predictable elevation in CKD, known association with adverse outcomes, and reduction with high doses of folic acid (25). Lastly, advanced atherosclerosis related to abnormal vascular calcification driven by an elevated calcium–phosphorous product (CPP) is an attractive hypothesis in ESRD, where recent studies suggest that not only is CPP related to coronary calcification, but that lowering of the CPP may reduce or stabilize the coronary calcification process (26). Importantly, the most acute short-term result of this vascular pathobiology is paradoxical intrarenal vasoconstriction and ischemic renal injury when exposed to iodinated contrast (9). This phenomenon is now a major therapeutic target for RCN prevention, as will be discussed.

PATHOPHYSIOLOGY OF RADIOCONTRAST NEPHROPATHY

There are three core elements in the pathophysiology of RCN: (a) direct toxicity of iodinated contrast to nephrons, (b) micro showers of atheroemboli to the kidneys, and (c) contrast- and atheroemboli-induced intrarenal vasoconstriction (27). Direct toxicity to nephrons with iodinated contrast has been demonstrated and appears to be related to the osmolality of the contrast (28). Hence, low-ionic or nonionic, and low-osmolar or isoosmolar, contrast agents have been shown to be less nephrotoxic *in vitro*. Micro showers of cholesterol emboli are thought to occur in about 50% of percutaneous interventions where a guiding catheter is passed through the aorta (29). Most of these showers are clinically silent. However, in approximately 1% of high-risk cases, an acute cholesterol emboli syndrome can develop manifested by acute renal failure, mesenteric ischemia, decreased microcirculation to the extremities, and, in some cases, embolic stroke. Because acute renal failure occurs after coronary artery bypass surgery with nearly the same risk predictors as in patients undergoing contrast procedures, it is thought that atheroembolism is a common pathogenic feature of both causes of renal failure (30). Finally, intrarenal vasoconstriction as a pathological vascular response to contrast media and, perhaps, as an organ response to cholesterol emboli is a final hypoxic/ischemic injury to the kidney during PCI (31). Hypoxia triggers activation of the renal sympathetic nervous system and results in a reduction in renal blood flow (31). It is important to note that there is disagreement concerning the direct vasoconstrictor or vasodilator effects of contrast agents in the kidney when given to animals (32,33). It is likely that in completely normal human renal blood vessels, contrast agents provoke a vasodilation and an osmotic diuresis. However, when there is vascular disease, endothelial dysfunction, and glomerular injury, contrast and the multifactorial insult of renal hypoxia provoke a vasoconstrictive response, and hence mediate in part an ischemic injury. The most important predictor of RCN is underlying renal dysfunction. The "remnant nephron" theory postulates that after sufficient chronic kidney damage has occurred and the eGFR is reduced to less than 60 mL per minute per 1.73 m^2, the remaining nephrons must pick up the remaining filtration load, have increased oxygen demands, and are more susceptible to ischemic and oxidative injury. Understanding the pathophysiology is key to devising a preventive strategy for RCN.

PREVENTION OF RADIOCONTRAST NEPHROPATHY

For patients with significant CKD, that is, a baseline eGFR of less than 60 mL per minute per 1.73 m^2, an RCN prevention strategy should be employed. In general, at an eGFR of 30 mL per minute per 1.73 m^2, the expected rate of RCN is 30% to 40%, and the rate of acute renal failure requiring dialysis is approximately 2% to 8% (Fig. 26.2) (9). There are four basic concepts in RCN prevention: (a) hydration, (b) choice and quantity of contrast, (c) pre-, intra-, and postprocedural end-organ protection with pharmacotherapy, and (d) postprocedural monitoring and expectant care.

Hydration with intravenous (IV) normal or one-half normal saline is reasonable starting 3 to 12 hours prior to the procedure at a rate of 1 to 2 mL per kg per hour (34–36). A simple IV rate to remember from clinical trials of hydration is 150 mL per hour. In those at risk, at least 300 to 500 mL of IV hydration should be received before contrast is administered. If there are any concerns regarding volume overload or heart failure, a right heart catheterization is strongly recommended for management during and after the case. A urine output of 150 mL per hour should be the target for hydration after the procedure. Importantly, if patients have more than a 150-mL per hour diuresis, they should have replacement of extra losses with more IV fluid. In general, this strategy calls for hydration orders of normal or one-half normal saline at 150 mL per hour for at least 6 hours after the procedure. When adequate urine flow rates were achieved in a clinical trial setting, there was a 50% reduction in the rate of RCN observed (36).

As discussed, the lower the ionicity and osmolality of the contrast agent, the less renal toxicity is expected. This has

now been confirmed in two large-scale, double-blind randomized controlled trials. In the Iohexol Cooperative Study, $n=1,196$, iohexol (Omnipaque) was found to be superior to high-ionic contrast (diatrizoate meglumine [Hypaque-76]) in patients with diabetes and baseline CKD (38). In the recently completed Nephrotoxicity in High-Risk Patients Study of Iso-Osmolar and Low-Osmolar Non-Ionic Contrast Media Study, iodixanol (Visipaque), a nonionic, isoosmolar contrast agent, was proven to be superior to iohexol, with lower rates of RCN observed (39). Iodixanol has also been demonstrated to be less thrombogenic than other contrast agents in the Randomized Trial of Contrast Media Utilization in High Risk PTCA with a 45% reduction in major adverse cardiac events compared to ioxaglate meglumine (Hexabrix); hence, iodixanol is the contrast agent of choice in patients at high renal risk undergoing intervention (40). Although it is desirable to limit contrast to the smallest volume possible in any setting, there is disagreement on a "safe" contrast limit (37). This is primarily due to the fact that the lower the eGFR, the smaller is the contrast needed to cause RCN. In general, it is desirable to limit contrast to less than 100 mL for any procedure (9,11). If staged procedures are planned, it is desirable to have more than 10 days between the first and second contrast exposures if RCN has occurred on the first contrast exposure (41).

There have been more than 35 randomized trials testing various strategies in the prevention of RCN (9). The majority of these trials were small and underpowered, and did not find the preventive strategy under investigation to be better than placebo. A few lessons have been learned from these trials: (a) Diuretics in the form of loop diuretics or mannitol can worsen RCN if there is inadequate volume replacement for the diuresis that follows; (b) low-dose or "renal dose" dopamine cannot be achieved despite its popularity in practice, given the counterbalancing forces of intrarenal vasodilation via the dopamine-1 receptor, and the vasoconstricting forces of the dopamine-2, alpha, and beta receptors, and (c) renal toxic agents including nonsteroidal antiinflammatory agents, aminoglycosides, and cyclosporin should not be administered in the periprocedural period. There are no approved agents for the prevention of RCN. The most popular strategy at the time of this writing is optimal hydration, iodixanol as the contrast agent of choice, and oral or intravenous N-acetylcysteine (NAC), a cytoprotective agent against oxidative injury. In brief, there is one supportive, double-blind randomized trial of fenoldopam versus placebo demonstrating improved renal blood flow after contrast exposure (42). A large confirmatory trial of fenoldopam in similar cases has been completed; unfortunately, no benefit was found with this agent (41). With NAC, there are now ten trials completed; five trials are positive and five trials are neutral, with an overall edge in favor of NAC (Table 26.1). Hence, there is almost complete equipoise on this agent. Most operators believe, given the seriousness of RCN as a complication, the relative safety of the strategies used, and the evolution of clinical trials shaping our practice, that the combination of hydration, use of iodixanol, and NAC is a reasonable three-pronged

TABLE 26.1. *Randomized, double-blind placebo controlled trials of N-acetylcysteine in the prevention of radiocontrast nephropathy[a, b]*

Study	Year	N	NAC dose	RCN definition	NAC RCN rate	Placebo RCN rate	p
Tepel (43)	2000	83	600 mg po bid	>0.5 mg/dL	1/41 (2.4)	9/42 (21.4)	0.01
Diaz-Sandoval (44)	2002	54	600 mg po bid (one dose pre-PCI)	>0.5 mg/dL or >25% rise	2/26 (8.0)	12/28 (45.0)	0.005
Shyu (45)	2002	121	400 mg po bid	>0.5 mg/dL	2/60 (3.3)	15/61 (24.6)	<0.0001
Kay (46)	2003	200	600 mg po bid	>25%	4/102 (3.9)	12/98 (12.2)	0.03
Durham (47)	2002	79	1,200 mg 1 hr pre- and 3 hr post-PCI	>0.5 mg/dL	10/38 (26.3)	9/41 (22.0)	>0.05
Briguori (48)	2002	183	600 mg po bid	>25%	6/92 (6.5)	10/91 (11.0)	0.22
Allaqaband (49)	2002	84	600 mg po bid	>0.5 mg/dL	8/45 (17.7)	6/39 (15.3)	0.92
Loutrianakis (50)	2003	47	600 mg po bid	>0.5 mg/dL or >25% rise	6/24 (25.0) 8/24 (33.3)	3/23 (13.0) 2/23 (8.7)	0.20 0.04
RAPPID (51)	2003	80	150 mg/kg over 30 min pre- and 50 mg/kg over 4 hr post-PCI	>0.5 mg/dL or >25% rise	2/41 (4.9)	8/39 (20.5)	0.05
Goldenberg (52)	2003	80	600 mg po tid	0.5 mg/dL	4/41 (9.8)	3/39 (7.7)	0.52
Total weighted proportions		1,011	Various	Various	45/510 (8.8)	85/501 (17.0)	0.00001

[a]Radiocontrast nephropathy (RCN) is defined as a rise in serum creatinine >25% from baseline or by an absolute >0.5-mg/dL increase from baseline prior to contrast exposure.
[b]NAC, N-acetylcysteine; po, orally; bid, twice daily; PCI, percutaneous coronary intervention; RAPPID, Rapid Protocol for the Prevention of Contrast-Induced Renal Dysfunction; tid, three times a day.

approach to minimize RCN and the risk of acute renal failure requiring dialysis.

Postprocedural monitoring is an issue in the modern era of shortstays and outpatient procedures. In general, high-risk patients in the hospital should have hydration started 12 hours before the procedure and continued at least 6 hours afterward. A serum creatinine should be measured 24 hours after the procedure. For outpatients, particularly those with eGFR

TABLE 26.2. *Ten-step checklist for radiocontrast nephropathy (RCN) risk stratification and prevention for patients at risk undergoing percutaneous coronary intervention (PCI)[a]*

1. Calculate eGFR (creatinine clearance)? High risk if <60 mL/min/1.73 m^2
2. Check diabetic status? Fivefold higher risk if diabetic
3. Discuss RCN risk in informed consent process
4. Discontinue NSAIDS and other renal toxic drugs
5. Nephrology consult for eGFR <15 mL/min for dialysis planning after PCI
6. Hydration NS or 1/2 NS 150 mL/hr 3 hr pre- and 6 hr postprocedure
7. Ensure urine flow rate >150 mL/hr after PCI
8. Iodixanol preferred contrast agent
9. Limit contrast volume to <100 mL
10. NAC 600 mg in 30 cc of ginger ale, two doses orally bid before and two doses orally bid after PCI

[a]eGFR, Estimated glomerular filtration rate; NSAIDS, nonsteroidal antiinflammatory agents; NS, normal saline; NAC, N-acetylcysteine.

of less than 60 mL per hour, either an overnight stay or discharge to home with 48-hour follow-up and creatinine measurement is advised. It has been demonstrated that those individuals who develop severe RCN have a rise of Cr greater than 0.5 mg per dL in the first 24 hours after the procedure. Hence, for those who have not had this degree of Cr elevation, and otherwise have had uneventful courses, discharge to home may be considered.

In summary, for RCN risk assessment and prevention, the items in Table 26.2 are advised. It is important that in the consent process RCN risks are discussed. For those with eGFR less than 30 mL per minute per 1.73 m^2, the possibility of dialysis should be mentioned. In those with eGFR less than 15 mL per minute per 1.73 m^2, nephrology consultation is advised with possible planning for dialysis after the procedure.

CONCLUSION

Chronic kidney disease is the most important factor in predicting adverse short- and long-term outcomes after PCI. Hence, the rationale for renal end-organ protection is based on chronic renal protection, avoidance of additive renal insults, and a comprehensive RCN prophylaxis. The pathogenesis of RCN goes beyond serum Cr and involves a unique vascular pathobiology, which interrelates both the renal and CVD outcomes. Through intense and systematic study of these unique mechanisms, new diagnostic and therapeutic targets will be discovered, which will enhance the cardiac care of patients with CKD, and, it is hoped, reduce the elevated risks and adverse outcomes associated with RCN.

REFERENCES

1. Lewis CE, Jacobs Jr DR, McCreath H, et al. Weight gain continues in the 1990s: 10-year trends in weight and overweight from the CARDIA study. Coronary Artery Risk Development in Young Adults. *Am J Epidemiol* 2000;151:1172–1181.
2. Bakris GL, Williams M, Dworkin L, et al. Preserving renal function in adults with hypertension and diabetes: a consensus approach. National Kidney Foundation Hypertension and Diabetes Executive Committees Working Group. *Am J Kidney Dis* 2000;36:646–661.
3. National Kidney Foundation. Clinical practice guidelines for chronic kidney disease: evaluation, classification, and stratification. *Am J Kidney Dis* 2002;2[Suppl 1]:S46–S75.
3a. MedRules. Clinical prediction rules for palm OS handhelds. Available at http//pbrain.hypermart.net/medrules.html
4. McCullough PA, Soman SS, Shah SS, et al. Risks associated with renal dysfunction in patients in the coronary care unit. *J Am Coll Cardiol* 2000;36:679–684.
5. Beattie JN, Soman SS, Sandberg KR, et al. Determinants of mortality after myocardial infarction in patients with advanced renal dysfunction. *Am J Kidney Dis* 2001;37:1191–2000.
6. Chertow GM, Lazarus JM, Christiansen CL, et al. Preoperative renal risk stratification. *Circulation* 1997;95:878–884.
7. Szczech LA, Best PJ, Crowley E, et al. Bypass Angioplasty Revascularization Investigation (BARI) Investigators. Outcomes of patients with chronic renal insufficiency in the bypass angioplasty revascularization investigation. *Circulation* 2002;105:2253–2258.
8. Keane WF, Eknoyan G. Proteinuria, albuminuria, risk, assessment, detection, elimination (PARADE): a position paper of the National Kidney Foundation. *Am J Kidney Dis* 1999;33:1004–1010.
9. McCullough PA, Manley HJ. Prediction and prevention of contrast nephropathy. *J Interv Cardiol* 2001;14:547–558.
10. McCullough PA. Cardiorenal risk: an important clinical intersection. *Rev Cardiovasc Med* 2002;3:71–76.
11. McCullough PA, Wolyn R, Rocher LL, et al. Acute renal failure after coronary intervention: incidence, risk factors, and relationship to mortality. *Am J Med* 1997;103:368–375.
12. Mangano CM, Diamondstone LS, Ramsay JG, et al. Renal dysfunction after myocardial revascularization: risk factors, adverse outcomes, and hospital resource utilization. The Multicenter Study of Perioperative Ischemia Research Group. *Ann Intern Med* 1998;128:194–203.
13. Rihal CS, Textor SC, Grill DE, et al. Incidence and prognostic importance of acute renal failure after percutaneous coronary intervention. *Circulation* 2002;105:2259–2264.
14. The sixth report of the Joint National Committee on prevention, detection, evaluation, and treatment of high blood pressure. *Arch Intern Med* 1997;157:2413–2446.
15. Garg J, Bakris GL. Angiotensin converting enzyme inhibitors or angiotensin receptor blockers in nephropathy from type 2 diabetes. *Curr Hypertens Rep* 2002;4:185–190.
16. Pitt B, Segal R, Martinez FA, et al. Randomised trial of losartan versus captopril in patients over 65 with heart failure (Evaluation of Losartan in the Elderly Study, ELITE). *Lancet* 1997;349:747–752.
17. Toto R. Angiotensin II subtype 1 receptor blockers and renal function. *Arch Intern Med* 2001;161:1492–1499.
18. Brenner BM, Cooper ME, de Zeeuw D, et al. Effects of losartan on renal and cardiovascular outcomes in patients with type 2 diabetes and nephropathy. *N Engl J Med* 2001;345:861–869.
19. Lewis EJ, Hunsicker LG, Clarke WR, et al. Renoprotective effect of the angiotensin-receptor antagonist irbesartan in patients with nephropathy due to type 2 diabetes. Renoprotective effect of the angiotensin-receptor antagonist irbesartan in patients with nephropathy due to type 2 diabetes. *N Engl J Med* 2001;345:851–860.
20. Parving HH, Lehnert H, Brochner-Mortensen J, et al. The effect of irbesartan on the development of diabetic nephropathy in patients with type 2 diabetes. *N Engl J Med* 2001;345:870–878.
21. Dahlof B, Devereux RB, Kjeldsen SE. Cardiovascular morbidity and mortality in the Losartan Intervention For Endpoint reduction in hypertension study (LIFE): a randomised trial against atenolol. *Lancet* 2002 23;359:995–1003.
22. Mann JF, Gerstein HC, Pogue J, et al. Renal insufficiency as a predictor of cardiovascular outcomes and the impact of ramipril: the HOPE randomized trial. *Ann Intern Med* 2001;134:629–636.
23. Agodoa LY, Appel L, Bakris GL, et al. Effect of ramipril vs amlodipine on renal outcomes in hypertensive nephrosclerosis: a randomized controlled trial. *JAMA* 2001;285:2719–2728.
24. Silverberg DS, Wexler D, Sheps D, et al. The effect of correction of mild anemia in severe, resistant congestive heart failure using subcutaneous erythropoietin and intravenous iron: a randomized controlled study. *J Am Coll Cardiol* 2001;37:1775–1780.
25. Friedman AN, Bostom AG, Selhub J, et al. The kidney and homocysteine metabolism. *J Am Soc Nephrol* 2001;12:2181–2189.
26. Chertow GM, Burke SK, Raggi P, et al. Sevelamer attenuates the progression of coronary and aortic calcification in hemodialysis patients. *Kidney Int* 2002;62:245–252.
27. Margulies K, Schirger J, Burnett Jr J. Radiocontrast-induced nephropathy: current status and future prospects. *Int Angiol* 1992;11:20–25.
28. Andersen KJ, Christensen EI, Vik H. Effects of iodinated x-ray contrast media on renal epithelial cells in culture. *Invest Radiol* 1994;29:955–962.
29. Keeley EC, Grines CL. Scraping of aortic debris by coronary guiding catheters: a prospective evaluation of 1,000 cases. *J Am Coll Cardiol* 1998;32:1861–1865.
30. Chertow GM, Lazarus JM, Christiansen CL, et al. Preoperative renal risk stratification. *Circulation* 1997;95:878–884.
31. Denton KM, Shweta A, Anderson WP. Preglomerular and postglomerular resistance responses to different levels of sympathetic activation by hypoxia. *J Am Soc Nephrol* 2002;13:27–34.
32. Uder M, Humke U, Pahl M, et al. Nonionic contrast media iohexol and iomeprol decrease renal arterial tone: comparative studies on human and porcine isolated vascular segments. *Invest Radiol* 2002;37:440–447.
33. Rauch D, Drescher P, Pereira FJ, et al. Comparison of iodinated contrast media-induced renal vasoconstriction in human, rabbit, dog, and pig arteries. *Invest Radiol* 1997;32:315–319.
34. Mueller C, Buerkle G, Buettner HJ, et al. Prevention of contrast media-associated nephropathy: randomized comparison of 2 hydration regimens in 1620 patients undergoing coronary angioplasty. *Arch Intern Med* 2002;162:329–336.
35. Solomon R, Werner C, Mann D, et al. Effects of saline, mannitol, and furosemide to prevent acute decreases in renal function induced by radiocontrast agents. *N Engl J Med* 1994;331:1416–1420.
36. Stevens MA, McCullough PA, Tobin KJ, et al. A prospective randomized trial of prevention measures in patients at high risk for contrast nephropathy: results of the P.R.I.N.C.E. Study. Prevention of Radiocontrast Induced Nephropathy Clinical Evaluation. *J Am Coll Cardiol* 1999;33:403–411.
37. Manske CL, Sprafka JM, Strony JT, et al. Contrast nephropathy in azotemic diabetic patients undergoing coronary angiography. *Am J Med* 1990;89:615–620.
38. Rudnick MR, Goldfarb S, Wexler L, et al. Nephrotoxicity of ionic and nonionic contrast media in 1196 patients: a randomized trial. The Iohexol Cooperative Study. *Kidney Int* 1995;47:254–261.
39. Aspelin P, Aubry P, Fransson SG, et al. Nephrotoxicity in High-Risk Patients Study of Iso-Osmolar and Low-Osmolar Non-Ionic Contrast Media Study Investigators. Nephrotoxic effects in high-risk patients undergoing angiography. *N Engl J Med* 2003;348:491–499.
40. Davidson CJ, Laskey WK, Hermiller JB, et al. Randomized trial of contrast media utilization in high-risk PTCA: the COURT trial. *Circulation* 2000;101:2172–2177.
41. Stone GW, Tumlin JA, Madyoon H, et al. Design and rationale of CONTRAST—a prospective, randomized, placebo-controlled trial of fenoldopam mesylate for the prevention of radiocontrast nephropathy. *Rev Cardiovasc Med* 2001;2 [Suppl 1]:S31–S36.
42. Tumlin JA, Wang A, Murray PT, et al. Fenoldopam mesylate blocks reductions in renal plasma flow after radiocontrast dye infusion: a pilot trial in the prevention of contrast nephropathy. *Am Heart J* 2002;143:894–903.
43. Tepel M, van der Giet M, Schwarzfeld C, et al. Prevention of radiographic-contrast-agent-induced reductions in renal function by acetylcysteine. *N Engl J Med* 2000;20;343:180–184.

44. Diaz-Sandoval LJ, Kosowsky BD, Losordo DW. Acetylcysteine to prevent angiography-related renal tissue injury (the APART trial). *Am J Cardiol* 2002;89:356–358.

45. Shyu KG, Cheng JJ, Kuan P. Acetylcysteine protects against acute renal damage in patients with abnormal renal function undergoing a coronary procedure. *J Am Coll Cardiol* 2002;16;40:1383–1388.

46. Kay J, Chow WH, Chan TM, et al. Acetylcysteine for prevention of acute deterioration of renal function following elective coronary angiography and intervention: a randomized controlled trial. *JAMA* 2003;289:553–558.

47. Durham JD, Caputo C, Dokko J, et al. A randomized controlled trial of N-acetylcysteine to prevent contrast nephropathy in cardiac angiography. *Kidney Int* 2002;62:2202–2207.

48. Briguori C, Manganelli F, Scarpato P, et al. Acetylcysteine and contrast agent-associated nephrotoxicity. *J Am Coll Cardiol* 2002;40:298–303.

49. Allaqaband S, Tumuluri R, Malik AM, et al. Prospective randomized study of N-acetylcysteine, fenoldopam, and saline for prevention of radiocontrast-induced nephropathy. *Catheter Cardiovasc Interv* 2002;57:279–283.

50. Loutrianakis E, Stella D, Hussain A, et al. Randomized comparison of fenoldopam and N-acetylcysteine to saline in the prevention of radio-contrast nephropathy. *J Am Coll Cardiol* 2003;41:327A.

51. Baker CS, Wragg A, Kumar S, et al. A rapid protocol for the prevention of contrast-induced renal dysfunction (RAPPID Study). *J Am Coll Cardiol* 2003;41:39A.

52. Goldenberg I, Jonas M, Matetzki S, et al. Contrast-associated nephropathy and clinical outcome of patients with chronic renal insufficiency undergoing cardiac catheterization: lack of additive benefit of acetylcysteine to saline infusion. *J Am Coll Cardiol* 2003;41:537A.

CHAPTER 27

Pre- and Postoperative Management of Cardiovascular Diseases and Risks in Patients with Peripheral Vascular Disease

Debabrata Mukherjee and Kim A. Eagle

Key Points

- Patients with peripheral vascular disease often have coexistent coronary artery disease, and those who require vascular surgery appear to have a significantly increased risk for cardiac complications.
- The urgency of noncardiac surgery should be determined. In many cases, patient or surgery-specific factors dictate immediate surgery, which may not allow further cardiac assessment or treatment. Perioperative medical management, surveillance, and postoperative risk stratification is appropriate in these cases.
- Patients with coronary artery bypass grafting in the last 5 years or percutaneous coronary intervention from 6 months to 5 years previously and who are free of clinical evidence of ischemia may generally have surgery without further testing, particularly if they are functionally very active.
- Patients with favorable invasive/noninvasive testing in the last 2 years need no further cardiac work-up if they have been asymptomatic since the test and are functionally very active.
- Patients with unstable coronary syndrome, decompensated heart failure, significant arrhythmias, or severe valvular heart disease scheduled for elective noncardiac surgery should have surgery canceled or delayed until the cardiac problem has been clarified and treated.
- Patients with one or more intermediate clinical predictors of cardiac risk and moderate or excellent functional capacity can generally undergo low- or intermediate-risk surgery with low event rates.
- Poor functional capacity or a combination of high-risk surgery and moderate functional capacity in a patient with intermediate clinical predictors of cardiac risk (especially if there are two or more) often requires further noninvasive cardiac testing.
- Patients with minor or no clinical predictors or risk and moderate or excellent functional capacity can safely undergo noncardiac surgery.
- Results of noninvasive testing can be used to define further management including intensified medical therapy, proceeding directly with surgery, or cardiac catheterization. Cardiac catheterization may lead to coronary revascularization and is especially appropriate if it significantly improves the patient's long-term prognosis.
- In the absence of contraindications, beta-blocker therapy should be given to all patients at high risk for coronary events who are scheduled to undergo noncardiac surgery.

INTRODUCTION

The prevalence of cardiovascular disease is increasing in the United States (1), and the number of noncardiac surgical procedures performed is also increasing. Atherosclerosis is a generalized process, and patients with peripheral vascular disease often have coexistent coronary artery disease (CAD). Ashton et al. (2) and others have shown that patients who require vascular surgery appear to have an increased risk for cardiac complications because many of the risk factors contributing to peripheral vascular disease (e.g., diabetes mellitus, tobacco use, hyperlipidemia) are also risk factors for CAD. The usual symptoms of CAD in these patients may be obscured by exercise limitations due to advanced age or intermittent claudication. Another factor leading to increased complications with vascular surgery is that major arterial operations are time-consuming and may be associated with substantial fluctuations in extravascular fluid volumes, cardiac filling pressures, systemic blood pressure, heart rate, and thrombogenicity (3). Preoperative risk assessment is an important step in reducing perioperative morbidity and mortality in this high-risk group. A few basic questions regarding general health, functional capacity, cardiac risk factors, co-morbid conditions, and type of operation can assist in evaluating risk. Good communication among physicians, anesthesiologists, and surgeons is crucial to minimizing risk.

Cardiac complications account for 50% to 65% of the morbidity and mortality seen after vascular surgery, and appropriate preoperative measures may significantly reduce risk. In a selective review of several thousand vascular surgical procedures (carotid endarterectomy, aortic aneurysm resection, and lower extremity revascularization) reported in the literature from 1970 to 1987, Hertzer found that cardiac complications were responsible for about half of all perioperative deaths, and that fatal events were nearly five times more likely to occur in the presence of standard preoperative indicators of CAD (4). Furthermore, the late (5-year) mortality rate for patients who were suspected to have CAD was twice that for patients who were not (approximately 40% vs. 20%).

OBJECTIVE

The purpose of preoperative evaluation is not to clear patients for surgery, but to assess medical status and cardiac risks posed by the surgery planned, and recommend strategies to reduce risk. Evaluation must be tailored to the circumstances that have prompted the consultation and the nature of the surgical illness. This might also be the opportunity to affect long-term treatment of a patient with significant CAD. The overall goals of the preoperative evaluation in patients with peripheral vascular disease are the same as those with any other patient, with the added caveat that these patients, by definition, are presenting with vascular disease, which has a strong association with coronary artery disease. A complete perioperative assessment in these patients includes history, physical examination, and appropriate laboratory tests.

CLINICAL EVALUATION

The history and physical examination should be focused on identification of cardiac risk factors and current cardiac status. The goal is to identify cardiac conditions such as recent myocardial infarction (MI), decompensated heart failure (HF), unstable angina, significant arrhythmias, and valvular heart disease. One should also identify serious comorbid conditions such as diabetes, stroke, renal insufficiency, and pulmonary disease, as these illnesses also affect periprocedural outcomes. The history should elicit functional capacity (the ability to climb stairs, do one's own housework, etc.). An individual's functional capacity (Table 27.1) has significant short-term and long-term prognostic implications. However, claudication in patients with peripheral vascular disease may make it difficult to assess the individual's functional capacity.

The physical examination should include general appearance (cyanosis, pallor, dyspnea during conversation/minimal activity, Cheyne–Stokes respiration, poor nutritional status, obesity, skeletal deformities, tremor, and anxiety), blood pressure in arms, carotid pulses, extremity pulses, and ankle–brachial indices. Jugular venous pressure and positive hepatojugular reflex are reliable signs of hypervolemia in chronic HF, and pulmonary rales and chest x-ray evidence of pulmonary congestion correlate better with acute HF.

TABLE 27.1. *Assessment of functional capacity and estimated energy requirements for various activities*[a]

1 MET
  Eat, dress, use the toilet
  Walk indoors around the house
  Walk on level ground at 2 mph
  Light housework such as washing dishes
4 METs
  Climb a flight of stairs
  Walk on level ground at 4 mph
  Run short distance
  Use a vacuum cleaner or lift heavy furniture
  Play golf or doubles tennis
>10 METs
  Swimming
  Singles tennis
  Basketball
  Skiing

[a]MET, Metabolic equivalent.
Modified from Eagle KA, Brundage BH, Chaitman BR, et al. Guidelines for perioperative cardiovascular evaluation for noncardiac surgery. Report of the American College of Cardiology/American Heart Association Task Force on Practice Guidelines. Committee on Perioperative Cardiovascular Evaluation for Noncardiac Surgery. *Circulation* 1996;93:1278–1317; and Eagle KA, Berger PB, Calkins H, et al. ACC/AHA guideline update for perioperative cardiovascular evaluation for noncardiac surgery-executive summary. A report of the American College of Cardiology/American Heart Association Task Force on Practice Guidelines (Committee to Update the 1996 Guidelines on Perioperative Cardiovascular Evaluation for Noncardiac Surgery). *J Am Coll Cardiol* 2002;39:542–553; with permission.

TABLE 27.2. *Clinical predictors of increased perioperative cardiovascular risk*

Major predictors
    Acute or recent myocardial infarction[a] with evidence of ischemia based on symptoms or noninvasive testing
    Unstable or severe[b] angina (Canadian class III or IV)[c]
    Decompensated heart failure
    High-grade atrioventricular block
    Symptomatic ventricular arrhythmias with underlying heart disease
    Supraventricular arrhythmias with uncontrolled ventricular rate
    Severe valvular heart disease
Intermediate predictors
    Mild angina pectoris (class 1 or 2)
    Prior myocardial infarction by history or Q waves
    Compensated or prior heart failure
    Diabetes mellitus (particularly insulin dependent)
    Renal insufficiency (creatinine ≥ 2.0 mg/dL)
Minor predictors
    Advanced age
    Abnormal electrocardiogram (left ventricular hypertrophy, left bundle-branch block, ST–T abnormalities)
    Rhythm other than sinus (e.g., atrial fibrillation)
    Low functional capacity (inability to climb one flight of stairs with a bag of groceries)
    History of stroke
    Uncontrolled systemic hypertension

[a]Recent myocardial infarction is defined as >7 days but ≤ 1 month; acute myocardial infarction is within 7 days.
[b]May include stable angina in patients who are usually sedentary.
[c]See ref. 42.
Adapted from Eagle KA, Berger PB, Calkins H, et al. ACC/AHA guideline update for perioperative cardiovascular evaluation for noncardiac surgery-executive summary. A report of the American College of Cardiology/American Heart Association Task Force on Practice Guidelines (Committee to Update the 1996 Guidelines on Perioperative Cardiovascular Evaluation for Noncardiac Surgery). *J Am Coll Cardiol* 2002;39:542–553, with permission.

Auscultation for cardiac rhythm and heart sounds (murmurs, gallops) and abdominal examination for aneurysm should also be performed. The physical exam can also alert the team to the presence of a pacemaker or implantable defibrillator. Patients with a significant aortic stenosis murmur, elevated jugular venous pressure, pulmonary edema, and/or a third heart sound are at high surgical risk. Clinical predictors of increased perioperative cardiovascular risk are summarized in Table 27.2.

Although individual clinical factors and risk indices are an important part of the evaluation of patients, clinical evidence of coronary artery disease may be obscured in patients with peripheral vascular disease. Thus, risk classifications based exclusively on clinical criteria may not prove to be as helpful when applied to patients with peripheral vascular disease as compared to a general population. Figure 27.1 demonstrates a stepwise approach to cardiac risk assessment prior to noncardiac surgery.

TYPE OF SURGERY

The type of surgery has significant implications for perioperative risk. Table 27.3 categorizes surgery into high, intermediate, and low risk. Patients undergoing major vascular surgery constitute a particular challenge (i.e., high-risk operations in a patient population with a high prevalence of significant CAD). Several studies have attempted to stratify the incidence of perioperative and intermediate-term outcomes according to the type of vascular surgery performed. In a prospective series of 53 aortic procedures and 87 infrainguinal bypass grafts for which operative mortality rates were nearly identical (9% and 7%, respectively), Krupski et al. found that the risk for fatal/nonfatal MI within a 2-year follow-up period was 3.5 times higher (21% vs. 6%) among patients who received infrainguinal bypass grafts (5). This difference probably is related to the fact that diabetes mellitus (44% vs. 11%) and a history of previous MI (43% vs. 28%), angina (36% vs. 15%), or HF (29% vs. 9%) all were significantly more prevalent in the infrainguinal bypass group. Fleisher et al. analyzed a 5% sample of Medicare claims from 1992 to 1993 of patients undergoing major vascular surgery (6). A total cohort of 2,865 individuals underwent aortic surgery, with a 7.3% 30-day mortality rate and an 11.3% 1-year mortality rate. A total cohort of 4,030 individuals underwent infrainguinal surgery, with a 5.8% 30-day mortality rate and a 16.3% 1-year mortality rate. This work further confirms that aortic and infrainguinal surgery continues to be associated with high 30-day and 1-year mortality, with aortic surgery being associated with the highest short-term and infrainguinal surgery being associated with the highest long-term mortality rates (6). L'Italien et al. presented comparable data regarding the perioperative incidence of fatal/nonfatal MI and the 4-year event-free survival rate after 321 aortic procedures, 177 infrainguinal bypass grafts, and 49 carotid endarterectomies (7). Slight differences in the overall incidence of MI among the three surgical groups, which may have been related to the prevalence of diabetes mellitus, were exceeded almost entirely in significance by the influence of discrete cardiac risk factors (previous MI, angina, HF, fixed or reversible thallium defects, and ST–T depression during stress testing) (7). These and other studies (8) suggest that the clinical evidence of CAD in a patient who has peripheral vascular disease appears to be a better predictor of subsequent cardiac events than the particular type of peripheral vascular operation to be performed.

CRITERIA FOR ESTIMATING RISK

Several criteria, including the Goldman criteria (9), the Detsky criteria (10), the Eagle criteria (11), and the Lee criteria (12), have been developed to estimate periprocedural cardiovascular risk. The Goldman criteria use nine variables that independently predict perioperative risk with point value assigned to each based on outcomes in a general surgical population (9). The Detsky criteria (10) are a modification of the

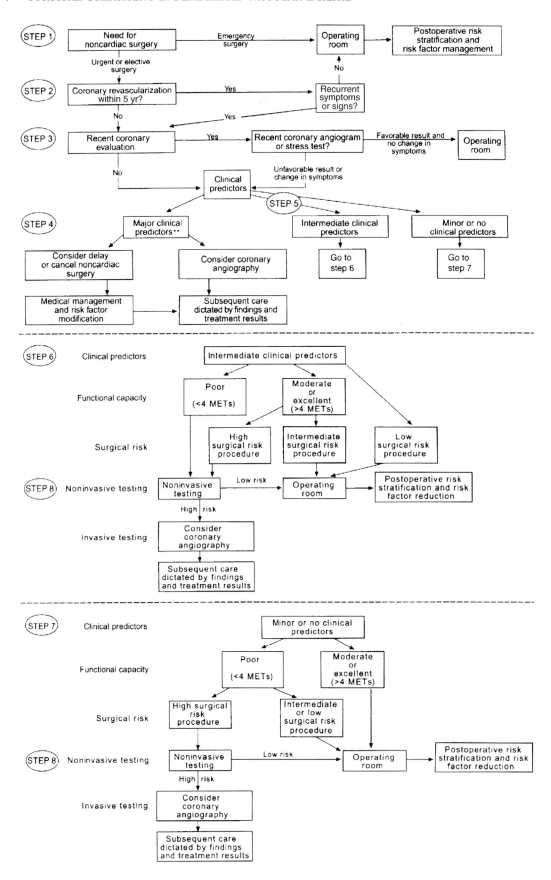

TABLE 27.3. *Cardiac risk stratification for different types of surgical procedures*

High risk (reported cardiac risk[a] >5%)
   Emergency major operations, particularly in the elderly
   Aortic, major vascular, and peripheral vascular surgery
   Extensive operations with large volume shifts/and or blood loss
Intermediate risk (reported cardiac risk <5%)
   Intraperitoneal and intrathoracic
   Carotid endarterectomy
   Head and neck surgery
   Orthopedic
   Prostate
Low risk[b] (reported cardiac risk <1%)
   Endoscopic procedures
   Superficial biopsy
   Cataract
   Breast surgery

[a]Combined incidence of cardiac death and nonfatal myocardial infarction.
[b]Do not generally require further preoperative cardiac testing.
Adapted from Eagle KA, Berger PB, Calkins H, et al. ACC/AHA guideline update for perioperative cardiovascular evaluation for noncardiac surgery-executive summary. A report of the American College of Cardiology/American Heart Association Task Force on Practice Guidelines (Committee to Update the 1996 Guidelines on Perioperative Cardiovascular Evaluation for Noncardiac Surgery). *J Am Coll Cardiol* 2002;39:542–553, with permission.

TABLE 27.4. *Lee criteria for prediction of cardiac risk of major noncardiac surgery*

High-risk surgery
Ischemic heart disease
History of heart failure
History of cerebrovascular disease
Insulin therapy for diabetes
Serum creatinine ≥2.0 mg/dL
Cardiac risk is related to the number of risk factors:
   No factors, >0.4% complications
   One factor, >0.9% complications
   Two factors, >7% complications
   Three or more factors, >11% complications

Adapted from Lee TH, Marcantonio ER, Mangione CM, et al. Derivation and prospective validation of a simple index for prediction of cardiac risk of major noncardiac surgery. *Circulation* 1999;100:1043–1049, with permission.

Goldman criteria to address the severity of coronary artery disease and heart failure in a general surgical population. The Lee criteria use six variables that independently predict perioperative risk in a general surgical population (Table 27.4 and Fig. 27.2) (12). The Eagle criteria (11) use clinical markers and stress imaging results to stratify risk in patients undergoing vascular surgery and are thus more applicable to patients with peripheral vascular disease (Table 27.5).

DIAGNOSTIC TESTING

Routine laboratory tests such as serum creatinine, hemoglobin, platelets, potassium, liver profile, and oxygen saturation are important in risk stratification. Arterial blood gas analysis is useful in patients with advanced pulmonary disease. A 12-lead electrocardiogram (ECG) provides important prognostic information. Patients who are at low risk based on history, physical examination, and routine laboratory tests may need no further evaluation. Noninvasive testing is useful in intermediate-risk patients. The preoperative guidelines are fairly straightforward about recommendations for patients about to undergo emergency surgery, the presence of prior cardiac revascularization, and the occurrence of major cardiac predictors. However, the majority of patients have either intermediate or minor clinical predictors of increased perioperative cardiovascular risk. Table 27.6 presents a short-cut approach to a large number of patients in whom the decision to recommend testing before surgery can be difficult. Essentially, if two of the three listed factors in Table 27.6 are true, the guidelines recommend consideration of the use of noninvasive cardiac testing as part of the preoperative evaluation. In any patient with an intermediate clinical predictor, the presence of either a low functional capacity or a high surgical risk should lead the physician to consider noninvasive testing. In the absence of intermediate clinical predictors, noninvasive testing should be considered when both the surgical risk is high and the functional capacity is low. Clinical predictors are defined in Table 27.2.

FIG. 27.1. Stepwise approach to preoperative cardiac assessment. MET, Metabolic equivalent. Major clinical predictors: unstable coronary syndromes, decompensated congestive heart failure, significant arrhythmias, severe valvular disease. Intermediate clinical predictors: mild angina pectoris, prior myocardial infarction, compensated or prior congestive heart failure, diabetes mellitus, renal insufficiency. Minor clinical predictors: advanced age, abnormal electrocardiogram, rhythm other than sinus, low functional capacity, history of stroke, uncontrolled systemic hypertension. (Adapted from Eagle KA, Brundage BH, Chaitman BR, et al. Guidelines for perioperative cardiovascular evaluation for noncardiac surgery. Report of the American College of Cardiology/American Heart Association Task Force on Practice Guidelines. Committee on Perioperative Cardiovascular Evaluation for Noncardiac Surgery. *Circulation* 1996;93:1278–1317; and Eagle KA, Berger PB, Calkins H, et al. ACC/AHA guidelines update for perioperative cardiovascular evaluation for noncardiac surgery-executive summary. A report of the American College of Cardiology/American Heart Association Task Force on Practice Guidelines (Committee to Update the 1996 Guidelines on Perioperative Cardiovascular Evaluation for Noncardiac Surgery). *J Am Coll Cardiol* 2002;39:542–553; with permission.)

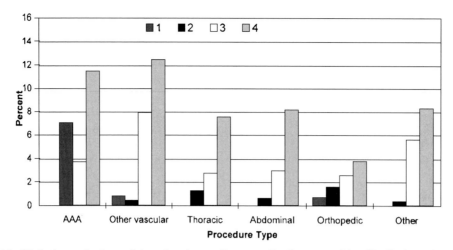

FIG. 27.2. Six independent correlates of major cardiac complications were identified in the cohort. These variables included high-risk type of surgery, ischemic heart disease, congestive heart failure, history of cerebrovascular disease, insulin therapy for diabetes, and preoperative serum creatinine >2.0 mg/dL. Patients with no, one, two, or more factors were assigned to classes I, II, III, or IV, respectively. Bars represent rate of major cardiac complications for patients in Revised Cardiac Risk Index classes according to type of procedure performed. AAA, Abdominal aortic aneurysm. Note that, by definition, patients undergoing AAA, thoracic, and abdominal procedures were excluded from class I. In all subsets except patients undergoing AAA, there was a statistically significant trend toward greater risk with higher risk class. (Adapted from Lee TH, Marcantio ER, Mangione CM, et al. Derivation and prospective validation of a simple index for prediction of cardiac risk of major noncardiac surgery. *Circulation* 1999;100:1043–1049, with permission.)

TABLE 27.5. *Cardiac risk stratification using clinical markers and perfusion imaging for patients undergoing vascular surgery*[a]

Clinical predictors
  Age >70 years
  Q-waves on an electrocardiogram
  Diabetes mellitus
  Ventricular arrhythmias necessitating treatment
  History of angina or congestive heart failure

Dipyridamole thallium
  Without thallium redistribution
  With thallium redistribution

Three or more risk factors, >50% rate of complications
One to three risk factors with abnormal thallium, >30% rate of complications
One to three risk factors with normal thallium, >3.2% rate of complications
No risk factors, >3.1% rate of complications

Patients with one or two clinical predictors and without thallium redistribution, 3.2% rate of complications (95% CI-0%–8%)
Patients with one or two clinical predictors and with thallium redistribution, 29.6% rate of complications (95% CI-16%–44%)

[a]CI, Confidence interval.
Adapted from Eagle KA, Coley CM, Newell JB, et al. Combining clinical and thallium data optimizes preoperative assessment of cardiac risk before major vascular surgery. *Ann Intern Med* 1989;110:859–866, with permission.

In most ambulatory patients, the test of choice is exercise ECG testing, which can provide an estimate of both functional capacity and detect myocardial ischemia through changes in the ECG and hemodynamic response. The ability to exercise moderately beyond 4 to 5 metabolic equivalents (METs) without symptoms defines low risk. Patients who can achieve greater than 85% of maximum predicted heart rate without ECG changes are at lowest risk. Patients with an abnormal ECG response at greater than 70% of predicted

TABLE 27.6. *Guide to noninvasive testing in preoperative patients if any two factors are present*

1. Intermediate clinical predictors (Canadian class I or II angina, prior myocardial infarction based on history or pathological Q waves, compensated or prior heart failure, or diabetes)
2. Poor functional capacity (<4 metabolic equivalents)
3. High-surgical-risk procedure (emergency major surgery[a] aortic repair or peripheral vascular, prolonged surgical procedures with large fluid shifts or blood loss)

[a]Emergency major operations may require immediately proceeding to surgery without sufficient time for noninvasive testing or preoperative interventions.
Adapted from Eagle KA, Berger PB, Calkins H, et al. ACC/AHA guideline update for perioperative cardiovascular evaluation for noncardiac surgery-executive summary. A report of the American College of Cardiology/American Heart Association Task Force on Practice Guidelines (Committee to Update the 1996 Guidelines on Perioperative Cardiovascular Evaluation for Noncardiac Surgery). *J Am Coll Cardiol* 2002;39:542–553, with permission.

TABLE 27.7. *Prognostic gradient of ischemic response during an exercise electrocardiogram test[a]*

High risk (ischemia at <4 METs, or heart rate <100 bpm, or <70% age predicted)
    Horizontal or downsloping ST depression >0.1 mV
    ST-segment elevation >0/1 mV in noninfarct lead
    Five or more abnormal leads
    Persistent ischemic response >3 min after exertion
    Typical angina
Intermediate risk (ischemia at 4–6 METs, or heart rate 100–130 bpm, or 70% to 85% age predicted heart rate)
    Horizontal or downsloping ST depression >0.1 mV
    Typical angina
    Persistent ischemic response >1–3 min after exertion
    Three to four abnormal leads
Low risk (no ischemia or ischemia at >7 METs, heart rate >130 bpm, or >85% age predicted)
    Horizontal or downsloping ST depression >0.1 mV
    Typical angina
    One or more abnormal leads
Inadequate test
    For patients undergoing noncardiac surgery, inability to exercise to at least the intermediate-risk level without ischemia

[a]MET, Metabolic equivalent; bpm, beats per minute.
Adapted from Eagle KA, Berger PB, Calkins H, et al. ACC/AHA guideline update for perioperative cardiovascular evaluation for noncardiac surgery-executive summary. A report of the American College of Cardiology/American Heart Association Task Force on Practice Guidelines (Committee to Update the 1996 Guidelines on Perioperative Cardiovascular Evaluation for Noncardiac Surgery). *J Am Coll Cardiol* 2002;39:542–553, with permission.

heart rate are at intermediate risk, and those with abnormal ECG response at less than 70% of predicted heart rate are at highest risk. The high-risk features on an exercise ECG test are summarized in Table 27.7. It must be emphasized that although routine ECG stress testing has a sensitivity to identify one vessel CAD of just 55% to 60%, its sensitivity for left main or advanced three-vessel disease is far higher, in the 85% to 90% range. Thus, for the purposes of identifying the highest risk population, it is quite reasonable.

In patients with important abnormalities on their resting ECG (e.g., left bundle-branch block, left ventricular hypertrophy with "strain" pattern, or digitalis effect), other techniques such as exercise echocardiography, exercise myocardial perfusion imaging, or pharmacologic stress imaging may be indicated. Pharmacologic stress or perfusion imaging is indicated in patients undergoing orthopedic, neurosurgical, or vascular surgery who are unable to exercise or have left bundle-branch block (LBBB)/paced rhythm. The sensitivity and specificity of exercise thallium scans in the presence of LBBB are low, and overall diagnostic accuracy varies from 36% to 60% (13,14). In contrast, the use of vasodilators in such patients has a sensitivity of 98%, a specificity of 84%, and a diagnostic accuracy of 88% to 92% (15–17). Exercise should not be combined with dipyridamole in such patients because catecholamines can also yield false-positive

results (18). Thus, in patients with LBBB, dipyridamole or adenosine–thallium imaging are the preferred methods.

In patients unable to perform adequate exercise, such as most patients with peripheral vascular disease (PVD), a nonexercise stress test should be used. In this regard, dipyridamole myocardial perfusion imaging testing and dobutamine echocardiography are the most commonly used tests. Intravenous dipyridamole should be avoided in patients with significant bronchospasm, critical carotid disease, or a condition that prevents their being withdrawn from theophylline preparations. Dobutamine should not be used as a stressor in patients with serious arrhythmias or severe hypertension or hypotension. For patients in whom echocardiographic image quality is likely to be poor, a myocardial perfusion study is more appropriate. If there is an additional question about valvular diseases, the echocardiographic stress test may be more useful. In many instances, either stress perfusion or stress echocardiography is appropriate. In a meta-analysis of dobutamine stress echocardiography, ambulatory electrocardiography, radionuclide ventriculography, and dipyridamole–thallium scanning in predicting adverse cardiac outcome after vascular surgery, all tests had a similar predictive value, with overlapping confidence intervals (19). Another meta-analysis of 15 studies demonstrated that the prognostic value of noninvasive stress imaging abnormalities for perioperative ischemic events is comparable among available techniques, but that the accuracy varies with coronary artery disease prevalence (20). The expertise of the local laboratory in identifying advanced coronary disease is more important in choosing the appropriate test. Figure 27.3 illustrates an algorithm for choosing the most appropriate stress test in various situations.

There is clinical evidence supporting the use of dipyridamole–thallium stress testing to risk-stratify patients with suspected CAD before vascular surgery. Boucher et al. reported on the utility of dipyridamole–thallium imaging in the preoperative assessment of cardiac risk in patients with peripheral vascular diseases (21). Forty-eight patients with suspected CAD were evaluated before they underwent vascular surgery; 16 of these patients had thallium redistribution. All 8 perioperative cardiac events occurred in patients who had preoperative thallium redistribution. Leppo et al. performed dipyridamole–thallium imaging in 100 consecutive patients admitted for elective peripheral vascular surgery, and determined that the presence of thallium redistribution was the most significant predictor of serious nonfatal MI or cardiac death (22). The odds for a serious cardiac event were 23 times greater in a patient with thallium redistribution than in a patient without redistribution, which strongly suggests that myocardial imaging may be used as a primary screening test before elective vascular surgery (22). The findings of these early papers have been confirmed by many subsequent studies. A recently published meta-analysis by Shaw et al. analyzed the results of ten articles and 1,994 vascular surgery candidates over a 9-year period (20). Cardiac death or nonfatal MI occurred in 1%, 7%, and 9% of

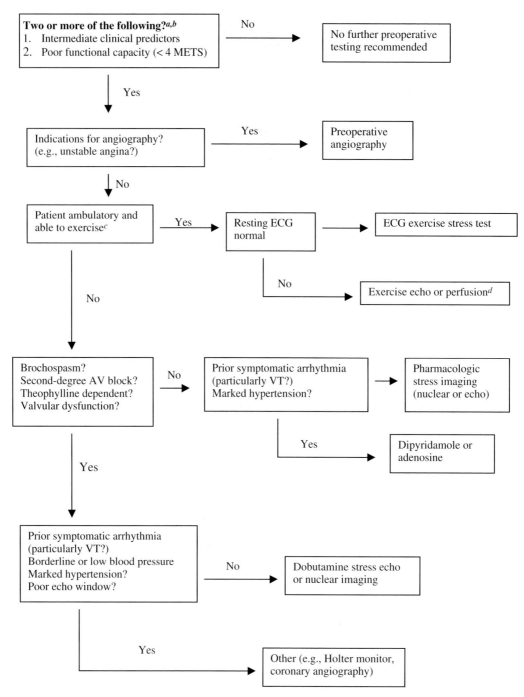

FIG. 27.3. Supplemental preoperative evaluation: When and which test? ECG, Electrocardiogram; VT, ventricular tachycardia; METS, metabolic equivalents; AV, atrioventricular. [a]Testing is only indicated if the results will impact care. [b]Refer to Table 27.1 for the metabolic equivalents, Table 27.2 for a list of clinical predictors, and Table 27.3 for the definition of high-risk surgical procedures. [c]Able to achieve ≥85% maximum predicted heart rate. [d]In the presence of left bundle-branch block, vasodilator perfusion imaging is preferred. (Adapted from Eagle KA, Brundage BH, Chaitman BR, et al. Guidelines for perioperative cardiovascular evaluation for noncardiac surgery. Report of the American College of Cardiology/American Heart Association Task Force on Practice Guidelines. Committee on Perioperative Cardiovascular Evaluation for Noncardiac Surgery. *Circulation* 1996;93:1278–1317, with permission.)

patients with normal results, fixed defects, and reversible defects on thallium scans, respectively, demonstrating the utility of dipyridamole–thallium scintigraphy for preoperative risk stratification.

The extent and severity of perfusion defects play a significant role in adverse perioperative events: The more extensive the perfusion abnormalities or the finding of cavity dilation or thallium lung uptake, the worse is the perioperative prognosis. Although the immediate purpose of preoperative examination is to assess the risk associated with the planned

TABLE 27.8. *American College of Cardiology/American Heart Association recommendations regarding coronary angiography before/after noncardiac surgery*

Class I: Patients with suspected or known coronary artery disease
  Evidence for high risk of adverse outcome based on noninvasive test results
  Angina unresponsive to adequate medical therapy
  Unstable angina, particularly when facing intermediate-risk or high-risk noncardiac surgery
  Equivocal noninvasive test results in patients at high clinical risk undergoing high-risk surgery
Class IIa
  Multiple markers of intermediate clinical risk and planned vascular surgery (noninvasive testing should be considered first)
  Moderate to large ischemia on noninvasive testing, but without high-risk features and lower left ventricular ejection fraction
  Nondiagnostic noninvasive test results in patients of intermediate clinical risk undergoing high-risk noncardiac surgery
  Urgent noncardiac surgery while convalescing from acute myocardial infarction
Class IIb
  Perioperative myocardial infarction
  Medically stabilized class III or IV angina and planned low-risk or minor surgery
Class III
  Low-risk noncardiac surgery with known coronary artery disease and no high-risk results on noninvasive testing
  Asymptomatic after coronary revascularization with excellent exercise capacity (≥7 metabolic equivalents)
  Mild stable angina with good left ventricular function and no high-risk noninvasive test results
  Noncandidate for coronary revascularization due to concomitant medical illness, severe left ventricular dysfunction (e.g., left ventricular ejection fraction <0.20), or refusal to consider revascularization
  Candidate for liver, lung, or renal transplant >40 years old as part of evaluation for transplantation, unless noninvasive testing reveals high risk for adverse outcome

Adapted from Eagle KA, Berger PB, Calkins H, et al. ACC/AHA guideline update for perioperative cardiovascular evaluation for noncardiac surgery-executive summary. A report of the American College of Cardiology/American Heart Association Task Force on Practice Guidelines (Committee to Update the 1996 Guidelines on Perioperative Cardiovascular Evaluation for Noncardiac Surgery). *J Am Coll Cardiol* 2002;39:542–553, with permission.

surgical procedure, the determination of long-term prognosis may be valuable in the overall management of a patient with known or suspected coronary artery disease.

Dobutamine stress echocardiography has also been used successfully to identify patients at risk for cardiac complications of surgery, with very high negative predictive values. In a meta-analysis, patients with no dobutamine-induced wall motion abnormalities had a very low event rate (0.4%), compared with a 23.4% event rate in patients who developed new wall motion abnormalities during dobutamine infusion. Dobutamine stress echocardiography has also been shown to provide prognostic value for predicting late events after vascular surgery. Furthermore, like dipyridamole–thallium imaging, the most useful role for stress echocardiography appears to be in patients at intermediate clinical risk.

For patients at high risk, it may be appropriate to proceed with coronary angiography rather than perform a noninvasive test. In patients with unstable angina or evidence of residual ischemia after recent MI, direct coronary angiography may be indicated. In general, indications for preoperative coronary angiography are similar to those identified for the nonoperative setting (Table 27.8).

COMBINED CLINICAL AND SCINTIGRAPHIC ASSESSMENT

Although the sensitivity of dipyridamole–thallium imaging for detecting patients at increased risk is excellent, one of its limitations for preoperative screening is its low specificity and positive predictive value. To improve the value of risk stratification, many reports have suggested utilization of the combination of clinical markers and noninvasive test results. Eagle et al. first reported on using assessment of clinical markers (history of angina, MI, congestive heart failure, diabetes, and Q wave on ECG) and thallium redistribution to identify a low-risk subset of patients (11). The authors demonstrated that patients without any of these clinical markers did not require dipyridamole–thallium testing. However, thallium redistribution had a significant predictive value in patients with one or two clinical risk factors. Within this group, 2 of 62 (3.2%; 95% confidence interval [CI]=0% to 8%) patients without thallium redistribution had events, compared with 16 events in 54 patients (29.6%; 95% CI=16% to 44%) with thallium redistribution (11). Recently, L'Italien et al. reported the results of a Bayesian model for perioperative risk assessment that combined clinical variables with dipyridamole–thallium findings (23). This analysis examined the type of procedure, specific institutional complication rates, and other clinical factors in a sequential manner followed by the addition of the dipyridamole–thallium findings. The addition of dipyridamole–thallium data reclassified greater than 80% of the moderate-risk patients into low-risk (3%) and high-risk (19%) categories ($p<0.0001$), but provided no stratification for patients classified as low or high risk according to the clinical model. Despite the findings of several of these papers and the suggestion to employ noninvasive testing only in patients of intermediate clinical risk, the identification of truly low risk patients may be difficult based on clinical variables alone in patients with peripheral vascular disease. It has also been shown that even in patients at low risk clinically, a finding of ischemia with dipyridamole–thallium testing increases the risk of myocardial infarction by ten fold.

MEDICAL THERAPY

Beta-Blockers

The effectiveness of beta-blockers in reducing perioperative cardiac risk has been evaluated in several studies. The first randomized, placebo-controlled study used atenolol in 200 high-risk patients scheduled to undergo noncardiac surgery (24). Atenolol was administered either intravenously or orally 2 days preoperatively and continued for 7 days postoperatively. The incidence of perioperative ischemia was significantly lower in the atenolol group than in the placebo group (24,25). There was no difference in the incidence of perioperative myocardial infarction or death from cardiac causes, but the rate of event-free survival at 6 months was higher in the atenolol group.

Poldermans et al. studied the perioperative use of bisoprolol in elective major vascular surgery (26). Bisoprolol was started at least 7 days preoperatively, the dose adjusted to achieve a resting heart rate of less than 60 beats per minute (bpm), and continued for 30 days postoperatively. The study was confined to patients who had at least one cardiac risk factor (a history of congestive heart failure, prior myocardial infarction, diabetes, angina pectoris, heart failure, age greater than 70 years, or poor functional status) and evidence of inducible myocardial ischemia on dobutamine echocardiography. Patients with extensive regional wall-motion abnormalities were excluded. Bisoprolol was associated with a 91% reduction in the perioperative risk of myocardial infarction or death from cardiac causes in this high-risk population. Because of the selection criteria used in this trial, the efficacy of bisoprolol in the group at highest risk, those in whom coronary revascularization or modification would be considered or for whom the surgical procedure might ultimately be canceled, cannot be determined. The rate of events in the standard-care group of 34% suggests that all but the patients at highest risk were enrolled in the trial. Urban et al. evaluated the role of prophylactic beta-blockers in patients undergoing elective total knee arthroplasty (27). One hundred seven patients were preoperatively randomized into two groups, control and beta-blockers, who received postoperative esmolol infusions on the day of surgery and metoprolol for the next 48 hours to maintain a heart rate less than 80 bpm. The number of ischemic events (control, 50; beta-blockers, 16) and total ischemic time (control, 709 minutes; beta-blocker, 236 minutes) were significantly lower with esmolol compared to the control group. In this study, prophylactic beta-adrenergic blockade administered after elective total knee arthroplasty was associated with a reduced prevalence

and duration of postoperative myocardial ischemia detected with Holter monitoring (27).

Alpha 2-Adrenergic Agonists

The effect of α_2-adrenergic agonists has also been studied in the perioperative period. Several small, randomized studies comparing clonidine with placebo failed to demonstrate that clonidine was effective in reducing the rates of myocardial infarction and death from cardiac causes (28,29). Mivazerol, an intravenous α_2-adrenergic agonist administered by continuous infusion, was compared with placebo in patients with known coronary disease or risk factors for it and who underwent major vascular or orthopedic procedures. Mivazerol was found to have no overall effect on the rates of cardiac complications (30). However, in the predefined subgroup of patients with known coronary artery disease who underwent major vascular surgery, mivazerol was associated with a significantly lower incidence of myocardial infarction and death from cardiac causes.

REVASCULARIZATION

Percutaneous Revascularization

No randomized trials of preoperative coronary revascularization have been performed, but several retrospective cohort studies have been published. Percutaneous coronary intervention (PCI), primarily balloon angioplasty, has been evaluated in three studies of patients who were undergoing noncardiac surgery (31–33). The indications for PCI were not well described in the studies, but most likely included the need to relieve symptomatic angina or reduce the perioperative risk of ischemia identified by noninvasive testing. All three studies had a low incidence of cardiac complications after noncardiac surgery, but no comparison groups were included.

One study used an administrative database of patients who were undergoing noncardiac surgery in the State of Washington. As compared with patients who did not undergo PCI preoperatively, those who did undergo the procedure had a lower incidence of perioperative cardiac complications (34). The benefit of revascularization was most apparent in the group that underwent PCI at least 90 days before noncardiac surgery. In contrast, when revascularization was performed within 90 days before noncardiac surgery, PCI was not associated with an improved outcome. This finding would suggest that PCI should not be used solely as a means of reducing perioperative risk. Coronary stents are now used in more than 80% of PCI, and use of stents during PCI presents unique challenges because of the risk of coronary thrombosis and bleeding during the initial recovery phase. In a cohort of 40 patients who received stents within 30 days of noncardiac surgery, all 8 deaths and 7 myocardial infarctions, as well as 8 of 11 bleeding episodes, occurred in patients who had undergone surgery within 14 days after stent placement (35). The complications appeared to be related to serious bleeding resulting from postprocedural anticoagulant therapy or to coronary thrombosis in those who did not receive 4 full weeks of antithrombotic therapy after stenting. These results suggest that it is prudent to wait at least 2 weeks, and preferably 4 weeks, after coronary stenting to perform noncardiac surgery, to allow complete endothelization and a full course of antiplatelet therapy to be given. Poststenting therapy includes a combination of aspirin and clopidogrel for 4 weeks, followed by aspirin for an indefinite period.

Coronary Artery Bypass Grafting

Coronary artery bypass grafting (CABG) has also been recommended to reduce the incidence of perioperative cardiac complications. Evidence of a potential protective effect of preoperative coronary artery bypass grafting comes from follow-up studies of randomized trials and/or registries comparing medical and surgical therapy for coronary artery disease. The largest study included 3,368 noncardiac operations performed within a 10-year period among patients assigned to medical therapy or CABG in the Coronary Artery Surgery Study (36). Prior successful CABG had a cardioprotective effect among patients who underwent high-risk noncardiac surgery (abdominal, thoracic, vascular, or orthopedic surgery) (36). The perioperative mortality rate was nearly 50% lower in the group of patients who had undergone CABG than in those who received medical therapy (3.3% vs. 1.7%, $p<0.05$). There was no difference in the outcome of patients undergoing low-risk procedures such as breast and urologic surgery. Fleisher et al. used Medicare claims data to assess 30-day and 1-year mortality after noncardiac surgery according to the use of cardiac testing and coronary interventions such as CABG and PCI within the year before noncardiac surgery (6). Preoperative revascularization significantly reduced the 1-year mortality rate for patients undergoing aortic surgery, but had no effect on the mortality rate for those undergoing infrainguinal surgery. Finally, an analysis of the Bypass Angioplasty Revascularization Investigation evaluated the incidence of postoperative cardiac complications after noncardiac surgery among patients with multivessel coronary disease who were randomly assigned to undergo PCI or CABG for severe angina (37). At an average of 29 months after coronary revascularization, both groups had similar low rates of postoperative myocardial infarction or death from cardiac causes (1.6% in each group). These data suggest that prior successful coronary revascularization, when accompanied by careful follow-up and therapy for subsequent coronary symptoms or signs, is associated with a low rate of cardiac events after noncardiac surgery (37).

The guidelines of the American College of Physicians support the use of preoperative testing and coronary therapies in high-risk patients who are undergoing major vascular surgery (38). An addendum suggests that all high-risk patients should also receive perioperative beta-blocker therapy. CABG or PCI should be limited to patients who have a clearly defined need for the procedure that is independent of the need for non-cardiac surgery (39). This includes patients who have poorly controlled angina pectoris despite maximal medical therapy and patients with one of several high-risk coronary characteristics, that is, clinically significant stenosis (greater than 50%) of the left main coronary artery, severe two- or three-vessel coronary artery disease (greater than 70% stenosis) with involvement of the proximal left anterior descending coronary artery, easily induced myocardial ischemia on preoperative stress testing, and left ventricular systolic dysfunction at rest.

POSTOPERATIVE THERAPY

Evaluation during noncardiac surgery should be used as an opportunity for assessment and management of modifiable risk factors for coronary artery disease, heart failure, hypertension, stroke, and other cardiovascular diseases. Assessment for hypercholesterolemia, smoking, hypertension, diabetes, physical activity, peripheral vascular disease, cardiac murmurs, arrhythmias, conduction abnormalities, and perioperative ischemia may lead to evaluation and treatments that reduce future cardiovascular risk. Patients who experience repetitive postoperative myocardial ischemia and/or sustain a perioperative MI are at substantially elevated long-term cardiac risk and should be a particular focus for risk factor interventions and future risk stratification and therapy.

CONCLUSIONS

Most patients with peripheral vascular disease have concomitant coronary artery disease, and cardiac complications account for 50% to 65% of the morbidity and mortality seen after vascular surgery. Comprehensive preoperative evaluation and appropriate therapy may significantly improve periprocedural outcomes. In addition to improving periprocedural outcomes, this is also an opportunity to modify cardiovascular risk factors and institute appropriate therapy to improve long-term prognosis.

REFERENCES

1. American Heart Association. *2002 heart and stroke statistical update.* Dallas, TX: Author, 2002.
2. Ashton CM, Petersen NJ, Wray NP, et al. The incidence of perioperative myocardial infarction in men undergoing noncardiac surgery. *Ann Intern Med* 1993;118:504–510.
3. Mangano DT. Perioperative cardiac morbidity. *Anesthesiology* 1990; 72:153–184.
4. Hertzer NR. Basic data concerning associated coronary disease in peripheral vascular patients. *Ann Vasc Surg* 1987;1:616–620.
5. Krupski WC, Layug EL, Reilly LM, et al. Comparison of cardiac morbidity rates between aortic and infrainguinal operations: two-year follow-up. Study of Perioperative Ischemia Research Group. *J Vasc Surg* 1993;18:609–615; discussion, 607–615.
6. Fleisher LA, Eagle KA, Shaffer T, et al. Perioperative and long-term mortality rates after major vascular surgery: the relationship to preoperative testing in the medicare population. *Anesth Analg* 1999;89:849–855.
7. L'Italien GJ, Cambria RP, Cutler BS, et al. Comparative early and late cardiac morbidity among patients requiring different vascular surgery procedures. *J Vasc Surg* 1995;21:935–944.

8. Roger VL, Ballard DJ, Hallett JW, Jr., et al. Influence of coronary artery disease on morbidity and mortality after abdominal aortic aneurysmectomy: a population-based study, 1971–1987. *J Am Coll Cardiol* 1989;14: 1245–1252.

9. Goldman L, Caldera DL, Nussbaum SR, et al. Multifactorial index of cardiac risk in noncardiac surgical procedures. *N Engl J Med* 1977;297:845–850.

10. Detsky AS, Abrams HB, McLaughlin JR, et al. Predicting cardiac complications in patients undergoing non-cardiac surgery. *J Gen Intern Med* 1986;1:211–219.

11. Eagle KA, Coley CM, Newell JB, et al. Combining clinical and thallium data optimizes preoperative assessment of cardiac risk before major vascular surgery. *Ann Intern Med* 1989;110:859–866.

12. Lee TH, Marcantonio ER, Mangione CM, et al. Derivation and prospective validation of a simple index for prediction of cardiac risk of major noncardiac surgery. *Circulation* 1999;100:1043–1049.

13. DePuey EG, Guertler-Krawczynska E, Robbins WL. Thallium-201 SPECT in coronary artery disease patients with left bundle branch block. *J Nucl Med* 1988;29:1479–1485.

14. Larcos G, Gibbons RJ, Brown ML. Diagnostic accuracy of exercise thallium-201 single-photon emission computed tomography in patients with left bundle branch block. *Am J Cardiol* 1991;68:756–760.

15. Rockett JF, Wood WC, Moinuddin M, et al. Intravenous dipyridamole thallium-201 SPECT imaging in patients with left bundle branch block. *Clin Nucl Med* 1990;15:401–407.

16. O'Keefe Jr JH, Bateman TM, Barnhart CS. Adenosine thallium-201 is superior to exercise thallium-201 for detecting coronary artery disease in patients with left bundle branch block. *J Am Coll Cardiol* 1993;21:1332–1338.

17. Hirzel HO, Senn M, Nuesch K, et al. Thallium-201 scintigraphy in complete left bundle branch block. *Am J Cardiol* 1984;53:764–769.

18. Tighe DA, Hutchinson HG, Park CH, et al. False-positive reversible perfusion defect during dobutamine–thallium imaging in left bundle branch block. *J Nucl Med* 1994;35:1989–1991.

19. Mantha S, Roizen MF, Barnard J, et al. Relative effectiveness of four preoperative tests for predicting adverse cardiac outcomes after vascular surgery: a meta-analysis. *Anesth Analg* 1994;79:422–433.

20. Shaw LJ, Eagle KA, Gersh BJ, et al. Meta-analysis of intravenous dipyridamole–thallium-201 imaging (1985 to 1994) and dobutamine echocardiography (1991 to 1994) for risk stratification before vascular surgery. *J Am Coll Cardiol* 1996;27:787–798.

21. Boucher CA, Brewster DC, Darling RC, et al. Determination of cardiac risk by dipyridamole–thallium imaging before peripheral vascular surgery. *N Engl J Med* 1985;312:389–394.

22. Leppo J, Plaja J, Gionet M, et al. Noninvasive evaluation of cardiac risk before elective vascular surgery. *J Am Coll Cardiol* 1987;9:269–276.

23. L'Italien GJ, Paul SD, Hendel RC, et al. Development and validation of a Bayesian model for perioperative cardiac risk assessment in a cohort of 1,081 vascular surgical candidates. *J Am Coll Cardiol* 1996;27:779–786.

24. Mangano DT, Layug EL, Wallace A, et al. Effect of atenolol on mortality and cardiovascular morbidity after noncardiac surgery. Multicenter Study of Perioperative Ischemia Research Group. *N Engl J Med* 1996;335:1713–1720.

25. Wallace A, Layug B, Tateo I, et al. Prophylactic atenolol reduces postoperative myocardial ischemia. McSPI Research Group. *Anesthesiology* 1998;88:7–17.

26. Poldermans D, Boersma E, Bax JJ, et al. The effect of bisoprolol on perioperative mortality and myocardial infarction in high-risk patients undergoing vascular surgery. Dutch Echocardiographic Cardiac Risk Evaluation Applying Stress Echocardiography Study Group. *N Engl J Med* 1999;341:1789–1794.

27. Urban MK, Markowitz SM, Gordon MA, et al. Postoperative prophylactic administration of beta-adrenergic blockers in patients at risk for myocardial ischemia. *Anesth Analg* 2000;90:1257–1261.

28. Ellis JE, Drijvers G, Pedlow S, et al. Premedication with oral and transdermal clonidine provides safe and efficacious postoperative sympatholysis. *Anesth Analg* 1994;79:1133–1140.

29. Stuhmeier KD, Mainzer B, Cierpka J, et al. Small, oral dose of clonidine reduces the incidence of intraoperative myocardial ischemia in patients having vascular surgery. *Anesthesiology* 1996;85:706–712.

30. Oliver MF, Goldman L, Julian DG, et al. Effect of mivazerol on perioperative cardiac complications during non-cardiac surgery in patients with coronary heart disease: the European Mivazerol Trial (EMIT). *Anesthesiology* 1999;91:951–961.

31. Allen JR, Helling TS, Hartzler GO. Operative procedures not involving the heart after percutaneous transluminal coronary angioplasty. *Surg Gynecol Obstet* 1991;173:285–288.

32. Elmore JR, Hallett Jr JW, Gibbons RJ, et al. Myocardial revascularization before abdominal aortic aneurysmorrhaphy: effect of coronary angioplasty. *Mayo Clin Proc* 1993;68:637–641.

33. Gottlieb A, Banoub M, Sprung J, et al. Perioperative cardiovascular morbidity in patients with coronary artery disease undergoing vascular surgery after percutaneous transluminal coronary angioplasty. *J Cardiothorac Vasc Anesth* 1998;12:501–506.

34. Posner KL, Van Norman GA, Chan V. Adverse cardiac outcomes after noncardiac surgery in patients with prior percutaneous transluminal coronary angioplasty. *Anesth Analg* 1999;89:553–560.

35. Kaluza GL, Joseph J, Lee JR, et al. Catastrophic outcomes of noncardiac surgery soon after coronary stenting. *J Am Coll Cardiol* 2000;35:1288–1294.

36. Eagle KA, Rihal CS, Mickel MC, et al. Cardiac risk of noncardiac surgery: influence of coronary disease and type of surgery in 3368 operations. CASS Investigators and University of Michigan Heart Care Program. Coronary Artery Surgery Study. *Circulation* 1997;96:1882–1887.

37. Hassan SA, Hlatky MA, Boothroyd DB, et al. Outcomes of noncardiac surgery after coronary bypass surgery or coronary angioplasty in the Bypass Angioplasty Revascularization Investigation (BARI). *Am J Med* 2001;110:260–266.

38. Palda VA, Detsky AS. Perioperative assessment and management of risk from coronary artery disease. *Ann Intern Med* 1997;127:313–328.

39. Eagle KA, Guyton RA, Davidoff R, et al. ACC/AHA guidelines for coronary artery bypass graft surgery: a report of the American College of Cardiology/American Heart Association Task Force on Practice Guidelines (Committee to Revise the 1991 Guidelines for Coronary Artery Bypass Graft Surgery). American College of Cardiology/American Heart Association. *J Am Coll Cardiol* 1999;34:1262–1347.

40. Eagle KA, Brundage BH, Chaitman BR, et al. Guidelines for perioperative cardiovascular evaluation for noncardiac surgery. Report of the American College of Cardiology/American Heart Association Task Force on Practice Guidelines. Committee on Perioperative Cardiovascular Evaluation for Noncardiac Surgery. *Circulation* 1996;93:1278–1317.

41. Eagle KA, Berger PB, Calkins H, et al. ACC/AHA guideline update for perioperative cardiovascular evaluation for noncardiac surgery-executive summary. A report of the American College of Cardiology/American Heart Association Task Force on Practice Guidelines (Committee to Update the 1996 Guidelines on Perioperative Cardiovascular Evaluation for Noncardiac Surgery). *J Am Coll Cardiol* 2002;39:542–553.

42. Campeau L. Letter: grading of angina pectoris. *Circulation* 1976;54:522–523.

CHAPTER 28

Surgery for Peripheral Vascular Disease

Glenn M. LaMuraglia and Giuseppe R. Nigri

Key Points

- Noncoronary atherosclerotic vascular disease has two major pathologies: obstructive disease and aneurysm.
- Decisions regarding reconstructive surgery for obstructive disease (not involving carotids) are centered around the clinical presentation and the examination.
- Carotid endarterectomy is the preferred treatment for patients with high-grade stenosis.
- Noninvasive carotid evaluation is more pervasive for preoperative patient evaluation, given the increased risk of invasive procedures in the diagnostic process.
- Treatment algorithms vary for lower extremity occlusive disease and are divided into acute versus chronic conditions.
- Lower extremity bypass with vein conduit is regarded as the gold standard.
- The size of an aortic aneurysm is considered the single most important risk for rupture.

The surgical management of noncoronary atherosclerotic vascular disease (NCAVD) is a very varied topic, which has filled many textbooks. Vascular medicine has not congealed as a well-defined specialty in the United States, which has resulted in the tradition of vascular and general surgeons providing the majority of these patients' evaluation and management, and development of the therapeutic plan.

The two major vascular pathologies that are considered in the therapy of NCAVD can be readily divided into obstructive atherosclerosis and aneurysm disease. The major impetus of treating obstructive atherosclerotic disease is the reversal of its natural course to restore adequate circulation to the affected end organ and prevent tissue necrosis, or death. The objective of treating peripheral aneurysms is to avoid their thrombosis with ensuing ischemia or rupture with possible exsanguination. Thus, the major questions relating to the surgical management of NCAVD are as follows: (a) Does the patient's clinical problem warrant a reconstructive procedure? (b) Do the findings provide the indication to undertake a reconstruction? (c) Can the optimal method be identified for achieving that goal? and (d) What are some of the technical alternatives that may be appropriate in the treatment of this patient? Therefore, other than for carotid disease, the decision for undertaking a reconstructive procedure for obstruc-

tive atherosclerotic disease is the clinical presentation of the patient and not the specific anatomic findings that can be identified. Once the decision is made that a reconstruction is indicated, the type of intervention is based not solely on anatomic findings, but also on the extent of the patient's symptomatology, presentation, general health, and comorbidities. Another important factor to consider is the specific outcome of the patient undergoing surgical treatment for NCAVD. Therefore, in addition to the indications for the operation, the expertise and the results of the surgeon and the institution where the surgery is performed are becoming recognized as an important determinant in the decision to undertake a reconstuction. This is to ensure that the morbidity and mortality of the procedure undertaken always remain significantly lower than the natural course of the treated disease process.

Despite the diversity of problems that the vascular surgeon confronts, the topics addressed here are limited to NCAVD, and divided into extracranial cerebrovascular disease, lower extremity occlusive disease, and aneurysmal disease.

EXTRACRANIAL CEREBROVASCULAR DISEASE

The purpose of carotid endarterectomy for the treatment of significant carotid stenotic lesions is to prevent stroke in asymptomatic or symptomatic patients. Symptomatic patients include those manifesting transient ischemic attacks or transient monocular blindness, and those patients evolving an acute, small stroke without hemorrhagic complications. Carotid endarterectomy is still the preferred method of treatment for symptomatic and asymptomatic patients who have a high-grade carotid stenosis. Multiple prospective multicenter randomized trials have confimed that medical management alone is not an adequate alternative to manage patients with significant carotid stenosis. These trials have determined that operative intervention is indicated in patients with symptomatic stenoses of greater than 50%, and asymptomatic lesions between 60% and 99% (1,2). Although there has been a concern of reduced efficacy for carotid endarterectomy in women who have an asymptomatic lesion of 60% to 99%, which may result from a smaller number of women entered in the trial, most clinicians do not discriminate between the sexes (3). In addition to the degree of stenosis, data have emerged from these trials that plaque ulceration is associated with a nearly twofold increase in neurological events when there is a stenosis present as well (1,2). Therefore, the presence of a significant stenosis/ulceration in either symptomatic or asymptomatic patients should low the threshold for recommending carotid endarterectomy (Table 28.1).

Contraindications for carotid endarterectomy include patients with an acute hemorrhagic or major stroke, without good neurological or reasonable cognitive function, and with anatomically inaccessible lesions, and the rare patient with comorbidities severe enough to significantly shorten his or her life expectancy or make anesthesia prohibitive. There is also a subset of patients with severe extracranial cerebrovascular disease who have been classified as "high-risk" patients: those with major comorbidities, a prior carotid endarterectomy (4) resulting in restenosis, a "hostile neck" including a prior radical neck dissection, radiation therapy, or very severe cervical arthritis. However, it should be noted that these "high-risk" patients do undergo successful, safe carotid endarterectomy in the hands of a skilled, experienced surgeon with similar outcomes to the normal patient population.

Proper evaluation to reliably quantify the severity of carotid disease is of paramount importance in determining whether a patient should undergo surgical intervention. Imaging procedures such as angiography that may result in a complication such as stroke should have this morbidity added to the outcome of the intervention because it occurred as a result of initiation to treat the patient. Therefore, noninvasive evaluation has become more pervasive in preoperative evaluation of patients with severe carotid stenosis, and the use of catheter-based carotid arteriography has been limited to a small group of patients. Duplex ultrasound (5), magnetic resonance imaging, and computed tomography (CT) angiography have emerged as viable alternatives for diagnostic imaging in the evaluation of patients with carotid stenosis. An important issue relating to duplex imaging of carotid arteries that must be emphasized is that not all noninvasive laboratories are very accurate, and the general trend is to overcall the degree of stenosis. It is therefore imperative that the clinician know the reliability of the laboratory where the study was performed.

Duplex ultrasonography is known to overestimate the degree of stenosis in patients who have severe or occluded carotids on the contralateral side, as well as those who have had a prior carotid endarterectomy. In those instances, further imaging utilizing magnetic resonance arteriography (MRA) or CT angiogram is indicated (6).

The surgical procedure for carotid endarterectomy is relatively straightforward, but must be done with a perfect tolerance. Exposure is through an oblique neck incision, and the arteries are controlled. A standard longitudinal incision through the common and internal carotid artery has been standard for many years (Fig. 28.1). Under specific circumstances, the utilization of a patch reconstruction of the arteriotomy with either greater saphenous vein or other prosthetic material has gained wide acceptance. Another technique of carotid surgery with similar short- and long-term outcomes is eversion endarterectomy, which utilizes transection and eversion of the internal carotid artery with removal of the plaque *in toto* (Fig. 28.2).

The controversy relating to the optimal method of cerebral protection during carotid clamping and endarterectomy is still widely debated. Regional anesthesia and neurological assessment of the awake patient, routine intraluminal shunting at the time of clamping, utilization of electroencephalogram monitoring and selective shunting, and stump pressure measurements all have been shown to have excellent results in centers of excellence.

An important determinant relating to those treating patients with carotid endarterectomy surgery is that they need to know their outcomes. The multiple trials that have been undertaken to evaluate the efficacy of surgery all indicate that the combined stroke and mortality rate for the symptomatic patient should be less than 5%, and for the asymptomatic patient it should be less than 3%, to achieve a true benefit for the patient undergoing a carotid endarterectomy (2,3,7). Therefore, it is imperative to carefully assess the patient for longevity in addition to comorbidities because the patient needs to live long enough to benefit from the perioperative risk of the procedure, even in skilled surgical hands (8).

TABLE 28.1. *Indications for carotid endarterectomy*

Symptomatic
    Transient ischemic attack (>50% stenosis)
    Transient monocular blindness (>50% stenosis)
    Stroke in evolution (>50% stenosis)
    Stroke, small and nonhemorrhagic (>50% stenosis)
    Global ischemia (>70% carotid stenosis) with
        contralateral or veretebrobasilar disease
    Symptoms with large plaque ulceration (>40% stenosis)
Asymptomatic
    Anatomy: >70% stenosis
    Large plaque ulceration and >50% stenosis
    Patient <80 yr old with expected longevity 2–3 yr
    Patient >80 yr old with expected longevity 2–3 yr with
        good cardiac risk stratification

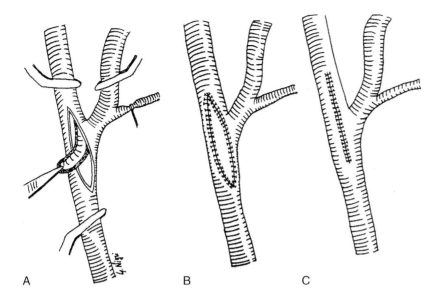

FIG. 28.1. Carotid endarterectomy. **A:** The proximal common, internal, and external carotid arteries are controlled with clamps. The arteriotomy is performed longitudinally along the artery, extending distally into the internal carotid artery beyond the atherosclerotic plaque. The endarterectomy is begun using a Freer elevator entering the subadventitial plane. After the endarterectomy, the arteriotomy is closed (**B**) with or (**C**) without a patch.

LOWER EXTREMITY OCCLUSIVE DISEASE

The evaluation and management of patients with upper or lower extremity ischemia should be based on their symptoms and their physical findings, and not solely on the anatomy of their obstructions. Although generalizations are difficult to make, one of the only indications for preemptive surgery for lower extremity occlusive disease should be that for correc-

tion of asymptomatic bypass graft stenosis. This is based on the well-documented findings that assisted primary patency of lower extremity bypass grafts have significantly better long-term patency, approaching that of primary patency, compared to secondary patency of these grafts (9).

Ischemia of the lower extremity may be easily divided into acute and chronic categories. Severe acute ischemia of the lower extremities still carries a high mortality of up to 20% in modern clinical series, and may require an amputation rate as high as 10% to 20% (10). The management of the acutely ischemic lower extremity remains a challenge and must be carefully assessed for both severity and likely etiology. The traditional six findings of pulselessness, pallor, pain, poikilothermy, paresthesias, and paralysis are paramount for identifying the problem and determining its severity. In patients who have lost distal sensation and/or motor function especially in the presence of muscle tenderness, the temporal window of tolerable ischemia is limited, and the limb viability is considered severely threatened, resulting in a surgical emergency. Etiologies such as an embolus or a thrombotic occlusion (of either a primary vessel or, more commonly, a peripheral bypass graft) or acute thrombosis of an aneurysm are common etiologies in addition to iatrogenic complications from a percutaneous intervention.

The treatment algorithm for these patients is dictated by multiple factors. These include the severity and the duration of ischemia of the presenting patient, the suspected etiology of the ischemia, and the resources available to the individual at the time of presentation. In a severely threatened limb, the patient may need to go emergently to the operating room for an attempted embolectomy or thrombectomy. The luxury of obtaining a standard arteriogram to define the anatomy may not be possible depending on the condition of the patient and the amount of time required to obtain the study. Often the surgeon may supplement the intraoperative evaluation with a single-shot on-table arteriogram to help identify the necessary anatomy for performing a reconstruction. In

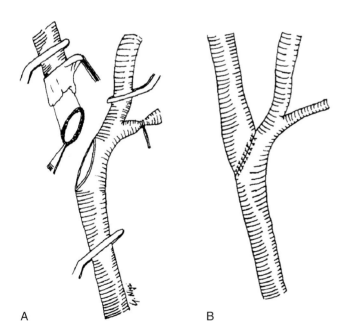

FIG. 28.2. Eversion carotid endarterectomy. **A:** The internal carotid artery (ICA) is transected obliquely. Endarterectomy of the ICA is begun by circumferentially elevating the adventitia from the arterial wall (intima and media). The adventitia is then rolled until all the disease is removed. **B:** After the endarterectomy of the plaque in the external and common carotid arteries, the ICA is anastomosed to the common carotid artery with a continuous suture.

the situation when the limb is ischemic but its viability not acutely threatened and the etiology is undefined, angiography with possible thrombolytic therapy may be a consideration. Expeditious evaluation of the patient can be undertaken with noninvasive vascular testing and adequate imaging studies (either an MRA or contrast arteriogram depending on renal function and availability) prior to going to the operating room for thromboembolectomy or other reconstruction.

The algorithm for specific surgical intervention is dictated by whether there is adequate inflow to the common femoral artery. In the acute setting when full evaluation in not feasible, the adequacy of the femoral pulse and the rest of the pulse examination is very important. In the presence of good inflow (which can be verified in the operating room with transducing pressure measurements), improvement in the outflow beyond the femoral artery is the goal in utilizing thromboembolectomy or a distal reconstruction (chronic ischemia is discussed in what follows).

As the presentation of acute or subacute ischemia of the lower extremity becomes less severe, the clinical approach becomes similar to that for the patient presenting with chronic lower extremity ischemia necessitating reconstruction. The indications for subacute or chronic lower extremity ischemia are strictly based on presentation and symptomatology, and are not based on anatomy. The mild- to increased-severity stratification of patients with chronic lower extremity ischemia includes claudication, disabling claudication, rest pain, and tissue loss (without healing). Indications for treatment should be based on the severity in symptomatology at the time of presentation. Because the majority of the determination is made on clinical criteria and not by testing, careful evaluation by a thorough history and physical exam are imperative in these patients. The patient who presents with claudication should be started on a defined exercise program of walking, to the point of developing claudication symptoms to reverse the physical deconditioning that has occurred with the limitations in ambulation, and to help the development of collateral systems. Other medical management at this point includes the modification of present risk factors for atherosclerosis, and overweight patients should be started on a weight reduction program, which can dramatically improve claudication. These patients can be conservatively managed over a 4- to 6-month program, which can result in a significant improvement. In many elderly patients, this becomes adequate for their lifestyle expectations. Disabling claudication can be defined as symptoms of lower extremity claudication that preclude the patient from earning his or her livelihood or prevent the patient from adequately caring for himself or herself, and other major lifestyle alterations that are disabling to the patient.

Rest pain or numbness of the lower extremities is generally first noted at night when the patient is recumbent, with symptoms in the forefoot that may require the patient to get up at night to walk and obtain gravitational augmentation of the lower extremity perfusion to reverse the symptoms of aching or numbness of the foot. When the presentation per-

sists during the day, it is indicative that the perfusion to the lower extremities is inadequate for normal homeostasis of the tissues in the foot. Surgical intervention on these patients generally does not require major reconstructive procedures, because a modest correction of the lower extremity perfusion and the use of an exercise program may be adequate to correct these symptoms. These patients will also have symptoms of claudication when they walk. As collaterals develop, these symptoms may improve. However, when these symptoms occur relatively acutely in a patient who did not have symptoms of claudication, the possibility of an embolus must be considered.

The most severe state of lower extremity ischemia is when tissue loss is present and there is vascular lab criteria to verify that perfusion is inadequate to heal the wound. In these circumstances, expeditious imaging and revascularization are indicated. Wounds that should heal based on vascular lab criteria but do not regardless of both adequate correction of local infection and wound care may require revascularization.

Proper evaluation for lower extremity reconstruction requires functional tests as well as an anatomic delineation of patent vessels, stenoses, and occlusions. The combination of an endovascular treatment with open surgery is common and often indicated; however, the focus of this chapter is limited to open surgical interventions. The guiding principle for lower extremity reconstruction includes first the establishment of good inflow to the common femoral artery. With good inflow and no significant femoral artery disease, an outflow reconstruction, or improving the perfusion down the lower extremity, is required. A major requirement of lower extremity reconstruction is to ensure that a stenosis or proximal occlusion of the profunda femoris artery is always repaired, because long-term viability of the lower extremity is often dependent on the patency of this artery.

Inflow disease of the lower extremities can be reconstructed "in-line," or "extraanatomic," in their configuration. In-line reconstruction for inflow disease would include an endarterectomy or bypass surgery parallel to the obstruction. This may include the aortoiliac segment, common, or external iliac arteries. Generally, a patch reconstruction is utilized for closure of the arterial segment when an endarterectomy is undertaken. The extent of the endarterectomy is dictated by the location of the disease; however, this is reserved primarily for focal disease segments such as the external iliac artery and the common femoral artery. In patients undergoing endarterectomy of the aorta and common iliac segments, long-term patency is excellent and equivalent to bypass graft procedures. However, when this endarterectomy is extended to include the external iliac arteries, long-term patency is not as good as bypass grafting. Therefore, with extensive aortoiliac disease, endarterectomy is generally not a good option, and aortofemoral bypass is preferable. Endarterectomy should not be considered in patients who have even modest aneurysmal changes in their aorta and iliac segments, because these vessels can further degenerate into aneurysms over time.

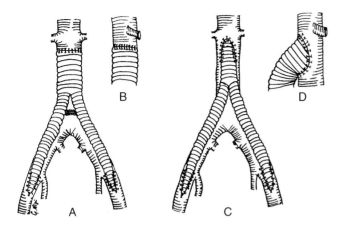

FIG. 28.3. The two types of proximal anastomoses of aortobifemoral bypass grafts. **A:** Aortobifemoral bypass performed in an end-to-end proximal anastomosis. **B:** Lateral view. **C:** Aortobifemoral bypass performed in an end-to-side proximal anastomosis. **D:** Lateral view.

In-line bypass surgery for inflow disease is achieved by either aortofemoral bypass or iliofemoral bypass. When the surgery is performed for occlusive disease, it is generally ill advised unless there are other pressing considerations. To perform a bypass between the aorta and the iliac system and not bring the bypass to the femoral vessels (even if the external iliacs are without significant disease) is not desirable because in patients with occlusive disease, the recurrent disease process is generally at the distal anastomosis. Thus, should a secondary reconstruction be required, access to the groin is much easier than at the iliac level, which is in the retroperitoneum. Aortofemoral bypasses can be performed either in an end-to-end proximal anastomosis (Fig. 28.3A, B) or an end-to-side proximal anastomosis (Fig. 28.3C, D). Although there may be some surgeon preference for this, an end-to-side proximal anastomosis for aortofemoral graft is generally utilized for patients who have severe occlusive disease in the external iliac artery. This provides preservation of pelvic flow in antegrade fashion. For an end-to-end proximal aortic anastomosis, pelvic flow can only be reconstituted by retrograde flow up the external iliac artery through the hypogastric arteries. The importance of these two types of aortic anastomoses have implications for catheter manipulations and placement of intraaortic balloon pumps. The long-term patency for aortofemoral bypass grafts is excellent, and is 85% to 90% at 5 years and 70% to 75% at 10 years (10–12).

Extraanatomic bypass for inflow to the femoral artery can include the axillary artery or the contralateral common femoral artery. Although these are both good options for inflow reconstruction, they are generally reserved for an emergent reconstruction, or patients who have either a hostile abdomen or a prior surgical intervention, or are deemed poor surgical candidates to undergo major aortic or abdominal surgery. The 5-year patency for axillofemoral bypass is improved with concomitant femoral–femoral artery bypass and

is 75% to 85% at 5 years (13–15). Femoral–femoral bypasses also are an excellent option for a more limited procedure, but the donor iliac system has to be large enough to provide perfusion to both lower extremities.

With inflow procedures, it is also important to ensure that the common femoral and the profunda femoris artery remain intact without significant stenoses at the time of reconstruction. The progression of disease is primarily in the superficial femoral artery, which is generally the first lower extremity vessel to occlude in nondiabetic patients with peripheral vascular disease.

When superficial femoral artery occlusion occurs due to progressive atherosclerosis, it is generally a benign process. When isolated, a superficial femoral artery occlusion results in claudication, for which studies have shown there is only a 10% to 15% requirement for further reconstruction because of progression of disease. For lower extremity outflow reconstructions, it is very important to view the hemodynamic studies and correlate them to the areas of anatomic obstructive disease. This review is critical because there is often multilevel disease, and hemodynamic studies can help determine the impact of the various stenoses and occlusions. Another major consideration when considering surgical options of the lower extremity is the availability of conduit. Lower extremity bypass with vein conduit is the gold standard. Vein grafts can be placed either in an *in situ* configuration, which includes the need to lyse the venous valves and ligate the side branches, or a reverse configuration. Long-term patency is equivalent and is 74% at 5 years (16–19). Close long-term follow-up is critical to maintaining primary patency in vein graft because assisted primary patency in the vein graft approaches that of primary patency, whereas secondary patency of vein grafts approach the long-term patency of prosthetic grafts (81% at 5 years) (18). Prosthetic bypasses have to be utilized for lower extremity reconstruction when there is no adequate vein conduit. The use of prosthetic bypasses to the above-knee popliteal artery with good distal runoff (two or three patent tibials to the ankle) has good long-term patency (primary patency 59% at 5 years and secondary patency 74% at 5 years) (20–22). However, in circumstances when prosthetic grafts can be the only conduit, vein cuff/patch methods have been devised at the distal anastomosis to significantly improve patency. These patients who have disadvantaged outflow or prosthetic bypass grafts to distal popliteal or tibial vessels need to be maintained on long-term coumadin anticoagulation to provide improved long-term patency.

Upper extremity treatment and revascularization follow similar principles to lower extremity revascularization. However, because of the significantly better collateral network to the upper extremity, it is rare that significant claudication or limb salvage procedures need to be undertaken for the upper extremity. Exceptions include patients with prior trauma or radiation therapy. The workload and wear and tear for the upper extremity is also not the same as for the lower extremities, which are used for ambulation, and therefore symptoms are generally mild and more easily tolerated. A notable exception is ischemia that can result in a patient who has had the construction of an arteriovenous fistula for dialysis access where a "steal" phenomenon can occur from the venous anastomoses. The reversal of flow in a vertebral artery in an otherwise asymptomatic patient is not an uncommon finding with proximal subclavian obstructions and should not be considered an indication for surgical or interventional correction on its own merit. However, when the subclavian artery occlusive disease is proximal to an internal mammary artery bypass to the coronary circulation, the merits of its reconstruction by a carotid subclavian bypass are self-evident. These procedures are easy to perform, are well tolerated, and have excellent long-term patency (94% at 5 years) (23,24).

ANEURYSMAL DISEASE

Abdominal aortic aneurysms can be considered significant when they reach a size of 4.5 to 5 cm in diameter. The major risk factors associated with the development of abdominal aortic aneurysms include advanced age, a positive history of smoking, hypertension, low high-density-lipoprotein cholesterol, and a positive family history. The size of the aortic aneurysm is considered the single most important risk factor for aneurysm rupture, but other factors have also been recognized. These include an expansion rate of greater than 0.6 cm per year, severe chronic obstructive pulmonary disease, especially with the use of steroids, a positive family history, poorly controlled blood pressure, a saccular versus a fusiform shape, and female gender.

The estimated annual risk of rupture of abdominal aortic aneurysm is mostly determined by its size. For aneurysms between 4 and 5 cm, the annual rupture risk is approximately 0.5% to 5% per year (25), but the decision for intervention has many considerations. Life expectancy is an important consideration when evaluating a patient for possible repair of abdominal aortic aneurysm, because the long-term life expectancy of patients with aortic aneurysms is lower than that of the general population. Factors that appear to be important for early mortality included age over 75 years, a previous history of coronary artery disease (especially congestive heart failure), renal failure with a creatinine of greater than 2.0, and chronic obstructive pulmonary disease (26,27). The patient's medical comorbidities also play an important role in the decision for intervention.

Operative intervention can be undertaken by either open abdominal aortic aneurysm repair or by an endovascular approach. The decision of repair procedure is in part determined by the patient's anatomy, but consideration should also be given to the patient's general medical condition and life expectancy. Risk factors that lead to higher operative mortality and morbidity have been shown to be greatest with patients in renal failure (creatinine greater than 1.8), followed by factors including a history of congestive heart failure, ischemia on electrocardiogram, pulmonary dysfunction, advanced age, and, to a lesser extent, female gender. Most centers of excellence have reported 30-day perioperative mortality rates for open abdominal aortic aneurysm repair to be

less than 2%. This helps to verify that such surgery can be performed at lower risk by skilled, experienced surgeons; however, it is also well documented in national databases that a higher mortality in the 4% to 8% range is not uncommon. In younger patients with no major comorbid conditions, open surgical reconstruction has been shown to have excellent long-term results, and should be the primary consideration for these types of patients. In older, more infirm patients with lower life expectancy, should surgery be considered and their anatomy be favorable, an endograft aneurysm repair through groin incisions is clearly the preferable method.

Proper imaging studies are important for abdominal aortic aneurysm reconstruction. The optimal method for screening patients for aneurysm and for tracking its size is ultrasonography. This can provide accurate measurements of the cross-sectional diameter of the aorta, is easily obtained, and is relatively inexpensive. When the decision has been made to treat a patient with an aortic aneurysm, CT scans performed with CT angiographic technique and three-dimensional reconstructions are very useful. With fine cuts and intravenous contrast, three-dimensional images can be undertaken on computer workstations, which provide very detailed and accurate delineation of the aortic aneurysm and its size, neck diameter, angulation, and length, and the status of the iliac vessels. The use of intravenous contrast also provides very important information regarding the arterial wall calcium, and the presence, quantity, and character of the intraluminal filling defects. This is critical to determining a suitable location for aortic clamp placement to avoid microembolization or other perioperative complications. The CT scan also provides very important information with respect to whether the aneurysm has an inflammatory component, whether there are penetrating aortic ulcers or venous abnormalities that may affect the surgical approach, as well as whether there is presence of horseshoe kidneys, lymphadenopathy, or other intraabdominal pathology. If the patient has a symptomatic aneurysm, and the question relates to whether a rupture is present, the use of intravenous contrast is not essential, and may contribute to perioperative renal dysfunction in patients who are likely to sustain shock. In patients who have significant renal compromise, magnetic resonance imaging (MRI) with gadolinium can be a reasonable substitute; however, patients with metallic implants, pacemakers, or severe claustrophobia are unsuitable for utilization of this modality. MRI is also not as suitable for preoperative evaluation because it does not provide information regarding arterial wall calcium, and it is not as accurate as a CT scan in measuring sizes. Catheter-based arteriography may also be helpful in specific situations, but it is rarely used in diagnostic purposes in preoperative evaluation of abdominal aortic aneurysms.

Because the endograft approach of abdominal aortic aneurysm is covered in Chapter 29, we discuss the open surgical procedures. There are two major approaches for open surgical repair of abdominal aortic aneurysms: the transperitoneal approach and the retroperitoneal approach. Although there is surgeon preference between these two surgical approaches, each has its advantages and disadvantages. The transabdominal approach provides the most flexibility for an open surgical repair of abdominal and iliac artery aneurysms provided that the proximal infrarenal aortic neck is of adequate size and surgically accessible. The right iliac system and the right renal artery can easily be exposed because the patient is supine. The advantage of the retroperitoneal approach is that it provides significant flexibility for dealing with difficult proximal aortic aneurysm necks, and facilitates the approach for para-, juxta-, or suprarenal aneurysms. It also appears to be better tolerated by patients with chronic obstructive lung disease, and the recovery of the patient from ileus appears to be superior to the transperitoneal approach. The retroperitoneal approach facilitates exposure in very obese patients because the pannus and intestinal contents are easily retracted to the side while the patient is in the right lateral decubitus position. However, in this position, access to the right renal artery is rarely possible, and exposure of the right iliac system is particularly difficult.

Open aortic aneurysm repair requires the anticoagulation of the patient prior to clamping of the aorta above the aneurysm. Sometimes, temporary clamping of the suprarenal or supraceliac aorta is necessary while the proximal anastomosis is undertaken. If the aortic aneurysm involves the renal arteries or the visceral vessels, occasionally a bypass to these vessels may be undertaken to exclude the aneurysm from the circulation. Bypass to the renal arteries can also be undertaken for occlusive disease at the time of aortic surgery. In selected cases, should there be significant occlusive disease in the visceral and/or renal arteries, a visceral and renal transaortic endarterectomy may be performed with excellent long-term results. It must be noted that these procedures require specific expertise and experience by the surgeon to be performed successfully.

Iliac aneurysms occur primarily in conjunction with aortic aneurysms. They may also occur primarily as an isolated problem; however, this is rare. Their repair is generally performed in conjunction with repair of the aorta because even in cases where the aortic aneurysm may not be large enough as a primary indication, the need to reconstruct the iliac aneurysm requires concurrent repair of the aorta as well. The threshold size for repair of an iliac aneurysm is not as clear-cut as it is for the aorta. However, iliac artery aneurysms that are 2.5 cm or greater should be evaluated and considered for surgery, and those greater than 3 cm should be reconstructed unless there is a significant contraindication. Surgery involving the iliac arteries for aneurysmal disease generally undertakes a distal anastomosis either at the iliac bifurcation or into the external iliac artery. Unless concomitant significant occlusive disease is present, the surgery for aneurysmal disease will rarely require a bypass to the femoral artery in the groin.

AORTIC DISSECTION

Aortic dissection is the most common acute calamity that involves the aorta, with an incidence similar to that of ruptured

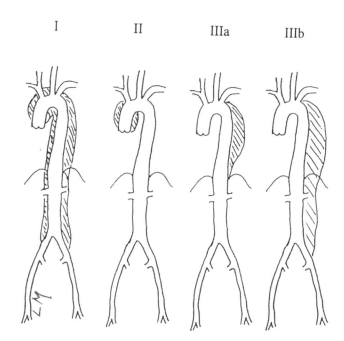

FIG. 28.4. The DeBakey classification of aortic dissections. (**I**) commencing in the ascending aorta and terminating at the aortic bifurcation; (**II**) limited to the ascending aorta; (**IIIA**) commencing distal to the left subclavian and confined to the chest; (**IIIB**) commencing distal to the subclavian and terminating at the aortic bifurcation.

abdominal aortic aneurysms. Although acute aortic dissection can occur in a dilated aorta, it can also occur in a normal-diameter aorta in otherwise young and healthy people. The early mortality of aortic dissection remains quite significant at around 27% (28). The acute mortality in aortic dissection is primarily a result of proximal complications of aortic rupture, cardiac tamponade, aortic valvular insufficiency, and coronary artery obstruction. This complication occurs only with a type I or a type II dissection, which involves the ascending aorta (Fig. 28.4). Rupture of the aorta is uncommon in patients who have more distal dissections (type III), unless they occur at the site of original intimal tear, or if the dissection occurs in already aneurysmal degenerated aorta (Fig. 28.4).

The majority of patients who develop an acute aortic dissection present with an acute excruciating back or chest pain that migrates caudally. This pain is very pronounced and noticeable, generally referred to as the worst shearing or tearing pain the patient has experienced. Although occasionally mistaken for myocardial pain, this pain associated with dissection is rarely described as pressure or angina-like symptoms. The majority of patients who have aortic dissection have a history of systemic hypertension and can occasionally present with aortic insufficiency and subsequent myocardial ischemia, usually involving the right coronary artery. Stroke, abdominal pain, and limb ischemia can also be presentations, but are not as common. It should be noted that the outcome for patients with aortic dissection is time related, and therefore the diagnosis should be considered and evaluation should be undertaken early in the patient's course of presentation.

The diagnosis of aortic dissection is best performed by a fine-cut CT scan with and without intravenous contrast. This can provide the characteristic double-barrel appearance of the aorta and provide the diagnosis even when the aorta is of normal diameter. Dynamic CT scan can also be valuable for determining the presence of branch vessel compromise as well as perfusion of one or both kidneys. With careful observation and reconstructions, the origin of the major visceral vessels off of the true or false lumen can generally be determined.

Initial mainstay of patients presenting with the diagnosis of aortic dissection is systemic blood pressure control. Once this can be undertaken, and the wall tension reduced to help obviate a rupture, full evaluation and determination of the extent of the aortic dissection is imperative.

Proximal aortic dissections (type I and type II) are treated by cardiac surgical reconstruction with either an aortic root replacement or composite root replacement involving the aortic valve. These patients are generally operated on emergently, and often with cerebral cooling (29). Should the patient be hemodynamically stable and in the rare instance have significant renal or visceral ischemia, repair of the renal or mesenteric circulation may need to be undertaken first or concomitantly with the ascending aortic reconstruction.

Patients with a type III aortic dissection are generally followed in the acute setting and do not undergo proximal aortic repair unless aortic rupture occurs. Although there are studies at comparing medical therapy with stent graft obliteration of the aortic tear site, there is no evidence that interventional therapy at the aortic tear site changes the natural course of the disease. Patients who have an aortic branch compromise, sometimes referred to as malperfusion syndrome, can be treated by a directed approach to the ischemic end organ (30). This can be achieved by an infrarenal or paravisceral surgical fenestration, a surgical bypass to the ischemic vessel, an endovascular fenestration within an aortic stent, or an ostial branch stent (Fig. 28.5).

It is important to understand the pathophysiology of aortic dissection and distal branch compromise. It is important to identify the longitudinal extent of the dissection of the aorta, the presence of distal reentry sites, the percentage of the aortic circumference encompassed by the false lumen, and the specific anatomy of the branch takeoffs, by inspecting the more distal portion of the vessel relating to the dissection or tearing process. This can be best undertaken with careful examination of a chest and abdominal CT angiogram to follow the true and the false lumen as they propagate down the aorta. These patterns can raise the index of suspicion that there is renal, visceral, or lower extremity ischemia, and, in accordance with the clinical picture, dictate whether surgical or percutaneous intervention should be rapidly undertaken (31). It is important to remember that good femoral pulses do not exclude the possibility that renal or visceral ischemia is concomitantly present.

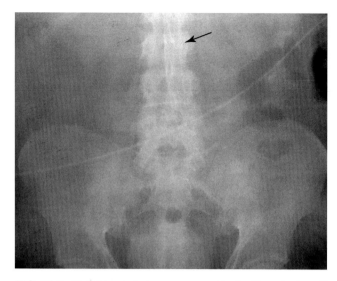

FIG. 28.5. Flat film of abdomen on a patient with a stent graft following aortic dissection. A 55-year-old man presented with chest pain and right lower extremity ischemia requiring amputation followed by renal failure and abdominal pain. Renal artery stents were also deployed. Arrow demonstrates aortic and iliac segments of the stent graft.

It should also be remembered that the aortic dissection flap is a dynamic process, which can change considerably when hearing the systolic and diastolic cycle of a heart. The dynamic changes can also cause obstruction at the level of the orifice of the vessel in question. Generally, the false lumen tends to be larger than the thoracic aorta, and it is not uncommon that this will compress the true lumen, resulting in significant distal ischemia of branch vessels coming off of the true lumen. An angiographic injection in the true lumen can also give the false impression that the side branches have adequate perfusion; however, suspicion of compromise of blood flow from the vessel origin should also be considered based on the topography of the findings. It is therefore because of this dynamic obstruction that reasonable reduction of the blood pressure can result in actual improvement in end-organ perfusion. However, if the clinical picture indicates renal dysfunction despite the fact that renal artery anatomy suggests adequate perfusion, careful evaluation of the anatomy should also be considered with the extent of iodinated contrast administered to the patient for evaluation and possible therapy. Intravascular ultrasound as an adjunct to planned angiographic intervention or therapy can be an invaluable tool in these patients for identifying the necessary anatomic configuration, real-time assessing the dynamic obstruction of the vessel orifices, and minimizing the administration of iodinated contrast.

It is generally accepted that the mortality of distal vascular compromise of aortic dissections can occur from treatment delays or missed diagnosis. Open surgical repair in these instances may be life saving; however, as interventional therapy improves, prospective and retrospective studies need to help delineate the optimal care of these very difficult patients.

REFERENCES

1. MRC European Carotid Surgery Trial: interim results for symptomatic patients with severe (70–99%) or with mild (0–29%) carotid stenosis. European Carotid Surgery Trialists' Collaborative Group. *Lancet* 1991;337:1235–1243.
2. North American Symptomatic Carotid Endarterectomy Trial. Methods, patient characteristics, and progress. *Stroke* 1991;22:711–720.
3. Endarterectomy for asymptomatic carotid artery stenosis. Executive Committee for the Asymptomatic Carotid Atherosclerosis Study. *JAMA* 1995;273:1421–1428.
4. Hobson 2nd RW, Goldstein JE, Jamil Z, et al. Carotid restenosis: operative and endovascular management. *J Vasc Surg* 1999;29:228–235; discussion, 235–238.
5. Eliasziw M, Streifler JY, Fox AJ, et al. Significance of plaque ulceration in symptomatic patients with high-grade carotid stenosis. North American Symptomatic Carotid Endarterectomy Trial. *Stroke* 1994;25:304–308.
6. Gertler JP, Cambria RP, Kistler JP, et al. Carotid surgery without arteriography: noninvasive selection of patients. *Ann Vasc Surg* 1991;5:253–256.
7. Barnett HJ, Taylor DW, Eliasziw M, et al. Benefit of carotid endarterectomy in patients with symptomatic moderate or severe stenosis. North American Symptomatic Carotid Endarterectomy Trial Collaborators. *N Engl J Med* 1998;339:1415–1425.
8. Biller J, Feinberg WM, Castaldo JE, et al. Guidelines for carotid endarterectomy: a statement for healthcare professionals from a special writing group of the Stroke Council, American Heart Association. *Circulation* 1998;97:501–509.
9. Bandyk DF, Schmitt DD, Seabrook GR, et al. Monitoring functional patency of *in situ* saphenous vein bypasses: the impact of a surveillance protocol and elective revision. *J Vasc Surg* 1989;9:286–296.
10. Dormandy JA, Rutherford RB. Management of peripheral arterial disease (PAD). TASC Working Group. TransAtlantic Inter-Society Concensus (TASC). *J Vasc Surg* 2000;31:S1–S296.
10a. Brewster DC, Perler BA, Robison JG, et al. Aortofemoral graft for multilevel occlusive disease. Predictors of success and need for distal bypass. *Arch Surg* 1982;117:1593–1600.
11. Crawford ES, Bomberger RA, Glaeser DH, et al. Aortoiliac occlusive disease: factors influencing survival and function following reconstructive operation over a twenty-five-year period. *Surgery* 1981;90:1055–1067.
12. Nevelsteen A, Wouters L, Suy R. Aortofemoral dacron reconstruction for aorto-iliac occlusive disease: a 25-year survey. *Eur J Vasc Surg* 1991;5:179–186.
13. Harris Jr EJ, Taylor Jr LM, McConnell DB, et al. Clinical results of axillobifemoral bypass using externally supported polytetrafluoroethylene. *J Vasc Surg* 1990;12:416–420; discussion, 420–421.
14. Passman MA, Taylor LM, Moneta GL, et al. Comparison of axillofemoral and aortofemoral bypass for aortoiliac occlusive disease. *J Vasc Surg* 1996;23:263–269, discussion, 269–271.
15. Criado E, Farber MA. Femorofemoral bypass: appropriate applica-

tion based on factors affecting outcome. *Semin Vasc Surg* 1997;10:34–41.
16. Taylor Jr LM, Edwards JM, Porter JM. Present status of reversed vein bypass grafting: five-year results of a modern series. *J Vasc Surg* 1990;11:193–205; discussion, 205–206.
17. Belkin M, Knox J, Donaldson MC, et al. Infrainguinal arterial reconstruction with nonreversed greater saphenous vein. *J Vasc Surg* 1996;24:957–962.
18. Sarac TP, Huber TS, Back MR, et al. Warfarin improves the outcome of infrainguinal vein bypass grafting at high risk for failure. *J Vasc Surg* 1998;28:446–457.
19. Gupta AK, Bandyk DF, Cheanvechai D, et al. Natural history of infrainguinal vein graft stenosis relative to bypass grafting technique. *J Vasc Surg* 1997;25:211–220; discussion, 220–225.
20. Quinones-Baldrich WJ, Prego AA, Ucelay-Gomez R, et al. Long-term results of infrainguinal revascularization with polytetrafluoroethylene: a ten-year experience. *J Vasc Surg* 1992;16:209–217.
21. Veith FJ, Gupta SK, Ascer E, et al. Six-year prospective multicenter randomized comparison of autologous saphenous vein and expanded polytetrafluoroethylene grafts in infrainguinal arterial reconstructions. *J Vasc Surg* 1986;3:104–114.
22. Sterpetti AV, Schultz RD, Feldhaus RJ, et al. Seven-year experience with polytetrafluoroethylene as above-knee femoropopliteal bypass graft. Is it worthwhile to preserve the autologous saphenous vein? *J Vasc Surg* 1985;2:907–912.
23. Vitti MJ, Thompson BW, Read RC, et al. Carotid–subclavian bypass: a twenty-two-year experience. *J Vasc Surg* 1994;20:411–417; discussion, 417–418.
24. Schardey HM, Meyer G, Rau HG, et al. Subclavian carotid transposition: an analysis of a clinical series and a review of the literature. *Eur J Vasc Endovasc Surg* 1996;12:431–436.
25. Hallett Jr JW, Naessens JM, Ballard DJ. Early and late outcome of surgical repair for small abdominal aortic aneurysms: a population-based analysis. *J Vasc Surg* 1993;18:684–691.
26. Mortality results for randomised controlled trial of early elective surgery or ultrasonographic surveillance for small abdominal aortic aneurysms. The UK Small Aneurysm Trial Participants. *Lancet* 1998;352:1649–1655.
27. Brown PM, Pattenden R, Vernooy C, et al. Selective management of abdominal aortic aneurysms in a prospective measurement program. *J Vasc Surg* 1996;23:213–220; discussion, 221–222.
28. Suzuki T, Mehta RH, Ince H, et al. Clinical profiles and outcomes of acute type B aortic dissection in the current era: lessons from the International Registry of Aortic Dissection (IRAD). *Circulation* 2003; 108[10 Suppl 1]:II312–II317.
29. Kaji S, Akasaka T, Katayama M, et al. Prognosis of retrograde dissection from the descending to the ascending aorta. *Circulation* 2003; 108[10 Suppl 1]:II300–II306.
30. Koschyk DH, Wolf W, Knap M, et al. Value of intravascular ultrasound for endovascular stent-graft placement in aortic dissection and aneurysm. *J Card Surg* 2003;18:471–477.
31. Lauterbach SR, Cambria RP, Brewster DC, et al. Contemporary management of aortic branch compromise resulting from acute aortic dissection. *J Vasc Surg* 2001;33:1185–1192.

CHAPTER 29

Stent Grafts for Abdominal Aortic Aneurysm

Zvonimir Krajcer

> **Key Points**
>
> - Surgical repair of abdominal aortic aneurysm (AAA) is the second most commonly performed vascular procedure in the United States.
> - Complications in elderly patients dramatically increase the perioperative death rate up to 60%.
> - Endovascular stent graft prosthesis for the treatment of AAA is receiving increasing attention as an alternative to standard surgical repair.
> - Endovascular treatment of AAA offers the potential to avoid significant morbidity and mortality associated with surgical repair.

EPIDEMIOLOGY OF ABDOMINAL AORTIC ANEURYSM

Abdominal aortic aneurysm (AAA) is a serious vascular disorder characterized by a permanent dilatation of the abdominal aorta having a diameter of at least 50% greater than normal. Men are five times more frequently affected than women (1,2). More than 90% of cases are secondary to atherosclerosis, and 89% are located in the infrarenal aorta (1–4).

The generally accepted diameter of AAA at which repair is indicated is 5 cm (1–5). There is a 90% mortality rate associated with an out-of-hospital AAA rupture, with the mortality rate decreasing to 50% for those who undergo emergency surgery (1–5).

To prevent this devastating event, more than 40,000 surgical repairs of AAA are performed in the United States annually, making this the second most commonly performed vascular surgical procedure (1). The current standard of treatment is replacement of the diseased aorta with a prosthetic graft. Surgical mortality in younger, asymptomatic patients undergoing elective resection is 3% to 5% (1).

Because of general anesthesia, large laparotomy, aortic clamping, and frequent need for blood transfusion, this procedure in an elderly population is associated with high morbidity. For patients with previous abdominal surgery, severe pulmonary, cardiovascular, or renal disease, the risk of perioperative death may be between 20% and 60%, and they may often be denied surgery because its risk exceeds the benefit (1,5,6). The prognosis of these patients denied surgery is poor, with 72% dying within 2 years, 43% of them from aneurysm rupture (6).

ENDOVASCULAR STENT GRAFT SYSTEMS

In the last decade, no area of treatment of peripheral vascular disease has attracted more enthusiasm than has the endovascular exclusion of AAA. It is estimated that as of year 2003, well more than 60,000 endoluminal AAA repairs had been performed with various stent graft devices worldwide. The use of stent grafts for endoluminal repair of AAA captured the interest of vascular surgeons, interventional radiologists, and interventional cardiologists. Whereas grafting had previously been the domain of the vascular surgeon, more recent developments in transcatheter delivery of vascular prostheses allowed nonsurgical specialties to use these devices for treatment of a variety of vascular defects.

The first endoluminal treatment of AAA in a clinical setting was introduced in 1990 and reported in 1991 by Parodi et al. (7). Initially, these devices were used in patients with comorbid illnesses or other conditions that increased the risk of conventional surgical procedure (7). More recently, the use of endoluminal grafts has been proposed for patients without comorbid illnesses (8–13).

Because endovascular stent grafting is minimally invasive procedure and therefore avoids these risks, it has gained increasing popularity with both physicians and patients. Although the technology is still in its infancy, substantial improvements have been recently made in the design and delivery of stent grafts.

The first-generation endovascular grafts were tubular grafts. Later aortouniiliac, one-piece, and bifurcated construction was introduced. The early prostheses were relatively inflexible and required a femoral artery sheath of 24 French or larger internal diameter (7). They are now more flexible and available in smaller diameters (14–20). Endovascular stent grafts have been developed to avoid major abdominal surgery and the related morbidity and mortality (21,22). The lower degree of invasiveness of endovascular stent grafts is particularly important because of coexisting morbid conditions in many patients presenting with AAA, and provides a therapeutic alternative for those who are not surgical candidates. Although long-term success of endoluminal stent grafts has yet to be demonstrated, a growing number of manufacturers and clinicians continue to evaluate the ever-expanding number of stent grafts.

Design Characteristics of Stent Grafts

Various graft designs and configurations have been tested in the laboratory and in clinical trials. The degree to which endovascular grafts differ from the characteristics of a surgically placed graft vary widely with respect to method and mechanism of fixation, mechanical properties of the stent graft, graft material, anatomic configuration, and delivery systems.

Stainless steel or nitinol stent technology has been used in conjunction with various graft materials, such as polyester (Dacron), and polytetrafluoroethylene (PTFE). All endovascular stent graft devices, however, fall within one of three categories: unibody in bifurcated design, modular (multicomponent), and aortomonoiliac. The last is combined with surgical placement of femoral–femoral crossover prosthesis and occlusion of the contralateral iliac artery.

What could be considered the ideal endovascular stent graft is in a state of evolution. The advantages and disadvantages of current endoluminal grafts are under debate and will probably remain debated for a number of years. Guidelines for the development, reporting standards, and use of endografts was established by the Endovascular Graft Committee, with input from the Society of Vascular Surgery, the International Society for Cardiovascular Surgery, and the Society of Cardiovascular and Interventional Radiology (23,24).

There are currently three commercially available endograft systems in the United States.

Ancure Device

The Ancure device (Fig. 29.1) is a unibody, unsupported graft, which means that the entire device is loaded on a

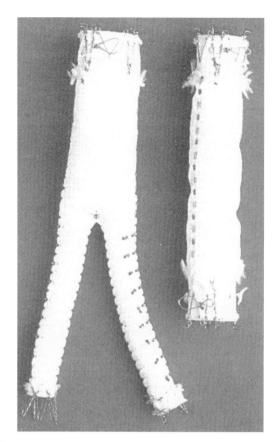

FIG. 29.1. The Ancure bifurcated and tube graft systems. (Courtesy of Guidant Corp., Menlo Park, CA.)

delivery system and there is no structural support of the woven polyester graft fabric. This device was available in bifurcated, and aortoiliac configurations. The main device was delivered through a 24 French introducer sheath, and a 12 French sheath was required to facilitate the deployment of the contralateral limb in the bifurcated device. A snaring maneuver of the wire that was incorporated in the delivery device is used for contralateral limb deployment.

The attachment system includes four independent V-shaped hooks, which penetrate the arterial wall for fixation. There are separate attachments at the proximal and distal ends of the graft. The hooks are positioned transmurally and are affixed by low-pressure balloon dilatation, which is incorporated in the delivery device. The radiopaque markers are located on the body of the graft for correct alignment and positioning. The use of the unibody design eliminates the endoleaks that can originate in the overlaps between various components of modular endografts. Tortuous anatomy and narrowed, calcified iliac arteries, however, can make the deployment of this stiff, one-piece system very difficult. Several investigators have reported that fewer than 30% of patients who were referred to their institutions for endoluminal AAA repair were candidates for the Ancure device (25–29).

This adds to the complexity and the duration of the procedure. Because of the increasing number of clinical

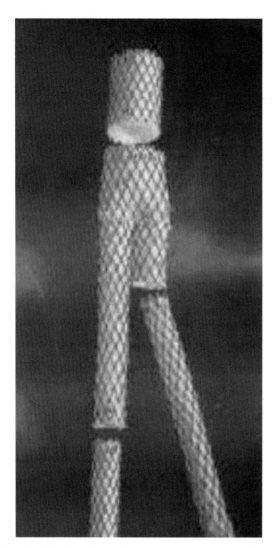

FIG. 29.2. The AneuRx modular stent graft system. (Courtesy of Medtronic AVE, Sunnyvale, CA.)

complications with Ancure, in April 2001 the manufacturer announced a voluntary recall of the endograft and halted the production until these problems were resolved. This device was again released for clinical use in August 2001, but in July 2003, Guidant voluntarily halted production of the stent graft system and withdrew it from the market because of in-

creased competition after the release of two new endograft systems.

AneuRx

The AneuRx device (Fig. 29.2) is a bifurcated, modular, fully supported stent graft with nitinol exoskeleton, which is lined with a thin-walled polyester fabric. The self-expanding nitinol exoskeleton provides flexibility and strength and is easily visible under fluoroscopy. Distinct radiopaque markers are located at critical endpoints to facilitate visualization of various endograft components during deployment. The two-piece system consists of a main bifurcation segment, which is housed in a 21 French delivery device, and a contralateral limb, which is housed in a 16 French delivery device. Aortic fixation of this endograft is accomplished by radial force at the attachment sites, which causes a frictional seal. The aortic neck of the bifurcated stent graft ranges from 20 to 28 mm in diameter and from 13.5 to 16.5 cm in length. The iliac limb ranges from 12 to 16 mm in diameter and from 8.5 cm to 11 cm in length. Additional modular components include aortic and iliac extender cuffs. The iliac and aortic extender cuffs allow the user to make the appropriate length adjustments by overlapping these components with already deployed segments until the AAA is completely excluded from the arterial circulation.

Description of Other Stent Graft Devices

There are several other stent graft devices that are currently being investigated and two systems that have received recent Food and Drug Administration (FDA) approval (Table 29.1). Many of the various endograft designs incorporate a nitinol framework for support and some degree of radial force for anchoring. This is seen in the Talent (World Medical/Medtronic, Sunrise, FL), and EXCLUDER (Gore, Sunnyvale, CA).

Zenith

The Zenith graft (Cook, Inc., Bloomington, IN), which is the most recent stent graft system to be approved for use, is a fully

TABLE 29.1. *Types of stent grafts*

Device (company)	Stent type	Deployment mode	Graft material[a]	Means of attachment	Special features
Zenith (Cook)	Barbed Gianturco Z stent	Self-expanding	Woven noncrimped Dacron	Barbs, active fixation	Full support
AneuRx (Medtronic)	Nitinol	Self-expanding	Lightweight woven Dacron	Friction radial force	Full support modular
Talent (Medtronic)	Nitinol	Self-expanding	Lightweight Dacron	Friction radial force	Full support modular
Excluder (Gore)	Nitinol	Self-expanding	ePTFE	Friction radial force	Full support Full support
PowerLink (Endologix, Bard)	Elgiloy wire	Self-expanding	ePTFE	Friction radial force	Full support, Y-design

[a]ePTFE, Expanded polytetrafluoroethylene.

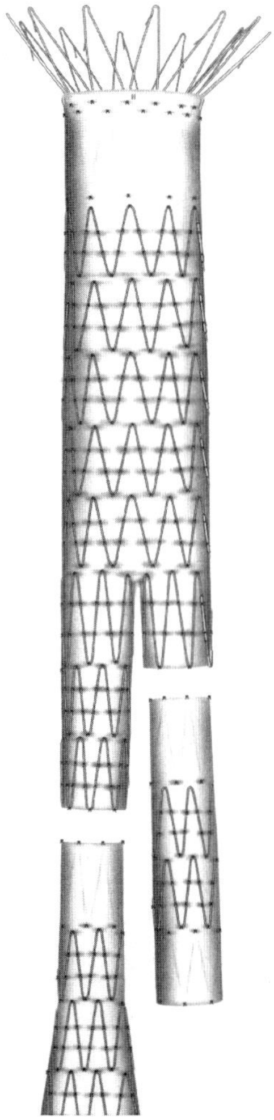

FIG. 29.3. The Zenith abdominal aortic aneurysm endovascular graft bifurcated three-component system. (Courtesy of Cook, Inc., Bloomington, IN.)

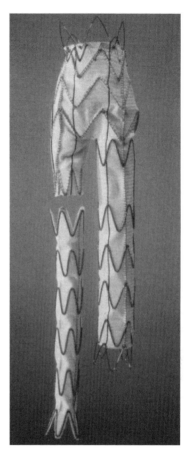

FIG. 29.4. The Talent graft. (Courtesy of World Medical/ Medtronic, Sunrise, FL.)

supported, modular, bifurcated system, which incorporates a polyester fabric on a network of Z-stents (Fig. 29.3). This endograft utilizes a series of suprarenal barbs, which, when released, are designed to mimic a surgical anastomosis. A study of 528 patients treated with the Zenith endograft reported successful implantation in all but 4 patients (18). The study also reported an overall endoleak rate of 15%, with 4% of those patients requiring urgent treatment. At 2 years, there were eight endograft migrations, three late conversions, and two ruptures.

Talent

The Talent graft (World Medical/Medtronic, Sunrise, FL) is a self-expanding, modular stent graft system composed of serpentine-shaped nitinol stents inlaid in woven polyester fabric (Fig. 29.4). The stents are spaced along a full-length nitinol spine, which provides longitudinal strength to an otherwise flexible graft that can accommodate tortuous aortoiliac angulations. The delivery system is composed of a

coaxial sheath with an internal pusher rod and a compliant polyurethane balloon, which is sequentially inflated to maximize apposition of the graft to the vessel wall. The main bifurcated component is configured with a 15-mm-long, uncovered stent at the proximal end to allow transrenal or suprarenal fixation. In the phase I and II clinical trials, the 30-day technical success rate was 96%. The Talent stent graft is the only device capable of addressing AAA necks larger than 28 mm in diameter (15,29). To the date of this writing this stent graft has not been released for clinical use.

EXCLUDER

The EXCLUDER endograft (Gore and Associates, Sunnyvale, CA) was approved for use in November 2002 and is a self-expanding modular component system. The EXCLUDER consists of expanded PTFE on the luminal surface and a nitinol-supporting frame on the outer surface (Fig. 29.5). The components are premounted on separate delivery catheters and constrained using lacing suture, which courses the length of the catheter and is attached to a deployment knob at the operator end. When the knob is loosened and pulled back, it releases the suture and the stent graft component expands immediately. A 18 French sheath is used to

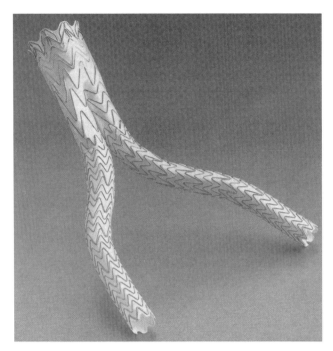

FIG. 29.5. The 20 French bifurcated EXCLUDER endoprosthesis. (Courtesy of W.L. Gore and Associates, Sunnyvale, CA.)

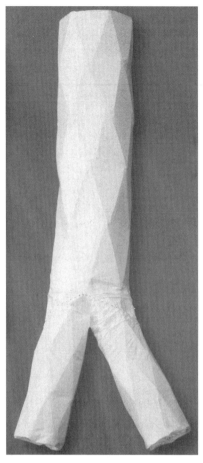

FIG. 29.6. The PowerLink. (Courtesy of Endologix, Irvine, CA.)

advance the bifurcated aortic, and a 12 French is used for the contralateral limb.

The PowerLink System

The PowerLink System (Endologix, Irvine, CA) is a self-expanding, unibody, bifurcated endograft (Fig. 29.6). The cage is made of single-wire stainless steel that are interconnected without the use of sutures. This endoskeleton is covered by extremely strong PTFE material and is delivered through a 21 French delivery system. The device is available for infrarenal and suprarenal fixation, with wide variety of neck and limb diameters.

The PowerLink has been tested in almost 500 patients worldwide and is currently being studied in phase II FDA trial in the United States. Thus far, in phase II trial report revealed a 98% success rate and a 30-day endoleak rate of 2%. There have been no deaths related to this device (22,23).

EndoFit

The EndoFit system (ENDOMED, Inc., Phoenix, AZ) is in phase I clinical trials. It is also a self-expanding stent graft, which is loaded over a vascular dilator and inside an introducer cartridge. The stent graft consists of two layers of expanded PTFE, which encapsulate individual nitinol wire stents. This system can accommodate larger proximal neck diameters than the other systems and has suprarenal fixation.

It is intended for use in patients with AAA, and thoracic aneurysms.

IMAGING TECHNOLOGY FOR DETERMINING PATIENT SELECTION

The simplest and most inexpensive noninvasive test available to confirm the presence of AAA is abdominal ultrasound. This test has been shown to be a reliable method of evaluation before contemplating a surgical AAA repair (9,34). Spiral computed tomography (CT) with three-dimensional reconstruction with intravenous contrast injection has been an essential method of preprocedural and postprocedural evaluation after endovascular AAA repair (9,34) (Fig. 29.7). This evaluation is of great benefit for determining whether iliac arteries are of adequate size to accommodate the endoprosthesis and whether any interventional procedure such as percutaneous transluminal angioplasty and/or stenting is necessary prior to the endovascular repair.

Preoperative preparation for endovascular AAA repair is essentially different from the open surgical repair. Correct selection of the diameter and length of the endograft is a key factor in minimizing most common complications

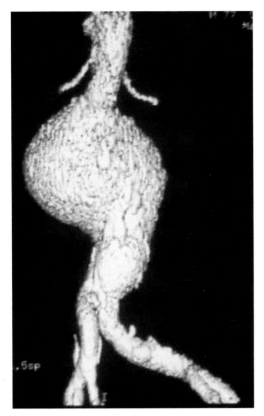
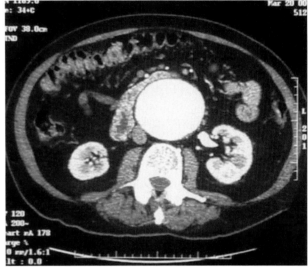

FIG. 29.7. A spiral computed tomographic image scan with three-dimensional reconstruction, with contrast of the abdomen and pelvis, revealing a large abdominal aortic aneurysm with appropriate length and diameter of the infrarenal neck and iliac arteries.

related to endovascular repair, which are graft-related endoleaks and stent graft migration. The successful implantation of endografts is predicated on sophisticated preoperative evaluation utilizing a combination of spiral CT scanning, three-dimensional reconstruction, and contrast arteriography with calibrated marker catheter. CT scanning produces axial "cuts" or slices, allowing accurate measurement of anatomic structures. CT scanning, however, is unsuitable for length sizing because of the underestimation of necessary length sizing of the endograft. Therefore, length sizing of the aorta and iliac arteries is most accurately performed using a calibrated marker catheter and contrast arteriography.

RESULTS OF ENDOLUMINAL REPAIR OF ABDOMINAL AORTIC ANEURYSM WITH ANCURE STENT GRAFT

Since Parodi's initial report, several studies have shown that endovascular treatment of AAAs can be preformed safely, resulting in lower morbidity rates and equal or lower mortality rates than with open surgical repair (8–13).

Of the 870 patients enrolled in the phase I and II clinical trials with Ancure endograft, deployment was successful in 96% of the cases, and mortality rates were similar to those concurrently enrolled to open surgical repair. In those same patients, 2.7% had type I endoleaks at 1 year and 1.3% had type I endoleaks at 2 years (25). The manufacturer has reported, however, observation of a 20% incidence of type II endoleak (branch flow) after 2 years of follow-up. The reduction of maximal diameter of the aneurysm in this study was seen in 51% of patients at 1 year and in 69% at 2 years. Interestingly, 13% of patients showed evidence of proximal neck enlargement, and that proportion increased to 21% at 2 years. The presence of endoleak, neck length, and aneurysm size, however, had no clear effect of neck enlargement (25). Conversion rates to an open surgical repair with the Ancure, however, have been higher than those associated with other devices, presumably due to technical complexities with the deployment of this device. To the date of this writing, there are no reports of aneurysm rupture with the current generation of this device (25). Several problems with the system have been identified, and include delivery system problems, kinking or external compression of the unsupported material, and narrowing in areas of atherosclerotic disease, which leads to graft thrombosis. To prevent this complication, the interventionists must frequently perform balloon angioplasty throughout the entire endograft and also place self-expandable stents in both iliac limbs.

RESULTS OF ENDOLUMINAL REPAIR OF ABDOMINAL AORTIC ANEURYSM WITH ANEURX STENT GRAFT

In a multicenter clinical trial, nearly 1,200 patients were treated with the AneuRx stent graft (14). The technical success rate in the AneuRx phase II clinical trial in 405 patients was 97.6% (14). The serious adverse events were 50% less frequent in the stent graft group than in the surgical group. In the AneuRx trial, the stent graft group had shorter duration of anesthesia, shorter duration of the procedure, less blood loss, less requirement for blood transfusion, shorter duration to endotracheal extubation, shorter time to unassisted ambulation, and earlier resumption of normal diet than a surgical group. Kaplan–Meier analysis of clinical trials patients treated with the AneuRx device revealed survival rate at 1 year was 93%, at 2 years was 88%, and at 3 years was 86%. The perioperative mortality was not different between the AneuRx and surgical groups; however, the late mortality was lower in the stent graft Group (14).

The same analysis showed that freedom from conversion to open repair was 98% at 1 year, 97% at 2 years, and 93% at 3 years. The freedom from secondary procedures was 94% at 1 year, 92% at 2 years, and 88% at 3 years. The incidence of endoleak after 4 years of follow-up in phase II clinical trial for AneuRx patients was 13.7%. These findings are of considerable concern because endoleak can lead to AAA expansion and rupture, and they clearly indicate a failure of the procedure. There were 10 (0.8%) ruptures reported among AneuRx phase II and III clinical trial patients. The incidence of AAA rupture reported among 36,000 patients with AneuRx stent graft worldwide is 0.22%.

RESULTS OF PERCUTANEOUS REPAIR OF ABDOMINAL AORTIC ANEURYSM WITH ANEURX STENT GRAFT

One limiting factor for the use of the current generation of stent grafts is their large-bore delivery devices, which require open surgical access to the femoral artery, and general or epidural anesthesia. This increases the invasiveness of the procedure and the risk of complications.

In 1996, we showed that endoluminal repair of AAA can be safely performed in the cardiac catheterization laboratory, with the use of Wallstent PTFE stent graft, local anesthesia, and 16 French sheath (21,22).

In an effort to decrease the invasiveness of this procedure, a technique was developed to percutaneously repair femoral artery entry sites after enduluminal repair of AAAs for large-bore sheaths. This was achieved with the use of a Prostar XL (Perclose, Inc., Redwood City, CA) percutaneous suture device and a 16 French sheath under local anesthesia in a cardiac catheterization lab (Fig. 29.8) (35,36). Between October 1995 and May 1998, 33 high-risk patients for surgical repair underwent infrarenal AAA exclusion with this device (21).

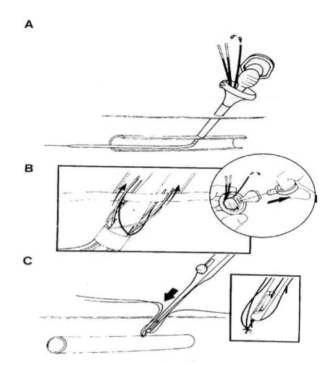

FIG. 29.8. The Prostar XL surgical suture method of areriotomy closure. (Courtesy of Perclose, Inc., Redwood City, CA.)

PERCUTANEOUS FEMORAL ARTERY ACCESS AND CLOSURE FOR ENDOLUMINAL REPAIR OF ABDOMINAL AORTIC ANEURYSM WITH ANEURX STENT GRAFT

Through December 2003, a total of 659 endoluminal AAA repairs had been performed at our institution. Percutaneous access and closure of the common femoral artery (CFA) after placement of the bifurcated component to deliver the AneuRx, Excluder and Zenith stent graft was performed in the last 195 patients. Percutaneous access and closure of the CFA after placement of a contralateral limb was performed in 98% of patients. The bilateral closure technique was successfully accomplished in 94.4% of patients. Figures 29.9A–D show the Perclose technique with 16 and 22 French sheaths.

The bilateral CFA access and closure technique has significantly shortened patient anesthesia time, intubation time, and procedure time. It has also reduced blood loss, need for transfusion, and number of groin complications compared with open femoral artery access and repair.

ENDOLUMINAL REPAIR OF ABDOMINAL AORTIC ANEURYSM IN HIGH-RISK PATIENTS

Of 475 patients treated with AneuRx stent graft for AAA repair at our institution, 58% were American Society of Anesthesiologists grade IV. This group was considered a high surgical risk. The majority (73%) of the patients were

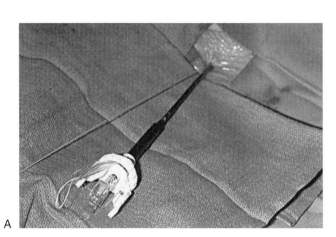

A

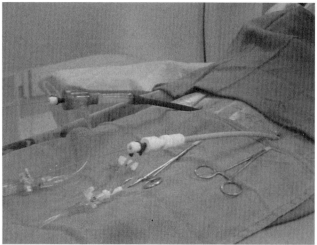

B

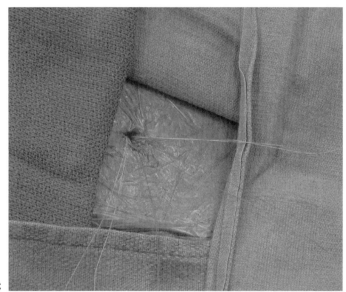

C

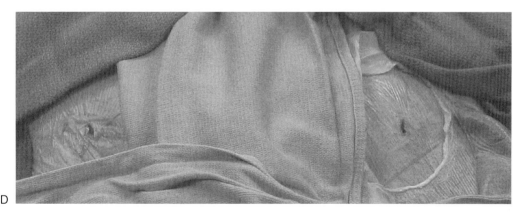

D

FIG. 29.9. A: The Prostar XL (Perclose, Inc., Redwood City, CA) is deployed prior to inserting the 16F sheath. **B:** A 22 French sheath with the CheckFlow valve (Cook, Inc., Bloomington, IN.) in the right femoral artery and a 16 French extra large introducer in the left femoral artery. **C:** After completion of the procedure, the sheath is pulled and the ProstarXL sutures are tied with a sliding knot technique. **D:** After the repair of bilateral arterial access sites.

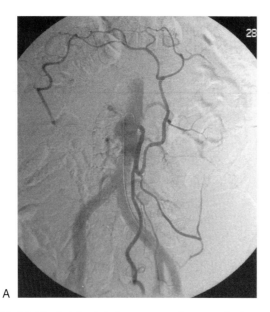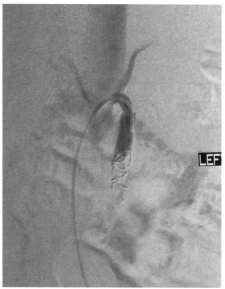

A   B

FIG. 29.10. A: The inferior mesenteric artery before exclusion. **B:** Occluded inferior mesenteric artery after coil embolization.

men, 44% had history of previous myocardial infarction, 39% had congestive heart failure, 23% had chronic renal failure and 23% had a "hostile abdomen." Procedural success was 99.2%. Complications include 1 patient who suffered non-Q myocardial infarction 24 hours after successful AAA exclusion and 1 patient who went for elective surgical repair 1 week after attempted endovascular exclusion because of an inability to advance the AneuRx device through the tortuous anatomy. There was no in-hospital or 30-day mortality, rupture, or surgical conversion. The mean length of hospital stay was 2.3 ± 3.3 days. On follow-up (15 ± 7 months), 10 late deaths occurred; none were device related or due to aneurysm rupture. This study revealed that endoluminal repair of AAA with AneuRx stent graft in high-risk patients offers a high procedural success rate and a very low complication rate.

PRESENT CONCERNS AND FUTURE IMPLICATIONS

Several aspects of endovascular grafting for AAAs have improved. Better imaging techniques, more experienced endovascular interventionalists, and enhanced device technology have facilitated more accurate endograft placement. The frequency of open surgical approach will continue to decline as other minimally invasive techniques such as laparoscopy-assisted and minilaparotomy incisions for AAA repair are refined.

As experience has been gained, a variety of difficulties have been encountered, including fabric erosion, fractures of stents grafts perforations, and graft rupture resulting in death. Such difficulties have tempered the enthusiasm of investigators, who have become reluctant to use endograft technology in younger or asymptomatic patients without comorbid conditions. Unlike the surgical patient, in whom the follow-up after resection and graft placement is minimal, those who receive endografts require closer long-term surveillance.

ENDOLEAK

Perigraft flow or endoleak, defined as flow outside the graft lumen, but contained within the aneurysm, is the most common complication of stent graft repair. They are classified into four types: (I) proximal or distal perigraft leak, usually related to poor attachment or seal; (II) collateral backflow, usually related to patent inferior mesenteric or lumbar arteries into the aneurismal sac; (III) fabric tear, poor seal, or modular disconnection; and (IV) graft-wall fabric porosity. Proximal or distal endoleaks occur at the respective ends of the device because of suboptimal sealing of the stent graft at the aortic or iliac segments. This can occur if the device is

FIG. 29.11. A: Aortogram immediately post exclusion. **B:** Aortogram 2 years post exclusion, revealing type III endoleak due to separation of the aortic extension cuff and the bifurcated segment of the AneuRx stent graft. **C:** Fluroscopy of the AneuRx stent graft in the lateral orientation. Modular separation and misalignment between the aortic cuff (*A*) and the upper portion of the bifurcated stent graft (*B*) is seen. Severe deformity and misalignment of the upper portion of the bifurcated segment in relation to the lower portion of the bifurcated segment can be seen (*C*).

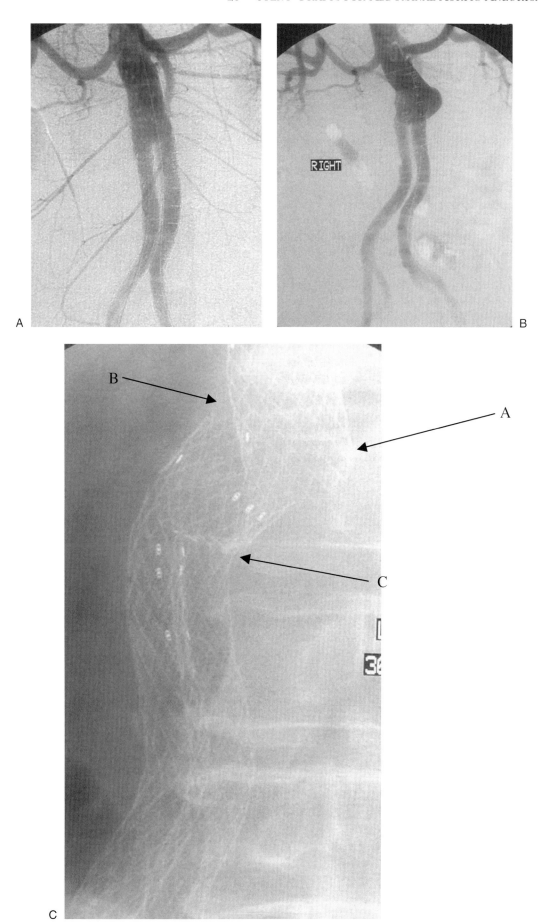

undersized in relationship to the aorta or iliac arteries. It can also be due to presence of severe tortuosity, calcifications, or thrombus in these regions. Type I endoleaks can be avoided by appropriate CT measurements prior to the procedure (Fig. 29.7). Collateral backflow to the aneurysm is a relatively common and bothersome occurrence after stent graft procedure. It can be avoided by preprocedural coil embolization of a large inferior mesenteric or lumbar artery (Fig. 29.10). Type II endoleak can be the best visualized on spiral CT. It usually opacifies through iliolumbar arteries or through the marginal artery of Drummond (a communication between the superior mesenteric and the inferior mesenteric arteries) (Fig. 29.10). Coil embolization of these branches can be a cumbersome and time-consuming procedure. The interventionist has to pay attention to anatomic findings because occlusion of these arteries can cause ischemic bowel injury. Fabric tear, modular disconnection, or poor seal can be treated with balloon angioplasty and placement of additional modular components (aortic or iliac extension cuffs) (Fig. 29.11).

The importance of endoleak stems from the realization that a persistent leak into the native aneurysm can potentate aneurysm growth and increase intraaneurysmal pressure, both of which can result in AAA rupture and death (37). Because of a considerable risk of endoleak with the current generation of stent graft devices and the potential risk of AAA rupture, this procedure should be reserved for patients who are at high risk for a conventional surgical repair and have AAAs that are larger than 5 cm in maximal diameter.

Further refinements in the design and the size of these devices are needed to expand the indications of this procedure. The future efforts to reduce the size of the delivery devices will offer the opportunity to repair the great majority of AAAs with the use of local anesthesia and percutaneous techniques.

REFERENCES

1. Chen JC, Hildebrand HD, Salvin AJ, et al. Predictors of death in ruptured and non-ruptured abdominal aortic aneurysms. *J Vasc Surg* 1996;24:491–499.
2. Johnston KW, Scobie TF. Canadian Society for Vascular Surgery Study Group. Nonruptured abdominal aortic aneurysm: six-year follow-up results from the multicenter prospective Canadian aneurysm study. *J Vasc Surgery* 1994;20:163–170.
3. Lawrence PF, Gozak C, Bhirangi L, et al. The epidemiology of surgically repaired aneurysms in the United States. *J Vasc Surg* 1999;30:632–640.
4. Ernst CB. Abdominal aortic aneurysm. *N Engl J Med* 1993;328:1167–1173.
5. Dardik A, Lin JW, Gordon TA, et al. Results of elective abdominal aortic aneurysm repair in the 1990's: a population based analysis of 2335 cases. *J Vasc Surg* 1999;30:985–995.
6. Zarins CK, Haris EJ. Operative repair for aortic aneurysms: the gold standard. *J Endovasc Surg* 1997;4:232–241.
7. Parodi JC, Palmaz JC, Barone HD. Transfemoral intraluminal graft implantation for abdominal aortic aneurysms. *Ann Vasc Surg* 1991;5:491–499.
8. Krajcer Z, Howell M. Update on endovascular treatment of peripheral vascular disease: new tools, techniques, and indications. *Tex Heart J* 2000;27:369–385.
9. Beebe HG. Imaging modalities for aortic endografting. *J Endovasc Surg* 1997;4:111–123.
10. Balm R, Eikleboom BC, van Leewen MS, et al. Spiral CT-angiography of the aorta. *Eur J Vasc Surg* 1994;8:544–551.
11. May J, White GH, Yu W, et al. Concurrent comparison of endoluminal repair versus no treatment for small abdominal aortic aneurysms. *Eur J Vasc Endovasc Surg* 1997;13:472–476.
12. Moore WS, for the EVT Investigators. The EVT tube and bifurcated endograft systems: technical considerations and clinical summary. *J Endovasc Surg* 1997;4:182–194.
13. Zarins C, White R, Schwarten D, et al. AneuRx stent graft versus open surgical repair of abdominal aortic aneurysms: multicenter prospective clinical trial. *J Vasc Surg* 1999;29:292–308.
14. Zarins CK, White RA, Moll FL, et al. The AneuRx stent graft: four-year results and worldwide experience 2000. *J Vasc Surg* 2001;33:S135–S145.
15. Craido FJ, Wilson EP, Fairman RM, et al. Update on the Talent aortic stent-graft: a preliminary report from United States phase I and II trials. *J Vasc Surg* 2001;33:S146–S149.
16. Matsummura JS, Katzen BT, Hollier LH, et al. Update on the bifurcated EXCLUDER endoprosthesis: phase I results. *J Vasc Surg* 2001;33:S150–S153.
17. White RA. Clinical and design update on the development and testing of a one-piece, bifurcated, polytetrafluoroethylene endovascular graft for abdominal aortic aneurysm exclusion: the Endologix device. *J Vasc Surg* 2001;33:S154–S156.
18. Greenberg RK, Lawrence-Brown M, Bhandari G, et al. An update of the Zenith endovascular graft for abdominal aortic aneurysms: initial implantation and mid-term follow-up data. *J Vasc Surg* 2001;33:S157–S164.
19. May J, White GH, Waugh R, et al. Improved survival after endoluminal repair with second generation prostheses compared with open repair in the treatment of abdominal aortic aneurysms: a 5-year concurrent comparison using life table method. *J Vasc Surg* 2001;33:S21–S26.
20. Bush RL, Lumsden AB, Dodson TF, et al. Mid-term results after endovascular repair of the abdominal aortic aneurysm. *J Vasc Surg* 2001;33:S70–S76.
21. Krajcer Z, Diethrich E. Successful endoluminal repair of arterial aneurysms by Wallstent prosthesis and PTFE graft: preliminary results with a new technique. *J Endovasc Surg* 1997;4:80–87.
22. Howell M, Zaqua M, Villareal R, et al. Endoluminal exclusion of abdominal aortic aneurysms: initial experience with stent-grafts in cardiology practice. *Tex Heart Inst J* 2000;27:136–145.
23. Veith FJ, Abbott WM, Yao JST, et al. Guidelines for the development and use of transluminally placed endovascular prosthetic grafts in the arterial system. *J Vasc Surg* 1995;21:670–685.
24. Ahn SS. Reporting standards for infrarenal endovascular abdominal aortic aneurysm repair. Ad Hoc Committee for Standardized Reporting Practices in Vascular Surgery of the Society for Vascular Surgery/International Society for Cardiovascular Surgery. *J Vasc Surg* 1997;25:405–410.
25. Makaroun MS. The Ancure endografting system: an update. *J Vasc Surg* 2001,33:S129–S134.
26. Makaroun MS, Deaton DH, for the Endovascular Technologies Investigators. Is proximal aortic neck dilatation after endovascular aneurysm exclusion a cause for concern? *J Vasc Surg* 2001;33:S39–S45.
27. Cuypers PW, Laheij RJ, Buth J. Which factors increase the risk of conversion to open surgery following endovascular abdominal aortic aneurysm repair? The EUROSTAR Collaborators. *Eur J Vasc Endovasc Surg* 2000;20:183–189.
28. Buth J, Laheij RJF, on behalf of the EUROSTAR Collaborators. Early complications and endoleaks after endovascular abdominal aortic aneurysm repair: report of a multicenter study. *J Vasc Surg* 2000;31:134–146.
29. Velazquez OC, Larson RA, Baum RA, et al. Gender-related differences in infrarenal aortic aneurysm morphpologic features: issues relevant to Ancure and Talent endografts. *J Vasc Surg* 2001;33:S77–S84.
30. Beebe HG, Cronenwett JL, Katzen BT, et al. Results of an aortic endograft trial: impact of device failure beyond 12 months. *J Vasc Surg* 2001;33:S55–S63.
31. Hölzenbein TJ, Kretschmer G, Thurnher S, et al. Midterm durability of abdominal aortic aneurysm endograft repair: a word of caution. *J Vasc Surg* 2001;33:S46–S54.

32. Deithrich EB. AAA stent grafts: current developments. *J Invasive Cardiol* 2001;5:383–390.
33. White RA. Clinical and design update on the development and testing of a one-piece, bifurcated, polytetrafluoroethylene endovascular graft for abdominal aortic aneurysm exclusion: the Endologix device. *J Vasc Surg* 2001;33:S154–S156.
34. Prinssen M, Wever JJ, Mali WP, et al. Concerns for the durability of the proximal abdominal aortic aneurysm endograft fixation from a 2-year and 3-year longitudinal computed tomography angiography study. *J Vasc Sirg* 2001;33:S64–S69.
35. White RA, Donayre CE, Walot I, et al. Computed tomography assessment of abdominal aortic aneurysm morphology after endograft exclusion. *J Vasc Surg* 2001;33:S1–S10.
36. Krajcer Z, Howell M. A novel technique using the Percutaneous Vascular Surgery Device to close the 22 French femoral artery entry site used for percutaneous abdominal aortic aneurysm exclusion. *Cathet Cardiovasc Interv* 2000;50:356–360.
37. Howell M, Villareal R, Krajcer Z. Percutaneous access and closure of femoral artery access sites associated with endoluminal repair of abdominal aortic aneurysms. *J Endovasc Ther* 2001;8:68–74.

CHAPTER 30

Surgical Treatment in Peripheral Vascular Disease and Foot Care Management

Zeeshan S. Husain, Charles G. Kissel, and Michael S. Schey

Key Points

- Lower extremity reconstruction and management in the vascular-compromised patient are implemented to preserve bipedal ambulation.
- Noninvasive vascular studies are a quick, cheaper alternative to arteriograms to determine whether revascularization is necessary.
- The diabetic patient population is prone to neuropathy, and wound healing may be compromised due to peripheral vascular disease.
- Almost 80% of all amputations begin with foot ulcerations.
- Noninfective osteolytic and arthritic changes can make osteomyelitis difficult to diagnose accurately.
- The goal of amputation is to remove nonviable tissue while retaining the greatest amount of function as possible.
- Brain and spinal cord lesions due to stroke, tumor, degenerative process, trauma, or birth injury affect lower extremity function.
- Recognition of early clinical signs is vital to preserving bipedal ambulation.

INTRODUCTION

The goal of lower extremity reconstruction and management in vascular-compromised patients is to preserve bipedal ambulation. Thirty thousand major lower extremity amputations are performed in the United States annually, with a significant number of these patients having peripheral vascular disease (PVD) and ulcerations often related to diabetes mellitus (1). Neuropathic and ischemic ulcers frequently lead to pedal infections requiring amputation for treatment. Skin grafts, local tissue transfers, partial foot, midfoot and rearfoot amputations, and joint fusions are salvage attempts to preserve lower extremities and their function before a below-knee amputation is needed. Often, patients with poor lower extremity circulation can have concurrent neuropathy, mostly secondary to diabetes mellitus, making these patients at high risk for developing ulcerations prone to osteomyelitis. Revascularization is often essential for successful conservative and surgical management of the foot and ankle complications associated with PVD.

COMMON PITFALLS WITH NONINVASIVE TESTING OF PERIPHERAL VASCULAR DISEASE IN PEDAL PATHOLOGY

Reliance on classic intermittent claudication (IC) symptoms may be misleading and may grossly underestimate the prevalence of IC (2). Achy, progressive pain in one or both lower extremities occurring with exertion and resolving with rest are the typical symptoms used, but these symptoms may not be realized in neuropathic patients. Noninvasive studies used alone in patients exhibiting signs of peripheral arterial disease (PAD) have shown poor correlation (3,4). Still, noninvasive studies are the primary diagnostic tools in patients with diabetes mellitus (DM); atherosclerosis; claudication; signs of critical ischemia; skin changes, or gangrene; absent or diminished pedal pulses; or femoral bruits (5,6). PAD frequently progresses to significant tissue ischemia, ulceration, or necrosis. Patients with lower extremity PAD symptoms, without more dramatic atherosclerotic disease like coronary artery disease, tend to receive less intensive treatment of atherosclerotic risk factors despite studies showing diminished 5-year survival rates due to concomitant generalized cardiovascular involvement (7,8). Failure to identify these patients and treat PAD effectively may prevent patients from receiving potentially beneficial therapies in the office setting before more complex and risky interventions become necessary.

Noninvasive studies are extremely valuable in assessing PAD of the lower extremities, but there are specific limitations that should be noted. Medial calcinosis or Mönckeberg's sclerosis (calcification of the tunica media that does not narrow the lumen, but causes artery stiffening), atherosclerosis (calcification in the lumen and media of the artery, causing stiffness), fear, anxiety, cold, discomfort, and an ill-fitting pressure cuff can all lead to falsely elevated ankle–brachial indicies (ABI) despite 71.2% sensitivity, 91.3% specificity, and 48.7% positive predictive value (9–11). Table 30.1 correlates the range of ischemic symptoms and pathology. High ABI values can give a false sense of security if not confirmed by another noninvasive test. An ABI of 1.0 with a good flow pattern in the dorsalis pedis and posterior tibial arteries only document adequacy at the ankle level. There still may be distal occlusions or perfusion problems. If a patient has a history of claudication and a normal ABI, then the patient should be evaluated by treadmill exercise to unmask arterial lesions that are not flow limiting at rest, but become evident as flow demand increases. Systolic toe pressures are not affected by medial calcinosis and provide a more accurate depiction of digital skin perfusion. An algorithm has been developed for the use of noninvasive vascular testing in assessing the healing potential of foot ulcers (Fig. 30.1).

Prior to surgical intervention, lower extremity vascular studies are paramount. Noninvasive vascular studies are a quick, cheaper alternative to arteriograms to determine whether revascularization is necessary. An ABI below 0.45 is typically used as a cutoff in determining when revascular-

ization is indicated. Other positive predictors include serum albumin (greater than 3.0 g per dL) to measure tissue nutrition and total lymphocyte count (greater than 1,500 per mm^3) to assess immunocompetence (14,15). Traditional indications for distal arterial reconstruction in the ischemic leg have included rest pain, severe claudication, and ulceration. This list now includes wounds secondary to trauma, previous surgery or neuropathy and monophasic blood flow at the ankle level.

To avoid unnecessary revascularization, limbs may also be assessed for distal perfusion with photoplethysmography (PPG), toe pressures (normal is 30 mm Hg or higher) and transcutaneous partial pressure of oxygen (TcPO$_2$) to confirm the ABI values (16–18). These parameters are more useful tests to determine whether lesions have the potential to heal or succeed following digital amputations. PPG transmits infrared light from an emitting diode into tissues, and reflected light varies with the blood content of the microcirculation. TcPO$_2$ (normal is 40 mm Hg or higher) are used in evaluating wound healing potential, monitoring effectiveness of hyperbaric therapy (greater than 10 mm Hg increase), and determining amputation level. If these parameters are poor, then vascular reconstruction is essential for surgical success if limb salvage is to be entertained. Recognizing the limitations of ABI alone and combining it with other basic diagnostic tests may prevent false diagnoses and provide better-directed treatment.

NEUROPATHY AND PERIPHERAL VASCULAR DISEASE

Sixteen million Americans have DM, 2.4 million of whom will develop foot ulcers which cost an average $36,000 for each ulcer treated (19). Diabetics are 15 times more likely to have peripheral vascular disease and 22 times more likely to have foot ulceration or gangrene than nondiabetics. Diffuse vascular disease is the most important factor leading to mortality and morbidity in patients with DM. Diabetes is the seventh-leading cause of death in the United States and is the most frequent cause of nontraumatic amputations due to neuropathic and ischemic ulcers. In fact, 20% of diabetics who enter the hospital are admitted for foot problems and 50% to 70% of U.S. amputations come from this population, accounting for 70,000 amputations annually (20). Furthermore, after an amputation, there is a 50% incidence of contralateral limb amputation within 2 years and a 33% incidence after 3 years (21). The 5-year mortality rate after below-knee amputation is 39% to 65% (19). The socioeconomic, physical, and psychological well-being of patients is significantly effected by amputations (see Chapters 5 & 10).

The diabetic patient population is prone to neuropathy and wound healing may be compromised due to PVD (22). Repeated low-level mechanical stress in insensate patients with deformities can cause neuropathic ulcerations (Fig. 30.2). These ulcerations typically present on weightbearing plantar surfaces. With continued pressure to these superficial ulcers subdermal hemorrhage can occur, indicating dermal

TABLE 30.1. *Correlation of ankle–brachial index (ABI) with peripheral arterial disease (PAD) (12)*

ABI index	Pathology
1.0–1.2	Normal
≤0.9	PAD present, patient may be asymptomatic
<0.8	Claudication likely
<0.5	Significant multilevel disease, poor or no skin lesion healing
<0.4	Ischemic rest pain
<0.15	Critical limb ischemia
0.0	Irreversible ischemia
>1.3	Suggests noncompressible vessels (elderly, claudication)

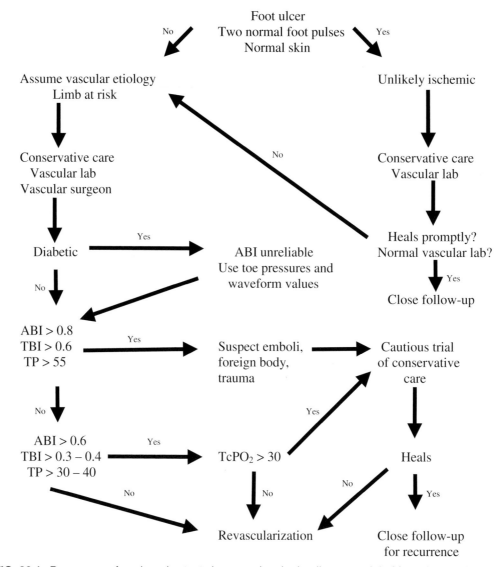

FIG. 30.1. Proper use of noninvasive tests in assessing the healing potential of foot ulcers. ABI, Ankle–brachial index; TP, toe pressure in mm Hg; TBI, toe–brachial index; TcPO₂, transcutaneous partial pressure of oxygen in mm Hg (13).

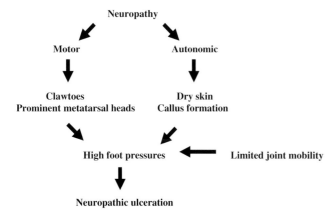

FIG. 30.2. Repetitive pressure points in the neuropathic patient can lead to ulceration.

breakdown from compromised nutrition supply. Offloading with accommodative padding, total contact casting, specialized gait-assisting devices (cane, walker, crutches, wheelchair, Camwalker, or Charcot restraint orthotic walker), or prophylactic surgery must be instituted early before these ulcers become clinically infected and require amputation for management. The University of Texas diabetic ulcer classification system (Table 30.2) aids in determining treatment protocol based on the level of the ulcer and underlying vascular impairment and neuropathy (23).

One of the most commonly misdiagnosed conditions in the neuropathic patient is Charcot neuroarthropathy. It is a noninfectious, destructive bone and joint fracture and/or dislocation associated with peripheral neuropathy. Charcot joint disease is most commonly due to DM (0.3% incidence in the diabetic population), tabes dorsalis (5% to 10% of this

TABLE 30.2. *The University of Texas diabetic ulcer classification system correlating ulcer with neuropathy and vascular compromise*

	0	1	2	3
A	Preulcerative lesion completely epithelialized	Superficial wound	Wound penetrating to tendon or capsule	Wound penetrating to bone or joint
B	With infection	With infection	With infection	With infection
C	With ischemia	With ischemia	With ischemia	With ischemia
D	With infection and ischemia	With infection and ischemia	With infection and ischemia	With infection and ischemia

[a]Risk of amputation increases as the grade and the stage increase (23).

population develop Charcot mostly in the knee, hip, ankle, shoulder, and elbow), and syringomyelia (20% to 25% of the population develop Charcot in the upper extremities) (24,25). Early intervention is vital to preventing advanced joint and structural destruction. Cast immobilization and offloading are essential to shorten the acute destructive Charcot phase. Once the foot has entered the remodeling phase, surgical intervention may be indicated. The neurotraumatic theory attributes repetitive microtrauma of an insensate joint leading to joint collapse and destruction (26).

Although the early stages of Charcot foot can be subtle, clinical diagnosis must be suspected in the high-risk neuropathic patient who presents with a warm, edematous joint even in the absence of a major traumatic event (Fig. 30.3). This appearance mimics cellulitis sometimes even with an elevated white blood cell (WBC) count. Plain films will show loss of the medial arch, bone hypertrophy, and lateral foot deviation. In this scenario, the neuropathic patient should be treated as presenting with an acute Charcot foot.

In the absence of an infection, total contact casting (TCC) remains the gold standard in offloading neuropathic ulcers by reducing vertical and horizontal forces on plantar surfaces while maintaining the ability to ambulate. The casts are changed weekly to ensure no further skin deterioration. TCC used to treat 21 neuropathic ulcers showed adequate healing (forefoot ulcers in 35 ± 12 days, midfoot ulcers in 73 ± 28 days, and rearfoot ulcers in 90 ± 12 days) even in the presence of fixed deformities (27). Similar studies using prefabricated pneumatic walking braces have shown comparable results in healing neuropathic ulcers (28,29).

If there is an ulcer present, osteomyelitis must also be considered. Magnetic resonance imaging (MRI) and WBC-labeled bone scans have shown promising results in differentiating these two different entities, because plain films can appear similar. Bone biopsy remains the gold standard for a definitive diagnosis. A true Charcot joint will exhibit cartilage cells in the pathology slides, whereas cartilage cells are usually not seen in an osteomyelitic joint. Both reports will typically show bone marrow edema and neutrophil infiltration, indicating an inflammatory response. Correlating plain films and biopsy results to the clinical appearance helps to recognize the acute Charcot foot versus the septic or the cellulitic foot. Upon diagnosing an acute or active Charcot joint, the goal should be to arrest the destruction with immobi-

lization primarily through bed rest and/or TCC. Pamidronate (90 mg intravenous infusion) has shown the ability to reduce Charcot joint temperatures ($3.4 \pm 0.7°C$ to $1.0 \pm 0.5°C$) in the affected foot and decrease alkaline phosphatase activity ($25 \pm 3\%$) to curtail the destructive Charcot phase (30,31).

CONSERVATIVE ULCER MANAGEMENT

Approximately 80% of all amputations begin with foot ulcerations. Impediments to wound healing are wound hypoxia (impair collagen synthesis), nutrition (serum albumin 3.0 g per dL or less), environmental factors (shearing forces), and metabolic disorders (DM or lymphedema). The presence of an ulcer does not automatically mean an infection is present (Fig. 30.4). Although superficial contamination may be present, clinical diagnosis is based on quantitative culture of greater than 10^5 bacteria. Decreasing the weight-bearing forces and debriding necrotic tissue optimizes ulcer healing. Debridement can be performed with various commercially available chemical or enzymatic debriding agents, mechanical debridement with dressing changes, and sharp debridement. The goal with debridement is to convert chronic wounds into acute wounds that can heal via secondary closure with direct epithelialization and wound contractures.

Ischemic ulcers are due to lack of perfusion, which creates an environment that lacks the vital nutrients for healing (Fig. 30.5). These ulcers are largely due to macrovascular disease, and require vascular reconstruction for adequate treatment (32). Clinical examination should include palpating pedal pulses and checking capillary fill time. Noninvasive testing should be required. These ulcers generally are extremely painful, have a gangrenous appearance with a central eschar, have hyperemic surrounding tissue, lack bleeding, and lack hair growth in the extremity. Bed-ridden patients place extreme pressures on sacral and posterior heel regions, which can create decubitus ulcers (a local form of ischemic ulcer). Because of the nature of these ulcers, ischemic ulcers should never be aggressively debrided until reestablishing vascular flow and offloading any pressure sources. Decubitus heel ulcers can be effectively treated with pressure-relieving ankle–foot orthosis devices. If the ulcer probes to the calcaneus, then a partial calcanectomy may be performed to remove any osteomyelitis and allow adequate room for delayed primary

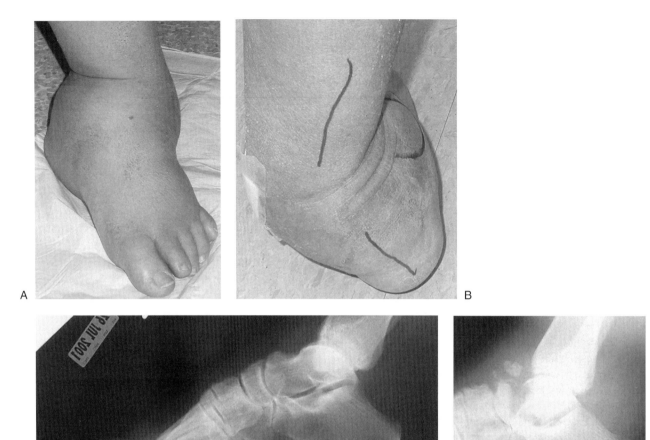

FIG. 30.3. Progressing Charcot stages following a minor ankle sprain. **A, B:** Typical clinical presentation of a suspected Charcot foot with warmth, edema, and erythema with significant ankle malposition (presentation after 1 year from initial ankle sprain). **C, D:** Sequential radiographs taken 5 months apart between initial ankle injury and above presenting clinical appearance (note the destructive changes in the talar neck due to lack of immobilization and protection).

closure. Table 30.3 lists the initial conservative care for ischemic foot ulcers.

Venous ulcerations are very common in patients with lower extremity edema. Patients who have undergone bypass surgeries are also prone to developing venous stasis ulcerations. These ulcers have irregular borders and hyperpigmented skin, and are commonly found on bony prominences of the lower legs (Fig. 30.6). Early breakdown of the skin results in weeping superficial ulcers. Controlling edema is the primary goal for treating venous ulcerations. Unna boots, edema-controlling dressings, and topical wound care products can be combined for treatment. Prophylactic compression stockings can prevent reulcerations. Vein ligation may also be considered to prevent recurrence.

Adjunctive therapies for chronic wounds include hyperbaric oxygen therapy, commercially available dermal grafts

(Apligraf, Organogenesis, Inc., Canton, MA; Dermagraf, Advanced Tissue Sciences, Inc., LaJolla, CA), vacuum-assisted closure systems, commercially available platelet-derived growth factors (becaplermin; Regranex, Ortho-McNeil Pharmaceutical, Inc., Raritan, NJ), segmental compression devices, and electrical stimulation. With favorable TcPO$_2$ values (40 mm Hg or greater), nonhealing wounds have shown 70% potential to heal (33).

Noninfected ulcers may be superficial or deep, and can be frequently treated on an outpatient basis. The treatment goal is to reduce infection rates. If acute ulcers become infected and are less than 4 weeks old, then antibiosis should be aimed at gram-positive organisms, mainly *Staphylococcus* and *Streptococcus* (oral: cephalexin, clindamycin; parental: cefazolin, clindamycin). Older ulcers should be treated for polymicrobial organisms (oral: amoxicillin+clavulanate,

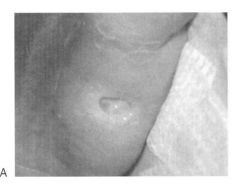 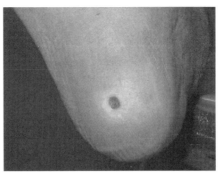 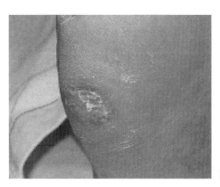

A

B,C

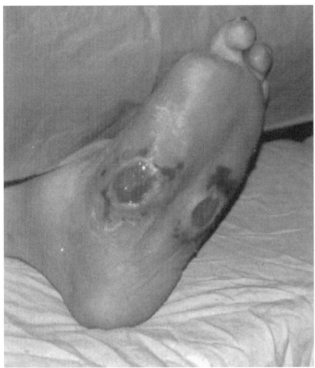 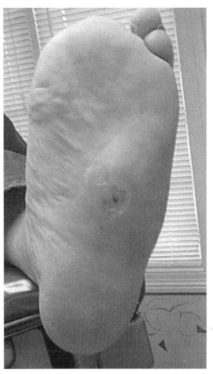

D

FIG. 30.4. Clinical presentation of an ulcer healing. **A:** Wagner grade 3 ulcer with clinical signs of infection (pus and colonization). **B:** Resolving ulcer with clean granular base and viable margins. **C:** Superficial hyperkeratotic ulcer with no opening (pressure-relieving devices will prevent recurrent breakdown). **D:** Plantar ulcerations due to Charcot collapsed foot.

clindamycin+ciprofloxacin; parental: ticarcillin+clavulanate, piperacillin+tazobactam, clindamycin+ciprofloxacin, cefazolin+aminoglycoside, cefepime+clindamycin) (34). If ulcers deteriorate and develop acute abscesses or osteomyelitis, surgical incision and debridement are essential.

The objectives for ulcer debridement are to remove all devitalized tissues, open the wound widely for inspection, remove all foreign material, and control the bleeding (35). When encountering muscle, muscle contractility, consistency, and bleeding are the best indicators of muscle viability (36). Muscle color is the least reliable sign of viability. Periosteum should not be sacrificed unless it is severely comminuted. Primary wound closure should be performed after 3 to 4 days

following the initial incision and drainage or when stabilized. Once ulcers have been stabilized and cleared of infection, prophylactic surgery can be performed to reduce reulceration rates.

OSTEOMYELITIS

Plain films can show osteomyelitic changes after 10 to 14 days. However, noninfective osteolytic and arthritic changes can make osteomyelitis difficult to accurately diagnose. Three-phase bone scans can be used to diagnose inflammatory reactions and areas of osteoclastic activity. Although highly sensitive, bone scans remain quite nonspecific. The first phase shows dynamic blood flow to the areas of

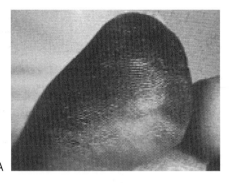
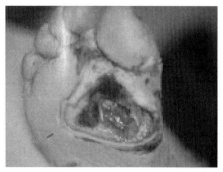
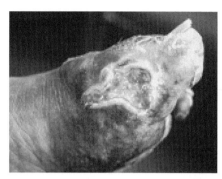

A

B,C

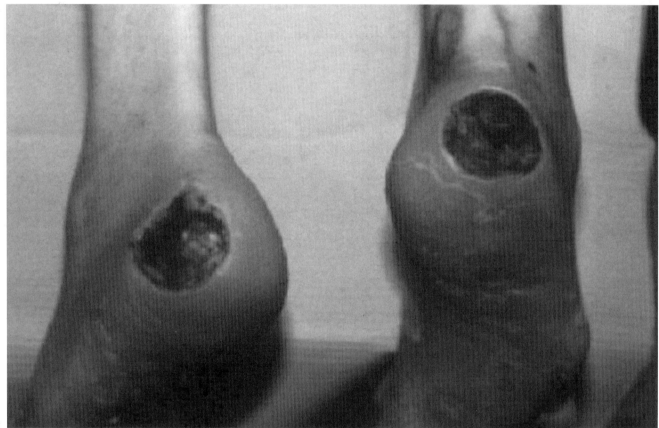

D

FIG. 30.5. Clinical presentation of ischemic and gangrenous ulcers. **A:** Superficial gangrenous changes with no open ulcers (not necessary for immediate amputation, can wait for vascular testing or resolution). **B:** Ischemic ulcer with signs of inadequate healing (can wait for revascularization unless underlying osteomyelitis or abscess is present). **C:** Deep gangrenous forefoot will likely need amputation upon vascular clearance. **D:** Decubitus heel ulcers.

inflammatory response. Cellulitis and osteomyelitis are visualized in the second phase (5 to 10 minutes after injection). Areas of uptake in the delayed phase signify osteoclastic activity such as osteomyelitis. White blood cells labeled with indium (WBC-In^{111}) are somewhat more specific for osteomyelitis than other inflammatory activities and can localize the infection. Patients with poor vasculature or renal impairment are not good candidates for bone scans, but they can be assessed by MRI to determine areas of inflammation and bone marrow edema. Caution should be taken not to base a definitive diagnosis on a positive bone scan or an MRI re-

port alone because chronic arthritic joints or active Charcot joints can present with similar findings. No large studies have been performed to determine whether an MRI alone correctly diagnoses osteomyelitis with high accuracy, but some studies show supporting data (37–39). Most institutions are relying more on MRI testing in differentiating osteomyelitis. Correlating plain films and clinical findings remain the primary diagnostic tools, with the gold standard remaining bone biopsy, a more cost-effective method, for definitive diagnosis.

Surgical excision of osteomyelitis in the vascularly compromised patient should begin with a vascular assessment

TABLE 30.3. *Initial conservative care of ischemic ulcers (13)*

Assessment	Estimate extent of problem and component of ischemia and infection by history, physical, vascular lab, culture, and radiographs; ulcerations and skin lesions measured perpendicularly to nearest millimeter for later comparison
Risk factor control	Stop smoking and control hypertension, blood glucose, and lipids; optimize nutritional, cardiac, pulmonary, renal, and hepatic functions
Debridement	Define extent of infection, identify specific pathogens, decompress abscesses, and removal necrotic tissue
Protection	Eliminate pressure, rest limb, and reduce edema
Medications	Antiplatelet agents and pentoxifylline are often added to enhance small vessel circulation
Wound care	Many dressing, ointments, and antibiotics are available; each has unique advantages and none is appropriate for all situations
Close follow-up	Early and frequent assessment of response to therapy is critical

to determine whether the foot has adequate circulation for antibiotic delivery as well as healing. Once vascular clearance is obtained or a bypass is performed, surgical planning for removal of all infected bone is done. The initial goal is to remove all nonviable tissue. For diagnosed osteomyelitis, wide excision of 5 mm or more has shown significant reduction of recurrence (40). In addition, the bone should be inspected for cortical density and appearance. Culturing the bone just proximal to the excision site will aid in determining resection of adequate bone. Punctate bleeding of hard bone proximal to the resection site minimizes the chance of recurrence. A definitive amputation can then be planned in 3 to 4 days or when stabilized. Foot length should be preserved as much as possible, because more proximal amputations decrease gait velocities. Intravenous antibiotics may be needed depending on the confidence of the surgeon that all infected bone was removed. Long-term intravenous antibiotics should be chosen and monitored by the infectious disease specialist. Recurrence of osteomyelitis should be closely monitored with repeated plain films.

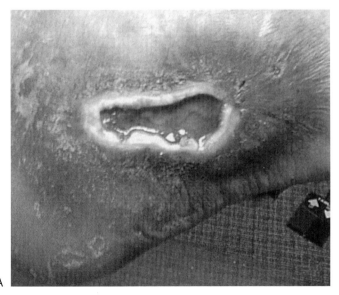

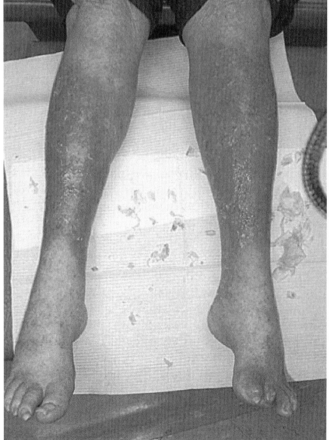

FIG. 30.6. Clinical presentation of venous stasis ulcerations. **A:** Stable superficial venous stasis ulcer over the lateral malleolus with hyperpigmented surrounding skin and fibrogranular base (edema control is paramount to ulcer healing). **B:** Chronic venous stasis changes to lower extremities prone to ulcerations.

SURGICAL AMPUTATIONS

Amputation is an unpleasant intervention, but one that is intended to improve the quality of life for a patient with a diseased or unsalvageable lower extremity. The goal of amputation is to remove nonviable tissue while retaining the greatest amount of function as possible. DM is the most common cause of nontraumatic lower limb amputations, and its associated PVD may greatly determine the level of amputation because of healing potential. Patient selection for surgical intervention should also be considered to avoid unnecessary risks. Medical risks associated with severe coronary artery disease may contraindicate longer surgical procedures due to prolonged anesthesia. These patients and nonambulatory patients may benefit from a primary proximal amputation, which is more cost-effective and equally efficacious (41). Furthermore, patients must understand compliancy issues with maintaining nonweightbearing, elevation, and proper wound care. Extreme precaution should also be given to the neuropathic foot, otherwise surgical success rates will diminish and the patient may require further surgical care. With proper evaluation and preparation, however, many limbs may be salvaged with partial foot amputations, thus dramatically affecting the risk to the contralateral foot, and the costs involved with maintaining patients with prostheses.

The principles of amputation include creating a site able to withstand friction from prostheses/shoes, avoiding unnecessary procedures to improve cosmetic outcome, balancing tendons to minimize equinovarus deforming forces, creating flaps under minimal tension, and controlling hemostasis. Determining the amputation level is very important from a biological and functional point of view. The biological amputation level is the most distal level that will heal. The functional amputation level is the level at which the patient is able to perform the activities of daily living either with a prosthesis or in a wheelchair. It is also a level that will resist additional ulcerations and need for further amputation. The success of limb salvage is to attain the most distal level amputation for preserving biomechanical function and reducing metabolic expense for postoperative gait.

Skin Grafts

Wounds that do not heal despite adequate perfusion may benefit from free tissue transfer techniques. Vascularized flaps have been shown to increase wound antibiotic delivery, improve wound oxygen tension, augment neutrophil wound activity, and assist treatments of chronic infections in ischemic regions (42).

Skin grafts are usually adequate for nonweightbearing surfaces plantarly. However, Charcot patients have collapsed longitudinal and transverse arches, which may require concurrent resection of plantar prominences. Without distal revascularization, midfoot amputations have shown 83% incidence of going to a below-knee amputation, which can be attributed to poor tendon balancing and poor perfusion (43).

Forefoot plantar grafts are rarely performed because of the high success of transmetatarsal amputations (TMA). TMA permits adequate skin coverage for closure for most forefoot ulcers, removes prominent metatarsal heads that could lead to future reulceration, and preserves stable biomechanics of the foot for ambulation.

Muscle flaps covered with skin grafts are the tissue of choice for weightbearing hindfoot ulcers (heel pad). Fasciocutaneous flaps can slide over the calcaneus during walking and reulcerate secondary to the shear stresses.

Hallux Amputation

Preservation of the hallux proximal phalanx base reduces the probability of sesamoid displacement (Fig. 30.7). The first ray plantarflexes to stabilize the hallux against the weightbearing surface in preparation for the propulsive phase of the gait. When the hallux is absent, excessive ground-reactive forces develop under the first metatarsal head and contraction of the lesser digits is exaggerated, thus placing the remaining foot structures at risk (44). Hallux amputation is not a benign procedure, and when necessary, should be performed as distally as possible to maintain appropriate loading of the remaining foot segments.

Lesser Digital Amputations

Digital amputations are indicated for distal osteomyelitis, gangrene, and PVD (Fig. 30.7). The terminal Syme's amputation resects the distal half of the distal phalanx and leaves an adequate flap for closure. Normal gait and the intrinsic tendon balance are retained. Furthermore, migration of adjacent digits and the plantar plate can be minimized. If all the phalanges of a digit need to be excised, focal pressures to the metatarsal head need to be addressed.

Partial Ray Resections

When ulcers under metatarsal heads yield osteomyelitis to the metatarsophalangeal joint, a partial ray resection is indicated where the entire digit and the affected metatarsal segment are surgically excised (Fig. 30.8). Isolated partial ray resections can be performed, but transfer lesions again need to be offloaded. If two or more adjacent rays have been partially resected, then the surgeon should strongly consider a TMA as a prophylactic procedure to maintain a functional level.

Transmetatarsal Amputations

The TMA is one of the most common forefoot amputations mainly due to its low complication rate (Fig. 30.9). Proper technique includes beveling the distal one-third metatarsal from dorsal–distal to plantar–proximal and creating a smooth parabola, with the second being the longest. The first metatarsal should be angled distal–lateral to proximal–medial to prevent any medial prominences. Similarly, the fifth

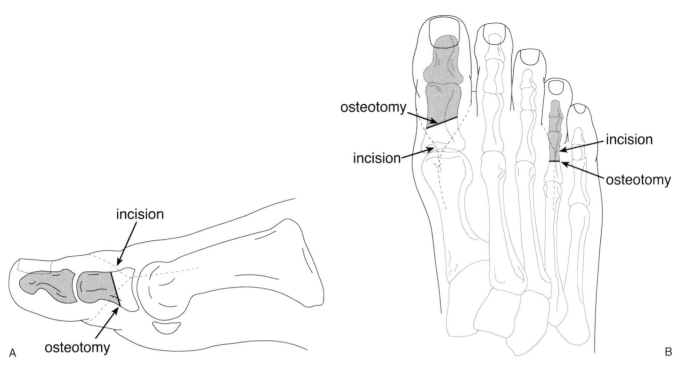

FIG. 30.7. Hallux and digital amputations. Partial proximal phalanx hallux amputation to preserve tendons at the base of the proximal phalanx and prevent sesamoid migration and similar amputation of a lesser digit to preserve plantar plate position under metatarsal heads. Dashed lines designate incision planning, and osteotomies are beveled to avoid plantar prominences.

metatarsal should be angled from distal–medial to proximal–lateral. The plantar flap should be preserved for the stump. With good preoperative incision planning, plantar ulcers can be concurrently excised with this procedure. Electrocautery and deep closure levels are discouraged. Patients with a TMA are able to return to ambulation with an ankle–foot orthosis (AFO), a custom-molded shoe with a toe filler, or a rocker-bottom shoe. If there is a significant equinovarus deformity present, a tendo-Achilles lengthening or split tibialis anterior tendon transfer can be performed to prevent plantar–lateral ulceration. Often, a TMA is performed at a level that is marginally vascularized. It is imperative in these cases to treat the patient with a minimum of 3 weeks of posterior splinting and total nonweightbearing for incision healing. This protocol will improve the success rates.

LisFranc Amputations

If a more proximal amputation is needed than a TMA, an amputation through the tarsometatarsal joints can be completed in a similar fashion (Fig. 30.10). The base of the second metatarsal may be cut to maintain a parabola. The lateral, medial, and plantar edges are beveled and smoothed. The base of the fifth metatarsal should be preserved due to the attachment of the peroneus brevis tendon. An equinovarus deformity is commonly seen with this amputation, which may be counteracted by a tendo-Achilles lengthening or split tibialis anterior tendon transfer. The LisFranc amputation is less stable than

the TMA due to compromise of the tibialis anterior and posterior tendon attachments and is prone to lateral ulcerations.

Chopart Amputations

The Chopart amputation, performed through the talonavicular and calcaneocuboid joints, has been criticized for muscle imbalance and equinus deformity (Fig. 30.11). Transferring the extensor tendon into the talar neck, lengthening the tendo-Achilles, and excising bony prominences may be performed to counter these problems (45). The equinus deformity is reduced by transferring the long extensors, peroneals, and tibialis anterior tendons to the distal stump. Patients remain nonweightbearing until complete stump healing before being fitted with a "clamshell" prosthetic. Heel ulcers, unsteady gait and poor balance, and the inability to fit into a prosthesis that can allow toe-off without stump overload are disadvantages of the Chopart amputation.

Syme's Amputations

The Syme's amputation involves an ankle disarticulation with removal of the malleoli and forward rotation of the heel pad over the residual tibia to create a limb that can still weight-bear and offer normal propulsion with a prosthesis. This amputation level avoids the equinovarus tendon imbalance created with a LisFranc or Chorparx amputation. The distal tibia serves to bear full extremity weight and the heel pad

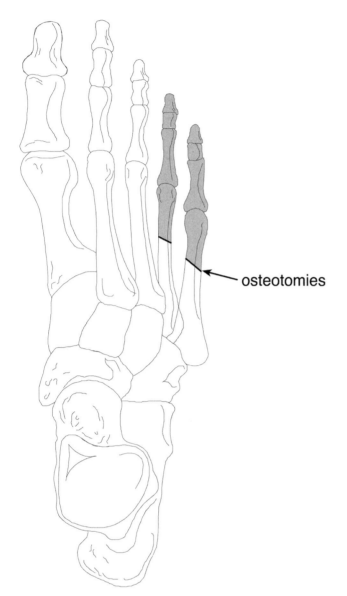

FIG. 30.8. Partial fourth- and fifth-ray resections. Partial fifth-ray resection with preservation of the base and the peroneus brevis tendon insertion (osteotomy beveled to prevent ulceration laterally).

is preserved for cushioning. The Syme's amputation creates adequate space beneath the extremity for a prosthetic that has less energy consumption with ambulation compared to the midfoot amputations. In the presence of infection, this amputation can be staged. In the first stage, the ankle is disarticulated and the infection is stabilized with several months of intravenous antibiotics. The definitive procedure is completed with malleoli resection. Care is taken to preserve the plantar fat pad, and the Achilles tendon is detached distally. Both structures are anchored to the tibia distally. Technical points to maintain include transecting the tibia just proximal to the articular cartilage parallel to the ground and preserving as much of the tibia as possible for weightbearing. Patients usually progress to weightbearing 10 to 14 days postopera-

tively in a TCC with a rubber walking heel. The patient is then fitted for a prosthetic, with little need for physical therapy for gait training. Like the Chopart amputation, the Syme's amputation may have complications due to marginal perfusion.

Below-Knee and Above-Knee Amputations

These amputation levels are reserved for nonsalvageable limbs or failed reconstructive cases. The limb may have extensive osteomyelitis or poor revascularization, making any salvaging attempt too risky. Patients who are nonambulatory and have severe lower extremity contractures and/or decubitus ulcers are good candidates for these proximal amputations. The level of amputation depends on which level is most optimal for healing. Even with a below-knee amputation, patients may regain ambulatory capability quite quickly with a prosthesis.

Survival rates for below-knee and above-knee amputations are 78% at 1 year and 55% at 3 years, with a 10% mortality rate at 30 days (46). Compared to normal walking speed, major proximal amputees (proximal to midfoot amputations) function at approximately 80% of their cardiac capacity (47). Normal walking speed and cadence decrease as oxygen consumption increases with more proximal amputations. At more proximal amputation levels, the capacity to walk short or long distances is greatly impaired, contributing to the low survival rates.

Complications to Amputations and Role of Prosthetics

The immediate postoperative goal is to reduce edema and maximize incision healing. In the larger amputation procedures, drains may be placed to avoid hematoma formations. Extremity elevation may help to reduce postoperative edema. The incisions should be carefully monitored for signs of infection or dehiscence. Tendon balancing should be performed to avoid equinovarus and lateral ulceration. Tendo-Achilles lengthening may be required after a TMA and more proximal amputations. If the peroneus brevis tendon insertion is sacrificed, then the tibialis anterior tendon may be transferred laterally to prevent varus deformity of the distal stump. After incision healing, tendon balancing is performed in those patients who demonstrate the need for it. Patients are slowly progressed into weightbearing with an appropriate prosthetic and physical therapy gait training.

Prosthetics attempt to restore gait following amputation. Often, toe fillers are used after digital and ray amputations to avoid digital migration, which predisposes the patient to new ulcerations. Shoe fillers and an AFO are commonly used for transmetatarsal and LisFranc amputations. An AFO is used to prevent lateral ulceration from the equinovarus deformity. A firmer AFO is needed for a LisFranc amputation to compensate for less anatomic support. Rocker-bottom shoes may be helpful for a smoother gait pattern.

A shoe is not sufficient for a Chopart amputation. Amputation at this level requires a semiflexible carbon attachment.

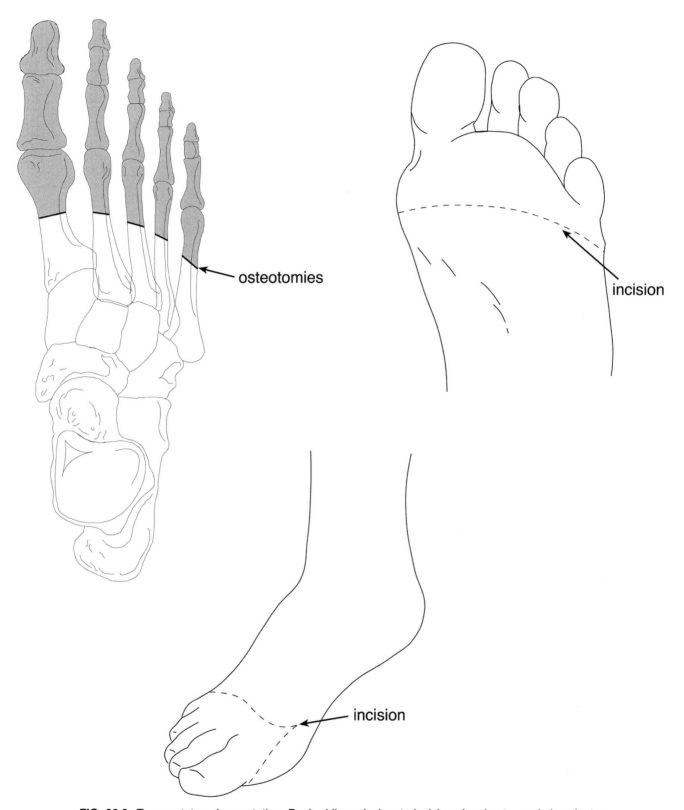

osteotomies

incision

incision

FIG. 30.9. Transmetatarsal amputation. Dashed lines designate incision planning to maximize plantar flap for closure. Osteotomies are beveled to minimize plantar, medial, and lateral prominences.

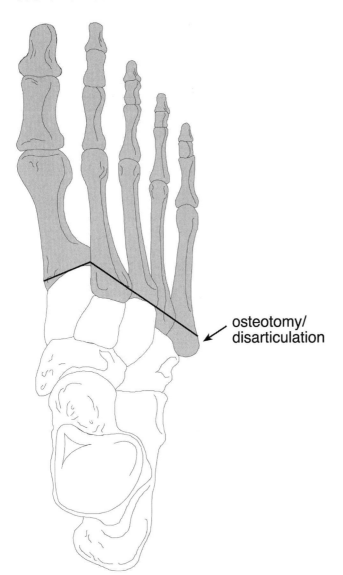

FIG. 30.10. LisFranc amputation. A smooth, bony parabola created with adequate incision planning. This amputation is unstable due to loss of peroneus longus insertion at the first metatarsal base plantarly. The peroneus brevis insertion should be preserved at the fifth metatarsal base.

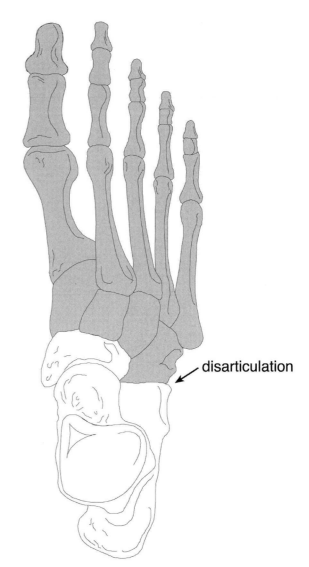

FIG. 30.11. Chopart amputation. This is the most unstable midfoot amputation due to the loss of the tibialis anterior and posterior tendons and peroneal tendons.

A Syme's prosthesis includes a durable liner with a medial or posterior window. Prosthesis should be reevaluated periodically for fit to ensure minimal stump irritation. Modern prosthetics incorporate strong, lightweight materials and provide more anatomic gait. This approach has reduced the effort and compensatory stresses on the remaining limb as well as provided more functional bipedal ambulation (48).

Arthrodesis Procedures

Rigid contractures from spastic equinus or tendon imbalance and joint instability from Charcot destruction may benefit from joint arthrodesis. The goal is to create a rigid plantigrade foot in an attempt to preserve bipedal gait. The most

common joints affected are the first metatarsophalangeal, tarsometatarsal, subtalar, and ankle joints. The purpose of an arthrodesis is to stabilize an otherwise unstable or malpositioned joint or to eliminate painful gait. Before operating on the Charcot foot, care must be taken to ensure that the acute destructive phase has resolved, because otherwise any internal fixation used is doomed to failure with continued bony collapse. The ankle and midfoot joints are commonly affected, creating a painful, unstable deformity. Infection, PVD, and active Charcot conditions are contraindications to surgery. Patients with a smoking history also have a higher incidence of nonunion rates compared to nonsmokers (18.6% vs. 7.1%) (49).

Numerous forms of fixation exist, each with its advantages and disadvantages. Internal fixation with screws, plates, and intramedullary rods can be utilized for rigid fixation providing compression and promoting primary bone healing.

Extensive dissection, wound dehiscence, nonunion or pseudoarthrosis, malunion, avascular necrosis, joint arthritis, and infection are complications encountered with internal fixation. Dissection should utilize atraumatic technique, minimal tissue handling, and avoidance of neurovascular and tendon structures. Joint preparation should use minimal resection to avoid excessive shortening. Nonunion rates of the Charcot ankle have been reported between 33% and 40% (50,51). Figure 30.12 illustrates arthrodesis procedures.

External fixation is used in complex situations for multiplanar correction and times when bone density is not optimal for internal fixation. Studies have found lower union rates using external fixation (78% to 83%) compared to internal fixation (95% to 100%) (52–54). Because of exposed pin tracts, infection rates are increased.

Patients should be kept nonweightbearing until radiographic union is noted (10 to 12 weeks). Patients are slowly allowed to increase weightbearing with physical therapy for gait training. AFO bracing and a solid-ankle, cushioned-heel, rocker-bottom shoe may be needed.

EFFECTS OF CEREBROVASCULAR ACCIDENTS ON LOWER EXTREMITY FUNCTION

Paracentral lobule lesions affect lower extremity function with particular patterns. Upper motor neuron lesions may occur at the level of the brain or spinal cord. Most brain lesions are due to cerebrovascular accidents (CVA), tumor, degenerative process, trauma, or birth injury. In acute events leading to a brain lesion, the first symptoms that will be seen are those of spinal shock (flaccid paralysis, hypotonia, areflexia, vasomotor paralysis, and paralysis of bowel and bladder). Within 4 to 6 weeks, these symptoms are replaced by symptoms that are directly associated with upper motor neuron damage. Six primary clinical signs can be associated with upper motor neuron lesions. These signs can also be appreciated in the upper extremities.

1. *Hyperreflexia.* Deep tendon reflexes are increased due to uninhibited reflex loop with lower motor neurons.
2. *Hypertonia.* Increased muscle tone is exhibited by fixed posture of the limbs and increased resistance to manipulation of the limbs.
3. *Spastic paralysis.* The muscles are without voluntary control in a state of increased muscular tone (hypertonia) and exaggeration of tendon reflexes (hyperreflexia).
4. *Clonus.* As a tendon is maintained in extension (dorsiflexion of the ankle), there is a series of rhythmic jerks (contractions followed by relaxations) by the flexors (posterior leg muscles).
5. *Clasp–knife.* There is rigidity of the extensor muscles of a joint such that the muscles offer resistance to passive flexion up to a point and then give away. This response and clonus are due to the exaggerated stretch reflex.
6. *Abnormal superficial reflex.* Contraction of skeletal muscle following cutaneous stimulation is a superficial reflex.

In the foot, a normal plantar reflex of digital plantarflexion occurs after the skin on the plantar surface of the foot is stimulated with a blunt handle of a percussion hammer (usually from the heel to the fifth metatarsal head and then across to the first metatarsal head). Upper motor neuron lesions are characterized by a Babinski sign (pathological), which is dorsiflexion of the hallux and fanning of the lesser toes.

CVA events involving the cerebellum can be separated into midline and lateral zones of the cerebellum. The cerebellum provides information about an intended movement and corrections in relation to the current activity to be relayed back to the cortex. The midline zone of the cerebellum may involve disorders of stance and gait in which broad-based walking in tandem (walking heel to toe alternating) is difficult. Ocular disturbance (nystagmus), titubation (rhythmic body or head tremor), and tilted head posture may also be seen in midline zone lesions. Lateral zone lesions can cause decomposition of movement where voluntary motor acts are jerky. Again, a broad-based stance with unsteady gait is seen accompanied by limb ataxia (uncoordinated limb movement). Hypotonia is exhibited due to decreased resistance to passive manipulation of the limbs. Patients are unable to arrest a muscular movement at a desired point (dysmetria). An intention tremor is seen in patients when they are asked to run their heel of one foot down the shin of the other leg.

Observational gait assessment identifies poor coordination and dysfunctional movement patterns. Dropfoot, ankle and knee instability, loss of forward progression, and significant asymmetry lead to decreased walking velocities, often 30% to 40% of normal speeds (55). Limited load transfer through the affected limb places increased demands on the uninvolved side. An extensor synergy emerges with hypertonicity and presents with (a) hip extension, adduction, and internal rotation; (b) knee extension; and (c) ankle plantarflexion and inversion. The equinovarus posturing is usually present throughout swing and stance phases on the involved limb. With hypotonicity, a flexor synergy emerges with (a) hip flexion, abduction, and external rotation and (b) knee flexion and ankle dorsiflexion and eversion. Both profiles present gait impedance factors such as altered posture, decreased functional mobility, joint pain, and predisposition to contracture formation (55).

Management consists of early, aggressive physical therapy and orthotic (AFO) treatment programs during the initial phases of in- and outpatient rehabilitation. Dropfoot can originate from neuromuscular disease (Charcot–Marie–Tooth disease, multiple sclerosis, myotonic dystrophy, and peripheral neuropathies) or spinal cord trauma, which is commonly treated with an AFO. Occasionally, surgical interventions may be required for the release of longstanding contractures or muscle–tendon transfer procedures for improved joint dynamics. Patients with spastic deformities or fixed varus deformities are less likely to be accommodated for ambulation with an AFO. Those in whom the limiting factor for

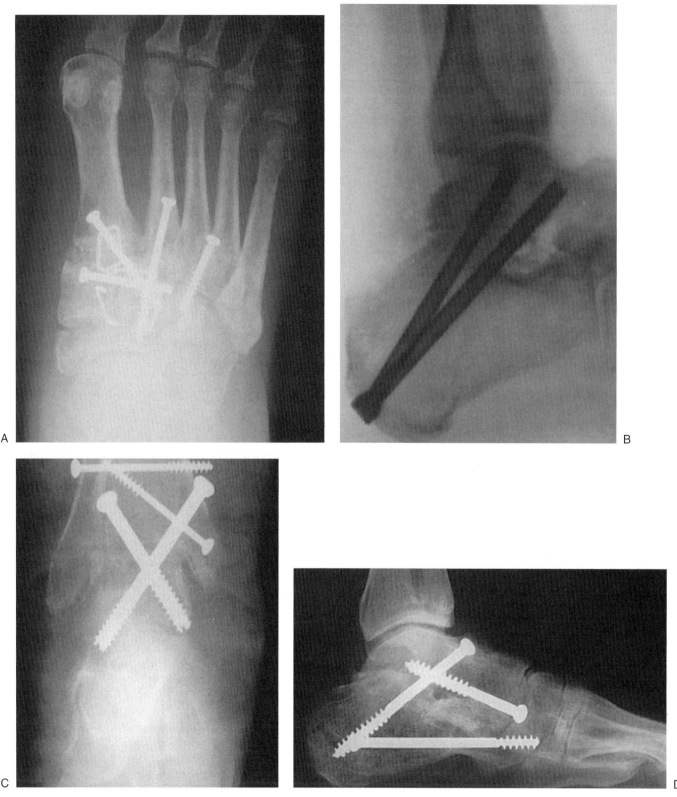

FIG. 30.12. Arthrodesis procedures for foot and ankle stabilization. **A:** Midfoot arthrodesis. **B:** Subtalar joint arthrodesis. **C:** Ankle joint arthrodesis. **D:** Triple arthrodesis (fusion of ankle, subtalar, and calcaneocuboid joints). (*continued*)

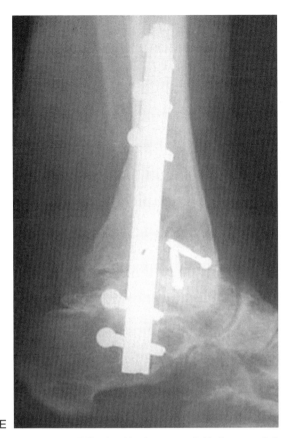
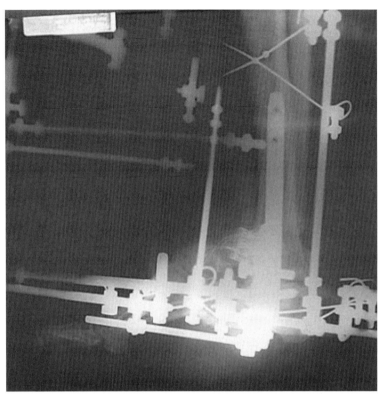

E

F

FIG. 30.12. (*Continued*) **E:** Intramedullary nail calcaneotalotibial arthrodesis. **F:** External fixator with intramedullary nail ankle and midfoot arthrodeses.

ambulation remains their pedal deformity are candidates for tendon lengthenings or transfers or joint fusions to prevent future contractures and prevent plantar ulcerations. Generally, most CVA patients are managed effectively without surgical procedures.

CONCLUSION

Foot management in the vascularly compromised patient poses great challenges. Proper care is best managed in a team-oriented fashion. First, the primary treating physician must monitor and address poor lower extremity perfusion as well as other underlying pathologies and comorbidities. Second, a vascular assessment will ensure adequate flow for healing and repair. All treating physicians should be in the habit of inspecting the feet and lower extremities *routinely* especially in high-risk patient populations. The surgical team (podiatric, plastic, orthopedic, and/or vascular surgeons) must monitor patients closely postoperatively through their rehabilitation period for long-term success. Recognition of early clinical signs of increased weightbearing pressures, ulcerations, deformities secondary to contractures, and destructive infective processes is vital to preserving bipedal ambulation. If surgical amputation or reconstruction is required, then the outcome result is highly dependent on the level and type of

amputation, proper shoegear, appropriate prosthetic fitting, and accommodative offloading techniques.

REFERENCES

1. Barber GG, McPhail NV, Scobie TK, et al. A prospective study of lower limb amputations. *Can J Surg* 1983;26:339–341.
2. Rose G. The diagnosis of ischaemic heart pain and intermittent claudication in field surveys. *Bull WHO* 1962;27:645–658.
3. McDermott MM, Mehta S, Greenland P. Exertional leg symptoms other than intermittent claudication are common in peripheral arterial disease. *Arch Intern Med* 1999;159:387–392.
4. Criqui MH, Fronek A, Barrett-Connor E, et al. The prevalence of peripheral arterial disease in a defined population. *Circulation* 1985;71:510–515.
5. Hafner J, Schaad I, Schneider E, et al. Leg ulcers in peripheral arterial disease: impaired wound healing above the threshold of chronic critical limb ischemia. *J Am Acad Dermatol* 2000;43:1001–1008.
6. Santilli JD, Santilli SM. Chronic critical limb ischemia: diagnosis, treatment, and prognosis. *Am Fam Physician* 1999;59:1899–1908.
7. McDermott MM, Mehta S, Ahn H, et al. Atherosclerotic risk factors are less intensively treated in patients with peripheral arterial disease than in patients with coronary artery disease. *J Gen Intern Med* 1997;12:209–215.
8. Hirsch AT. Claudication as an "orphan disease": rationale and goals of drug therapy for peripheral arterial disease. *Vasc Med* 1996;1:37–42.
9. McDermott MM, Greenland P, Liu K, et al. The ankle brachial index is associated with leg function and physical activity: the walking and leg circulation study. *Ann Int Med* 2002;136:873–883.
10. McDermott MM, Kerwin DR, Liu K, et al. Prevalence and

significance of unrecognized lower extremity peripheral artery disease in general medicine practice. *J Gen Intern Med* 2001;16:384–390.

11. Greenland P. Clinical significance, detection, and medical treatment for peripheral arterial disease. *J Cardiopulm Rehabil* 2002;22,73–79.

12. Transatlantic Inter-Society Concensus (TASC) Working Group. Management of peripheral arterial disease. *J Vasc Surg* 2000;31:S1–S296.

13. Sykes MT, Godsey JB. Vascular evaluation of the problem diabetic foot. *Clin Podiatr Med Surg* 1998;15:49–83.

14. Pinzur MS, Sage R, Stuck R, et al. Transcutaneous oxygen as a predictor of wound healing in amputations of the foot and ankle. *Foot Ankle* 1992;13;271–273.

15. Dickaut SC, DeLee JC, Page CP. Nutritional status: importance in predicting wound-healing after amputation. *J Bone Joint Surg* 1984; 66A:71–75.

16. Wyss CR, Matsen FA, Simmons CW, et al. Transcutaneous oxygen tension measurements on limbs of diabetic and nondiabetic patients with peripheral vascular disease. *Surgery* 1984;95:339–346.

17. Ramsey DE, Manke DA, Sumner DS. Toe blood pressure: a valuable adjunct to ankle pressure measurement for assessing peripheral arterial disease. *J Cardiovasc Surg* 1983;24:43–48.

18. Bacharach JM, Rooke TW, Osmundson PJ, et al. Predictive value of transcutaneous oxygen pressure and amputation success by use of supine and elevation measurements. *J Vasc Surg* 1992;15,558–563.

19. Glover JL, Weingarten MS, Buchbinder DS, et al. A 4-year outcome-based retrospective study of wound healing and limb salvage with chronic wounds. *Adv Wound Care* 1997;10:33–38.

20. National Diabetes Fact Sheet. *National estimates and general information on diabetes in the United States.* Atlanta, GA: Department of Health and Human Services, Centers for Disease Control and Prevention, 1997.

21. Fabrin J, Larsen K, Holstein PE. Long-term follow-ups in diabetic Charcot feet with spontaneous onset. *Diabetes Care* 2000;23:796–800.

22. Levin ME. Preventing amputation in the patient with diabetes. *Diabetes Care* 1995;18:1383–1394.

23. Armstrong DG, Lavery LA, Harkless LB. Classification of diabetic foot wounds. *J Foot Ankle Surg* 1996;35:528–531.

24. Kucan JO, Robson MC. Diabetic foot infections: fate of the contralateral foot. *Plast Reconstr Surg* 1986;77:439–441.

25. Bodily DC, Burgess EM. Contralateral limb and patient survival after leg amputation. *Am J Surg* 1983;146:280–282.

26. Eloesser L. On the nature of neuropathic affectations of the joints. *Ann Surg* 1917;66:201.

27. Sinacore DR. Healing times of diabetic ulcers in the presence of fixed deformities of the foot using total contact casting. *Foot Ankle Int* 1998;19:613–618.

28. Fleischli JG, Lavery LA, Vela SA, et al. Comparison strategies for reducing pressure at the site of neuropathic ulcers. *J Am Podiatr Med Assoc* 1997;87:466–472.

29. Baumhauer JF, Wervey R, McWilliams J, et al. A comparison study of plantar foot pressure in a standardized shoe, total contact cast, and prefabricated pneumatic walking brace. *Foot Ankle Int* 1997;18: 26–33.

30. Jude EB, Boulton AJM. Medical treatment of charcot's arthropathy. *J Am Podiatr Med Assoc* 2002;92:381–383.

31. Selby PL, Young MJ, Boulton AJ. Bisphosphonates: a new treatment for diabetic charcot neuroarthropathy. *Diabet Med* 1994;11:28–31.

32. LoGerfo FW, Gibbons GW. Vascular disease of the lower extremities in diabetes mellitus. *Endocrinol Metab Clin North Am* 1996;25:439–445.

33. Grolman RE, Wilkerson DK, Taylor J, et al. Transcutaneous oxygen measurements predict a beneficial response to hyperbaric oxygen therapy in patients with nonhealing wounds and critical limb ischemia. *Am Surg* 2001;67:1072–1079.

34. Dow G, Browne A, Sibbald G. Infection in chronic wounds: controversies in diagnosis and treatment. *Ostomy Wound Manage* 1999;45:23–40.

35. Hoover NW, Ivins JC. Wound debridement. *AMA Arch Surg* 1959;79: 701–710.

36. Scully RE, Artz CP, Sako Y. An evaluation of the surgeon's criteria for determining the viability of muscle during debridement. *AMA Arch Surg* 1956;73:1031–1035.

37. Umans H, Haramati N, Flusser G. The diagnostic role of gadolinium enhanced MRI in distinguishing between acute medullary bone infarct and osteomyelitis. *Magn Reson Imaging* 2000;18:255–262.

38. Morrison WB, Schweitzer ME, Bock GW, et al. Diagnosis of osteomyelitis: utility of fat-suppressed contrast-enhanced MR imaging. *Radiology* 1993;189:251–257.

39. Unger E, Moldofsky P, Gatenby R, et al. Diagnosis of osteomyelitis by MR imaging. *Am J Roentgenol* 1988;150:605–610.

40. Simpson HRW, Deakin M, Latham JM. Chronic osteomyelitis. *J Bone Joint Surg* 2001;83B:403–407.

41. Cronenwett JL, Colen LB. Ischemic limb salvage by revascularization and free tissue transfer. In: Yao JST, ed., *Ischemic extremity: advances in treatment.* New York: McGraw-Hill, 1995;405–418.

42. Eshima I, Mathes SJ, Paty P. Comparison of the intracellular bacterial killing activity of leukocytes in musculocutaneous and random-pattern flaps. *Plast Reconstr Surg* 1990;86:541–547.

43. Wieman TJ, Griffith GD, Polk HC. Management of diabetic midfoot ulcers. *Am J Surg* 1992;215:627–632.

44. Poppen NK, Mann RA, O'Konski M, et al. Amputation of the great toe. *Foot Ankle* 1981;6:333–337.

45. Letts MD, Pyper AL. The modified Chopart's amputation. *Clin Orthop* 1990;256:44–49.

46. Nehler MR, Coll JR, Hiatt WR, et al. Functional outcome in a contemporary series of major lower extremity amputations. *J Vasc Surg* 2003;38:7–14.

47. Pinzur MS, Gold J, Schwartz D, et al. Energy demands for walking in dysvascular amputees as related to the level of amputation. *Orthopedics* 1992;15:1033–1037.

48. Pinzur MS, Cox W, Kaiser J, et al. The effect of prosthetic alignment on relative limb loading in persons with trans-tibial amputation: a preliminary report. *J Rehabil Res Dev* 1995;32:373–377.

49. Johnson JE. Surgical treatment for neuropathic arthropathy of the foot and ankle. *Instr Course Lect* 1999;48:269–277.

50. Ishikawa SN, Murphy GA, Richardson EG. The effect of cigarette smoking on hindfoot fusions. *Foot Ankle Int* 2002;23:996–998.

51. Simon SR, Tejwani SG, Wilson DL, et al. Arthrodesis as an early alternative to nonoperative management of Charcot arthropathy of the diabetic foot. *J Bone Joint Surg* 2000;82A:939–950.

52. Marks RM, Parks BG, Schon LC. Midfoot fusion technique for neuroarthropathic feet: biomechanical analysis and rationale. *Foot Ankle Int* 1998;19:507–510.

53. Monroe MT, Beals TC, Manoli A. Clinical outcome of arthrodesis of the ankle using rigid internal fixation with cancellous screws. *Foot Ankle Int* 1999;20:227–231.

54. Maenpaa H, Lehto MU, Belt EA. What went wrong in triple arthrodesis? An analysis of failures in 21 patients. *Clin Orthop* 2001;391:218–223.

55. Goldie PA, Matyas TA, Evans OM. Deficit and change in gait velocity during rehabilitation after stroke. *Arch Phys Med Rehabil* 1996;77:1074–1082.

CHAPTER 31

Vascular Concepts in Wound Healing

William J. Ennis and Patricio Meneses

Key Points

- Macrovascular flow alone cannot provide adequate blood supply for healing.
- Fetal would healing is rapid and noninflammatory and may serve as a model to reduce scaring and end-organ destruction.
- Chronic wounds are those that fail to proceed through an orderly and timely process.
- "Stunned wound" is similar to stunned myocardium and implies viable tissue with limited perfusion.
- Angiogenesis is inhibited in most normal adults and may be due in part to cyclooxygenase-2 inhibitors and angiotensin-converting enzyme inhibitors.
- Wound healing has three phases: (a) the inflammatory phase, (b) the proliferative phase, and (c) the remodeling phase.
- The critical clinical pathway for would healing is accurate diagnosis.
- The microcirculatory net starts at about 100 mm below the skin surface.
- Noninvasive techniques for measuring microcirculation include (a) intravital capillarosocopy, (b) laser Doppler perfusion imaging, (c) transcutaneous oxygen measurements, and (d) laser Doppler flowmetry.

INTRODUCTION

Wound healing is inextricably linked to the vascular system. Without adequate blood flow with its supply of nutrients and oxygen, the repair process of adult tissue would be impossible. Because of the tremendous growth and interest in the field of vascular medicine, a bias has developed toward the diagnosis and treatment of macrovascular problems. Interventional procedures and surgical techniques have been perfected giving many patients a chance at limb salvage and wound healing that were not available even a few years ago. Macrocirculation refers to the named vessels that can be seen with the unaided eye and are amenable to interventional or surgical manipulation. As a result of the emphasis placed on the macrovascular system, there is a misconception that the presence of adequate macrovascular flow alone will result in successful healing or limb salvage. Recently, wound care clinicians have been turning their attention to the status of the microcirculation to predict healing. The microcircula-

tion refers to an enormous "web" of microscopic vessels and their communications, which the skin and other organs are dependent on for nutrients and oxygen (1). Studying wound healing along this paradigm requires a refocusing of traditional views from a macro level to the micro or cellular level. At this level, there are many commonalities across tissue types in relation to inflammatory responses and repair processes. Karl Weber (2) proposed that there was a "common ground" when he asked the question, "What characteristics of tissue are common to most organs?" His theory eloquently describes the common ground at the organ (stroma and mesenchymal cells), cellular (fibroblast-like cells), and molecular levels (genes that govern phenotypic expression) (2). This chapter explores the wound healing process, factors affecting healing, macro and microcirculation, and common vascular-based wound etiologies. Each wound type is discussed with attention to pathophysiology, patient work-up, and treatment options. Throughout this chapter an emphasis is placed on the role of the microcirculation as it relates to wound healing, tissue preservation, and ultimately limb salvage.

WOUND HEALING

Most mature human tissues heal through the process of repair. In this process, the wounded tissue is replaced with connective tissue (scar) at the expense of structural integrity. The resultant scar tissue demonstrates a reduced tensile strength and energy absorption (3,4). A replacement with structurally identical tissue is known as tissue repair. The epidermis, liver, and gastrointestinal tract are a few examples of adult human tissues that have retained this capability. There has been recent interest in limiting the inflammatory phase of healing to minimize scar tissue formation and attempt to emulate tissue regeneration (5). An area of interest for wound care clinicians has been the healing process in fetal tissue. Fetal wound healing is rapid and proceeds without an inflammatory response (6). This unique wound healing response is a result of several conditions. The fetus lives in a sterile environment, which is rich in hyaluronic acid and growth factors (7). In addition, the fetal immune system is immature and underdeveloped (8). Fetal tissue is hypoxic, but this does not seem to have the same adverse effect as in the adult (9). The fetus also has a low collagen concentration and undetectable level of transforming growth factor-β (TGF-β). Shah et al., working with rats, showed that an inhibition of TGF-β1, which alters the relative amounts of the three TGF-β subunits, permits skin regeneration with less scarring than in controls (10). Another finding is the decreased quantity of collagen deposited in the wound site at the initial stage of healing. A high level of fetal steroids and a low quantity of neutrophils might be factors that give rise to the diminished inflammatory response in the fetal wound healing process. Current research is aimed at utilizing the lessons learned from fetal healing to address some chronic wound healing problems.

PHASES OF HEALING

A chronic wound has been defined as one that fails to proceed through an orderly and timely process to produce anatomic and functional integrity, or one that proceeds through the repair process without establishing a sustained anatomic and functional result (11). There is little agreement in the literature concerning time frames for the healing of various wound etiologies. Some authors feel that with a consistent clinical work-up and treatment protocol, wounds of various etiologies will heal with along a similar time course (12).

The wound healing process is a continuum from time of injury to complete wound healing, but for the sake of discussion and training, it is traditionally divided into three overlapping phases, which occur in sequence (inflammatory phase, proliferative phase, remodeling phase) (13). Inflammation can be defined as a localized protective tissue response elicited by injury or destruction of tissues, which serves to destroy, dilute, or wall off both the injurious agent and the injured tissues (14). There are two significant responses in the inflammatory phase. The first is the vascular response, in which platelets assist with initial hemostasis and release critical growth factors. The cellular response refers to the influx of polymorphonuclear cells, which release enzymes and cytokines, and remove bacteria and debris through the process of phagocytosis. Monocytes are transformed into tissue macrophages when they move into the tissues from the capillaries. Macrophages are considered the most critical cells in the healing process (15). These cells perform additional phagocytosis, and release enzymes and growth factors in large quantities. The hypoxic condition noted centrally in most wounds induces a proangiogenic response, which is initiated by the tissue macrophage (16). This neovasularization process is central to the concepts developed throughout this chapter.

The proliferative phase follows and somewhat overlaps the inflammatory phase moving down the healing cascade. The proliferative phase of healing consists in the processes of fibroplasias (reinforcement of injured tissue), neovascularization (establishment of appropriate blood supply), and reepithelialization (17). Angiogenesis is fundamental to tissue repair and wound healing, but when excessive, can result in disease states (e.g., tumor growth, diabetic retinopathy) (18). Angiogenesis is inhibited in most normal adult tissues (19). Recent work in the field of antiangiogenesis (oncology research) has led wound clinicians to investigate the drug history of chronic wound patients because medications known to inhibit angiogenesis such as cyclooxygenase-2 inhibitors and angiotensin-converting enzyme inhibitors may have an impact on the clinical healing potential (20,21). Abnormal vascular morphogenesis may result in deficient microperfusion despite angiogenesis. The wound healing benefits of topically applied platelet-derived growth factor may in part be a result of stabilizing the newly formed microvasculature (22). A novel approach in wound healing borrows from the innovative cardiac research of Isner (23,24). Endothelial cell precursors from bone marrow are being evaluated as a potential therapy for chronic wounds in early, small, phase 1 trials.

The remodeling phase represents the last phase of healing along the continuum, but this process continues long after the surface undergoes reepithelialization. A continual process of deposition and remodeling occurs. A large family of enzymes known as matrix metalloproteinases (MMPs) participate in this controlled tissue degradation process (25). Attempts at modifying the quantity and relative ratios of the 20 known MMPs have been the focus of numerous wound healing experiments in recent years (26,27).

FACTORS AFFECTING HEALING

Many patients fail to proceed through the traditional phases of healing and end up with chronic, nonhealing wounds. The term chronic wound seems to imply a definite temporal relationship with fixed time points. In fact, the terms acute and chronic carry a somewhat different meaning in wound care compared to other areas of medicine (e.g., acute and chronic renal failure). As previously described, a chronic wound fails to heal within an expected time frame for the underlying

TABLE 31.1. *The overall healing rate and the mean and median time to healing from two sources*

	Hospital-based outpatient clinic (140)	Christ Hospital outpatient clinic
Number of wounds	303	344
Wounds healed	225 (74%)	252 (73%)
Kaplan–Meier-derived mean time to healing	14 ± 1	12 ± 1
Kaplan–Meier-derived median time to healing	9 ± 1	9 ± 1

Ennis WJ, Meneses P., Clinical Evaluation:Outcomes, benchmarking, introspection and quality improvement. *Ostomy Wound Manage* 1996;42(10A):40S–47S.

etiology (11). Implicit in this definition is the need for published agreed-on healing times for various wound etiologies, which are not readily available in the literature. Standard healing rates could lead to the use of advanced wound healing technologies earlier in the course of therapy as the wounds begin to deviate from their projected healing curves (28).

Despite the well-accepted theory that wounds heal at different rates related to their underlying etiology, a review of our own data failed to reveal any statistically significant differences in Kaplan–Meier-derived survival time healing curves for any wound etiology (Tables 31.1 and 31.2). The data were generated from both a community hospital and a tertiary care facility, and implied that even case mix may not play as important a role as previously anticipated. This finding exemplifies the importance of taking an evidence-based approach to practice. Because a universal diagnostic and therapeutic approach (the Least Common Denominator Model, William J. Ennis, DO) was applied when diagnosing and treating these wounds, it is interesting that similar healing rates were achieved for the various wound etiologies (Table 31.3). These findings raise the question of whether there are truly significant wound healing rate variations in the literature and clinical practice, or simply wide practice variations. This concept explains the difficulty in performing wound care meta-analysis studies.

Factors Impeding Healing

Articles and textbook chapters traditionally divide factors that impede healing into three distinct categories. (a) Lo-

TABLE 31.3. *Least common denominator model*

Tissue oxygenation
Infection
Nutrition/immune status
Infection
Psychosocial
Pressure/neuropathy

cal factors are those that impede the healing process at the wound bed level. These factors include, but are not limited to, the presence of bacteria, circulation defects, foreign bodies, moisture, nutrients, and oxygen levels. (b) Systemic factors are those that affect the patient as a whole and therefore affect the wound from a systemic level. Comorbid illnesses, nutrition, obesity, and advancing age are examples of systemic factors. (c) The third category refers to iatrogenic, or clinician-induced, factors. Medications prescribed, dressings applied, and modalities utilized all affect the healing process and are under the control of the clinician.

Overlap Theory

We have proposed a unifying "overlap model" to more accurately reflect the factors that affect the wound healing process. This model implies there is wide overlap among the three traditional categories (29). Although it is helpful to use the traditional categories for teaching purposes, it does not reflect clinical reality. A 70-year-old diabetic patient with peripheral vascular disease and a leg ulcer has systemic factors including age and diabetes that affect healing. The ischemia, at a macrocirculatory level, translates into a microcirculatory defect with its associated paucity of nutrients and cellular oxygen. The use of insulin and medications such as pentoxyfilline are clinician-induced therapies, which have specific effects on the healing process systemically and locally. The overlap model attempts to break down each of the items noted in the three traditional categories into their least common denominator at a cellular level. This theory is in alignment with our therapeutic approach and eliminates the need for complicated wound-specific diagnostic and treatment algorithms.

Of particular interest in wound healing is a phenomenon we have referred to as the "stunned wound" (30). This term

TABLE 31.2. *Healing times for the wound types analyzed from two different sources (Kaplan–Meier computations)[a]*

	Hospital-based outpatient clinic (12)			Christ Hospital outpatient clinic		
	n	Mean	Median	*n*	Mean	Median
Venous	82	13 ± 2	8 ± 1	126	10 ± 1	8 ± 1
Arterial	15	13 ± 3	10 ± 2	33	16 ± 3	12 ± 1
Diabetic	63	10 ± 2	6 ± 1	37	15 ± 1	14 ± 3
Pressure	39	9 ± 1	9 ± 2	55	12 ± 1	10 ± 1
Postoperative	33	9 ± 1	7 ± 2	35	13 ± 1	10 ± 2
Traumatic	75	9 ± 1	7 ± 1	46	11 ± 1	8 ± 1
Collagen	13	13 ± 4	9 ± 2			
Other	9	11 ± 4	6 ± 1			
Lymphedema				12	11 ± 1	9 ± 1

[a]The values calculated for the wound type were not significant for any of these clinics.

is used to describe a wound that initially follows a "normal" healing trajectory, but subsequently plateaus and becomes recalcitrant. The concept is similar to the physiological phenomenon in cardiology known as "stunned myocardium," a syndrome that occurs post-myocardial ischemia (31). Although "stunned" tissue does not display normal cellular activity, the process is reversible with aggressive, rapid resuscitative efforts. There is evidence of increased microvascular permeability in stunned tissue (32). The exact mechanism responsible for stunning is unclear, but may involve changes in the calcium ion flux and/or the production of free radicals (33). There are conflicting ^{31}P nuclear magnetic resonance spectroscopy reports concerning levels of phosphocreatine, ATP, and inorganic phosphates found in stunned myocardium (34,35). These same phosphate-containing biochemicals have been measured in chronic wounds and skin using the same technology (36,37). Regardless of the responsible biochemical mechanism, the tissue will remain viable but dormant (hibernating) if perfusion remains inadequate. Perfusion that does not meet cellular demands over time will eventually lead to cellular death. The analogies to dermal wound healing are numerous.

Most clinicians have witnessed, to their surprise, rapid reepithelialization across a wound surface that had been stagnant for a long period of time. Often, the clinician is unable to identify a therapeutic modality, patient compliance factor, or other exogenous influence to explain this fortunate, yet surprising finding. Why on week 7, for example, did the wound progress toward healing? What triggers were now present that, if identified, could possibly have been added by the provider to jump start this process earlier?

LEG ULCERS

Building on the previous information about the wound healing process with an emphasis on the cellular mechanisms involved, a process for the diagnosis and treatment of some common leg ulcers will be described. Many of the necessary vascular testing procedures have been reviewed elsewhere in this book, and therefore only wound care-specific applications will be discussed in detail (see Chapters 15 & 17).

The most important aspect of any wound healing clinical pathway is to ensure an accurate diagnosis. Although this sounds obvious, there are many clinical tenets regarding wound care that are inaccurate and based on experience, preference, and training without much scientific validity. As with all areas of medicine, the history and physical exam form the basis for a preliminary diagnosis and treatment plan. Specific to wound care, the clinician must determine when the ulcer started, the initial appearance, speed of development, influencing factors (i.e., pain with elevation, timing of pain, etc.), prior history of ulcers, previous treatments and responses, and the location of the wound. General historical information includes the traditional categories of past medical, surgical, psychosocial, and family history and a complete review of the patient's medications including over-the-counter, herbal, and

all treatments considered "alternative." The physical exam needs to be complete with the examiner assessing the actual wound at the end of the exam. The wound dressing should not be removed until the entire history and physical exam are completed. If the wound bed is examined at the onset, the examiner can be biased toward an initial diagnosis that blunts his or her senses to picking up subtle physical findings that could otherwise change the initial diagnostic impression. The clinician should be knowledgeable about the history and physical exam findings associated with conditions that impair healing (38). Roenigk and Young presented a leg ulcer classification scheme utilizing seven distinct categories (39) (vascular, vasculitis, hematologic, infectious, neurotrophic, metabolic, and malignant). Despite the large list of differential diagnoses, the vast majority of patients in a clinic setting will have either venous, ischemic, or diabetic ulcerations.

Based on the previously described Least Common Denominator Model (Table 31.3), a systematic approach to the work-up of a patient with a lower extremity ulceration will be described. The most important aspect of the work-up centers around the adequacy of tissue perfusion. It is imperative that tissue perfusion is analyzed within the paradigm of both the macro and microvascular status. The initial evaluation focuses on the macrocirculation with the palpation of peripheral pulses. Ankle pulses are, however, not sufficient to detect impaired arterial circulation, and additional testing is always required for the patient with leg ulcerations (40). Performing an ankle–arm index is useful not only for wound healing prediction, but as an overall marker for cardiovascular health (41,42). Only about 10% of patients presenting to an outpatient wound clinic will have isolated arterial disease as an etiology for their leg ulcer (43). Arterial duplex, segmental pressures, pulse volume recordings, and magnetic resonance angiography are other noninvasive macrocirculation studies that may be ordered. An interventional angiogram is still considered the gold standard. After a complete assessment of the macrocirculation, the clinician's attention must turn to the status of the microcirculation. It is postulated that pathology within this circulatory bed is the common endpoint for many wound etiologies.

MICROCIRCULATION

A brief description of the thickness and distribution of the blood vessels in the various skin layers will help explain the noninvasive instruments available to study the microcirculation. A superficial (subpapillary) plexus and deep horizontal plexus of arterioles and venules are present within the dermis (44). Most of the microcirculation is found 1 to 2 μm below the epidermal surface in the upper, papillary dermis. The deep plexus is formed from the perforating vessels of the underlying muscle and subcutaneous fat. The outer layer of nonviable keratin known as the stratum corneum has a depth between 10 and 20 μm. The epidermis has a depth between 40 and 150 μm. The microcirculatory net therefore starts at about the 100-μm level. The second layer of skin, the dermis, has a depth between 1,000 and 4,000 μm. This means that communicating vessels, which emanate from the papillary dermis at about the 200- to 500-μm level, have a variable length (45,46). It is the superficial plexus that gives rise to the "capillary loop" into the papillary system (47), which represents the source of nutrition for the skin and the surface area for the exchange of gases and molecules between the skin tissue and blood. Each papilla contains one to three terminal capillary loops innervated by sympathetic, parasympathetic, and sensory nerve endings (48). Despite the lack of agreement on the presence of parasympathetic fibers, most studies strongly suggest that the skin microcirculation is regulated by sensory and autonomic fibers (49). There are specialized arteriovenous shunts (glomus bodies), which allow blood to bypass the capillary bed. These shunts represent the thermoregulatory function of the skin. This system is dominant, representing 85% of the total blood flow, whereas the nutritive bed represents only 15%. The nutritive capillaries are responsible for tissue viability by providing oxygen, nutrients, and fluid exchange. The capillary density determines the diffusion distance for gases and nutrients to dissolve through the tissues (50). The distinction between nutritive and nonnutritive flow is difficult to assess with indirect techniques. It is therefore critical to know the depth of penetration for any instrument when assessing the skin microcirculation. Instruments that sample at 500 μm or less are measuring the nutritive cutaneous flow, whereas studies beyond this mark are analyzing shunted (nonnutritive) flow. Intravital capillaroscopy and laser Doppler perfusion imaging (LDPI) are noninvasive techniques that sample only the nutritive capillary bed, whereas transcutaneous oximetry and laser Doppler flowmetry (LDF) detect deeper levels of the skin microcirculation (51).

NONINVASIVE TECHNIQUES FOR MEASURING MICROCIRCULATION

Intravital Capillaroscopy

Intravital capillaroscopy is a noninvasive technique used to identify nutrient capillaries. It consists of an optical microscope with epiillumination, which is applied to the nail fold capillaries. The capillaries lie parallel to the skin surface in the nail fold. This anatomic distribution of the loop creates an ideal place to measure capillary blood flow velocity (52,53).

A modification to intravital capillaroscopy using indocyanine green dye and a camera with an infrared microchip was able to detect capillary aneurysms in patients with collagen vascular disease and microangiopathy (54). Further advances to this technique have been introduced with orthogonal polarization spectral imaging, which works without the fluorescent dye and gives more flexibility to the analyses. The resolution obtained by this instrument reaches 1 μm per pixel, and the target surface can be reached at a 1.0 mm depth. *In vivo*, the usual depth is 200 μm (55,56). As a result, this technique has made possible the analysis of other tissues such as brain tumors, liver, burn wounds, gut, and the skin of neonates (49). With this technology, it is possible to measure the capillary blood cell velocity, capillary density (capillaries per mm^2) and the diameter of the erythrocyte column (48).

Laser Doppler Perfusion Imaging

LDPI is a recently developed technique, which utilizes a low-intensity laser (helium–neon) light. The device measures the backscattering created by moving red blood cells over a specific rectangular area, analyzing up to 4,096 individual points. The wavelength of this monochromatic light is 670 nm with a maximum accessible power of 1 mW. Two parameters of the returning laser light from the skin are analyzed. The first is the number of shifted photons, which relates to the concentration of moving red blood cells. The second is the mean Doppler shift of these photons, which relates to the blood cell velocity. These Doppler shift results are accumulated and translated into numeric values expressed in volts and in an image-colored map. Colors range from dark blue to burnt red and indicate minimum and maximum perfusion, respectively.

The laser Doppler flux is a value that results from the multiplication of these two parameters and is expressed in arbitrary units (Au) (53). The penetration of the laser beam reaches 500 μm when applied to intact skin; however, penetration can reach 2.5 times greater in other nonskin tissues like granulation tissue (46). Kernick and Shore reported that hematocrit, scanner head height, and Brownian motion are all factors that affect LDPI measurements (57). Several studies have utilized this technique for the assessment of skin microcirculation. Pellaton et al. found that perfusion values in older patients with a history of cigarette use, and were significantly lower than the values for nonsmokers during hyperemia (58). Cigarette smoking decreases the vasorelaxing capacity of skin microcirculation. Other studies have evaluated the possible pathways for vasodilation and the effect of surgical revasularization on the microcirculation (59,60). LDPI also has been applied to measure burn depth, healing time, and treatment responses (61–63). In our clinic, we have been analyzing the progression of wound healing using LDPI (Lisca, Perimed) on wound bed granulation tissue formation after stimulation with a collagen-based biological dressing. Increases in laser flux measurements correlate with increases in granulation tissue and subsequent healing (Figs. 31.1 and 31.2). These observations have been validated through a published correspondence by Blot and Monstrey (64) and in a clinical study by Nayeri et al. (65).

Transcutaneous Oxygen Measurements

Transcutaneous oximetry (TcPO$_2$) is a technique widely used to detect the skin oxygen tension. A dime-sized, Clarke-type, solid-state polarographic electrode containing a platinum cathode with a reference electrode of silver chloride is housed in a probe tip along with a heater and thermistor (66).

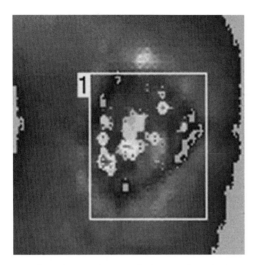

FIG. 31.1. (See Color Fig. 31.1.) A laser Doppler image perfusion scan of a diabetic foot ulcer wound bed on the first day of biological collagen dressing.

The tip of the probe is covered with a permeable membrane. An electrolyte solution fills the reservoir inside the probe. The reduction of oxygen at the cathode generates a current, which is then fed into the PO_2 channel of a monitor and converted into a voltage and digitized. The electrode is attached via a fixation device to the immediate periwound skin and heated to 43°C to 45°C, which induces hyperemia and the dissolution of keratin lipids, thereby increasing gas permeability. This procedure evaluates total microcirculation without the ability to differentiate the nutritive from the nonnutritive flow. To standardize the process and account for variations in overall tissue oxygenation, a regional perfusion index is calculated. This index is a calculated value taken from the periwound measurement divided by a chest wall control value. $TcPO_2$

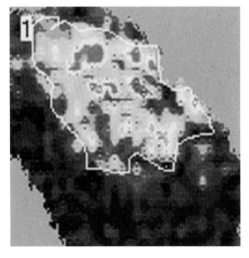

FIG. 31.2. (See Color Fig. 31.1.) Increase in angiogenesis in the wound bed after 21 days of biological collagen dressing therapy.

testing has been largely used in patients undergoing hyperbaric oxygen therapy and is useful in evaluating the effect of this therapy on the microcirculation (67,68).

Laser Doppler Flowmetry

This technology, used since the 1970s, is the basis for LDPI. It consists of a He–Ne low-intensity laser at 638 nm transmitted by a fiber optic to a terminal provided with a heater and thermistor to maintain a temperature constant. Measurements are done at a single point after a set temperature is achieved, similar to $TcPO_2$ testing. Like $TcPO_2$ measurements, total microcirculation is evaluated instead of isolating the nutritive flow. Measuring only one site results in inconsistent results due to the heterogeneity of microcirculation (51). The concepts and mechanisms behind this technology are similar to those described in the section on LDPI.

ISCHEMIC ULCERS

Well-defined criteria are available for the diagnosis of chronic critical limb ischemia, and wound healing is not possible in these patients without some form of revascularization (69). A more difficult clinical scenario is a patient with a non-healing leg ulcer above the threshold of chronic critical limb ischemia. Treatment suggestions in the literature include a trial of not more than 8 weeks of conservative wound care followed by revascularization in the recalcitrant case (70). Ischemic ulcers occur on the toes, foot, and ankle, often at the lateral malleoli. The wounds appear punched out and pale, and demonstrate little granulation tissue or exudation. The wounds are small initially and gradually enlarge over time. Pain can be severe. Often the wound bed is covered with a gray/yellow fibrinous debris or a firm black eschar. Microcirculatory testing is appropriate for confirmation of the diagnosis, as a baseline study before revascularization, and when revascariztion is either contraindicated or will only be utilized if healing is not achieved with local measures. The decision to proceed with amputation is often a difficult one in the nonreconstructable vascular patient. Recently recommendations for limb salvage versus amputation in the nonreconstructable vascular patient were generated through the analysis of three microcirculatory tests (laser Doppler, transcutaneous oxygen, and capillaroscopy) (71). This type of quantitative analysis could result in a more cost-effective, reproducible approach for patients. Skin perfusion pressures utilizing laser Doppler have been shown to correlate with toe pressures, and may provide another testing option when toe pressures are not available (72).

The gold standard of care is the reestablishment of flow to the wound bed whenever possible. The location of the wound, however, must be kept in mind when reviewing the angiogram and planning the proposed revascularization. A wound 2 cm above the lateral malleoli will not likely respond to a femoral posterior tibial bypass placed at the bifurcation of the medial and lateral branches. Collateral flow, the patency of the pedal arch, and the condition of the microcirculation will all play a role in the overall success of the revasculariztion. A multidisciplinary approach with vascular surgery, interventionalists, internists, and wound care specialists can help optimize outcomes. Transcutaneous oxygen measurements can be used to follow the success of percutaneous angioplasty procedures. In a study of claudicants, macrovascular improvement (ankle–brachial pressure) was immediate, but microcirculatory improvements were noted several weeks later (73). Recent data indicate that because of endothelial trauma, tissue edema, autoregulation of sympathetic stimuli, and surgical soft tissue trauma, a postrevascularization $TcPO_2$ study should be delayed until at least 3 days after the procedure (74). Animal studies have proven that this phenomenon is not solely due to edema (75).

Nonsurgical approaches include risk factor modification for atherosclerosis, pharmacologic therapy, and local wound care therapies and modalities. Risk factor modification has been described throughout this book and will not be discussed further (see Chapters 8, 12 and 13). Pharmacologic therapy for ischemic ulcers mirrors the therapies for generalized atherosclerosis (see Chapter 32) (76). Recently, a report was published describing wound healing responses with the use of cilostazol in five patients (77). Topical therapy must be approached with the knowledge of the vascular supply. If adequate perfusion is present, then the use of moist healing products, which augment autolytic debridement, can be utilized. Care should be taken when considering any occlusive dressings for the ischemic ulcer. A dry, stable eschar should be treated with protective dry dressings if adequate perfusion is lacking. Debridement of the intact eschar may result in exposure of deep structures and increase the risk of infection and further soft tissue loss.

When adequate perfusion is present, the usual spectrum of wound care products can be used. Acceleration of granulation tissue can sometimes be achieved with novel growth factor therapies (65,78). Laser Doppler-derived skin perfusion pressures and skin blood flow were found to be predictive of healing in a study using topical platelet-derived growth factors to treat ischemic leg ulcers (79). Wound healing modalities such as electrical stimulation and negative pressure therapy and the use of bioengineered tissues can be used in sequence or in combination to stimulate angiogenesis and thereby augment the microcirculation (80–82). The increasing awareness of transcutaneous testing has led to a renewed interest in the concepts of spinal cord stimulation to augment microcirculatory flow in ischemic limb patients (83,84).

VENOUS ULCERS

Accurate prevalence information is difficult to obtain because the diagnosis of venous disease is so imprecise (85). A total of 2.5 million people in the United States have venous ulcers, resulting in 2 million lost work days at a cost of 2 to 4 billion dollars for treatment (86). The problem will continue to escalate because 20% of the U.S. population will be over

65 years by 2010 (86). There is a 62% predominance of women suffering with venous ulcers, many of whom have had their ulcers for greater than 1 year (87). The literature states that only 50% to 60% of venous ulcers will heal within 6 months of therapy (88,89).

Despite the fact that 66% of the circulating blood is located on the venous side of the circulation at any one time, there is a paucity of definitive information concerning the pathophysiology of venous disease. Most of the focus has been placed on the diagnosis and treatment of arterial disorders. Reasons for this discrepancy include vascular surgeon interest, funding opportunities, fewer available venous diagnostic studies, general awareness of atherosclerosis and heart disease in the general population, and the mistaken concept that there is a lack of life- or limb-threatening sequelae of venous diseases. Another limitation has been the difficulty in developing an adequate animal model to study venous disorders (90).

The term "stasis" is actually a misnomer. The concept has been disproved in the literature, but the term is still frequently used (91). It has actually been shown that venous blood has a normal or increased oxygen level and the flow characteristics failed to demonstrate stasis (92). The increased pressures previously described in chronic venous insufficiency have been shown to propagate all the way back to the nutritive capillaries (93).

There are numerous theories to describe the underlying pathophysiology that results in a venous ulceration (94–108). A complete examination of the extremity should include checking pulses and assessing for secondary signs of venous insufficiency (hemosiderin deposits, eczematous dermatitis, atrophie blanche, lipodermatosclersois, varicose veins, and edema) (109,110). Wound biopsy is an often neglected step in the standard work-up of a venous ulcer patient. Biopsy should be considered as part of the work-up if the wounds are greater than 6 months to 1 year in duration or have an irregular appearance, or when concerns exist for underlying inflammatory conditions or carcinoma. Not infrequently, a patient who was treated with a provisional diagnosis of venous disease turns out to have another condition (e.g., lymphoma, rheumatoid arthritis, etc.) (111). The classic appearance of a venous ulcer involves a medial-leg, irregularly shaped, partial-thickness ulcer with well-defined borders surrounded by erythematous or hyperpigmented skin (112). The wounds are classically located on the medial aspect of the leg in the "gaiter" distribution. There is no classic wound bed appearance for venous ulcers, with any combination of fibrin and granulation tissue being possible. The amount of wound exudate is variable, but frequently there is a significant quantity. Pain that is eliminated with elevation of the legs is a classic history, although many patients fail to demonstrate this phenomenon, and some actually obtain relief with a dependent position. Telangiectatic veins are often present along the medial ankle, which is known as a corona phlebectatica. Arterial disease, which can exist in up to 30% of cases, must be ruled out. This can be done easily in the office by performing an ankle–brachial index (85). In the absence of arterial insufficiency and a normal sensory exam, venous disease is confirmed in the majority of cases with a typical-appearing ulcer. An initial classification system was developed by a subcommittee of the Society for Vascular Surgery and the International Society of Cardiovascular Surgery in 1988 (113). Because of the tremendous increase in diagnostic testing options and a broader understanding of venous disorders, a consensus statement was released by the American Venous Forum in 1994. The new classification system grouped venous patients into four categories known as CEAP (clinical, etiology, anatomic, pathophysiological) (114,115). Although the system is somewhat cumbersome, it is thorough and allows for a uniform language to help compare research findings and communicate with other clinicians on venous disease issues. As clinical procedures continue to develop (e.g., subfascial endoscopic perforator surgery) the system will undergo modifications, but it appears to be clinically sound and an accepted standard (115).

There are many pathological findings in the microcirculation of venous ulcer patients. Using capillaroscopy, it has been noted that there is a great deal of capillary proliferation. The introduction of fluorescein dye to the technique resulted in the identification of a pericapillary halo, which was later attributed to microedema, which may impair the exchange of materials at the tissue level (53). This technique also detected the presence of thrombotic capillaries further worsening tissue perfusion. Capillaroscopic studies comparing ischemic wounds with venous wounds show that the microcirculation in both conditions is very similar with no statistically significant differences in the nongranulation tissue area of the wound and in the adjacent skin area. Significant differences were obtained in the granulation tissue area, where the capillary density was lower in ischemic wounds, and in the distant skin area, where the capillary density was higher in the ischemic patient. The similarities found in the nongranulation tissue and adjacent skin area support the idea that both types of ulcers have the same genesis from the microcirculation standpoint. This finding was corroborated by LDPI and LDF (116).

VASCULITIC WOUNDS

This category of wounds is frequently described in the wound literature as an "atypical wound." The index of suspicion should rise when the patient gives a history of a rapidly progressing wound, severe pain, unusual location, unusual appearance, or recent change in medications, or has numerous comorbid conditions known to have cutaneous manifestations. One of the more common conditions seen in a wound center are small vessel-hypersensitivity vasculitic wounds secondary to leukocytoclasis. Palpable purpura on the lower extremities is the hallmark finding for this disorder. These lesions may evolve into pustules, plaques, vesicles, or bullae (117). Inflammation involving the superficial dermal plexus results in oval purpura, whereas involvement of the deeper plexus can result in a larger infarct region of the skin. Moist

wound therapy is appropriate, but the key to effective treatment is antiinflammatory/immune-suppressive therapy either topically or locally as the clinical situation dictates, and the elimination of the offending agent. The history and physical examination should help guide the diagnosis. Vasculitic ulcers secondary to autoimmune disorders are seen frequently in referral-based wound centers. Of patients with rheumatoid arthritis, 8% to 9% suffer from leg ulcerations (118). These patients may have underlying arterial and/or venous disease, and a careful work-up is needed so that the patient is not inappropriately labeled a "rheumatoid ulcer" case. The treatment for an arterial or venous etiology is the same as previously described. A true rheumatoid ulcer is usually smooth, undulating, and often painful, and can be in unusual locations on the legs. In addition to standard moist wound healing, bioburden management, debridement when needed and pain control, systemic corticosteroids, and immune-suppressive agents are often needed. Skin grafting becomes necessary in a large number of cases. Recently, our clinic has used debridement, negative pressure therapy for wound bed preparation, and autologous split thickness skin grafting.

Although not a true vasculitic lesion, pyoderma gangrenosum (PG) is a clinical entity that can be associated with rheumatoid arthritis, but is more often associated with inflammatory bowel disease (119). In up to 50% of cases, there is no identified underlying systemic disease responsible for PG (120). The disease presents with chronic, recurring, destructive skin lesions. The lesions often develop in areas of prior skin trauma; this phenomenon is known as pathergy. The lesions typically begin as small, painful nodules or pustules, which then rapidly expand. The wound bed is moist and can have fibrin, eschar, and dusky granulation tissue (Fig. 31.3). The edges of the wound are undermined and irregular, and there is a violaceous color to the wound perimeter. Biopsy is nondiagnostic, but is often needed to rule out other differential diagnoses. These lesions are very painful, and fail to respond to standard wound care dressings and

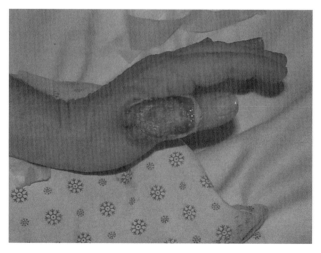

FIG. 31.3. Pyoderma gangrenosum lesion of the thumb.

treatments. Systemic therapy is usually required with steroids. Frequently, immunosuppressives are required as well. Recently, topical tacrolimus has been used with a fair amount of success (121,122). Recently, the Mayo clinic experience with PG was published and their conclusion was that PG is frequently overdiagnosed (123). As with all wound treatment regimens, if an adequate response is not achieved within 4 weeks, the process of history, physical, and noninvasive testing must be repeated to ensure an accurate provisional diagnosis. All treatment regimens must be critically reviewed and patient compliance ensured. With experience, the diagnosis can be made clinically. Our treatment protocol includes steroid therapy followed by debridement. Initial debridement can lead to extension of the lesions as previously mentioned. Wound bed preparation includes electrical stimulation, topical tacrolimus, and either bioengineered tissue grating when possible or autologous skin grafting. Growth factors and systemic therapy with infliximab have recently been reported as well (124,125).

Other systemic disorders associated with vasculitic leg ulcers that must be considered are systemic lupus, scleroderma, Sjogren's syndrome, and Bechet's disease. These conditions all have classic historical, physical, and laboratory findings, but share in common atypical appearing leg ulcers. As with the PG and rheumatoid arthritis, moist wound healing, modalities that increase angiogenesis, and systemic therapy for the underlying disorder must all be in place to achieve successful healing outcomes.

LEG ULCERS SECONDARY TO HEMATOLOGIC DISORDERS

As with the previously described ulcerations, this group of conditions has a microvascular disorder as the common endpoint for ulceration. The red blood cell disorders of sickle cell disease, thalassemia, and polycythemia all have characteristic microvascular vasoocclusion. Sickle cell disease (SCD) affects 1 in 600 African Americans and can result in painful, small, fibrin-filled ulcerations, recalcitrant to therapy (126). As with other wound etiologies, the primary therapy is aimed at the underlying disorder. Specific issues need to be addressed with the sickle cell patient, however. The use of hydroxyurea is approved for therapy in adults with SCD. It should be noted that leg ulcers have also been reported as a complication of hydroxyurea use (127,128). Wound bed pain can be disabling in this condition. The use of occlusive gel sheet dressings has proven quite useful not only for pain management, but also to aid with the autolytic debridement of the gelatinous necrosis that is frequently seen in the wound bed of patients with SCD. Gelatinous necrosis refers to a yellow/gray film on the surface of the wound bed, which is composed of collagen and tissue macromolecules, which can be pealed off painlessly. Often, the underlying wound bed is granular. With exposure and dessication of the underlying granulation tissue, however, the return of severe pain is rapid, and a gel sheet should be applied quickly. Bioengi-

neered human skin equivalents have proven to be effective in our center for wound bed stimulation and pain control. Recently, some authors have reported an increased frequency of venous valvular incompetence with SCD, suggesting that compression bandaging should be included in the treatment regimen (129). In cryoglobulinemia and cryofibrinogenemia, immunoglobulins reversibly precipitate in the cold (130). Painful superficial ulcers can arise in a netlike configuration. Biopsy and serum levels are diagnostic. Moist wound healing dressings and systemic therapy are necessary for treatment. Patients who have recurrent venous ulcerations, deep vein thrombosis, or a family history should be worked up for protein C, protein S, antithrombin 3, antiphospholipid antibody disease, and factor V Leiden mutations. There is a higher prevalence of these disorders in the venous ulcer population, and wound care clinicians need to have a higher index of suspicion (131).

LEG ULCERS: INFECTIOUS, METABOLIC, MALIGNANT

Infectious etiologies for leg ulcers include fungal, mycobacterial, atypical mycobacterial, syphilitic, leprosy, and bacterial infections. With an increasing population of immune-suppressed patients, these etiologies need consideration if the history is compatible with high risk. Bacterial infections are usually secondary and rarely the primary cause of a leg ulcer. Metabolic diseases with cutaneous manifestations include gout, diabetes, Gaucher's disease, porphyria, and pyoderma, which has previously been described in this chapter. An underlying cancer may present with a cutaneous metastatic lesion as the first sign of the malignancy (132). A wound biopsy should always be considered if the wound has been present for more than 6 months to 1 year, or if the wound has an atypical appearance.

NEUROTROPHIC ULCERS

This diabetic foot ulcer is the prototype for this category, but the wound care professional must remember tabes dorsalis, leprosy, polio, and traumatic and toxic neuropathies, Charcot–Marie–Tooth disease and inherited sensory neuropathies are on the list of differentials. The diabetic foot has been described elsewhere in this text and only a few brief comments will be made. Although macrovascular disease plays an important role in the etiology and healing of diabetic foot ulcers, neuropathy is the most prevalent disorder leading to the breakdown of tissue (133). Akbari and LoGerfo noted that the pathology in the microcirculation of the diabetic patient is not occlusive, but maldistributed with a lack of vasodilatory capabilities (134). Surgical revascularization does not repair the defect in the microcirculation, which explains why some patients fail to heal their diabetic ulcers despite patent bypass grafts (135). Less invasive, interventional procedures may be of benefit when the desired endpoint is healing a wound (136). In addition, the vascular testing for the diabetic patient must include an assessment of the microcirculation. It is well known that the ankle–brachial index is falsely elevated in the diabetic patient and that a toe pressure is more reliable (137). Recently modifications to the toe pressure measurement have been introduced, which utilize pulse oximeter-derived toe values (138). Transcutaneous oxygen testing may provide the best predictor, however, for diabetic ulcer healing (139). In addition to standard moist wound healing, the clinician must provide bioburden control, adequate offloading of the ulcer, and tight glucose control as part of an overall treatment program.

SUMMARY

In this chapter, we reviewed the healing process and factors that impede healing with an emphasis on cellular activity and the microcirculation. We described the more common leg ulcer conditions and reviewed our standard approach to such patients. Recently, our clinic has been analyzing microcirculation before, immediately after, and then 1 to 2 weeks postoperatively to plot changes seen with bypass, angioplasty, physical therapy wound modalities, supplemental nasal oxygen, pain control, and edema. We hope to create an improved treatment protocol to help achieve limb salvage for these complex patients by analyzing their complete vascular system.

REFERENCES

1. Ennis WJ, Meneses P. Technologies for assessment of wound microcirculation. In: Krasner D, Rodeheaver G, Sibbald G, ed.,*Chronic wound care,* 3rd ed. Wayne, PA: HMP, 2001:469–482.
2. Weber KT. In search of common ground. In: Weber KT, ed., *Wound healing in cardiovascular disease.* Armonk, NY: Futura, 1995:295–307.
3. Forrester JC. Mechanical, biochemical, and architectural features of surgical repair. *Adv Biol Med Phys* 1973;14:1–3.
4. Bryant R. Wound repair: a review. *J Enterostomal Ther* 1987;14:262–266.
5. Wilgus TA, Vodovotz Y, Vittandini E, et al. Reduction in scar tissue formation in full thickness wounds with topical celcoxib treatment. *Wound Repair Regen* 2003;11(1):25–34.
6. Roswell AR. The intrauterine healing of fetal muscle wounds: experimental studies in the rat. *Br J Plast Surg* 1984;37(4):635–642.
7. Bleacher JC, Adolph VR, Dillon PW, et al. Fetal tissue repair and wound healing. *Dermatol Clin* 1993;11(4):677.
8. Cates K, Rowe J, Ballow M. The premature infant as a compromised host. *Curr Prob Pediatr* 1983;13(8):1–63.
9. Pritchard J, McDonald P, Gant N. The morphological and functional development of the fetus. In: Pritchard J, McDonald P, Gant N, eds., *Williams obstetrics.* Norwalk, CT: Appleton-Century-Croft, 1985:145.
10. Shah M, Foreman DM, Ferguson MW. Control of scarring in adult wounds by neutralising antibody to transforming growth factor β. *Lancet* 1992;339:213–214.
11. Lazarus GS, Cooper DM, Knighton DR, et al. Definitions and guidelines for assessment of wounds and evaluation of healing. *Arch Dermatol* 1994;130:489–493.
12. Ennis WJ, Meneses P. Wound healing at the local level: the stunned wound. *Ostomy Wound Manage* 2000;46[Suppl 1]:39S–48S.
13. Ennis WJ, Meneses P. Leg ulcers: a practical approach to the leg ulcer patient. *Ostomy Wound Manage* 1995;41[7A]:52S–62S.
14. Calvin M. Cutaneous wound repair. *Wounds* 1998;10(1):12–32.
15. Leibovich SJ, Ross R. The role of the cacrophage in wound repair; a study with hydrocortisone and antimacrophage serum. *Am J Pathol* 1975;78:71–100.
16. Knighton D. Regulation of wound-healing angiogenesis: effect on oxygen gradients and inspired oxygen gradients. *Surgery* 1981;90:262–270.
17. Kirsner RS, Bogensberger G. The normal process of healing. In: Kloth LC, McCulloch J, eds., *Wound healing: alternatives in management.* Philadelphia: FA Davis 2001:3–34.
18. Morrison WA, Mitchell GM, Barker JE, et al. Angiogenesis in wound healing and surgery. In: Fan TPD, Kohn EC, ed., *The new angiotherapy.* Totowa, NJ: Humana Press, 2001:105–113.
19. Fidler IJ. Angiogenesis and cancer metastasis. *Cancer J* 2000;[Suppl 2]:S134–S141.
20. Masferrer J. Approach to angiogenesis inhibition based on cyclo-oxygenase-2. *Cancer J* 2001;7(3):S144–S150.
21. Qiu JG, Factor S, Chang TH, et al. Wound healing: captopril, an angiogenesis inhibitor, and *Staphylococcus aureus* peptidoglycan. *J Surg Res* 2000;92(2):177–185.
22. Hellstrom M, Gerhardt H, Kalen M, et al. Lack of pericytes leads to endothelial hyperplasia and abnormal vascular morphogenesis. *J Cell Biol* 2001;153:543–553.
23. Murayama T, Tepper OM, Silver M, et al. Determination of bone marrow-derived endothelial progenitor cell significance in angiogenic growth factor-induced neovascularization *in vivo. Exp Hematol* 2002;30(8):967–972.
24. Isner J, Kalka C, Kawamoto A, et al. Bone marrow as a source of endothelial cells for natural and iatrogenic vascular repair. *Ann N Y Acad Sci* 2001;953:75–84.
25. Ovington L, Cullen B. Matrix metalloprotease modulation and growth factor protection. *Ostomy Wound Manage* 2002;48(6):2–13.
26. Edwards JV, Yager DR, Cohen IK, et al. Modified cotton gauze dressings that selectively absorb neutrophil elastase activity in solution. *Wound Repair Regen* 2001;9(1):50–58.
27. Klein SA, Anderson GL, Kennedy AB, et al. The effects of a broad-spectrum matrix metalloproteinase inhibitor on characteristics of wound healing. *J Invest Surg* 2002;15(4):199–207.
28. Marks J, Hughes LE, Harding KG, et al. Prediction of healing time as an aid to the management of open granulating wounds. *World J Surg* 1983;7(5):641–645.
29. Ennis WJ, Meneses P. Factors impeding wound healing. In: Kloth L, McCulloch J, eds.,*Wound healing alternatives in management,* 3rd ed. Philadelphia: CPR Press, 2002:68–96.
30. Ennis WJ, Meneses P. Wound healing at the local level: the stunned wound. *Ostomy Wound Manage* 2000;46[Supp1 A]:39S–48S.
31. Bolli R, Marban E. Molecular and cellular mechanisms of myocardial stunning. *Physiol Rev* 1999;79(2):609–634.
32. Chen JM, Gong XQ, Zhong JG, et al. The role of microvascular permeability in the mechanism for stunned myocardium in rats. *Microvasc Res* 1997;54(3):214–220.
33. Bolli R, Zughaib M, Li XY, et al. Recurrent ischemia in the canine heart causes recurrent bursts of free radical production that have a cumulative effect on contractile function. A pathophysiological basis for chronic myocardial stunning. *J Clin Invest* 1995;96(2):1066–1084.
34. Geshi E, Sordahl LA, Ito S, et al. Simultaneous evaluations of contractility and energy metabolism of stunned myocardium using ^{31}P magnetic resonance spectroscopy. *Jpn Heart J* 1998;39(6):791–807.
35. Martin C, Schulz R, Rose J, et al. Inorganic phosphate content and free energy charge of ATP hydrolysis in regional short-term hibernating myocardium. *J Cardiovasc Res* 1998;39:318–326.
36. Ennis WJ, Driscoll DM, Meneses P. A preliminary study on ^{31}P NMR spectroscopy: a powerful tool for wound analysis using high-energy phosphates. *Wounds* 1994;6(5):166–173.
37. Ennis WJ, Meneses P. ^{31}P NMR spectroscopic analysis of wound healing. The effect of hydrocolloid therapy. *Adv Wound Care* 1996;9(3):21–26.
38. Seamen S. Considerations for the global assessment and treatment of patients with recalcitrant wounds. *Ostomy Wound Manage* 2000;46[1A]:10S–29S.
39. Roenigk HH, Young J. Leg ulcers. In: Young J, Olin JW, Bartholomew JR, ed.,*Peripheral vascular diseases,* 2nd ed. St. Louis, MO: Mosby–Year Book, 1996:637–668.
40. Moffat C. Ankle pulses are not sufficient to detect impaired arterial circulation in patients with leg ulcers. *J Wound Care* 1995;4(3):134–138.
41. Newman AB, Shemanski L, Manolio TA, et al. Ankle–arm index as a

predictor of cardiovascular disease and mortality in the cardiovascular health study. *Arterioscler Thromb Vasc Biol* 1999;19:538–545.

42. Wutschert R, Bounameaux H. Predicting healing of arterial leg ulcers by means of segmental systolic pressure measurements. *Vasa* 1998;27:224–228.

43. Baker SR, Stacey MC, Singh G, et al. Aetiology of chronic leg ulcers. *Eur J Vasc Surg* 1992;6:245–251.

44. Jakubovic HR, Ackerman B. Structure and function of skin: development, morphology, and physiology. In: Moshella H, eds., *Dermatology*, 3rd ed. Philadelphia: WB Saunders, 1992:3–79.

45. Kochevar IE, Pathak MA, Parrish JA. Photophysics, photochemistry, and photobiology. In: Fitzpatrick TB, et al., eds., *Dermatology in general medicine.* New York: McGraw-Hill, 2003:1267–1275.

46. Kolarova H, Dritichova D, Wagner J. Penetration of laser light into the skin *in vitro. Lasers Surg Med* 1999;24:231–235.

47. Braverman IM, Yen A. Capillary loops of the dermal papillae. *J Invest Dermatol* 1977;68:44–52.

48. Abbink EJ, Wollersheim H, Netten PM, et al. Reproducibility of skin microcirculatory measurements in humans, with special emphasis on capillaroscopy. *Vasc Med* 2001;6:203–210.

49. Ruocco I, Cuello AC, Parent A, et al. Skin blood vessels are simultaneously innervated by sensory, sympathetic, and parasympathetic fibers. *J Comp Neurol* 2002;448:323–336.

50. Hern S, Mortimer PS. Visualization of dermal blood vessels—capillaroscopy. *Clin Exp Dermatol* 1999;24:473–478.

51. Christ F, Bauer A, Brugger D. Different optical methods for clinical monitoring of the microcirculation. *Eur Surg Res* 2002;34:145–151.

52. Pazos-Moura CC, Moura EG, Bouskela E, et al. Nailfold capillaroscopy in non-insulin dependent diabetes mellitus: blood flow velocity during rest and post-occlusive reactive hyperaemia. *Clin Physiol* 1990;10:451–461.

53. Coleridge Smith PD. The microcirculation in venous hypertension. *Vasc Med* 1997;2:203–213.

54. Bollinger A, Saesseli B, Hoffmann U, et al. Intravital detection of skin capillary aneurysms by video microscopy with indocyanine green in patients with progressive systemic sclerosis and related disorders. *Circulation* 1991;83:546–551.

55. Groner W, Winkelman JW, Harris AG, et al. Orthogonal polarization spectral imaging: a new method for study of the microcirculation. *Nat Med* 1999;5:1209–1213.

56. Langer S, Born F, Hatz R, et al. Orthogonal polarization spectral imaging versus intravital fluorescent microscopy for microvascular studies in wounds. *Ann Plast Surg* 2002;48:646–653.

57. Kernick DP, Shore AC. Characteristics of laser Doppler perfusion imaging *in vitro* and *in vivo. Physiol Meas* 2000;21:333–340.

58. Pellaton C, Kubli S, Feihl F, et al. Blunted vasodilatory responses in the cutaneous microcirculation of cigarette smokers. *Am Heart J* 2002; 144 (2):269–274.

59. Newton DJ, Khan F, Belch JJF. Assessment of microvascular endothelial function in human skin. *Clin Sci* 2001;101:567–572.

60. Rora S, Pomposelli F, LoGerfo FW, et al. Cutaneous microcirculation in the neurophatic diabetic foot improves significantly but not completely after successful lower extremity revascularization. *J Vasc Surg* 2002; 35 (3):501–505.

61. Kloppenberg FW, Beerthuizen GI, ten Duis HJ. Perfusion of burn wounds assessed by laser doppler imaging is related to burn depth and healing time. *Burns* 2001;27(4):359–363.

62. Brown RFR, Rice P, Bennett NJ. The use of laser imaging as an aid in clinical management decision making in the treatment of vesicant burns. *Burns* 1998;24:692–698.

63. Droog EJ, Steenbergen W, Sjoberg F. Measurement of depth of burns by laser Doppler perfusion imaging. *Burns* 2001;27:561–568.

64. Blot SI, Monstrey SJ. The use of laser Doppler imaging in measuring wound healing progress. *Arch Surg* 2001;136(1):116.

65. Nayeri F, Stromberg T, Larsson M, et al. Hepatocyte growth factor may accelerate healing in chronic leg ulcers: a pilot study. *J Dermatol Treat* 2002;13(2):81–86.

66. Sheffield PJ. Measuring tissue oxygen tension: a review. *Undersea Hyperb Med* 1998;25(3):179–188.

67. Kalani M, Jorneskog G, Naderi N, et al. Hyperbaric oxygen (HBO) therapy in treatment of diabetic foot ulcers long term follow up. *J Diabetes Complications* 2002;16(2):153–158.

68. Ratliff CR. TCOMs as a screening tool for hyperbaric oxygen therapy. *Plast Surg Nurs* 200;20(1):15–17.

69. Second European Consensus. Second European Consensus document on chronic critical leg ischemia. *Circulation* 1991;84:1–26.

70. Hafner J, Schaad I, Schneider E, et al. Leg ulcers in peripheral arterial disease (arterial leg ulcers): impaired wound healing above the threshold of chronic critical limb ischemia. *J Am Acad Dermatol* 2000;43:1001–1008.

71. Ubbink DT, Geert HJJ, Spincemaille, et al. Prediction of imminent amputation in patients with non-reconstructible leg ischemia by means of microcirculatory investigations. *J Vasc Surg* 1999;30:14–21.

72. Tsai FW, Tulsyan N, Jones DN, et al. Skin perfusion pressure of the foot is a good substitute for toe pressure in the assessment of limb ischemia. *J Vasc Surg* 2000;32:32–36.

73. Stalc M, Poredos P. The usefulness of transcutaneous oximetry in assessing the success of percutaneous transluminal angioplasty. *Eur J Endovasc Surg* 2002;24:528–532.

74. Arroyo CI, Tritto VG, Buchbinder D, et al. Optimal waiting period for foot salvage surgery following limb revascularization. *J Foot Ankle Surg* 2002;41(4):228–232.

75. Friedman HI, Smith K, Magee J. The effect of subcutaneous edema on transcutaneous oximetry. *J Invest Surg* 1998;11:21–27.

76. Hiatt WR. Pharmacologic therapy for peripheral arterial disease and claudication. *J Vasc Surg* 2002;36:1283–1291.

77. Dean SM, Vaccaro PS. Successful pharmacologic treatment of lower extremity ulcerations in 5 patients with chronic critical limb ischemia. *J Am Board Fam Pract* 2002;15(1):55–62.

78. Saba AA, Freedman BM, Gaffiedl JW, et al. Topical platelet-derived growth factor enhances wound closure in the absence of wound contraction: an experimental and clinical study. *Ann Plast Surg* 2002;49(1):62–66.

79. Chleboun JO, Martins R, Rao S. Laser Doppler velocimetry and platelet growth factor as prognostic indicators for the healing of ulcers and ischaemic lesions of the lower limb. *Cardiovasc Surg* 1995;3(3):285–290.

80. Kloth L. Physical modalities in wound management: UVC, therapeutic heating and electrical stimulation. *Ostomy Wound Manage* 1995;41(5):18–20, 22–24, 26–27. Review.

81. Argenta L, Morykwas M. Vacuum assisted closure. A new method for wound control and treatment. Clinical experience. *Ann Plast Surg* 1997;38(6):563–576: discussion S77.

82. Long RE, Falabella AF, Valencia I, et al. Treatment of refractory, atypical lower extremity ulcers with tissue engineered skin (Apligraf). *Arch Dermatol* 2002;137(12):1660–1661.

83. Petrakis IE, Sciacca V. Transcutaneous oxygen tension in the testing period of spinal cord stimulation in critical limb ischemia of the lower extremities. *Int Surg* 1999;84:122–128.

84. Ghajar AW, Miles JB. The differential effect of the level of spinal cord stimulation on patients with advanced peripheral vascular disease in the lower limbs. *Br J Neurosurg* 1998;12(5):402–408.

85. Milestones, pebbles, and grains of sand. In: Browse N, Burnand K, Wilson N, Irvine A, eds., *Diseases of the veins.* London: Arnold, 1999:1–2.

86. Kerstein MD, Gahtan V. Outcomes of venous ulcer care: results of a longitudinal study. *Ostomy Wound Manage* 2000;46(6):22–29.

87. Sibbald RG. Venous leg ulcers. *Ostomy Wound Manage* 1998;44(9): 52–64.

88. Falanga V, Margolis D, Alvarez O, et al. Rapid healing of venous ulcers and lack of clinical rejection with allogeneic cultured human skin equivalent. *Arch Dermatol* 1998;134:293–300.

89. Lyon RT, Veith FJ, Bolton L, et al. Clinical benchmark for healing of chronic venous ulcers. *Am J Surg* 1998;176:172–175.

90. Dalsing MC, Ricotta JJ, Wakefield T, et al. Animal models for the study of lower extremity chronic venous disease: lessons learned and future needs. *Ann Vasc Surg* 1998;12:487–498.

91. Schwartzberg JB, Kirsner RS. Stasis in venous ulcers: a misnomer that should be abandoned. *Dermatol Surg* 2000;26:683–684.

92. Dormandy JA. Pathophysiology of venous leg ulceration-an update. *Angiology* 1997;48(1):71–75.

93. Junger M, Hahn M, Klyscz T, et al. Microangiopathy in the pathogenesis of chronic venous insufficiency. In: Ramelet HJ, Brunner SW, eds., *Management of leg ulcers.* Basel: Karger, 1999:124–129.

94. Browse NL, Burnand KG. The cause of venous ulceration. *Lancet* 1982;2(8292):243–245.

95. Falanga V, Kirsner R, Katz MH, et al. Pericapillary fibrin cuffs in

venous ulceration. Persistence with treatment and during ulcer healing. *J Dermatol Surg Oncol* 1992;18(5):409–414.

96. Falanga V, Eaglstein WH. The trap hypothesis of venous ulceration. *Lancet* 1993;341:1006–1008.

97. Higley HR, Ksander GA, Gerhardt CO, et al. Extravasation of macromolecules and possible trapping of transforming growth factor-β in venous ulceration. *Br J Dermatol* 1995;132:79–85.

98. Coleridge Smith PD, Thomas P, Scurr JH, et al. Causes of venous ulcerations: a new hypothesis. *Br Med J* 1988;296:1726–1727.

99. Thomas P, Nash GB, Dormandy JA. White cell accumulation in dependent legs of patients with venous hypertension: a possible mechanism for trophic changes in the skin. *Br Med J* 1988;296:1693–1695.

100. Moyses C, Cederholm-Williams SA, Michel CC. Haemoconcentration and accumulation of white cells in the feet during venous stasis. *Int J Microcirc Clin Exp* 1987;5:311–320.

101. Salim AS. The role of oxygen-derived free radicals in the management of venous (varicose) ulceration: a new approach. *World J Surg* 1991;15:264–269.

102. Kaminski MV, Cordts PR. Gut-derived oxidative stress: a pathological factor in leg ulcers with and without chronic venous insufficiency. *Wounds* 1998;10(1):33–37.

103. Falanga V, Kruskal J, Franks JJ. Fibrin- and fibrinogen-related antigens in patients with venous disease and venous ulceration. *Arch Dermatol* 1991;127:75–78.

104. Margolis DJ, Kruithof EKO, Barnard M, et al. Fibrinolytic abnormalities in two different cutaneous manifestations of venous disease. *J Am Acad Dermatol* 1996;34:204–208.

105. Maessen-Visch MB, Hamulyak K, Tazelaar DJ, et al. The prevalence of factor V Leiden mutation in patients with leg ulcers and venous insufficiency. *Arch Dermatol* 1999;135:41–44.

106. Munkvad S, Jorgensen M. Resistance to activated protein C a common anticoagulant deficiency in patients with venous leg ulceration. *Br J Dermatol* 1996;134:296–298.

107. Grossman D, Heald PW, Wang C, et al. Activated protein C resistance and anticardiolipin antibodies in patients with venous leg ulcers. *J Am Acad Dermatol* 1997;37:4.9–4.13.

108. Hasan A, Murata H, Falabella A, et al. Dermal fibroblasts from venous ulcers are unresponsive to the action of transforming growth factor-β1. *J Dermatol Sci* 1997;16:595–566.

109. Rowland J. Intermittent pump versus compression bandages in the treatment of venous leg ulcers. *Aust N Z J Surg* 2000;70:110–113.

110. McCulloch JM, Marler KC, Neal MB, et al. *Adv Wound Care* 1994;7(4):22–25.

111. Pekanmäki K, Kolari PJ, Kiistala U. *Clin Exp Dermatol* 1987;12:350–353.

112. Falanga V. Venous ulceration; assessment, classification and management. In: Kane D, Krasner D, eds., *Chronic wound care*, 2nd ed. Wayne, PA: HMP, 1997:165–171.

113. Porter JM, Rutherford RB, Clagett GP, et al. Reporting standards in venous disease. *J Vasc Surg* 1988;8:172–181.

114. Beebe HG, Bergan JJ, Bergqvist D, et al. Classification and grading of chronic venous disease in the lower limbs. *Dermatol Surg* 1995;21:642–647.

115. Beebe HG, Bergan JJ, Bergqvist D, et al. Classification and grading of chronic venous disease in the lower limbs. *Vasc Surg* 1996;30(1):5–11.

116. Gschwandtner ME, Ambrozy E, Maric S, et al. Microcirculation is similar in ischemic and venous ulcers. *Microvasc Research* 2001;62:226–235.

117. Ouahes N, Phillips TJ. Leg ulcers. *Curr Prob Dermatol* 1995;7:113–137.

118. Thurtle OA, Cawley MID. The frequency of leg ulcerations in rheumatoid arthritis. *J Rheumatol* 1983;10:507–509.

119. Magro CM, Crowson AN. The spectrum of cutaneous lesions in rheumatoid arthritis: a clinical and pathological study of 43 patients. *J Cutan Pathol* 2003;30(1):1–10.

120. Powell FC, Su WPD, Perry HO. Pyodrma gangrenosum: classification and management. *J Am Acad Dermatol* 1996;34:395–409.

121. Lyon CC, Stapelton M, Smith AJ, et al. Topical tacrolimus in the management of peristomal pyoderma gangrenosum. *J Dermatol Treat* 2001;12(1):13–17.

122. Lazarous MC, Kerdel FA. Topical tacrolimus protopic. *Drugs Today* 2002;38(1):7–15.

123. Weenig RH, Davis MD, Dahl PR, et al. Skin ulcers misdiagnosed as pyoderma gangrenosum. *N Engl J Med* 2002;347:1412–1418.

124. Freedman BM, Oplinger EH. Use of becaplermin in progressive limb-threatening pyoderma gangrenosum. *Adv Skin Wound Care* 2002;15(4):180–182.

125. Grange F, Djilali-Bouzina F, Weiss AM, et al. Corticosteroid resistant pyoderma gangrenosum associated with Crohn's disease: rapid cure with infliximab. *Dermatology* 2002;205(3):278–280.

126. Fixler J, Styles L. Sickle cell disease. *Pediatr Clin North Am* 2002;49(6):1193–1210.

127. Charache S, Terrin ML, Moore RD. Effect of hydroxyurea on the frequency of painful crises in sickle cell anemia. *N Engl J Med* 1995;332:1317–1322.

128. Yeh H. Hydroxyurea induced cutaneous ulceration in older patients. *J Am Geriatr Soc* 2000;48(2):232.

129. Clare A, FitzHenley M, Harris J, et al. Chronic leg ulceration in homozygous sickle cell disease: the role of venous imcompetence. *Br J Hematol* 2002;119(2):567–571.

130. Choucair MM, Fivenson DP. Leg ulcer diagnosis and management. *Dermatol Clin* 2001;19(4):659–678.

131. Maessen-Visch MB, Hamulyak K, Tazelaar DJ, et al. The prevalence of factor V Leiden mutation in patients with leg ulcers and venous insufficiency. *Arch Dermatol* 1999;135:41–44.

132. Tumman J, Coggins R. A case of mistaken identity: primary cutaneous lymphoma presenting as venous ulceration. *Hosp Med* 1999;60(10):761.

133. Boulton AJ, Meneses P, Ennis WJ. Diabetic foot ulcers: a framework for prevention and care. *Wound Repair Regen* 1999;7:7–16.

134. Akbari CM, LoGerfo FW. Limb salvage strategies for the high risk foot. *Wounds* 2000;12[Suppl 6]:778–818.

135. Arora S. Pomposelli F, LoGerfo FW, et al. Cutaneous microcirculation in the neuropathic diabetic foot improves significantly but not completely after successful lower extremity revascularization. *J Vasc Surg* 2002;35:501–505.

136. Faglia E, Mantero M, Caminite M, et al. Extensive use of peripheral angioplasty particularly infropopliteal, in the treatment of ischaemic diabetic foot ulcers: clinical results of a multicenter study of 221 consecutive diabetic subjects. *J Intern Med* 2002;252:225–232.

137. Brooks B, Dean R, Patel S, Wu B, et al. TBI or not TBI? That is the question. Is it better to measure toe pressure than ankle pressure in the diabetic patients? *Diabet Med* 2001;18:528–532.

138. Johansson KEA, Marklund BRG, Fowelin JHR. Evaluation of a new screening method for detecting peripheral arterial disease in a primary health care population of patients with diabetes mellitus. *Diabet Med* 2002;19:307–310.

139. Kalani M, Brismar K, Fagrell B, et al. Transcutaneous oxygen tension and toe blood pressure as predictors for outcome of diabetic foot ulcers. *Diabetes Care* 1999;22:147–151.

140. Ennis WJ, Meneses P. Wound Healing at the local level: The Stunned wound. *Ostomy Wound Manage* 2000;46(Supp 1A):39S–48S.

CHAPTER 32

Management of Patients with Lower Extremity Ulcers

Catherine R. Ratliff

Key Points

- Arterial ulcers are less common, but more difficult to treat than venous ulcers because of underlying ischemic process.
- The identified risk factors of lower extremity arterial disease (LEAD) include diabetes, smoking, advanced age, dyslipidemia, hypertension, obesity, hyperhomocysteinemia, cardiovascular disease, cardiovascular surgery, and sickle-cell anemia.
- Ulceration due to arterial insufficiency is punched out and often with a dry, pale wound bed at external pressure sites, whereas ulcers from venous disease are exudative, not pale, but with pink granulation tissue, and edema is usually present.
- Pain is often the first symptom of LEAD.
- Hemosiderosis and dermatitis are characteristic skin changes associated with venous disease.
- Common methods to diagnose venous ulcers include Doppler ultrasonography, photoplethysmography, air plethysmography, and duplex ultrasonography, although often they are diagnosed based on clinical assessment alone. The aims of therapy in venous ulcer management include reduction of edema, improvement of pain, ulcer healing, and prevention of recurrence.

INTRODUCTION

It is estimated that leg ulcers affect approximately 2.5 million people in the United States (1). Approximately 2 million workdays are lost each year in the United States because of leg ulcers. The per-patient cost of ulcer care by home health nurses has been estimated at $40,000, and patients report out-of-pocket expenses of $1,000 per year (1). The best treatment for any leg ulcer is dependent on accurate diagnosis. The etiology, pathogenesis, diagnosis, and treatment of arterial and venous leg ulcers are discussed in this chapter.

PATIENTS WITH LOWER EXTREMITY ARTERIAL ULCERS

Arterial ulcers are much less common than ulcers of venous origin, but are more difficult to treat because of the underlying ischemic process (Fig. 32.1). They have a prevalence rate of approximately 30% in people over age 65 years (2). Elderly patients may present with a history of cardiac or cerebrovascular disease, leg claudication, and pain in the distal foot (3). There are many terms that refer to arterial ulcers, including ischemic ulcers, peripheral vascular disease, peripheral arterial occlusive disease, and peripheral arterial disease, but the one that is becoming more recognized is lower extremity arterial disease (LEAD) (4).

The incidence of LEAD increases with age and is greater among men. Approximately 10% of people older than 55 years have asymptomatic disease, 5% have symptomatic disease (intermittent claudication), and 1% have rest pain or gangrene. The presence of disease (intermittent claudication) is less than 2% among men under 50 years of age, but increases to 6% among those 70 years or older. Prevalence for women follows the same pattern, but with a 10-year delay (80 years or

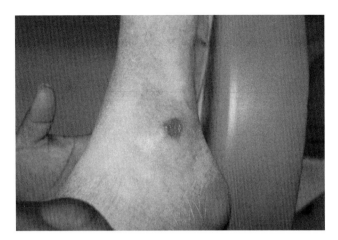

FIG. 32.1. Arterial ulcer. Typical punched-out appearance of arterial ulcer with thinning of the epidermis and loss of hair growth on the leg.

older) (5). In patients with intermittent claudication, worsening occurs in about 16%, bypass surgery is required in about 7%, and amputation is required in about 4% (6).

Etiology

Atherosclerosis is the most common cause of LEAD. The identified risk factors are diabetes, smoking, advanced age, dyslipidemia, hypertension, obesity, hyperhomocysteinemia, cardiovascular disease with cardiovascular surgeries, and sickle-cell anemia (4). In the young adult, arterial disease is typically due to premature atherosclerotic disease or to thromboangiitis obliterans (Buerger's disease or arteriosclerosis obliterans) and is strongly associated with smoking (5).

Pathophysiology

Arterial occlusion due to any cause can result in ischemia, with could lead to ulceration. Peripheral vascular disease due to atherosclerosis, diabetes with microvascular or macrovascular disease, and/or vasculitis can lead to ischemia with ulceration (7). There is often overlap, and the exact cause cannot always be identified.

Atherosclerotic disease typically occurs between the abdominal aorta and the distal vessels and is most common at the bifurcation sites. The initial triggering event is thought to be lipid accumulation and endothelial injury, which result in plaque formation and enlargement. Contributing factors include increased blood viscosity and coagulability and increased smooth muscle tone within the vessel. The result is a reduction in blood flow to the tissues and a loss of the ability to respond to increased metabolic demands with increased blood flow (5).

Rose (8) found that when arteries become narrowed, an increased pressure gradient occurs across the stenosis. Although blood flow changes can be detected at a 30% stenosis

downstream from the occlusion, critical compromise generally occurs with a 50% reduction in the diameter of the vessel. When peripheral arterial occlusion becomes severe, the mechanism of peripheral vasodilation is inadequate to meet the needs of the skin, muscle, and nerves of the extremity, even at rest. The resulting symptoms of ischemia may manifest as rest pain, ulcers, and gangrene.

Risk Factors

Risk factors for LEAD are the same as for coronary artery disease, with smoking being the most predictive. Nicotine and its metabolite, cotinine, affect the vessels in a number of ways. They can cause primary endothelial injury with sloughing of the endothelial cells and thickening of the arterial wall, enhance the growth of arthromatous plagues, increase smooth muscle tone (vasoconstriction), and increase the blood viscosity (5). Elevated lipoproteins and homocysteine levels are also risk markers, as are reduced high-density lipoproteins (4).

Hypertension, particularly systolic hypertension, is a common risk factor for LEAD. The link is thought to be related to the vessel wall changes. Vessel wall changes seen with hypertension include increased production of smooth muscle, activation of the renin–angiotensin–aldosterone system, increased arteriolar sodium transport, high intracellular calcium levels, increased production of factors contributing to vasoconstriction, and increased interaction between the endothelium and the circulating blood elements (5).

Diabetes is another important risk factor. Diabetes can cause increased plaque formation, increased red blood cell rigidity, increased blood viscosity and coagulability, hypertrophy of the smooth muscle, and increased vascular resistance. Hyperinsulinemia and insulin resistance may also contribute to hypertrophy of smooth muscle (5). Diabetics with LEAD typically exhibit more severe and advanced disease at earlier ages, and the risk of ulceration, gangrene, and amputation is significantly increased. The most commonly involved vessels are the infrapopliteal (tibial and peroneal). Multisegmental occlusions and multivessel disease are common. Disease is usually bilateral and these patients are usually poor candidates for angioplasty because of the small vessels.

Assessment

The assessment goals of a patient with LEAD are to determine the severity of the LEAD and identify potential contributing factors, interventions to minimize these factors, and methods to assess for healing (see Fig. 32.2). Patient history should include questions such as risk factors for LEAD, past and present tobacco use, and history of hypertension, diabetes, elevated cholesterol levels with treatment, angina, myocardial infarction, or cerebrovascular accident. In addition, one needs to elicit a wound history. Descriptions of the wound, its onset and course, and previous therapies are important components to include. The physical examination must include a

Common Characteristics
- Typical wound appearance
    - Round punched-out appearance of wound edges
    - Dry, pale, or necrotic ulcer base
    - Granulation tissue minimal or absent
    - Wound size usually small; may be deep
    - Minimal exudate
    - Gangrene (wet or dry); necrosis common
- Located on the tips of toes, over phalangeal heads, web spaces, proximal to lateral malleolus, areas exposed to repetitive trauma or rubbing of footwear, midtibia
- Small to moderate exudate
- Pain maybe severe with intermittent claudication, rest pain
- Dependent rubor and pallor on elevation

Establish Etiology
- Assessment of risk factors (diabetes, smoking, hypertension, atherosclerosis)
- Leg(s) assessment (thick toe nails, hair loss on legs, skin shiny and taut, pitting or dependent edema)
- Ankle–brachial index <0.8
- Diminished or absent pulses/cool skin temperature
- Assessment of wound (edema, exudate, odor, size, tissue, and periwound)

Optimize Perfusion
- Vascular consult for revascularization, and/or wet gangrene
- Smoking cessation
- Regular exercise program
- Control of diabetes
- Avoidance of cold, caffeine
- Weight control

Moisturize Intact Skin
- If dry gangrene present, then keep wound dry to prevent bacterial growth
- Use topical therapy with moisture-retentive dressings

FIG. 32.2. Arterial ulcer (lower extremity arterial disease) algorithm.

through assessment of the lower extremities to determine the perfusion status.

Pain is often the first symptom of LEAD. Questions regarding the presence of pain and its location and characteristics are important. Patients may report aching, heaviness, fatigue, or numbness when walking that is usually relieved with a few minutes of rest. The pain usually occurs in the muscle group just distal to the level of the obstruction. The frequent complaint of calf pain is because the gastrocnemius muscle has the greatest oxygen consumption of any muscle group in the leg during ambulation.

Intermittent claudication is the pain that occurs with moderate to heavy activity and is relieved by 2 to 5 minutes of rest. This typically occurs with 50% occlusion of the involved vessel (9). Treadmill exercise testing is one method of determining functional disability related to intermittent claudication.

Nocturnal pain develops as the occlusion worsens. This type of pain occurs when the patient is in bed and is caused by leg elevation and reduced cardiac output. Rest pain refers to pain that occurs in the absence of activity and with the legs in a dependent position, often resulting in edema. Rest pain signals advanced, often multilevel occlusive disease. In general, pain occurs one joint distal to the occlusion. Intermittent claudication is typically described as "cramping," whereas rest pain is usually referred to as a "constant deep aching" pain in the toes or forefoot, or as a severe, nagging, burning pain when in bed. Often, patients with severe nocturnal or rest pain sleep sitting in a chair. In the diabetic patient with neuropathy, rest pain may not be present.

The physical assessment is geared to the lower extremity for its perfusion status. Leg appearance should be compared to the contralateral leg to identify skin changes. To assess color changes with leg elevation and dependence, one places the patient supine and raises leg to a 60-degree angle for 15 to 60 seconds while assessing for a visible color change (pallor in fair-skinned individuals and gray hues in dark-skinned individuals). The leg is then placed in a dependent position and one observes for the development of rubor caused by the pooling of blood within the chronically dilated arterioles. Dependent rubor or a bluish red color shows evidence of maximal arteriolar dilation. Pallor occurring within 25 seconds of elevation generally indicates severe occlusive disease, as does dependent rubor (5).

To assess for venous filling time, one elevates the limb to provide venous drainage and then places the leg in a dependent position. The amount of time (seconds) required for venous filling is recorded. Normal filling time is 10 to 15 seconds. Prolonged venous filling time is independently predictive of LEAD. A filling time of more than 20 seconds usually indicates severe arterial occlusive disease (5).

Pulses should be compared with the contralateral pulse and should be assessed in a proximal-to-distal fashion. Diminished or absent pedal pulses are predictive of arterial disease. Palpation of a normal dorsalis pedis or posterior tibialis pulse is considered normal. The absence of both a dorsalis pedis and a posterior tibial pulse is evidence of arterial disease. A handheld Doppler can be used to auscultate when both pulses are nonpalpable.

Capillary refill is measured by pressing against the toe pad firmly to empty the blood vessels and then monitoring the time for the tissue to regain color. Normal refill time is considered to be less than 3 seconds. The patient with arterial disease may have normal capillary refill because the emptied vessels may refill in a retrograde fashion from the surrounding veins even if arterial inflow is impaired (9).

The ankle–brachial index (ABI) is a comparison of perfusion pressures in the lower leg with those in the upper arm. The ABI is used to screen for significant arterial insufficiency and to identify patients who need further work-up. It can also be used to detect stenosis after revascularization. An ABI of less than 0.9 is diagnostic of LEAD, 0.6 to 0.8 shows borderline perfusion, and less than 0.5 is indicative of severe ischemia. Patients with arterial insufficiency should have the ABI checked periodically because it may decrease over time (4).

ABI is only an indirect measure and cannot be considered accurate in patients with noncompressible vessels (such as the diabetic with vessel calcification), where the ABI may be falsely elevated. Therefore, diabetic patients who have evidence of ischemia but normal or elevated ABIs should be referred for toe pressures or transcutaneous oxygen measurements.

Toe pressures are generally more accurate in diabetics and those with atherosclerosis because the blood vessels in their toes are less likely to be calcified. This procedure is performed in exactly the same manner as the ABI except that a toe cuff is placed around the great toe and the Doppler probe is placed against the distal toe surface to monitor the signal. A normal toe pressure is greater than 0.6 times (i.e., 60% of) the brachial artery pressure (5).

Transcutaneous oxygen ($TcPO_2$) measurements can be done on patients with diabetes, history of smoking, or hypercholesterolemia to assess the adequacy of oxygen delivery to the skin. $TcPO_2$ of less than 40 mm Hg is associated with impaired wound healing. Angiography or arteriography may also be done on those patients with $TcPO_2$ less than 40 mm Hg or an ABI less than 0.8 in nondiabetic patients to rule out significant arterial occlusive disease in whom surgical intervention is planned.

Vascular studies may be needed to further assess the perfusion status. Studies include pulse volume recordings, segmental pressure analysis, and color-flow duplex scanning. The pulse volume recording provides a reflection of actual perfusion volume over the course of the cardiac cycle. Normal vessels are described as triphasic; with moderately occlusive disease, the waveform may be monophasic, and with severe disease, it becomes blunted. Segmental pressure recordings are used to determine the level of the occlusion. Differences of greater than 20 mm Hg between cuffs indicate an occlusion. Color duplex imaging provides both anatomic (presence of plaques or stenosis) and functional (direction and velocity of blood flow) analysis of the arteries in the legs. It has begun to replace arteriography because it is noninvasive, and arteriography only provides anatomic information (5).

Lower Extremity Arterial Disease Ulcer Characteristics

These ulcers can be present almost anywhere on the leg, and are usually distal to the impaired arterial blood supply. Most of these ulcers are located between toes or tips of toes, over phalangeal heads, around lateral malleolus, or in an area of trauma or rubbing from footwear. These ulcers are relatively small, with well-defined, round or punched-out borders. The wound bed is usually pale, gray, or yellow with no evidence of new granulation tissue, and tendons may be exposed. Necrosis or cellulitis may be present. There is minimal exudate because of the decreased blood flow to the area. The periwound may appear blanched or purpuric and also may have a shiny appearance.

Clinical Management of the Patient with Lower Extremity Arterial Disease

These ulcers often require months to heal because of the co-existing disease processes. The prognosis for wound healing is directly correlated with the patient's ability to deliver sufficient oxygen and nutrients to support the repair process. Perfusion and oxygenation can be improved with surgical techniques, pharmacologic agents, and lifestyle changes such as smoking cessation and weight reduction.

The patient with LEAD and an ABI of less than 0.5 is very unlikely to heal without surgical revascularization. Surgical intervention should also be considered for patients with an ABI greater than 0.5 who are surgical candidates and fail to respond to pharmacologic and behavioral therapy. Options include bypass grafting using the saphenous vein, angioplasty for minimal occlusive disease, and placement of stents.

Long-term patency rates from angioplasty have been disappointing, but sometimes can be improved with administration of anticoagulants or by placement of stents into the stenotic area immediately after angioplasty (9). Patients with prior deep vein thrombosis (DVT) may also be poor candidates for bypass grafting, because studies have shown that they may be unlikely to heal even with a patent bypass graft (10).

Amputation is reserved as last resort, and is usually indicated for patients with irreversible ischemia and gangrene. A preoperative TcPO$_2$ of greater than 20 mm Hg is associated with greater success in healing amputation sites.

Traditional outcomes following revascularization usually look at limb retention and hemodynamic results. Generally, health-related quality of life is not measured. Tretinyak et al. (11) looked at 46 patients, and found a mild improvement in functional status postoperatively, but overall quality of life was slow to show improvement following revascularization. Health-related quality of life should be an important outcome when considering the risks and benefits of revascularization in this patient population. Patients also need to be educated that revascularization surgery is not necessarily sufficient for lifelong management and additional surgeries may be required in the future.

The mainstay of pharmacologic therapy includes medications to reduce the risk of thrombotic events, hemorrheologic agents, and analgesics. Aspirin in doses of 75 to 325 mg a day may help to prevent disability and death from stroke and myocardial infarction. Cilostazol, an antiplatelet and antithrombotic drug, improves intermittent claudication and appears to be a good option for improving the walking distances of patients with intermittent claudication. Cilostazol in doses of 100 mg twice a day has been shown to be significantly better than pentoxifylline or placebo for increasing walking distance in patients with intermittent claudication, but was associated with a greater frequency of side effects such as headaches and diarrhea. Benefits of the drug are dose related and may be lost with discontinuation of the medication. Cilostazol also modifies plasma lipoproteins in patients with arterial disease. Although pentoxifylline is the most commonly prescribed drug for LEAD, there are no data to support it in the treatment of LEAD. Prostaglandins (PGE-1 and PGE-2), ciprostine, and serotoninergic blocking agents have not been proven to be beneficial (4).

Analgesics may be required to relieve the chronic pain and improve quality of life. Pain control also prevents vasoconstriction caused by sympathetic stimulation. Systemic vasodilators are generally contraindicated because the vasodilation may divert blood from the affected area. Frequently, these patients may need to be referred to a chronic pain clinic for management of the ischemic pain.

The ability to improve tissue perfusion and promote wound healing depends on the patient's willingness to make appropriate lifestyle changes to modify correctable risk factors. The patient should be educated on the benefits of a walking program. A typical walking program involves 30 to 60 minutes of walking 4 to 5 days a week at a rate of 2 miles per hour. In addition, the patient should be counseled about ceasing smoking and normalizing blood pressure, cholesterol, and glucose levels. The patient should maintain hydration status to reduce blood viscosity, avoid cold, caffeine, and constrictive clothes to reduce the vasoconstriction, and practice weight control to reduce the workload of the ischemic extremity (4).

Topical wound therapy for LEAD is based on the overall principles for chronic wound care including debridement, identification and eradication of infection, filling of dead space, maintenance of a moist wound environment, and protection from mechanical trauma. No significant difference in overall healing rates or outcomes has been found among the various moist wound dressings for patients with LEAD ulcers (12). Caregiver time, ease of use, availability, and cost need to be considered when selecting a dressing. In addition, the type of dressing may change over time as the wound heals or deteriorates. Ulcers need to be assessed at dressing changes, and modifications in the treatment plan implemented based on this assessment.

All chronic wounds contain bacterial flora, and so it is important to distinguish among contamination, colonization, and infection. The prompt identification and treatment of any infection is important when managing an infection. Because the ischemic wound is less able to manage an inflammatory response, an absence of progress toward healing over 2 to 4 weeks may signal an infection. Other indicators of infection may be increased pain, increased necrosis, fluctuance of the periwound, increased drainage, and a faint halo of erythema surrounding the wound. Management of infected ulcers includes debridement of all necrotic tissue and treatment with antimicrobials.

Debridement of necrotic tissue is important to reduce bacterial bioburden and promote healing. However, the one exception is dry, black eschar on the feet. Although necrotic tissue is a potential medium for bacteria, a dry, intact eschar can also serve as a bacterial barrier. This is advantageous when managing a poorly perfused wound, in which any bacterial invasion is likely to result in clinical infection. Current opinion supports the maintenance of dry, black eschar when the leg is clearly ischemic with limited or no potential for healing (4).

Traditionally there has been concern about the use of sustained, continuous high-compression bandages (30 to 40 mm Hg) in patients with an ABI of less than 0.8 due to the possibility of ischemia. However, little evidence exists to support this concern. In patients with mixed arterial/venous disease and edema, omission of compression complicates the treatment of the venous component of the disease. For patients with mixed disease and moderate arterial insufficiency (ABI greater than 0.5 but less than 0.8) who present with ulcers and edema, a trial of a modified, reduced compression bandaging to a level of 23 to 30 mm Hg at the ankle may reduce edema and thereby promote healing. Close supervision by health care professionals is required, and more frequent bandaging may be needed to assess for complications and patient tolerance (4).

MANAGEMENT OF WOUNDS IN LOWER EXTREMITY VENOUS DISEASE

Venous ulcers (also known as venous insufficiency ulcers, stasis ulcers, venous leg ulcers, or varicose ulcers) account for 70% to 90% of all leg ulcers (Fig. 32.3). In the United States, approximately 7 million people have venous insufficiency, with approximately one in seven, or 1 million people, progressing to develop ulceration (13). The refractory nature of these ulcers affects quality of life, and the high costs of long-term therapy make them a major health problem. The cost of venous leg ulcers is estimated to be $1 billion per year in the United States, with the average cost per patient over a lifetime exceeding $40,000 (13). Women seem to develop these ulcers more than men and they are more common with increasing age.

Venous ulcers significantly affect one's life because of the inability to work, social isolation, and frequent clinic visits. They also have a major economic impact from loss of productivity and the cost of dressings and health care. In addition, recurrence rates of 57% to 97% have been reported, reflecting the chronicity of the condition and the failure to effectively manage the underlying problem.

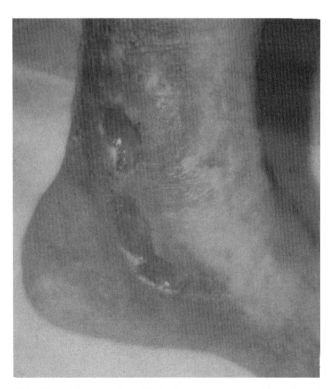

FIG. 32.3. Venous ulcer. Typical appearance and location of venous ulcer with hemosiderin staining of surrounding tissue and ruddy red color of the wound bed.

Etiology

Venous hypertension, sustained elevation of the venous pressure in the legs on ambulation, is the primary culprit of the disease. Venous hypertension is caused by one of three pathologies: reflux or valve dysfunction, obstruction of the deep veins, and failure of the calf muscle pump such as from paralysis. Valve dysfunction may be due to congenital weakness or secondary to previous thrombophlebitis (DVT). Obstruction of the venous system in the legs can result from obesity and pregnancy. Occupations that involve standing and sitting for prolonged periods of time also place patients at increased risk for developing venous hypertension with possible ulceration. Varicose veins, previous vein stripping, and sclerotherapy also suggest abnormalities of the venous system that may contribute to the development of venous ulceration. Varicosities on the leg's surface may be due to superficial disease alone or combine with perforator and/or deep venous ulceration (14).

Risk Factors

The most common cause of venous outflow obstruction is DVT (see Fig. 32.4). DVT is present in up to 75% of patients with lower extremity venous disease. Other factors that may impede venous flow include pregnancy, obesity, congestive heart failure, congenital abnormalities, edema, ascites, trauma, and tumors to the leg. When obstruction occurs, the veins distal to the obstruction become distended and venous pressures rise, resulting in venous stasis. The severity of the obstruction and the resulting stasis is determined by the extent of the venous obstruction and the development of collateral circulation (5).

Pathophysiology

The venous system of the leg includes three major vein components: deep veins, superficial veins, and perforator veins. The deep veins include the posterior and anterior tibial and the peroneal veins. The superficial venous system, visible beneath the skin, is referred to as the saphenous system because it comprises the greater and lesser saphenous veins. It is located in the subcutaneous fat and within the fascia of the muscle compartments. The deep veins lie within the muscle compartments of the leg and are paired and are located next to the arteries. The perforator or communicating veins connect the superficial with the deep veins. There are more than 90 perforating veins in each leg. At the medial malleolus, the perforating veins are not surrounded by fascia and are in direct contact with the skin. Increased venous pressure is transmitted through the perforating vein to the skin, leading to superficial varicosities and ulcerations (15).

The causes of valvular incompetence are not fully understood. It is theorized that valve leaflets are damaged by venous distention, venous hypertension, and DVT. Valvular impairment allows reflux and pooling of blood in the legs. Venous

Common Characteristics

- Medial lower leg
- Large ulcer(s) with irregular shaped borders
- Lipodermatosclerosis (thickening of skin)
- Periwound hyperpigmentation
- Moderate to heavy serous exudate
- Pain relieved by elevation
- Associated with dermatitis

Establish Etiology

- Assessment of risk factors (DVT, obesity, pregnancy, leg trauma, smoking, CHF, vascular surgeries, family history)
- Leg(s) assessment (edema, varicosities, "bowling pin"-shaped leg)
- Ankle-brachial index >0.8
- Palpation of pulses/skin temperature normal
- Doppler examination
- Venous duplex studies

Arterial Component

Vascular consult
for
revascularization

No/Minimal Arterial Component

Optimize venous return

- Compression (Unna boots, compression wraps, stockings, pumps)
- Exercise (walking)
- Weight management
- Smoking cessation
- Surgery
- Topical therapies

FIG. 32.4. Venous ulcer (lower extremity venous disease) algorithm.

insufficiency is a disease of the cutaneous microcirculation as seen with the skin capillaries (atrophie blanche) together with the changes in the microlymphatics. In patients with venous incompetence, venous pressure does not decrease during exercise as it does in normal subjects, but remains elevated.

Various causation theories have been proposed such as pericapillary fibrin cuff deposition, abnormalities of the fibrinolytic system, leukocyte plugging of the vessels in the legs, and growth factor-trapping theories. There is also a growing recognition that excessive proteolytic activity by proteases, especially the matrix metalloproteinases and fibrinolytic factors of the plasminogen activation system, may be a key feature in the development of venous leg ulcers (7).

Assessment

The history should include a screen for etiologic factors including prior surgeries, pregnancies, leg trauma, family history of venous disease, and a history of DVT. A family history of venous disease is important because there is a strong familial predisposition. The history of the current ulcer should include description, onset and course, and treatments that have been tried and their effectiveness. The patient should specifically be asked whether compression therapy was used, and, if it was, what type, the patient's tolerance/compliance, and

the response to the therapy. The physical assessment should focus on edema, skin changes, characteristics of ulcer(s), and periulcer skin.

Venous ulcers may be characterized by a dull, aching pain or sensation accompanied by heaviness. Patients may report that it typically worsens during the day as a result of prolonged dependency and is usually alleviated by leg elevation. The presence of concomitant arterial disease may also be responsible for pain. Arterial pain is aggravated by leg elevation and may produce intermittent claudication with walking. Up to 25% of patients with venous ulcers may have concomitant arterial disease (3).

Lower leg edema is common in the patient with venous disease and may be present to varying degrees. Edema occurs because the elevated venous pressures push fluid through the distended and permeable capillary membrane into the surrounding tissue. Sudden onset of edema is associated with DVT, trauma, and cellulitis. In contrast, venous insufficiency is accompanied by a gradual onset of pitting edema that worsens with prolonged standing and diminishes after rest in a recumbent position with the legs elevated. Chronic venous insufficiency is associated with edema that is persistent despite periods of leg elevation. Furthermore, the initial pitting edema may become "nonpitting" or "brawny" as more fibrin and fluid leak into the tissues (4).

Hemosiderosis and dermatitis are characteristic skin changes associated with venous disease. Hemosiderosis is a grayish-brown hyperpigmentation caused by extravasation of red blood cells into the tissues. The subsequent breakdown of red blood cells causes the deposition of hemosiderin, an iron-containing pigment, into the dermis. Eczema or "stasis dermatitis" may appear and is characterized by erythema, edema, pruritis, scaling, and weeping of the lower leg. The term "stasis" is an incorrect term because true stasis of blood does not exist, but pooling of fluid and extravasation of red blood cells leads to the irritation of the skin (5,14).

The combination of chronic edema, fibrin deposits, and the presence of inflammatory mediators causes lipodermatosclerosis. It involves sclerosing of the dermis and the subcutaneous tissues and is indicative of longstanding venous disease. On palpation, the leg may have the feel of woody induration and appear hyperpigmented around the ankle. Edema above and below the gaiter (ankle) area creates the appearance of an inverted bottle.

Accompanying this is the appearance of atrophie blanche seen in about one-third of patients. It presents as white areas of extremely thin skin dotted with tiny blood vessels. The skin here is very thin and fragile, and ulcers may develop even after minor trauma (14). These changes in the skin also create small breaks in the skin and can lead to increased absorption of topically applied substances. Consequently, the patient becomes quickly sensitized to topical agents and is at an increased risk for developing contact dermatitis (5).

Varicosities are another prevalent finding in venous insufficiency. Dilated varicose veins may be observed in the calf and along the thighs. Another common finding is a sunburst pattern of small venous channels inferior and distal to the medial malleolus known as the ankle venous flare.

Ulcer Characteristics

Although these ulcers can occur anywhere between the knee and the ankle, the medial malleolus is the classic location for venous ulcers. This location is the point of highest pressure within the venous system because the medial malleolus represents the most distal point along the hydrostatic column of pressure, is distal to the calf pump, and is near the endpoints of the lesser saphenous vein. The ulcers typically have irregular edges, and may be limited to dermis or shallow subcutaneous tissue. They may be single or multiple, and can involve the entire circumference of the leg. The wound bed may be beefy red granulation tissue with yellow adherent or loose slough present. Necrosis or exposed tendon is rare, and, if present, one should look at other causes. Undermining or tunneling is uncommon. Typically, moderate to heavy amounts of exudates are present.

Diagnostic Evaluation

In many cases of venous ulcers, diagnosis may be made by clinical assessment alone. Diagnostic testing can provide a definitive diagnosis specifying the functional or anatomic vessel abnormality. The tourniquet test used to identify the level of vascular incompetence in superficial venous insufficiency and to assess whether the deep venous system is involved. The patient lies in a supine position with the leg elevated 45 degrees to drain the blood from the saphenous vein, which takes approximately 30 seconds. Tourniquets are applied to the upper and the lower thigh, below the knee, and above the ankle. The patient stands and the tourniquets are sequentially removed while the examiner observes for distention of the superficial veins at each level. If the saphenous vein fills in less than 20 seconds, venous insufficiency either superficial or deep is present (14).

Doppler ultrasonography is used to verify pulses when the presence of edema makes palpation difficult. It can also be used to auscultate venous reflux and to obtain ABI measurements. For patients with an ABI greater than 0.5 but less than 0.8, reduced compression bandages of 23 to 30 mm Hg should be used at the ankle. Compression should not be used in patients with an ABI of less than 0.5 (4).

Photoplethysmography uses an infrared light and a transducer probe to measure venous reflux and venous filling times. In venous hypertension, it takes less than 20 to 25 seconds for the venous system to refill (normally it takes about 35 to 45 seconds) (5).

Air plethysmography can differentiate between superficial and deep venous disease, and assess valvular insufficiency and the efficiency of the calf muscle. It is conducted by placing an air-filled cuff around the calf and measuring the calf muscle volume, venous reflux and refill, calf muscle pumping capacity, and ambulatory venous pressures. Normal venous function is characterized by high intravenous standing pressure and low walking pressures. Venous hypertension is characterized by sustained high walking pressures (5).

Duplex ultrasonography imaging with or without color has become the standard diagnostic tool for assessing venous disease and has replaced venography. Duplex imaging produces images of blood flow and its direction through vessels, pinpointing the anatomic site of reflux or obstruction, thickened, abnormal vein walls, and the presence and age of a thrombus. Duplex scanning can be used to calculate the superficial venous pressures and allows for quantification of venous reflux and valve closure times.

Clinical Management of Venous Ulcers

The goals of therapy in venous ulcer management include reduction of edema, improvement of pain, ulcer healing, and prevention of recurrence. The easiest method to improve venous return and reduce edema is bed rest with leg elevation. Elevation of the legs above the heart for 30 minutes three or four times a day and during the night allows the edema to subside and improves venous circulation.

Surgical and nonsurgical treatment of venous insufficiency with ulceration includes surgical obliteration or ligation of veins, valvular repair, compression therapy, pharmacologic therapy, and bioengineered tissue replacements.

Surgical Management

Vascular surgeons can now ligate incompetent perforator veins using fiber-optic instruments to perform subfascial endoscopic perforator surgical procedures, and is usually reserved for patients who are compliant and do not respond to more conservative therapies. This procedure is replacing the Linton procedure, where the entire medial aspect of the leg is opened to remove the saphenous vein.

Compression Therapy

Compression dressings can be categorized as either static (stockings and wraps) or dynamic compression (pneumatic pump devices). Static compression devices can be further subdivided into elastic products, including short and long stretch wraps, and inelastic products including Unna boots and orthotic devices.

Short-stretch bandages provide sustained compression and calf muscle support. They are advantageous in that they can be washed and reused multiple times. However, they are relatively inelastic, which means that they are less conformable and more likely to slip out of place. The contracting calf muscle exerts a high pressure against the bandage. This pressure drives the blood in the veins upward, and when the calf mus-

cle relaxes, the bandage does not exert pressure. Short-stretch bandages then require the patient to be ambulatory.

Elastic or long-stretch bandages are popular because of their ability to maintain high compression over several days up to a week. Because of the elasticity, they continue to exert compression even when the leg is elevated.

Layered bandage systems (usually three or four layers) combine inelastic and elastic layers to provide calf muscle support and sustained compression. The combined effects of layering and tension, with circumference and width being relatively constant, afford effective subbandage pressures that can be maintained for up to 1 week.

There are several zinc-based paste products used to create a nonconformable inelastic boot around the extremity. The generic term for these dressings is the Unna boot, named for the physician, Dr. P. G. Unna, who originated the concept. Most of these products comprise wrap gauze bandages impregnated with zinc oxide and glycerin, and some also contain calamine (Fig. 32.5). The bandage should be applied from the ball of the foot to 1 in. below the knee in a spiral fashion with 50% to 75% overlap and consistent slight tension. An outer wrap of elastic bandage or self-adherent wrap should be applied over the paste bandage from the base of the toes to the knees. Unna's boot is most appropriate for ambulatory patients because it works primarily by providing static support of the calf muscle pump. As edema decreases and limb circumference decreases, the boot loses its therapeutic effect as a result of its inability to continue to conform to the leg.

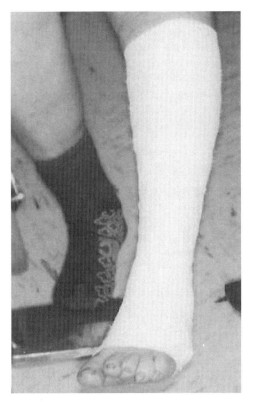

1. Assemble equipment.

2. Wash your hands and put on nonsterile gloves.

3. Wash the affected leg and cleanse ulcers.

4. Pat the leg dry.

5. Apply a moisture barrier to affected leg(s).

6. If an ulcer is draining a lot, you may apply foam pad over it to absorb the drainage.

7. Apply the Unna boot, beginning just above toes. In a circular fashion, wrap it up to bend of knee. When you are finished wrapping, the Unna boot must be smooth with no wrinkles or creases.

8. Cover the Unna boot with elastic bandage, applying pressure while wrapping.

9. Remove weekly or twice weekly as indicated by drainage, edema, and/or patient preference.

FIG. 32.5. Unna boot paste bandage wrapped from the toes to the bend of the knee.

Regular boot changes can occur weekly, and in some cases every 2 weeks.

The CircAid Thera-Boot orthotic device provides both sustained compression and calf pump support by assisting with calf pump function in addition to providing a continuous compression. It consists of multiple Velcro straps, which can be adjusted for comfort. The ability to remove and reapply the device permits more frequent bathing and wound care.

Therapeutic support stockings are most commonly used in patients with venous hypertension to prevent ulceration. They may also be used for patients with an existing ulcer once the edema has been controlled and the limb circumference has stabilized. They offer various levels of compression from mild to high and are available in a variety of sizes, colors, and styles. To determine the correct size, the leg is measured at the ankle, at the calf, and from the ankle to the knee. Noncompliance is a major issue, with reasons for the noncompliance being cost, difficulty of application, comfort issues, and simply forgetting to put them on. Compression stockings will become nontherapeutic because of loss of elasticity over the course of 3 to 6 months. Adequate compression beyond this time cannot be guaranteed. The cost of the stockings should be emphasized to the patient as offsetting the greater costs associated with managing recurrences. Patients should be fit with two pairs of support stockings so that they can wear one pair while the other is being cleaned. Stockings are removed when going to bed and reapplied as soon as the patient awakens and before dangling legs over the side of the bed. Antiembolism hose provides subtherapeutic levels of compression and are not considered therapeutic compression.

Pneumatic compression devices may be useful as an adjunct to bandaging whether used alone or as an alternative to bandaging or stockings in patients who are relatively immobile and so unable to activate the calf muscle. The dynamic pneumatic compression sleeves consist of powered devices applied to the legs to propel venous blood upward. Intermittent pneumatic pumps and sequential gradient compression devices are examples of dynamic therapy. Most of the dynamic devices consist of a limb sleeve with one or more chambers, which inflate intermittently and/or sequentially to create a positive pressure gradient (30 to 60 mm Hg), which propels blood out of the leg and back to the heart. Patients commit 2 to 4 hours a day for therapy.

Whatever compression system is chosen, it must create a pressure gradient from the ankle to the knee. The law of Laplace mathematically relates the bandage tension and the number of layers to the inverse of the radius of the leg and the bandage width. Thus, if the bandage tension is constant as one winds the bandage up the leg, a compression gradient will develop because the ankle diameter is smaller. Larger diameters are encountered up the leg, resulting in lesser degrees of compression given a constant bandage tension. This provides support against venous hypertension at the ankles when the patient is standing. A therapeutic level of compression is commonly considered to be 30 to 40 mm Hg at the ankle (14).

In conclusion, research has shown that compression therapy increases the ulcer healing as compared to no compression, and high compression is more effective than low compression and should be used only in the absence of significant arterial disease. No difference from different types of compression systems (multilayer and short-stretch bandages, Unna's boot) have been shown. Intermittent and pneumatic compression appears to be a useful adjunct to bandaging (16). Caution should be used in bandaging patients with congestive heart failure because there is a risk of causing fluid volume overload by shifting fluid out of the tissues into the vascular system and potentially contributing to acute pulmonary edema. This is of particular concern with the dynamic devices because shifts can occur rapidly. In addition, compressing a leg with an active thrombus can result in dislodgement and free embolism.

Pharmacologic Therapy

The hemorrheologic agent pentoxifylline (Trental) has shown the most promise for venous ulcers. It decreases blood viscosity and white cell adhesion while increasing fibrinolysis. Several studies report that doses of 400 to 800 mg taken orally three times a day can accelerate the healing of venous ulcers. Stanozolol has also been shown to reduce areas affected by lipodermatosclerosis.

Topical Therapy

Topical therapy for venous ulcers should follow the same principles of topical therapy for any chronic wound, which are aimed at optimizing the wound bed including debridement, control of infection, exudate absorption, and maintenance of a moist wound environment. Eczematous dermatitis may require topical steroid ointments. Excessive exudate may require the use of barrier creams containing zinc oxide to protect the skin. Thick hyperkeratosis may require the addition of keratolytics (e.g., urea) (15).

Adjunctive Therapies

There is emerging evidence that bioengineered skin products or skin substitutes may be helpful in the treatment of venous ulcers when used in conjunction with compression bandaging. Other biological agents such as growth factors and cytokines are being evaluated for their efficacy.

Factors That Affect Healing

Although compression therapy is considered to be the gold standard for venous ulcers, it is not always successful. It is important to be knowledgeable about risk factors associated with failure of the ulcer to heal so that the health care provider can modify these risks whenever possible. Margolis and et al. (17) did a retrospective cohort study of 260 patients with chronic venous ulcers, and defined several risk factors that were associated with the failure of a patient's ulcer to heal within 24 weeks while using compression therapy. These included increased wound area, increased wound duration, ABI less than 0.8, history of vein ligation or stripping, history of hip or knee replacement surgery, inability to walk one block, undermining wound margins, and the presence of fibrin on greater than 50% of the wound.

CONCLUSION

The treatment of lower leg ulcers has progressed within the last decade. Improved patient outcomes have been facilitated by the emergence of wound care teams within many practice settings. These wound care practitioners are demanding better ways to diagnose and treat these ulcers, resulting in improved healing.

REFERENCES

1. Phillips T, Stanton B, Provan A, et al. A study of the impact of leg ulcers on quality of life: financial, social, and psychological implications. *J Am Acad Dermatol* 1994;31:49.
2. Hirsch A, Crigu M, Treat-Jacobson D, et al. Peripheral arterial disease detection, awareness, and treatment in primary care. *JAMA* 2001;286:1317–1324.
3. Araujo de T, Valencia I, Federman D. Managing the patient with venous ulcers. *Ann Intern Med* 2003;138:326–334.
4. Bonham P, Flemister B. *Guideline for the management of wounds in patients with lower-extremity arterial disease.* Glenview, IL: WOCN, 2002.
5. Doughty D, Waldrop J, Ramundo J. Lower-extremity ulcers of vascular etiology. In: Bryant R, ed., *Acute and chronic wounds: nursing management.* St. Louis, MO: Mosby–Year Book, 2000:265–295.
6. Halperin, JL. Evaluation of patients with peripheral vascular disease. *Thromb Res* 2002;106:V303–V311.
7. Sarkar PK, Ballantyne S. Management of leg ulcers. *Postgrad Med J* 2000;76:674–682.
8. Rose, S. Noninvasive vascular laboratory for evaluation of peripheral arterial occlusive disease: Part I. Hemodynamic principles and tools of the trade. *J Vasc Interv Radiol* 2000;11:1107–1114.
9. Cantwell-Gab K. Identifying chronic peripheral arterial disease. *Am J Nurs* 1996;96(7):40–46.
10. Treiman GS, Copland S, McNamara RM, et al. Factors influencing ulcer healing in patients with combined arterial and venous insufficiency. *J Vasc Surg* 2001;33:1158–1164.
11. Tretinyak AS, Lee ES, Kuskowski MA, et al. Revascularization and quality of life for patients with limb-threatening ischemia. *Ann Vasc Surg* 2000;15:84–88.
12. Nelson EA, Bradley MD. Dressings and topical agents for arterial leg ulcers. *Cochrane Database Syst Rev* 2003;1:CD001836.
13. Valencia IC, Falabella A, Kirsner R, et al. Chronic venous insufficiency and venous leg ulcerations. *J Am Acad Dermatol* 2001;44:401–421.
14. Kunimoto B, Cooling M, Gulliver W, et al. Best practices for the prevention and treatment of leg ulcers. *Ostomy Wound Manage* 2001;47:34–46, 48–50.
15. Choucair MM, Fivenson DP. Leg ulcer diagnosis and management. *Dermatol Clin* 2001;19:659–678.
16. Cullum N, Nelson EA, Fletcher AW, et al. Compression for venous ulcers. *Cochrane Database Syst Rev* 2001;2:CD00265.
17. Margolis DJ, Berlin JA, Strom BL. Risk factors associated with the failure of a venous leg ulcer to heal. *Arch Dermatol* 1999;135:920–926.

CHAPTER 33

Excimer Laser Revascularization for Peripheral Arterial Disease

Technology, Interventional Techniques, and Clinical Outcomes

John R. Laird

Key Points

- Excimer laser revascularization has the advantage of less collateral thermal injury than the use of continuous laser wavelengths.
- Comparison studies between the excimer laser and balloon angioplasty demonstrate that the laser significantly reduced the need for stenting.
- Potential benefits for the use of the excimer laser include treatment of long total superficial femoral artery occlusions and less distal embolization.
- In critically ischemic limbs, the excimer laser allows crossing of total flush occlusions even when guidewire crossing fails.

INTRODUCTION

Two decades after the clinical introduction of percutaneous transluminal angioplasty (PTA) as a recanalization technique in the femoropopliteal and infragenicular arteries, a number of factors affecting the primary and long-term success of the procedure have been identified. Long lesion length, occlusion, poor peripheral runoff, symptoms of limb-threatening ischemia, and the presence of diabetes all correlate with diminished primary success and long-term patency (1–4). In many institutions, PTA has been abandoned for the treatment of long occlusions and diffuse disease due to the poor long-term clinical outcomes. For such severe disease, treatment options have been limited to medical management, bypass surgery, or, at worst, amputation. Patients too fragile or unwilling to undergo the morbidity and mortality associated with bypass surgery have been left to live with their pain, or face amputation. With advances in laser catheter design and refinement of recanalization techniques, improved results have been seen with laser-assisted angioplasty of complex peripheral arterial disease. There has been renewed interest in excimer laser angioplasty for the treatment of patients with long total occlusions and diffuse disease who otherwise would have limited options for treatment.

Continuous wave, hot-tipped lasers were evaluated and abandoned for peripheral interventions in the late 1980s due to a high complication rate caused by thermal damage to surrounding tissue (5–9). In contrast, excimer laser angioplasty of the leg arteries has been practiced commercially in Europe since 1994 (10). The 308-nm excimer laser utilizes flexible fiber-optic catheters to deliver intense bursts of ultraviolet (UV) energy in short pulse durations (Fig. 33.1). The advantages of UVB light lie in its short penetration depth of 50 μm and its ability to break molecular bonds directly, by a photochemical, rather than thermal, process. A unique feature of using UV light is its direct lytic action. In addition, excimer laser catheters remove a tissue layer of about 10 μm with each pulse of energy. Tissue is ablated only on contact without a consequent rise in temperature to surrounding tissue. Consequently, clinical outcomes with the excimer laser

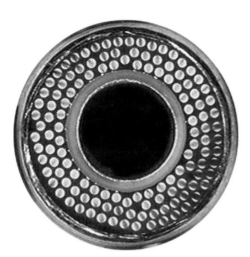

FIG. 33.1. Excimer laser catheter with central guidewire lumen and multiple laser fibers circumferentially distributed around the guidewire lumen. (Courtesy of Spectranetics, Colorado Springs, Co.)

to treat long superficial femoral artery (SFA) occlusions and disease below the knee are very good.

EXCIMER LASER IN LONG TOTAL SUPERFICIAL FEMORAL ARTERY OCCLUSIONS

Scheinert et al. analyzed the data of 318 consecutive patients (mean age 64 ± 10.7 years) who underwent excimer laser-assisted recanalization of chronic SFA occlusions (number of lesions 411, mean occlusion length 19.4 ± 6.0 cm) during a 1-year period ending December 31, 1996 (11). The primary approach (crossover 89.7%, antegrade 6.6%, transpopliteal 3.6%) to crossing the occlusion with a multifiber excimer laser catheter was successful in 342 of 411 lesions (83.2%). A secondary attempt was performed in 44 cases, including use of the transpopliteal approach in 39 cases. Despite the treatment of very long occlusions, the total technical success rate was 372 of 411 (90.5%).

The step-by-step technique (Fig. 33.2) was applied in the majority of cases to initially cross the occluded vessel segment. This technique was particularly beneficial for entering flush occlusions without visible proximal stump or for passing a segment resistant to guidewire crossing. The routine use of this technique may have contributed to the low rate of occlusive arterial wall dissections with a resultant stent frequency of only 7.3%. Relevant interventional complications were acute reocclusion (1.0%), perforation (2.2%), and embolization/distal thrombosis (3.9%). Postinterventionally, 219 patients (68.8%) were in clinical category 0; 53 patients (16.6%) were in category 1; and 26 patients (8.2%) in were category 2 (Rutherford classification). Based on a standard life-table analysis including primary interventional failures, the primary patency rate after 1 year was 20.1%. Repeat balloon angioplasty was performed on restenoses, resulting in a primary assisted patency rate of 64.6% after 1 year. The performance of repeat recanalization procedures on reoccluded arteries resulted in a 75.1% secondary patency rate.

THE PERIPHERAL EXCIMER LASER ANGIOPLASTY STUDY

The Peripheral Excimer Laser Angioplasty (PELA) study was a multicenter, prospective, randomized trial comparing excimer laser-assisted PTA versus PTA alone to treat long, total SFA occlusions. Two hundred and fifty-one patients with claudication (Rutherford category 2 through 4) of greater than 6 months duration and total occlusions of 10 cm or greater in the SFA were randomized (50% laser+PTA, 50% PTA alone) at 13 U.S. sites and six German sites. Stenting was optional, but discouraged. Clinical success was defined as primary patency (50% diameter stenosis or less at 1 year by ultrasound with no reintervention) and no serious adverse event (SAE: death, myocardial infarction, vascular surgical repair, amputation, bypass, acute limb ischemia). Patient enrollment was completed in December 2001, and 12-month follow-up was completed in December 2002.

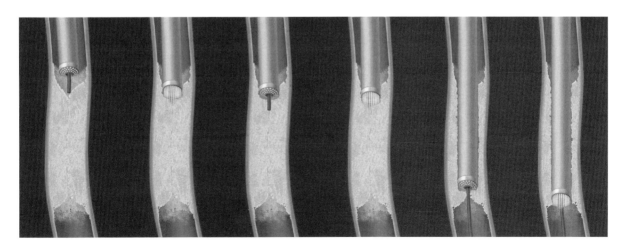

FIG. 33.2. The step-by-step technique for crossing total occlusions. The laser catheter is advanced together with the guidewire through the occlusion.

TABLE 33.1. *Excimer laser series comparison—superficial femoral artery occlusions*

Series	Scheinert et al. (16)	PELA Laser	PELA Balloon	p
Patient and lesion characteristics				
Patients	318	101	88	NS
Mean age (yr)	64	66	65	NS
Men (%)	65	75	77	NS
Occlusion length (cm)	19.4	20.2	20.8	NS
Acute procedural results				
Procedural success (%)	91	85	91	NS
Stent implanted (%)	7	42	59	0.02
Procedural complications				
Death	0	0	0	
Amputation	0	0	0	
Surgical intervention	0	1[b] (0.9%)	0	
Acute reocclusion	4 (1.3%)	1 (0.9%)	0 (0%)	
Perforation	9 (2.2%)	9 (8.9%)	3 (3.4%)	
Embolization	16 (3.9%)	2 (2.0%)	7 (8.0%)	
12-month results				
Vessel patent without reintervention (%)	21	49	49	NS
Functional status improvement at follow-up (% stable/improved Rutherford category)	100	88	90	NS

[a]PELA, Peripheral excimer laser angioplasty study.
[b]Pseudoaneurysm repair at puncture site.

Acute procedural results from a preliminary analysis of 189 PELA study patients were similar in both laser and balloon groups. Procedural success was 85% in the laser group and 91% in the PTA group. Total procedural complications were 12.8% and 11.4%, respectively. The only significant difference between the two groups was in the number of stents used. Stents were implanted in 42% of patients in the laser group and in 59% of the stent group. The 12-month patency rates and functional status were also similar in both groups (12).

The acute results from the preliminary PELA analysis are similar to results reported in the Scheinert et al. series of 411 patients. In both series, procedural success rates were high, complication rates were low, and there was significant clinical improvement at follow-up (Table 33.1). The combination of excimer laser technology with current interventional devices and advanced recanalization techniques offers advantages over standard PTA techniques. First, in similarly complex lesions, excimer laser debulking prior to PTA results in the need for fewer stents (Fig. 33.3). In-stent restenosis is much more difficult clinical problem to treat than simple balloon angioplasty of focal restenosis in a native vessel. With a similar restenosis rate, the therapy that reduces the number of stents is desirable to minimize the risk of in-stent restenosis and procedural costs. Second, excimer laser recanalization of long, total SFA occlusions may result in a significantly

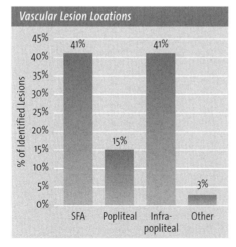
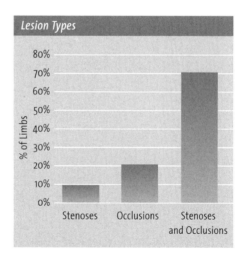

FIG. 33.3. Lesion types and locations treated in the laser angioplasty for critical limb ischemia phase 2 trial.

lower rate of distal embolization. Although perforations were higher in the laser group of the PELA study, they can be sealed with balloons and stents with virtually no clinical sequela. In contrast, distal embolization cannot be treated, and the long-term consequences of this complication are potentially more severe (13). Irrespective of technique, restenosis is relatively higher after recanalization of very long chronic SFA occlusions than stenoses and short occlusions. However, with an aggressive surveillance program including functional clinical testing as well as color-coded duplex ultrasound, restenosis can be detected at an early stage. Timely reintervention on the target lesion can be performed in the majority of cases on an outpatient basis, resulting in high secondary patency rates.

LASER ANGIOPLASTY FOR CRITICAL LIMB ISCHEMIA PHASE 2

The Laser Angioplasty for Critical Limb Ischemia (LACI) phase 2 clinical study protocol evolved from a 25-patient phase 1 registry so that it harmonized with the recommendations of the TransAtlantic Inter-Society Consensus document (14). In LACI 2, critical limb ischemia (CLI) patients (Rutherford category 4 through 6) who were poor bypass candidates and had culprit lesions in the SFA, popliteal, and/or infrapopliteal arteries were enrolled. Poor surgical candidacy was determined if one or more of three conditions were met: no venous conduit was available for creating a bypass, no suitable distal anastomosis site existed, and comorbid conditions placed the patient in American Society of Anesthesiologists class 4 or higher. As in phase 1, treatment consisted of excimer laser angioplasty plus PTA plus optional stent, with the primary endpoints being limb salvage and total survival at 6 months.

LASER ANGIOPLASTY FOR CRITICAL LIMB ISCHEMIA PHASE 2 RESULTS

At 15 sites in the United States and Germany, the LACI 2 enrolled 145 patients with 155 critically ischemic limbs and 423 lesions. Patient and limb characteristics were typical of patients with systemic vascular disease, with a high incidence of diabetes, hypertension, and cardiac disease (Table 33.2). LACI patients presented with severe and diffuse vascular disease typical of critical limb ischemia. In the 423 lesions, 41% were in the SFA, 15% were in the popliteal artery, and 41% were in infrapopliteal arteries. Furthermore, 70% of the patients had a combination of stenoses and occlusions, making treatment very complex (Fig. 33.4).

Use of the excimer laser led to an increase in the ability to treat this very complex patient population. Despite a failed guidewire crossing in 8% of the cases, laser treatment was delivered in 99% of the cases, with adjunctive balloon angioplasty successfully performed in 96% of the cases (Fig. 33.5). By utilizing the step-by-step laser technique to cross an occlusion, the initial crossing success was improved by 7% and the ability to deliver balloon angioplasty was improved by 4% (Table 33.3). In-hospital SAEs were extremely low in this very fragile patient group. There were no deaths, perforations, or bypasses as a result of the procedure, and no patient had acute limb ischemia postintervention. Reintervention procedures to reopen stenosed or occluded lesions were expected, given the complexity of the disease. SAEs during the 6-month enrollment period included 10% mortality, almost exclusively from cardiac causes. Major amputation was required in 11 cases, and 4 limbs received surgical revascularization. No patient died in the first 30 days after the index procedure, but 15 patients died during follow-up and another 11 withdrew or were lost to follow-up.

At 6 months, 10% of the patients died and 34% survived with persistent CLI. However, in poor surgical candidates with a high probability of amputation, LACI resulted in a limb salvage rate of 93% in survivors at 6 months. Only 2% of LACI patients required surgical intervention during follow-up. Furthermore, of surviving legs, 69% improved in Rutherford category, 27% maintained the same Rutherford category, and only 4% declined in Rutherford category.

The LACI study shows that the excimer laser-assisted endovascular intervention in CLI results in a higher limb salvage

TABLE 33.2. *Laser angioplasty for critical limb ischemia phase 2 patient and limb characteristics*

Characteristics			
Patients (145)		Limbs (155)	
Mean age (yr)	72 ± 10 (45–91)	Rutherford category (%)	
Men (%)	53	3	29
Duration of CLI[a] (weeks)	25 ± 37 (1–261)	5 or 6	71
Risk factors (%)		Reasons for poor surgical candidacy (%)	
Smoking	53	Absence of Venous Graft	32
Coronary artery disease	50	Poor/no distal vessel	68
Prior stroke	21	High surgical risk	46
Diabetes mellitus	66	Only one reason	61
Hypertension	83	Any two reasons	33
Dyslipidemia	56	All three reasons	6
Obesity	35		

[a]CLI, Critical limb ischemia.

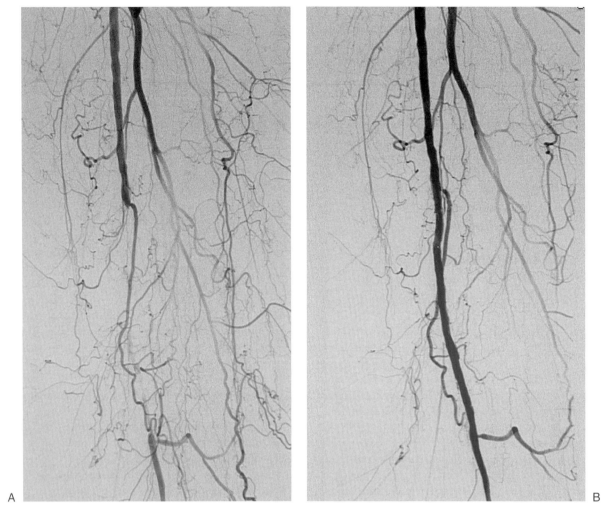

A   B

FIG. 33.4. A: Baseline angiogram showing occlusion of the superficial femoral artery. **B:** Following laser-assisted recanalization, an excellent result without the need for stenting.

rate than could be expected for poor surgical candidates. The treatment can be delivered to a fragile patient population with a high incidence of comorbid disease without increasing risks over other established therapies for CLI.

OTHER POTENTIAL LASER APPLICATIONS

Potential applications for excimer lasers in peripheral interventions include debulking of in-stent restenosis, stent-supported recanalization of chronic iliac artery occlusions, and thrombus removal for acute limb ischemia and ischemic stroke. Scheinert et al. studied 212 consecutive patients with chronic unilateral iliac artery occlusions (mean length 8.9 ± 3.9 cm) who were treated with excimer laser-assisted recanalization with stent implantation (16). A total of 527 stents were implanted. Technical success was achieved in 190 (90%) patients. There was a low complication rate of 1.4%, and primary patency rates were 84% at 1 year, 81% at 2 years, 78% at 3 years, and 76% at 4 years. A new potential for laser treatment of ischemic events such as acute limb ischemia, acute

stroke, and acute ischemic cerebral syndromes has emerged (17,18). The excimer laser is effective in treating fresh coronary thrombus. The underlying principle of thrombus dissolution with the laser is that a thrombus absorbs light of wavelengths 400 to 600 nm without adversely affecting surrounding structures. Studies evaluating laser-induced thrombolysis are ongoing.

The fundamental merit of the excimer laser lies in its ability to evaporate and debulk tissue. The 308-nm excimer laser facilitates the successful treatment of the most severe peripheral disease by ablating and removing thrombus and other obstructive material. Excimer laser debulking transforms a diffuse, polymorphous lesion into a more easily ballooned stenosis with fewer complications. By removing the thrombus burden common to diffuse disease, the laser reduces the potential for distal embolization. Furthermore, the laser may reduce the number of dissections, resulting in the need for fewer stents. Excimer laser catheters and techniques have improved dramatically since the mid 1990s, resulting in the effective removal of obstructive disease with a very low

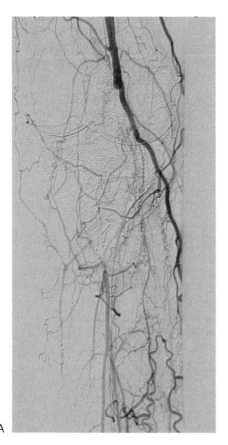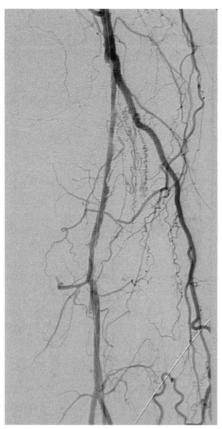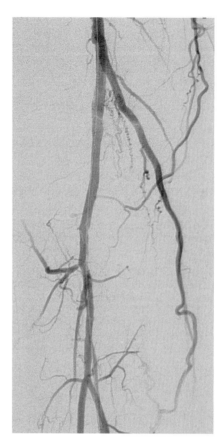

A   B,C

FIG. 33.5. A: Baseline angiogram showing total occlusion of the popliteal artery in a patient with critical limb ischemia. **B:** Following debulking with a 2.0-mm excimer laser catheter. **C:** Final result after adjunctive balloon angioplasty.

TABLE 33.3. *Procedure results and serious adverse events (SAEs) in the laser angioplasty for critical limb ischemia phase 2 trial*

Procedure results

Guidewire crossing success	92%
Laser treatment delivered	99%
Adjunctive balloon	96%
Stent placement	45%
Procedure success ($<$50% residual stenosis)	85%
Straight-line flow established	89%
Mean hospital stay	3 days

Adjudicated SAEs

	In-hospital	All follow-up	Total
Death	0	15	15
Major amputation	2	9	11
Nonfatal myocardial infarction or stroke	0	2	2
Reintervention	1	23	24
Hematoma with surgery	1	0	1
Acute limb ischemia	0	1	1
Perforation with surgery	0	0	0
Bypass	0	0	3
Endarterectomy	0	0	1

Forty-eight (33%) patients experienced one or no SAE.

complication rate and good clinical outcomes as shown in the PELA and LACI trials.

REFERENCES

1. Dormandy JA, Rutherford RB. Management of peripheral arterial disease (PAD). TASC Working Group. TransAtlantic Inter-Society Concensus (TASC). *J Vasc Surg* 2000;31(1 Pt 2):S1–S296. Review.
2. Capek P, McLean GK, Berkowitz HD. Femoropopliteal angioplasty: factors influencing long-term success. *Circulation* 1991;83[Suppl I]:I70–I80.
3. Johnston KW, Rae M, Hogg-Johnston SA, et al. Five-year results of a prospective study of percutaneous transluminal angioplasty. *Ann Surg* 1987;206:403–413.
4. Pentacost MJ, Criqui MH, Dorros G, et al. Guidelines for peripheral percutaneous transluminal angioplasty of the abdominal aorta and lower extremity vessels. *Circulation* 1994;89:511–531.
5. Wollenek G, Laufer G. Comparative study of different laser systems with special regard to angioplasty. *Thorac Cardiovasc Surg* 1998;36 [Suppl 2]:126–132.
6. Seeger JM, Kaelin LD. Limitations and pitfalls of laser angioplasty. *Surg Annu* 1993;25:177–192.
7. White RA, White GH, Mehringer MC, et al. A clinical trial of laser thermal angioplasty in patients with advanced peripheral vascular disease. *Ann Surg* 1990;212:257–265.
8. AbuRahma AF, Robinson PA, Kennard W, et al. Intraoperative peripheral Nd:YAG laser-assisted thermal balloon angioplasty: short-term and intermeidate-term follow-up. *J Vasc Surg* 1990;12:566–572.
9. McAlpin GM, Rama K, Berg RA. Thermal laser assisted balloon angioplasty in lower extremity occlusive disease. *Am Surg* 1991;57:558–565.
10. Visona A, Perissinotto C, Lusiana L, et al. Percutaneous excimer laser angioplasty of lower limb vessels: results of a prospective 24-month follow-up. *Angiology* 1998;49:91–98.
11. Scheinert D, Laird JR, Schroder M, et al. Excimer laser-assisted recanalization of long, chronic superficial femoral artery occlusions. *J Endovasc Ther* 2001;8:156–166.
12. Laird JR. *Peripheral Excimer Laser Angioplasty (PELA) trial results.* Presented at Late Breaking Clinical Trials, TCT Annual Meeting, September 2002.
13. Biamino G, Scheinert D. Excimer laser treatment of SFA occlusions. *Endovasc Today* 2003;May/June:45–48.
14. Gray BH, Laird JR, Ansel GM, et al. Complex endovascular treatment for critical limb ischemia in poor surgical candidates: a pilot study. *J Endovasc Ther* 2002;9:599–604.
15. Laird JR. *Laser angioplasty for critical limb ischemia (LACI): results of the LACI phase 2 clinical trial.* Presented at ISET Annual Meeting, January 2003.
16. Scheinert D, Schröder M, Ludwig J, et al. Stent supported recanalization of chronic iliac artery occlusions. *Am J Med* 2001;110(9):708–715.
17. Ansel GM, Botti CF, Silver MJ. Mechanical devices and acute limb ischemia. *Endovasc Today* 2003;March:45–48.
18. Topaz ON. Laser. In: Topal EJ, ed., *Textbook of interventional cardiology,* 4th ed. Philadelphia: WB Saunders, 2003:675–703.

CHAPTER 34

Stent Selection for Iliac and Superficial Femoral Artery Interventions

Elie Hage-Korban and Malcolm T. Foster, III

Key Points

- Most stents are made of one of the following metals: stainless steel, nitinol, tantalum, platinum, cobalt, and various alloys.
- The two fundamental stents designs are balloon-expandable stents and self-expanding stents.
- Balloon-expandable stents are made from materials that can be deformed by balloon inflation. These include the Palmaz (Cordis), Intrastent (Boston Scientific), Bridge (Medtronic), VistaFlex (Angiodynamics), OMNILINK (Guidant), Express (Boston Scientific), and Genesis (Cordis) stents.
- Self-expanding stents are manufactured in the expanded form and then compressed and fitted to a delivery system. These include the Wallstent (Boston Scientific), SMART (Cordis), Memotherm Flexx (Bard), Symphony (Boston Scientific), DYNALINK (Guidant), Intracoil (EV3), and Protégé (EV3) stents.
- Balloon-expandable stents offer some advantage over self-expanding stents in terms of precision of placement.
- Self-expanding stents that are crush recoverable are preferred for extremity arteries and vessels with extreme tortuosity, varying diameters, or significant tapering.
- Nitinol strut fractures have been observed after superficial femoral artery stenting, but the clinical significance of this finding is uncertain.
- Drug-eluting stents may have a similar impact in superficial femoral artery and infrapopliteal intervention as coronary drug-eluting stents, but the data are preliminary.

INTRODUCTION

The past decade has witnessed a major expansion in percutaneous interventions for the treatment of peripheral arterial occlusive disease. Catheter-based intervention has advanced from an investigational status to an effective, widely used, minimally invasive method of treating stenotic and occlusive lesions in the peripheral arterial system. The introduction of stents has improved the results of angioplasty and minimized complications such as dissection and threatened abrupt occlusion. Stents are based on a concept of intravascular scaffolding that buttresses the arterial wall and maintains lumen patency. In this chapter we describe and compare the different types of stents used to treat obstructive lesions in the iliac arteries and superficial femoral arteries (SFA).

BACKGROUND

Treatment of stenotic or occluded arteries is indicated in symptomatic patients. The main indications for percutaneous endovascular treatment are the following (1):

1. Ischemic rest pain or tissue necrosis of an extremity
2. Lifestyle-limiting claudication refractory to medical therapy
3. Insufficient inflow for a distal bypass graft

4. Renal transplant (pelvic kidney)
5. Vasculogenic impotence

The guidelines for iliac percutaneous transluminal angioplasty established by the Joint Council of the American Heart Association are the following (1):

- Category 1: noncalcified, concentric stenosis less than 3 cm in length
- Category 2: stenosis 3 to 5 cm in length that is calcified, or eccentric stenosis less than 3 cm in length
- Category 3: stenosis 5 to 10 cm in length, or chronic occlusions less than 5 cm in length after thrombolytic therapy
- Category 4: stenosis greater than 10 cm in length, chronic occlusion greater than 5 cm in length after thrombolytic therapy, extensive aortoiliac disease, and iliac stenosis in a patient with abdominal aortic aneurysm

Lesions in the first and second categories have the best clinical outcomes following percutaneous intervention. Stents may best be reserved for category 3 and 4 lesions.

A lesion is considered hemodynamically significant if the vessel is narrowed by more than 50% (2,3). Another way to determine the significance of a stenosis is the translesion pressure gradient. A peak-to-peak systolic pressure gradient of 10 mm Hg or greater or a mean gradient of 5 mm Hg at rest is considered hemodynamically significant. A translesion gradient greater than 15 mm Hg after vasodilator therapy, or a mean gradient greater than 10 mm Hg after vasodilator therapy, is also considered significant, even in the absence of a significant gradient at rest (4–6).

A major indication for stent placement is failed angioplasty, defined as a significant dissection, a residual stenosis of more than 30%, or a residual mean translesional gradient of more than 5 mm Hg. Primary stenting is usually reserved for total occlusions. The lowered risk of distal embolization in treating stenoses with primary stenting versus percutaneous angioplasty (PTA) is a theoretical advantage yet to be proven (7,8). This strategy has been validated in the treatment of total occlusions where primary stenting was associated with less distal embolization (9–13).

Several studies have compared the safety and the efficacy of PTA and primary stenting (1,14). Bosch et al. performed a meta-analysis of 14 studies, which included more than 2,000 patients, comparing the results of primary stenting with balloon angioplasty in the iliac arteries (15). The initial technical success was higher for the primary stenting group versus PTA (96% vs. 91%) (16,17). However, this was not statistically significant. The 4-year patency rate was higher in the stent group. The authors concluded that stent placement in the iliac interventions reduced long-term restenosis by 39%. However, some prospective studies failed to confirm this finding (18,19). Another study found a complication rate of 6% after stent placement in the iliac arteries. Primary and secondary 5-year patency rates ranged from 58% to 82% and from 78% to 91%, respectively. These results compare favorably to the outcomes of surgical aortoiliac bypass grafting (20,21).

No randomized prospective trial has been published comparing the results of different types of stent. In the meta-analysis performed by Bosch et al., 4-year primary patency rate was 80% for the Palmaz stent, 70% for the Wallstent, and 64% for the Strecker stent (15). This has not been reproduced in other series (22).

The Food and Drug Administration (FDA) has defined the indications for iliac and SFA stent placement as follows (23):

1. Suboptimal result of angioplasty: (a) residual dissection, (b) residual pressure gradient
2. Total occlusion
3. Recurrent stenosis after angioplasty

In clinical practice, iliac and SFA stenting have become more widely applied, particularly with off-label use of approved devices (e.g., biliary stents). Operators have expanded the use of stents based on peer-reviewed data as well as favorable experiences with coronary stenting. The evolution of iliac and SFA stent design has followed two parallel paths: balloon-expandable stents and self-expanding stents.

The Palmaz design, a tubular slotted stent, was the prototype for balloon-expandable stents (24). The Wallstent, a steel mesh, was the prototype for self-expanding stents. There are more than 100 stents with varying designs, materials, and mechanical properties. As a general concept, most stents have been used between the clavicle and the femoral ligament, including the iliac arteries. Crush-recoverable, self-expanding

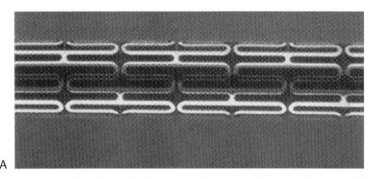
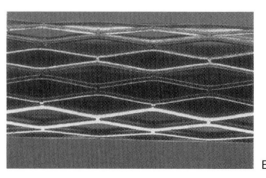

A   B

FIG. 34.1. A: Palmaz stent (Cordis) prior to deployment. **B:** Same stent following balloon expansion. (Courtesy of Cordis Corp., Warren, NJ.)

stents are preferred in the neck and extremities, including the superficial femoral arteries.

Most stents are made of one of the following metals: stainless steel, nitinol, tantalum, platinum, and cobalt (25). A multitude of technological methods have been used to manufacture stents, including laser cutting, water jet cutting, photoetching, coiling, and various wire-forming techniques.

BALLOON-EXPANDABLE (ILIAC) STENTS

Balloon expandable stents are made from materials that are deformed by the inflation of the supporting balloon. After deflation, the mechanical memory preserves the stent in the expanded shape, except for recoil, which is intrinsic to the elastic properties of the metal used. The ideal metal should have a low expansion yield, high elastic modulus, and high expansion strength (hoop strength). Stents are manufactured in the compressed state to enhance deliverability. The most widely used material is stainless steel, typically 316L, a particularly corrosion-resistant material with a low content of carbon. Alternative materials include tantalum, platinum, and cobalt chromium. The balloon-expandable stents are manufactured in the small-diameter, deliverable configuration and balloon-dilated to the expanded shape at the target site within the vessel.

The following is a select list of balloon-expandable (iliac) stents in the United States:

- Palmaz (Cordis): FDA iliac approved (Fig. 34.1)
- Intrastent (EV3)
- AVE Bridge (Medtronic)
- VistaFlex (Angiodynamics)
- OMNILINK (Guidant)
- Express (Boston Scientific) (Fig. 34.2)
- Genesis (Cordis)

SELF-EXPANDING (ILIAC AND SUPERFICIAL FEMORAL ARTERY) STENTS

Self-expanding stents are manufactured in the expanded form and then compressed and fitted to a delivery system. On release from the delivery system, the stent expands to a preset diameter. The chronic outward force of the stent prevents recoil. One of the advantages of self-expanding stents is the conformability to varying diameters within the artery. Another advantage is immediate recovery from crush. Stainless steel and nitinol are the metals most often used for this type of stent design.

The following is a select list of self-expanding (iliac and SFA) stents:

- Wallstent (Boston Scientific): FDA iliac approved (Fig. 34.3)
- SMART stent (Cordis): FDA iliac approved (Fig. 34.4)
- Memotherm Flexx (Bard)

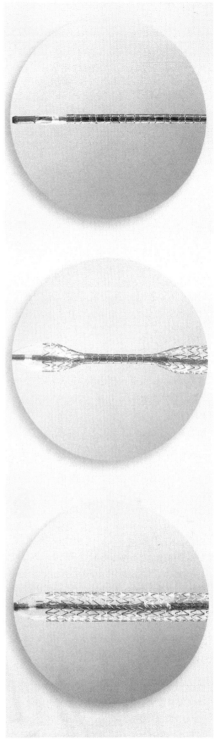

FIG. 34.2. Express stent (Boston Scientific). **Top:** Stent loaded on balloon catheter prior to deployment. **Middle:** During deployment. **Bottom:** Fully deployed stent with inflated balloon. (Courtesy of Boston Scientific Corp., Natick, MA.)

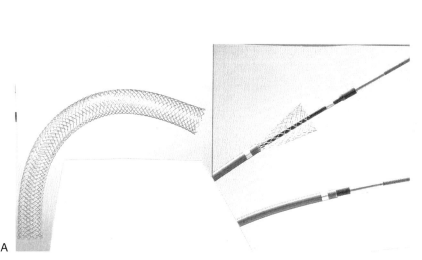
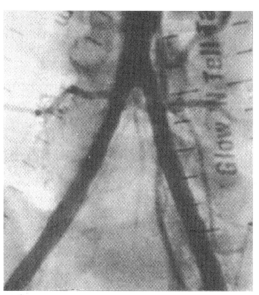

A   B

FIG. 34.3. A: Wallstent (Boston Scientific). This self-expanding stent has great flexibility, and as the sheath is pulled back **(right, bottom)**, the stent is deployed and expands **(right, top)**. **B.** Angiogram of left-iliac artery following stent deployment. (Courtesy of Boston Scientific, Natick, MA.)

- Symphony (Boston Scientific) (Fig. 34.5)
- DYNALINK (Guidant)
- Intracoil (EV3)
- Protégé (EV3)

The following is a select list of covered stents:

- Wallgraft (Boston Scientific): Wallstent and polyethylene teryltolate
- Corvita (Boston Scientific): Wallstent and polyurethane
- Hemobahn (Gore): nitinol and polytetrafluorethylene (PTFE)
- Aneurex (Medtronic): nitinol and PTFE
- Precedent (Boston Scientific): nitinol and PTFE
- aSpire (Vascular Architects): nitinol and PTFE
- Jostent (JoMED): balloon-expanded stainless steel and PTFE

COMPARISON OF STENTS

Given the recent introduction of stents to peripheral intervention, there is a paucity of data comparing the results of different stents. Following the approval of the Palmaz stent and the Wallstent, the SMART stent satisfied a noninferiority standard required by the FDA to obtain an iliac indication. In many circumstances, operators rely on the specific properties of available stents to determine the most appropriate choice for an iliac or SFA intervention.

A number of variables may be considered, including the following (26–31):

1. Radial force/hoop strength
2. Flexibility
3. Trackability
4. Radiopacity
5. Magnetic resonance imaging compatibility
6. Size of delivery system
7. Conformability

Selection of Iliac Stents

The iliac Wallstent (Fig. 34.3), the Palmaz 308 (Fig. 34.1), and the SMART (Fig. 34.4) stent are approved for the treatment of appropriate iliac lesions. The stents that have the most data regarding long-term patency are the Wallstent (11,32), the Palmaz 308 stent, and the Strecker stent. Given the diversity in design of these stents, the choice of the stent may not be critical for the success of an iliac intervention. Nonetheless, some generalizations can be made regarding the suitability of specific stents. Lesion characteristics, access site, introducer size, vessel tortuosity, and lesion location are factors that influence the choice of a stent (33,34).

Short focal lesions can be treated with balloon-expandable or self-expanding stents. Occlusions and long lesions are best treated with long, balloon-expanded stents. The same applies for treating a calcified fibrous lesion with significant recoil. The Palmaz stent is well suited for this type of lesion. Based on the available data, the AVE Bridge Flexible stent may have comparable hoop strength and flexibility. Newer stents like the the Genesis, Intrastent, OMNILINK, Express, and Assurant stents offer advantages with respect to more user-friendly delivery systems, crossing profile, flexibility, expansion ratio, and foreshortening characteristics (35–37).

The Express LD stent is a Boston Scientific balloon-expandable stent (Fig. 34.6). It has a tandem stent design of micro and macro elements that are constructed in tandem

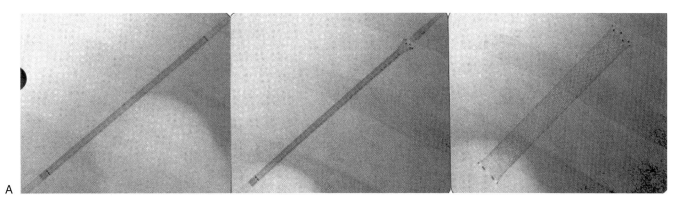

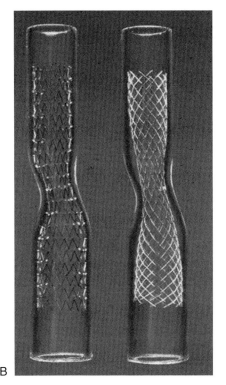

FIG. 34.4. A: The SMART stent (Cordis) is approved for iliac stenosis. It is made from a single laser-cut metal piece. This self-expanding stent is shown under fluoroscopy before, during, and following full deployment. **B:** The SMART stent in the left glass tube is snugly approximated to the wall, whereas another self-expanding stent appears to leave a space between the struts and the wall. (Courtesy of Cordis Corp., Warren, NJ.)

to increase flexibility, conformability, radiopacity and radial strength. It is compatible to a 6 French delivery system over a 0.035-in. wire.

The OMNILINK stent is a Guidant balloon-expandable stent; it is made of stainless steel and has an open-cell design. It is delivered over a 0.035-in. wire via a 6 French system. The stent is premounted on a balloon. It has two radiopaque markers located underneath the balloon, which fluoroscopically mark the working length of the balloon.

The Bridge Assurant is a Medtronic balloon-expandable stent made of 316L stainless steel material. It has an eight-crown open-cell design, which can be delivered over a 0.035-in. guidewire. The Bridge, OMNILINK, and Express stents are not fully connected. They represent a somewhat open-cell design (Table 34.1).

The Genesis (later-generation Palmaz) is a Cordis balloon-expandable stent (9,24,38,39). It is compatible with 4 and 6 French delivery sheath systems. It has a closed-cell de-

sign that prevents tissue prolapse, and provides cells of a consistently size and shape throughout the length of the circumference. The Genesis has an 86% open area. It has seven cells per circumference. It is designed in flex segments, which increase its flexibility and its conformability to the vessel bends, increasing its predeployed as well as its postdeployed conformability. Differential expansion and contraction of the flex segments preserve scaffolding even in tortuous anatomy. The Genesis is mounted on the balloon with Stent Securement technology, creating two to three times greater stent retention than conventional mounting and allowing for a lower delivery profile. The Genesis can be delivered over 0.014-in., 0.018-in., and 0.035-in. wires. It is laser cut from a single tube of stainless steel with no welds. This design confers minimal stent shortening. The stent is adjacent to balloon marker bands, allowing for precise positioning. The Palmaz-based stent is a tubular, slotted, stainless steel stent, fully connected. The Genesis is a

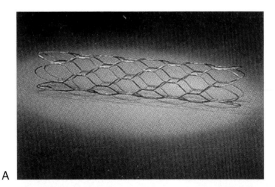

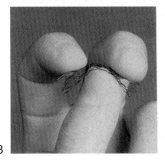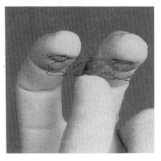

FIG. 34.5. A: The Symphony stent (Boston Scientific) is a self-expanding stent. **B:** After compression (**left**), it resumes its normal architecture. (Courtesy of Boston Scientific, Natick, MA.)

third-generation Palmaz design with undulating longitudinal connectors.

Calcified, aortic bifurcation lesions are best treated by a "kissing stent" technique to prevent compromise of the contralateral iliac artery ostium by plaque shifting. The type of stent for this location remains controversial. Most experts recommend balloon-expandable stents, which limit the elastic recoil of the vessels at the bifurcation, whereas some advocate self-expanding stents to reduce the risk of hemolysis and thrombus formation by the stiff metallic struts.

The VistaFlex (Angiodynamics) is a woven, balloon-expandable stent comparable to laser-cut nitinol stents. It is extremely flexible and demonstrates good vessel conformability. It is a bridge between the self-expanding and the balloon-expandable designs.

SELECTION OF SUPERFICIAL FEMORAL ARTERY STENTS

Self-expanding stents have an advantage when treating lesions in extremities (e.g., the SFA). Self-expanding stents are crush recoverable and generally more flexible than balloon-expandable stents (40). With tortuous vessels, balloon-expandable stents must be used with caution. Kinking of the vessel at the end of a stiff stent may increase the risk of vessel rupture and/or restenosis. The self–expanding nitinol stents such as the SMART, Luminex, Protégé, DYNALINK, Bridge SE, and Zilver stents, which are laser cut from a single nitinol tube, are appropriate for such types of lesions and vessels.

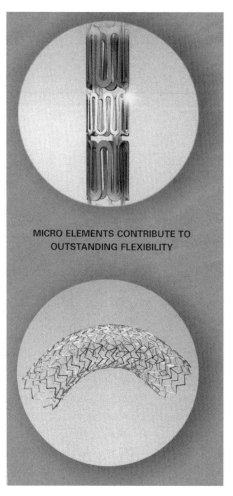

MICRO ELEMENTS CONTRIBUTE TO OUTSTANDING FLEXIBILITY

FIG. 34.6. The Express LD stent (Boston Scientific) is a balloon-expandable stent mounted in a 6-Fr delivery system over a 0.035-in. wire. The stent has micro and macro elements to provide strength and flexibility. (Courtesy of Boston Scientific, Natick, MA.)

Nitinol stents, because they easily conform to the vessel size and shape, are particularly well suited for vessel segments that transition abruptly in size (e.g., from a 10-mm common iliac to a 7-mm external iliac). Unlike the nitinol designs, the Wallstent, a nonsegmented steel mesh, does not conform to all aspects of the irregularly shaped vessel, resulting in some areas of malapposition where the metal does not come in contact with the vessel wall.

Balloon-expandable stents offer some advantage over the self-expanded stents in terms of precision of placement. This is related to the delivery system of the stents as well as the foreshortening characteristics. Some of the nitinol stents, such as the Symphony, SMART, Luminex, and Zilver stents, have radiopaque markers attached to the stent ends to improve visibility and facilitate more precise deployment.

The Intracoil stent from Sulzer is the only stent approved in the United States for SFA intervention. The Intracoil is a nitinol wire coil. In clinical trials, the stent provided an 85% clinical patency rate at 9 months follow-up (41). In another

TABLE 34.1. *Manufacturer and type of stents used in peripheral arteries*

Name	Manufacturer	Diameter (mm)	Length (mm)	Type[a]	Material
Zilver	Cook	6, 7, 8, 9, 10	20, 30, 40, 60, 80	SE	Nitinol
Symphony	Boston Scientific	6, 7, 8, 10, 12, 14	20, 22, 23, 40, 60	SE	Nitinol
Luminex	Bard	6, 7, 8, 9, 10, 12	20, 30, 40, 50, 60, 80, 100, 120	SE	Nitinol
Wallstent	Boston Scientific	5, 6, 7, 8, 10, 12, 14, 16, 18, 20	20, 40, 55, 45, 60, 80, 90, 94		Nitinol
Genesis	Cordis	4–10	12–79	BE	316L Stainless steel
SMART	Cordis	6–14	20–80	SE	Nitinol
PRECISE	Cordis	5–10	20, 30, 40	SE	Nitinol
Express LD	Boston Scientific	6–10	17–57	BE	316L Stainless steel
OMNILINK	Guidant	5–10	18–58	BE	316L Stainless steel
Bridge	Medtronic	6–10	20–60	BE	316L Stainless steel

[a]SE, Self-expandable; BE, balloon-expandable.

study, the primary patency rate of the Intracoil stent was 86% (42).

The Symphony stent is a Boston Scientific stent (Fig. 34.5). Its hexagonal architecture results in a unique self-expanding design that is both flexible and strong. It has three radiopaque markers on each stent end, which provide clear visualization of stent margins during deployment and postprocedure follow-up. It is delivered via a 7 French catheter system over a 0.035-in. guidewire. The Symphony does not possess the same ability to conform to varying vessel diameters as the segmented nitinol stents. The Symphony tends to straighten tortuous arterial segments. The stent consists of welded nitinol filaments, increasing its rigidity compared to the segmented designs.

The Zilver stent (Cook) is a self-expanding nitinol stent with multiple gold markers on each end for precise placement (Fig. 34.7). The stent is preloaded in a 7 French introducer, designed to provide maximum flexibility without kinking or compressing. It is delivered via a 7 French sheath or a 9 French guiding catheter. The stent displays excellent kink resistance

within tortuous anatomy without lumen reduction. Z-stent design ensures optimal wall apposition while maintaining a strong, equally distributed radial force throughout the lumen. Gold markers enhance visibility during fluoroscopy. The Zilver has minimal foreshortening during deployment.

The Luminex stent, from Bard (Fig. 34.8), is a nitinol self-expanding stent delivered via a 6 French sheath over a 0.035-in. guidewire. The SAFE version has a novel catheter with tip-to-outer catheter configuration. It is a softer atraumatic tip, and the StentLoc Plus Delivery Control System facilitates positioning and stent delivery. The Luminex has radiopaque tantalum markers at the edge of the stent. It has less than 2% stent shortening.

The Wallstent (11,32), from Boston Scientific (Fig. 34.3), is a steel mesh self-expanding stent with 6 French sheath and 0.035-in. guidewire compatibility for up to 10 mm in diameter. Its exclusive HALO technology provides significant fluoroscopic visibility. The reconstrainability with up to 87% of the stent deployed allows a unique opportunity to reposition the stent for proper placement. Primary patency at 6 months

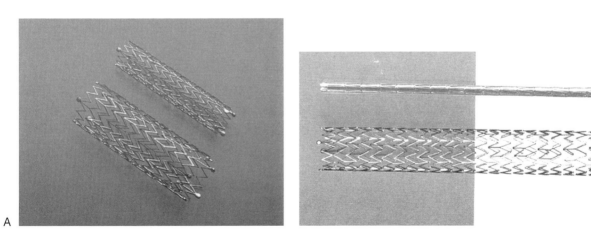

FIG. 34.7. A: The Zilver stent (Cook) is a self-expanding stent made by laser cutting from a single nitinol metal tube. It has gold markers at the ends to help in precise placement. **B, Top:** Stent mounted on balloon. **Bottom:** Fully expanded stent. (Courtesy of Cook, Bloomington, IN.)

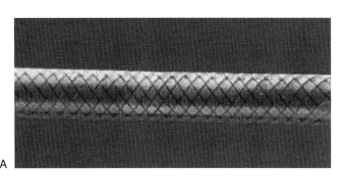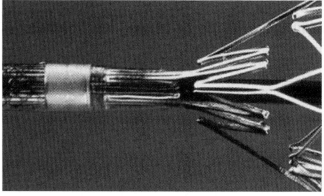

FIG. 34.8. A: The Luminexx stent (Bard) is a nitinol self-expanding stent. It has tantalum markers at the edges for precise placement. **B:** Stent in partial deployment. It is loaded on a 0.35-in. guidewire and delivered via a 6-Fr sheath. (Courtesy of C. R. Bard, Inc., Murray Hill, NJ.)

was 93%, at 12 months was 88%, and at 36 months was 77%. Secondary patency at 6 months was 98%, at 12 months was 98%, and at 36 months was 92%.

The SMART stent is a Cordis self-expanding stent (Fig. 34.4). It is a nitinol-based stent laser cut from one piece of tube, minimizing the weak points that might result from welding. It is also based on a segmented design, which enhances conformability and contourability. Its MicroMarker Technology creates distinctive line configurations that represent the proximal and distal ends of the stent for better placement precision. This facilitates the identification of the predeployment, initial release, and postdeployment stages of stent delivery. The stent has less than 8% foreshortening from the proximal stent end only, minimizing the need for repositioning or the need for double stenting. It is compatible with a 7 French sheath or a 9 French guide system over a 0.035-in. guidewire.

The PRECISE stent is another Cordis self-expanding nitinol stent, similar to the SMART stent, but with a smaller delivery system. The PRECISE is compatible with a 6 French sheath or an 8 French Guide over a 0.014-in. or a 0.018-in. guidewire. The design allows better contrast flow and enhanced trackability and crossability. Its novel TruMark technology of unique coil construction reduces system compressibility.

The DYNALINK stent by Guidant is a nitinol self-expanding stent. The stent is available in diameters ranging from 5 to 14 mm, and up to 100 mm in length. The delivery systems are 0.018-in. and 0.035-in. compatible, using 6 to 8 French intoducers. The ACCULINK investigational version of the DYNALINK stent is tapered from the proximal end of the stent to the distal end. The tapered stent was used in the ACCULINK for Revascularization of Carotids in High Risk patients trial of carotid stenting for stroke prevention in high-risk patients. The ACCULINK stent is also being evaluated in the National Institutes of Health-sponsored randomized Carotid Revascularization Enderectomy versus Stent Trial of carotid stenting versus surgical endarterectomy (43).

STRUT FRACTURES

In a recent trial comparing sirolimus-eluting SMART stents to bare nitinol SMART stents for SFA lesions, a number of strut fractures were noted. A preliminary analysis of the data implicated areas of overlapping metal where two stents had been placed. The significance of the finding is uncertain. The rate of target lesion revascularization was zero in both arms of the study (44). In a retrospective analysis, Singh observed a 14% rate of fracture in nitinol stents placed in the SFA. The overall rate of restenosis in the series was 14%. The rate of restenosis in the fractured stents was 7% (45). Although no unusual consequences were reported, other operators have observed pseudoaneurysms and arterial–venous fistulas (Craig Walker, MD, Homa LA, personal communication, 2003).

SUMMARY

A number of balloon-expandable and self-expanding stents are currently used for iliac and SFA intervention. Most stents are used off label, with the exception of the Wallstent, the Palmaz 308, and the SMART stent, each of which has an indication for iliac use after suboptimal angioplasty or opening an occlusion. Primary and secondary patency rates after iliac stenting have been excellent, generally regardless of stent design. Lesion characteristics, vessel size, tortuosity, and varying diameters (such as a highly tapering vessel) may influence stent selection.

For SFA intervention, self-expanding stents that immediately recover from crush are recommended, although a number of series demonstrated acceptable results with balloon-expandable stents such as the Palmaz. Patency rates appear to be worse than with iliac stenting, but the morbidity of infrainguinal surgery is sufficiently high that many operators prefer stenting, with surgery as a fallback if restenosis is a problem. Data directly comparing nitinol stents to steel mesh stents for SFA intervention are lacking. Furthermore, preliminary favorable data with drug-eluting stents may render the comparison moot. For now, flexibility, trackability, precise placement, and small delivery systems dictate the choice of stent.

REFERENCES

1. Pentecost MJ, Criqui MH, Doros G, et al. Guidelines for peripheral percutaneous transluminal angioplasty of the abdominal aorta and lower extremity vessels. A statement of health professionals from a special writing group of the Councils on Cardiovascular Radiology, Atherosclerosis, Cardiothoracic and Vascular Surgery, Clinical Cardiology, and Epidemiology and Prevention, the American Heart Association. *Circulation* 1994;89:511–531.
2. Berne FA, Lawrence WP, Carlton WH. Roentgenographic measurements of arterial narrowing. *AJR Am J Roentgenol* 1970;110:757–759.
3. May AG, Van de Berg L, DeWeese J, et al. Critical arterial stenosis. *Surgery* 1963;54:250–259.
4. Kinney TB, Rose SC. Intraarterial pressure measurements during angiographic evaluation of peripheral vascular disease: techniques, interpretation, applications and limitations. *AJR Am J Roentgenol* 1996;166:277–284.
5. Tetteroo E, Haaring C, van der Graff Y, et al. Intraarterial pressure gradients after randomized angioplasty or stenting of iliac artery lesions. Dutch Iliac Stent Trail Study Group. *Cardiovasc Intervent Radiol* 1996;19:411–417.
6. Brewster DC, Waltman AC, O'Hara PJ, et al. Femoral arterial pressure measurements during aortography. *Circulation* 1979;60:120–124.
7. Bosch JL, Hunink MGM. Meta-analysis of the results of percutaneous transluminal angioplasty and stent placement for aortoiliac occlusive disease. *Radiology* 1997;204:87–96.
8. Tetteroo E, van der Graff Y, Bosch JL, et al. Randomized comparison of primary stent placement versus primary angioplasty followed by selective stent placement in patients with iliac artery occlusive disease. *Lancet* 1998;351:1153–1159.
9. Vorwerk D, Guenther RW, Schurmann K, et al. Aortic and iliac stenoses: follow-up and results of stent placement after insufficient balloon angioplasty in 118 cases. *Radiology* 1996;198:45–48.
10. Strecker EP, Boos IB, Hagen B. Flexible tantalum stents for the treatment of iliac artery lesions: long-term patency, complications, and risk factors. *Radiology* 1996;199:641–647.
11. Murphy TP, Webb MS, Lambiase RE, et al. Percutaneous revascularization of complex iliac artery stenoses and occlusions with use of Wallstents: three-year experience. *J Vasc Interv Radiol* 1996;7:21–27.
12. Dyet JF, Gaines PA, Nicholson AA, et al. Treatment of chronic iliac artery occlusions by means of percutaneous endovascular stent placement. *J Vasc Interv Radiol* 1997;8:349–353.
13. Henry M, Amor M, Echevenor G, et al. Percutaneous endoluminal treatment of iliac occlusions: long-term follow-up in 105 patients. *J Endovasc Surg* 1998;5:228–235.
14. Ballard JL, Sparks SR, Taylor PC, et al. Complications of iliac stent deployment. *J Vasc Surg* 1996;24:545–555.
15. Bosch JL, Tetteroo E, Mali WP, et al. Iliac arterial occlusive disease: cost-effectiveness analysis of stent placement versus percutaneous transluminal angioplasty. Dutch Iliac Stent Trial Study Group. *Radiology* 1998;208:641–648.
16. Long AL, Sapoval MR, Beyssen BM, et al. Strecker stent implantation in the iliac arteries: patency and predictive factors for long-term success. *Radiology* 1995;194:739–744.
17. Palmaz JC, Garcia OJ, Schatz RA, et al. Placement of balloon-expanded intraluminal stents in iliac arteries: first 171 procedures. *Radiology* 1990;174:969–975.
18. Timaran CH, Stevens SL, Freeman MB, et al. External iliac and common iliac artery angioplasty and stenting in men and women. *J Vasc Surg* 2001;34:440–446.
19. Saker MB, Oppat WF, Kent SA, et al. Early failure of aortoiliac kissing stents: histopathologic correlation. *J Vasc Interv Radiol* 2000;11:333–336.
20. Lanuner J, Dake MD, Bleyn J, et al. Peripheral arterial obstruction: prospective study of treatment with a transluminally placed self-expanding stent-graft. *Radiology* 2000;217:95–104.
21. Mendelsohn RO, Santos RM, Crowley JJ, et al. Kissing stents in the aortic bifurcation. *Am Heart J* 1998;136:600–605.
22. Kadir S, White Jr RI, Kauffman SL, et al. Long-term results of aortoiliac angioplasty. *Surgery* 1983;94:10–14.
23. Sigwart U, Puel J, Mirkovitch V, et al. Intravascular stents to prevent occlusion and restenosis after transluminal angioplasty. *N Engl J Med* 1987;316:701–706.
24. Palmaz JC, Balloon-expandable intravascular stent. *AJR Am J Roentgenol* 1988;150:1263–1269.
25. Rabkin DJ, Lang EV, Brophy DP. Nitinol properties affecting uses in interventional radiology. *J Vasc Interv Radiol* 2000;11:343–350.
26. Lossef SV, Lutz RJ, Mundorf J, et al. Comparison of mechanical deformation properties of metallic stents with use of stress–strain analysis. *J Vasc Interv Radiol* 1994;5:341–349.
27. Dyet JF, Watts WG, Ettles DF, et al. Mechanical properties of metallic stents: how do these properties influence the choice of stent for specific lesions. *Cardiosvasc Intervent Radiol* 2000;23:47–54.
28. Duda SH, Wiskirchen J, Tepe G, et al. Physical properties of endovascular stents; an experimental comparison. *J Vasc Interv Radiol* 2000;11:645–654.
29. Schrader SC, Beyar R. Evaluation of the compressive mechanical properties of endoluminal metal stents. *Cathet Cardiovasc Diagn* 1998;44:179–187.
30. Lenhart M, Volk M, Manke C, et al. Stent appearance at contrast-enhanced MR angiography: *in vitro* examination with 14 stents. *Radiology* 2000;217:173–178.
31. Meyer JM, Buecker A, Schuermann K, et al. *In vitro* tests of 22 metallic stents and the possibility of determining their patency by MR angiography. *Interv Radiol* 2000;35:739–746.
32. Martin EC, Katzen BT, Benenati JF, et al. Multicenter trial of the Wallstent in the iliac and femoral arteries. *J Vasc Interv Radiol* 1995;6:843–849.
33. Rutherford RB, Becker GJ. Standards for evaluating and reporting the results of surgical and percutaneous therapy for peripheral arterial disease. *J Vasc Interv Radiol* 1991;2:169–174.
34. Murphy TP. The role of stents in aortoiliac occlusive disease. In: Becker GJ, Perler BA, eds. *Vascular disease: surgical and interventional management.* New York: Thieme, 1998;111–135.
35. Marin ML, Veith FJ, Cynamon J, et al. Effect of polytetrafluoroethylene covering of Palmaz stents on the development of intimal hyperplasia in human iliac arteries. *J Vasc Interv Radiol* 1996;7:651–656.
36. Henry M, Amor M, Henry I, et al. Percutaneous endovascular treatment of peripheral aneurysms. *J Cardiovasc Surg* 2000;41:871–883.
37. Palmaz JC, Encarcacion CE, Garcia OJ, et al. Aortic bifurcation stenosis: treatment with intravascular stents. *J Vasc Interv Radiol* 1991;2:319–323.
38. Palmaz JC, Laborde JC, Rivera FJ, et al. Stenting of the iliac arteries with the Palmaz stent: experience from a multicenter trial. *Cardiovasc Intervent Radiol* 1992;15:291–297.
39. Murphy KD, Encarcacion CE, Le VA, et al. Iliac artery stent placement with the Palmaz stent: follow-up study. *J Vasc Interv Radiol* 1995;6:312–329.
40. Dotter CT, Buschmann RW, McKinney MK, et al. Transluminal expandable nitinol coil stent grafting: preliminary report. *Radiology* 1983;147:259–260.
41. http://fdagov.sitesearch.google.com/fdagov?client=fdagov&q=cache%3Ahttp%3A%2F%2Fwww%2Efda%2Egov%2Fohrms%2Fdockets%2Fac%2F01%2Fbriefing%2F3747b1ʹ01%2Epdf+Sulzer%20stent
42. Jahnke T, Voshage G, Stefan MH, et al. Endovascular placement of self-expanding nitinol coil stents for the treatment of femoropopliteal obstructive disease. *J Vasc Interv Radiol* 2002;13:257–266.
43. Transcatheter Cardiovascular Therapeutics. Presentation, Washington, D.C., September 24–28, 2002.
44. Duda SH, Pusich B, Richter G, et al. Sirolimus-eluting stents for the treatment of obstructive superficial femoral artery disease: six-month results. *Circulation* 2002;106:1505–1509.
45. Rocha-Singh. Nitinol stent fractures in the superficial femoral artery. *JACC* 2003;41:6(Supp. A):79A.

CHAPTER 35

Technical Requirements for Cardiovascular Training in Peripheral Vascular Disease

Elie Hage-Korban, Joel M. Cohn, and George S. Abela

Key Points

- There are three levels of competency for the peripheral vascular disease care provider. These levels dictate the level of care a provider may give and the actual requirements needed.
- A peripheral vascular disease care provider must undergo a comprehensive training program, which includes didactics, laboratory experience, and invasive and interventional experience.
- A key component to the training process is completion of the general competencies as defined by the Accreditation Council of Graduate Medical Education.

INTRODUCTION

The discipline of vascular medicine is becoming an integral part of modern medicine. Its resurgence has been attributed to multiple factors, which include the technological leap in endovascular medicine, the overwhelming success achieved with intracoronary interventions, and the shift in public interest from survival advantage to improved quality of life. The natural consequence has been a shortage in available personnel, resulting in the need to train more peripheral vascular specialists. Vascular medicine training is still achieved as part of an established training program in cardiology, radiology, or general surgery. This has resulted in several training standards published by the various medical societies, including the Society of Cardiovascular and Interventional Radiology, the American College of Radiology, the American Heart Association, the American College of Cardiology, the Society of Cardiac Angiography and Intervention, and the Society of Vascular Surgery (Table 35.1) (1–8). These standards are, ironically, quite variable and based primarily on expert opinions rather than evidence-based educational guidelines. Furthermore, the published standards have been heavily focused on endovascular procedural volume rather than on fundamental understanding of vascular medicine.

Standards in the medical field are designed to improve the quality of care and to make physicians accountable for their practice and the type of care they provide to their patients. This may be perceived in a negative manner as an intrusion into the particulars of the profession to limit competition. This chapter focuses on the technical requirements in training fellows in peripheral vascular disease at progressively increasing levels of clinical and technical complexity. Many of the clinical elements have already been well described in other chapters including physical exam, noninvasive and invasive examination, and medical and surgical treatment.

In this chapter, we propose a system for training cardiovascular fellows in vascular medicine that is based on competency-based education applied to the training guidelines adopted by the American College of Cardiology Core Cardiology Training Symposium (ACC-COCATS) (9). However, the education should be largely based on the assessment of specific competencies (10,11). Competency in any discipline should be determined by acquiring the basic knowledge related to that field, applying it appropriately to clinical scenarios, and then performing the appropriate invasive procedure with adequate success and acceptable complication rates. Hence, the aim of our system is to provide the trainee with a broad base of knowledge and experience in the

442

TABLE 35.1. *Credentialing standards[a]*

Organization	Diagnostic angiography[b]	Number of arterial lysis	PTA
SCVIR (1)	200	0	25
AHA (2)	100 (50)	10	50 (25)
SCAI (1990) (3)	100 (50)	15	50 (25)
SCAI (1999) (4)	0	0	3
SVS (1993) (5)	50[c]	0	10–15
SVS (1999) (6)	100 (50)[d]	0	38 (17)[e]
ACC (7)	100 (50)	10	50 (25)

[a]PTA, percutaneous transluminal angioplasty; SCVIR, Society of Cardiovascular and Interventional Radiology; ACC, American College of Cardiology; SVC, Society of Vascular Surgery; SCAI, Society of Cardiovascular Angiography and Intervention; AHA, American Heart Association.

[b]Number in parentheses represent primary operator cases.

[c]Includes intraoperative angiogram.

[d]75 arterial, 25 percutaneous arterial punctures; each vessel selected is an additional angiogram.

[e]Includes multiple interventions at the same site.

Adapted from Sacks D, Becker GJ, Matalon TAS. Credentials for peripheral angioplasty: comments on Society of Cardiac Angiography and Intervention Revisions. *J Vasc Interv Radiol* 2001;12:277–280, with permission.

diagnosis, treatment, and prevention of vascular diseases. We hope to provide a comprehensive system that will be adopted by various cardiovascular training programs.

In this chapter, we adopt the multilevel approach proposed by the ACC-COCATS to train cardiology fellows in peripheral vascular disease (PVD) (9). Each of the three levels of competence and training includes a defined required knowledge base and skills that must be mastered by the trainee. We address the proposed requirements for each level after going through the general curriculum.

Training in cardiovascular medicine should be comprehensive and must include the following:

• Didactic sessions that encompass the different aspects of knowledge and training
• Noninvasive vascular laboratory experience
• Invasive diagnostic experience
• Interventional vascular experience

DIDACTIC TEACHING

The curriculum should be stratified into multiple sessions. These sessions should be structured in a conference pattern either distributed throughout the core conference curriculum or presented in an intensive peripheral month, as currently required. The topics covered should include at least the following:

1. Anatomy of the vascular system
2. Physiological principles governing the peripheral vascular system (PVS)
3. Pathophysiological states of the peripheral system
4. History taking in the PVS
5. Physical examination of the PVS
6. Differential diagnosis of PVD
7. Screening for PVD

8. The appropriate selection of the diagnostic tools for PVD
9. Treatment modalities for PVD
10. Principles of angiography for PVD
11. Selection of the best treatment modalities tailored to the specific findings of the invasive or noninvasive studies: medical treatment versus percutaneous intervention versus surgical approach
12. Cardiovascular disease and its association with vascular disease in other conditions
13. Upper and lower extremity acute and chronic occlusive disease
14. Aortoiliac occlusive disease
15. Vascular trauma (penetrating injuries, blunt trauma)
16. Mesenteric vascular disease (renovascular and chronic splanchnic occlusive disease)
17. Aneurysmal disease
18. Venous disease
19. Lymphatic system

NONINVASIVE LABORATORY EXPERIENCE

Any trainee interested in the management of vascular patients should have exposure to the noninvasive diagnostic tools available for screening and diagnosis of different PVD states (Table 35.2). The trainee should spend a minimum of 1 month in the vascular lab getting acquainted with the various studies, primarily carotid arterial studies, ankle–brachial index (resting and exercise), segmental arterial waveform analysis, renal and abdominal ultrasound, venous duplex, and upper extremities and lower extremities arterial studies. This training must be performed under the direct supervision of a credentialed interpreting physician. By the end of that period, the fellow in training should be able to interpret such studies independently. This level of competency should be assessed by keeping a log of the studies that the

TABLE 35.2. *Summary of training requirements for different levels in peripheral vascular disease care programs* [a]

Level	Cumulative period of training (months)	Components of training + clinic	Number of procedures
1	2	1 mo noninvasive lab 8 half-days vascular clinic	50 (25) carotid US 50 (25) renal US 50 (25) venous US 50 (25) limb arterial US 50 (25) ABI/PVR
2	12	2–3 mo vascular service 3 mo noninvasive lab 12 half-days vascular clinic 1 mo PVD catheterization lab	Noninvasive, as in level 1 25 diagnostic peripheral angiograms 25 peripheral interventions 8 mo catherization suite (coronary and PVD)
3	12	1 mo vascular service 1 mo noninvasive lab 9 mo peripheral vascular catherization suite 1 half-day vascular clinic per week	Noninvasive and diagnostic angiograms as in level 2 50 (25) peripheral interventions 10 peripheral thrombolytics

[a]US, ultrasound; ABI, ankle–brachial index; PVR, pulse volume recording; PVD, peripheral vascular disease.

Modified from Beller GA, Bonow RO, Fuster V, et al. ACC revised recommendations for training in vascular medicine and peripheral catheter-based interventions, Task force 11: training in vascular medicine and peripheral catheter-based interventions. *J Am Coll Cardiol* 2002;39:1242–1246, with permission.

trainee observed, with a minimum of 100 studies in each category and a minimum of 25 studies interpreted independently by the trainee and confirmed by the supervising physician. Some exposure to newer modalities including magnetic resonance angiography and computerized tomographic angiography should also be obtained during the vascular laboratory experience.

INVASIVE DIAGNOSTIC EXPERIENCE

All physicians participating in a vascular training program should have some exposure to the peripheral angiography suite with the degree of involvement tailored to the level of expertise they are seeking (Table 35.2). The minimum requirement is 1 day a week in the angiography suite during that month period, where the trainee can assist in the performance of these procedures or just observe the primary operator. The trainee should spend a total of 8 months in the angiography suite as part of his or her primarily training performing coronary and noncoronary procedures. For a trainee to be certified in the performance of peripheral angiography, he or she has to assist in the performance of 50 procedures and be the primary operator in another 25. However, no trainee should be allowed to independently perform these invasive procedures unless approved by the supervising physician, who must be a certified operator. Moreover, the physician should be exposed to the different vascular access techniques. Complication rates should be within the accepted community standards. By the end of this rotation, the fellow must be able to understand the limitations of peripheral angiography, management of complications, and interpretation of angiographic studies.

PERCUTANEOUS INTERVENTIONAL TRAINING

Training in peripheral endovascular procedures should not be limited to the technical portion of the procedure. Any physician who is interested in the performance of percutaneous transluminal angioplasty (PTA) should fulfill the minimum training requirements as stated previously (Table 35.2). This means that the performing physician should have fulfilled steps 1, 2, and 3. In addition, the trainee should assist in at least 25 peripheral interventions and be the primary operator in another 25. These must be documented, signed by the supervising interventionalist, and include an accurate report of the complications. Moreover, given the more intricate nature of the peripheral interventions, the trainee should be familiar with multiple vascular access and approaches to different lesions with documentation (Table 35.2).

Level 1 Training

This includes basic training in peripheral vascular disease. Level 1 is the minimum amount of training required for any cardiovascular specialist to graduate. The duration of the training is a 1-month period spent in the noninvasive laboratory as stated previously. In addition, the fellow should spend

TABLE 35.3. *General competency items*

1. Patient care
2. Medical knowledge
3. Practice-based learning and improvement
4. Interpersonal and communication skill
5. Professionalism
6. System-based practice

TABLE 35.4. *Scoring of general competency items*

Fellow Name: _____ Evaluator's Initials: _____ Date of Evaluation: _____

Patient Care (a)	1 = Poor 5 = Average 9 = Superior
Able to integrate diagnostic findings into provisional diagnosis and treatment plan	123/ 456/ 789 NO
Adequately prepares for invasive procedures	123/ 456/ 789 NO
Appreciates the onset of complications	123/ 456/ 789 NO
Appropriate antibiotic selection	123/ 456/ 789 NO
Appropriately interprets lab, x-ray, and other ancillary studies	123/ 456/ 789 NO
Appropriately orders lab, x-ray, and other ancillary studies	123/ 456/ 789 NO
Appropriately uses precatheterization intravenous fluids	123/ 456/ 789 NO
Appropriately orders studies for preoperative assessment	123/ 456/ 789 NO
Demonstrates caring and empathy	123/ 456/ 789 NO
Demonstrates critical decision making	123/ 456/ 789 NO
Detects early wound infection and institutes prompt treatment	123/ 456/ 789 NO
Detects early hematoma at access site complication and institutes prompt treatment	123/ 456/ 789 NO
Develops a reasonable treatment plan based on the patient's clinical presentation	123/ 456/ 789 NO
Discusses issue of health promotion (e.g., lipid and blood pressure control, smoking cessation, diet, exercise, etc.)	123/ 456/ 789 NO
Discusses injury control strategies with patients (e.g., postcatheterization instructions to increase healing and decreased risk of healing)	123/ 456/ 789 NO
Effectively manages postcatheterization care (e.g., fluid management, follow-up labs)	123/ 456/ 789 NO

Medical Knowledge (b)	
Able to integrate diagnostic findings into provisional diagnosis and treatment plan	123/ 456/ 789 NO
Accurately interprets laboratory studies	123/ 456/ 789 NO
Accurately interprets lab, x-ray, and other ancillary studies	123/ 456/ 789 NO
Accurately interprets ultrasound and Dopler studies	123/ 456/ 789 NO
Adequate and accurate physical examination	123/ 456/ 789 NO
Appreciates the onset of complications in the catheterization lab and clinical setting	123/ 456/ 789 NO
Appropriately orders laboratory studies	123/ 456/ 789 NO
Demonstrates a mastery of vascular anatomy	123/ 456/ 789 NO
Demonstrates an understanding of the nutrition	123/ 456/ 789 NO
Demonstrates appropriate pharmacologic management	123/ 456/ 789 NO
Demonstrates solid general medical knowledge	123/ 456/ 789 NO
Develops a broad differential diagnosis	123/ 456/ 789 NO
Effectively manages postcatheterization complications (i.e., hypo- and hypertension, arrhythmias)	123/ 456/ 789 NO
Performs adequate history and physical examination	123/ 456/ 789 NO
Provides adequate pain management	123/ 456/ 789 NO
Recognizes critical conditions	123/ 456/ 789 NO
Understands evidence-based medicine (e.g., epidemiology, clinical rules, clinical guidelines)	123/ 456/ 789 NO

Practice-based Learning and Improvement (c)	
Accepts advice and/or criticism appropriately	123/ 456/ 789 NO
Adequately prepares for procedures	123/ 456/ 789 NO
Anticipates barriers to patient throughput times	123/ 456/ 789 NO
Applies pretest and posttest probabilities when integrating test results into patient care	123/ 456/ 789 NO
Attends post-mortem examinations	123/ 456/ 789 NO
Attends the research conference	123/ 456/ 789 NO
Attends catheterization conferences, grand rounds, journal club, research conference, basic science conference	123/ 456/ 789 NO
Contributes helpful discussion on rounds	123/ 456/ 789 NO
Integrates feedback into future situations (does not make the same mistake twice)	123/ 456/ 789 NO
Procedure logs are complete and current	123/ 456/ 789 NO
Resident acknowledges limitations and readily seeks advice	123/ 456/ 789 NO
Resident follows up on admitted and discharged patients	123/ 456/ 789 NO

Interpersonal and Communication Skills (d)	
Communicates effectively with patient and family	123/ 456/ 789 NO
Communicates condition with primary care physicians on admissions	123/ 456/ 789 NO
Communicates effectively and with sensitivity to a diverse patient population	123/ 456/ 789 NO
Medical records are complete	123/ 456/ 789 NO
Catheterization and other procedural reports are are complete	123/ 456/ 789 NO

Continued

TABLE 35.4. *Continued*

Professionalism (e)	
Acts as an advocate for the patient	123/ 456/ 789 NO
Adheres to ethical principles in cardiovascular medicine	123/ 456/ 789 NO
Fairly assesses patients on issues of competency and mental capacity	123/ 456/ 789 NO
Systems-based Practice (f)	
Able to integrate diagnostic findings into provisional diagnosis and treatment plan	123/ 456/ 789 NO
Able to use system resources to provide optimal care	123/ 456/ 789 NO
Adopts a multidisciplinary model in patient care	123/ 456/ 789 NO
Appropriately applies and uses technology in the context of patient care (e.g., uses handheld computers, Internet access, access of the library, and evidence-based medicine)	123/ 456/ 789 NO
Appropriately orders laboratory studies	123/ 456/ 789 NO
Appropriately orders other studies (electrocardiogram, ultrasound, Doppler, etc.)	123/ 456/ 789 NO
Arranges proper follow-up to correct attending	123/ 456/ 789 NO
Interacts appropriately with referring physician and multidisciplinary physician group	123/ 456/ 789 NO
Interacts with nursing appropriately	123/ 456/ 789 NO

Core Competency Composite Score

Mean Score	Category
_____	a = patient care
_____	b = medical knowledge
_____	c = practice-based learning and improvement
_____	d = interpersonal and communication skills
_____	e = professionalism
_____	f = systems-based practice

Adapted from Reisdorff EJ, Hayes OW, Carlson DJ, et al. Assessing the new general competencies for resident education: a model from an emergency medicine program. *Acad Med* 2001;76:753–757.

one half-day period in the outpatient vascular clinic alternating between cardiologists and vascular surgeons. An equivalent of eight clinics should be sufficient for this level. All cardiovascular fellowship candidates should spend at least 4 months in the cardiac angiography laboratory. They should be involved in the assistance of 25 noncardiac angiographic procedures. This level is not qualified to independently perform such invasive procedures.

Level 2 Training

This is intended for physicians interested in focusing on peripheral vascular disease as a career plan. The trainee should fulfill both the noninvasive and the invasive requirements as stated previously (Table 35.2). In addition, he or she should spend a total of 12 half-days in clinic alternating between cardiovascular specialists and vascular surgeons. Moreover, he or she should spend 1 month on the vascular inpatient service with both percutaneous and surgical teams. At this level, the trainee should be able to perform and interpret various noninvasive and invasive diagnostic procedures, manage patients with wide array of peripheral vascular pathology, perform the pre- and postcatherization management of these patients, perform risk stratification, and discuss risk factor modification.

Level 3 Training

This is intended for physicians interested in the complete spectrum of managing patients with PVD. This includes per-

cutaneous treatment of various vascular stenotic lesions. The physician should spend at least 12 months in the management of patients with vascular diseases. He or she must meet both the level 1 and level 2 training. In addition, he or she should assist in the performance of 25 peripheral interventions and be the primary operator in another 25 procedures. The trainee should fulfill the previously mentioned criteria for performing peripheral interventions. It is not necessary to combine this training with a full year dedicated for interventional training (coronary and noncoronary). The 12-month period dedicated for peripheral interventions should be adequate to fulfill these requirements, with a minimum of 8 months spent in the angiography suite.

COMPETENCY ASSESSMENT

Fellow evaluation is an integral part of a successful educational program. Fellow performance must be assessed in accordance with the Accreditation Council of Graduate Medical Education (ACGME) recommendations based on the recently introduced General Competency (GC) modules (10). We propose some modifications to fit our proposed model of training. Six GCs have been identified (Table 35.3). We believe that the attitudes, skills, and knowledge expressed in the GCs are already an integral part of the training program. It is the responsibility of the program to assess the fellow's achievement of the GCs by using a dependable set of measures. Each item of the GC module should be scored as indicated in Table 35.4, and then a derived score for every GC is calculated (11). The general assumption is that the trainee's performance is an implicit indicator of the quality of training, and the scores provide a two-way improvement tool. Also, curricula defining the various competencies will be provided to the trainees as a guideline for the expected behaviors.

The foregoing proposed model is being used at our institution, and its usefulness in monitoring acquisition of ACGME general competencies is effective and objective.

REFERENCES

1. Spies JB, Bakal CW, Burke DR, et al. Standards for interventional radiology. Standards of Practice Committee of the Society of Cardiovascular and Interventional radiology. *J Vasc Interv Radiol* 1991;2:59–65.
2. Levin DC, Becker GJ, Dorros G, et al. Training standards for physicians performing peripheral angioplasty and other percutaneous peripheral vascular interventions. A statement for health professionals from the special writing group of the Councils on Cardiovascular Radiology, Cardio-Thoracic and Vascular Surgery, and Clinical Cardiology, the American Heart Association. *Circulation* 1992;86:1348–1350.
3. Wexler L, Dorros G, Levin D, et al. Guidelines for percutaneous transluminal angioplasty. The Society for Cardiac Angiography and Interventions, Interventional Cardiology Committee, Subcommittee on Peripheral Interventions. *Cathet Cardiovasc Diagn* 1990;21:128–129.
4. Babb JD, Collins TJ, Cowley MJ, et al. Revised guidelines for the performance of peripheral vascular intervention. *Catheter Cardiovasc Intervent* 1999;46:21–23.
5. White RA, Fogarty TJ, Baker WH, et al. Endovascular surgery credentialing and training for vascular surgeons. *J Vasc Surg* 1993;17:1095–1102.
6. White RA, Hodgson KJ, Ahn SS, et al. Endovascular interventions training and credentialing for vascular surgeon. *J Vasc Surg* 1999;29:177–186.
7. Spittell Jr JA, Nanda NC, Creager MA, et al. Recommendations for peripheral transluminal angioplasty: training and facilities. American College of Cardiology Peripheral Vascular Disease Committee. *J Am Coll Cardiol* 1993;21:546–548.
8. Sacks D, Becker GJ, Matalon TAS. Credentials for peripheral angioplasty: comments on Society of Cardiac Angiography and Intervention revisions. *J Vasc Interv Radiol* 2001;12:277–280.
9. Beller GA, Bonow RO, Fuster V, et al. ACC revised recommendations for training in adult cardiovascular medicine core cardiology training II (COCATS 2) (revision of the COCATS training statement). Task force 11: training in vascular medicine and peripheral catheter based interventions. *J Am Coll Cardiol* 2002;39:1242–1246.
10. Swing S. *GME outcomes project of the ACGME.* Presented at the Association for Hospital Medical Education 2000 Spring Educational Institute, St. Petersburg, Florida, May 11, 2000.
11. Reisdorff EJ, Hayes OW, Carlson DJ, et al. Assessing the new general competencies for resident education: a model from an emergency medicine program. *Acad Med* 2001;76:753–757.

CHAPTER 36

Training and Credentialing for Interventional Therapy for Peripheral Vascular Disease

Christopher J. White

Key Points

- Training of internal medicine and cardiovascular specialists in peripheral vascular disease is critical in the management of hypertension, congestive heart failure, and angina.
- Three levels of training are defined: level 1, basic exposure of 2 months of training during fellowship; level 2, 2 to 3 months of exposure including inservice and outpatient exposure including noninvasive lab; level 3, catheter-based interventions.
- Skills in coronary interventions do translate into peripheral vascular procedures.
- Clinical competencies for peripheral vascular percutaneous interventions include cognitive, technical, and clinical skills.

INTRODUCTION

There are compelling reasons for cardiologists to undertake a more global approach to patients with atherosclerotic diseases (1–3). Atherosclerosis is a systemic disease, which often involves several vascular beds, resulting in the common occurrence of both cardiac and noncardiac vascular problems (4,5). Noncardiac vascular disease directly affects the management of patients with heart disease. Renovascular hypertension is the most common cause of secondary hypertension in patients with atherosclerosis elsewhere. Coronary artery disease is the most common cause of morbidity and mortality in patients with atherosclerotic peripheral vascular disease. Peripheral vascular symptoms, such as claudication, impair the effectiveness of cardiovascular rehabilitation programs. Renovascular hypertension, causing medically resistant hypertension, negatively affects the medical management of angina pectoris and congestive heart failure.

CARDIOVASCULAR TRAINING PROGRAMS

The American Board of Internal Medicine's Subspecialty Board of Cardiovascular Diseases specifically requires training of fellowship candidates in the diagnosis and management of peripheral vascular diseases to qualify for cardiovascular medicine board certification. The American College of Cardiology has developed a core curriculum for vascular medicine training (6). Three levels of training in vascular medicine are described.

Level 1 is basic training in vascular medicine, which all cardiology fellows should receive. At least 2 months of the fellowship, either as dedicated rotations or in the aggregate, should be dedicated to vascular medicine. Instruction should include the evaluation and management of arterial, venous, and lymphatic diseases, such as peripheral arterial disease, acute arterial occlusion, carotid artery disease, renal artery stenosis, aortic aneurysm, vasculitis, vasospasm, venous thrombosis and insufficiency, and lymphedema. Training should also include instruction in the recognition and management of medical disorders associated with vascular diseases, including hypertension, hyperlipidemia, diabetes mellitus, and hypercoagulable states.

Trainees should be familiar with the noninvasive vascular laboratory and knowledge regarding vascular tests such as segmental pressure measurements, pulse volume recordings, and duplex ultrasonography, and the information that can be derived from such testing. The cardiology fellow should be cognizant of imaging techniques that can be used to further assess the aorta, vena cavae, and peripheral arteries and veins, such as computed tomographic angiography, magnetic resonance imaging, and digital substraction angiography, and recognize the indications for catheter-based interventions and surgical revascularization.

Level 2 training is additional training for fellows wishing to develop special expertise in evaluating and managing patients with vascular disease. This level does not include training in catheter-based interventions. Trainees who plan a vascular medicine track as part of their cardiovascular fellowship should spend at least 2 to 3 months on an inpatient vascular medicine consultation service, at least 1 day per week in the outpatient vascular medicine clinic, at least 3 months in the noninvasive vascular laboratory, and 2 months in the peripheral vascular catheterization laboratory. Additional rotations could be allocated to vascular surgery, hematology, neurology, and rheumatology, to acquire fundamental experience in these important areas as they relate to vascular medicine.

Level 3 training is training for noncoronary, catheter-based vascular interventions to ensure that the trainee develops both cognitive and technical skills necessary for appropriate decision making in patients with vascular disease. In addition cardiology fellows who plan to independently perform peripheral vascular arteriography and venography require additional training regarding vascular access, knowledge of the normal vascular anatomy and common variants, and knowledge of the common patterns of collateral formation. Specific training in noncardiac diagnostic angiography should include the techniques of antegrade femoral artery access, contralateral femoral artery access, and vascular closure devices.

Exposure to noncardiac angiography includes imaging of the aorta and its first-order branches. An example is aortography in patients suspected of aortic dissection including selective angiography of the aortic arch vessels, mesenteric vessels, renal arteries, and iliofemoral arteries. Another example of peripheral vascular angiographic training is selective angiography of the subclavian, internal mammary, and gastroepiploic arteries to determine suitability or patency of coronary bypass grafts.

Trainees planning to perform peripheral vascular interventional procedures must have knowledge of the indications, limitations, and complications of these procedures as well as an in-depth understanding of the alternative treatment methods. Those planning to practice interventional procedures must obtain experience in peripheral vascular intervention during a fourth year of interventional cardiology fellowship training.

FEASIBILITY OF CARDIOLOGISTS PERFORMING PERIPHERAL VASCULAR INTERVENTION

Our initial experience in performing peripheral angioplasty in 164 consecutive patients over a 20-month period revealed that coronary intervention skills transferred easily to peripheral vascular procedures (7). Prior to performing angioplasty, we observed the performance of peripheral angioplasty in several labortories performing high-volume peripheral angioplasty; we were proctored for our intial cases by a credentialed operator, and our initial cases were reviewed and discussed with a vascular surgeon. Lower extremity percutaneous transluminal angioplasty (PTA) was performed in 116 patients, upper extremity PTA in 30 patients, and renal artery PTA in 18 patients. Successful results were obtained in 92% (191/208) of the lesions attempted. In no patient did a failed attempt result in worsening of the patient's clinical condition or the need for emergency surgery. The overall major complication rate of 4.3% (7/164) was similar to other published studies.

Our experience suggests that experienced interventional cardiologists, working closely with vascular surgeons, possess the necessary technical skills to perform peripheral vascular angioplasty in a safe and effective manner. The expertise of our vascular surgery colleagues was relied on for guidance in patient and lesion selection, which contributed to our high rate of success and low incidence of complications. Our results did not demonstrate a learning curve. The percentage of patients with totally occluded vessels (25%) and the average lesion length (5.8 ± 8.0 cm) attest to the relatively difficult lesions we routinely accepted for treatment.

Achieving a success rate of 92% for all lesions and a 99% success rate for stenoses suggests that coronary angioplasty skills can be adapted to the treatment of noncoronary lesions quite effectively. These results are consistent with those of other investigators, in that success rates were higher for nontotal occlusions and lesions of shorter length.

POSTGRADUATE CERTIFICATION FOR PERIPHERAL VASCULAR INTERVENTION

Many physicians with specialty training and certification in internal medicine, cardiology, vascular surgery, and radiology are performing peripheral vascular interventional procedures. These physicians have received either formal training in accredited programs or practical on-the-job training. Unfortunately, there is no uniform standard by which physicians with an interest in performing peripheral vascular interventional procedures can be measured. An on-going turf war over the provision of these services between competing subspecialties in many hospitals is clearly not in the best interests of patient care. Several professional societies, including the American College of Cardiology, the American Heart Association, the American Society of Cardiovascular Interventionists, the Society of Cardiovascular Interventional Radiologists, the Society of Vascular Surgery, and the Society for Cardiac Angiography and Interventions, have published disparate guidelines for the performance of peripheral angioplasty (8–14).

TABLE 36.1. *Elements of competence for peripheral vascular disease*

Cognitive: The fund of knowledge required is derived from the specialties of vascular medicine and angiology. It includes the knowledge of the natural history of the disease, the anatomy and physiology of the affected organ systems, interpretation of noninvasive tests, and an understanding of the indications for treatment and expected outcomes (risks and benefits) of the treatment options.

Procedural: These skills involve the full range of invasive percutaneous cardiovascular techniques, including gaining vascular access, performing diagnostic angiography, performing angioplasty and intervention, administering thrombolytic agents, and recognizing and managing complications of these procedures.

Clinical: This category encompasses the skills necessary to manage inpatients and outpatients with noncardiac vascular diseases. It includes the ability to admit patients to the hospital and provide daily care. The ability to perform a complete history and physical examination and to integrate the patient's history, physical examination, and noninvasive laboratory data to make accurate diagnoses is required. Finally, it requires establishing a doctor–patient relationship and continuity of care to provide long-term care for this chronic disease.

The realization that there is a need to enable cardiologists to provide noncardiac vascular care to patients with concomitant peripheral vascular disease has required revision of prior guidelines which were not cardiology-specific (14). This was done to provide a more focused view of the role of the cardiologist, specifically the interventional cardiologist, in the management of these patients. Percutaneous peripheral angioplasty is being performed by cardiologists with widely varying backgrounds and clinical experience. Clinical competency to perform peripheral vascular percutaneous interventions can be broken down into cognitive, technical, and clinical skill sets (Table 36.1).

Previously published guidelines for the performance of peripheral vascular intervention have suffered from a lack of specificity for the cardiologist's needs, being consensus or compromise recommendations from multiple specialties, often requiring almost unachievable training requirements for the practicing physician. One solution to these problems is a tiered approach to clinical competency (14). This tiered approach would recognize specific strengths and weaknesses of cardiologists in attaining clinical competency in the field of peripheral vascular intervention. The first step in achieving competency is the establishment of criteria for the performance of a narrow range of procedures, termed "restricted certification." Physicians wishing to enter the field of peripheral vascular intervention would meet defined criteria for the performance of specific procedures. The second step of clinical competency is the establishment of criteria that would allow experienced physicians to participate in all areas of peripheral vascular intervention, which would be termed "unrestricted certification."

"RESTRICTED" CERTIFICATION TO PERFORM PERCUTANEOUS TRANSLUMINAL ANGIOPLASTY

Iliac Intervention

Interventional cardiologists have more day-to-day clinical experience with retrograde femoral–iliac artery vascular access than any other specialty. The treatment of iliac artery stenotic or occlusive lesions directly affects the treatment of coronary artery disease. The ability of the cardiologist to preserve vascular access sites for coronary interventions or hemodynamic support with intraaortic counterpulsation balloons is inarguably desirable. The interventionalists' familiarity with the iliac artery anatomy, their technical expertise with guidewires, balloons, and stents, and the relatively common occurrence of these lesions in patients with coronary atherosclerosis make a compelling argument for enabling them to treat these lesions. The following are proposed criteria for interventional cardiologists to achieve limited credentials for the performance of iliac artery angioplasty:

1. Active credentials for the performance of coronary interventions.
2. Attendance at a peripheral angioplasty demonstration course.
3. Proctoring of three cases by an "unrestricted credentials" proctor.

Renal Intervention

The treatment of systemic hypertension, including the evaluation of the secondary causes of hypertension such as renovascular hypertension, is a core element of cardiovascular specialty training. Vascular access sites (femoral or brachial) used for renal artery PTA are standard procedures for invasive/interventional cardiologists. The technique of renal angioplasty and stent placement is virtually identical to angioplasty and stent placement of lesions in saphenous vein coronary bypass grafts, currently performed on a routine basis by interventional cardiologists. The treatment of renovascular hypertension in the setting of refractory angina pectoris or congestive heart failure can allow patients who may be poor candidates or at high risk for coronary revascularization to be controlled with medical therapy (15). Once again, the increased frequency of renovascular disease in patients with coronary artery disease makes a very strong argument for enabling interventional cardiologists to diagnose and treat these patients (16). The following are proposed criteria for interventional cardiologists to achieve limited credentials for the performance of renal artery angioplasty:

1. Active credentials for the performance of coronary interventions.
2. Attendance at a peripheral angioplasty demonstration course.
3. Proctoring of three cases by an "unrestricted credentials" proctor.

"UNRESTRICTED" CERTIFICATION FOR PERCUTANEOUS TRANSLUMINAL ANGIOPLASTY

Interventional cardiologists may be eligible for unrestricted competency either by certification of their training program director after achieving competence in peripheral intervention during cardiology specialty training in an accredited 3-year cardiology fellowship, completion of a fourth-year angioplasty fellowship, or after proctorship by a practicing peripheral vascular interventionist. This experience should include training in the cognitive, procedural, and clinical skills necessary to practice peripheral intervention. Documentation of the candidate's experience, including types of cases performed, case volume, and major complication rates, is required, and should be attested to in writing from either the training program director or the proctor.

Candidates for unrestricted competency should have documented the performance of 100 peripheral diagnostic angiograms and participation in at least 50 peripheral angioplasty procedures. The candidate should be the primary operator for at least half of the cases. Included in this experience should be at least ten cases involving the administration of thrombolytic therapy or mechanical thrombectomy for peripheral arterial or venous disease. Candidates may accumulate their experience by combining fellowship experience, "limited" credentials procedures (i.e., iliac or renal procedures), and proctored cases to achieve the necessary threshold experience to merit "unrestricted" credentials.

CONCLUSION

The technical skills necessary to perform coronary angioplasty are transferable to the peripheral vasculature. However, an understanding of the natural history of peripheral disease, knowledge of patient and lesion selection criteria, and knowledge of other treatment alternatives are essential elements required to perform these procedures safely and effectively. For interventional cardiologists who are inexperienced in the treatment of peripheral vascular disease, appropriate preparation and training including a team approach that includes an experienced vascular surgeon are both desirable and necessary before attempting percutaneous peripheral angioplasty.

There are inherent advantages for patients when the interventionalist performing the procedure is also the clinician responsible for the pre- and postprocedure care, analogous to the vascular surgeon who cares for patients before and after surgical procedures. Judgments regarding the indications, timing, and risk-to-benefit ratio of procedures are enhanced by a long-term relationship between physician and patient. Finally, in view of the increased incidence of coronary artery disease in patients with atherosclerotic peripheral vascular disease, the participation of a cardiologist in their care is appropriate.

REFERENCES

1. Dzau VJ, Cooke JP. The time has come for vascular medicine. *Ann Intern Med* 1990;112:138–139.
2. Frye RL. Role of the cardiologist in peripheral vascular disease. *J Am Coll Cardiol* 1991;18:641–642.
3. Isner JM, Rosenfeld K. Redefining the treatment of peripheral artery disease. Role of percutaneous revascularization. *Circulation* 1993;88:1534–1557.
4. Criqui MH. Peripheral arterial disease and subsequent cardiovascular mortality: a strong and consistent association. *Circulation* 1990;82:2246–2247.
5. Hertzer NR. The natural history of peripheral vascular disease: implications for its management. *Circulation* 1991;83:I12–I19.
6. Beller GA, Bonow RO, Fuster V, et al. Revised recommendations for training in adult cardiovascular medicine core cardiology training II (COCATS 2) revision of the COCATS training statement. Task force 11: Training in vascular medicine and peripheral catheter-based interventions. *J Am Coll Cardiol* 2002;39:1242–1246.
7. White CJ, Ramee SR, Collins TJ, et al. Initial results of peripheral vascular angioplasty performed by experienced interventional cardiologists. *Am J Cardiol* 1992;69:1249–1250.
8. Levin DC, Becker GJ, Dorros G, et al. Training standards for physicians performing peripheral angioplasty and other percutaneous peripheral vascular interventions. *Circulation* 1992;86:1348–1350.
9. Spies JB, Bakal CW, Burke DR, et al. Guidelines for percutaneous transluminal angioplasty. *Radiology* 1990;177:619–626.
10. Wexler L, Levin D, Dorros G, et al. Training standards for physicians performing peripheral angioplasty: new developments. *Radiology* 1991;178:19–21.
11. Cowley JM, King III SB, Baim D, et al. Guidelines for performance of peripheral percutaneous transluminal angioplasty. *Cathet Cardiovasc Diagn* 1988;21:128–129.
12. Pentecost MJ, Criqui MH, Dorros G, et al. Guidelines for peripheral percutaneous transluminal angioplasty of the abdominal aorta and lower extremity vessels. A statement for health professionals from a special writing group of the Councils on Cardiovascular Radiology, Arteriosclerosis, Cardio-Thoracic and Vascular Surgery, Clinical Cardiology, Epidemiology and Prevention, of the American Heart Association. *Circulation* 1994;89:511–531.
13. Spittell JA, Nanda NC, Creager MA, et al. Recommendations for peripheral transluminal angioplasty: training and facilities. American College of Cardiology Peripheral Vascular Disease Committee. *J Am Coll Cardiol* 1993;21:546–548.
14. Babb JD, Collins TJ, Cowley MJ, et al. Revised guidelines for the performance of peripheral vascular intervention. *Cathet Cardiovasc Interv* 1999;46:21–23.
15. Khosla S, White CJ, Collins TJ, et al. Effects of renal artery stent implantation in patients with renovascular hypertension presenting with unstable angina or congestive heart failure. *Am J Cardiol* 1997;80:363–366.
16. Jean WJ, Al-Bittar I, Xwicke DL, et al. High incidence of renal artery stenosis in patients with coronary artery disease. *Cathet Cardiovasc Diagn* 1994;32:8–10.

CHAPTER 37

Deep Vein Thrombosis

Risks and Management

Alok Maheshwari, Avanti Mehrotra, Richard Henry, George S. Abela,
and Alejandro R. Prieto

Key Points

- Deep vein thrombosis (DVT) is a common disorder commonly associated with disability from postphlebitic syndrome and frequently complicated by pulmonary embolism.
- History and physical examination findings may not always be reliable in the diagnosis of DVT.
- A positive result of D-dimer testing is common, has no diagnostic significance, and always requires confirmatory objective testing.
- In most clinical centers, color-flow Duplex scanning is the imaging test of choice for patients with suspected DVT.
- An etiology for venous thrombosis can now be identified in greater than 60% of patients. The most common cause of inherited thrombophilia is factor V Leiden (activated protein C resistance), which accounts for 40% to 50% of selected cases.
- Approximately 50% of untreated individuals with DVT develop pulmonary embolism within days or weeks of the event. Anticoagulant therapy is the mainstay of therapy for patients with symptomatic proximal DVT.

INTRODUCTION

Deep vein thrombosis (DVT) is an important cause of morbidity and mortality, and its annual incidence in the developing countries is 1 in 1,000 people (1). DVT most commonly affects the lower extremities, although it may also occur in the veins of the arms, cerebral sinus, retina, and mesentery. The importance of DVT as a disease entity stems from the fact that it is commonly associated with disability from postphlebitic syndrome and frequently complicated by pulmonary embolism (PE), which can be fatal in approximately 10% of hospitalized patients.

INITIAL APPROACH

Clinical Diagnosis

Swelling, pain, and discoloration in the involved extremity are the classic symptoms of DVT, although they are often un-

reliable in diagnosis, and a wide differential diagnosis exists for these complaints (Table 37.1). In study of 160 patients with suspected DVT but negative venograms, the causes of leg pain that mimicked DVT were identified as muscle strain, tear, or twisting injury to the leg (40%); swelling in a paralyzed limb (9%); lymphangitis or lymph obstruction (7%); venous insufficiency (7%); popliteal cyst (5%); cellulitis (3%); knee abnormalities (2%); and unknown (26%) (2).

Broadly, the causes of the DVT can be classified into two categories: hereditary and acquired (Table 37.2). History should focus on the known risk factors for DVT, including immobilization or prolonged hospitalization/bed rest, recent surgery, obesity, prior episode(s) of venous thrombosis, lower extremity trauma, malignancy, use of oral contraceptives or hormone replacement therapy, postpartum status, and stroke. A positive family history may suggest the presence of a hereditary defect.

TABLE 37.1. *Mimics of deep vein thrombosis*

Superficial thrombophlebitis
Chronic venous valvular insufficiency
Venous obstruction
Cellulitis
Lymphedema
Popliteal (Baker's) cyst
Internal derangement of the knee
Drug-induced edema
Calf muscle pull or tear
Immobilization
Congestive heart failure
Hyperhomocysteinemia
Antiphospholipid antibody syndrome
Myeloproliferative disorders: polycythemia vera, essential
  thrombocythemia
Paroxysmal nocturnal hemoglobinuria
Inflammatory bowel disease
Nephrotic syndrome
Hypervoscosity: Waldenstrom's macroglobulinemia, multiple
  myeloma
Marked leukocytosis in acute leukemia
Sickle cell anemia

Obstetric history in women of recurrent fetal loss suggests the possible presence of an inherited thrombophilia or antiphospholipid antibodies. History of collagen-vascular disease, myeloproliferative disease, atherosclerotic disease, or nephrotic syndrome and drugs that can induce antiphospholipid antibodies (hydralazine, procainamide, and phenothiazines) may be pertinent in some cases.

Physical Examination

Physical examination findings are often nonspecific. Described signs of ipsilateral edema, warmth, and Homan's sign have been shown to be of little value in diagnosis (3). One must look for possible underlying malignancy, heart failure,

TABLE 37.2. *Causes of deep vein thrombosis*

Inherited
  Factor V Leiden mutation
  Prothrombin gene mutation
  Protein S deficiency
  Protein C deficiency
  Antithrombin deficiency
  Rare: heparin cofactor II deficiency, plasmingen
    deficiency, dysfibrinogenemia, factor XII deficiency,
    increased factor VII coagulant activity
  Congenital venous anomalies
Acquired
  Malignancy: tissue factor, cancer procoagulant
  Surgery, especially orthopedic
  Trauma
  Pregnancy
  Oral contaceptives, hormone replacement therapy,
    tamoxifen

signs of hepatic vein thrombosis, and nephrotic syndrome whenever clinically indicated.

Laboratory Testing

The initial laboratory evaluation should include a complete blood count, coagulation studies (prothrombin time, activated partial thromboplastin time, D-dimer, fibrinogen), serum chemistries including liver and renal function tests, and urinalysis. Prostate-specific antigen measurement may be considered in men over the age of 50 years. However, it is neither warranted nor cost effective to do a routine search for malignancy.

Some simple observations can often provide a clue to the underlying etiology of DVT. Polycythemia vera or essential thrombocythemia may be suspected if there are elevations in the hematocrit or platelet count. Secondary polycythemia or secondary (reactive) thrombocytosis may point toward an occult neoplasm. A leukoerythroblastic picture with nucleated red blood cells and immature white cells suggests the possibility of bone marrow involvement by myeloproliferative disorder or a tumor. The development of thrombocytopenia and thrombosis in patients on heparin therapy should prompt a consideration of heparin-induced thrombocytopenia. Antiphospholipid antibody syndrome may be suggested by an otherwise unexplained prolongation of the activated partial thromboplastin time that does not correct on 1:1 dilution with normal plasma.

DIAGNOSIS OF DEEP VEIN THROMBOSIS

Table 37.3 lists the tests for diagnosing DVT. We discuss these in turn.

D-Dimer Test

D-dimer is a specific degradation product of cross-linked fibrin (4–7). Because concurrent production and breakdown of clot characterizes thrombosis, patients with thromboembolic disease have elevated levels of D-dimer. The two older tests for measuring D-dimer are the enzyme-linked immunoabsorbent assay (ELISA) and a rapid, but less sensitive, latex agglutination. These tests have a low specificity of 15% to 38% in DVT and PE. The most useful assay is the whole-blood agglutination test (SimpliRED) (8,9). This is a 10-minute bedside test that is both rapid and sensitive. Studies

TABLE 37.3. *Tests for the diagnosis of deep vein thrombosis*

D-dimer test
Contrast venography
Venous ultrasonography (duplex scan or compression
  ultrasonography)
Plethysmography
Magnetic resonance imaging

TABLE 37.4. *False-positive D-dimers*

Recent surgery or trauma
Recent myocardial infarction or stroke
Disseminated intravascular coagulation
Pregnancy or recent delivery
Infection
Active collagen vascular disease
Metastatic cancer

have shown it has a sensitivity of 93% for proximal DVT and 70% for calf DVT, and an overall specificity of 77%. All D-dimer tests are more sensitive for proximal than distal clot, and may miss up to 30% of calf DVTs. False-positive D-dimers can occur in certain patient populations (Table 37.4).

D-dimer levels below 500 ng per mL by ELISA or a negative SimpliRED assay in conjunction with a low clinical probability or other negative noninvasive tests may be useful in excluding DVT (10). However, a negative D-dimer assay may be insufficient as a stand-alone test in patient populations with a moderate or high clinical suspicion of venous thromboembolism. D-dimer is of no use for patients developing suspected DVT/PE during their hospitalization, and therefore the test should not be requested for inpatients. D-dimer is of no use in patients already on warfarin, heparin, or low-molecular weight heparin (LMWH). In pregnant women, D-dimer is of questionable value, and it has been recommended that it not be used to make diagnosis of DVT/PE. All patients with suspected recurrent DVT should have pretest probability assessment, D-dimer assay, *and* imaging study. DVT can be ruled out only if the imaging study is unequivocally normal and the D-dimer test is negative. The D-dimer test should be requested and used only in conjunction with pretest probability scoring for outpatients presenting with symptoms or signs of DVT. A positive result of D-dimer testing is common, has no diagnostic significance, and always requires confirmatory objective testing.

Venography

Venography is the gold standard modality for the diagnosis of DVT (11). However, this is an invasive test and is not always technically possible, and there is a risk of side effects including phlebitis in 2% to 5% of patients and a risk of allergic reactions (12). For this reason, ultrasound has supplanted venography for the initial evaluation of the patient with suspected DVT. If the ultrasound is equivocal or unavailable, venography may be useful. Venography is also useful if the patient has a high clinical probability of thrombosis and a negative ultrasound, and it is also valuable in symptomatic patients with a history of prior thrombosis in whom the ultrasound is nondiagnostic. In these patients, it usually can distinguish between acute events and chronic changes seen on ultrasound. A contrast study can delineate occlusion, recanalization, and collateral channels.

Duplex Ultrasonography

In most clinical centers, color-flow duplex scanning is the imaging test of choice for patients with suspected DVT (Fig 37.1). This test is inexpensive, noninvasive, and widely available. In several studies that have compared it against venography, the average sensitivity and specificity for the diagnosis of proximal DVT is 97% (13). However, its sensitivity for the diagnosis of calf vein DVT is as low as 75% (13) see Chapter 15.

The three techniques used are compression ultrasonography, duplex ultrasonography, and color flow duplex imaging, often in conjunction with each other. Noncompressibility of the vascular lumen under gentle ultrasound probe pressure is the simplest criterion for diagnosing DVT. The B-mode, or two-dimensional ultrasound, provides a two-dimensional image of the vein and surrounding structures. The pulsed Doppler is used to evaluate the blood flow characteristics. In a normal vein, the blood flow is spontaneous and phasic with respiration and can be augmented with distal compression. The flow is described as continuous when there is loss of phasic pattern, and this indicates venous outflow obstruction. In color flow sonography, pulsed Doppler signals are used to produce images, which can easily identify veins. In addition, the sonographer can distinguish a fresh clot from an old clot based on echogenicity, homogeneity, and collateral flow. Ultrasound can also distinguish other causes of leg swelling, such as tumor, popliteal cyst, abscess, aneurysm, and hematoma.

However, ultrasound does have its clinical limitations. High-sensitivity testing requires sophisticated diagnostic equipment. Scans are very reader dependent, and duplex scanning is less sensitive for clots below the knee. Suprainguinal veins are also hard to visualize. Duplex scans are less likely to detect nonoccluding thrombi. During the second half of pregnancy, ultrasound becomes less specific because the gravid uterus compresses the inferior vena cava, thereby changing Doppler flow in the lower extremities. However, an experienced sonographer may still detect a clot in a pregnant patient by demonstrating a noncompressible vein.

Plethysmography

Plethysmography measures change in lower extremity volume in response to certain stimuli. By using a tourniquet and respiratory variation, the operator can detect changes in leg volume as a function of venous outflow. Changes in such objective variables as calf circumference, cutaneous blood flow, and electrical resistance occur when there is obstruction of venous return. Photoplethysmography is based on the absorption of light by the hemoglobin in the red blood cells (14). Strain gauge plethysmography is based on the measurement of changes in the calf dimensions when the venous outflow is occluded by the inflation of the thigh cuff (15). Impedance plethysmography (IPG) is based on changes in electrical resistance, and is the most widely used and accurate form of

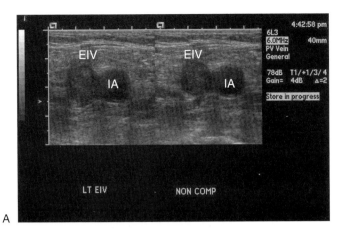

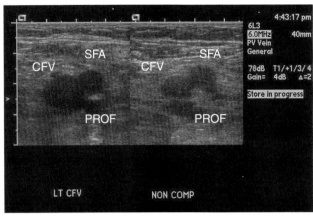

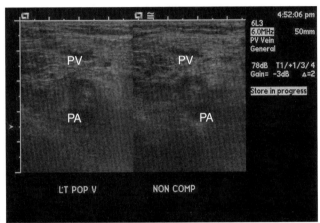

FIG. 37.1. Use of compression ultrasound to demonstrate thrombus in the venous system of a patient with deep venous thrombosis. In each figure, the left images are a normal ultrasound examination. The artery is seen pulsating during the examination, but typically the vein is larger than the artery. In each figure, the right images show that in the presence of thrombus, the vein is not compressible. **A, Left:** External iliac vein (EIV) with thrombus (Thr) in the lumen of the vein (transverse view) visualized at baseline ultrasonography. **Right:** Same images demonstrating lack of vein compression. **B, Left:** Common femoral vein (CFV) and adjacent superficial femoral artery (SFA) above and profunda (PROF) below. **Right:** Same images demonstrating lack of vein compression. **C, Left:** Popliteal vein (PV) is superior to the popliteal artery (PA). **Right:** Same images demonstrating lack of vein compression. (Courtesy of Dr. James Zito, Thoracic Cardiovascular Institute, Lansing, MI.)

plethysmography. IPG is very operator dependent, and early literature displayed a 95% correlation with venography for proximal DVT. However, recent literature shows that the sensitivity of IPG is generally around 65% to 70% (13). Because any impairment of venous outflow affects plethysmography results, many false positives occur (Table 37.5).

Magnetic Resonance Imaging

Magnetic resonance venography represents a significant advance in the diagnosis of DVT. It detects leg, pelvis, and pulmonary thrombi, and is more than 95% sensitive and specific for DVT (16–19). It distinguishes a mature from an immature clot. Because it is expensive and requires significant patient cooperation, it should not replace ultrasound as the primary screening tool. It is most useful in the second and third trimester of pregnancy, when ultrasound becomes less accurate. It is safe in all stages of pregnancy.

TABLE 37.5. *Plethysmography false positives*

Postphlebitic syndrome
Abdominal tumors
Pregnancy
Congestive heart failure

The diagnosis of DVT is established in patients with a first episode of DVT with a positive noninvasive study, with positive predictive values for compression ultrasonography and impedance plethysmography of 94% (95% confidence interval: 87% to 98%) and 83% (95% confidence interval: 75% to 90%), respectively. A repeat study should be obtained on days 5 to 7 if the initial study is negative and the clinical suspicion is high (20). Venography is used only when the results are equivocal or noninvasive testing is not clinically feasible.

SCREENING FOR A HYPERCOAGULABLE STATE

An etiology for venous thrombosis can now be identified in greater than 60% of patients. Inherited thrombophilia is a genetic predisposition to the development of venous thromboembolism. The most common cause of inherited thrombophilia is factor V Leiden (activated protein C resistance), which accounts for 40% to 50% of selected cases (i.e., thrombosis at less than 45 years of age, a positive family history of venous thrombosis, or recurrent thrombosis). The second-most-common cause is the prothrombin gene mutation and deficiencies in protein S, protein C, and antithrombin; rarely, some dysfibrinogenemias account for the remaining cases (21,22). Furthermore, more than one factor is often at play in a given patient. A thrombophilic state leading to venous thrombosis can be inherited or acquired, and there is no clear consensus regarding screening for these conditions. Clinically, however, it may be prudent to screen the patients who develop venous thrombosis without an immediately identified risk factor, particularly if they are younger, have recurrent thrombosis, or have a family history of venous thromboembolism. Other important clinical scenarios that may increase the yield of this screening are DVT with oral contraceptive use or pregnancy, thrombosis in unusual vascular beds such as portal, hepatic, mesenteric, or cerebral veins, a history of warfarin-induced skin necrosis, and unprovoked upper extremity venous thrombosis.

The timing of testing is an important consideration in the laboratory evaluation of factor V Leiden, antithrombin, protein C, or protein S deficiency. Acute thrombosis, comorbid illness, and anticoagulant therapy influence the concentrations of these plasma proteins, and potentially erroneous diagnoses can be made. Testing is usually recommended for these deficiency states at least 2 weeks after completing the initial 3- to 6-month course of oral anticoagulant therapy following a thrombotic event. However, a deficiency of these proteins is essentially excluded if the plasma levels of antithrombin, protein C, and protein S are normal at presentation. A low concentration, on the contrary, must be confirmed by repeat testing after anticoagulation is discontinued. The second-generation assay for activated protein C resistance, methods to detect the prothrombin gene mutation, and assays for antiphospholipid antibodies or homocysteine are not affected by anticoagulation.

UPPER EXTREMITY DEEP VEIN THROMBOSIS

DVT of the upper extremities has become increasingly common secondary to an increased number of patients on prolonged central venous access. The conditions that are associated with an increased risk for upper extremity DVT are shown in Table 37.6. Upper extremity DVT has been shown to have a rate of PE approaching that in the lower extremity DVT in recent studies (23). Long-term effects include a severe postphlebitic syndrome in the upper extremity, and a functional disability in the affected extremity in 25% to 40% of patients with untreated subclavian–axillary vein thrombosis (24).

Imaging modalities, including duplex sonography (somewhat limited in the central innominate and superior vena cava segments), venography, contrast-enhanced computed tomography scanning, and magnetic resonance venography, often in combination with cross-sectional magnetic resonance imaging, can be used to establish the diagnosis.

As in lower extremity DVT, anticoagulation is the mainstay of therapy. However, in the presence of symptomatic acute severe thrombosis, thrombolytic therapy is a useful approach (25). The preferred means of thrombolysis in this setting is catheter-directed infusion directly in the proximity of the thrombosis. Urokinase was used most frequently in the past, but alteplase and reteplase are the preferred thrombolytics. The results with catheter-based thrombolysis are very impressive, and in as many as 72% to 88% of cases, there is a near complete resolution of the thrombus (25). The major determinant of the success of this therapy is the chronicity of the thrombosis.

Definitive management of patients with underlying anatomic abnormalities can be undertaken after the acute thrombus is resolved. This is often dictated by factors such as etiology, presence of malignancy, and other patient-specific factors. Patients with primary subclavian axillary vein thrombosis resulting from extrinsic compression at the thoracic outlet are treated with surgical decompression after the initial thrombolytic and anticoagulation therapy. Secondary causes of central venous obstruction and thrombosis can be treated with balloon angioplasty and stent implantation.

TREATMENT OF DEEP VEIN THROMBOSIS

The goals of DVT treatment are to prevent acute complications such as thrombosis extension, recurrence, and pulmonary embolism, as well as to prevent late complications, including postphlebitic syndrome and chronic thromboembolic pulmonary hypertension. Approximately 50% of untreated individuals develop pulmonary embolism within days or weeks of the event. Anticoagulant therapy is the mainstay of therapy for patients with symptomatic proximal DVT.

Elastic compression stockings should be used in DVT and may reduce the rate of postthrombotic syndrome, as shown in one study of 194 patients, where the use of graded compression stockings reduced the rate of postthrombotic syndrome by 50% (26).

The following general recommendations for the treatment of acute DVT are based on the Sixth ACCP Consensus Conference on Antithrombotic Therapy (27,28) and those of the American Heart Association/American College of Cardiology (29).

The acute treatment of patients with DVT is with subcutaneous low-molecular weight heparin (LMWH), or

TABLE 37.6. *Conditions associated with increased risk for upper extremity deep vein thrombosis*

Extrinsic subclavian vein compression as in thoracic outlet syndrome
Acquired scarring or compression in the central venous system: multiple central venous caths, ipsilateral arteriovenous fistula, thoracic adenopathy and/or malignancy, fibrosing mediastinitis
Chronically indwelling central lines or pacemaker/defibrillator leads
Recent chest or neck surgery
First rib and clavicle fracture
Hypercoagulable states and vasculitides

Adapted from Sharafuddin MJ, Sun S, Hoballah JJ. Endovascular management of venous thrombotic diseases of the upper torso and extremities. *J Vasc Interv Radiol* 2002;13: 975–990; with permission.

unfractionated heparin given either intravenously or as a weight-adjusted subcutaneous dose.

LMWH dosing is individualized for each patient. LMWH offers a more consistent and predictable anticoagulant response and is administered subcutaneously without the need to monitor activated partial thromboplastin time (aPTT). It is at least as effective as unfractionated heparin, and reduces the incidence of major bleeding during initial treatment and overall mortality at follow-up (30). The advent of LMWH has made the outpatient treatment of DVT possible. Trials of home treatment with LMWH have shown that it is cost effective, preferred by patients, and does not result in more complications when compared with the inpatient treatment in the initial phase of DVT (31).

Unfractionated heparin dose should be adjusted to prolong aPTT to 1.5 to 2.5 times the mean of the control value, or the upper limit of the normal aPTT range. It has been shown that weight-based nomograms are a safe and cost effective strategy for unfractionated heparin dosing. In general, the treatment with LMWH or heparin should continue for at least 5 days, and oral anticoagulation should overlap with LMW heparin or unfractionated heparin for 4 to 5 days. Warfarin can usually be initiated at the same time as heparin, at an initial dose of 5 to 10 mg. Heparin can be discontinued on day 5 or 6 if therapeutic international normalized ratio (INR) has been obtained for 2 consecutive days.

Platelet count should be done on days 3 to 5 of therapy to monitor for heparin-induced thrombocytopenia. In the event of continuation of heparin, another platelet count should be done on days 7 to 10, and another one at day 14. Heparin should be discontinued if there is a rapid or sustained decrease in the platelet count, or a platelet count of less than 100,000 per μL.

Oral anticoagulation with warfarin should target at an INR of 2.5 (range 2.0 to 3.0). Long-term therapy with either LMWH or adjusted-dose unfractionated heparin may be used if there is a contraindication to oral anticoagulants.

Thrombolytic agents are controversial in the management of DVT. They are best used in patients with pulmonary embolism and hemodynamic instability or those with massive iliofemoral thrombosis.

Inferior vena caval (IVC) filters (32) are indicated in individuals with a contraindication to the use of anticoagulant therapy or a significant complication with its use, or those with a recurrent thromboembolic event despite adequate anticoagulation. Some of the relative indications for IVC filters are (a) large, free-floating iliocaval thrombus; (b) chronic thromboembolic disease (undergoing pulmonary embolectomy); (c) thromboembolic disease with limited cardiopulmonary reserve; (d) poor compliance; (e) prophylactic (e.g., massive trauma, history of thromboembolism with upcoming surgery); (f) DVT thrombolysis; and (g) renal cell cancer with renal vein or IVC involvement. Complete IVC thrombosis or an inability to gain access to IVC are the only absolute contraindications of IVC filter placement. Several different filters are available, and there are no direct prospective comparative

studies between these filters to allow comment on their relative efficacy. In a recent review of the various studies on IVC filters (32), the authors concluded that these filters are easy and safe to insert, and appear to be effective in the short-term and, likely, the long-term recurrences of pulmonary embolism. However, they may result in IVC thromboses and a higher incidence of recurrent lower extremity DVT than anticoagulation alone.

The duration of treatment with DVT is at least 3 months with a first thromboembolic event with an identifiable reversible risk factor, whereas a minimum of 6 months of treatment should be offered in an idiopathic first event. Patients with recurrent idiopathic DVT or those with an ongoing risk factor (e.g., malignancy, anticardiolipin antibody syndrome) should receive treatment for 12 months or longer.

Alternatives to Low-Molecular Weight Heparin and Heparins

In the last decade, several new anticoagulants have been developed (Table 37.7) (33). These agents specifically target individual components of the coagulation pathway, which offers a theoretical advantage over the heparins and LMWHs, which act at multiple targets. Many of these agents have several different attractive properties, including improved pharmacodynamics, total chemical synthesis, once-daily dosing, no need for monitoring, and oral administration.

DEEP VEIN THROMBOSIS PROPHYLAXIS

DVT prophylaxis is the ideal method of preventing the complication of pulmonary embolism in the hospital setting. The need for DVT prophylaxis will depend on the patient's clinical condition, the contemplated surgical procedure, and the presence of known risk factors for DVT. High-risk surgical procedures include extensive pelvic or abdominal surgery for malignant disease, major orthopedic surgery on lower limbs, and general surgery in patients older than 40 years with recent history of DVT or PE (34). These patients must receive DVT prophylaxis consisting of a combination of graduated compression stockings and low-dose unfractionated heparin or LMWH. In lower-risk patients where DVT may still be a concern, such as in elderly patients admitted for stroke, malignancy, or cardiac disease, and lower-risk general surgical procedures, DVT prophylaxis may comprise either one of the aforementioned prophylactic approaches.

Prophylaxis for DVT should be started before the surgery and be continued until the patient is fully ambulatory. For total knee or hip replacement, a minimum of 7 to 10 days of therapy is recommended (35). Studies have shown the need to continue DVT prophylaxis for 28 to 42 days after total hip replacement, although the data on total knee replacement beyond 10 days are not as convincing (36). Enoxaparin given for 4 weeks has also been shown to be superior to that for 1 week in patients undergoing major abdominal or pelvic cancer surgery (37). Acute spinal cord injury with

TABLE 37.7. *Newer anticoagulants[a]*

Drug	Indication/study area	Comments
Direct thrombin inhibitors		
Lepirudin	HITTS	Recombinant hirudin
Argatroban	HITTS	Small synthetic arginine analogue
Bivalirudin	Acute coronary syndrome for percutaneous intervention	Semisynthetic, previously known as Hirulog
Ximelagatran	VTE, chronic atrial fibrillation	Oral prodrug in phase 3 trials, metabolizes to melagatran
Factor Xa inhibitors		
Fondaparinux	VTE prevention in hip replacement, and major hip and knee surgery	Synthetic pentasaccharide
Danaparoid sodium	VTE prevention in hip replacement	Predominant factor Xa inhibitor
Tissue factor VIIa inhibitors		
Nematode anticoagulant peptide c2	VTE	Given subcutaneously every 2 days, in phase 3 trials
Tissue factor pathway inhibitor	Severe sepsis	Phase 3 trials
Oral heparin		
SNAC/heparin	VTE	Rapid clearance, phase 3 trials
Factors Va and VIIIa cleavage		
Activated protein C	Severe sepsis	

[a]HITTS, Heparin-induced thrombocytopenia thrombosis syndrome; VTE, venous thromboembolism, SNAC, sodium-N-[8(2-hydroxylbenzoyl)amino]caprylate.

Adapted from Hyers TM. Management of venous thromboembolism: past, present, and future. *Arch Intern Med* 2003;163:759–768, with permission.

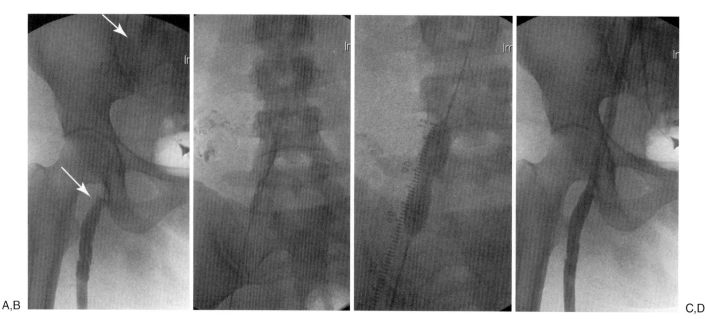

A,B   C,D

FIG. 37.2. Angiogram demonstrating complete thrombotic occlusion of the right common iliac vein (CIV) in a patient with May–Thurner syndrome. After local thrombolysis therapy and stenting of the right CIV, there was complete restoration venous patency. **A:** Total thrombotic occlusion of the right CIV (*arrows*). **B:** Catheter crossing the thrombotic occlusion for lytic treatment. **C:** Balloon inflation and stent placement at the site of vein compression. **D:** Widely patent CIV following thrombolysis and stenting. (Courtesy of Dr. Michael Ouimette, Sparrow Hospital, Lansing, MI.)

paralysis is also a high-risk situation, and LMWH is most effective in this condition. In general medical patients, there is no convincing evidence of decrease in mortality with DVT prophylaxis, although it is often recommended for high-risk medical patients, including those with congestive heart failure, pulmonary infections, ischemic strokes, and lower limb paresis.

Ximelagetran, an oral direct thrombin inhibitor, does not require monitoring of coagulation levels or dose adjustment, and was recently shown to be superior to warfarin for prevention of venous thromboembolism in patients admitted for total hip replacement. Several studies are being performed to confirm the effectiveness of ximelagetran in this setting as well as for the treatment of DVT (38).

DEEP VEIN THROMBOSIS THROMBOLYTIC THERAPY

Catheter-based thrombolytic therapy has been an emerging treatment for DVT. This treatment option provides more complete and rapid dissolution of thrombus than to heparin-based therapy and less bleeding complications than systemic thrombolytics due to a reduced dose. Bleeding, however, remains a concern, and this has limited the use of this therapy to patients with either multilevel DVT or cases of massive DVT (phlegmasia cerulea dolens), particularly in young individuals, who are at higher risk for morbidity from lifelong chronic venous insufficiency (39,40). Figure 37.2 demonstrates the combined use of thrombolytic therapy with stenting of the common iliac vein in a patient with May–Thurner syndrome. The common iliac vein is compressed by the iliac artery, leading to obstruction of venous flow and thrombosis (41,42). In this case, lysis and stenting were used to reestablish venous flow in a situation that would have otherwise required extensive vascular surgery.

REFERENCES

1. Carter CJ. Epidemiology of venous thromboembolism. In: Hull RD, Pineo GF, eds. *Disorders of thrombosis.* Philadelphia: WB Saunders, 1996:159–174.
2. Hull RD, Hirsh J, Sackett DL, et al. Clinical validity of a negative venogram in patients with clinically suspected venous thrombosis. *Circulation* 1981;64:622–625.
3. Ebell MH. Evaluation of the patient with suspected deep vein thrombosis. *J Fam Pract* 2001;50:167–171.
4. Aschwanden M, Labs KH, Jeanneret C, et al. The value of rapid D-dimer testing combined with structured clinical evaluation for the diagnosis of deep vein thrombosis. *J Vasc Surg* 1999;30:929–935.
5. Kearon C, Ginsberg JS, Douketis J, et al. Management of suspected deep venous thrombosis in outpatients by using clinical assessment and D-dimer testing. *Ann Intern Med* 2001;135:108–111.
6. Ginsberg JS, Kearon C, Douketis J, et al. The use of D-dimer testing and impedance plethysmographic examination in patients with clinical indications of deep vein thrombosis. *Arch Intern Med* 1997;157:1077–1081.
7. Kelly J, Rudd A, Lewis RR, et al. Plasma D-dimers in the diagnosis of venous thromboembolism. *Arch Intern Med* 2002;162:747–756.
8. Pittet JL, de Moerloose P, Reber G, et al. VIDAS D-dimer: fast quantitative ELISA for measuring D-dimer in plasma. *Clin Chem* 1996;42:410–415.
9. Wells PS, Brill-Edwards P, Stevens P, et al. A novel and rapid whole-blood assay for D-dimer in patients with clinically suspected deep vein thrombosis. *Circulation* 1995;91:2184–2187.
10. Bounameaux H, de Moerloose P, Perrier A, et al. Plasma measurement of D-dimer as diagnostic aid in suspected venous thromboembolism: an overview. *Thromb Haemost* 1994;71:1–6.
11. Lensing AW, Buller HR, Prandoni P, et al. Contrast venography, the gold standard for the diagnosis of deep-vein thrombosis: improvement in observer agreement. *Thromb Haemost* 1992;67:8–12.
12. Heijboer H, Cogo A, Buller HR, et al. Detection of deep vein thrombosis with impedance plethysmography and real-time compression ultrasonography in hospitalized patients. *Arch Intern Med* 1992;152:1901–1903.
13. Tovey C, Wyatt S. Diagnosis, investigation, and management of deep vein thrombosis. *BMJ* 2003;326:1180–1184.
14. Tan YK, daSilva AF. Digital photoplethysmography in the diagnosis of suspected lower limb DVT: is it useful? *Eur J Vasc Endovasc Surg* 1999;18:71–79.
15. Maskell NA, Cooke S, Meecham Jones DJ, et al. The use of automated strain gauge plethysmography in the diagnosis of deep vein thrombosis. *Br J Radiol* 2002;75:648–651.
16. Carpenter JP, Holland GA, Baum RA, et al. Magnetic resonance venography for the detection of deep venous thrombosis: comparison with contrast venography and duplex Doppler ultrasonography. *J Vasc Surg* 1993;18:734–741.
17. Moody AR, Pollock JG, O'Connor AR, et al. Lower-limb deep venous thrombosis: direct MR imaging of the thrombus. *Radiology* 1998;209:349–355.
18. Fraser DG, Moody AR, Morgan PS, et al. Diagnosis of lower-limb deep venous thrombosis: a prospective blinded study of magnetic resonance direct thrombus imaging. *Ann Intern Med* 2002;136:89–98.
19. Fraser DG, Moody AR, Davidson IR, et al. Deep venous thrombosis: diagnosis by using venous enhanced subtracted peak arterial MR venography versus conventional venography. *Radiology* 2003;226:812–820.
20. Birdwell BG, Raskob GE, Whitsett TL, et al. Clinical validity of normal compression ultrasonography in outpatients suspected of having deep vein thrombosis. *Ann Intern Med* 1998;128:1–7.
21. Mateo J, Oliver A, Borrell M, et al. Laboratory evaluation and clinical characteristics of 2,132 consecutive unselected patients with venous thromboembolism—results of the Spanish Multicentric Study on Thrombophilia (EMET-Study). *Thromb Haemost* 1997;77:444–451.
22. Margaglione M, Brancaccio V, Giuliani N, et al. Increased risk for venous thrombosis in carriers of the prothrombin G G20210A gene variant. *Ann Intern Med* 1998;129:89–93.
23. Hingorani A, Ascher E, Lorenson E, et al. Upper extremity deep venous thrombosis and its impact on morbidity and mortality rates in a hospital-based population. *J Vasc Surg* 1997;26:853–860.
24. Ellis MH, Manor Y, Witz M. Risk factors and management of patients with upper limb deep vein thrombosis. *Chest* 2000;117:43–46.
25. Sharafuddin MJ, Sun S, Hoballah JJ. Endovascular management of venous thrombotic diseases of the upper torso and extremities. *J Vasc Interv Radiol* 2002;13:975–990.
26. Brandjes DP, Buller HR, Heijboer H, et al. Randomised trial of effect of compression stockings in patients with symptomatic proximal-vein thrombosis. *Lancet* 1997;349:759–762.
27. Hyers TM, Agnelli G, Hull RD, et al. Antithrombotic therapy for venous thromboembolic disease. *Chest* 2001;119(1 suppl):176S–193S.
28. Hirsh J, Lee AY. How we diagnose and treat deep vein thrombosis. *Blood* 2002;99:3102–3110.
29. Hirsh J, Fuster V, Ansell J, et al. American Heart Association/American College of Cardiology Foundation guide to warfarin therapy. *J Am Coll Cardiol* 2003;41:1633–1652.
30. Van den Belt AGM, Prins MH, Lensing AWA, et al. Fixed dose subcutaneous low molecular weight heparins versus adjusted dose unfractionated heparin for venous hromboembolism. In: *Cochrane Library, Issue 1.* Oxford: Update Software, 2002.
31. Schraibman IG, Milne AA, Royle EM. Home versus in-patient treatment for deep vein thrombosis. *Cochrane Library, Issue 1.* Oxford: Update Software, 2002.
32. Kinney TB. Update on inferior vena cava filters. *J Vasc Interv Radiol* 2003;14:425–440.
33. Hyers TM. Management of venous thromboembolism: past, present, and future. *Arch Intern Med* 2003;163:759–768.
34. Hirsh J, Crowther MA. Venous thromboembolism. In: Hoffman R,

Benz Jr EJ, Shattil SJ, et al., eds. *Hematology. Basic principles and practice,* 3rd ed. Philadelphia: Churchill Livingston, 2000:2074–2087.

35. Geerts WH, Heit JA, Clagett GP, et al. Prevention of thromboembolism. *Chest* 2001;119(1 suppl):132S–175S.

36. Eikelboom J, Quinlan DJ, Douketis JD. Extended-duration prophylaxis against venous thromboembolism after total hip or knee replacement: a meta-analysis of the randomized trials. *Lancet* 2001;258(9275):105–109.

37. Bergqvist D, Agnelli G, Cohen AT, et al. The ENOXACAN II Investigators. Duration of prophylaxis against venous thromboembolism with enoxaparin after surgery for cancer. *N Engl J Med* 2002;346:975–980.

38. Francis CW, Berkowitz SD, Comp PC, et al. Comparison of ximelagatran with warfarin for the prevention of venous thromboembolism after total knee replacement. *N Engl J Med* 2003:349:1762–1764.

39. Sharafuddin MJ, Sun S, Hoballah JJ, et al. Endovascular management of venous thrombotic and occlusive disease of the lower extremities. *J Vasc Interv Radiol* 2003;14:405–423.

40. Forster AJ, Wells PS. The rationale and evidence for the treatment of lower-extremity deep venous thrombosis with thrombolytic agents. *Curr Opin Hematol* 2002;9:437–442.

41. Patel NH, Stookey KR, Ketcahm DB, et al. Endovascular management of acute extensive iliofemoral deep venous thrombosis caused by May–Thurner syndrome. *J Vasc Interv Radiol* 2000;11:1297–1302.

42. Lamont JP, Pearl GP, Patetsios P, et al. Prospective evaluation of endoluminal venous stents in the treatment of the May–Thruner syndrome. *Ann Vasc Surg* 2002;16:61–64.

CHAPTER 38

Pulmonary Embolism

Diagnosis and Treatment

Alejandro R. Prieto and John Penner

Key Points

- Pulmonary embolism (PE) is the third-leading cause of mortality in the United States and also may lead to long-term complications.
- Venous thrombi often are formed in patients who have a contributing genetic predisposition.
- Large emboli may lodge and attach to the larger veins as well as the right cardiac chambers.
- The clinical presentation of a PE usually varies depending on the size and the type of embolus present.
- Chest x-ray, electrocardiography, blood gases, laboratory markers, echocardiography, ventilation–perfusion scan, spiral computed tomography, and angiography are useful techniques in the diagnosis of PE.
- Anticoagulant therapy is the mainstay in the management of PE.
- Heparin therapy is used in acute PE to inhibit thrombus propagation and prevent recurrent emboli.
- Traditionally given only in cases of massive PE, thrombolytic therapy may also benefit patients with echocardiographic evidence of thrombus or right ventricular dysfunction.
- Embolectomy is a rapidly evolving treatment option.

INTRODUCTION

Pulmonary embolism (PE) is the third-most-common cause of death in the United States, and is the sole or major contributing cause of acute hospital deaths in about 10% of adults (1). Although it is a condition often addressed primarily by internists and pulmonary specialists, it is intimately linked to the cardiovascular specialty, essentially representing a disorder of the peripheral vascular system. By reason of its presenting symptoms, which include chest discomfort, shortness of breath, and light-headedness, is often confused with other cardiovascular disease entities (2). The hemodynamic complications of PE including right ventricular failure are most appropriately managed by cardiologists. Furthermore, cardiologists are well acquainted with the variety of treatment options, including thrombolytic therapy, and are most apt to properly evaluate echocardiograms, which recently have been an indispensable component in the risk stratification of patients with PE.

The presenting symptoms of PE are nonspecific, and therefore its diagnosis requires a high index of suspicion. Most deaths from PE are not due to a therapeutic failure, but rather from a prophylactic oversight or diagnostic error. A deep vein thrombosis (DVT) is the most common source of pulmonary embolism, and symptoms of DVT always should be sought in a patient suspected of having PE. However, two-thirds of patients with proven PE do not have symptoms of DVT, and conversely, half of patients with proven DVT and

461

without symptoms of PE have undiagnosed pulmonary emboli of significant size (1,3). Because clinical judgment is not consistently reliable, specific diagnostic tests are essential and must be instituted early when PE is suspected.

Anticoagulant therapy is the mainstay for the management of PE, and it must be administered early in order to be effective. Delaying therapeutic anticoagulation for only 24 hours increases the risk of recurrent embolism from 4% to 23%, with a fivefold increase in the likelihood of death within 1 year (1,4). The use of thrombolytic agents in acute pulmonary embolism remains controversial. Thrombolytics, however, are indicated in the presence of hemodynamic collapse, right ventricular dysfunction, or echocardiographic evidence of mobile cardiac thrombi in transit.

PATHOPHYSIOLOGY

In more than 95% of instances, venous emboli originate where deep leg vein thrombi have been identified above the level of the knee (5). Other less common sources of venous emboli include the axillosubclavian vein, the right heart chambers, and the pulmonary artery itself. Above-the-knee thrombi usually originate from propagating calf vein thrombi. However, they also may form *de novo,* particularly in cases of hip or pelvic trauma. Below-the-knee thrombi by themselves infrequently are associated with embolism unless they extend proximally to the popliteal veins or above.

Venous thrombi often are formed in patients who have a contributing genetic predisposition. Such hypercoagulable states (Table 38.1) result from genetic mutations, which lead to quantitative or qualitative defects, reducing the effectiveness of several of the naturally occurring anticoagulants (anti-thrombin III, protein C, protein S) (6). The factor V

TABLE 38.1. *Risk factors for thromboembolism*

Inherited
  Prothrombin 20210A mutation
  Factor V Leiden mutation (activated protein C resistance)
  Antithrombin III deficiency
  Protein C and protein S
  Familial plasminogen deficiency
  Hyperhomocysteinemia (may be acquired)
Acquired
  Surgery (knee, hip, and major or prolonged surgery)
  Trauma (major trauma and hip fracture)
  Advanced age
  Obesity
  Immobilization
  Oral contraceptives/pregnancy and the postpartum period
  Cerobrovascular accident and spinal cord injury
  Malignancy
  Congestive heart failure
  Prior venous thromboembolism
  Antiphospholipid antibodies (anticardiolipin antibodies and lupus anticoagulant)
  Indwelling venous infusion catheters and venous pacemakers
  Initial days of warfarin therapy

Leiden and the prothrombin G20210A mutation are unique because they are not true genetic defects; rather, they exhibit nucleotide substitutions that permit an escape from their natural inhibitors, thus promoting coagulation processes. These latter mutations are common in the general populations of white descent, and are associated with a moderate, but increased risk for venous thromboembolism (7). A precipitating environmental stress usually is necessary to initiate a thrombotic event when patients carry these mutations. Such acquired risk factors include obesity, oral contraceptive use, pregnancy, malignancy, acute ischemic stroke, spinal cord injury and an indwelling central venous catheter (2). Commonly, in a person with an existing congenital hypercoagulable state, the presence of an acquired risk factor will increase the inherent predisposition for venous thromboembolism.

Once deep vein thrombosis occurs, a portion or all of the thrombus can detach as an embolus and flow through the venous system toward the pulmonary arterial circulation, the first significant barrier to the forward flow of the emboli (4). A large embolus, however, may lodge and attach to the larger veins as well as the right cardiac chambers. A smaller embolus may then dislodge from these sites in a similar manner to initiate a PE.

When an embolus occludes one or more of the major pulmonary vessels, numerous pathophysiological effects occur. A physiological alveolar dead space may be created if there is a total obstruction of the pulmonary vasculature, resulting in compensatory hyperventilation manifested clinically by dyspnea and tachypnea. Through various mechanisms, pulmonary vascular resistance increases, which leads to a rise in pulmonary arterial and right ventricular pressure. If an embolus is large enough to occlude flow into an area that is served by at least two lobar arteries (massive PE), right-sided failure and hemodynamic collapse may ensue (1). The presence of a preexisting cardiopulmonary condition such as heart failure or chronic obstructive pulmonary disease (COPD) may exaggerate the hemodynamic effects of a smaller pulmonary vascular obstruction (4).

Finally, there are various degrees of ventilation–perfusion mismatching due to misdistribution of blood flow in the pulmonary circulation. This creates a pseudoshunt in areas with normal or unobstructed flow wherein a large portion of blood passes through the pulmonary vascular bed in a very rapid manner, allowing less time for alveolar gas equilibration. Several other proposed mechanisms are involved, but the ones just discussed explain most of the respiratory abnormalities encountered with PE (1).

The clinical sequelea of small acute emboli in the pulmonary artery, as in deep vein thrombosis, is complete loss of function if anatomic resolution is not accomplished either by lyses or organization (4). In cases of a larger or recurrent embolus, however, recanalization of the affected artery may not be complete, and gas exchange will remain impaired. Pulmonary vascular resistance also will continue to be elevated due to a reduction in the distensibility of the recanalized vessel. If the obstruction persists, chronic cor pulmonale may then develop and cardiac output may not be sufficient to meet the metabolic demands of the body particularly during exercise. Death often ensues within a few years in severe cases (1).

CLINICAL PRESENTATION

As in the case of pulmonary embolism, the clinical diagnosis of deep vein thrombosis is unreliable. Even with the presence of classical findings such as pain, erythema, edema, tenderness, and a palpable cord, only 50% of those presenting will actually have a DVT. Conversely, at least 50% of patients with DVT lack any of these findings (1). A Homan's sign (calf pain with flexion of the knee and dorsiflexion of the ankle) may be elicited in a minority of patients, but is a nonspecific finding. Moses's sign (pain with calf compression against the tibia) is likewise a nonspecific finding. Because DVT often cannot be diagnosed or excluded on the basis of clinical findings, diagnostic tests should be sought for any unexplained diffuse leg pain or swelling.

Diagnostic Assays

There is a wide variety of tests available for diagnosing DVT. The traditional gold standard is contrast phlebography (8). As is the case with other gold standard tests, however, it is costly, invasive, and not universally available. It also may be nondiagnostic at times, as in cases of a massive leg DVT, where the contrast material may not reach the obstruction (9). Venous ultrasonography, which detects the loss of venous compressibility, has been the diagnostic test of choice in most centers. It is reliable in diagnosing upper leg DVT and is generally more accurate than impedance plethysmography (which measures changes in the electrical resistance caused by obstruction to venous flow) (10). It must be noted, however, that as many as half of patients with PE have no imaging evidence of DVT, and therefore a negative diagnostic test for DVT, although helpful, cannot not rule out the presence of a PE (11).

The clinical presentation of a PE usually varies depending on the size and the type of embolus present (12). Dyspnea and tachypnea are present universally, but in cases of a massive PE, syncope and hypotension requiring pressor support predominate. If a pulmonary infarction is present, pleuritic chest pain and hemoptysis may occur. A pleural rub also may be heard as small emboli lodge in the peripheral pulmonary arterial tree, in close proximity to the pleura (13).

Most patients who do not have a massive PE or a pulmonary infarction present with very nonspecific findings, and, as mentioned earlier, a high index of suspicion is required to make a diagnosis. In the Prospective Investigation of Pulmonary Embolism Diagnosis (PIOPED) trial, 32% of patients with a high probability of having a PE based on history, physical examination, chest radiography, arterial blood gas analysis, and electrocardiographic findings did not have angiographic evidence of pulmonary emboli. Among the patients in whom the clinical probability of pulmonary embolism was considered to be low, 9% had positive angiograms (14). Clinical probability, therefore, was much more useful

in excluding the diagnosis of PE rather than in confirming it (4). Unfortunately, most patients entered into the trial fell into a clinically indeterminate group in whom the incidence of angiographically confirmed embolism was 30%.

Another interesting finding from the PIOPED trial was that dyspnea was not present in 27% of patients and tachypnea was not present in 30% of patients ultimately proven to have embolism. Furthermore, clinically apparent venous thrombosis was found in only 11% of patients. The problem of diagnosing a PE is confounded by the presence of cardiac or other lung disease in several patients who are at risk. Congestive heart failure, myocardial infarction, aortic dissection, COPD, and pneumonia may either be coexistent or need to be included in the differential diagnosis. Due to the nonspecific clinical presentation of a PE and its associated high mortality risk, the threshold for ordering a confirmatory diagnostic test must be low to avoid underdiagnosis.

DIAGNOSIS

Chest X-ray

The diagnostic tests for PE that are available in the clinical setting have evolved over time (Table 38.2). There are various nonspecific tests, which may point to a possible diagnosis of this condition. The chest radiograph, although usually abnormal, cannot reliably discriminate between the diagnosis of a PE and many other conditions. It will help point to a diagnosis of pneumonia or congestive heart failure with a typical infiltrate or pulmonary edema, respectively, or to a diagnosis of

TABLE 38.2. *Procedures used in the diagnosis of pulmonary embolism (PE)*

Procedure	Comment
Chest x-ray	Findings are nonspecific, but may be helpful in diagnosing pneumonia or congestive heart failure
12-lead electrocardiogram	Usually nonspecific, but helpful in diagnosing myocardial infarction; some findings such as the S1Q3T3 pattern may help confirm the diagnosis of PE
Arterial blood gas analysis	Insensitive in diagnosing PE
D-dimer	Nonspecific; however, is useful in ruling out PE if the test is negative (high negative predictive value)
Troponin T and I	A marker of right ventricular dysfunction; may be helpful in prognostication
Echocardiogram	Nonspecific, may help in the risk stratification of patients
Ventilation–perfusion scan	Results fall in the low-probabiltiy/intermediate range in about 50% of patients
Spiral computed tomography	Noninvasive test of choice in most tertiary institutions
Angiography	Usually reserved for indeterminate results after noninvasive testing

PE with a focal area of avascularity (Westermark's sign), or a wedged-shaped density, especially when abutting a pleural surface (Hampton's hump). These findings, however, are not mutually exclusive, and the most useful chest x-ray finding is in fact a completely normal study, which excludes non-PE causes of dyspnea and tachypnea. Furthermore, a normal chest x-ray also will improve the diagnostic accuracy of a ventilation–perfusion scan.

Electrocardiography

Similar to the chest x-ray, the electrocardiographic (ECG) findings in PE usually are nonspecific. These findings include sinus tachycardia and minor ST-segment and T-wave changes. Due to an acute cor pulmonale, a large pulmonary embolus may present with ECG changes most notably affecting lead III, and include an increase in the size of the normal Q wave in this lead, slight ST-segment elevation, and a shallow inversion of the T wave. These changes may mimic an acute inferior infarction pattern; however, leads II and aVF are minimally affected if ever in cases of PE. In the precordial leads (Fig. 38.1), elevated ST segments and inverted T waves sometimes are seen over the right ventricle, whereas S waves may become more prominent over the left ventricle. In other cases, lead V1 may have the typical changes of a right bundle-branch block (RBBB) pattern (15). A previously normal QRS complex in this lead would be very

helpful in alerting a physician to the potential diagnosis of an acute PE.

Blood Gases

The arterial blood gas (ABG) analysis is a blood test frequently ordered by physicians when trying to rule out PE. This test, however, has been proven to be of no discriminatory value in the evaluation of a patient suspected to have a PE. The partial pressure of oxygen varies widely in patients with PE and is normal in most patients with a small embolus as well as in up to 20% of patients with a massive embolus. The A–a gradient, which is the difference between the measured arterial oxygen and the alveolar oxygen, is a more sensitive measure of pulmonary gas exchange. It is, however, also insensitive for the detection of PE, as small pulmonary emboli do not impair pulmonary gas exchange, and nearly every type of pulmonary pathology can affect the A–a gradient (1,16). Therefore, the ABG should not be relied on as a confirmatory test for diagnosing PE. It may help in discriminating patients who may need supplemental oxygen; however, pulse oximetry is sufficient in this regard.

Laboratory Markers

Serological markers have also been investigated as a possible confirmatory test for diagnosing a PE. Among these

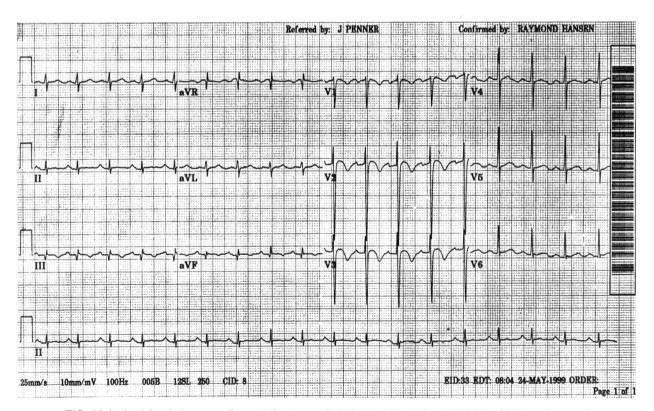

FIG. 38.1. A 12-lead electrocardiogram demonstrating sinus tachycardia, with an S1Q3T3 pattern and T-wave inversion on leads V1 to V3 consistent with acute right ventricular pressure overload.

markers, the plasma D-dimer assay holds the most promise. The D-dimer, a fibrinolytic digestion product of fibrin, usually is elevated when thrombi are undergoing lysis. Almost any acute systemic illness such as the postoperative state, sepsis, or a myocardial infarction can increase the D-dimer level. Therefore, a positive test lacks specificity. A low D-dimer level obtained using the more sensitive enzyme-linked immunosorbent assay, on the other hand, was useful for ruling out a PE with a sensitivity of 84.8% in one blinded study (17). With the availability of a rapid clinical assay, the D-dimer test should be added to the diagnostic algorithm for evaluating suspected cases of PE.

Cardiac troponins, which are reliable indicators of myocardial injury, have also been shown to be elevated in cases of PE. It is thought that they become elevated due to right ventricular dysfunction, which ensues after an embolic event. Although one study demonstrated that it is an insensitive test, like the D-dimer assay, it has a high negative predictive value (18). Furthermore, in a recent study by Konstantinides et al., cardiac troponins were demonstrated to be significantly associated with right ventricular dysfunction and the risk for in-hospital complications as well as overall mortality (19).

Echocardiography

Although not specifically a diagnostic test for PE per se, echocardiography has recently been shown to be a valuable tool for prognostication and risk stratification of patients with PE. It also may help in the diagnosis of PE if a suspected patient is noted to have increased right ventricular volumes. A particular regional pattern of right ventricular hypokinesis has been noted in patients with PE. This pattern of hypokinesis involves the base and free wall of the right ventricle, but spares the apex (20). The finding of right ventricular dysfunction confers a worse prognosis than does normal right ventricular function after PE (21). Furthermore, the finding of moderate to severe right ventricular dysfunction in one study was associated with a more favorable response to thrombolytic therapy rather than heparin (22). Another important although less often seen finding derived from two-dimensional echocardiography is a right-sided thrombus-in-transit (Figs. 38.2 through 38.4). Although not studied as extensively as right ventricular dysfunction, this finding is probably another indication for thrombolytic therapy. This was suggested by a clinical series of eight patients with a right-sided thrombus and documented PE, all of whom received 100 mg of recombinant tissue plasminogen activator with resolution of the thrombus in 1 to 4 hours (23). Finally, a repeat two-dimensional echocardiogram approximately 6 weeks after treatment can identify patients with persistent pulmonary hypertension and/or right ventricular dysfunction, which is a marker of poor long-term outcome (24).

Ventilation–Perfusion Scan

The ventilation–perfusion (VQ) scan was formerly the initial diagnostic test of choice ordered by physicians to rule out the

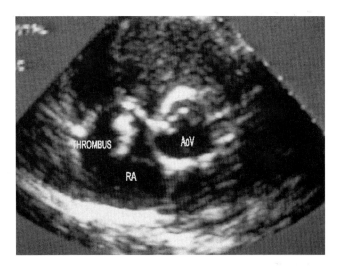

FIG. 38.2. A short-axis transthoracic echocardiograph image revealing a thrombus in the right atrium (RA). AoV, Aortic valve.

presence of a PE. This test has now been largely supplanted by the more accurate spiral computed tomography in most tertiary institutions. Despite certain limitations, the VQ scan remains a valuable tool for diagnosing PE when interpreted properly. The perfusion scan is performed by intravenous infusion of radioisotope-labeled microaggregates of albumin; and measures the distribution of blood flow through the pulmonary arterial tree; the ventilation scan measures the distribution of radioactive gas or aerosol as it washes through the bronchoalveolar tree. A normal ventilation scan coupled with an abnormal perfusion scan manifested by a perfusion defect is interpreted as a VQ scan mismatch. The two extremes in the diagnostic interpretation of a VQ scan are a

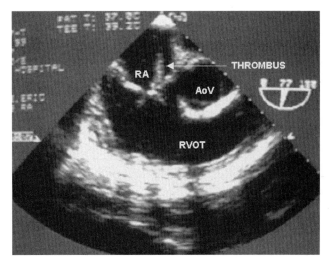

FIG. 38.3. A transesophageal echocardiograph short-axis view at the level of the aortic valve (AoV), confirming the presence of the thrombus detected on the transthoracic echocardiograph. RA, Right atrium; RVOT, right ventricular outflow tract.

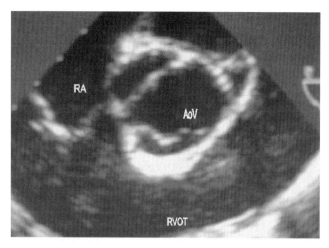

FIG. 38.4. Follow-up transesophageal electrocardiograph after thrombolytic therapy demonstrating the successful dissolution of the thrombus. RA, Right atrium; AoV, aortic valve; RVOT, right ventricular outflow tract.

negative perfusion scan, which rules out the diagnosis of pulmonary embolism with the same degree of certainty as a negative pulmonary angiogram, and a high-probability scan (Fig. 38.5) (characterized by multiple, segmental, mismatched defects), which is associated with embolism in approximately 87% of patients. When coupled with a high clinical probability of embolism, the positive predictive value of a high-probability scan is increased to 96% (4).

The main difficulty with the interpretation of a VQ scan lies in the fact that approximately 50% of patients will have either an intermediate-probability or a low-probability scan (33% and 16%, respectively, in the PIOPED study) (14). The results of lung scans falling in these two categories are by

and large indeterminate, and therefore a more definitive test is required depending on the index of suspicion. Patients with COPD are even more problematic because a higher proportion of their scans fall into the indeterminate category (25). The results of a VQ scan therefore are only definitive when interpreted as normal or high probability. As long as this important limitation is kept in mind, potential problems of misdiagnosis can be avoided.

Spiral Computed Tomography

Contrast-enhanced spiral computed tomography (CT) or spiral CT angiography (Fig. 38.6) is the latest diagnostic study to be utilized for the noninvasive detection of pulmonary emboli. Initially, spiral CT was touted to have a 100% sensitivity and a 96% specificity for centrally located PE when compared to pulmonary angiography (26). When the more peripheral or fifth-order branches were included, however, there was a significant drop-off in the accuracy of the test, and it was not certain whether this modality would be incorporated into the diagnostic algorithm for the detection of PE. Despite of the fact that subsegmental emboli may be missed by spiral CT, however, it still has a better sensitivity, specificity, and interobserver agreement than a VQ scan (27–29). Furthermore, Goodman and colleagues demonstrated that the risk of a pulmonary embolus after a negative helical CT is low and comparable to a normal or low-probability VQ scan (30). A negative ultrasound examination of the legs is further reassurance in those patients still suspected to have PE despite a negative spiral CT. The value of a spiral CT is further enhanced by its ability to detect other parenchymal lung disease as well as aortic dissection, which may be primarily responsible for the patient's symptoms. In our institution, our diagnostic algorhythm begins with a spiral CT in suspected cases of PE, followed by an ultrasound of the legs if

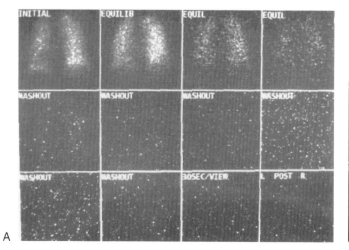

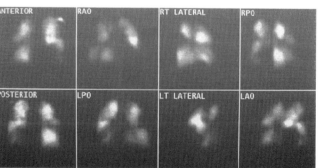

FIG. 38.5. A normal ventilation scan (**A**) and an abnormal perfusion scan (**B**) revealing large bilateral segmental and subsegmental mismatched defects.

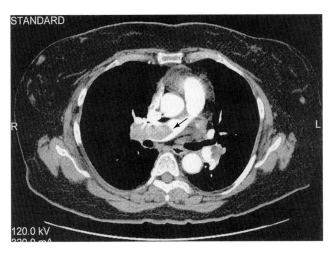

FIG. 38.6. Spiral computed tomography demonstrating a filling defect (*arrow*) consistent with a large thrombus within the right pulmonary artery.

the spiral CT results are negative. A negative ultrasound may be followed by a pulmonary angiogram if a high index of suspicion for PE is still present. The VQ scan may still be used if a pulmonary angiogram or spiral CT is contraindicated mainly due to intravenous contrast dye allergy or renal insufficiency.

Angiography

When the diagnosis of a PE remains uncertain after a negative or equivocal finding in one or two of the noninvasive diagnostic modalities, a pulmonary angiogram may be required. In experienced hands, the pulmonary angiogram is relatively safe and outweighs the risk of a missed diagnosis of PE. Although highly regarded as the gold standard for diagnosing PE, the pulmonary angiogram has limitations as well. Similar to a coronary angiogram, a filling defect or vessel cutoff may be missed, depending on the interpreter, the technical adequacy of the images, and the location of the emboli. An adequate angiogram usually consists of good vessel opacification with digital acquisition in the ipsilateral posterior oblique and ipsilateral anterior oblique view (2). Additional (e.g., anteroposterior) or magnified views may sometimes be required if the diagnosis remains uncertain. It must be noted that a completely normal pulmonary angiogram may still miss small and distal emboli, which are usually responsible for pulmonary infarcts. If done properly, however, the positive predictive value of a pulmonary angiogram approaches 100%, whereas a negative technically adequate pulmonary angiogram can rule out PE with a more than 90% certainty (1). It should be noted that small emboli may undergo lysis within a 24-hour period, and thus angiography delayed for more than 24 hours may fail to identify significant pulmonary emboli (see Fig 40.4).

MANAGEMENT

Hemodynamic Stabilization

A wide range of treatment options is available for both the treatment of PE and the prevention of future recurrences. Assessment of the overall respiratory and hemodynamic status of the patient is important for initial risk stratification and early institution of potentially life-saving measures such as mechanical ventilation and inotropic agents. In the hypotensive patient, dobutamine is a good first choice to improve right ventricular systolic function and decrease right ventricular afterload. With frank shock, however, norepinephrine is the preferred first-line agent to rapidly increase blood pressure. Volume loading in general is not advisable because it may worsen the already elevated right ventricular afterload. In more stable patients, attention should be given to adequate oxygenation and pain relief.

Anticoagulant Therapy

In hemodynamically stable patients suspected to have a PE, anticoagulation with intravenous unfractionated heparin within the first 24 hours is essential. The role of heparin in acute PE is to inhibit thrombus propagation and prevent recurrent emboli. In the presence of heparin, the natural fibrinolytic system acting within the clot can slowly reduce the size and extent of the existing thrombus. Because heparin works by binding and enhancing the activity of antithrombin III, those patients who have a significant anti-thrombin III deficiency (less than 50%) on a congenital basis or as a result of increased utilization will respond best to a direct thrombin inhibitor for effective anticoagulation. To be maximally effective, heparin should be administered as early as possible even while the diagnosis of PE is still in question. Low-molecular weight heparin (LMWH) has replaced standard unfractionated heparin in several clinical settings such as DVT treatment and prevention. LWMH is a more ideal anticoagulant because it has a greater bioavailability, a more predictable dose response, and a longer half-life than unfractionated heparin (31). However, there are insufficient data to warrant the use of LMWH as opposed to standard heparin for the treatment of PE (32).

After the diagnosis of a PE has been established, and heparin is continued generally for 7 to 10 days, outpatient anticoagulation for postembolic prophylaxis must be instituted. Warfarin has been the drug of choice for this task and must be started while heparin is still being given. The reason for this is twofold. First, warfarin, which is a vitamin K antagonist, requires approximately 3 to 5 days to achieve full anticoagulant effect. Second, warfarin has an initial procoagulant effect, which becomes more apparent during a prothrombotic state. This early procoagulant effect is due to a decline in the levels of protein C and protein S, which are naturally occurring anticoagulants. Patients with inherited deficiency and low stores of protein C or protein S will thus be more susceptible to thrombosis during the first few days of warfarin therapy, and therefore continuation of heparin is warranted until a sufficient decline in other vitamin K proteases is achieved.

After successful initiation of warfarin therapy, the duration of postembolic prophylaxis remains controversial and should probably be individualized. A comparison of 6 weeks versus 6 months of oral anticoagulant therapy by Schulman et al. revealed a 50% reduction in recurrent thromboembolism in the 6-month anticoagulation group (33). After cessation of anticoagulation, however there was a linear increase in the cumulative risk, corresponding to 5% to 6% annually (33). Therefore the duration of anticoagulation may need to be extended particularly in patients who have permanent risk factors for venous thromboembolism, venous insufficiency, systemic lupus erythromatosus, and idiopathic venous thromboembolism. Furthermore, prolonged or even lifelong oral anticoagulation should be considered for patients with an irreversible acquired or genetic predisposition to venous thrombosis, major ventilation–perfusion scan defects, or a history of recurrent thromboembolic events, even though such a strategy is associated with an increased risk of hemorrhagic complications (34).

Vena Caval Filters

Another method of postembolic prophylaxis is the implantation of an inferior vena caval filter. Although vena caval filters prevent large thrombi from passing upward into the pulmonary arteries, they do not prevent smaller pulmonary emboli from reaching the pulmonary circulation. Rarely, large emboli may bypass the filters or may originate above the filter (1). If anticoagulation is omitted, vena caval filters do not prevent DVT.

For these reasons and the invasiveness of the implantation procedure itself, vena caval filters are not first-line alternatives for postembolic prophylaxis. They are, however, indicated in patients who have had a PE and have contraindications for anticoagulation or have had a thromboembolic episode while on anticoagulation. Patients who are at a high mortality risk if a recurrent episode of PE occurs (e.g., chronic thromboembolic pulmonary hypertension) also may benefit from these devices.

Thrombolytic Agents

A controversial treatment option for patients with an acute PE is the use of a thrombolytic agent. Alteplase, streptokinase, and urokinase are the Food and Drug Administration-approved thrombolytic agents for this condition. Their benefits over heparin include a more rapid and complete resolution of pulmonary vascular obstruction; superior hemodynamic improvement, as measured by right atrial, right ventricular, and pulmonary arterial pressures; and fewer PE recurrences

(1,35,36). The Achilles heel of thrombolytic agents, however, is the possible risk of bleeding, most notably intracranial hemorrhage, which can occur in 1% to 2% of cases. The mortality of a PE episode despite heparin therapy should therefore be high enough to warrant the use of these agents. In routine PE cases without hemodynamic instability, this may not be the case. In those patients with PE and hemodynamic compromise, rapid dissolution of the thrombus is vital, and therefore thrombolysis is indicated. Other, more controversial indications include cases of PE with right ventricular dysfunction and the two-dimensional echocardiogram finding of a mobile cardiac thrombus-in-transit. There have been case reports and small randomized studies proving the efficacy of thrombolytic agents in this subset of cases, and they are probably beneficial when these echo findings are associated with a large PE, which is commonly the case (35,37–39).

Embolectomy

Another controversial treatment option in acute PE is pulmonary embolectomy. This is a surgical procedure wherein thrombus is extracted through an arteriotomy in the main pulmonary artery (40). Although this treatment option is appealing, because to the associated high surgical morbidity and mortality rates, it is only indicated in cases of massive PE wherein patients have an existing contraindication to the use of a thrombolytic agent. Surgical embolectomy also has been successfully performed in patients who have failed thrombolytic therapy (41).

Percutaneous approaches to pulmonary embolectomy are being investigated (42,43). These approaches involve removal of thrombus either by suctioning it or by fragmenting it using a mechanical device. One such device is the Amplatz thrombectomy device (ATD). The ATD is driven by high air pressure from an external air source (50 to 100 psi) and mediates mechanical clot fragmentation. A rapidly spinning encapsulated impeller (150,000 rpm) creates an aspirating vortex, which agitates and pulls the thrombus toward its distal tip (44). In one study in humans, the use of this device successfully decreased thrombus in the pulmonary artery and improved pulmonary arterial pressure. Adjunctive fibrinolytic therapy, however, was required to decrease the pulmonary arterial pressure significantly. Another disadvantage of this particular device was its lack of steerability and torque control (45). Further advances in this and other devices are anticipated, and in the foreseeable future, patients may be undergoing primary percutaneous intervention for removal of thrombus similar to primary angioplasty for myocardial infarctions.

SUMMARY

Pulmonary embolism is an important cause of acute hospital death and also may lead to long-term complications such as chronic cor pulmonale. Due to its nonspecific clinical presentation, the diagnosis of PE requires a high index of suspicion. The D-dimer assay is a useful laboratory marker for excluding the diagnosis of PE. Cardiac troponins may also be helpful in assessing right ventricular function and overall in-hospital risk. For a more definitive diagnosis, spiral CT has supplanted the older VQ scan in most tertiary centers due to a higher overall accuracy rate. An echocardiogram is a very useful tool in risk-stratifying patients as well as for excluding right ventricular dysfunction and right-sided thrombi. Anticoagulant therapy is the mainstay in the management of PE. Thrombolytic agents are indicated in cases of PE accompanied by hemodynamic instability, and, although more controversial, are probably also indicated when right ventricular dysfunction or a right-sided thrombus is found on echocardiography. Embolectomy is a rapidly evolving treatment option, which at this stage of its development is only indicated in patients with massive PE and an existing contraindication to the use of a thrombolytic agent.

REFERENCES

1. Feied CF. Venous thrombosis and pulmonary embolism. In: Marx JA, ed., *Rosen's emergency medicine: concepts and clinical practice,* 5th ed. St. Louis, Mosby, 2002:1210–1234.
2. Goldhaber SZ. Pulmonary embolism. In: Braunwald E, Zipes DP, Libby P, et al., eds., *Heart disease: a textbook of cardiovascular medicine,* 6th ed. Philadelphia: WB Saunders, 2001:1886–1907.
3. Meignan M, Rosso J, Gauthier H, et al. Systematic lung scans reveal a high frequency of silent pulmonary embolism in patients with proximal deep venous thrombosis. *Arch Intern Med* 2000;160:159–164.
4. Fedullo PF. Pulmonay embolism. In: Murray JF, Nadel JA, eds., *Textbook of respiratory medicine,* 3rd ed. Philadelphia: WB Saunders, 2000:1503–1521.
5. Kobzik L. The lung. In: Cotran RS, Kumar V, Collins T, eds. *Robbins pathologic basis of disease,* 6th ed. Philadelphia: WB Saunders, 1999:697–755.
6. Subar M. Clinical evaluation of hypercoagulable states. *Clin Geriatr Med* 2001;17:57–70.
7. Martinelli I. Risk factors in venous thromboembolism. *Thromb Haemost* 2001;86:395–403.
8. Rabinov K, Paulin S. Roentgen diagnosis of venous thrombosis in the leg. *Arch Surg* 1972;104:134–144.
9. Couson F, Bounameaux C, Didier D, et al. Influence of variability of interpretation of contrast venography for screening of postoperative deep venous thrombosis on the results of a thromboprophylactic study. *Thromb Haemost* 1993;70:573–575.
10. Heijboer H, Buller HR, Lensing AWA, et al. A comparison of real-time compression ultrasonography with impedance plethysmography for the diagnosis of deep-vein thrombosis in symptomatic outpatients. *N Engl J Med* 1993;329:1365–1369.
11. Turkstra F, Kuijer PMM, van Beek EJR, et al. Diagnostic utility of ultrasonography of leg veins in patients suspected of having pulmonary embolism. *Ann Intern Med* 1997;126:775–781.
12. Stein PD, Terrin ML, Hales CA, et al. Clinical, laboratory, roentgenographic, and electrocardiographic findings in patients with acute pulmonary embolism and no pre-existing cardiac or pulmonary disease. *Chest* 1991;100:598–603.
13. Wagenvoort CA. Pathology of pulmonary thromboembolism. *Chest* 1995;107:10S–17S.
14. The PIOPED Investigators: value of the ventilation/perfusion scan in acute pulmonary embolism: Results of the Prospective Investigation

Of Pulmonary Embolism Diagnosis (PIOPED). *JAMA* 1990;263:2753–2759.
15. Wagner WS, ed. *Marriott's practical electrocardiography,* 10th ed. Philadelphia: Lippincott Williams & Wilkins, 2001:214–215.
16. Stein PD. Arterial blood gas analysis in the assessment of suspected acute pulmonary embolism. *Chest* 1996;109:78–81.
17. Ginsberg JS, Wells PS, Kearon C, et al. Sensitivity and specificity of a rapid whole-blood assay for D-dimer in the diagnosis of pulmonary embolism. *Ann Intern Med* 1998;129:1006–1011.
18. Dieter RS, Ernst E, Ende DJ, et al. Diagnostic utility of cardiac troponin-I levels in patients with suspected pulmonary embolism. *Angiology* 2002;53:583–585.
19. Konstantinidis S, Geibel A, Olschewski M, et al. Importance of cardiac troponins I and T in risk stratification of patients with acute pulmonary embolism. *Circulation* 2002;106:1263–1268.
20. McConnell MV, Solomon SD, Rayan ME, et al. Regional right ventricular dysfunction detected by echocardiography in acute pulmonary embolism. *Am J Cardiol* 1996;78:469–473.
21. Lualdi JC, Goldhaber SZ. Right ventricular dysfunction after acute pulmonary embolism: pathophysiologic factors, detection, and therapeutic implications. *Am Heart J* 1995;130:1276–1282.
22. Goldhaber SZ, Haire WD, Feldstein ML, et al. Alteplase versus heparin in acute pulmonary embolism: randomised trial assessing right-ventricular function and pulmonary perfusion. *Lancet* 1993;341:507–511.
23. Cuccia C, Campana M, Franzoni P, et al. Effectiveness of intravenous rTPA in the treatment of massive pulmonary embolism and right heart thromboembolism. *Am Heart J* 1993;126:468–472.
24. Ribeiro A, Lindmarker P, Johnson H, et al. Pulmonary embolism: one-year follow-up with echocardiography Doppler and five year survival analysis. *Circulation* 1999;99:1325–1330.
25. Lesser BA, Leeper KV, Stein PD, et al. The diagnosis of acute pulmonary embolism in patients with chronic obstructive lung disease. *Chest* 1992;102:17–22.
26. Remy-Jardin M, Remy J, Wattinne L, et al. Central pulmonary thromboembolism: diagnosis with spiral volumetric CT with single breath hold technique: comparison with pulmonary angiography. *Radiology* 1992;185:381–387.
27. Goodman LR, Curtin JJ, Mewissen, et al. Detection of pulmonary embolism in patients with unresolved clinical and scintigraphic diagnosis: helical CT versus angiography. *AJR Am J Roentgenol* 1995;164:1369–1374.
28. Remy-Jardin M, Remy J, Deschildre F, et al. Diagnosis of pulmonary embolism with spiral CT: comparison with pulmonary angiography and scintigraphy. *Radiology* 1996;200:699–706.
29. Rossum AB, Pattynama PMT, Ton, ERTA, et al. Pulmonary embolism: validation of spiral CT angiography in 149 patients. *Radiology* 1996;201:467–470.
30. Goodman LR, Lipchik RJ, Kuzo RS, et al. Subsequent pulmonary embolism: risk after a negative helical CT pulmonary Angiogram–prospective comparison with scintigraphy. *Radiology* 2000;215:535–542.
31. Weitz JI. Low-molecular-weight heparins. *N Engl J Med* 1997;337:688–698.
32. Goldhaber SZ. Unsolved issues in the treatment of pulmonary embolism. *Thromb Res* 2001;103:V245–V255.
33. Schulman S, Sofie-Rhedin A, Lindmarker P, et al. A comparison of six weeks with six months of oral anticoagulant therapy after a first episode of venous thromboembolism. *N Engl J Med* 1995;332:1661–1665.
34. Schulman S, Granqvist S, Holmstrom M, et al. The duration of oral anticoagulant therapy after a second episode of venous thromboembolism. *N Engl J Med* 1997;336:393–398.
35. Goldhaber SZ, Haire WD, Feldstein ML, et al. Alteplase versus heparin in acute pulmonary embolism: randomised trial assessing right-ventricular function and pulmonary perfusion. *Lancet* 1993;341:507–511.
36. Konstantinides S, Geibel A, Olschewski M, et al. Association between thrombolytic treatment and the prognosis of hemodynamically stable patients with major pulmonary embolism: results of a multicenter registry. *Circulation* 1997;96:882–888.
37. Wolfe MW, Lee RT, Feldstein ML, et al. Prognostic significance of right ventricular hypokinesis and perfusion lung scan defects in pulmonary embolism. *Am Heart J* 1994;127(5):1371–1375.

38. Casazza F, Bongarzoni A, Centonze F, et al. Prevalence and prognostic significance of right-sided cardiac mobile thrombi in acute massive pulmonary embolism. *Am J Cardiol* 1997;79:1433–1435.

39. Cuccia C, Campana M, Franzoni P, et al. Effectiveness of intravenous rTPA in the treatment of massive pulmonary embolism and right heart thromboembolism. *Am Heart J* 1993;126:468–472.

40. Aklog L, Williams CS, Byrne JG, et al. Acute pulmonary embolectomy: a contemporary approach. *Circulation* 2002;105:1416–1419.

41. Doerge HC, Schoendube FA, Loeser H, et al. Pulmonary embolectomy: review of a 15-year experience and role in the age of thrombolytic therapy. *Eur J Cardiothorac Surg* 1996;10:952–957.

42. Goldhaber SZ. Integration of catheter thrombectomy into our armamentarium to treat acute pulmonary embolism. *Chest* 1998;114:1237–1238.

43. Cho KJ, Dasika NL. Catheter technique for pulmonary embolectomy or thrombofragmentation. *Semin Vasc Surg* 2000;13:221–235.

44. Bildsoe MC, Moradian GP, Hunter DW, et al. Mechanical clot dissolution: new concept. *Radiology* 1989;171:231–233.

45. Muller-Hulsbeck S, Brossman J, Jahnke T, et al. Mechanical thrombectomy of major and massive pulmonary embolism with use of the Amplatz thrombectomy device. *Invest Radiol* 2001;36:317–322.

CHAPTER 39

Recognizing, Understanding, and Treating Chronic Venous Insufficiency

Patricia Thorpe

Key Points

- Chronic venous insufficiency (CVI) describes the changes in physiology and appearance of the leg due to elevated ambulatory venous pressures related to valve incompetence or reflux (90%) and venous obstruction (10%).
- About 25 million U.S. adults have varicose veins, and 7 million have significant clinical symptoms.
- Approximately 70% of leg ulcers are venous.
- Factors predisposing to varicose veins include obesity, pregnancy, physical position (such as standing for a long time), age, and smoking.
- The clinical symptoms related to venous stasis and varicose veins include tiredness, ache, heaviness, restless legs, nocturnal cramps, tightness or fullness, pruritis, and dry skin.
- Color duplex and B-mode ultrasound are the preferred diagnostic tools for investigating acute and chronic venous disease.
- Symptomatic reflex can be treated with great saphenous vein removal or "stripping," catheter ablation with radiofrequency or laser, or foam sclerotherapy.
- Physicians must observe limbs for signs and symptoms of venous disease to treat or refer patients for further care.

INTRODUCTION

Cardiologists may encounter a significant amount of venous disease. Signs of chronic venous insufficiency (CVI) include leg swelling, skin discoloration, dematitis, and dermatosclerosis as well as stasis ulcer. However, the signs may go unreported (by the patient) and unnoted (by the physician). Various socioeconomic and cultural factors govern this behavior. For instance, except in tropical climates, most people conveniently cover varicose veins (VV), spider veins, and leg edema. When skin changes secondary to venous disease are painless, most people do not complain. In general, leg discomfort is regarded as a normal part of aging, working long hours, and being "out of shape." Edema from venous hypertension is easy to dismiss because it improves overnight instead of becoming steadily worse. There is a common perception that venous disease occurs in old age, and mostly in women. Leg swelling has been associated with elderly women, and most of us recall seeing unsightly "granny" stockings, giving everyone a generally negative view of compression hose. Although the incidence of venous disease does increase with age, young people can be affected by either valve reflux or obstruction. Young women and men with early appearance of varicose veins find little empathy, and their concerns can be regarded as vanity. However, the appearance of spider veins and minor varicosities are true signs of venous insufficiency. In fact, chronic venous insufficiency is the most common problem in vascular medicine and affects all age groups (1). Nearly 25 million adults in the United States have varicose veins, and approximately 7 million have

TABLE 39.1. *Clinical signs and differentiating disorders* [a]

Signs	DVT	Reflux	Lymphedema	PVD	CHF
Thigh edema	X		X		
Calf edema	X	X	X		
Ankle edema	X	X	X		X
Toe edema			X		
Telangectasia		X			
Pigmentation	X	X			
Malleolar ulcer	X	X	X		
Toe ulcer				X	
Heel ulcer				X	
Shiny skin + hard edema				X	
Dependent discoloration	X				

[a]DVT, Deep vein thrombosis; PVD, peripheral vascular disease; CHF, congestive heart failure.

significant clinical symptoms (2). Epidemiologic studies in Europe suggest that nearly 15% of men and 25% of women have visible varicose veins (3). It is estimated that 3% of the Medicare population will experience a venous ulcer and undergo multiple physician visits for skin care. This component of the disease is estimated to cost the U.S. taxpayers approximately 200 million dollars annually (4).

Insurance data on the Mutual of Omaha website (www.mutualofomaha.com) suggest two-thirds of the nearly 1.5 million venous treatments recorded annually for insured working individuals are related to symptomatic greater saphenous vein reflux and varicose veins. Although the prevalence increases with age, a surprising number of young individuals have venous problems. Many young men and women manifest varicose veins on one or both limbs as early as their late

teen-age years. For young adults, the motivation to seek treatment includes a concern about appearance, discomfort with activity, and, quite often, an understandable concern about the risk of phlebitis and stasis ulcers. There is equal prevalence by gender for thrombotic states as well as varicose veins. However, with VV, women are five times more likely to seek evaluation and intervention than men. Approximately 70% of leg ulcers are venous. In a peripheral vascular ambulatory care clinic, at least 20% of patients will have mixed arterial and venous disease. Overall, the prevalence of venous disease is thought to be ten times greater than arterial disease, but, as a culture, we tend to focus on symptoms of arterial disease and ignore venous conditions.

We can reassure patients that, for the most part, varicose veins do not lead to thromboembolic disease. However, varicosities occasionally thrombose and cause a painful phlebitis, which is treated with topical and systemic antiinflammatory agents and analgesics. On the other hand, deep vein thrombosis (DVT) does not invariably result in superficial varicose veins. Whereas venous reflux is seen at all ages, thromboembolic disease has a bimodal population distribution. Deep vein thrombosis and symptomatic postthrombotic conditions are often seen in a younger population (20 to 45 years) when the underlying etiology is a hypercoagulability issue, and more frequently in an older population when immobilization from surgery or malignancy are risk factors for DVT.

In a clinical cardiology practice, most of the patients will be older than 50 years of age. If the clinician is observant, a significant amount of venous disease can be detected. Distinguishing bilateral ankle edema caused by congestive failure from venous insufficiency and/or lymphedema combines careful history taking, a search for certain physical characteristics (Table 39.1), and a few pertinent questions that can

TABLE 39.2. *Clinical patterns and differentiating disorders* [a]

Condition	CHF	Reflux incompetence	Obstruction DVT	Lymphedema	Severe PVD
Edema unchanged in a.m.				+	+
Edema less in a.m.	+	+	+		No
Edema worse in p.m.	+	+	+	+	No
Diuretics effective	+	No	Limited	Limited	+
Dependent discoloration			Reddish/purple	No	+
Hyperpigmentation		+	++	Lichinification	No
Varicosities		+	Possibly		No
Medial malleolar ulcer		+	+		No
Toe or heal ulcer	+				+
Toe edema				+	No
Compression effective	Yes	Yes	Yes	Yes	Contraindicated
Discomfort increases with standing or sitting; feels better moving around	NC	Yes	No, may get worse	No	No
Discomfort increases with standing or sitting; worse with activity	NC	No	Yes	May	+
Feels better with legs elevated	Maybe	Maybe	Yes	Maybe	No, feels worse

[a]CHF, Congestive heart failure; DVT, deep vein thrombus; PVD, peripheral vascular disease.

TABLE 39.3. *Peripheral vascular ulcers: arterial versus venous*

Characteristics	Ischemic ulcer	Venous ulcer
Size	↓	↑
Margin	Regular	Irregular
Pain	++	—
Base of ulcer	Clean	Fibrin and Debris
Discharge	Dry	Wet
Infection	↓	↑
Location (common)	Lateral malleolus distal toe	Medial malleolus

help separate the clinical patterns of different disorders. Lymphedema is often a perplexing diagnosis of exclusion. The leg edema characteristically extends to ankles, feet, and toes, unlike other conditions. It does not respond to elevation as well as edema caused by venous hypertension. The painless edema and skin changes of lymphatic stasis do, however, respond to compression. Clinical clues that help distinguish disorders with lower extremity edema are listed in Table 39.2. It is particularly important to clearly discern between stasis ulcers from venous hypertension and ischemic ulcers secondary to arterial disease. Table 39.3 should aid in determining the etiology of distal ulcers.

CHRONIC VENOUS INSUFFICIENCY: PATHOPHYSIOLOGY

Chronic venous insufficiency is a term used to describe changes in physiology and appearance of the leg due to elevated ambulatory venous pressures related to the following:

- Valve incompetence or reflux (90%), which may be primary, as in the case of varicose veins, or secondary, due to postthrombotic damage to valves. Reflux involves the superficial veins more commonly than the deep veins. Varicose veins are related to incompetence of valves in the superficial system (Fig. 39.1).
- Venous obstruction (10%), which results from residual blockage following thrombosis.

Factors that predispose to varicose veins include obesity, pregnancy, position during work (such as standing for long periods), age, and smoking. Spider veins can result from local trauma as well. A familial tendency can predispose an individual to varicose veins. The inheritance pattern is not clearly established. There is a strong influence of hormones, as seen by the increase in pelvic pressure and appearance of varicose veins during pregnancy. In most cases, the VV appear in the first trimester. The hereditary and hormonal factors are tendencies influenced by gravity and venous pressure increases due to incompetent valves (5). Subdermal and superficial veins subjected to constant increase in hydrostatic pressure elongate and dilate. This causes additional local valve failure and additional pressure. Treatment with compression counteracts the pathological pressure asserting forces on the

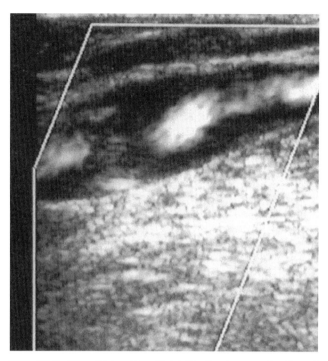

FIG. 39.1. (See Color Fig. 39.1.) Duplex image of reflux at the saphenofemoral valve. This is the cause of the prominent medial thigh varicosity.

superficial veins. Removal or sclerosis of the abnormal veins may cause the limb to look better, but this does not address the underlying pathology of the incompetent valve and venous hypertension. Removal or ablation of the vein(s), which transmits the abnormal pressure below the failed valve(s), has been shown to effectively remove the hydrodynamic force causing the problems (6).

VARICOSE VEINS: HISTORICAL INSIGHTS

Varicose veins are unique to bipedal human beings. There is no readily studied animal model for venous insufficiency because this is a well-documented clinical problem peculiar to humans. The history of early venous interventions is detailed in Friedman's *A History of Vascular Surgery* (7:141–156). Sushruta, an Indian surgeon who preceded Hippocrates by several centuries, first described aneurysms of the veins in a medical compendium entitled *Sushruta Samhita*. Hundreds of years later, Hippocrates offered understanding of the pathophysiology of venous hypertension. He recognized the peril of excising varicosities, noting that ulcers could result. He recommended compression bandages, which have remained the mainstay of traditional, conservative treatment of venous insufficiency for several thousand years. Linen wraps and plaster bandages were used as early as the first century A.D., according to historical accounts of Celsus. A century later, Galen introduced an intervention for varicose veins that differs little from modern practice. He described performing phlebectomy using varicele hooks and local ligation in a manner similar to contemporary technique. The supposed metaphysical relationship of varicosities to "bad humors" has never really been completely dispelled. Some myths dating back to Hippocrates remarked about the inverse relationship of baldness to varicose veins. In 1579, Ambrose Pare wrote about varicose veins, "It is best not to meddle with such as are inveterate; for of such being cured there is to be feared a reflux of the melancholy bloud to the noble parts, whence there may be imminent danger of malign ulcers, a cancer, madness or suffocation." From Pare's remarks, we can gather that some may have recognized an association of varicosities with manifestations of venous thrombosis, including pulmonary embolism. However, in 1868, John Gay, a British surgeon, noted that varicose ulcer was a misnomer. He realized that ulcers were not always associated with varicosities, so perhaps the term "venous ulcer" would be more accurate. The fact that even in 2003 no single theory is universally accepted as an explanation of the etiology of varicose veins substantiates the prevailing mystery of this ubiquitous condition.

Treatment of varicose veins and venous disease has really only evolved in the last 100 years. Recent endovascular treatments have made a significant impact on clinical conditions that have been known for centuries with little treatment other than compression. In 1896, the Unna boot was one of the first innovations since Hippocrates introduced compression therapy. Paul Unna was a German dermatologist, who began the practice we still use today of using a simple plaster boot for treating stasis ulcers.

The surgical treatment of venous disease initially focused on varicose vein treatment. Even today, although endovascular techniques have evolved over the last 10 to 15 years, the great majority of interventions for venous insufficiency consist of surgical treatment of varicosities and their recurrence. Early in the twentieth century, Alexis Carrel and Charles Guthrie experimented with venous grafts. The excision of the saphenous vein for treatment of varicosities was introduced by Friedrich Trendelenburg and expanded upon by John Homans, who noted the importance of also identifying and ligating perforating veins in attempts to reduce the incidence of recurrence. In the 1930s and 1940s, Robert Linton made important contributions to surgical management of venous disease particularly with respect to the role of communicating veins. Treatment of reflux disease by "vein stripping" and ligation became the standard treatment for symptomatic and unsightly varicose veins and stasis ulcer disease. In the mid 1990s, endoscopic perforator vein ligation was introduced as a less invasive technique for treatment of recalcitrant venous ulcers. Interestingly, patients failing to respond to this treatment were generally found to have undiagnosed deep venous obstruction.

J. Berberich and S. Hirsch first reported imaging veins with x-rays and contrast in 1923. Phlebography performed with pedal infusion of contrast, with and without tourniquets, continued throughout the century until the popularization of noninvasive ultrasound imaging in the mid 1980s. Strandness, Nicolaides, and colleagues greatly advanced understanding of duplex imaging of venous disease and noninvasive physio-

logical testing of valve reflux and ambulatory venous hypertension (8,9). Now, in addition to duplex imaging with color flow and Doppler, magnetic resonance imaging can provide noninvasive investigation of the deep axial veins capable of demonstrating compression or thrombus. Standing duplex, plethysmography, and descending venography, however, remain the primary tools for evaluating valve competence (10).

VARICOSE VEINS: CLINICAL ASSESSMENT

The recent evolution of minimally invasive endovascular approaches for varicose veins has increased public interest in seeking interventional treatment (11). Treating patients seeking consideration for laser or radiofrequency ablation requires knowledge of anatomy and the pathophysiology of venous hypertension. Sclerotherapy and ambulatory phlebectomy are adjunctive treatments required for treating this disease.

Although varicose veins are generally visible, patients can also present with complaints of progressive daily swelling or discomfort. Clinical evaluation of varicose veins is commonly prompted by the following:

- Concern about appearance.
- Symptomatic relief of aching and discomfort associated with VV.
- Concern about progressive worsening of VV and complications associated with "vein problems." Many are confused about the relationship of thrombosis or "blood clots" and varicose veins, and therefore seek advice regarding the risk of thrombotic complications.

The symptoms are very general, and there is poor correlation with severity of pathology. Epidemiologic surveys have shown that most leg symptoms have a nonvenous cause, and that about 50% of adults have such complaints with or without VV (12). The clinical symptoms related to venous stasis and VV include the following:

- Tiredness
- Ache that increases as the day progresses or with activity
- Heaviness
- Restless legs
- Nocturnal cramps
- Tightness or fullness
- Pruritis and dry skin (tightness and histamine release)

PHYSICAL EXAM AND DIAGNOSTIC TESTING

It is important to obtain ultrasound documentation of reflux, as well as exclusion of deep vein thrombosis, plus a pertinent physical exam and clinical history Diagnostic classifications have evolved to aid clinicians in evaluating venous disease. The CEAP classification represents the collective effort of an ad hoc committee of physicians to establish a system whereby venous disease can be described and followed after intervention (13,14). The basic elements of the CEAP classification include the clinical condition (C), the

TABLE 39.4. *Clinical severity score for chronic venous disease*[a]

Condition	Absent = 0	Mild = 1	Moderate = 2	Severe = 3
Pain	None	Variable	Daily occasional analgesics	Daily, limits activities, regular analgesics
Varicosities	None	Few with competent GS/LS	Multiple with reflux GS/LS	Extensive multisegmental
Edema	None	Evening ankle	Afternoon edema above ankle	Morning edema leg elevation
Skin pigmentation	None or focal light	Diffuse, not expanding	Diffuse over lower third calf	Wider distribution, newer
Inflammation	None	Mild cellulitis periulcer margin	Diffuse over lower third calf	Severe cellulites or venous eczema
Induration	None	Focal <5 cm	Medial of lateral	Entire lower third calf
Number ulcers all	0	1	2–4	>4
Open ulcer duration	None	<3 mo	>3 mo to <1 year	Not healed after >1 year
Open ulcers size	None	<2 cm diameter	2–4 cm	>4 cm
Compression therapy	Not worn or noncompliant	Intermittent use	Wears most days	Wears full time + leg elevation

[a]GS, Greater saphenous; LS, lesser saphenous.
Modified from Rutherford RB, Padberg Jr FT, Comerata AJ, et al. Venous severity scoring: an adjunct to venous outcome assessment. *J Vasc Surg* 2000;31:1307–1312.

etiology (E), the anatomic location of the problem (A), and the pathophysiology (P) such as reflux or obstruction. The Venous Clinical Severity Score provides a means of assessing the patient's condition in the clinic (15,16). A summary version of the scoring system is given in Table 39.4. Baseline assessment of venous disease, like that of arterial disease, allows the clinician to document initial severity of the patient's condition as well as the outcome of therapy.

In the clinic, recognizing venous disease leads to the need for noninvasive testing to confirm reflux and ruleout deep vein thrombosis. For the most part, patients will present with chronic signs and symptoms that may not be their primary concern on the visit to their cardiologist. A relatively simple and inexpensive tool available to the physician is the same handheld Doppler used for obtaining ankle–brachial indices on patients with peripheral arterial disease. With some training and effort, the clinician can use this tool to evaluate venous disease as well. With the handheld Doppler, different audible signal patterns characterize venous flow in obstructed and unobstructed veins. A phasic signal that changes with distal or proximal augmentation indicates a patent vein. A weak signal may come from a recanalized segment or a collateral, and there will be less or a phasic pattern. If the segment above the test level is indeed obstructed, there will be no phasicity because the distal transmission of the cardiac rhythm will be blocked (see Chapter 15).

Detecting valvular incompetence is an acquired skill. With the patient standing, the Doppler wand is placed at the common femoral level, where a Valsalva maneuver will produce retrograde flow through the incompetent valve. If there is a competent valve above the test level, there will be cessation of flow with the Valsalva. Limb compression is used to detect incompetent valves below the inguinal level. Compression stops flow, and competent valves do not leak or reflux. Therefore, no signal is heard. If the intervening valve is incompetent, however, the flow is reversed with compression,

and this has a different sound than the forward rush of blood that occurs when the compression is released. This produces the typical "to-and-fro" sound indicating reflux. This is a simple screening tool, and requires some knowledge of venous anatomy. Furthermore, it is not quantitative and can be confusing if there are duplicated segments or large collaterals. Use of the handheld Doppler is a quick and readily available technique to complement the acquisition of ankle–brachial indices in the clinic.

Color duplex and B-mode ultrasound are the preferred diagnostic tools for investigating acute and chronic venous disease. This has replaced phlebography as the gold standard in venous diagnosis. The studies, however, are operator dependent. In particular, standing reflux is an exam not performed everywhere. Ideally, a step-stool stand of two steps, with a small platform, allows the patient to be elevated for the comfort and ease of the technologist. The patient stands with weight on the unaffected limb as the valves are checked with and without compression. With regard to deep vein obstruction and evaluation for chronic occlusion, one must specifically request examination of the pelvic veins. This is, in fact, an abdominal exam, for which the patient must remain without eating for about 6 hours prior to the study. We record velocities in the axial segments and pay attentions to the waveform. The loss of phasicity is a clue to more proximal blockage. In a thin person, very high velocities, similar to those seen with an arterial stenosis, may detect the left iliac compression.

OUTPATIENT MANAGEMENT OF VARICOSE VEINS

The unsightly appearance of varicose veins prompts many patients to seek intervention. However, the promise of minimally invasive techniques has resulted in advances in multiple areas of venous therapy (17). In warm seasons or climates,

TABLE 39.5. *Treatment options for varicose veins*

Noninvasive treatment options
    Leg elevation
    Compression
    Topical therapy
    Oral medication
Minimally invasive treatment options
    Sclerotherapy
    Ambulatory phlebectomy
    Catheter ablation saphenous vein
    Subfascial endoscopic perforator ligation
Invasive treatment options
    Skin grafting
    Saphenous stripping and ligation
    Open subfascial perforator ligation
    Valvuloplasty

dress habits make legs more visible. The simplicity of an outpatient catheter-directed therapy with cosmetic results appeals to many people who would not consider surgery. Vein stripping and catheter ablation share the same clinical indication, which is treatment of chronic venous hypertension. The severity of a patient's condition determines the treatment options. Symptomatic reflux can be treated with greater saphenous vein removal or "stripping," catheter ablation with radiofrequency or laser, or foam sclerotherapy. This is usually done in conjunction with "stab" or ambulatory phlebectomy to remove protruding varicosities and injection sclerotherapy for treatment of associated spider and reticular veins. Treatment options for venous nonobstructive venous insufficiency are listed in Table 39.5.

COMPRESSION THERAPY

Myths and darkness surround the realm of compression stockings, which have been considered a fundamental therapy for centuries. The public has a fairly negative opinion of compression stockings gathered from seeing aged relatives in hot, bulky, sagging socks. Furthermore, patients placed in white, thigh-high T.E.D. hose in the hospital find them less satisfactory at home. Antiembolic stockings, designed for immobilized patients, are not designed to provide therapeutic compression during ambulation. They are designed for patients who are at rest because they exert less than 20 mm Hg pressure at the ankle. Therapeutic stockings are designed to provide ankle pressures of 20 to 30 mm Hg in class I, 30 to 40 mm Hg in class II, 40 to 50 mm Hg in class III, and 50 to 60 mm Hg in class IV. Class I and II stockings are readily available in knee-high, thigh-high, and pantyhose styles. New fabrics make them easier to put on and not as hot in warm weather compared to older, bulkier designs. Class III and IV stockings are special-order items for severely symptomatic individuals. Most patients with edema related to reflux benefit from knee-high stockings, which help control calf swelling. Thigh swelling is more common in obstructive disease involving iliofemoral vein segments.

The most important factors determining patient compliance with stockings are the fit and the patient's ability to actually put the stockings on. Thus, measurements need to be taken in the morning, before edema develops. Stocking education, in the clinic, is important. A nurse can teach the patient or spouse the tricks of getting stockings on before he or she gives up the struggle. For this reason, knee-high stockings are effective because they provide needed compression at the ankle and are easier to wear than thigh-high stockings or pantyhose. Stockings must be renewed every 4 to 6 months if worn regularly. The Circaid legging system (Circaid Medical Products, San Diego, CA) is a unified combination of Velcro straps, which provide sustained compression and ease of vestment compared to stockings. They are bulkier than stockings, but the Velcro does not expand with edema, and therefore better daily compression can be achieved with minor interval adjustments (Fig. 39.2). Less agile or obese patients find the legging easier to wear, and very athletic individuals often prefer the Circaid legging for

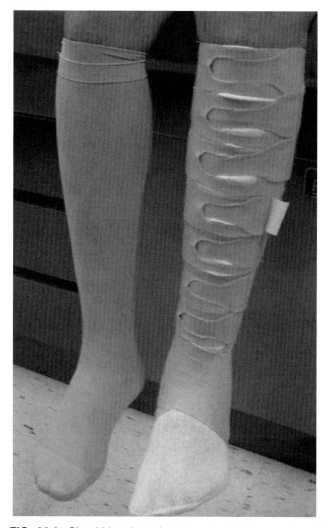

FIG. 39.2. Circaid legging, shown on the right, over class I stockings for added compression.

TABLE 39.6. *Compression therapy resources*

Company name	Product	Headquarters
Sigvaris, Inc.	Compression stockings	1119 Highway 74S Peachtree City, GA 30269
Venosan North America, Inc.	Compression stockings	PO Box 1067, Asheboro NC 27204
Beiersdorf-Jobst, Inc.	Compression stockings	5825 Carnegie Blvd. Charlotte, NC 28209
Medi USA	Compression stockings	6481 Franz Warner Parkway, Whitsett, NC
Juzo	Compression garments	PO Box 1088, Cuyahoga Falls, OH 44223
Circaid Medical Products	Sustained, nonelastic Velcro compression	9323 Chesapeake Drive, Suite B2, San Diego, CA 92123
Biocompression Systems, Inc.	Sequential gradient lymphedema pumps	120 West Commercial Avenue, Moonachie, NJ 07074
Kendall	Compression devices, T.E.D. stockings	15 Hampshire Street, Mansfield MA 02048

the added support. The market for compression stockings is enormous, and companies are eager to work with clinicians and pharmacies to establish support for venous patients (Table 39.6).

SCLEROTHERAPY

Injection of spider veins and smaller reticular veins is part of the art of medicine. Sclerotherapy of VV had its origins in World War I, when cosmetic results accompanied antisyphilis injections when given in large veins. Sotradecol became the first sclerosing agent in the United States in 1946. The sclerosing agents can vary from alcohol-based products to hypertonic saline solutions. They are divided into groups based on chemical configuration and effect, and are listed in Table 39.7. Sclerotherapy success is highly dependent on physician judgment. The vein size, skin color, and solution strength are variables to consider in treating a limb. Larger varicosities are preferentially treated with surgical phlebectomy. Sclerotherapy for the office practice is prudently confined to telangectasia and small (less than 1 mm) reticular veins. Guidelines for sclerotherapy have been published under the auspices of the American Venous Forum (18).

As with other treatments, patient selection is important, and common indications and contraindications are listed in Table 39.8. Cosmetic concerns lead many patients to seek sclerotherapy, and knowing it is not covered by insurance, they willingly pay for the service. Depending on the number of sites, the process can be staged into several office visits. Weiss and Weiss give a good discussion of techniques and

TABLE 39.7. *Sclerotherapy guidelines*

Solution	Category	Vessel	Pros[a]	Cons[a]
Polidocanol 0.25%–1.0%	Detergent	Small–medium	Painless, low complication	Awaits FDA approval
Sotradecol (sodium tetradecyl sulfate)	Detergent	All sizes	FDA approved, painless if not extravascular	Ulcerogenic at high concentration
Scleromate (sodium morrhuate)	Detergent	Small	FDA approved	Very allergenic
Ethano-lin (ethanolamine oleate)	Detergent			Not FDA approved
Hypertonic saline 11.5%–23.4%	Hyperosmolar	Small, reticular	Not allergenic	Painful, but less than with lidocaine; ulcers and pigmentation rare
Sclerodex (hypertonic saline–dextrose)	Hyperosmolar	Small	Complications rare, can mix own solution	Commercial agent, not FDA approved
Scleremo (chromated glycerine)	Chemical irritant	Small and tiny	Complications rare	Weak sclerosant, not FDA approved
Varigloban (polyiodinated iodine)	Chemical irritant	Large	Very corrosive in large veins	Not FDA approved, not for use if iodine allergy is present

[a]FDA, Food and Drug Administration.

precautions in their chapter in the *Handbook of Venous Disorders* (19). The procedure differs slightly for reticular veins and telangectasia. It involves use of a 3-cc syringe and a 27- to 30-gauge needle bent 10 to 30 deg. With the patient recumbant, the needle is inserted into a blue reticular vein and aspirated to confirm intravascular position. The injection volume is confined to 0.5 cc per site unless the reticular system is extensive. The sclerosant is injected slowly, and one can see the blood disappear. Patients must be able to wear temporary compression stockings after sclerosis of veins larger than tiny telangectasia. Compression stockings or elastic wraps suffice. It is important to be aware of possible complications and not trivialize cosmetic vein injections. A small risk of permanent discoloration due to pigmentation is possible and difficult to predict. Hyperpigmentation occurs in 10% to 30% of patients and is more frequent with Sotradecol than saline. The discoloration is due to deposition of hemosiderin in the perivascular space. It naturally dissipates in 70% of patients over 3 to 6 months. When it does not, there is no good way to lessen the discoloration, although many techniques have been tried. Another side effect is the appearance of new telangectasia adjacent to the treated site. This is called talangectasia matting. It occurs in about 15% of patients, and the risk is increased with estrogen therapy, obesity, and trauma. Most of the matting disappears with time. The worst complication is ulceration of focal necrosis. This relates to extravasation of the sclerosing agent. When it is recognized, treatment is injection of normal saline and massage at the site to dilute the subcutaneous stasis of the agent. Superficial thrombophlebitis can occur and can be treated with analgesics such as aspirin and nonsteroidal antiinflammatory medications. The tender, warm errythematous swelling should not be confused with the normal nodular fibrosis that occurs after sclerotherapy of a 4- to 8-mm varicose vein. Deep vein thrombosis and pulmonary embolism are very rare with injection of small veins. They have been associated with sclerotherapy of large veins with a large dose. Perhaps the worst complication is that of unintended arterial injection causing immediate thrombosis. Inordinate pain and ischemic blanching rapidly progressing to sharply demarcated cyanosis are the signs and symptoms indicating arterial injection. Emergency treatment aims at containing the agent (ice) and irrigation of the vessel with heparinized saline or heparin and consideration of longer-term anticoagulation (20).

Foam sclerotherapy is a relatively new and exciting form of treatment of venous disease. Foaming the sclerosing permits controlled injection with ultrasound guidance, with less risk of escape injury and more efficient closure of veins due to uniform vessel–wall contact with the agent. The procedure can be performed with ultrasound guidance and may be extended to treatment of the saphenous vein in the near future. A 10-year prospective, randomized, controlled trial with surgery and standard sclerotherapy suggests foam technique may be an acceptable alternative with comparable long-term results (21).

A brief mention of laser therapy will help address questions from patients with visible venous disease. This is not a treatment for venous hypertension caused by reflux. Some patients have a phobia of needles, and laser treatment is an alternative therapy for cosmetic ablation of telangectasia and small reticular veins. The safety and efficacy of 1,064-nm neodymium:yttrium aluminum garnet laser with 10- to 20-msec pulses have shown this approach to have promise. It penetrates up to 5 mm for treatment of reticular veins and has an affinity for deoxyhemoglobin represented by the purplish spider veins. The ideal site for laser/pulsed light is small, shallow, oxygenated telangectasia on the face. Although epidermal injury is less with the 1,064-nm wavelength, evolution of this treatment option is ongoing. Injection of sclerosing agent remains quicker, albeit invasive (19).

AMBULATORY PHLEBECTOMY

Surgical phlebectomy has long been combined with high ligation of the saphenous vein with and without saphenous removal. It is now combined with catheter-directed therapies as the same adjunctive technique for removal of veins too large for schelrotherapy. The practice of mini incisions and stab avulsion phlebectomy was introduced 1975, and since then, many instruments have been designed by various surgeons for percutaneous removal of varicosities (22). The varicose veins are marked on the skin with permanent ink while the patient is standing. With the patient in Trendelenburg position, 2- to 3-mm incisions are made with an 11 blade parallel to the axis of the vein to prevent entering it. The flat side of the hook is passed under the vein until the hook can be rotated toward the skin. The vein is pulled toward the opening with countertension placed on the surface. Gentle tugging and a twisting motion allow avulsion of the vein while the internal ends retract. Focal compression is applied, and compression stockings or firm elastic wraps are maintained for several weeks. Local anesthesia can be used, and antibiotics are not indicated. Bruising and pain are minimized with compliant compression stocking use after the procedure.

SAPHENOUS VEIN ABLATION

Minimally invasive endovascular intervention has proven safe and effective for elimination of the incompetent greater

TABLE 39.8. *Patient selection for sclerotherapy[a]*

Contraindications	Indications
Pregnancy (first and second trimesters)	Pain
Allergy to a given sclerosant	Cosmetic
Obesity	Selected perforator reflux
Deep vein thrombosis or trauma	Tributaries of GSV or LSV
Arterial ischemia peripheral vascular disease	Lateral system webs 1–2 mm
Reflux at the SFJ	
Nonambulatory patient	

[a]GSV, Greater saphenous vein; LSV, lesser saphenous vein; SFJ, saphenofemoral junction.

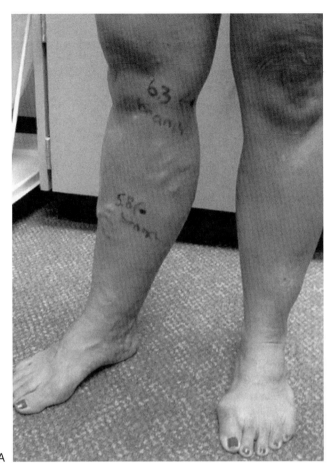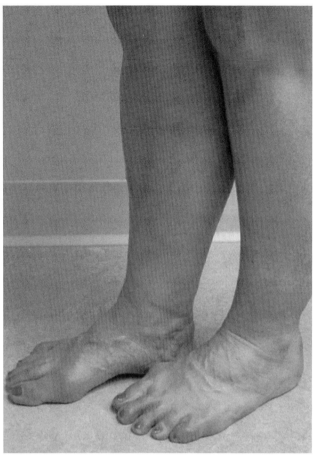

A   B

FIG. 39.3. (A) Before and **(B)** 1-year follow-up images of painful, medial calf varicosities treated with radiofrequency ablation procedure in a 36-year-old aerobics instructor.

saphenous vein (23). Catheter-directed ablation is considered an alternative to surgical vein stripping in carefully selected patients (Fig. 39.3) (24,25). Large, randomized studies have not been performed. It appears that patient preference for minimally invasive therapies is a significant factor in the number of interventions performed. Patients undergoing saphenous vein removal or ablation without preoperative evaluation to exclude venous obstruction can develop complications including intractable stasis ulcers. If postthrombotic venous insufficiency is present, the performance of subfascial endoscopic perforator vein surgery and saphenous ablation remains controversial (26). The procedures are now combined with perforator ligation and/or ambulatory phlebectomy as clinically indicated. Advantages over traditional surgery include less bruising and discomfort, prompt return to normal activities, and outpatient status for a relatively short procedure performed with conscious sedation and local anesthesia (27).

There are two Food and Drug Administration-approved devices for this procedure. The radiofrequency device is the Closure System (VNUS Medical Technologies Inc., San Jose, CA). This is a dedicated, computer-controlled, bipolar generator with sheath-contained electrode probes on a 6 or 8 French catheter. Chandler et al. reported on nearly 300

radiofrequency-treated limbs with a mean follow-up of 4.9 months (25). Twenty-one of 290 successfully treated veins (7.2%) had recanalization of greater than 5 cm of the vein, but there was only a 3.8% incidence of reflux (25). They also noted that the average 3- to 5-year incidence of recurrent varicosities and reflux after surgery was 28% and 26%, respectively, following saphenectomy, and 64% and 49%, respectively, following high ligation. Therefore, reduction in the incidence of recurrent reflux and varicosities are the key clinical outcomes to monitor to gauge success of these new procedures. Weiss and Weiss reported excellent patient acceptance and clinical results with 2-year follow-up (27).

The laser device is the Endovascular Laser Venous System (ELVS; Angiodynamics Inc., Queensbury, NY). The system employs a Precision 810 and a Precision 980 fiber-coupled diode laser, which delivers 15 W of optical power. Min reported on the evolution of laser ablation (28). At the 28th annual meeting of the Society of Interventional Radiology, Min reported on 305 patients who underwent laser ablation of the greater saphenous vein. Successful closure was achieved in 97%, and 298 of 304 (98%) had documented closure at 3- to 30-month follow-up (29). Both systems claim advantages over traditional surgery including short procedure time and prompt return to normal activities after an outpatient procedure performed in the clinic or angiography suite with conscious sedation and local anesthesia. There is reportedly less postoperative pain, bruising, and scarring than with traditional surgical vein stripping (25,27,28).

Veins that measure between 2 and 15 mm in supine diameter can be treated. The Closure catheter can be used over the wire or with a guiding sheath. Alternatively, each catheter can be separately passed through the saphenous vein through a short introducer sheath placed near the ankle or below the knee. Most procedures are performed with ultrasound guidance, but fluoroscopic localization of the proximal valve and starting point is available and easier in some labs. When the starting point just below the saphenofemoral valve is located, the probe is engaged and slowly pulled back to treat the saphenous vein to the level of the medial condyle. Tumescent anesthesia, with in the saphenous fascia, is used to cushion the dermis and the nerve from the heat. The techniques vary, with some using Esmarch compression wraps and others using just tumescent anesthesia. The goal is complete collapse of the vein with no flow and no thrombus. This can be confirmed immediately after withdrawal of the catheter. Following removal of the sheath, class II compression panty-

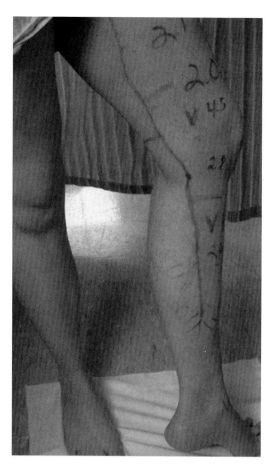

FIG. 39.5. Mapping of greater saphenous with ultrasound prior to percutaneous ablation outpatient procedure.

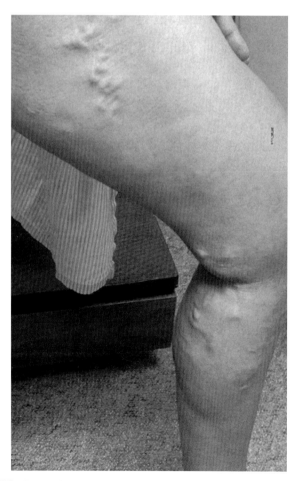

FIG. 39.4. Medial varicose veins due to greater saphenous reflux.

hose is worn for 1 to 2 weeks. Both legs can be treated at one sitting if necessary. The systems cost about $30,000 to $35,000 for the generator and between $600 and $1,000 for the disposable catheter. Insurance reimbursement for the procedure is available through Medicare and private third-party payors.

Selecting a patient for catheter ablation requires documentation of saphenofemoral reflux, determination of large tributaries, and exclusion of DVT (Figs. 39.4 and 39.5). Patients without a history of DVT, but a known hypercoagulable state, such as factor V Leiden, may be treated prophylactically with low-molecular weight heparin. Very large patients are not good candidates because it is harder to obtain sufficient compression of the upper thigh to assure proper vessel wall contact with the probe. Complications include bruising and discomfort, but these are both very mild compared to surgical stripping. Patients are immediately ambulatory and may return to normal activities. Follow-up ultrasound in 1 to 2 weeks is recommended to confirm ablation of the greater saphenous vein and absence of thrombus near the saphenofemoral junction. A low incidence of saphenous vein neuropathy will occur because 10% of the population has a duplicate or recurrent saphenous nerve that may be injured. The focal medial thigh numbness that accompanies this injury usually dissipates over time, but may persist in a minority of affected individuals.

SUMMARY

Management of venous disease is becoming a specialty among vascular interventionalists, but all physicians should recognize it. Unfortunately, they do not. It is common for patients to ignore venous disease as well. The medical community has not proactively treated venous disorders, and patients often accept leg discomfort and swelling as part of growing older and not exercising. The lower extremity heaviness and fatigue develop slowly and become familiar. Patients adjust their lifestyle and do not always recognize the impact of leg problems on their quality of life (30). This is seen with both arterial and venous conditions. As in all areas of vascular intervention, patient selection is a key to good clinical outcomes. If the clinician recognizes venous disease, even inexpensive, conservative treatment such as properly fitting compression stockings can significantly help patients with mild conditions. There is opportunity to provide an important clinical service by providing care for venous problems because they are so prevalent in an aging society. Clinicians must observe limbs for signs and symptoms of venous disease to treat or refer patients for further care. This is truly our responsibility given the immense socioeconomic impact of untreated venous disease.

REFERENCES

1. Ricotta JJ, Dalsing MC, Ouriel K, et al. Research and clinical issues in chronic venous disease. *Cardiovasc Surg* 1997;5:343–349.
2. Tran NT, Meissner MH. The epidemiology, pathophysiology, and natural history of chronic venous disease. *Semin Vasc Surg* 2002;15(1):5–12.
3. Callan, MJ. Epidemiology of varicose veins. *Br J Surg* 1994;81:167–173.
4. Hume M. Venous ulcers, the vascular surgeon and the Medicare budget. *J Vasc Surg* 1992;16:5:671–673.
5. Weiss, RA, Feided CF, Weiss M. *Vein diagnosis and treatment.* New York: McGraw-Hill, 2001.
6. Bergan JJ. Causes of venous varicosities and telangectasias; implications for treatment. *J Vasc Biol Med* 1995;85:1101–1106.
7. Friedman, SG. *A history of vascular surgery.* Mount Kisko, NY: Futura, 1989.
8. Killowich LA, Bedford GR, Beach KW, et al. Diagnosis of deep vein thrombosis. A prospective study comparing duplex scanning to contrast venography. *Circulation* 1989;79:810–814.
9. Nicolaides AN, Eklof B, Bergan JJ, et al. Classification and grading of chronic venous disease in the lower limbs: a consensus statement. *Phlebology* 1995;10:42–45.
10. Marston WA. PPG, APG, duplex: which noninvasive tests are most appropriate for the management of patients with chronic venous insufficiency? *Semin Vasc Surg* 2002;15(1):13–20.
11. Bradbury A, Evans C, Allan P, et al. What are the symptoms of varicose veins? Edinburgh Vein Study Cross Sectional Population Survey. *Br Med J* 1999;318:353–356.
12. Bergan JJ, Kumins NH, Owens EL, et al. Surgical and endovascular treatment of lower extremity venous insufficiency. *J Vasc Interv Radiol* 2002;13:563–568.
13. Porter JP, Rutherford RB, Clagett GP, et al. Reporting standards in venous disease. *J Vasc Surg* 1988;8:172–181.
14. Porter JP, Moneta GM, and an International Consensus Committee on Chronic Venous Disease. Reporting standards in venous disease: an update. *J Vasc Surg* 1995;21:635–645.
15. Rutherford RB, Padberg Jr FT, Comerota AJ, et al. Venous severity scoring: an adjunct to venous outcome assessment. *J Vasc Surg* 2000;31:1307–1312.
16. Meissner MH, Natiello C, Nicholls SC. Performance characteristics of the venous clinical severity score. *J Vasc Surg* 2002;36:889–895.
17. Bergan JJ. Prospects for minimal invasion in venous disease. *Vasc Surg* 1999;33:247–250.
18. Villavicencio JL. Sclerotherapy guidelines. In: Glovicski P, Yao JT, eds., *Handbook of venous disorders,* 2nd ed. New York: Oxford University Press, 2001:253–266.
19. Weiss RA, Weiss MA. Sclerotherapy of telangectasia. In: Glovicski P, Yao JT, eds., *Handbook of Venous Disorders,* 2nd ed., New York: Oxford University Press, 2001:268–277.
20. Goldman MP. Complications of sclerotherapy. In: Glovicski P, Yao JT, eds., *Handbook of Venous Disorders,* 2nd ed. New York: Oxford University Press, 2001:278–288.
21. Belcaro G, Cesarone MR, DiRenzo A, et al. Foam-sclerotherapy, surgery, sclerotherapy, and combined treatment for varicose veins: a 10-year, prospective, randomized, controlled trial (VEDICO Trial). *Angiology* 2003:54;307–315.
22. Bergan JJ. Varicose veins: hooks, clamps, and suction. Application of new techniques to enhance varicose vein surgery. *Semin Vasc Surg* 2002;15(1):21–26.
23. Harris EJ. Radiofrequency ablation of the long saphenous vein without high ligation versus high ligation and stripping for primary varicose veins: pros and cons. *Semin Vasc Surg* 2002;15(1):34–38.
24. Meissner MH. Overview: the management of lower extremity venous problems. *Semin Vasc Surg* 2002;15(1):1–4.
25. Chandler JG, Pichot O, Sessa C, et al. Treatment of primary venous insufficiency by endovenous saphenous vein obliteration. *Vasc Surg* 2000:34;201–214.
26. Kalra M, Gloviczki P. Subfascial endoscopic perforator vein surgery: who benefits? *Semin Vasc Surg* 2002;15(1):39–49.
27. Weiss RA, Weiss MA. Controlled radiofrequency endovenous occlusion using a unique radiofrequency catheter under duplex guidance to eliminate saphenous varicose vein reflux: 2-year follow-up. *Dermatol Surg* 2002;29:38–42.
28. Min RJ. Endovenous laser treatment of the incompetent greater saphenous vein. *J Vasc Interv Radiol* 2001;12:1167–1171.
29. Min RJ. Percutanous techniques for treatment of saphenous vein reflux: endovenous laser. *J Vasc Interv Radiol* 2003;S1–S197 14:12–13.
30. Lamping DL, Schroter S, Kurz X, et al. Evaluation of outcomes in chronic venous disorders of the leg: development of a scientifically rigorous, patient-reported measure of symptoms and quality of life. *J Vasc Surg* 2003;37:410–419.

CHAPTER 40

Pulmonary Arterial Hypertension

Vallerie V. McLaughlin

Key Points

- Pulmonary arterial hypertension is defined as a mean pulmonary artery pressure greater than 25 mm Hg, a pulmonary capillary wedge pressure less than 15 mm Hg, and a pulmonary vascular resistance greater than 3 Wood units.
- Pulmonary arterial hypertension results from endothelial proliferation and dysfunction, an imbalance of vasoconstrictors and vasodilators, and an imbalance of cell proliferation and apoptosis.
- Right ventricular function is the main determinant of survival in pulmonary arterial hypertension.
- Heart catheterization is required to establish the diagnosis, guide the appropriate therapy, and determine the prognosis.
- Continuous intravenous epoprostenol therapy improves symptoms, exercise tolerance, hemodynamics, and survival in patients with advanced pulmonary arterial hypertension.
- Oral endothelin antagonists improve exercise tolerance in patients with pulmonary arterial hypertension.

CLASSIFICATION AND EPIDEMIOLOGY OF PULMONARY HYPERTENSION

Pulmonary hypertension is a complex syndrome, which may result from a variety of different diseases. The classification of pulmonary hypertension has recently been revised by the World Health Organization (WHO), and is displayed in Table 40.1. (1). Category 1, pulmonary arterial hypertension (PAH), is the focus of this chapter. Diseases of the left heart, such as left ventricular dysfunction, hypertensive heart disease, and aortic or mitral valve disease, can elevate pulmonary artery pressure by raising left atrial pressure. This represents pulmonary venous hypertension, and treatment should be directed at the underlying left heart pathology. Although common, pulmonary venous hypertension is not the focus of this chapter and will not be discussed further. Diseases of lung parenchyma, such as emphysema and pulmonary fibrosis, may cause mild to moderate pulmonary hypertension, and constitute WHO category 3. The only treatment ade-

quately studied in this patient population is continuous oxygen therapy. Also included in WHO category 3 is sleep apnea, which is not uncommonly associated with pulmonary hypertension. Chronic thromboembolic pulmonary hypertension (WHO category 4) may present with symptoms and hemodynamic findings similar to pulmonary arterial hypertension. Chronic thromboembolic pulmonary hypertension is perhaps the one surgically curable form of pulmonary hypertension, and although the management of this disorder is beyond the scope of this chapter, the importance of evaluating pulmonary hypertension patients for thromboembolic disease will be emphasized. Disorders directly affecting the pulmonary vasculature such as schistosomiasis and sarcoidosis may also result in pulmonary hypertension.

Included in category 1 pulmonary arterial hypertension (PAH) is primary pulmonary hypertension (PPH). Primary pulmonary hypertension is a rare disease, with a prevalence of approximately two cases per million. In the National Institutes of Health (NIH) Registry on PPH, the ratio of women

TABLE 40.1. *Classification of pulmonary hypertension*

Pulmonary arterial hypertension
    Primary pulmonary hypertension
        Sporadic
        Familial
    Related to
        Collagen vascular disease
        Congenital systemic to pulmonary shunts
        Portal hypertension
        Human immunodeficiency virus infection
        Anorexigens
        Persistent pulmonary hypertension of the newborn
Pulmonary venous hypertension
Pulmonary hypertension associated with disorders of
    the respiratory system and/or hypoxemia
Pulmonary hypertension due to chronic thrombotic
    and/or embolic disease
Pulmonary hypertension due to disorders directly
    affecting the pulmonary vasculature

From Rich S, ed. Primary pulmonary hypertension, executive summary from the World Symposium, Primary Pulmonary Hypertension 1998. Available from the World Health Organization at http://www.who.int/ncd/cvd/pph.html, with permission.

to men was 1.7:1 and the mean age at the time of diagnosis was 36 ± 15 years (2). Although most cases are considered sporadic, the gene for familial PPH has recently been identified. It is located on chromosome 2 and encodes for the bone morphogenetic protein II receptor. The familial form of PPH has two unique features, genetic anticipation, with the disease occurring earlier and earlier with each generation, and variable penetrance, with a 10% to 20% chance of expressing the phenotype if the gene is inherited. In the NIH registry, 6% of cases were thought to be familial (2). More recent series have suggested that 12% of PPH patients are familial, and the true incidence is likely even higher (3).

The pulmonary vessel histopathology of PPH is indistinguishable from that of a number of known causes of pulmonary hypertension, such as congenital heart disease, anorexigen use, human immunodeficiency virus (HIV) infection, portopulmonary hypertension, and collagen vascular disease. Additionally, response to treatment of pulmonary hypertension in these disease entities is often similar to that in PPH. Therefore, these entities were placed in WHO category 1. The identical endothelial pathology strongly suggests that the changes in the pulmonary vessels are the final, common pathway for endothelial injury, which can be precipitated by a variety of causes, some of which are known and others of which are not. Pulmonary arterial hypertension may complicate the course of any collagen vascular disease; however, it occurs most frequently in limited scleroderma (the CREST variant). Pulmonary arterial hypertension may occur in association with any systemic to pulmonary shunts, such as atrial septal defects, ventricular septal defects, and patent ductus arteriosus. It may also complicate more complex congenital heart disease. In some cases, patients may present with PAH years after corrective surgery. The incidence of PAH is elevated in those with portal hypertension. Among patients being evaluated for liver transplantation, up to 4% have significant PAH. Because the perioperative mortality is substantial in such patients, preoperative identification of PAH in liver transplant candidates is essential. The incidence of PAH is also elevated in those infected with HIV. Epidemiologic studies have suggested that the incidence of PAH in the HIV population is in the range of 0.5% to 2%. Pulmonary arterial hypertension may complicate HIV at any stage in the course of the disease. Once PAH develops, prognosis is similar to the prognosis of PPH patients. The ingestion of anorexigens is clearly linked to the development of PAH, and the risk increases with the duration of anorexigen use. The causal agents, fenfluramines and dexfenfluramines, were taken off the market in the United States in September 1997.

PATHOGENESIS

The pathology of the pulmonary vessels in PAH is complex and poorly understood. Endothelial cell proliferation is a hallmark of the disease, but it is not known at what stage of the disease this process occurs. The reduction in endogenous vasodilators (nitric oxide and prostacyclin) and the increase in endogenous vasoconstrictors (endothelin and thromboxane) are integral to the pathogenesis of the disease, and represent the basis of available therapies. Researchers have demonstrated a loss of prostacyclin synthase enzyme and gene expression in the pulmonary vessels of patients with PPH, and it has been demonstrated that patients with PPH have decreased prostacyclin production (4). It is not clear whether this is a cause or an effect. Endothelial cell nitric oxide synthase production is also reduced, and correlates inversely with the extent and severity of the histologic lesions (5). Similarly, endothelin-1 expression is inversely related to nitric oxide synthase (6). Classically, PAH has been characterized by the presence of the plexiform lesion, which is a mass of disorganized vessels with proliferating endothelial cells, smooth muscle cells, myofibroblast, and macrophages. The voltage-regulated (Kv) potassium channel in smooth muscle has been demonstrated to be abnormal in the pulmonary arteries of patients with PPH, resulting in vasoconstriction (7).

In situ small-vessel thrombosis may be an additional contributing factor to the cause or propagation of PAH. Abnormalities in platelet activation and function occur, and biochemical markers of a procoagulant environment are present. Thrombosis may play an important role involving growth factors, platelets, and the vessel wall in many of the proposed processes in the cause and/or progression of the disease. Increased shear stress caused by elevated pressure and/or flow may initiate PAH, as seen in congenital cardiovascular shunts. Increased shear forces on the endothelial cell probably cause the release of mediators that induce vascular smooth

TABLE 40.2. *National Institutes of Health presenting symptoms from primary pulmonary hypertension*

	Initial (%)	Eventual (%)
Dyspnea	60	98
Fatigue	19	73
Chest pain	7	47
Near syncope	5	41
Syncope	8	36
Edema	3	37

muscle growth, which results in remodeling of the pulmonary arteries.

CLINICAL PRESENTATIONS

Pulmonary hypertension is an insidious killer. By the time symptoms occur, the disease is usually very advanced; without treatment, death often occurs in less than 3 years. Even when symptoms appear, they are often nonspecific, such as breathlessness and chest pain, and because the patients are often young and otherwise healthy, they are discounted by both patient and physician. The NIH registry recorded presenting symptoms in 187 patients diagnosed with PPH (Table 40.2) (2). Dyspnea was by far the most common presenting symptom, occurring in 60% of patients, and virtually all of the patients developed this symptom during the course of the disease. Fatigue, chest pain, and syncope were other common presenting symptoms. Peripheral edema and fatigue were present in patients who had advanced disease and were experiencing right heart failure. In addition, chest pain, syncope, and palpitations became more frequent as the disease progressed. The nonspecific nature of the symptoms is one reason the disease may go undiagnosed for months to years. In the NIH registry, the average time from the onset of symptoms until the diagnosis was more than 2 1/2 years.

The physical findings in early pulmonary hypertension are subtle, such as increased intensity in P2 and a right ventricular lift. As the disease advances, nearly all patients develop the murmur of tricuspid regurgitation. Pulmonary regurgitation is less common. A right-sided, fourth heart sound is quite common, and reflective of reduced right ventricular compliance. Reduced carotid pulse volumes are a result of low cardiac output. Once right ventricular failure ensues, peripheral edema is common, as is distension of the neck veins with prominent a and v waves in the jugular pulse. Late in the disease, a prominent right-sided third heart sound develops, and sometimes ascites occurs.

The natural history of PAH is generally one of progressive decline. Historically, predictors of poor survival include advance functional class, hemodynamic parameters such as high right atrial pressure, low cardiac output, high mean pulmonary artery pressure, and low exercise tolerance (8).

DIAGNOSTIC EVALUATION

A number of diagnostic modalities provide useful information about patients with PAH. Early in the disease process, the electrocardiogram (ECG) may be normal, but by the time the patient is symptomatic, the QRS complex usually demonstrates right axis deviation and right ventricular enlargement. Other ECG abnormalities include right atrial enlargement and right bundle-branch block (Fig. 40.1). Arrythmias are very uncommon in this disease, but occasionally supraventricular tachycardias are encountered.

When PAH is mild, the chest radiograph is often normal. Moderate pulmonary hypertension usually produces some enlargement of main and proximal pulmonary arteries. When the pulmonary hypertension is advanced, in addition to pulmonary artery dilation, the right atrium and ventricle are also enlarged, producing cardiomegaly. Right ventricular enlargement is most easily appreciated on the lateral chest radiograph as reduction in retrosternal air space. Extensive parenchymal

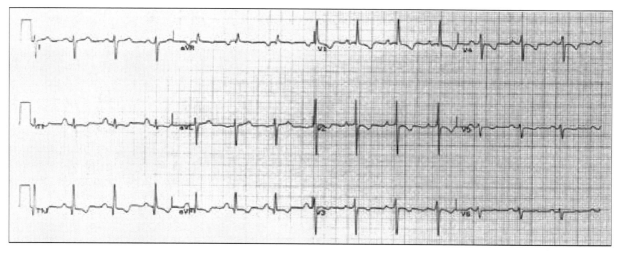

FIG. 40.1. Electrocardiogram demonstrating right atrial enlargement, right ventricular enlargement, right axis deviation, and right bundle-branch block.

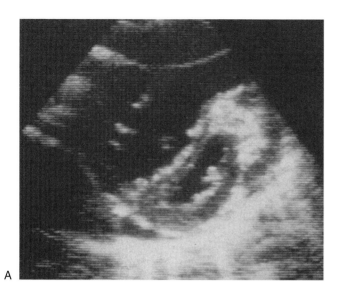
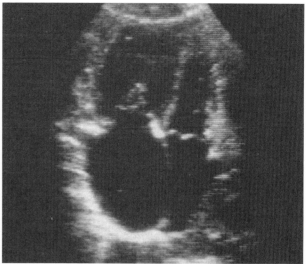

FIG. 40.2. A: Echocardiogram demonstrating right atrial and ventricular enlargement and flattening of the intraventricular septum; parasternal short axis view. **B:** Echocardiogram demonstrating right atrial and ventricular enlargement and flattening of the intraventricular septum; apical four-chamber view.

lung disease, especially fibrosis, indicates that it is the likely cause of the pulmonary hypertension. Massively enlarged pulmonary arteries may be associated with PAH related to a congenital systemic to pulmonary shunt.

Evaluating exercise performance is useful for objectively determining the effect of pharmacologic therapy and prognosis. The 6-minute walk is most commonly employed because of its ease of performance and lack of need for specialized equipment. The 6-minute walk test has served as the primary endpoint in the majority of the trials of pharmacologic agents in PAH. Modified treadmill protocols may also be useful, particularly in patients with less advance symptoms. Formal cardiopulmonary exercise testing with continuous measure of lung and arterial oxygen and carbon dioxide concentrations may also be useful, and correlates with survival (9).

Echocardiography is an extremely valuable diagnostic tool for evaluating the patient with suspected PAH. If there is significant elevation in pulmonary pressure, the right atrium and right ventricle are usually dilated (Fig. 40.2). The more severe the elevation of pressure and/or the longer it is present, the greater is the dilation. Flattening of the intraventricular septum during systole and diastole indicates right ventricular pressure and volume overload, respectively. Once pulmonary pressure is elevated, tricuspid regurgitation is nearly always present, and allows for calculation of the right ventricular systolic pressure. Errors in the echocardiographic assessment of pulmonary artery pressures may occur, and may result in both overestimation and underestimation of the pulmonary artery pressures. The echocardiogram is also useful for excluding left heart causes of the pulmonary hypertension, such as left ventricular dysfunction or mitral valve disease. It may also detect congenital cardiovascular shunts that may provoke PAH. The injection of intravenous agitated saline may uncover such a defect.

Radioisotope ventilation perfusion scanning or spiral computed tomography imaging is required for all patients with newly diagnosed pulmonary hypertension to exclude pulmonary thromboembolism as a cause. Symptomatic pulmonary hypertension due to thromboembolism is virtually always associated with a very abnormal lung scan, showing large areas of hypoperfusion (Fig. 40.3). Minor perfusion abnormalities are common in PAH, but are rarely confused with the large defects caused by thromboembolic disease (10). An abnormal ventilation perfusion scan warrants further evaluation with a pulmonary angiogram. Angiographic

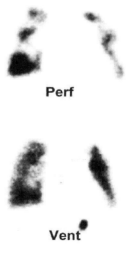

FIG. 40.3. Lung scan demonstrating multiple mismatched perfusion defects, typical of chronic thromboembolic disease. Vent, Ventilation; perf, perfusion.

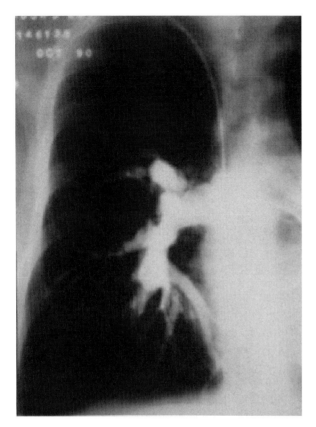

FIG. 40.4. Typical angiographic abnormalities in chronic thromboembolic pulmonary hypertension. Note abrupt cutoffs and webbing with poor distal perfusion.

signs of chronic thromboembolic disease include vessel cutoffs, webs, and pouching (Fig. 40.4). Patients with chronic thromboembolic pulmonary hypertension should be referred to a center with expertise in pulmonary thromboendarterectomy.

Pulmonary function testing should be performed as part of the initial evaluation of the patient with newly diagnosed pulmonary hypertension to exclude parenchymal lung disease as the cause. Pulmonary function tests are relatively normal in patients with PPH. Some patients may demonstrate mild-to-moderate reduction in diffusion capacity (2). Oxygen saturation is usually normal in patients with PPH. Significant desaturation suggests intracardiac shunting due either to congenital heart disease or a patent foramen ovale. Patients with PAH related to scleroderma tend to have a reduction in diffusing capacity of carbon monoxide, even before the onset of PAH symptoms. A reduction in diffusing capacity of carbon monoxide to vital capacity ratio suggests that pulmonary vascular disease is a more like cause of dyspnea than interstitial fibrosis in the scleroderma population.

Cardiac catheterization remains the cornerstone for making the diagnosis of PAH. Right heart catheterization documents the pulmonary artery pressure, cardiac output, and pulmonary vascular resistance. Right atrial pressure is also measured; this and cardiac output are the most important de-

terminants of prognosis (8). The NIH registry demonstrated that cardiac indices less than 2.0 L per minute per m² and right atrial pressures equal to or greater than 20 mm Hg were associated with an extremely shortened life expectancy. Cardiac catheterization also identifies any intracardiac shunts and evidence of other structural abnormalities. It is crucial to obtain an adequate pulmonary capillary wedge pressure, or, if necessary, a left ventricular end diastolic pressure. If elevated (greater than 15 mm Hg), the diagnosis is pulmonary venous hypertension, and the patient should be treated accordingly. At the time of diagnostic catheterization, it is important to test vascular reactivity because it is very useful in determining the best treatment strategy (11). Hemodynamic measurements are made before and during prostacyclin or adenosine infusion or nitric oxide inhalation. A substantial reduction in mean pulmonary artery pressure to near normal levels is considered to be a good indicator of a favorable response to oral calcium channel blocker therapy. A consensus on the definition of a "response" to an acute vasodilator has recently been agreed on and will be presented in upcoming guidelines from the European Society of Cardiology and the American College of Chest Physicians. A response is defined as a reduction in mean pulmonary artery pressure of at least 20% and at least 10 mm Hg, to a value of less than 35 mm Hg (12).

MANAGEMENT

Conventional Therapies

Diuretics are frequently used to reduce excessive edema in patients with right heart failure. They are particularly useful when hepatic congestion, ascites, and edema are present. In refractory cases, more than one diuretic is required. In some instances, patients must be treated with intravenous diuretics. Digoxin can increase cardiac output and reduce circulating neurohormones (13). It is sometimes used in those with a low cardiac output, but cannot be strongly recommended. Anticoagulant therapy has been associated with an improved survival in one prospective and one retrospective study (14,15). In patients who were nonresponders to calcium channel blockers, a significant improvement in survival was noted in those treated with anticoagulants, with a survival of 91%, 62%, and 47% after 1, 2, and 3 years, respectively, compared to 52%, 31%, and 31%, respectively, in patients who did not receive anticoagulants (15). Although the effectiveness of warfarin anticoagulation in patients with PAH has never been tested in a prospective randomized long-term trial, based on the known pathogenesis of PAH and the data, the use of low-dose warfarin maintaining an international normalized ratio of 2.0 to 2.5 times control is recommended. The benefit of warfarin is most clearly established in those with PPH; however, in the absence of a contraindication, it is commonly used in individuals with other forms of PAH. Patients with hypoxemia (oxygen saturation less than 90%), either at rest or with exercise, should receive supplemental oxygen.

Calcium Channel Blockers

Although many drugs have been utilized for vasodilation in the setting of PPH, calcium channel blockers have been most widely tested for this purpose, and have appeared to produce a more consistent reduction in pulmonary artery pressure and pulmonary vascular resistance than other vasodilators. The literature suggests that approximately 25% of patients with PPH will respond to calcium channel blockers; however, this is an overestimation. Response to calcium channel blockers is rare in patients with other types of PAH. Of a group of 17 patients who responded to high-dose calcium channel blockers, Rich et al. reported a 94% 5-year survival rate, compared to a 36% survival rate among patients who did not respond to therapy (15). Diltiazem and nifedipine were the calcium channel blockers used in this study. Calcium channel blockers with negative inotropic effects such as verapamil should be avoided. Because of the dramatic impact that this therapy has had on patients who respond, most patients with PPH should be considered for acute vasodilator testing to determine if calcium channel blockers would be warranted. Calcium channel blockers must be used with great caution. Some patients such as those who are clinically unstable should not be challenged. Calcium channel blockers should almost always be instituted with invasive hemodynamic guidance. An increase in right atrial pressure and/or a decline in cardiac output warrants discontinuation of therapy. When used without the benefit of hemodynamic monitoring, calcium channel blockers may worsen right ventricular failure and potentially cause premature death. Patients who respond should receive a long-term treatment with the appropriate dose of calcium channel blockers, but still require careful follow-up to monitor both the safety and the efficacy of treatment. Patients who initially tolerate calcium channel blockers but subsequently deteriorate should have them discontinued.

Prostacyclin (Epoprostenol) and Prostacylin Analogues

Prostacyclin is a metabolite of arachidonic acid, and is produced primarily in the vascular endothelium. Patients with PPH have a reduction in prostacyclin synthase (16). The major pharmacologic actions of prostacyclin include potent vasodilation of the pulmonary and systemic arterial and venous beds and inhibition of platelet aggregation. Chronic effects likely include pulmonary vascular remodeling and positive inotropic effects. Intravenous prostacyclin (epoprostenol, Flolan) is commercially available. Prostacyclin analogues include treprostinil, beraprost, and iloprost, which are administered by subcutaneous, oral, and inhalation routes, respectively.

Intravenous Prostacyclin (Epoprostenol, Flolan)

In 1996, Barst et al. reported the results of a prospective randomized, multicenter, open trial comparing the effects of continuous intravenous epoprostenol plus conventional ther-

apy with that of conventional therapy alone in 81 patients with New York Heart Association Functional class III or IV PPH (17). The primary endpoint of distance walked in 6 minutes improved in the 41 patients treated with epoprostenol (from 315 m at baseline to 362 m at 12 weeks), whereas it decreased in the 40 patients treated with conventional therapy alone (270 m at baseline compared to 204 m at 12 weeks). There were also improvements in hemodynamic parameters. Mean changes in pulmonary vascular resistance in the epoprostenol and control groups were –21% and +9%, respectively ($p > 0.001$). There was also a significant difference in survival; 8 patients died during the study, all of whom had been randomly assigned to the conventional therapy group ($p = 0.003$). A similar trial in patients with PAH related to the scleroderma spectrum of diseases also demonstrated an improvement in exercise tolerance and hemodynamics with epoprostenol (18). We reported our long-term results of epoprostenol therapy in 27 patients with PPH over a period of 16.7 months (19). Twenty-six patients had improvement in symptoms and hemodynamic parameters. The mean pulmonary artery pressure decreased by 20% and the pulmonary vascular resistance decreased by 53% compared to baseline. In addition, the long-term effects of epoprostenol exceeded the acute pulmonary vasodilator response achieved in all but 1 patient. Importantly, even patients with little or no response to acute vasodilator testing at the time of cardiac catheterization experienced a substantial reduction in pulmonary vascular resistance after long-term therapy with epoprostenol.

More recently, long-term survival data with epoprostenol therapy in the setting of PPH has been described in two large cohorts. We studied 162 consecutive patients diagnosed with PPH and treated with epoprostenol for a mean of 3 years (range 1 month to 10 years) (3). The observed survival with epoprostenol therapy at 1, 2, and 3 years was 87.8%, 76.3%, and 62.8%, respectively, and was significantly greater than the expected survival of 58.9%, 46.3%, and 35.4%, respectively, based on historical data from the NIH registry (Fig. 40.5). In a group of 178 patients with PPH treated with epoprostenol and followed for a mean of 26 months (range 0.5 to 98 months), Sitbon et al. observed a survival at 1, 2, and 3 years of 85%, 70%, and 63%, respectively (Fig. 40.6) (20). Both groups found the survival of patients who were functional class III at the time of institution of epoprostenol therapy to be significantly greater than that of patients who were functional class IV at the time of initiation of epoprostenol therapy. Univariate predictors of survival in our study included functional class, exercise test duration, baseline right atrial pressure, and change in pulmonary vascular resistance with vasodilator challenge. Both groups demonstrated that the response to epoprostenol after a short period of time (3 to 18 months) was predictive of long-term survival. Patients who had improved to functional class I or II with epoprostenol had an excellent subsequent long-term survival. The subsequent survival for patients who remained functional class III or IV despite therapy with epoprostenol was ominous.

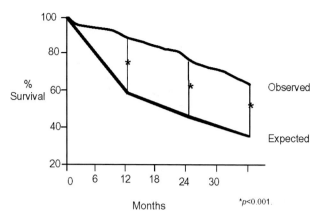

FIG. 40.5. Survival observed in 162 epoprostenol-treated primary pulmonary hypertension patients versus expected survival based on the National Institutes of Health registry equation. (Adapted from McLaughlin VV, Shillington A, Rich S. Survival in primary pulmonary hypertension: the impact of epoprostenol therapy. *Circulation* 2002;106:1466–1482, with permission.)

Epoprostenol is administered through a permanent intravenous catheter and delivered by an ambulatory infusion system. The delivery system is complex, and requires the patients to learn the techniques of sterile preparation of the medication, operation of the ambulatory infusion pump, and care of the permanent intravenous catheter. Side effects related to epoprostenol therapy are common and include headache, flushing, nausea, diarrhea, and an unusual type of jaw discomfort, which occurs with the first bite or two of a meal. Other chronic side effects include thrombocytopenia, weight loss, foot pain, gastropathy, and ascites. In most patients, the symptoms are minimal and well tolerated. Other complications related to epoprostenol therapy include infection of the central venous catheter and interruptions of therapy. The expected local central line infection rate is in the range of 0.22 to 0.68 per patient per year, and that of bacteremia is 0.14 to 0.39 per patient per year (3,17–20). Even a brief interruption in therapy can result in rebound pulmonary hypertension and has been fatal in some instances. Catheter thrombosis is a rare

event. Epoprostenol is very expensive. In the United States, the average cost is $60,000 per year.

Dosing of epoprostenol is problematic. Early on it was noted that tolerance to the beneficial effects of epoprostenol seemed to occur. This led to the practice of clinicians progressively increasing the dose in anticipation of symptoms. In 1999, we made the observation that patients treated with chronic epoprostenol therapy may suffer adverse effects related to high-cardiac output states (21). We studied 12 patients on chronic epoprostenol therapy with intolerable side effects and high cardiac output. All patients underwent successful reduction in the dose of epoprostenol (mean dose reduction 39%) without a change in pulmonary artery pressure. Although the cardiac output went down to the normal range, all patients retained their clinical benefit without a return intolerance of the drug. Importantly, patients had fewer side effects related to epoprostenol. Currently, we dose epoprostenol to attain a cardiac index of 2.5 to 4.0 L per minute per m^2.

Prostacyclin Analogues

Because of the complexity with delivery of intravenous epoprostenol, the risk of infections, which may sometimes be life threatening, and other potentially severe adverse events, an alternative mode of delivery is desirable. Clinical studies have suggested that subcutaneously delivered treprostinil (Remodulin) may also be efficacious in the treatment of PAH. A parallel, placebo-controlled 12-week trial in 470 patients with PAH (either primary or associated with collagen vascular or congenital heart disease) demonstrated improvements in 6-minute walk distance, symptoms, and hemodynamics in patients treated with treprostinil versus those treated with placebo (22). There was a significant improvement in the primary endpoint of 6-minute walk distance of 17 m with a reduction in the Borg Dyspnea Score (Fig. 40.7). Importantly, improvements in 6 minute walk distance were related to the dose of treprostinil. The mean dose at week 12 was 9.1 ng per minute. The group in the highest quartile of dose (13.8 ng per kg per minute) had a 35-m improvement in 6-minute walk distance. The treatment effect of treprostinil was also more impressive in patients who were functional class III

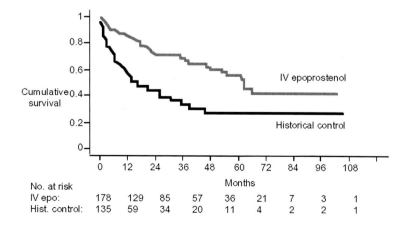

No. at risk									
IV epo:	178	129	85	57	36	21	7	3	1
Hist. control:	135	59	34	20	11	4	2	2	1

FIG. 40.6. Kaplan–Meier estimates of survival among 178 intravenously epoprostenol-treated (IV-epo) primary pulmonary hypertension patients versus historical controls (Hist. control) from the same center. (Adapted from Silbon O, Humbert M, Nunes H, et al. Long-term intravenous epoprostenol infusion in primary pulmonary hypertension. *J Am Coll Cardiol* 2002;40:780–788, with permission.)

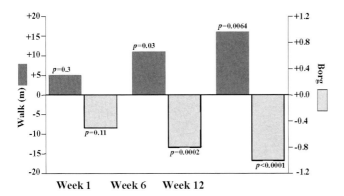

FIG. 40.7. Effect of treprostinil on 6-min walk on the Borg Dyspnea Scale during the 12-week placebo controls from the same center.

and IV at baseline than in patients who were functional class II and in those with lower 6-minute walk distances at baseline. Most patients experience pain and/or erythema at the site of the subcutaneous infusion. Numerous remedies have been used in an attempt to control this infusion site reaction. No therapy has emerged as uniformly successful to treat this problem; however, recommendations include local therapies such as warm and cold packs, topical agents, and nonsteroidal antiinflammatory agents. Narcotic opioids should not be used to control pain.

Beraprost is an orally active epoprostenol analogue, which has been used primarily in Japan for the treatment of pulmonary hypertension. Beraprost has a short half-life and must be given three to four times per day, preferably with food. A Japanese retrospective analysis suggested an improved survival in 24 patients treated with oral beraprost versus 34 patients treated with conventional therapy (23). The double-blind, randomized, controlled Arterial Pulmonary Hypertension and Beraprost European Trial (ALPHABET) recently evaluated beraprost in 130 patients with functional class II or III PAH (24). From baseline to week 12, the between-treatment group difference in the primary endpoint of distance walked in 6 minutes was 24 m. There were also favorable trends in hemodynamic parameters. The treatment effect was most prominent in the PPH group, with less significant improvements in those with PAH related to other disorders. The U.S. beraprost trial, although demonstrating improvement at 3 and 6 months, did not demonstrate a treatment benefit at 1 year (25). Inhaled iloprost has been studied in Europe. One uncontrolled, long-term observational study demonstrated an improvement in cardiopulmonary hemodynamics and exercise capacity with aerosolized Iloprost (26). The Aerosolized Iloprost Randomized Study Group recently reported the results of a placebo-controlled study with the inhalation of iloprost six to nine times per day versus placebo in patients with functional class III or IV PPH or pulmonary hypertension related to thromboembolic disease (27). At the end of a 12-week period, there were improvements in 6-minute walk distance, functional class, dyspnea, and quality of life in

patients treated with active iloprost. The magnitudes of these improvements were more impressive in patients with PPH. The cumbersome nature of this treatment, which requires inhalation six to nine times per day, may limit the practicality of its use. Although neither beraprost nor iloprost is commercially available in the United States, clinical trials with iloprost will begin soon.

Endothelin Receptor Antagonists

Endothelin-1 is a potent vasoconstrictor and smooth muscle mitogen. Plasma endothelin-1 levels are elevated in patients with PPH, and these levels correlate inversely with prognosis (28). Recently, the endothelin antagonists have been investigated in the setting of PAH. The first placebo-controlled study with the dual endothelin receptor antagonist bosentan (Tracleer) in 32 patients with PPH or PAH related to the scleroderma spectrum of disease demonstrated an improvement in exercise tolerance and hemodynamics (29). An international, multicenter, randomized, double-blind, placebo-controlled study was recently conducted in patients with PAH (30). Patients treated with bosentan experienced a significant improvement in 6-minute walk distance of 36 m as compared to a reduction of 8 m in patients treated with placebo, resulting in a mean treatment effect of 44 m in favor of bosentan ($p=0.0002$). Bosentan also improved the composite secondary endpoint of "time to clinical worsening," which was defined as death, lung transplantation, hospitalization or discontinuation due to worsening PAH, need for epoprostenol therapy, or need for atrial septostomy ($p=0.038$) (Fig. 40.8). The most concerning adverse effect associated with bosentan is increased incidence of abnormal liver function tests, which is dose related. Patients treated with this drug should undergo monthly liver function monitoring. Recommendations to either reduce the dose or discontinue the drug are based on the degree of transaminase elevations. The A-selective

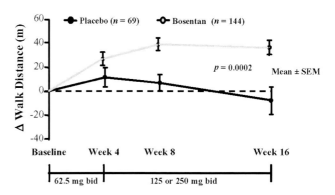

FIG. 40.8. Effect of bosentan on 6-min walk distance in the randomized, placebo-controlled Bostentan: Randomized Trial of Endothelin Receptor Antagonist Therapy-1. SEM, Standard error of the mean; bid, twice a day. (Adapted from Rubin L, Badesch D, Barst R, et al. Bosentan therapy for pulmonary arterial hypertension. *N Engl J Med* 2002;346:896–903, with permission.)

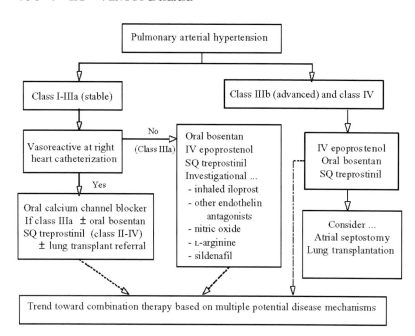

FIG. 40.9. A proposed algorithm for the treatment of primary pulmonary hypertension. IV, intravenous; SQ, subcutaneous. (Adapted from Tapson VF, McLaughlin VV, Robbins IM, et al. Treatment algorithm for pulmonary hypertension. *Adv Pulm Hypertens* 2002;1:6, with permission.)

endothelin receptor antagonist sitaxsentan has also been studied in patients with PAH. An open-label pilot study with this agent demonstrated a significant improvement in exercise tolerance as measured by the 6-minute walk and cardiopulmonary hemodynamics (31). There were two cases of acute hepatitis in this small cohort, one of them fatal, which may have been related to the large doses used in the trial. A large, double-blind, placebo-controlled trial with the agent has recently been completed, and results should be available soon. Another A-selective endothelial receptor antagonist, ambersantan, demonstrated encouraging results in a phase II clinical trial, and will be studied in a phase III clinical trial in the near future.

Phosphodiesterase Inhibitors

Phosphodiesterase-5 inhibitors produce pulmonary vasodilation by promoting an enhanced and sustained level of cyclic GMP, an identical effect to inhaled nitric oxide. When tested as a single oral agent, sildenafil has been shown to be a potent and selective pulmonary vasodilator with equal efficacy to inhaled nitric oxide in lowering pulmonary artery pressure and pulmonary vascular resistance (32). Sildenafil has a preferential effect on the pulmonary circulation because of the high expression of this phosphodiesterase-5 in the lung. Although many anecdotal reports appear in the published medical literature on the success of sildenafil as an oral therapy for patients with PPH, the safety and the efficacy of sildenafil as a treatment for PAH are under investigation.

Atrial Septostomy

A palliative form of therapy, graded atrial balloon septostomy, has received renewed interest. Sandoval *et al.* demonstrated

that graded or stepwise balloon dilation of the atrial septum can be done safely (33). Systemic saturations are monitored during the procedure, and further dilation is not performed when arterial saturation falls to 75% or the left ventricular diastolic pressure reaches 18 mm Hg. They demonstrated improved peripheral oxygen delivery, because the increased cardiac output more than compensates for the fall in hemoglobin saturation. In the United States, balloon septostomy is reserved for those patients who are deteriorating in spite of continuous intravenous epoprostenol and are candidates for lung transplantation. The procedure is not recommended for patients in the terminal stages of the disease (late class IV with advanced right heart failure) because of the high procedural mortality.

Lung Transplantation

Lung transplantation has been performed successfully in patients with PPH for more than a decade. Because these patients have severe right ventricular dysfunction, it was originally believed that heart–lung transplantation was the only transplantation option. More recently, bilateral lung transplantation and single-lung transplantation have been performed successfully in patients with PPH. The immediate reduction in pulmonary artery pressure and pulmonary vascular resistance is associated with an improvement in right ventricular function. Bilateral lung transplantation is preferred at most centers because there is greater pulmonary vascular reserve should the patient sustain a rejection or an infection. Single-lung transplantation may be preferred in some situations because the operation is technically less challenging and the wait time is shorter. As with any type of organ transplantation, the major long-term morbidity and mortality are related to the high incidence of rejection and opportunistic infections. In addition, lung transplantation carries a high risk of the development of bronchiolitis obliterans. In the era of epoprostenol, lung transplantation should be considered a treatment of last resort for PPH. However, due to the long wait time for lung transplantation at most institutions, it is prudent to evaluate and list a patient for transplantation at the time of diagnosis. If the patient responds well to medical therapy, he or she may go "inactive" on the transplantation list.

A proposed algorithm for the treatment of patients with PAH is displayed in Fig. 40.9.

SUMMARY

Great progress has been made over the last two decades in our understanding, diagnosis, and treatment of PAH. The anatomic–histologic changes are not pathognomonic for any specific etiology, but represent the final common pathway in response to endothelial injury. Molecular mechanisms related to endothelial cell function and response to injury are beginning to be understood. There is much greater awareness of diseases that cause or are associated with PAH, and therefore clinicians' threshold to utilize diagnostic tools, such as echocardiography, is lower. Consequently, the disease is being diagnosed earlier in its course. Finally, breakthroughs in treatment, particularly prostacyclins and endothelin receptor antagonists, have turned a dismal prognosis into a more hopeful one.

REFERENCES

1. Rich S, ed. *Primary pulmonary hypertension, executive summary from the World Symposium, Primary Pulmonary Hypertension 1998.* Available from the World Health Organization at http://www.who.int/ncd/cvd/pph.html
2. Rich S, Dantzker DR, Ayers SM, et al. Primary pulmonary hypertension—a national prospective study. *Ann Intern Med* 1987;107:216–223.
3. McLaughlin VV, Shillington A, Rich S. Survival in primary pulmonary hypertension: the impact of epoprostenol therapy. *Circulation* 2002;106:1477–1482.
4. Christman BW, McPherson CD, Newman JH, et al. An imbalance between excretion of thromboxane and prostacyclin metabolites in pulmonary hypertension. *N Engl J Med* 1992;327:70–75.
5. Giad A, Saleh D. Reduced expression of endothelial nitric oxide synthase in the lungs of patients with primary pulmonary hypertension. *N Engl J Med* 1995;333:214–221.
6. Stewart DJ, Levy RD, Cernacek P, et al. Increased plasma endothelin-1 in pulmonary hypertension: marker or mediator of disease? *Ann Intern Med* 1991;114:464–469.
7. Voelkel NF, Tuder RM, Weir EK. Patho-physiology of primary pulmonary hypertension: from physiology to molecular mechanisms. In: Rubin LJ, Rich S., eds., *Primary pulmonary hypertension.* New York: Marcel Dekker, 1997:83–133.
8. D'Alonzo GE, Barst RJ, Ayers SM, et al. Survival in patients with primary pulmonary hypertension: results from a national prospective registry. *Ann Intern Med* 1991;115:343–348.
9. Wensel R, Opitz CF, Anker SD, et al. Assessment of survival in patients with primary pulmonary hypertension: importance of cardiopulmonary exercise testing. *Circulation* 2002;106:319–324.
10. Rich S, Pietra G, Kieras K, et al. Primary pulmonary hypertension: radiographic and scintigraphic patterns of histologic subtypes. *Ann Intern Med* 1986;105:499–502.
11. Raffy O, Azarian R, Brenot F, et al. Clinical significance of the pulmonary vasodilator response during short-term infusion of prostacyclin in primary pulmonary hypertension. *Circulation* 1996;93:484–488.
12. Badesh DB, Abman S, Ahearn G, et al. Medical therapy for pulmonary arterial hypertension: ACCP evidence based guidelines for clinical practice. *Chest* 2004:in press.
13. Rich S, Seidlitz M, Dodin E, et al. The short-term effects of digoxin in patients with right ventricular dysfunction from pulmonary hypertension. *Chest* 1998;114:787–792.
14. Fuster V, Steel P, Edwards W, et al. Primary pulmonary hypertension: natural history and the importance of thrombosis. *Circulation* 1984;70:580–587.
15. Rich S, Kaufman E, Levy P. The effect of high doses of calcium-channel blockers on survival in primary pulmonary hypertension. *N Engl J Med* 1992;327:76–81.
16. Tuder R, Cool C, Geraci M, et al. Prostacyclin synthase expression is decreased in lungs from patients with severe pulmonary hypertension. *Am J Respir Crit Care Med* 1999;159:1925–1932.
17. Barst R, Rubin L, Long W, et al. A comparison of continuous intravenous epoprostenol (prostacyclin) with conventional therapy for primary pulmonary hypertension. *N Engl J Med* 1996;334:296–301.
18. Badesch DB, Tapson VF, McGoon MD, et al. Continuous intravenous epoprostenol for pulmonary hypertension due to the scleroderma spectrum of disease. A randomized, controlled trial. *Ann Intern Med* 2000;132:425–434.
19. McLaughlin V, Genthner D, Panella M, et al. Reduction in pulmonary vascular resistance with long-term epoprostenol (prostacyclin) therapy in primary pulmonary hypertension. *N Engl J Med* 1998;338:273–277.
20. Sitbon O, Humbert M, Nunes H, et al. Long-term intravenous epoprostenol infusion in primary pulmonary hypertension. *J Am Coll Cardiol* 2002;40:780–788.
21. Rich S, McLaughlin V. The effects of chronic prostacyclin therapy on cardiac output and symptoms in primary pulmonary hypertension. *J Am Coll Cardiol* 1999;34:1184–1187.
22. Simonneau G, Barst RJ, Galie N, et al. Continuous subcutaneous infusion of treprostinil, a prostacyclin analogue, in pateints with pulmonary arterial hypertension: a double-blind, randomized, placebo-controlled trial. *Am J Respir Crit Care Med* 2002;165:800–804.
23. Nagaya N, Uematsu M, Okano Y, et al. Effect of orally active prostacyclin analogue on survival of outpatients with primary pulmonary hypertension. *J Am Coll Cardiol* 1999;34:1188–1192.
24. Galie N, Humber M, Vachiery JL, et al. Effects of beraprost sodium, an oral prostacyclin analogue, in patients with pulmonary arterial hypertension: a randomized, double-blind, placebo-controlled trial. *J Am Coll Cardiol* 2002;39:1496–1502.
25. Barst RJ, McGoon M, McLaughlin V, et al. Beraprost therapy for pulmonary arterial hypertension. *J Am Coll Cardiol* 2003;41:2119–2125.
26. Hoeper M, Schwarze M, Ehlerding S, et al. Long-term treatment of primary pulmonary hypertension with aerosolized iloprost, a prostacyclin analogue. *N Engl J Med* 2000;342:1866–1870.
27. Olschewski H, Simonneau G, Galie N, et al. Inhaled iloprost for severe pulmonary hypertension. *N Engl J Med* 2002;347:322–329.
28. Galie N, Grigioni F, Bacchi Reggiani L, et al. Relation of endothelin-1 to survival in patients with primary pulmonary hypertension. *Eur J Clin Invest* 1996;26(Suppl 1):A48 (Abstract 273).
29. Channick RN, Simonneau G, Sitbon O, et al. Effects of the dual endothelin receptor antagonist bosentan in patients with pulmonary hypertension: a randomised placebo-controlled study. *Lancet* 2001;358:1119–1123.
30. Rubin L, Badesch D, Barst R, et al. Bosentan therapy for pulmonary arterial hypertension. *N Engl J Med* 2002;346:896–903.
31. Barst RJ, Rich S, Widlitz A, et al. Clinical efficacy of sitaxsentan, an endothelin-A receptor antagonist, in patients with pulmonary arterial hypertension: open-label pilot study. *Chest* 2002;121:1860–1868.
32. Michelakis E, Tymchak W, Lien D, et al. Oral sildenafil is an effective and specific pulmonary vasodilator in patients with pulmonary arterial hypertension. *Circulation* 2002;105:2398–2403.
33. Sandoval J, Gaspar J, Pulido T, et al. Graded balloon dilation atrial septostomy in severe primary pulmonary hypertension. A therapeutic alternative for patients nonresponsive to vasodilator treatment. *J Am Coll Cardiol* 1998;32:297–304.

CHAPTER 41

The Economic Impact of Peripheral Vascular Disease

Terry L. Woodward

Key Points

- Federal funding for cardiovascular disease research has historically been lower than that for other diseases, and very few studies have directly analyzed the costs of peripheral vascular disease (PVD).
- PVD is high in Western Europe and North America, with symptomatic PVD prevalence as high as 5% in people older than age 50 years.
- The greatest risk factor for PVD is age, with the disease dramatically increasing in people older than 65 years. The number of people older than 65 years is expected to double by 2030 in the United States.
- Other risk factors are less clear, but cigarette smoking and diabetes are correlated with PVD.
- Although there are limited data on PVD costs, direct procedural costs for PVD treatment and diagnosis probably represent several billion dollars in the United States.
- PVD incidence and costs are likely to increase with an aging population.

INTRODUCTION

Peripheral vascular disease (PVD) is broadly defined as any disease of the blood and lymph vessels, excluding the heart and thoracic aorta (1). Most studies reviewed here have concentrated on PVD as defined by abnormal pressure gradients (indicated by the ankle–brachial index) and/or symptomatic PVD such as intermittent claudication. Unlike cardiovascular disease (CVD), there have been few epidemiologic, economic, or quality-of-life studies specifically examining PVD. Additionally, there is little valid information on trends in the incidence of PVD (2), and PVD studies outside of Western Europe and the United States are lacking. PVD data from CVD studies and several regional studies of PVD in Western countries will be reviewed and the potential direct costs of PVD discussed.

In the United States, federal funding of CVD research has historically been lower on a per-patient basis than that for other major serious diseases. For example, the National Institutes of Health (NIH) spends approximately $40 per heart disease patient per year, compared to $338 per cancer patient and $2,100 per HIV/AIDS patient (3). Despite the disproportionate spending, the NIH-approved budget for heart, lung, and blood research is not trivial at $2.58 billion, ranking second only to cancer research ($4.19 billion). The substantial budget has enabled comprehensive epidemiologic as well as socioeconomic studies. In contrast, there have been few studies examining epidemiologic and socioeconomic factors in PVD. Instead, most published epidemiologic reports on PVD have been adjuncts to studies on coronary heart disease (2). The lack of comprehensive PVD studies is not surprising given that CVD claims approximately 950,000 lives in the United States, or 40.6% of all deaths, and is a contributing cause of nearly 70% of all U.S. deaths, whereas PVD only directly causes 17,000 deaths (4,5). Although rarely life-threatening, PVD can seriously affect quality of life and causes a significant financial burden to developed countries, especially if indirect costs such as lost work time are considered.

INCIDENCE

The incidence of PVD is likely increasing due to both an aging population and the better management and survival of patients with CVD (6), although definitive studies examining trends in PVD are lacking (2). The prevalence of intermittent claudication in adults was studied in three European populations with patients at least 45 years old. The lowest prevalence of intermittent claudication, at 2.7%, was found in adults aged 45 to 74 years in Maastricht, Holland (7). An investigation of a Swedish population of adults aged 50 to 89 years revealed a 4.1% prevalence, and a Scottish study found 4.6% of adults aged 55 to 74 years presented with intermittent claudication (8,9). A U.S. study of men aged 65 years or older reported a prevalence of 3% (10). These data suggest that, if intermittent claudication is used as the sole presenting indication of PVD, approximately 2.5% to 5% of the population in Western Europe and the United States older than age 50 years have symptomatic PVD. The U.S. Census Bureau estimated the population of the United States to be 288 million in 2002, with approximately 80 million adults over the age of 50 years (11); this indicates that in the United States alone, 2 to 4 million patients have PVD and the presenting symptom of intermittent claudication.

Intermittent claudication is frequently used to estimate the prevalence of PVD, but the prevalence of intermittent claudication underestimates the presence of PVD by 200% to 500% (12). To examine all PVD, including asymptomatic patients, the most commonly used measure is the ankle–brachial index, a measurement of the ratio of systolic blood pressure at the ankle to that at the arm. A normal ankle–brachial index value is 0.95 to 1.5, whereas in clinical practice an ankle–brachial index of less than 0.9 is greater than 90% sensitive and specific in identifying arterial narrowing in PVD (2,13). Severe PVD has been classified as a ratio of less than 0.6 (14). Comparison of two studies, one measuring all PVD (7) and the other only measuring patients with symptomatic PVD (15), demonstrates that PVD prevalence may be substantially underrepresented if asymptomatic disease is not included (Table 41.1).

RISK FACTORS

The American Heart Association has two classifications of risk factors in CVD, major risk factors and contributing risk factors. Major risk factors are those that research has shown

significantly increase the risk of heart and blood vessel disease (16). Contributing risk factors include factors associated with increased risk of CVD, but the significance or prevalence of which has not been conclusively determined. Major cardiovascular risk factors include increasing age, gender (men have a greater risk of heart disease earlier in life), heredity, and race. Additionally, there are several major cardiovascular risk factors associated with lifestyle, including smoking tobacco, high blood cholesterol, high blood pressure, physical inactivity, obesity, and diabetes mellitus.

Although studies have suggested that most CVD major risk factors are also associated with PVD, conclusive data are less clear. However, at least two major risk factors have emerged for PVD: age and cigarette smoking.

Age and Smoking

The greatest risk factor for PVD is age, with the disease prevalence increasing as much as tenfold between patients younger than 60 years compared with those greater than 75 years old (17). Cigarette smoking has been reported to be a more important risk factor for PVD than for CVD (18). A longitudinal study of more than 5,200 men and women in Framingham, Massachusetts, indicated that cigarette smoking was more closely correlated with the risk of development of intermittent claudication than any other risk factor (19). The Edinburgh Artery Study reported that more than 90% of patients referred to vascular clinics in hospital had a history of cigarette smoking (18). Although a correlation between PVD and cigarette smoking has not directly been demonstrated, experts clearly support the relationship (20).

Diabetes Mellitus

Diabetes is a leading cause of limb amputations, nephropathy, and blindness (diabetic retinopathy). All three outcomes are largely considered to be manifestations of impaired peripheral microvascular circulation. Several studies have demonstrated a twofold to fourfold increase in the risk of developing PVD or intermittent claudication in diabetics (21–23). The Framingham Study demonstrated that the relative risk for intermittent claudication was greater than the relative risk for coronary heart disease in diabetics (20). A recent review by Fowkes pointed to several other studies that refuted the idea that diabetes is a more important risk factor for PVD than CVD (2). Nonetheless, uncontrolled diabetes appears to be correlated with PVD, as determined by the ankle–brachial index ratio. Beks and colleagues found that 7% of diabetics with normal glucose tolerance had abnormal ankle–brachial ratios (24). The ratio increased to 20.9% in poorly regulated patients requiring multiple medications to regulate glucose. Risk of amputations, nephropathy, and blindness are less accurate indicators of PVD because diabetes may increase other factors that directly or indirectly affect these conditions (2). Although there are conflicting reports on whether diabetes is a stronger risk factor for PVD than CVD, there is much

TABLE 41.1. *Prevalence of peripheral vascular disease (PVD)*

Age (years)	Symptomatic PVD (%) (17)	Age (years)	All PVD (%) (7)
<40	0%–2.0		
50	0.5%–2.5	<60	2.5
60	1.0%–4.5	60–69	8.3
70	2.0%–9	>70	18.8

stronger agreement that uncontrolled diabetes appears to be a significant risk factor in PVD.

Other Risk Factors

Hypertension, gender, dyslipidemia, and other factors have been associated with PVD risk. Epidemiologic studies have demonstrated that dyslipidemia, especially elevated triglycerides and low-density-lipoprotein cholesterol, are risk factors for PVD (2) Hypertension is associated with a two- to threefold increased risk of claudication (25). It is unclear, however, whether high blood pressure contributes to PVD or is a result of PVD. Additionally, antihypertensive studies have not determined whether a reduction in blood pressure causes a decrease in PVD incidence (26). Gender-related prevalence of PVD is less clear than gender prevalence of CVD. Although two studies have shown that severe PVD or symptomatic PVD has a higher prevalence in men than in women, data are not conclusive on total incidence of PVD by gender (7,15,27).

COST

No studies have fully evaluated the overall costs of treating this disease (1) or determined indirect costs associated with PVD. Data on incidence and cost in specific geographic regions or for treatment of specific PVD conditions have been reported. PVD has been estimated to account for nearly 10% of all cardiovascular events (4). In the United States alone, the disease results in approximately 777,000 office visits each year, with 63,000 requiring hospital admission (4). Approximately 17,400 deaths are directly related to PVD per year in the United States.

One of the most comprehensive regional assessments of PVD costs came from a detailed survey of direct costs of critical limb ischemia in PVD patients in the United Kingdom (28, also reviewed in 27). The survey was used to estimate total costs for critical limb ischemia in the United Kingdom (Fig. 40.1). The study focused on direct costs, including consultations, prescriptions, in- and outpatient costs, and diagnostics, and ambulatory procedures (procedural costs). Total direct procedural costs for critical limb ischemia were estimated to be approximately 214 million pounds in 1994, with more than two-thirds of these costs represented by bypass surgery, amputation, and treatment of leg ulcers. In 1994, the British pound was approximately equal to $1.56 U.S. Assuming that incidence and treatment costs were similar in the United Kingdom and the U.S., we find the direct procedural inflation-adjusted costs of critical limb ischemia to be close to $2 billion U.S. today. A study of PVD in Maryland estimated that the yearly direct cost of patients with symptomatic PVD was approximately $30.5 million in 1989 (29). Assuming that the incidence and the treatment of symptomatic PVD in Maryland are similar to those in the entire United States, we find that these data indicate direct inflation-adjusted treatment costs for symptomatic PVD exceed $2.6 billion per year in

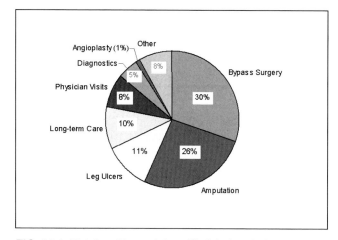

FIG. 41.1. Total cost for peripheral limb ischemia in the United Kingdom. (Adapted from Hart WM, Guest JF. Critical limb ischaemia: the burden of illness in the UK. *Br J Med Econ* 1995;8:211–221, with permission.)

the United States alone. However, demographics differences within the United States are likely to result in different PVD prevalence as well as costs.

Estimation of PVD costs by studies conducted 10 years ago or longer or studies that have concentrated on severe symptomatic PVD likely significantly underrepresent the total costs associated with the disease. For example, analysis of cost pools in the U.K. study (Fig. 41.1) indicates that of is likely that total costs as well as cost distribution have changed in the last decade. For instance, angioplasty only represented approximately 1% of the total cost for critical limb ischemia in this study. Angioplasty, however, has increased since the early 1990s, without a corresponding decrease in bypass surgery. At least one study has demonstrated significant increase in angioplasty for PVD, increasing from 14 per 100,000 in 1989 to 33 per 100,000 in 1995. Coronary angioplasty data demonstrate that angioplasty may have increased significantly even after 1995, as transluminal coronary angioplasty increased by nearly 50% between 1993 and 1998 (5). Therefore, these data probably underrepresent the angioplasty cost component in treatment of PVD.

Critical limb ischemia is a serious and costly outcome of progressive PVD. However, PVD results in substantial costs outside of critical limb ischemia. Critical limb ischemia occurs infrequently and is therefore difficult to reliably measure. A consensus group in Europe has calculated that 500 to 1,000 people in a population of 1 million have critical limb ischemia, based on (a) the percentage of critical limb ischemia patients who require major amputations, (b) the percentage of the total number of amputations that are related to critical limb ischemia, and (c) the percentage of amputations in the general population (30). Table 41.2 demonstrates that critical limb ischemia occurs infrequently among the general population with PVD and compared to other conditions associated with PVD. In fact, critical limb ischemia occurs at

TABLE 41.2. *Prevalence and incidence of peripheral vascular disease and related complications in the general population*[a]

Indication	Incidence (I) or prevalence (P)/million	Percentage
Critical limb ischemia	I: 300/year P: 500–1000	I: 0.03%/year (30) P: 0.05%–0.1%
Claudicants	P: 19,000 P: 14,500 I: 2,000/year	P: 1.9 % (31) P: 1.45% (32) I: 0.2%/year (31)
Asymptomatic	P: 40,000 P: 36,000	P: 4.0 % (31) P: 3.6% (32)
Asymptomatic abdominal aneurysm	P: 9,000	P: 0.9 % (31)
Deaths from aortic aneurysm	I: 260/year	I: 0.026 %/year (31)

[a]Data from U.S. and U.K. studies.

approximately one-fifth the incidence of symptomic claudication, and 1/10 to 1/25 as often as PVD. Clearly, there is a substantial market for PVD treatment. It is likely that direct costs in the treatment of more severe PVD exceed $2 to $3 billion dollars in the United States, whereas total costs have not been determined. Worldwide direct costs may exceed $5 billion because the incidence of CVD is similar in Western Europe to the that in the United States. Successful treatment of CVD, especially by stents, angioplasty, and bypass surgery, will extend patient life, but may increase the incidence of symptomatic PVD.

Importantly, the numbers of persons with the risk factors most closely correlated with PVD are increasing, including persons older than 65 years of age, persons with diabetes, and persons smoking. A study based on information from the World Health Organization and the U.S. Census Bureau has estimated that the number of persons 65 years or older in the United States will more than double from 35 million in 2000 to 71 million in 2030, representing an increase from 12.4% to 19.6% of the U.S. population (33). Worldwide, the population older than 65 years is expected to increase from 420 million to 973 million from 2000 to 2030. Although smoking incidence is falling in developed countries at about 1.5% per year, it is rising in developing countries at about 1.7% per year (34). The number of U.S. adults with diagnosed diabetes is expected to double by 2050, and type II diabetes in children and teens is growing even faster (35). The substantial increase in these key risk factors of PVD will increase the demand for early diagnosis, prophylactic therapies, and substantially improved treatment modalities for PVD in the coming decades.

REFERENCES

1. Langley PC, Coons SJ. Peripheral vascular disorders. A pharmacoeconomic and quality-of-life review. *Pharmacoeconomics* 1997;11:225–236.
2. Fowkes FGR. Epidemiological research on peripheral vascular disease. *J Clin Epidemiol* 2001;54:863–868.
3. Istook E, Porter JE. Should disease prevalence determine NIH fund allocations? *Physicians Weekly* 1998;15:23.
4. Kannel WB. The demographics of claudication and the aging of the American population. *Vasc Med* 1996;1:60–64.
5. Woodward TL, Abela GS, Briefs N. Percutaneous myocardial revascularization: financial potential and market acceptance. In: Abela GS, ed., *Myocardial revascularization: novel percutaneous approaches.* New York: Wiley-Liss, 2002:263–268.
6. Bajwa TK, Shalev YA, Gupta A, et al. Peripheral Vascular disease, Part 1. *Curr Probl Cardiol* 1998;23:245–297.
7. Stoffers HEJH, Rinkens PELM, Kester ADM, et al. The prevalence of asymptomatic and unrecognized peripheral arterial occlusive disease. *Int J Epidemiol* 1996;25:282–290.
8. Fowkes FGR, Housley E, Cawood EHH, et al. Edinburgh Artery Study: prevalence of asymptomatic and symptomatic peripheral arterial disease in the general population. *Int J Epidemiol* 1991;20:384–392.
9. Skau T, Jonsson B. Prevalence of symptomatic leg ischemia in a Swedish community—an epidemiological study. *Eur J Vasc Surg* 1993;7:432–437.
10. Mittelmark MB, Psaty BM, Rautaharju PM, et al. Prevalence of cardiovascular diseases among older adults. The Cardiovascular Health Study. *Am J Epidemiol* 1993;137:311–317.
11. U.S. Census Bureau 2002. Available at http://www.census.gov
12. Criqui MH. Peripheral arterial disease—epidemiological aspects. *Vasc Med* 2001;6:3–7.
13. Carter SA. Indirect systolic pressures and pulse waves in arterial occlusive disease of the lower extremities. *Circulation* 1968;37:624–638.
14. Criqui MH, Denenberg JO. The generalized nature of atherosclerosis: how peripheral arterial disease may predict adverse events from coronary artery disease. *Vasc Med* 1998;3:241–245.
15. Dormandy JA, Rutherford RB. Management of peripheral arterial disease (PAD). TASC Working Group. TransAtlantic Inter-Society Concensus (TASC). *J Vasc Surg* 2000;31:S1–S296.
16. American Heart Association. *Heart and stroke statistical update.* Dallas, TX: Author, 2001.
17. Criqui MH, Fronek A, Barrett-Connor E, et al. The prevalence of peripheral arterial disease in a defined population. *Circulation* 1985;71:510–515.
18. Fowkes FGR, Housley E, Riemersma RA, et al. Smoking, lipids, glucose intolerance, and blood pressure as risk factors for peripheral atherosclerosis compared with ischaemic heart disease in the Edinburgh Artery Study. *Am J Epidemiol* 1992;135:331–340.
19. Kannel WB, Shurtleff D. The Framingham Study. Cigarettes and the development of intermittent claudication. *Geriatrics* 1973;28:61–68.
20. Regensteiner JG, Hiatt WR. Treatment of peripheral arterial disease. *Clin Cornerstone* 2002;4:26–40.
21. Kannel WB, McGee DL. Diabetes and cardiovascular disease. The Framingham Study. *JAMA* 1979;241:2035–2038.
22. Kannel WB, D'Agostino RB, Wilson PW, et al. Diabetes, fibrinogen, and risk of cardiovascular disease: the Framingham experience. *Am Heart J* 1990;120:672–676.
23. Newman AB, Siscovick DS, Manolio TA, et al. Ankle–arm index as a marker of atherosclerosis in the Cardiovascular Health Study.

Cardiovascular Heart Study (CHS) Collaborative Research Group. *Circulation* 1993;88:837–845.

24. Beks PJ, Mackaay AJ, de Neeling JN, et al. Peripheral arterial disease in relation to glycaemic level in an elderly Caucasian population: the Hoorn study. *Diabetologia* 1995;38:86–96.

25. Murabito JM, D'Agostino RB, Silbershatz H, et al. Intermittent claudication. A risk profile from the Framingham Heart Study. *Circulation* 1997;96:44–49.

26. Makin A, Lip GY, Silverman S, et al. Peripheral vascular disease and hypertension: a forgotten association? *J Hum Hypertens* 2001;15:447–454.

27. Meijer WT, Hoes AW, Rutgers D, et al. Peripheral arterial disease in the elderly: the Rotterdam Study. *Arterioscler Thromb Vasc Biol* 1998;18:185–192.

28. Hart WM, Guest JF. Critical limb ischaemia: the burden of illness in the UK. *Br J Med Econ* 1995;8:211–221.

29. Tunis SR, Bass EB, Steinberg EP. Use of angioplasty, bypass surgery, and amputation in the management of PVD. *N Engl J Med* 1991;325:556–562.

30. Second European consensus document on chronic critical leg ischemia. *Circulation* 1991;84(4 Suppl):IV1–26.

31. Fowkes FGR. Peripheral vascular disease, 2002. Healthcare needs assessment epidemiological program. Available at http://hcna.radcliffe-online.com/pvdframe.htm

32. Golomb BA, Criqui MH, Bundens WP. Peripheral arterial disease. In: Hiatt WA, Hirsch AT, Regensteiner JG, eds., *Peripheral arterial disease handbook*. Boca Raton, FL: CRC Press, 2001:57–79.

33. Goulding MR. Public health and aging: trends in aging—United States and worldwide. *Morbid Mortal Weekly Rep* 2003;50:101–106; available at www.cdc.gov/mmwr/preview/mmwrhtml/mm5206a2.htm

34. World Health Organization. Health hazards of tobacco, 1996. Available at www.who.int/archives/ntday/ntday96/pk96__3.htm

35. Koplan, JP. Diabetes: disabling, deadly, and on the rise. At a Glance. 2003. Available at http://www.cdc.gov/nccdphp/aag/aag__ddt.htm

CHAPTER 42

Billing and Coding for Peripheral Vascular Disease

Mary A. Metler, Linda K. East, Terence Whiteman, and Patricia M. Dear

---

Key Points

- Billing and coding is a dynamic process, which requires constant attention and updating. Physicians need to become familiar with this aspect of practice.
- Documentation in the medical record is the key that supports medical necessity, for billing/coding, reimbursement, and passing an audit. All physician offices should periodically conduct a medical record audit to ensure that billing is in line with documented visits/procedures.
- Peripheral vascular procedures may be performed in conjunction with or separate from coronary angiography. When performed independently, peripheral vascular procedures must include multiple codes.
- When choosing diagnostic codes, all diagnoses should be included, and preferably those codes should be enumerated for clarification of the primary diagnosis. Symptom-related diagnoses may be included (i.e., chest pain); however, if a more specific diagnosis is available (i.e., acute myocardial infarction), that should be the primary diagnosis.

It is not possible to be overeducated with regard to the reimbursement process. Physicians spend enormous amounts of time and money on their education before they ever open or join a medical practice. Primary education of medical students, interns, residents, and fellows deals with patient care, procedures, and learning the technology of equipment and research, but not how to make financial arrangements with insurance carriers, how to code procedures or diagnoses, and how to document patient care to ensure maximum reimbursement. Accordingly, most physicians are educated in medicine, but not in practice management. Just as education is important in treating the patient, education is also vital in creating and maintaining a profitable and efficient medical practice. A physician may be an excellent clinician, treat a high volume of patients, and have very good outcomes, but if he or she is not educated regarding business, reimbursement, contractual agreements, malpractice insurance, clinical guidelines, practice aging reports, or the rules for billing each insurance provider, all efforts will go unrewarded.

The realm of billing and coding is a dynamic one. Every physician should make an effort to understand the Evaluation and Management section and the codes in the *Physicians' Current Procedural Terminology* (CPT) code book, as well as the procedural sections relevant to his or her area of specialty or practice (e.g., the Cardio Surgery section and the Radiology section) (1). It is important to remember that these codes are modified each year (with new codes added and old ones deleted), which requires that the practices' coding and billing procedures and forms (e.g., superbills or encounter forms) be reviewed and updated regularly. The physicians' CPT codebook is a systematic listing *of all codes* for physician-related procedures and services. Each procedure or service is identified by a five-digit code, which is clearly defined and is inclusive (bundled), exclusive of related procedures or "add on's" to the procedure performed. For example, when a physician performs an angioplasty, he or she would bill for all components of the care including catheterization. However, if more than one vessel is angioplastied in the same session, it is not possible to bill this as another full procedure, but instead each is billed as an additional vessel.

Each code is assigned a resource-based relative value unit with a corresponding dollar amount for reimbursement by insurance carriers. In determining what fees to charge for the services provided, the physician may want to consider reviewing fees based on Medicare's reasonable and customary fees. Medicare sends out a fee schedule annually, which identifies codes and average reimbursement rates. Other insurance carriers may choose to participate with the physician through a variety of approaches such as fee schedule discounting or managed care contracting, so it is important to review the reimbursement style and expectation for the other carriers with whom one participates. In the decision-making process for establishing charges and billing amounts, it is important to do the homework required to determine the maximum fee schedule in one's region.

Another important aspect in understanding coding and billing is use of the *International Classification of Diseases* (ICD-9) (2). This book is the standard text utilized for identifying diagnostic codes. Each CPT current procedural terminology code must be linked to an ICD-9 diagnostic code from this listing for procedures and services rendered. In the case of the patient with multiple diagnostic codes, all codes should be included for the coder/biller to submit, with the primary diagnosis identified. For example, if a patient has undergone coronary artery bypass graft, one must include coronary artery disease as a diagnosis. Surely a patient would not undergo bypass surgery if he or she did not have coronary artery disease. By the same token, by including as many diagnoses possible, reimbursement is more likely to occur with the first submission. There are some procedural codes that are not payable with particular diagnostic codes. An example is echocardiography. This code is not payable for visual disturbance or to rule out emboli, but is payable for transient ischemic attacks or any type of valve disorder. One critical key to choosing a diagnostic code is to remember that screening, postoperative, or status postcodes, also known as V codes, are not payable as primary diagnoses. There must always be a primary diagnostic code prior to utilization of the V code (which is a patient status code and not always required). For example, when providing services for preoperative screening, it is acceptable to list V81.72 (preop screening), but there must also be a code that is the reason for the surgery and any additional symptoms or diseases that exist. The V code should be used as the final choice in a string of diagnoses.

In the case of billing evaluation and management services (E/M), documentation in the medical record is critical establishing the medical necessity of the services performed and the choice of an appropriate coding level. This is best achieved by utilizing a step-by-step fashion starting with the definition of a new patient versus an established patient. A new patient is defined as one who has not received any professional services from the physician or another physician in the same specialty who belongs to the same group practice, within the last 3 years. Therefore, if a patient has received *any* services from the physician or one of the partners in the practice in the last 3 years, the patient is considered an established patient. The exception would be if the group is a multispecialty group and one of the partners evaluated the patient for a condition unrelated to the specialty. The next step in the decision-making tree concerns the complexity of the patient encounter. The components required for appropriate billing include history, physical examination, medical decision making, and the average time spent in face-to-face contact with the patient. The first three of these components are key and include the documentation of either a problem focused, an expanded problem focused, or a detailed or comprehensive level of care. It must be noted that in the case of a comprehensive examination, the physician must perform an extended history of the present illness, a review of systems as related to the problem(s) identified in the history, and a review of all additional body systems as well as a complete past, family, and social history. In addition, a general multisystem examination or a complete examination of a single organ system is required. One must remember that although it is easier to look at the average time spent, as an indicator for choosing the appropriate E/M code, it is the documentation that supports this code, not the time spent. Time may only be used as an indicator if counseling or coordination of care dominates at least 50% of the visit. In addition, if an extended amount of time is spent with the patient discussing treatment options or other care issues, this additional time must be documented and may be billed by utilizing an extended time code.

Another area of confusion surrounds the understanding of billing E/M services for a consultation or a referral. One must remember that in the case of a consultation, the referring physician is asking for the opinion and advice of the consultant. The expectation is that the patient will be returned to the referring physician for treatment and management of the diagnosed condition. In the case of a consultation, the consultant must submit a final written report to the referring physician. This report must contain the opinion of the patient's condition. If the intention is to provide diagnosis and treatment of the patient, then billing the E/M services for a new patient with follow-up visits would be appropriate. One should remember the rules that apply to new patient visits as discussed previously.

In 1995, evaluation and management guidelines regarding documentation were established to provide all physicians direction when identifying the E/M services and codes they performed. The 1997 evaluation and management guidelines were established to provide physicians in certain specialties (e.g., cardiology) with a more specific and focused approach when documenting the evaluation and management of their patients. Understanding the differences and requirements of each should help physicians determine which would most accurately represent their work through their documentation. The area of coding for physician evaluation and management services continues to be refined and improved, and annual updates in this area are key to accuracy in reporting codes and correct reimbursement.

In the case of coding/billing procedural services such as with endovascular testing/procedures, the billing must correspond with appropriate documentation. In this case, a procedural or operative note would be appropriate documentation. For accurate documentation, the procedure notes should include the following components: patient name, date of procedure, diagnoses, procedure performed, and names of participating physicians. In addition, in the case of a surgical procedure, the note should include the patient position and draping, the administration of anesthesia (including conscious sedation), a detailed description of the procedure, the condition of the patient following the procedure, and the names of the physicians participating in the procedure, with the signature of the primary surgeon.

It is important to understand that with most procedures, but particularly with endovascular procedures, there are various components to the billing process. Physicians may bill for a total component (technical and professional), professional component only (supervision and interpretation), or interpretation alone. The vascular access portion of the study is "matched" with codes for the supervision and interpretation of the procedure. The key to determining the level of service performed is found in the documentation in the medical record. It is critical to remember that if there is inadequate or no documentation of any part of a procedure or office visit, the assumption is that the service was not provided. The documentation must stand alone as evidence for the services being billed. If the documentation does not support the level of billing and the practice undergoes an audit, the physician could be charged with fraud, resulting in penalties, fines, loss of medical licensure, and possible jail time. It is recommended that periodic chart audits be performed regularly to ensure that documentation standards are being adhered to. This can be accomplished by having a quality assurance practice in the professional office. If the physician qualifies as a high-volume specialist, insurance carriers may request a quality assurance audit. Different rules apply in different states. Additionally, it is often helpful to the reimbursement process to include the examination notes with the submission of the claim if the procedure is complex or not well understood. *Physicians often mistake services delivered with those that are documented and coded.* The documentation must reflect the medical necessity of the services and the care delivered to the patient with appropriate CPT and ICD-9 codes selected. There has been an enormous emphasis on documentation of E/M services, but the same rules apply to procedural billing as well. The lack of documentation or confusion about coding are the most common mistakes made in the billing process, and lead to medical necessity denials. It is vital to include the specific reason for the study, the specific findings and documentation of the physician's presence during the service, and specific details regarding the procedure itself (access site, approach, whether selective or nonselective, whether unilateral or bilateral, etc.). When all aspects of the case are clearly and concisely documented, there is no question on the part of the biller/coder or the insurance carrier. This will help to protect physicians and medical practices/clinics during an audit, and creates excellent documentation habits, which creates a win/win situation for physician, patient, practice, and health insurance carrier (3).

Billing, coding, and documentation of endovascular procedures has been and continues to be an evolutionary process.

An understanding of the language utilized is critical to understanding the billing procedure. For example, consider the difference between selective and nonselective angiography. During the course of an angiographic study, it is important to know that *nonselective* means the catheter does not advance beyond the vessel accessed, whereas *selective* refers to the catheter advancement to a subsequent first-order, second-order, or third-order vessel (how many intersections were crossed). The billing and subsequent reimbursement will depend on understanding this concept. If both nonselective and selective procedures are performed in the same session, then one would bill for the highest order (selective). By the same token, it is important to document whether a procedure was performed unilaterally or bilaterally. If there is no bilateral code provided for a service, but a bilateral service was performed, one should code the procedure utilizing the unilateral code twice. As is the case with coronary angiography, often a diagnostic procedure turns into an interventional one. When this scenario occurs, both the diagnostic codes and the interventional codes should be provided with all associated ICD-9 codes. By including all associated ICD-9 codes with each claim, there is an increased likelihood of reimbursement. Additionally, by providing the biller with an enumerated list of these codes by order of importance, there will be no reason for guessing which diagnostic code is primary, secondary, and so on. As noted earlier, one should never bill a V code (screening, postop, status post, or family history) as a primary code.

In understanding the billing and coding process for peripheral procedures, it is important to recognize that peripheral studies may be performed in conjunction with a coronary angiogram or as an individual service. In the case of combining studies, the billing codes for coronary angiogram apply as well as the additional codes when a catheter is positioned for peripheral studies. In the case of a renal study, the codes begin at 36245, which correspond to selective catheter placement, arterial system, including each first-order abdominal, pelvic or lower extremity artery branch within a vascular family branch. Additionally, the code 75724 would be used to describe bilateral renal angiography (selective) with supervision and interpretation. If there is no indication for coronary angiography and only peripheral studies are performed, multiple codes must be used to accurately report the procedure. In other words, all CPT codes for both procedures must be included for a combined service, and multiple codes corresponding to peripheral vascular studies completed independent of a coronary angiogram. Documentation for billing and coding of these procedures requires knowledge of the arterial access puncture site, catheter movement, and final position of the catheter. This is where the documentation of the procedure is critical for completion of the billing component. In addition to documentation of all of the foregoing (access site, etc.), there must be clear notes regarding what angiograms were performed and at what location during the catheter manipulation process injections were completed.

When reporting these procedures, one needs to remember that there are five vascular systems. These include arterial, venous, pulmonary, portal, and lymphatic systems. It must be specified which vascular system is being studied, followed by a description of the primary branch. The most highly selective vessel catheterized in a vascular branch determines the level of coding. If the documentation regarding final catheter placement for injection is incomplete or unclear, reimbursement may be lower or compromised.

For many invasive procedures, the patient is provided with medication for inducement of conscious sedation. It is important to document the medications given (including doses and frequency given during the procedure) to induce this state and to bill for these services (99141 and 99142). These codes are to be utilized for physicians administering conscious sedation other than anesthesiologists or nurse anesthetists. If there is another physician present to administer the sedative and monitor the patient, one should not bill for this service. In some cases, the conscious sedation is bundled into the procedure code. Careful review of these codes will determine whether additional coding is required.

To this point, the procedures discussed are those performed in the hospital. It is important to recognize that physician services performed and documented in the hospital record are the basis of the hospital's reimbursement as well. The expression "not documented, not done" applies to both the physician and the site where the services were performed. Hospitals are dependent on the same complete, clear, and legible documentation in the medical record as is the physician practice. There are additional noninvasive vascular diagnostic studies, which may be performed either as an inpatient or in an outpatient department (physician office included). Perhaps one of the most common studies is an extremity arterial study. This may be performed on either the upper or lower extremities and may include ankle–brachial indices, Doppler waveform analysis, volume plethsmography, and/or transcutaneous oxygen tension measurement. Many handheld instruments are available for this purpose; however, to qualify for billing, there must be a printout of the results included in the medical record. If these services are performed without a documented printout of the testing, it is not permissible to submit billing for the procedure. There are more complex levels for extremity arterial studies, which include single-level studies or multiple-level studies. To qualify for a multiple-level study, there must be multiple segmental blood pressure measurements, segmental Doppler waveform analysis, segmental volume plethysmography, and/or segmental transcutaneous oxygen tension measurements. There must also exist measurements with postural provocative tests and the associated documentation of such. It is also possible to perform this testing at rest and following treadmill exercise. When performing such a service, one should not bill for cardiovascular stress testing alone (93015), because it is already bundled into the code (93926) that includes the peripheral vascular studies both at rest and following exercise.

Another common office procedure includes studies of the extremities for venous disease. These may be performed as either as a unilateral or a bilateral procedure, and may include impedence plethysmography, phleborheography, and/or Doppler waveform analysis with responses to compression or other maneuvers. It is also possible to perform complete bilateral duplex ultrasound scans of the extremity veins; one should make sure to report the indications for the scan, complete results, and the utilization of compression or other maneuvers during the scan.

Less common to the majority of general cardiology practices is the performance of cerebrovascular arterial studies and visceral vascular studies. It must be noted that these are acceptable studies with associated CPT billing codes; however, appropriate diagnostic (ICD-9) codes and complete documentation must be included for appropriate reimbursement.

There is no way to distill all the billing, coding, and documentation required into a neat and easy package. Attention to detail, diligence, and continuing education are key to successful reimbursement for services provided. Just as physicians participate in continuing medical education, so do they need to provide continuing billing education for themselves and the medical billers/coders who work for them. The use of coding software or a subscription to a coding newsletter is a good idea to keep up to date regarding billing and reimbursement for new and existing procedures. Often the rules change and if the office is unaware, payment may be denied or delayed unnecessarily. Documentation in the medical record cannot be stressed enough. If documentation is incomplete, unclear, or illegible and additional information is called for or an audit is performed, the physician billing for the services is at risk. One should not take this chance. The physician should document all he or she does, and if working with residents or fellows, ensure that the attending physician's participation is clearly provided for all key portions of the service. Commonly used language may be as follows: "A review of systems [ROS] was performed during the patient visit. Please see ROS form provided for this date of service. I performed a history and physical examination of the patient and discussed the patient management with the fellow/resident. I reviewed the fellow/resident note and agree with the documented findings and plan of care."

It is important to note that medical student notes cannot be used to cosign for services rendered as for residents and fellow notes. A complete note by the attending physician is required in the absence of a resident note.

In documenting procedures, one must be sure to include all components as described previously including access sites, catheter placement, and injection sites. One needs to provide the indications for the procedure, all events that occur during the procedure, the patient's condition at the completion of the procedure, and a complete note of the findings and recommendations. Finally, all appropriate diagnostic codes should be given for each encounter. By enumerating these codes, the physician is able to guide the biller and ensure that the primary diagnosis is coded as such. One should be as specific in the coding as possible; for example, in the case of a myocardial infarction, the site of the infarction should be noted (anterior, inferior, etc.) as well as the status (acute, recent, or old). One should not assume that the biller/coder will know which diagnostic codes to use; the physician should identify them. Perhaps the most important point to remember is that billing and coding is a team effort. The physician must provide the appropriate documentation, the coder must be able to identify and sequence the codes correctly, and the biller must be able to accurately report those services to the payor for accuracy in reimbursement. Understanding the vital connection of physician documentation, coding, and billing to reimbursement will go a long way in protecting and improving the reimbursement the physician and associated health care providers will ultimately receive.

REFERENCES

1. American College of Cardiology Foundation. *American College of Cardiology Foundation guide to CPT 2003: practical reporting of cardiovascular services and procedures.* Baltimore, MD: Author, 2003.
2. World Health Organization. *International classification of diseases,* 9th rev. Geneva: Author, 1978.
3. Grider DJ. *Medical record chart analyzer.* Chicago: American Medical Association, 2002.

APPENDIX

Nutrition and Exercise Guidelines

Mary Noel

Dietary components and their effects on the body[a]

Nutrient	Usual effects on body	Foods high in this nutrient (not an exclusive list)
Fats		
Saturated fats	↑ LDL ↑ Total blood cholesterol	Fats that are hard at room temperature, e.g., animal fats (meat, milk [whole, 2%], butter, ice cream, cream), cashews, macadamia nuts
Polyunsaturated fats	↓ LDL ↓ HDL ↓ Total blood cholesterol	Fats that are liquid at room temperature, e.g., vegetable oils such as safflower, corn oils, avocado
Trans fatty acids	↑ LDL	Vegetable fats that have been transformed by hydrogenation into hard fats at room temperature, e.g., margarines, shortening, and hydrogenated fats in processed foods
Monounsaturated fats	↓ LDL ↑ HDL No change total blood cholesterol	Olive oil, canola oil
Omega-3 and -6 fatty acids	↓ LDL ↑ HDL	Fish, fish oils (e.g., salmon, shell fish, cold water fish) and nuts
Carbohydrates		
Refined or simple carbohydrates	↑ Triglycerides	Soda pop, candy, table sugar, items containing sugars such as corn syrup, molasses, honey
High-glycemic-index	↑ Triglycerides ↑ blood glucose	Glucose, sucrose, honey bagels, sports drinks, soda pop, potatoes, bread, rice
Alcohol	↑ Triglycerides ↑ HDL	Beer, wine, bourbon, and other liquors
Vitamins		
Vitamin E	↑ Anticoagulation (particularly of cholesterol plaques)	Nuts, vegetable oil, margarine from vegetable oils, avocados
Folacin (folic acid)	↓ Homocysteine	Fruits (oranges are exceptionally high), vegetables (spinach is exceptionally high) whole grains, nuts, fortified breads and cereals
Minerals		
Sodium	↑ Blood pressure (population studies show this occurs only in around one-third of U.S. population)	Table salt, flavoring salts (such as onion salt), preserved meats (such as luncheon meats, ham, sausages), processed foods (such as prepared meals, packaged foods) sports drinks
Calcium	↓ Blood pressure (DASH study)	Dairy products, sardines, clams, oysters, kale, turnip greens, mustard greens, tofu
Magnesium	↓ Blood pressure (DASH study)	Whole-grain cereals, tofu, nuts, meat, milk, green vegetables, legumes, chocolate
Potassium	↓ Blood pressure (DASH study)	Fruits, milk, meat, cereal, vegetables, legumes
Fiber (U.S. recommendation 20–30 g/day)		
Soluble fiber	↑ Clearance of cholesterol	Gums: oat bran, legumes, guar, barley; pectins: apples, citrus fruits, strawberries, carrots (e.g., for fiber of 6 g/cooked 1/2 cup of kidney beans, baked beans, navy beans; 3 g/cooked 1/2 cup of lentils, peas, oat bran)
Insoluble fiber	↑ Fecal material with fiber as bulk agent	Cellulose: whole-wheat flour, bran (wheat), vegetables; hemicellose: bran (wheat), whole grains; lignan: mature vegetables, wheat, fruits, edible seeds (strawberries) (e.g., for fiber of 6 g/1 oz. serving of All Bran, Branbuds, 100% Bran; 3 g/1 oz. serving of Most, Honey Bran)

[a] LDL, Low-density lipoprotein; HDL, high-density lipoprotein; DASH, Dietary Approaches to Stop Hypertension.

GUIDANCE ON HOW TO UNDERSTAND AND USE THE NUTRITION FACTS PANEL ON FOOD LABELS

[Source: http://www.nutrition.gov]

People look at food labels for different reasons. Whatever the reason, many consumers would like to know how to use this information more effectively and easily. The following information was updated in July 2003 by the U.S. Food and Drug Administration (FDA), Center for Food Safety and Applied Nutrition, and is intended to make it easier to use nutrition labels to make quick, informed food choices that contribute to a healthy diet.

The Nutrition Facts panel has two parts: the main or top section (see 1–5 on the following sample nutrition label, which contains product-specific information (serving size, calories, and nutrient information), and varies with each food product; and the bottom part (see 6 on the following sample nutrition label), which contains a footnote. This footnote is only on larger packages and provides general dietary information about important nutrients.

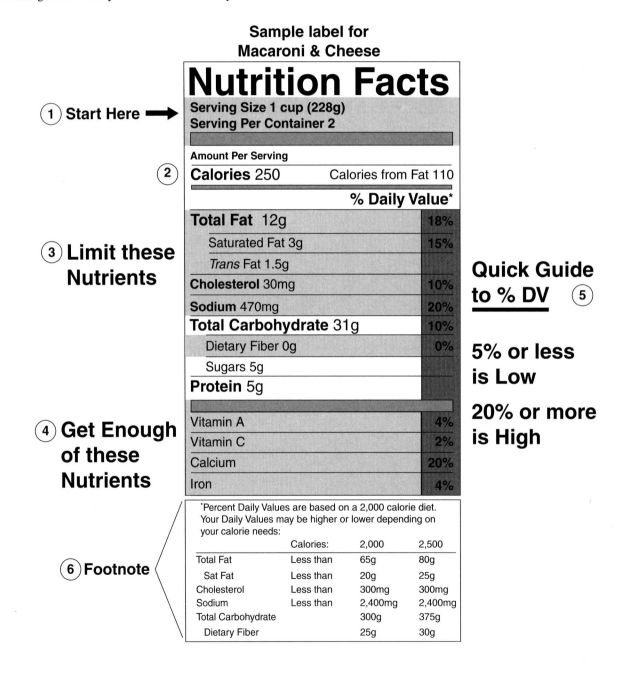

The Serving Size

Serving Size 1 cup (228g)
Serving Per Container 2

The first place to look on the Nutrition Facts panel is the part giving the serving size and the number of servings in the package (see 1 on the sample label). Serving sizes are provided in familiar units, such as cups or pieces, followed by the metric amount, for example, the number of grams. Serving sizes are based on the amount of food people typically eat, which makes them realistic and easy to compare to similar foods.

One should pay attention to the serving size, including how many servings there are in the food package, and compare it to how much one actually eats. The size of the serving on the food package influences all the nutrient amounts listed on the top part of the label. In the sample label shown here, one serving of macaroni and cheese equals one cup. If one ate the whole package, one would eat *two* cups. That doubles the calories and other nutrient numbers, including the percentage daily values (%DV), as follows (see subsequent discussion on calories and %DV for more information):

	Single serving	%DV	Double serving	%DV
Serving size	1 cup (228 g)		2 cups (456 g)	
Calories	250		500	
Calories from fat	110		220	
Total fat	12 g	18	24 g	36
Trans fat	1.5 g		3 g	
Saturated fat	3 g	15	6 g	30
Cholesterol	30 mg	10	60 mg	20
Sodium	470 mg	20	940 mg	40
Total carbohydrate	31 g	10	62 g	20
Dietary fiber	0 g	0	0 g	0
Sugars	5 g		10 g	
Protein	5 g		10 g	
Vitamin A		4		8
Vitamin C		2		4
Calcium		20		40
Iron		4		8

Calories and Calories from Fat

Amount Per Serving
Calories 250   Calories from Fat 110
% Daily Value*

Calories provide a measure of how much energy one gets from a serving of this food (see 2 on sample label). The label also indicates how many of the calories in one serving come from fat. In this example, there are 250 calories in a serving of this macaroni and cheese. Of these, 110 calories, almost half, come from fat. If one ate the whole package content, one would consume two servings, or 500 calories, and 220 calories would come from fat.

Eating too many calories per day is linked to overweight and obesity.

The Nutrients

The top section in the sample nutrition label (3 and 4) shows nutrients that are important for health and separates them into two main groups:

Limit These Nutrients

Total Fat 12g   **18%**
Saturated Fat 3g   **15%**
Trans Fat 1.5g
Cholesterol 30mg   **10%**
Sodium 470mg   **20%**

The nutrients listed first (see 3 on sample label) are the ones Americans generally eat in adequate amounts, or even too much of. They are identified on the chart as Limit These Nutrients. Eating too much fat, saturated fat, trans fat, cholesterol, or sodium may increase the risk of certain chronic diseases, like heart disease, some cancers, or high blood pressure. Eating too many calories is linked to overweight and obesity.

Health experts recommend that intake of saturated fat, trans fats, and cholesterol be kept as low as possible as part of a nutritionally balanced diet.

Nutrition Facts information obtained from http://www.nutrition.gov.

Get Enough of These

Dietary Fiber 0g	0%

Vitamin A	4%
Vitamin C	2%
Calcium	20%
Iron	4%

Americans often do not get enough dietary fiber, vitamin A, vitamin C, calcium, and iron in their diets. They are identified on the chart (4 on sample label) as Get Enough of These. Eating enough of these nutrients can improve health and help reduce the risk of some diseases and conditions. For example, getting enough calcium can reduce the risk of osteoporosis, in which bones become brittle and break as one ages (see calcium example in what follows).

One can use the food label not only to help limit the nutrients one wants to cut back on, but also to increase those nutrients one wants to consume in greater amounts.

The Percent Daily Value

18%
15%
10%
20%
10%
0%
4%
2%
20%
4%

This part of the Nutrition Facts panel states how much the nutrients (fat, sodium, fiber, etc.) in a serving of food contribute to the total daily diet.

The %DVs are based on recommendations for a 2,000-calorie diet. For labeling purposes, the FDA sets 2,000 calories as the reference amount for calculating %DVs. The %DV is the percentage of the recommended daily amount of a nutrient in a serving of food. Total daily intake of fat, saturated fat, sodium, and cholesterol (3 on the sample label) should be limited to less than 100%DV. One should have 100% of each of the essential nutrients like calcium, iron, and vitamins A and C as well as other components such as dietary fiber (4 on the sample label) each day.

*Percent Daily Values are based on a 2,000 calorie diet. Your Daily Values may be higher or lower depending on your calorie needs:

	Calories:	2,000	2,500
Total Fat	Less than	65g	80g
Sal Fat	Less than	20g	25g
Cholesterol	Less than	300mg	300mg
Sodium	Less than	2,400mg	2,400mg
Total Carbohydrate		300g	375g
Dietary Fiber		25g	30g

Determining the %DV: Example for Total Fat

Is 12 g of total fat high or low? In other words, does one serving (containing 12 g of fat) contribute a lot or a little total fat to a daily diet?

% Daily Value*	
Total Fat 12g	?
Saturated Fat 3g	?
Trans fat 1.5g	
Cholesterol 30mg	?
Sodium 470mg	?

According to the %DV on the label example, 12 g of fat corresponds to 18%DV. If one serving of macaroni and cheese contains 18%DV for total fat, 82% of the fat allowance is left for all the other foods eaten that day.

% Daily Value*	
Total Fat 12g	18%
Saturated Fat 3g	15%
Trans Fat 1.5g	
Cholesterol 30mg	10%
Sodium 470mg	20%

Nutrition Facts information obtained from http://www.nutrition.gov.

% fat allowance utilized

% fat allowance remaining

← 82% →

0%   18%   100%
total fat allowance

Quick Guide to %DV

| 18% |
| 15% |
| 10% |
| 20% |
| 10% |
| 0% |
| |
| |
| |
| 4% |
| 2% |
| 20% |
| 4% |

The general guide (5 on the sample label) indicates that 5%DV or less is low and 20%DV or more is high. This means that 5%DV or less is low for all nutrients, those one wants to limit (e.g., fat, saturated fat, cholesterol, and sodium) and those one wants to consume in greater amounts (fiber, calcium, etc). As the Quick Guide shows, 20%DV or more is high for all nutrients.

As an example, consider again at the amount of total fat in one serving listed on the sample nutrition label for macaroni and cheese. Is 18%DV contributing a lot or a little to the maximum fat limit of 100%DV? The Quick Guide to %DV shows that 18%DV is not high; however, if one ate the whole package (two servings), one would double that amount, eating 36% of the daily allowance for total fat. That would leave 64% of the fat allowance for *all* of the other foods eaten that day, snacks and drinks included.

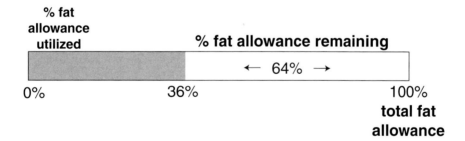

% fat allowance utilized

% fat allowance remaining

← 64% →

0%   36%   100%
total fat allowance

Comparisons

The %DV makes it easy to make comparisons. One can compare one product or brand to a similar product and see which is higher or lower in a nutrient because the serving sizes are generally consistent for similar types of foods. See comparison example 1.

Nutrient Content Claims

One can quickly distinguish one claim from another, such as reduced fat versus light or nonfat. By comparing the %DVs for total fat in each food product, one can see which is higher or lower in that nutrient, without having to memorize definitions. This works when comparing all nutrient content claims, for example, less, light, low, free, more, high, etc. See comparison examples 1 and 2.

Dietary Trade-Offs

The %DV can be used to help make dietary trade-offs with other foods throughout the day. A favorite food that is high in fat can be balanced with foods that are low in fat at other times of the day. By paying attention to how much one eats, the total amount of fat for the day can be kept below 100%DV.

Nutrition Facts information obtained from http://www.nutrition.gov.

Nutrients That Have No %DV

Trans fats, sugars, and protein have no listed %DV on the Nutrition Facts panel.

Trans Fats

Scientific reports link trans fat (and saturated fat) with raising low-density lipoprotein (LDL)-cholesterol ("bad cholesterol") levels, which increases the risk of coronary heart disease, a leading cause of death in the United States, However, experts have not provided a reference value for trans fat nor any other information that FDA believes is sufficient to establish a daily value or %DV.

Sugars

No daily reference value has been established because no recommendations have been made for the total amount of sugars to eat in a day. The sugars listed on the Nutrition Facts panel include naturally occurring sugars (like those in fruit and milk) as well as those added to a food or drink. The ingredient list gives specifics on added sugars.

Protein

A %DV is required to be listed if a claim is made for protein, such as "high in protein." Otherwise, unless the food is meant for use by infants and children younger than 4 years old, none is needed. Current scientific evidence indicates that protein intake is not a public health concern for adults and children older than 4 years of age.

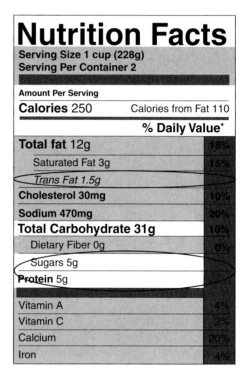

To limit nutrients that have no %DV, like trans fat and sugars, one should compare the labels of similar products and choose the food with the lowest amount.

Calcium

Experts advise consumers to consume adequate amounts of calcium in their daily diet. This guideline is given in forms of milligrams (mg), but the Nutrition Facts panel only lists a %DV for calcium. For consumers to know how the calcium they consume relates to expert advice, they need to do some simple math (this applies to calcium only).

Example: Experts advise adolescents, especially girls, to consume 1,300 mg and postmenopausal women 1,200 mg of calcium daily. To find the %DV that corresponds to 1,300 and 1,200 mg, we divide the number of mg by 10 (the DV for calcium on food labels is 1,000 mg). When converted to a percentage, this gives a factor of 10. Thus, the daily target for teenage girls, 1,300 mg, equals 130%DV, and the daily target for postmenopausal women, 1,200 mg, equals 120%DV.

To convert the %DV for calcium into milligrams, we multiply by 10. A container of yogurt might list 30%DV for calcium. To convert this to milligrams, we multiply by 10, which equals 300 mg of calcium for the yogurt.

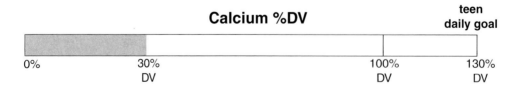

Equivalencies:

$$30\%DV = 300 \text{ mg calcium} = \text{one cup of milk}$$

$$100\%DV = 1,000 \text{ mg calcium}$$

$$130\%DV = 1,300 \text{ mg calcium}$$

Nutrition Facts information obtained from http://www.nutrition.gov.

The important thing to recall is that the %DV for calcium on the food package shows how much one serving contributes to the total amount one needs. See comparison example 2.

```
┌────────────────────────────────────────────┐
│ Nutrition Facts                             │
│ Serving Size 1 cup (236ml)                  │
│ Servings Per Container 1                    │
│ ━━━━━━━━━━━━━━━━━━━━━━━━━━━━━━━━━━━━━━       │
│ Amount Per Serving                          │
│ Calories 80          Calories from Fat 0    │
│ ━━━━━━━━━━━━━━━━━━━━━━━━━━━━━━━━━━━━━━       │
│                          % Daily Value*     │
│ Total Fat  0g                        0%     │
│   Saturated Fat 0g                   0%     │
│   Trans Fat 0g                              │
│ Cholesterol  Less than 5mg           0%     │
│ Sodium 120mg                         5%     │
│ Total Carbohydrate 11g               4%     │
│   Dietary Fiber 0g                   0%     │
│   Sugars 11g                                │
│ Protein 9g                          17%     │
│ ━━━━━━━━━━━━━━━━━━━━━━━━━━━━━━━━━━━━━━       │
│ Vitamin A 10%      •      Vitamin C 4%      │
│ Calcium 30% • Iron 0% • Vitamin D 25%       │
│ *Percent Daily Values are based on a 2,000  │
│ calorie diet. Your daily values may be higher│
│ or lower depending on your calorie needs:   │
└────────────────────────────────────────────┘
```

The Footnote, or Lower Part of the Nutrition Facts Panel

*Percent Daily Values are based on a 2,000 calorie diet. Your Daily Values may be higher or lower depending on your calorie needs:

		Calories:	2,000	2,500
Total Fat	Less than		65g	80g
Sal Fat	Less than		20g	25g
Cholesterol	Less than		300mg	300mg
Sodium	Less than		2,400mg	2,400mg
Total Carbohydrate			300g	375g
Dietary Fiber			25g	30g

The asterisk after the heading %Daily Value on the Nutrition Facts panel (6 on the sample label) refers to the footnote in the lower part of the nutrition label, which indicates that %DVs are based on recommendations for a 2,000-calorie diet. This statement must be on all food labels. The remaining information in the full footnote, however, may not be on the package if the size of the label is too small. When the full footnote does appear, it is always the same. It does not change from product to product because it shows dietary advice for all Americans—it is not about a specific food product.

The daily values are based on expert dietary advice about how much of some key nutrients one should eat each day depending on whether one eats 2,000 or 2,500 calories a day.

Example: The total fat information in the footnote states that a person who eats 2,000 calories per day should eat less than 65 g of fat in all the foods each day. A person doing this will follow nutrition experts' advice to consume no more than 30% of daily calories from fat. Because the DV for total fat is less than 65 g, this is the same thing as keeping total fat intake for the day below 100%DV.

*Percent Daily Values are based on a 2,000 calorie diet. Your Daily Values may be higher or lower depending on your calorie needs:

		Calories:	2,000	2,500
Total Fat	Less than		65g	80g
Sal Fat	Less than		20g	25g
Cholesterol	Less than		300mg	300mg
Sodium	Less than		2,400mg	2,400mg
Total Carbohydrate			300g	375g
Dietary Fiber			25g	30g

Nutrition Facts information obtained from http://www.nutrition.gov.

For a person who consumes 2,500 calories per day, the footnote shows how the daily values change for some nutrients but not for others. The daily values for cholesterol (300 mg) and sodium (2,400 mg sodium) remain the same no matter how many calories one eats, but recommended levels of intake for other nutrients depend on how many calories are consumed.

*Percent Daily Values are based on a 2,000 calorie diet. Your Daily Values may be higher or lower depending on your calorie needs:			
	Calories:	2,000	2,500
Total Fat	Less than	65g	80g
Sal Fat	Less than	20g	25g
Cholesterol	Less than	300mg	300mg
Sodium	Less than	2,400mg	2,400mg
Total Carbohydrate		300g	375g
Dietary Fiber		25g	30g

Recall that the %DVs listed on the top half of the food label are based on recommendations for a 2,000-calorie diet, not a 2,500-calorie diet.

Comparison Examples

Comparison Example 1

Which of the following kinds of milk has more calories? One is "reduced fat," the other is chocolate "nonfat" milk. Each serving size is one cup. Which is higher in fat and saturated fat?

Reduced Fat Milk
2% Milkfat

Nutrition Facts

Serving Size 1 cup (236ml)
Servings Per Container 1

Amount Per Serving

Calories 120   Calories from Fat 45

	% Daily Value*
Total Fat 5g	8%
Saturated Fat 3g	15%
Trans Fat 0g	
Cholesterol 20mg	7%
Sodium 120mg	5%
Total Carbohydrate 11g	4%
Dietary Fiber 0g	0%
Sugars 11g	
Protein 9g	17%

Vitamin A 10%   ·   Vitamin C 4%
Calcium 30%·Iron 0%·Vitamin D 25%
*Percent Daily Values are based on a 2,000 calorie diet. Your daily values may be higher or lower depending on your calorie needs:

Chocolate Nonfat Milk

Nutrition Facts

Serving Size 1 cup (236ml)
Servings Per Container 1

Amount Per Serving

Calories 80   Calories from Fat 0

	% Daily Value*
Total Fat 0g	0%
Saturated Fat 0g	0%
Trans Fat 0g	
Cholesterol Less than 5mg	0%
Sodium 120mg	5%
Total Carbohydrate 11g	4%
Dietary Fiber 0g	0%
Sugars 11g	
Protein 9g	17%

Vitamin A 10%   ·   Vitamin C 4%
Calcium 30%·Iron 0%·Vitamin D 25%
*Percent Daily Values are based on a 2,000 calorie diet. Your daily values may be higher or lower depending on your calorie needs:

Nutrition Facts information obtained from http://www.nutrition.gov.

Comparison Example 2

Which of the following kinds of milk has more calcium? One is "reduced fat," the other is chocolate "nonfat" milk. Each serving size is one cup.

Reduced Fat Milk
2% Milkfat

Chocolate Nonfat Milk

Nutrition Facts			Nutrition Facts		
Serving Size 1 cup (236ml)			Serving Size 1 cup (236ml)		
Servings Per Container 1			Servings Per Container 1		
Amount Per Serving			**Amount Per Serving**		
Calories 120	Calories from Fat 45		**Calories** 80	Calories from Fat 0	
		% Daily Value*			% Daily Value*
Total Fat 5g		**8%**	**Total Fat** 0g		**0%**
Saturated Fat 3g		**15%**	Saturated Fat 0g		**0%**
Trans Fat 0g			*Trans* Fat 0g		
Cholesterol 20mg		**7%**	**Cholesterol** Less than 5mg		**0%**
Sodium 120mg		**5%**	**Sodium** 120mg		**5%**
Total Carbohydrate 11g		**4%**	**Total Carbohydrate** 11g		**4%**
Dietary Fiber 0g		**0%**	Dietary Fiber 0g		**0%**
Sugars 11g			Sugars 11g		
Protein 9g		**17%**	**Protein** 9g		**17%**
Vitamin A 10% · Vitamin C 4%			Vitamin A 10% · Vitamin C 4%		
Calcium 30% ·Iron 0%·Vitamin D 25%			Calcium 30% ·Iron 0%·Vitamin D 25%		
*Percent Daily Values are based on a 2,000 calorie diet. Your daily values may be higher or lower depending on your calorie needs:			*Percent Daily Values are based on a 2,000 calorie diet. Your daily values may be higher or lower depending on your calorie needs:		

DO VITAMIN AND MINERAL SUPPLEMENTS SUCH AS POTASSIUM, CALCIUM, AND MAGNESIUM HELP LOWER BLOOD PRESSURE?

[Source: http://www.nhlbi.nih.gov]
Research has shown that potassium lowers blood pressure. Studies have not indicated that calcium and magnesium supplements prevent high blood pressure.

Potassium

Potassium helps to prevent and control blood pressure. Some good sources are various fruits, vegetables, dairy foods, and fish.

Foods high in potassium

Food	Serving size	Potassium (mg)
Apricots, dried	10 halves	407
Avocados, raw	1 oz	180
Bananas, raw	1 cup	594
Beets, cooked	1 cup	519
Brussel sprouts, cooked	1 cup	504
Cantaloupe	1 cup	494
Dates, dry	5	271
Figs, dry	2	271
Kiwi fruit, raw	1 medium	252
Lima beans	1 cup	955
Melons, honeydew	1 cup	461
Milk, fat free or skim	1 cup	407
Nectarines	1	288
Orange juice	1 cup	496
Oranges	1	237
Pears (fresh)	1	208
Peanuts dry roasted, without salt	1 oz.	187
Potatoes, baked, flesh and skin	1	1081
Prune juice	1 cup	707
Prunes, dried	1 cup	828
Raisins	1 cup	1089
Spinach, cooked	1 cup	839
Tomato products, canned, sauce	1 cup	909
Winter squash	1 cup	896
Yogurt plain, skim milk	8 oz.	579

Source: Values were obtained from the U.S. Department of Agriculture Nutrient Database for Standard References, Release 15 for Potassium, K (mg) content of selected foods per common measure. Available at http://www.nal.usda.gov/fnic/foodcomp/Data/SR15/wtrank/wt_rank.html

Calcium and Magnesium

These nutrients have not been consistently shown to prevent high blood pressure, but are important nutrients for overall good health.

Good sources of calcium are dairy foods such as milk, yogurt, and cheese. Low-fat and nonfat dairy products have more calcium than the high-fat versions.

Foods high in calcium

Food	Serving/size	Calcium (mg)
Broccoli, raw	1 cup	42
Cheese, cheddar	1 oz	204
Milk, fat-free or skim	1 cup	301
Perch	3 oz	116
Salmon	3 oz	181
Sardine	3 oz	325
Spinach, cooked	1 cup	245
Turnip greens, cooked	1 cup	197
Tofu, soft	1 piece	133
Yogurt plain, skim milk	8 oz	452

Source: Values were obtained from the U.S. Department of Agriculture Nutrient Database for Standard References, Release 15 for Calcium, Ca (mg) content of selected foods per common measure. Available at http://www.nal.usda.gov/fnic/foodcomp/Data/SR15/wtrank/wt_rank.html

One can get enough magnesium by following a healthy diet. Magnesium is found in whole grains, green leafy vegetables, nuts, and dry peas and beans.

Nutrition Facts information obtained from http://www.nutrition.gov.

Foods high in magnesium

Food	Serving size	Magnesium (mg)
Beans, black	1 cup	120
Broccoli, raw	1 cup	22
Halibut	1/2 fillet	170
Nuts, peanuts	1 oz	64
Okra, frozen	1 cup	94
Oysters	3 oz	49
Plantain, raw	1 medium	66
Rockfish	1 fillet	51
Scallop	6 large	55
Seeds, pumpkin and squash	1 oz (142 seeds)	151
Soy milk	1 cup	47
Spinach, cooked	1 cup	157
Tofu	1/4 block	37
Whole-grain cereal, ready to eat	3/4 cup	24
Whole-grain cereal, cooked	1 cup	56
Whole-wheat bread	1 slice	24

Source: Values were obtained from the U.S. Department of Agriculture Nutrient Database for Standard References, Release 15 for Magnesium, Mg (mg) content of selected foods per common measure. Available at http://www.nal.usda.gov/fnic/foodcomp/Data/SR15/wtrank/wt_rank.html

MODERATE-LEVEL PHYSICAL ACTIVITIES

[Source: http://www.nhlbi.nih.gov]
Being physically active is one of the most important things one can do to prevent or control high blood pressure. It also helps to reduce the risk of heart disease.

One should engage in at least 30 minutes of moderate-level physical activity on most days of the week. Examples of such activities are brisk walking, bicycling, raking leaves, and gardening.

*Examples of moderate amounts of activity**

Washing and waxing a car for 45–60 minutes   **Less Vigorous, More Time***
Washing windows or floors for 45–60 minutes
Playing volleyball for 45 minutes
Playing touch football for 30–45 minutes
Gardening for 30–45 minutes
Wheeling self in wheelchair for 30–40 minutes
Walking 1¾ miles in 35 minutes (20 min/mile)
Basketball (shooting baskets) for 30 minutes
Bicycling 5 miles in 30 minutes
Dancing fast (social) for 30 minutes
Pushing a stroller 1½ miles in 30 minutes
Raking leaves for 30 minutes
Walking 2 miles in 30 minutes (15 min/mile)
Water aerobics for 30 minutes
Swimming laps for 20 minutes
Wheelchair basketball for 20 minutes
Basketball (playing a game) for 15–20 minutes
Bicycling 4 miles in 15 minutes
Jumping rope for 15 minutes
Running 1½ miles in 15 minutes (10 min/mile)   **More Vigorous, Less Time**
Shoveling snow for 15 minutes
Stairwalking for 15 minutes

*A moderate amount of physical activity is roughly equivalent to physical activity that uses approximately 150 calories of energy per day, or 1,000 calories per week.

**Some activities can be performed at various intensities; the suggested durations correspond to expected intensity of effort. NIH-NHLBL Clinical Guidelines Obesity 1998.

Nutrition Facts information obtained from http://www.nutrition.gov.

One can divide the 30 minutes into shorter periods of at least 10 minutes each. Examples are using stairs instead of an elevator, getting off a bus one or two stops early, or parking one's car at the far end of the lot at work. If one already engages in 30 minutes of moderate-level physical activity a day, one can get added benefits by doing more by engaging in moderate-level activity for a longer period each day or in a more vigorous activity.

Most people do not need to see a doctor before they start a moderate-level physical activity. One should check first with one's doctor if one has heart trouble or has had a heart attack, is older than age 50 years and is not used to moderate-level physical activity, has a family history of heart disease at an early age, or has any other serious health problem.

Index

Page numbers followed by *f* indicate a figure; *t* following a page number indicates tabular material